PRACTICAL NEUROLOGY
SECOND EDITION

PRACTICAL NEUROLOGY

SECOND EDITION

Editor

José Biller, M.D.

Professor and Chairman
Department of Neurology
Indiana University School of Medicine
Chief, Neurology Services
Indiana University Medical Center
Indianapolis, Indiana

LIPPINCOTT WILLIAMS & WILKINS
A **Wolters Kluwer** Company

Philadelphia · Baltimore · New York · London
Buenos Aires · Hong Kong · Sydney · Tokyo

Acquisitions Editor: Anne M. Sydor
Developmental Editor: Marc Bendian
Production Editor: Jonathan Geffner
Manufacturing Manager: Colin Warnock
Cover Designer: QT Design
Compositor: Circle Graphics
Printer: Maple Press

© 2002 by LIPPINCOTT WILLIAMS & WILKINS
530 Walnut Street
Philadelphia, PA 19106 USA
LWW.com

Printed in the USA

Library of Congress Cataloging-in-Publication Data

Practical neurology / [edited by] José Biller.—2nd ed.
    p. ; cm.
  Includes bibliographical references and index.
  ISBN 0-7817-3019-8
    1. Neurology. I. Biller, José.
    [DNLM: 1. Nervous System Diseases—diagnosis. 2. Nervous System
  Diseases—therapy. WL 141 P895 2002]
  RC346 .P685 2002
  616.8—dc21

2001038951

10 9 8 7 6 5 4

*to the memory of my parents,
Osías Biller and Elena Grinshpan*

CONTENTS

I. DIAGNOSIS

II. TREATMENT

CONTRIBUTING AUTHORS

Harold P. Adams, Jr., M.D.
Professor, Department of Neurology, University of Iowa College of Medicine; Director, Division of Cerebrovascular Diseases, University of Iowa Hospitals, Iowa City, Iowa

John C. Andrefsky, M.D.
Physician, Department of Neurology, Akron General Medical Center, Akron, Ohio

Martin J. Arron, M.D.
Assistant Professor, Department of Medicine, Division of General Internal Medicine, Northwestern University Medical School; Associate Staff, Department of Medicine, Division of General Internal Medicine, Northwestern Memorial Hospital, Chicago, Illinois

Marianna R. Beattie, D.D.S.
Dentist, University of Iowa College of Dentistry, Iowa City, Iowa

Xabier Beristain, M.D.
Assistant Professor, Department of Neurology, Indiana University School of Medicine; Attending Physician, Department of Neurology, Indiana University Medical Center, Indianapolis, Indiana

José Biller, M.D.
Professor and Chairman, Department of Neurology, Indiana University School of Medicine; Chief, Neurology Services, Indiana University Medical Center, Indianapolis, Indiana

Allison Brashear, M.D.
Associate Professor, Department of Neurology, Indiana University School of Medicine; Director, Mark L. Dyken, M.D. Neurology Outpatient Clinic, University Hospital, Indiana University Hospital, Indianapolis, Indiana

Paul W. Brazis, M.D.
Professor, Departments of Neurology and Ophthalmology, Mayo Clinic–Jacksonville, Jacksonville, Florida

Askiel Bruno, M.D.
Associate Professor, Department of Neurology, Indiana University School of Medicine, Indianapolis, Indiana

Bruce A. Cohen, M.D.
Professor, Department of Neurology, Northwestern University Medical School; Attending Neurologist, Department of Neurology, Northwestern Memorial Hospital, Chicago, Illinois

James J. Corbett, M.D.
McCarty Professor of Neurology and Professor of Ophthalmology, University of Mississippi Medical School; Chairman, Department of Neurology, University of Mississippi Medical Center, Jackson, Mississippi

James R. Couch, Jr., M.D., Ph.D.
Professor and Chairman, Department of Neurology, University of Oklahoma Health Sciences Center, Oklahoma City, Oklahoma

Edward C. Daly, M.D., Ph.D.
Assistant Professor, Department of Neurology, Indiana University Medical Center; Staff Neurologist, Neurology Service, Roudebush VA Medical Center, Indianapolis, Indiana

Natalie L. Denburg, Ph.D.
Assistant Research Scientist, Department of Neurology, University of Iowa College of Medicine; Staff Neuropsychologist, Department of Neurology, University of Iowa Hospitals and Clinics, Iowa City, Iowa

Kathleen B. Digre, M.D.
Professor, Departments of Neurology and Ophthalmology, University of Utah Medical School, Salt Lake City, Utah

David W. Dunn, M.D.
Associate Professor, Departments of Psychiatry and Neurology, Indiana University School of Medicine; Director, Outpatient Clinics, Department of Child and Adolescent Psychiatry, Riley Hospital, Indianapolis, Indiana

Mark Eric Dyken, M.D.
Associate Professor, Department of Neurology, University of Iowa College of Medicine; Director, Sleep Disorders Center, Department of Neurology, Division of Clinical Neurophysiology, University of Iowa Hospitals and Clinics, Iowa City, Iowa

Rodger J. Elble, M.D., Ph.D.
Professor and Chairman, Department of Neurology, Director, Center for Alzheimer Disease and Related Disorders, Southern Illinois University School of Medicine, Springfield, Illinois

M. Cara Erskine, M.Ed., CCC, SLP/A
Senior Speech Language Pathologist/Audiologist, Rehabilitation Services, University of Maryland, Baltimore, Maryland

Martin R. Farlow, M.D.
Professor and Vice Chairman for Research, Department of Neurology, Indiana University School of Medicine; Co-Director, Alzheimer Disease Clinic, University Hospital, Indianapolis, Indiana

James D. Fleck, M.D.
Clinical Assistant Professor, Department of Neurology, Indiana University School of Medicine, Indianapolis, Indiana

Jeffrey I. Frank, M.D.
Associate Professor, Department of Neuromedical/Neurosurgery, University of Chicago; Director, Neurosciences Critical Care, Chicago, Illinois

Bhuwan P. Garg, M.B.B.S.
Professor, Department of Neurology, Indiana University School of Medicine; Department of Neurology; James Whitcomb Riley Hospital for Children, Indianapolis, Indiana

Julius M. Goodman, M.D.
Clinical Professor, Department of Surgery, Section of Neurosurgery, Indiana University School of Medicine; Chairman, Department of Surgery, Section of Neurosurgery, Methodist/Clarian Hospital, Indianapolis, Indiana

David Lee Gordon, M.D.
Associate Professor of Clinical Neurology and Medicine, Director, Emergency Medical Skills and Neurology Training, Center for Research in Medical Education, University of Miami School of Medicine, Miami, Florida

Neill R. Graff-Radford, M.B.B.Ch.
Professor, Department of Neurology, Mayo Clinic, Jacksonville, Florida

Michael W. Groff, M.D.
Director of Spinal Surgery, Department of Surgery, Section of Neurosurgery, Indiana University School of Medicine; Neurosurgeon, Department of Surgery, Section of Neurosurgery, Indiana University Hospital, Indianapolis, Indiana

Gregory Gruener, M.D.
Associate Professor, Department of Neurology, Loyola University; Attending Physician, Department of Neurology, Loyola University Medical Center, Maywood, Illinois

Timothy C. Hain, M.D.
Associate Professor, Department of Neurology, Northwestern University; Director, Vestibular Laboratory, Department of Neurology, Northwestern Memorial Hospital, Chicago, Illinois

Ann Marie Hake, M.D.
Clinical Assistant Professor, Department of Neurology, Indiana University School of Medicine, Indianapolis, Indiana

Holli A. Horak, M.D.
Visiting Lecturer, Department of Neurology, Indiana University Medical Center, Indianapolis, Indiana

Aki Kawasaki, M.D.
Head of Research–Pupillography, Neuroophthalmology Unit, University Eye Clinic of Lausanne, Hopital Ophthalmique Jules Gonin, Lausanne, Swtzerland

John C. Kincaid, M.D.
Kenneth L. and Selma G. Ernest Professor, Department of Neurology, Indiana University School of Medicine, Indianapolis, Indiana

Oldrich J. Kolar, M.D., Ph.D.
Director, Indiana Center for Multiple Sclerosis and Neuroimmunopathologic Disorders, Indianapolis, Indiana

Marian P. LaMonte, M.D., M.S.N.
Associate Professor, Department of Neurology and Surgery, Division of Emergency Medicine, University of Maryland School of Medicine; Director, The Maryland Brain Attack Center, The University of Maryland Medical Center, Baltimore, Maryland

David S. Lefkowitz, M.D.
Associate Professor, Department of Neurology, Wake Forest University School of Medicine; Department of Neurology, Wake Forest University Baptist Medical Center, Winston-Salem, North Carolina

Bertrand C. Liang, M.D.
Medical Director, Department of Research and Development, Amgen, Inc., Thousand Oaks, California

Diane M. Liang, B.S.N., R.N.
LL Consulting, Newbury Park, California

Jeri A. Logemann, Ph.D.
Ralph and Jean Sundin Professor, Department of Communication Sciences and Disorders, Northwestern University, Evanston; Director, Speech, Language, Voice, and Swallowing Service, Northwestern Memorial Hospital, Chicago, Illinois

Betsy B. Love, M.D.
Clinical Associate Professor, Department of Neurology, Indiana University School of Medicine, Indianapolis, Indiana

Raúl N. Mandler, M.D.
Professor, Department of Neurology, George Washington University; Director, The George Washington ALS Center, Washington, DC

Omkar N. Markand, M.D.
Director, Clinical Neurophysiology, Professor, Department of Neurology, Indiana University School of Medicine; Neurology Staff, Director, EEG/Epilepsy Section, Department of Neurology, University Hospital, Indianapolis, Indiana

Gary J. Martin, M.D.
Vice Chairman and Professor, Department of Medicine, Northwestern University Medical School; Vice Chairman, Department of Medicine, Northwestern Memorial Hospital, Chicago, Illinois

David H. Mattson, M.D., Ph.D.
Professor, Department of Neurology, Indiana University School of Medicine; Director, Neuroimmunology/Multiple Sclerosis Program, Indiana University Medical Center, Indianapolis, Indiana

Bette G. Maybury, M.D.
Clinical Associate Professor, Department of Neurology, Indiana University School of Medicine; Physician, Department of Neurology, Indiana University Hospital, Indianapolis, Indiana

Michael P. McQuillen, M.D., M.A.
Professor, Department of Neurology, University of Rochester School of Medicine and Dentistry; Attending Physician, Department of Neurology, Strong Memorial Hospital, Rochester, New York

Galen W. Mitchell, M.D.
Associate Professor, Department of Neurology, University of Pittsburgh, Pittsburgh, Pennsylvania

Richard T. Miyamoto, M.D.
Arilla Spence DeVault Professor and Chairman, Department of Otolaryngology–Head and Neck Surgery, Indiana University School of Medicine; Co-Chief, Department of Otolaryngology–Head and Neck Surgery, Clarian Health Partners, Inc., Indianapolis, Indiana

Paul B. Nelson, M.D.
Chairman and Betsy Barton Professor of Neurologic Surgery, Department of Surgery, Section of Neurosurgery, Indiana University School of Medicine, Indianapolis, Indiana

Robert M. Pascuzzi, M.D.
Professor and Vice Chairman, Co-Director of Resident Education, Department of Neurology, Indiana University School of Medicine; Chief, Wishard Health Services Section, Department of Neurology, Wishard Health Services, Indianapolis, Indiana

Alok Pasricha, M.D.
Neurophysiology Fellow, Department of Neurology, Northwestern Univerity; Neurophysiology Fellow, Department of Neurology, Northwestern Memorial Hospital, Chicago, Illinois

Hema Patel, M.D.
Clinical Associate Professor, Department of Neurology, Section of Pediatric Neurology, Indiana University School of Medicine; Child Neurologist, Department of Neurology, Section of Pediatric Neurology, Riley Hospital for Children, Indiana University Medical Center, Indianapolis, Indiana

Rahman Pourmand, M.D.
Professor; Department of Neurology, Director, Neuromuscular Program, Chief, EMG Laboratory, State University of New York, Stony Brook, New York

R. Venkata Reddy, M.D.
Associate Professor, Department of Neurology, Indiana University School of Medicine; Chief, Neurophysiology Laboratories, Roudebush VA Medical Center, Indianapolis, Indiana

Robert L. Rodnitzky, M.D.
Professor, Department of Neurology, University of Iowa College of Medicine; Director, Movement Disorders Clinic, University of Iowa Hospitals and Clinics, Iowa City, Iowa

Karen L. Roos, M.D.
John and Nancy Nelson Professor of Neurology, Department of Neurology, Indiana School of Medicine, Indiana University Hospital, Indianapolis, Indiana

Shane J. Rose, M.D.
Resident, Department of Diagnostic Radiology, Indiana University Medical Center, Indianapolis, Indiana

Mark A. Ross, M.D.
Associate Professor, Department of Neurology, Kentucky Clinic; Associate Professor, Department of Neurology, Chandler Medical Center, Lexington, Kentucky

Jack M. Rozental, M.D., Ph.D.
Associate Professor, Department of Neurology, Northwestern University Medical School; Chief, Neurology Service, VA Chicago Health Services, Chicago, Illinois

Frank A. Rubino, M.D.
Professor, Department of Neurology, Mayo Clinic Jacksonville; Consultant, Department of Neurology, St. Luke's Hospital, Jacksonville, Florida

Daniel E. Rusyniak, M.D.
Assistant Professor, Department of Emergency Medicine, Division of Medical Toxicology; Adjunct Assistant Professor, Department of Neurology, Indiana University School of Medicine, Indianapolis, Indiana

Vicenta Salanova, M.D.
Associate Professor, Department of Neurology, Indiana University School of Medicine, Indianapolis, Indiana

Jeffrey L. Saver, M.D.
Associate Professor, Department of Neurology, University of California–Los Angeles Medical Center; Neurology Director, University of California–Los Angeles Stroke Center, Los Angeles, California

Scott A. Shapiro, M.D.
Professor, Department of Surgery, Section of Neurosurgery, Indiana University School of Medicine; Chief, Department of Surgery, Section of Neurosurgery, Wishard Memorial Hospital; Indiana University Medical Center, Indianapolis, Indiana

Muhammad A. Shoaib, M.D.
Fellow, Department of Neurology, University of Iowa College of Medicine, Iowa City, Iowa

Rodney A. Short, M.D.
Assistant Professor, Department of Neurology, University of Iowa, Iowa City, Iowa

Barbara E. Thomas, M.S., CCC–SLP
Senior Speech/Language Pathologist, Department of Rehabilitation Services, University of Maryland Medical Center, Baltimore, Maryland

Daniel Tranel, Ph.D.
Professor, Department of Neurology, University of Iowa College of Medicine; Chief of Neuropsychology, Department of Neurology, University of Iowa Hospitals and Clinics, Iowa City, Iowa

B. Todd Troost, M.D.
Professor and Chairman, Department of Neurology, Wake Forest University School of Medicine; Chief, Department of Neurology, North Carolina Baptist Hospital, Winston-Salem, North Carolina

Ergun Y. Uc, M.D.
Assistant Professor, Department of Neurology, University of Iowa; Staff Physician, Department of Neurology, University of Iowa Hospital, Iowa City, Iowa

Mohammad Kaleem Uddin, M.D.
Neurology Resident (PGY IV), Department of Neurology, Northwestern University, Chicago, Illinois

Michael W. Varner, M.D.
Professor, Department of Obstetrics and Gynecology, University of Utah School of Medicine, Salt Lake City, Utah

Steven J. Willing, M.D., M.B.A
Associate Professor, Department of Radiology, Indiana University School of Medicine, Indianapolis, Indiana

Joanne M. Wojcieszek, M.D.
Associate Professor, Department of Neurology, Indiana University School of Medicine, Indianapolis, Indiana

Michael K. Wynne, Ph.D.
Associate Professor; Department of Otolaryngology–Head and Neck Surgery, Indiana University School of Medicine; Audiologist, Department of Otolaryngology–Head and Neck Surgery, Riley Hospital for Children and University Hospital, Indianapolis, Indiana

Thoru Yamada, M.D.
Professor, Department of Neurology, University of Iowa College of Medicine; Chief, Division of Clinical Electrophysiology, University of Iowa Hospitals and Clinics, Iowa City, Iowa

Robert D. Yee, M.D.
Professor and Chairman, Department of Ophthalmology, Indiana University School of Medicine; Chairman, Department of Ophthalmology, Indiana University Hospital, Indianapolis, Indiana

Engin Y. Yilmaz, M.D., Ph.D.
Fellow, Department of Neurology, Indiana University School of Medicine, Indianapolis, Indiana

Phyllis C. Zee, M.D., Ph.D.
Professor, Department of Neurology, Northwestern University; Director, Sleep Disorders Center, Northwestern Memorial Hospital, Chicago, Illinois

PREFACE

This new edition of *Practical Neurology*, like the first edition, is intended to assist those medical students, residents, fellows, and practicing physicians involved in the care of patients with neurologic disorders. The text is divided into 58 chapters and one appendix, all written by well-established clinicians/educators. I am extremely grateful to all of the authors for their up-to-date contributions. The new edition consists of 35 chapters on diagnosis, 23 chapters on treatment—including "ABCs" of neurologic emergencies—and one appendix on the clinical signs and ancillary diagnostic studies of delirium. Much of the text has been rewritten, and new chapters and many new figures have been added. As in the first edition, we have deliberately tried to maintain balanced, practical, and nonencyclopedic discussions. Emphasis remains on addressing the more common neurologic disorders that a busy clinician is likely to encounter in practice.

José Biller, M.D.
June 2001

ACKNOWLEDGMENT

I am indebted to all my early neurology teachers from the School of Medicine in Uruguay, who personify all that is best in the practice of medicine, for stimulating my interest in clinical neurology and semiology. The editing and final production of this book are the result of the efforts of a dedicated team. I especially thank Anne Sydor, Marc Bendian, and Lippincott Williams & Wilkins for their encouragement, effort, and professionalism; and Phyllis Cowherd for her extraordinary patience in the production of this edition and for her wonderful secretarial and administrative support.

I. DIAGNOSIS

1. APPROACH TO THE PATIENT WITH ACUTE CONFUSIONAL STATE (DELIRIUM/ENCEPHALOPATHY)

John C. Andrefsky
Jeffrey I. Frank

Delirium is a syndrome characterized by confusion with inattention, alteration of arousal, disorientation, and global cognitive impairment. All patients with delirium should be promptly evaluated because of the progressive and potentially lethal nature of many of the etiologic factors as well as the danger these patients may pose to themselves. Management of the underlying cause leads to resolution in most circumstances. In this chapter, the terms *delirium* and *confusion* are used interchangeably.

All physicians encounter delirious patients during their careers, and knowing the patients at risk of delirium improves early recognition of the syndrome. The point prevalence of adults in the general population older than 55 years is 1.1%. Ten percent to 40% of the hospitalized elderly and 60% of nursing home patients older than 75 years are delirious. Patients with cancer, acquired immunodeficiency syndrome, or a terminal illness and those who have undergone bone marrow transplantation and other surgical procedures are at increased risk of delirium.

    I. Etiology. The common pathophysiologic mechanism of all causes of delirium is widespread dysfunction of both the cortical and the subcortical neurons, which leads to characteristic global, nonfocal neurologic manifestations in most cases. The causes can be structural in nature and affect a focal population of neurons or disrupt neuronal functioning diffusely through impairment of signals between neurons by means of a variety of pathophysiologic mechanisms. The neurotransmitters **acetylcholine** and **dopamine** are known to play a central role in the regulation and communication of large numbers of neurons and neuronal systems that subserve both focal and diffuse brain functioning.

    Cholinergic neuronal pathways serve almost all areas of the brain and participate in most executive brain functions, including those of a delirious patient. The important functions include cortical arousal, attention, learning and memory, mood, thought, perception, and orientation. Anticholinergic medications are known to induce hyperactivity and decrease the ability to selectively attend. **Dopaminergic neurons** are primarily found in the nigrostriatal, hypothalamic–pituitary, and ventral tegmental areas but diffusely project to the frontal and temporal areas responsible for delirious symptoms. Dopaminergic neurons contribute to normal cognitive functions such as **attention, mood, memory, thought,** and **perception.** Intoxication with dopamine agonists commonly causes delirium and neuroleptic agents with antidopaminergic actions are commonly used to manage delirium. Changes in the relative influences of these two systems on their neuronal populations determine to a large extent both the presence and severity of delirium.

    The spectrum of causes of delirium (Table 1.1) includes commonly encountered (e.g., metabolic derangements) and rare (e.g., acute intermittent porphyria) conditions, and many are reversible and carry an excellent prognosis if the patient is treated in a timely manner. Many delirious patients often have more than one diagnosis that contributes to the pathologic state. The following are the basic etiologic categories of delirium. Specific clinical features are outlined later and in the **Appendix.**

        A. Infection is one of the most common causes of delirium. Systemic infections always should be considered as a potential cause of confusion, especially in the care of elderly patients and those with previous brain damage, who are particularly prone to encephalopathy from systemic processes. Central nervous system (CNS) infections, although less commonly encountered than systemic infections, can cause severe brain damage if not recognized immediately and should be a primary consideration in the care of postoperative neurosurgical and immunosuppressed patients.

        B. Metabolic abnormalities are a common cause of delirium and often coexist with other precipitants of delirium, such as sepsis and uremia. Often, the metabolic derangement must be extreme to cause confusion, and individual susceptibilities frequently dictate which patients have symptoms of a given metabolic abnormality.

Table 1.1 Causes of delirium

Infection
  Outside central nervous system
    Sepsis
    Localized
  Central nervous system
    Meningitis
      Bacterial
      Tuberculous
      Cryptococcal
      Lyme disease
      Syphilitic
    Toxoplasmosis
    Tertiary syphilis
    Encephalitis
      Herpes simplex
    Progressive multifocal leukoencephalopathy
    Human immunodeficiency virus
    Abscess
      Brain
      Epidural
    Subdural empyema
    Subacute spongiform encephalopathy
    Whipple's disease
Autoimmune
  Acute disseminated encephalomyelitis
  Systemic lupus erythematosus
Metabolic abnormalities
  Electrolyte disorders
  Hyperosmolality, hypoosmolality
  Central pontine myelinolysis
  Hypernatremia, hyponatremia
  Hypokalemia
  Hypercalcemia
  Hypophosphatemia
  Hypermagnesemia, hypomagnesemia
  Acid–base disorders
    Acidosis
    Alkalosis
End-organ failure
  Hyperglycemia
    Diabetic ketoacidosis
      Hyperosmolar nonketotic hyperglycemia
  Hypoglycemia
  Hypercapnia
  Hypoxia
  Hypotension
  Uremia
  Hepatic encephalopathy
  Reye's syndrome
  Pancreatic encephalopathy
  Acute intermittent porphyria
Endocrinopathy
  Hyperthyroidism, hypothyroidism
  Cushing's syndrome
  Adrenal cortical insufficiency
  Pituitary failure

Table 1.1 (*continued*)

Nutritional deficiency
    Wernicke's encephalopathy
    Pellagra
    Vitamin B_{12} deficiency
Intoxication
    Acute alcohol intoxication
    Alcohol withdrawal
    Opioid intoxication
    Cocaine intoxication
    Amphetamine intoxication
    Phencyclidine intoxication
    Sedative–hypnotic intoxication
    Sedative–hypnotic withdrawal
    Barbiturate intoxication
    Barbiturate withdrawal
    Benzodiazepine intoxication
    Benzodiazepine withdrawal
    Lithium intoxication
    Carbon monoxide poisoning
Medications
Hemorrhage
    Intracranial hemorrhage
        Subarachnoid hemorrhage
            Aneurysm
            Arteriovenous malformation
            Disseminated intravascular coagulation
Central nervous system trauma
    Acute subdural hematoma
    Subacute subdural hematoma
    Epidural hematoma
    Subarachnoid hemorrhage
    Concussion
    Contusion
Vascular
    Transient ischemic attack
    Cerebral infarction
    Vasculitis
    Venous occlusion
Tumors
    Central nervous system
        Primary
        Metastatic
        Meningeal carcinomatosis
    Paraneoplastic
        Limbic encephalitis
Seizures
    Generalized
    Partial
    Postconvulsive
Miscellaneous
    Hypertensive encephalopathy
    Beclouded dementia
    Postoperative delirium
    Cardiac bypass
    Temperature dysregulation
    Sensory deprivation
    Sleep deprivation
    Hydrocephalus

C. **End-organ failure** manifests as striking abnormalities at general physical examination and usually is readily recognized. Failure to promptly control hypotension and hypoxia can allow patients to suffer severe brain damage. Liver and kidney failure can cause delirium alone or decrease the metabolism and excretion of certain medications and their metabolites, and delirium ensues.

D. **Endocrinopathy** manifests as abnormalities of multiple organ systems. It usually has a subacute onset but must be specifically considered to recognize the pattern of systemic involvement.

E. **Nutritional deficiencies** most often (in the United States) affect patients with alcoholism, those with systemic cancer, and those with malabsorption syndromes. If managed early, most of the neurologic sequelae can be prevented.

F. **Intoxication** with and **withdrawal** from illicit drugs and alcohol can be life-threatening and necessitate prompt recognition and timely intervention and support.

G. **Medications** cause delirium among patients who have impaired renal and liver function or interference with metabolism from other drugs. Inquiry should be made about use of medications such as antipsychotics, tricyclic antidepressants, levodopa, antihistamines, digoxin, theophylline, and corticosteroids because these drugs can precipitate or aggravate delirium. Particular attention should be paid to the anticholinergic and dopaminergic properties of medications the patient is taking.

H. **Hemorrhage and infarction** in the CNS that cause delirium usually are associated with focal neurologic signs and are an **emergency,** frequently necessitating neurosurgical intervention. Patients with right-sided cerebral infarcts are at an increased risk of delirium.

I. **CNS trauma** can cause concussion, brain contusion, and epidural and subdural hematoma, each potentially manifesting as a confused state with associated focal neurologic features. Confusion associated with traumatic hemorrhage can be immediate or delayed. The severity of the neurologic effects of brain contusion varies from transient loss of consciousness with minimal structural injury to progressive deterioration of mental status with severe, life-threatening edema.

J. **Vascular causes** usually manifest as focal neurologic signs. However, lesions localizing to particular areas of the posterior circulation and right hemisphere may manifest as confusional states with focal features only discernible by experienced neurologists. CNS vasculitis often is associated with headache, focal neurologic signs, and variable manifestations of systemic illness.

K. **CNS tumors,** malignant and benign, primary and metastatic, can cause prominent changes in mental status, including confusion, focal neurologic findings, headaches, and signs of increased intracranial pressure (ICP).

L. **Seizures** (absence and partial) and postconvulsive states (secondary to generalized tonic–clonic and partial seizures) are common causes of intermittent confusion.

M. **Hypertensive encephalopathy** must be managed promptly to prevent end-organ damage and should be considered in the care of patients with extreme hypertension, mental status changes, and papilledema.

N. **Beclouded dementia** and **postoperative delirium** are encountered frequently by physicians practicing in a general medical setting. Patients with dementia are particularly sensitive to infections, metabolic abnormalities, and medications that may cause delirium. Patients become confused postoperatively because of metabolic aberrations, impaired gas exchange, infection, side effects of medication, and the result of physiologic derangements such as hypothermia and global hypoperfusion.

II. **Clinical manifestations.**

A. **Mental status.** Examination of a delirious patient is challenging. Histories from patients with encephalopathy must be interpreted with skepticism. It is important to seek information from families and friends. Prodromal symptoms can develop abruptly or over hours to days, with resolution occurring in days to weeks. Almost all patients with delirium have hour to hour fluctuations in the degree of impairment of mental status. Understanding the premorbid functioning of patients may assist in the diagnosis and prognosis, especially if the patient has an underlying structural pathologic condition such as cerebral infarction or dementia or end-organ failure, in which resolution of delirium can take weeks.

The history and physical examination should be performed in a quiet room with few distractions or interruptions. Restraints should be avoided unless the safety of the patient or medical personnel is at risk. Much information regarding the mental status of the patient is obtained during the course of social interaction. Engage the patient in a friendly and polite manner. Note whether the patient readily engages in greetings and conversation and follows a logical progression of thoughts. Frequent topic changes can signify confusion. Avoid frustrating questions, which can sabotage patient cooperation in subsequent parts of the examination.

1. **Attention.** The hallmark of delirium is the inability to maintain selective attention to the environment and mental processes. Patients are easily distracted and often unable to engage in conversation or readily shift their attention from one task to another.

2. **Orientation.** Delirious patients often are disoriented to time and place but oriented to person.

3. **Arousal.** Changes in level of arousal are common, ranging from agitation with increased alertness to somnolence.

4. **Memory.** Because registration depends on the ability to focus attention, delirious patients frequently are unable to form new memories and do so only during lucid periods. Recall of recently learned material usually is impaired while remote memory is preserved.

5. **Perception.** Impairment of both qualitative and quantitative perception is common for delirious patients. Hallucinations usually are either visual or auditory. Illusions and delusions are prominent.

6. **Disordered thinking.** Abnormalities of cognitive processing and problem solving are common.

7. **Emotional disturbances.** Marked emotional lability and inappropriate emotional responses occur frequently but are not readily appreciated until the patient is engaged in conversation.

8. **Language abnormalities.** The inattention and distractibility of delirium challenges meaningful interaction and communication with others. The verbal output of delirious patients tends to be rambling and incoherent. Aphasia often is mistaken for confusion. Patients with focal disturbances of language (comprehension, repetition, expression, and naming) should be evaluated for focal processes.

9. **Disturbances of the sleep–wake cycle** are common. Patients may remain awake for most of the day and night with only brief naps or may reverse their normal sleep pattern. Many of the conditions that cause delirium also cause insomnia and restless leg syndrome. The nocturnal exacerbation of confusion ("sundowning") of a patient with dementia can be a source of frustration for caregivers.

B. **Other neurologic findings.**
1. **Papilledema** is a sign of increased ICP or hypertensive encephalopathy. However, its absence does not rule out an increase in ICP, because the funduscopic changes evolve over hours to days.
2. **Pupillary changes.**
   a. Fixed and dilated pupils occur with anticholinergic (e.g., atropine, scopolamine) intoxication.
   b. Enlarged but reactive pupils are present with increased sympathetic activity, intoxication with amphetamines or cocaine, and therapeutic use of epinephrine and norepinephrine as pressor agents.
   c. Midposition unreactive pupils can be caused by glutethimide overdose or focal midbrain dysfunction, often from distortion by an expanding supratentorial mass.
   d. Use of opioids is associated with constriction of the pupils (<2 mm).

   e. The presence of a unilaterally dilated pupil with or without the other components of third cranial nerve palsy is a sign of brainstem distortion. *This is a neurologic emergency* until proved otherwise and necessitates immediate diagnosis and treatment.

3. Abnormalities of **ocular motility** associated with confusion usually signal the presence of either increased ICP or brainstem distortion.

   a. Upgaze palsy suggests a lesion of the dorsal upper midbrain or distortion due to hydrocephalus.

   b. Unilaterally impaired eye adduction (with pupillary dilation) and diminished consciousness represent a third nerve palsy, a *neurologic emergency* necessitating immediate diagnosis and treatment until proved otherwise.

   c. Delirium with **quadriparesis** can occur as a result of central pontine myelinolysis, progressive multifocal leukoencephalopathy, and acute disseminated encephalomyelitis (ADEM).

   d. Delirium with **paraparesis** can occur with cryptococcosis, vitamin B_{12} deficiency, and ADEM.

   e. Cushing's disease and hypokalemia can manifest as **proximal muscular weakness.**

4. The presence of **abnormal limb movement** often is helpful in determining the cause of delirium.

   a. **Myoclonus** is asynchronous irregular twitching of a single muscle, groups of muscles, or entire limbs, usually with proximal predominance. It can be associated with metabolic abnormalities, hypoxic–ischemic injury, lithium intoxication, and CNS infection, including tertiary syphilis and subacute spongiform encephalopathy (SSE).

   b. **Asterixis** is recurrent brief lapses of posture observed with arms raised and elbows and wrists extended. It is a common manifestation of hepatic encephalopathy and uremia but can be associated with other forms of metabolic encephalopathy.

   c. The **tremor** most frequently observed with delirium is coarse and irregular, most prominent in the fingers of the extended arms and absent at rest, and most commonly associated with hyperthyroidism, intoxication with sympathomimetics (amphetamine, cocaine, phencyclidine), alcohol intoxication and withdrawal, and barbiturate and benzodiazepine withdrawal.

   d. **Gait ataxia** is prominent with intoxication, vitamin B_{12} deficiency, syphilis, and Wernicke's encephalopathy.

   e. **Seizures** can cause confusion and often signify a structural brain abnormality, metabolic abnormality, or intoxication or withdrawal state.

      (1) **Partial complex seizures** are the most common type of focal seizures that can cause confusion. Although rarely encountered, **epilepsia partialis continua** is a focal motor epilepsy whereby clonic movements of the face, arm, and leg recur intermittently for long periods of time. It can go unrecognized as seizures by an inexperienced clinician. The presence of epilepsia partialis continua implies an irritative structural lesion involving cerebral cortex by any process that can cause focal cortical damage (e.g., stroke, encephalitis, neoplasm).

      (2) **Generalized seizures** can cause confusion or postconvulsive encephalopathy. **Absence seizures** are generalized seizures that induce brief lapses of consciousness with prominent automatism. Children who endure frequent interruptions in consciousness can be misdiagnosed with confusion or learning disability without recognition of the underlying seizure disorder.

III. Evaluation. The neurologic findings of delirium are discussed in **II.B.**

   A. The **history** is the most important part of the evaluation and often yields information that helps tailor an efficient investigation strategy, frequently with more rapid diagnosis and resolution of symptoms. Often family members and other observers must be the primary historian for delirious patients. The **Appendix**

presents the characteristic clinical manifestations and laboratory and radiologic findings as a quick reference for specific causes of delirium.

1. **Headache.** Acute headache reported by a confused patient can signify a severe intracranial pathologic condition such as subarachnoid (SAH) or intraparenchymal hemorrhage, whereas progressive headaches are more suggestive of a CNS neoplasm, infection, or hydrocephalus.

2. **Previous brain damage.** Patients with cerebral infarction, progressive neurologic disease, psychiatric illness, head trauma, or previous neurosurgical procedures are predisposed to delirium, often in association with other neurologic signs.

3. **Preexisting medical conditions** such as cardiac and lung disease are risk factors for life-threatening conditions that cause delirium. Abnormal hepatic and renal function can impair metabolism and excretion of medication.

4. **Drug history.** When evaluating a delirious patient, the clinician should always obtain a detailed substance abuse history. Inquiries about the specific substance abused, frequency of usage, and interval since last used are important.

5. **Exposure history.** Inquiries should be made about exposure to meningitis, human immunodeficiency virus (HIV), carbon monoxide, and other potential CNS toxins.

6. **Medications.** Addition of new medications or changes of dosage frequently are associated with confusion. Medications high in anticholinergic or dopaminergic activity are particularly common culprits.

B. **General physical examination.**

1. **Abnormalities of vital signs** often herald a medical emergency.

   a. **Hypotension** from dehydration, sepsis, cardiac arrhythmia, or congestive heart failure must be recognized and controlled promptly to prevent further neurologic and other end-organ damage.

   b. **Tachycardia** can be a manifestation of infection, cardiac abnormality, hyperthyroidism, dehydration, withdrawal states, intoxication with sympathomimetic drugs, or sympathetic overactivity from delirium.

   c. **Hypoventilation** related to pneumonia or drug overdose can result in hypoxia or hypercapnia.

   d. **Increases in body temperature** are associated with infection, withdrawal states, and hyperthyroidism. Hypothermia is associated with sepsis and barbiturate overdose.

2. **Nuchal rigidity** is a sign of meningeal irritation as frequently occurs with CNS infection and SAH. **Meningitis, encephalitis,** and **SAH** should be pursued diagnostically in the presence of nuchal rigidity or if clinical suspicion is high even in its absence.

3. In all cases of confusion, there should be a search for **evidence of head trauma,** such as scalp laceration, depressed skull fracture, or hemotympanum. Signs of cerebrospinal fluid (CSF) leak are particularly important because they predispose patients to bacterial meningitis.

4. **Purulent drainage** from the nares or a **gray and immobile tympanic membrane** can represent sinusitis or otitis media, respectively. The nasal septum should be examined for erosions due to cocaine use.

5. The **skin** should be examined for cyanosis, hirsutism, hyperpigmentation, and scaly dermatitis. The clinician should inspect the skin of all patients for the presence of track or "pop" marks, which imply intravenous drug use.

6. **Examination of the heart** can reveal murmurs and irregular rhythms that predispose patients to cerebral circulatory compromise.

7. **Decreased or absent breath** sounds can be caused by congestive heart failure or pneumonia, the resulting hypoxia potentially contributing to delirium.

8. Patients with **abdominal tenderness** should be evaluated for intraabdominal infection. Neurosurgical patients with a ventriculoperitoneal shunt can have shunt infection that manifests as abdominal peritonitis.

9. Patients with delirium from hepatic failure can have **ascites, splenomegaly, spider telangiectasia, caput medusae, icteric sclera,** and **jaundice.**

C. Ancillary tests.

    1. Measurement of serum levels of **electrolytes, glucose, blood urea nitrogen,** and **creatinine, complete blood cell count** (with differential), **liver enzymes, prothrombin** and **partial thromboplastin times,** and **arterial blood gases** with arterial ammonia level cover all of the metabolic abnormalities that must be urgently identified.

    2. **A drug screen** and a **blood alcohol level** should be included.

    3. If the results of the foregoing laboratory tests are negative, **HIV, fluorescent treponemal antibody-absorption, thyroid function,** and **cortisol stimulation tests** are needed.

    4. An **electrocardiogram** to rule out arrhythmia and cardiac ischemia and a **chest radiograph** to rule out infections (e.g., pneumonia) that contribute to delirium or pulmonary processes that can compromise ventilation and oxygenation should be obtained.

D. Lumbar puncture. If meningitis or encephalitis is suspected, CSF analysis is mandatory. CSF examination also is indicated if findings at computed tomography (CT) of the brain are negative in cases of suspected SAH. Routine CSF analysis consists of white blood cell (WBC) count with differential and red blood cell (RBC) count, glucose and total protein, and Gram stain and culture. Often, patients with delirium need more than the basic CSF studies. Studies used to evaluate specific entities that cause delirium are presented in **Appendix.**

    1. Contraindications to lumbar puncture

        a. Coagulopathy or platelet count less than 50,000 mm^3

        b. Loss of cisternal spaces, evidence of brainstem distortion, absent or distorted fourth ventricle, and any posterior fossa mass on a CT scan

        c. Abscess over the lumbar puncture site

        d. Clinical suspicion of an intracranial mass lesion or increased ICP

    2. The **CSF WBC count** is considered abnormal when more than four WBCs of any type or one neutrophil are found. An increased WBC count suggests CNS infection.

        a. Neutrophils predominate in bacterial infection of the CNS and in early viral encephalitis, particularly that caused by enteroviruses.

        b. Lymphocytes predominate in tuberculous and cryptococcal meningitis, syphilitic infection, herpes simplex encephalitis, toxoplasmosis, and HIV infection.

    3. The presence of **any RBCs** in the CSF is abnormal and requires explanation. Traumatic tap is the most common cause.

        a. Two important pathologic processes that increase the RBC count include SAH and herpes simplex encephalitis. Cerebral infarction, brain tumor (primary and metastatic), traumatic hematoma, and nontraumatic intracerebral hemorrhage inconsistently increase the RBC in the CSF.

        b. **Xanthochromia** is yellow color caused by the presence of **oxyhemoglobin** and **bilirubin** from lysed RBCs in the supernatant of centrifuged CSF. Oxyhemoglobin reaches its peak level in about 36 hours and disappears in 7 to 10 days. Bilirubin appears in the CSF with SAH, reaches its maximum in approximately 48 hours, and disappears in 2 to 4 weeks.

    4. A normal **CSF glucose** level is greater than 50% of the serum glucose level. A low CSF glucose occurs with CNS infection, SAH, hepatic failure, and hypoglycemia.

    5. Increases in **CSF protein** level occur with CNS infection, hemorrhage, and obstruction of CSF flow. Acute intermittent porphyria, hypothyroidism, and Wernicke's encephalopathy are associated with increased protein levels.

        a. Assuming a normal concentration of serum proteins, CSF protein level increases 1 mg per 1,000 RBCs. If a higher ratio is present, the presence of a pathologic process should be suspected.

    6. **CSF Gram stain and cultures** should be performed on all CSF specimens. In cases of suspected bacterial meningitis, latex agglutination testing provides rapid identification of some common bacterial antigens.

7. **Polymerase chain reaction** analysis can assist with identification of CNS infection due to organisms not readily grown on culture media (e.g., viruses). This test is performed infrequently and usually at tertiary care centers.
8. **India ink CSF staining** can be used to rapidly determine the presence of cryptococci, but skepticism should be brought to a negative result of an India ink study when clinical suspicion is high. Fungal cultures are more sensitive.
9. **CSF glutamine** level is elevated in cases of hepatic encephalopathy, but in most cases of hepatic encephalopathy the diagnosis is self-evident without CSF examination. This test is rarely performed.
10. **CSF cytologic evaluation** is used to screen for carcinomatous meningitis, CNS lymphoma, and intracellular toxoplasmosis.

E. **Neuroimaging.**
1. **CT** can help identify most causes of delirium that involve structural damage to the brain, including intraparenchymal, epidural, subdural, and subarachnoid hemorrhage, tumors, infarction, hydrocephalus, and edema.
   a. The CT scan may be normal in cases of early cerebral infarction, meningitis, or hemorrhage of low volume or if the patient has severe anemia.
   b. Intravenous contrast material should be administered for cases of suspected brain abscess or tumor when the patient's condition is medically and neurologically unstable and immediate neurosurgical intervention may be required. If the patient's condition is stable, magnetic resonance imaging (MRI) should be performed instead of CT with contrast material.
2. **MRI of the brain** is useful in the evaluation of delirious patients with suspected herpes simplex encephalitis, white matter processes (e.g., ADEM), a posterior fossa mass, multiple lesions (e.g., metastasis, septic emboli), or immunosuppression. The length of time necessary for completion of MRI often precludes its use in evaluations of unstable and agitated patients.
3. **Magnetic resonance angiography (MRA)** and **venography (MRV)** of the brain are noninvasive diagnostic studies used to diagnose many conditions that affect the vasculature of the brain. Aneurysms, arteriovenous malformations, dissection of large vessels, cerebral venous sinus occlusion, and stenosis and occlusion of both intracranial and extracranial vessels often can be detected with MRA/MRV. Conventional angiography is more sensitive than is MRA/MRV for the diagnosis of CNS vascular disease.
4. **Angiography** should be considered when aneurysm, arteriovenous malformation, venous occlusive disease, or CNS vasculitis is suspected. Identification of the process affects therapeutic management decisions.

F. **Electroencephalography** (EEG) has a role in the evaluation of delirious patients.
1. Almost all patients with delirium have an abnormal EEG with either a posterior dominant rhythm frequency of less than 8 Hz or a relative decrease from an alpha wave of 12 to 10 Hz with mild encephalopathy. As the encephalopathy worsens, the background becomes disorganized, and high-voltage theta and delta activity (slowing) appears with loss of EEG reactivity at frequencies less than 5 to 6 Hz.
2. EEG helps in the diagnosis of complex partial status epilepticus and absence seizures and in identification of abnormal brain activity among patients with seizures.
3. Specific EEG patterns such as triphasic waves (often observed with metabolic derangements) or high-voltage slowing with sharp waves on a flat background (often observed with SSE) can help corroborate clinical diagnostic suspicions.

G. **Brain biopsy** is rarely indicated for the evaluation of delirium. It is necessary when histologic typing of CNS tumors will affect management and outcome and in cases of suspected CNS vasculitis or abscess if the risks of empiric therapy outweigh the risks of the procedure. The presence of encephalitis and SSE can be confirmed with brain biopsy.

Table 1.2 Differential diagnosis of delirium

Aphasia
Mania
Psychosis
Depression
Dementia
Transient global amnesia

IV. Differential diagnosis. Certain conditions can masquerade as delirium (Table 1.2), often requiring an experienced clinician to differentiate the actual process from delirium. Accurate diagnosis is imperative for proper prescription of therapy.

    A. Aphasia. Language formulation disturbance (aphasia) can be initially misdiagnosed as confusion. Because other focal abnormalities (e.g., visual field defects, hemiparesis, hemisensory loss) frequently accompany aphasia more than they do delirium, focal examination findings should drive a thorough "ruling-out" of aphasia. Patients with nonfluent aphasia have normal language comprehension and sensorium but decreased spontaneous speech or mutism with writing difficulty that parallels the verbal expressive deficit. A patient with nonfluent aphasia has a frustrated insight into the language problem. Differentiation of delirious patients from those with fluent aphasia can be difficult. Patients with fluent aphasia have severe comprehension problems but normal or slightly reduced spontaneous speech, often nonsensical without any meaningful content. A patient with fluent aphasia is unaware of the language problem and is frequently agitated, impairing interaction with others. Attention usually is normal.

    B. Psychiatric disorders usually are characterized by prominent changes in several aspects of the mental status examination. Examples include mania, depression, and schizophrenia. A manic patient has a consistently elevated mood, increased goal-directed activity, and grandiosity. In contrast, a delirious patient has emotional lability and is unable to complete tasks.

    C. Dementia. Patients with dementia have memory impairment out of proportion to other aspects of the mental status examination. Patients with dementia may have focal neurologic findings, such as aphasia, apraxia, and agnosia, that delirious patients typically do not have. Attention impairment usually occurs late in the course of dementia.

    D. Transient global amnesia usually occurs among middle-aged or elderly persons and is an acute, self-limited episode of amnesia that lasts for several hours. The memory deficit is for the present and recent past. The key features of delirium, such as inattention, disturbed language function, changes in level of consciousness, and impaired cognitive ability, are notably absent.

V. Diagnostic approach. In the evaluation of a patient with delirium, a logical, stepwise approach enables the clinician to rapidly and accurately diagnose the underlying cause. Figures 1.1, 1.2, 1.3, and 1.4 are algorithms for a practical guide to diagnosis.

    A. On presentation, consider causes such as hypotension and hypoxia that are an immediate threat to life.

    B. If oxygenation and circulation are adequate, a neurologic examination for signs of increased ICP, intracranial hemorrhage, or CNS infection should be performed. If the findings at examination are abnormal, emergency CT of the brain should be performed.

    C. On arrival, admission tests should be performed to rule out a metabolic, cardiac, or toxic cause.

    D. EEG should be performed to rule out ictal activity, if seizures are suspected.

    E. CT and EEG should be performed if all laboratory results are negative.

    F. A lumbar puncture should be performed, if there are no contraindications (see **III.D.**), if CT and EEG have not led to a diagnosis.

(*text continues on page 16*)

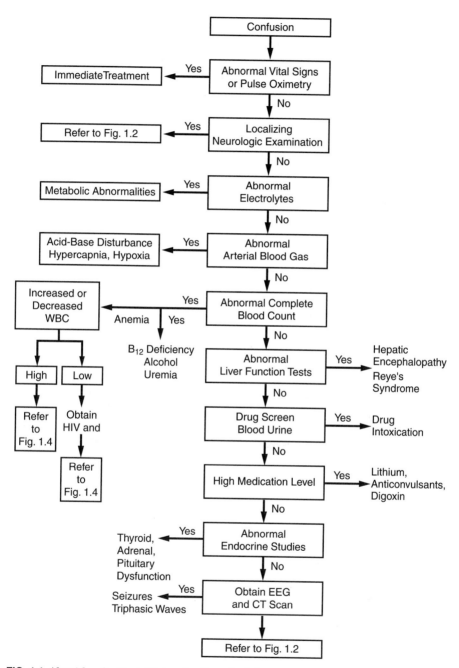

FIG. 1.1 Algorithm for the initial evaluation of a delirious patient. Conditions that require immediate diagnosis and treatment are included. *WBC,* white blood cell count; *HIV,* human immunodeficiency virus; *EEG,* electroencephalogram; *CT,* computed tomography.

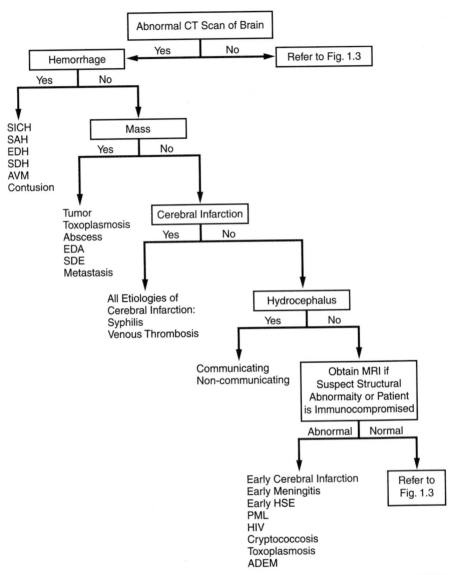

FIG. 1.2 Algorithm for structural intracranial disease. *CT*, computed tomography; *SICH*, spontaneous intracerebral hemorrhage; *SAH*, subarachnoid hemorrhage; *EDH*, epidural hematoma; *SDH*, subdural hematoma; *AVM*, arteriovenous malformation; *EDA*, epidural abscess; *SDE*, subdural empyema; *MRI*, magnetic resonance imaging; *HSE*, herpes simplex encephalitis; *PML*, progressive multifocal leukoencephalopathy; *HIV*, human immunodeficiency virus; *ADEM*, acute disseminated encephalomyelitis.

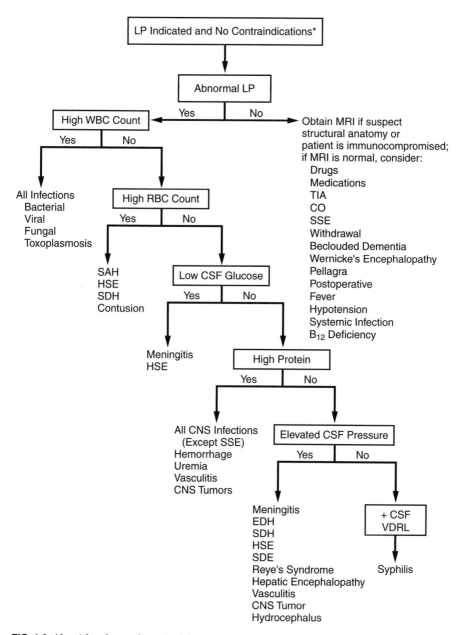

FIG. 1.3 Algorithm for cerebrospinal fluid examination. *LP*, lumbar puncture; *RBC*, red blood cell; *SAH*, subarachnoid hemorrhage; *HSE*, herpes simplex encephalitis; *SDH*, subdural hematoma; *CSF*, cerebrospinal fluid; *CNS*, central nervous system; *SSE*, subacute spongiform encephalopathy; *EDH*, epidural hematoma; *SDE*, subdural empyema; *MRI*, magnetic resonance imaging; *VDRL*, Venereal Disease Research Laboratory test; *TIA*, transient ischemic attack; *CO*, carbon monoxide.

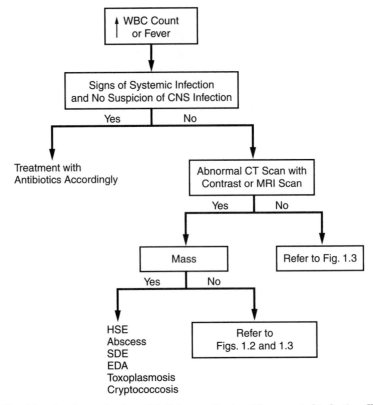

FIG. 1.4 Algorithm for the evaluation of delirious patients with suspected infection. *WBC*, white blood cell count; *CNS*, central nervous system; *CT*, computed tomography; *MRI*, magnetic resonance imaging; *HSE*, herpes simplex encephalitis; *SDE*, subdural empyema; *EDA*, epidural abscess.

     G. MRI should be performed if the clinician suspects that a structural lesion exists despite normal CT findings or if encephalitis, a white matter process, multiple lesions, or a posterior fossa mass is suspected or the patient is immunosuppressed.

     H. Figure 1.3 includes a list of entities to consider when all of the tests do not provide enough information for a diagnosis.

   VI. Criteria for diagnosis. The diagnosis of delirium or acute confusion is given to any patient for whom the predominate abnormalities at mental status examination are inattention and a decline in general cognitive functioning. The *Diagnostic and Statistical Manual of Mental Disorders–IV*[1] (*DSM-IV*) lists the following criteria for the diagnosis of delirium due to a general medical condition:

     A. Disturbance of consciousness (e.g., reduced clarity of awareness of the environment) with reduced ability to focus, sustain, or shift attention.

     B. A change in cognition (e.g., memory deficit, disorientation, language disturbance) or the development of a perceptual disturbance that is not better accounted for by preexisting, established, or evolving dementia.

[1]From the Diagnostic and Statistical Manual of Mental Disorders, Fourth Edition, revised. Washington, DC, American Psychiatric Association, 2000. Printed with permission from the American Psychiatric Association.

  C. A disturbance that develops over a short time, usually hours to days, and tends to fluctuate during the course of the day.

  D. Evidence from the history, physical examination, or laboratory findings that the disturbance is caused by the direct physiologic consequences of a general medical condition.

VII. Referral. If the cause of delirium has been firmly established and the proper treatment initiated, no referral is necessary.

  A. A **neurologic consultation** should be obtained for a suspected primary CNS process, when the diagnosis is unclear, or when neurologic decline continues despite seemingly appropriate management of the underlying cause of delirium. Any focal neurologic abnormality indicates a condition that warrants the advice of a neurologist.

  B. **Neurosurgical consultation** is specifically indicated for assistance with management of intracranial mass lesions (e.g., neoplasm, hemorrhage, edema) or for an invasive intracranial procedure (e.g., brain biopsy, placement of an ICP monitor).

  C. An **infectious disease consultation** is prudent when CNS infection is suspected or for complex systemic infections, as occur among immunosuppressed patients.

  D. **Rheumatologic consultation** can be helpful for assistance in the diagnosis and management of collagen vascular diseases and vasculitis.

Recommended Readings

Aurelius E, Johansson B, Skoldenberg B, et al. Rapid diagnosis of herpes simplex encephalitis by nested polymerase chain reaction assay of cerebrospinal fluid. *Lancet* 1990;337:189–192.

Britton CB, Miller JR. Neurological complications in acquired immunodeficiency syndrome (AIDS). *Neurol Clin* 1984;2:315–339.

Brown P, Cathala F, Castaigne P, et al. Creutzfeldt-Jakob disease: clinical analysis of a consecutive series of 230 neuropathologically verified cases. *Ann Neurol* 1986;20:597–602.

Brown TM. Drug-induced delirium. *Semin Clin Neuropsychiatry* 2000;5:113–124.

Busto U, Sellers EM, Naranjo CA, et al. Withdrawal reaction after long-term therapeutic use of benzodiazepine. *N Engl J Med* 1986;315:854–859.

Charness ME, Simon RP, Greenberg DA. Ethanol and the nervous system. *N Engl J Med* 1989; 321:442–454.

Fann JR. The epidemiology of delirium: a review of studies and methodological issues. *Semin Clin Neuropsychiatry* 2000;5:64–74.

Frey JL, Masferrer R. Postoperative encephalopathy. *BNI Q* 1990;6:30–34.

Greenlee JE. Progressive multifocal leukoencephalopathy. *Curr Clin Topics Infect Dis* 1989;10:140–156.

Griggs RC, Satran R. Metabolic encephalopathy. In: Rosenberg RN, ed. *Comprehensive neurology.* New York: Raven Press, 1991.

Horenstein S, Chamberlin W, Conomy J. Infarction of the fusiform and calcarine regions: agitated delirium and hemianopsia. *Trans Am Neurol Assoc* 1967;92:85–89.

Lipowski ZJ. Delirium in the elderly patient. *N Engl J Med* 1989;320:578–582.

Lockwood AH. Neurologic complications of renal-disease. *Neurol Clin* 1989;7:617–627.

Lowenstein DH, Massa SM, Rowbotham MC, et al. Acute neurologic and psychiatric complications associated with cocaine abuse. *Am J Med* 1987;83:841–846.

Mancall EL. Nutritional disorders of the nervous system. In: Aminoff MJ, ed. *Neurology and general medicine.* New York: Churchill Livingstone, 1989.

Medina JL, Rubino FA, Ross E. Agitated delirium caused by infarctions of the hippocampal formation and fusiform and lingual gyri. *Neurology* 1974;24:1181–1183.

Medina JL, Chokroverty S, Rubino FA. Syndrome of agitated delirium and visual impairment: a manifestation of temporo-occipital infarction. *J Neurol Neurosurg Psychiatry* 1977; 40:861–864.

Mesulam MM, Geschwind N. Disordered state in the post-operative period. *Urol Clin North Am* 1976;3:199–215.

Mesulam MM, Waxman SG, Geschwind N, et al. Acute confusional states with right middle cerebral artery territory infarctions. *J Neurol Neurosurg Psychiatry* 1976;29:84–89.

Mullally W, et al. Frequency of acute confusional states with lesions of the right hemisphere. *Ann Neurol* 1982;12:113.

Pousada L, Leipzig RM. Rapid bedside assessment of postoperative confusion in older patients. *Geriatrics* 1990;45:59–63.

Sterns RH, Riggs JE, Schochet SS Jr. Osmotic demyelination syndrome following correction of hyponatremia. *N Engl J Med* 1986;314:1535–1542.

Taylor D, Lewis S. Delirium. *J Neurol Neurosurg Psychiatry* 1993;56:742–751.

Thompson TL, Thompson WL. Treating postoperative delirium. *Drug Ther* 1983;13:30.

Trzepacz PT. Is there a final common neural pathway in delirium? Focus on acetylcholine and dopamine. Semin Clin Neuropsychiatry 2000;5:132–148.

Tune LE, Damlouji NF, Holland A, et al. Association of postoperative delirium with raised serum levels of anticholinergic drugs. *Lancet* 1981;2:651–653.

Whitley RJ, Soong SJ, Linneman C Jr, et al. Herpes simplex encephalitis: clinical assessment. JAMA 1982;247:317–320.

2. APPROACH TO THE PATIENT WITH DEMENTIA

Rodney A. Short
Neill R. Graff-Radford

In the *Diagnostic and Statistical Manual of Mental Disorders–IV (DSM-IV)* criteria, **dementia** is defined as a decline in memory and at least one other cognitive function (aphasia, apraxia, agnosia, or a decline in an executive function, such as planning, organizing, sequencing, or abstracting). This decline impairs social or occupational functioning in comparison with previous functioning. The deficits should not occur exclusively during the course of delirium and should not be accounted for by another psychiatric condition, such as depression or schizophrenia. Dementia is further defined by a possible, probable, or definite etiologic diagnosis.

   I. Incidence and prevalence of dementia. It is estimated that more than 4% of persons older than 65 years have dementia and that approximately 50% to 75% of patients with dementia have Alzheimer's disease. It is also noteworthy that the incidence of Alzheimer's disease and vascular dementia is age related; that is, the older one is, the greater is the chance of having one of these diseases. The prevalence of dementia is estimated to be 20% among persons older than 85 years. These data should be analyzed in the context of the aging population. For example, in the United States, 50% of persons are expected to live past the age of 75 years and 25% past the age of 85 years.
   II. Etiology. Table 2.1 lists many of the causes of dementia. In a review by Clarfield of more than 1,000 patients in 11 studies for which follow-up data were available, the dementia was partially reversed in 8% cases and completely reversed in 3%. Among the treatable patients, metabolic disease was thought to be the cause of dementia for 16%, depression for 26%, and drugs for 28%.
   III. Criteria for diagnosis. The following are the diagnostic guidelines for Alzheimer's disease (the most common cause of dementia), vascular dementia (the second most common cause of dementia), and Lewy body disease and frontotemporal lobar degeneration (the second and third most common causes of degenerative dementia). Also presented are the guidelines for diagnosis of mild cognitive impairment, which bridges the spectrum between dementia and normal cognition.
      A. The **National Institute of Neurological and Communicative Disorders and Stroke** and the **Alzheimer's and Related Diseases Association** criteria for the diagnosis of Alzheimer's disease are as follows:
         1. Criteria for the clinical diagnosis of **probable Alzheimer's disease**
            a. Dementia established by means of clinical examination and documented with the Mini-Mental State Examination, Blessed Dementia Rating Scale, or other similar examination and confirmed with neuropsychological tests.
            b. Deficits in two or more areas of cognition
            c. Progressive worsening of memory and other cognitive function
            d. No disturbance of consciousness
            e. Onset between the ages of 40 and 90 years, most often after 65 years.
            f. Absence of systemic disorders or other brain diseases that in and of themselves could account for the progressive deficits in memory and cognition
         2. Supporting findings in the diagnosis of **probable Alzheimer's disease**
            a. Progressive deterioration of specific cognitive functions such as aphasia, apraxia, or agnosia
            b. Impaired activities of daily living and altered patterns of behavior
            c. Family history of similar disorders, particularly if confirmed neuropathologically
            d. Laboratory results as follows:
               (1) Normal results of lumbar puncture as evaluated with standard techniques
               (2) Normal pattern or nonspecific electroencephalographic changes, such as increased slow-wave activity
               (3) Evidence of cerebral atrophy at computed tomography (CT) with progression documented by means of serial observation

Table 2.1 Causes of dementia

Degenerative	Psychiatric
Alzheimer's disease	*Depression*
Lewy body disease	*Alcohol abuse*
Parkinson's disease	*Drug-related disorder*
Frontotemporal lobar degeneration	*Personality disorder*
Frontotemporal dementia	*Anxiety disorder*
Progressive nonfluent aphasia	**Toxic/Metabolic**
Semantic dementia	*Vitamin B_{12} deficiency*
Progressive supranuclear palsy	*Thyroid deficiency*
Corticobasal degeneration	*System failure: liver, renal, cardiac,*
Multiple system atrophy	*respiratory*
Huntington's disease	*Heavy metals*
Olivopontocerebellar degeneration	*Toxins* (e.g., glue sniffing)
Vascular	**Traumatic**
Multiple infarction	*Subdural hematoma*
Single stroke	*Closed head injury*
Binswanger's disease	*Open head injury*
Vasculitis	Pugilistic brain injury
Subarachnoid hemorrhage	Anoxic brain injury
Infectious	**Tumors**
Fungal meningitis	*Glioblastoma*
Syphilis	*Lymphoma*
AIDS dementia	*Metastatic tumor*
Creutzfeldt–Jakob disease	**Other**
Post–herpes simplex encephalitis	*Symptomatic hydrocephalus*

Italics indicate the etiologic factor is at least partially reversible or treatable.

3. Other clinical features consistent with the diagnosis of **probable Alzheimer's disease,** after exclusion of causes of dementia other than Alzheimer's disease
   a. Plateaus in the course of progression of the illness
   b. Associated symptoms of depression; insomnia; incontinence; delusions; illusions; hallucinations; catastrophic verbal, emotional, or physical outbursts; sexual disorders; and weight loss.
   c. Other neurologic abnormalities for some patients, especially those with advanced disease, and including motor signs such as increased muscle tone, myoclonus, or gait disorder
   d. Seizures in advanced disease
   e. CT findings normal for age
4. Features that make the diagnosis of **probable Alzheimer's disease** uncertain or unlikely
   a. Sudden, apoplectic onset
   b. Focal neurologic findings such as hemiparesis, sensory loss, visual field deficits, and incoordination early in the course of the illness
   c. Seizures or gait disturbance at the onset or early in the course of the illness
5. Clinical diagnosis of **possible Alzheimer's disease**
   a. May be made on the basis of the dementia syndrome, in the absence of other neurologic, psychiatric, or systemic disorders sufficient to cause dementia and in the presence of variations in onset, presentation, or clinical course.
   b. May be made in the presence of a second systemic or brain disorder sufficient to produce dementia, which is not considered to be the principal cause of the dementia.
   c. Should be used in research studies when a single, gradually progressive severe cognitive deficit is identified in the absence of any other identifiable cause.

    6. Criteria for diagnosis of **definite Alzheimer's disease** are the clinical criteria for probable Alzheimer's disease and histopathologic evidence obtained from a biopsy or autopsy.

    7. Classification of Alzheimer's disease for research purposes should specify features that differentiate subtypes of the disorder, such as familial occurrence, onset before 65 years of age, presence of trisomy 21, and coexistence of other relevant conditions such as Parkinson's disease.

B. The **National Institute of Neurological Disorders** and **Stroke-Association Internationale pour la Recherche et L'Enseignement en Neurosciences** criteria for the diagnosis of **vascular dementia** are as follows:

    1. The criteria for **probable vascular dementia** include all of the following:

        a. Dementia defined similarly to *DSM-IV* criteria

        b. Cerebrovascular disease defined by the presence of focal signs on neurologic examination, such as hemiparesis, lower facial weakness, Babinski sign, sensory deficit, hemianopia, and dysarthria consistent with stroke (with or without history of stroke), and evidence of relevant cerebrovascular disease at brain imaging (CT or magnetic resonance imaging), including multiple large-vessel infarcts or a single strategically situated infarct (angular gyrus, thalamus, basal forebrain, or posterior or anterior cerebral artery territories), as well as multiple basal ganglia and white matter lesions and white matter lacunes or extensive periventricular white matter lesions, or combinations thereof.

        c. A relation between the two previous disorders manifested or inferred by the presence of one or more of the following: (1) onset of dementia within 3 months after a recognized stroke, (2) abrupt deterioration in cognitive functions, or (3) fluctuating, stepwise progression of cognitive deficits.

    2. Clinical features consistent with the diagnosis of **probable vascular dementia** include the following:

        a. Early presence of a gait disturbance

        b. History of unsteadiness and frequent, unprovoked falls

        c. Early urinary frequency, urgency, and other urinary symptoms not explained by urologic disease

        d. Pseudobulbar palsy

        e. Personality and mood changes, abulia, depression, emotional incontinence, or other subcortical deficits, including psychomotor retardation and abnormal executive functioning

    3. Features that make the diagnosis of **vascular dementia** uncertain or unlikely include the following:

        a. Early onset of memory and other cognitive functions, such as language, motor skills, and perception in the absence of corresponding lesions at brain imaging

        b. Absence of focal neurologic signs other than cognitive disturbance

        c. Absence of cerebrovascular lesions on CT scans or magnetic resonance images

    4. The term **Alzheimer's disease with cerebrovascular disease** should be reserved to classify the condition of patients fulfilling the clinical criteria for possible Alzheimer's disease and who also have clinical or brain imaging evidence of relevant cerebrovascular disease.

C. **Lewy body disease** is defined pathologically by the presence of cortical Lewy bodies and is part of a spectrum with Parkinson's disease, which has brainstem Lewy bodies. The **McKeith criteria** for the clinical diagnosis of Lewy body disease are as follows:

    1. Progressive cognitive decline interferes with normal social and occupational functioning.

    2. Deficits on tests of attention/concentration, verbal fluency, psychomotor speed, and visuospatial functioning often are prominent.

    3. Prominent or persistent memory impairment may not be present early in the course of illness.

    4. Two of the following core features are necessary for the diagnosis of **probable Lewy body disease** and one is necessary for **possible Lewy body disease**:
      a. Fluctuating cognition or alertness
      b. Recurrent visual hallucinations
      c. Spontaneous features of parkinsonism
    5. Features supportive of the diagnosis are repeated falls, syncope or transient loss of consciousness, neuroleptic sensitivity, systematized delusions, tactile or olfactory hallucinations, rapid eye movement sleep behavior disorder, or depression.
    6. The following features suggest a **disorder other than Lewy body disease:**
      a. Cerebrovascular disease evidenced by focal neurologic signs or cerebral infarcts present on neuroimaging studies
      b. Findings at examination or ancillary testing that another medical, neurologic, or psychiatric disorder sufficiently accounts for clinical features

D. Frontotemporal lobar degeneration involves focal atrophy of the frontal or temporal lobes or both, the distribution of atrophy determining the clinical presentation. The age at onset tends to be slightly younger (often before 65 years) than is that for Alzheimer's disease. Patients with frontotemporal lobar degeneration usually do not have Alzheimer's-type pathologic findings and usually are found to have either **dementia lacking distinctive histologic features** or **Pick's disease.** The three clinical phenotypes are frontotemporal dementia, progressive nonfluent aphasia, and semantic dementia. The **Neary criteria** for the clinical diagnosis of frontotemporal lobar degeneration are as follows:

    1. In **frontotemporal dementia,** character change and disordered social conduct are the dominant features initially and throughout the disease course. Instrumental functions of perception, spatial skills, praxis, and memory are intact or relatively well preserved. Core criteria are as follows:
      a. Insidious onset and gradual progression
      b. Early decline in social interpersonal conduct
      c. Early impairment in regulation of personal conduct
      d. Early emotional blunting
      e. Early loss of insight
    2. In **progressive nonfluent aphasia** expressive language is the dominant feature initially and throughout the disease course. Other aspects of cognition are intact or relatively well preserved. Core criteria are as follows:
      a. Insidious onset and gradual progression
      b. Nonfluent spontaneous speech with at least one of the following: agrammatism, phonemic paraphasias, anomia
    3. In **semantic dementia,** a semantic disorder (impaired understanding of word meaning or object identity) is the dominant feature initially and throughout the disease course. Other aspects of cognition, including autobiographical memory, are intact or relatively well preserved. Core criteria are as follows:
      a. Insidious onset and gradual progression
      b. Language disorder characterized by the following:
        (1) Progressive, fluent, empty spontaneous speech
        (2) Loss of word meaning manifested as impaired naming and comprehension
      c. Semantic paraphasia with or without **d.**
      d. Perceptual disorder characterized by one or both of the following:
        (1) Prosopagnosia—impaired recognition of identity of familiar faces
        (2) Associative agnosia—impaired recognition of object identity
      e. Preserved perceptual matching and drawing reproduction
      f. Preserved single-word repetition
      g. Preserved ability to read aloud and write to dictation of orthographically regular words
    4. Diagnostic exclusion features for **frontotemporal lobar degeneration** syndromes are abrupt onset with ictal events; head trauma related to onset; early, severe amnesia; spatial disorientation; logoclonic, festinant speech

with loss of train of thought; myoclonus; corticospinal weakness; cerebellar ataxia; choreoathetosis; brain images with predominant postcentral structural or functional deficit or multifocal lesions; or laboratory test results that indicate brain involvement of a metabolic or inflammatory disorder such as multiple sclerosis, syphilis, acquired immunodeficiency syndrome, and herpes simplex encephalitis.

E. Memory problems are common among the elderly but do not always herald the onset of dementia. Isolated memory impairment, or **mild cognitive impairment,** progresses to dementia at a rate of approximately 10% to 12% per year. Petersen et al. developed the following criteria for **mild cognitive impairment** among patients who underwent a complete neurologic and neuropsychological evaluation:

1. A memory problem
2. Normal activities of daily living
3. Normal general cognitive functioning
4. Abnormal memory functioning for age
5. No dementia according to *DSM-III-R* criteria

IV. Evaluation

A. History. It is essential that the history be obtained not only from the patient but also from an independent informant—the spouse, for example. In most the patient can be told, "I am now going to ask your spouse some questions, and if your spouse makes any errors, feel free to make corrections." Sometimes the informant may not want to speak openly in front of the patient, so the clinician may want to arrange a separate interview, perhaps while the patient is undergoing another test or later by telephone.

1. **Patient difficulties.** Determine what difficulties the patient is having and what family members have noticed. Commonly a patient with dementia may not know there is a memory difficulty or be able to give accurate details of the problem. Begin by asking the patient an open-ended question such as, "What problems are you having?" This often does not elicit the desired responses. Even with specific questions such as, "Are you having difficulty with your memory?" the clinician may not be told what the problems are. The informant may have to be asked specific questions, such as, "What can't the patient do now that he (or she) could do before?" or "Does the patient sometimes ask the same question more than once in the same conversation?"

2. **Time course.** The time the family first noticed problems and the course the disease has taken over time are critical factors in the evaluation. A disease that is slowly progressive time fits the profile of a degenerative disease such as Alzheimer's. A disease that starts suddenly or follows a stepwise progression would be more in keeping with vascular dementia. Rapidly progressive dementia (over a few months) suggests Creutzfeldt–Jakob disease.

3. **Functioning of the patient.** Determine how well the patient has been functioning at work and at home, including performance of the basic activities of daily living. Patients with mild cognitive impairment are by definition able to function well. Patients with progressive nonfluent aphasia or semantic dementia usually also are able to function well. Ask what the patient does to keep busy. Does he or she read the newspaper, watch the news on television, keep the checkbook, do the shopping, prepare the meals, take part in a sport or hobby? Knowing this information helps in the planning of questions to ask during the mental status part of the examination.

4. **Issues of safety.** Ask whether the patient drives. If so, has the patient ever become lost while driving or had any accidents, near-accidents, or traffic violations? If the patient prepares meals, has he or she ever left the stove on? Does the patient keep weapons, and if so, has this posed any danger to the patient or to others?

5. **Etiologically directed history.** Include a history of vascular disease and risk factors, head injury, toxic exposure, symptoms of infection or exposure to diseases such as tuberculosis, psychiatric history such as depression,

symptoms of depression (such as a change in weight, insomnia, crying, or anhedonia), medications, systemic illnesses, other past illnesses, and alcohol or tobacco use.

The following questions may bring out symptoms of Lewy body disease: Does the patient have good days and bad days? What specifically can't the patient do on bad days? Does the patient see things that are not there? Does the patient act out dreams at night? Look for personality and behavioral changes in frontotemporal dementia with specific questions such as, Does the patient drive recklessly, such as run stop signs or speed? Has the patient developed poor table manners such as eating excessively fast? Does the patient have rituals or do things repetitively?

6. **Family history.** Ask what the patient's parents died of and at what ages. Ask specifically whether there were memory problems in the later years. Then ask about the ages and health of the patient's siblings and children. Patients with late-onset Alzheimer's disease commonly have a family history of disease. A strong family history for a younger patient suggests an autosomal dominant disease such as familial Alzheimer's disease, familial frontotemporal lobar degeneration, Huntington's disease, or spinocerebellar ataxia.

B. **Physical examination.**
   1. Give a **standardized short mental state test,** such as the Folstein Mini-Mental State Examination (see Folstein et al., 1975). Asking about news events is a highly sensitive measure of recent memory. Be sure that the patient has been exposed to this information. Ask questions such as, Who is the president? What is his wife's name? Who was the last president? What is his wife's name? Note any evidence of aphasia, apraxia, or agnosia. Anomia with preservation of orientation suggests semantic dementia. Observe for lack of insight and disinhibited behaviors that occur in frontotemporal dementia.
   2. Look for **cardiovascular risk factors** such as hypertension, arterial bruits, arrhythmia, and heart murmur.
   3. Complete a **full neurologic examination.** Pay special attention to focal deficits such as visual field cuts, paresis, sensory loss, and ataxia. Alzheimer's disease occasionally begins as progressive visual dysfunction similar to that of Balint's syndrome. Evaluate for any extrapyramidal difficulties, such as hypokinesia, increased muscle tone, a masklike face, and micrographia. Determine whether the patient has any problem walking. This is often best undertaken in the hallway rather than in the examining room. Note the patient's step size, speed of walking, arm swing, and ability to turn. The palmomental reflex and snout reflex are not particularly helpful because they are common among healthy elderly. The grasp reflex occurs late in the course of the disease.

C. **Laboratory studies**
   1. **Recommended in all cases** are complete blood cell count, chemistry panel, erythrocyte sedimentation rate, thyroid function tests, vitamin B_{12} level, syphilis serologic testing, computed tomography or magnetic resonance imaging, and neuropsychological evaluation.
   2. **Recommended selectively** are electroencephalography, lumbar puncture, chest radiograph, acquired immunodeficiency syndrome test, drug screen, single photon emission computed tomography (SPECT) or positron emission tomography (PET), and heavy metal screen.
   3. **Electroencephalography** can be useful in diagnosing Creutzfeldt–Jakob disease, differentiating depression or delirium from dementia, evaluating for encephalitis, revealing seizures as causes of memory difficulties, and diagnosing nonconvulsive status epilepticus.
   4. **Lumbar puncture** is recommended if the patient has cancer, infection is a possibility, hydrocephalus is seen at imaging, the patient is younger than 55 years, the dementia is acute or subacute, the patient is immunosuppressed, or vasculitis or connective tissue disease is suspected.
   5. **PET** or **SPECT** can be useful in differentiating frontotemporal dementia from Alzheimer's disease. In one blinded study in which PET was used to

evaluate patients with and those without dementia, the sensitivity was only 38% and the specificity was 88%.

6. Numerous **diagnostic biomarkers** for degenerative diseases are becoming available; however, the positive predictive value of these biomarkers in a typical clinical scenario is uncertain. Cerebrospinal fluid amyloid β and τ protein levels are reported to be 90% sensitive and 80% specific for Alzheimer's disease. We use this test only when a lumbar puncture is being performed for other reasons, such as evaluation for hydrocephalus. Cerebrospinal fluid 14-3-3 protein is reported to be 94% sensitive and 93% specific for Creutzfeldt–Jakob disease compared with neurologic controls, but false-positive and false-negative results do occur (and are probably more likely in atypical cases, in which it would be the most useful). The ε4 allele of the apolipoprotein E gene (apoE4) is a well-established risk factor for Alzheimer's disease; however, the American Medical Association does not recommend apoE4 testing in the diagnosis of Alzheimer's disease or if the patient's condition is presymptomatic. Mutations in the presenilin-1, presenilin-2, and amyloid precursor protein genes can cause early-onset, autosomal dominant Alzheimer's disease. Only mutations in presenilin-1 are commercially available for testing, and genetic counseling is required before and after testing.

V. Differential diagnosis. Be aware of the possible causes of dementia in Table 2.1. The most important reversible causes include depression, medication, hydrocephalus, thyroid disease, vitamin B_{12} deficiency, fungal infection, neurosyphilis, subdural hematoma, and brain tumor.

Alzheimer's disease usually is a slowly progressive dementia without focal neurologic deficit but with prominent anterograde amnesia followed by naming difficulties and visuospatial problems. Patients with **Lewy body dementia** with or without Alzheimer's disease often have extrapyramidal deficits without a resting tremor and with prominent psychiatric symptoms that include psychosis and depression. **Vascular dementia** is characterized by a sudden onset, stepwise progression, a history of stroke risk factors (previous stroke, transient ischemic attack, hypertension, atrial fibrillation, and coronary artery disease), focal signs, and imaging studies showing strokes.

When a patient has a prominent change in behavior, perseverations, hyperphagia, poor insight, and, in the beginning, relative preservation of memory, suspect **frontotemporal dementia.** Progressive language difficulties with preservation of activities of daily living and orientation may lead to a diagnosis of **progressive nonfluent aphasia** or **semantic dementia. Corticobasal degeneration** is characterized by progressive asymmetric apraxia and rigidity and **progressive supranuclear palsy** by axial rigidity and vertical eye movement abnormalities. However, both can manifest as cognitive symptoms. **Creutzfeldt–Jakob disease** can manifest as a subacute course, myoclonus, visual changes, and ataxia. Look for **hydrocephalus** if the patient has gait abnormality, memory loss, preserved naming, a large head (approximately 10% of cases), and incontinence.

Much overlap exists clinically and pathologically with these various syndromes, for example, Alzheimer's disease and Lewy body disease. Frontotemporal lobar degeneration, corticobasal degeneration, and progressive supranuclear palsy also can have similar clinical and pathologic features.

Acknowledgment
This work was supported by National Institute of Aging grant P50 AG16574-02 and the State of Florida Alzheimer's Disease Initiative.

Recommended Readings
Alzheimer's Disease and Related Disorders Association (ADRDA), 919 North Michigan Avenue, #1000, Chicago, IL, 69611-1678, (800)272-3900.

Becker P, Feussner JR, Mulrow CD, et al. The role of lumbar puncture in the evaluation of dementia: the Durham Veterans Administration/Duke University Study. *J Am Geriatr Soc* 1985;33:392–396.

Clarfield A. The reversible dementias: do they reverse? *Ann Intern Med* 1988;109:476–486.

Consensus Report of the Working Group on Molecular and Biochemical Markers of Alzheimer's Disease. *Neurobiol Aging* 1998;19:109–116.

Corey-Bloom J, Thal LJ, Galasko D, et al. Diagnosis and evaluation of dementia. *Neurology* 1995;45:211–218.

Diagnostic and Statistical Manual of Mental Disorders. 4th ed. Washington, DC: American Psychiatric Association, 1994.

Folstein MF, Folstein SE, McHugh PR. "Mini-mental state": a practical method for grading the cognitive state of patients for the clinician. *J Psychiatr Res* 1975;12:189–198.

Graff-Radford NR, Godersky JC, Jones M. Variables predicting surgical outcome in symptomatic hydrocephalus in the elderly. *Neurology* 1989;39:1601–1604.

Heston L. Morbid risk in first-degree relatives of persons with Alzheimer's disease. *Arch Gen Psychiatry* 45:97–98, 1988.

McKeith IG, Perry EK, Perry RH. Report of the second dementia with Lewy body international workshop: diagnosis and treatment. Consortium on Dementia with Lewy Bodies. *Neurology* 1999;53:902–905.

McKhann G, Drachman D, Folstein M, et al. Clinical diagnosis of Alzheimer's disease: report of the NINCDS-ADRDA Work Group under the auspices of the Department of Health and Human Services Task Force on Alzheimer's Disease. *Neurology* 1984;34:939–944.

Morris JC, ed. *Handbook of dementing illnesses.* New York: Marcel Dekker, 1994.

Mortimer JA. The epidemiology of Alzheimer's disease: beyond risk factors. In: Iqbal I, et al., eds. *Research advances in Alzheimer's disease and associated disorders.* New York: John Wiley & Sons, 1995:3–11.

Neary D, Snowden JS, Gustafson L, et al. Frontotemporal lobar degeneration: a consensus on clinical diagnostic criteria. *Neurology* 1998;51:1546-1554.

Petersen RC, Smith GE, Waring SC, et al. Mild cognitive impairment: clinical characterization and outcome. *Arch Neurol* 1999;56:303–308.

Post SG, Whitehouse PJ, Binstock RH, et al. The clinical introduction of genetic testing for Alzheimer disease: an ethical perspective [Consensus Statement]. *JAMA* 1997;277:832–836.

Roman GC, Tatemichi TK, Erkinjuntti T, et al. Vascular dementia: diagnostic criteria for research studies: report of the NINDS-AIREN International Workshop. *Neurology* 1993;43:250–260.

3. APPROACH TO THE PATIENT WITH APHASIA

Jeffrey L. Saver

Aphasia is loss or impairment of language processing caused by brain damage. Language disorders are common manifestations of cerebral injury. Reflecting the centrality of language function in human endeavor, aphasia is a major source of disability.

I. **Pathophysiology**
   A. **Cerebral dominance.** The left hemisphere is dominant for language among approximately 99% of right-handed persons and 60% of left-handed persons.
   B. **Neuroanatomy.** A specialized cortical–subcortical neural system surrounding the sylvian fissure in the dominant hemisphere subserves language processing (Fig. 3.1). Circumscribed lesions in different components of this neurocognitive network produce distinctive syndromes of language impairment.

II. **Etiology**
   A. **Stroke.** Cerebrovascular disease is a frequent cause of aphasia. The perisylvian language zone is supplied by divisions of the middle cerebral artery, a branch of the internal carotid artery. The classic aphasic syndromes are most distinctly observed in ischemic stroke because vascular occlusions produce discrete, well-delineated brain lesions.
   B. **Other focal lesions.** Any focal lesion affecting the language cortices also produces aphasia, including primary and metastatic neoplasms and abscesses. **Primary progressive aphasia** is an uncommon neurodegenerative syndrome character-ized by slowly progressive, isolated language impairment in late life and focal atro-phy of dominant frontotemporal cortices. Persons with this disorder frequently have generalized dementia after the first 2 years of illness. Among the causes of pri-mary progressive aphasia are a focal variant of Alzheimer's disease, a focal variant of Pick's disease, and focal neuronal loss without specific histopathologic features.
   C. **Diffuse lesions.** Diseases producing widespread neuronal dysfunction disrupt language processing along with other cognitive and noncognitive neural func-tions. **Traumatic head injury** and **Alzheimer's disease** are epidemiologically common causes of aphasic symptoms, although not of isolated aphasia.

III. **Clinical manifestations**
   A. **Nonfluency versus fluency.** *Fluency* refers to the rate, quantity, and ease of speech production.
      1. In **nonfluent** speech, verbal output is meager (<50 words/min), phrase length is shortened (one to four words per phrase), production is effortful, articula-tion often is poor, and the melodic contour (prosody) is disturbed. Nonfluent speakers often preferentially use substantive nouns and verbs, eliding small connecting grammatical/functor words (telegraphic speech).
      2. In **fluent** speech, verbal output is generous (and may even be more abun-dant than is customary), phrase length is normal, production is easy, artic-ulation usually is preserved, and the melodic contour is intact.
      3. **Anatomic correlate.** Nonfluency indicates damage to the frontal language regions anterior to the fissure of Rolando. Fluency signals that these areas are intact.
   B. **Auditory comprehension impairment**
      1. Impaired ability to understand spoken language ranges from complete mys-tification by simple one-word utterances to subtle failure to extract the full meanings of complex sentences. In informal conversation, aphasic patients often capitalize on clues from gestures, tone, and setting to supplement their understanding of the propositional content of a speaker's utterances. Exam-iners may underestimate the extent of auditory comprehension impairment if they do not conduct formal testing of a patient's comprehension without nonverbal cues.
      2. **Anatomic correlate.** Comprehension impairment generally reflects damage to the temporoparietal language regions posterior to the fissure of Rolando. Preserved comprehension indicates that these areas are intact.

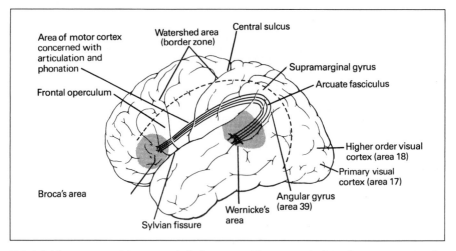

FIG. 3.1 The neurocognitive network for language. The core perisylvian language cortices lie within the *dashed line* and include Broca's area in the inferior frontal gyrus, the supramarginal and angular gyri in the parietal lobe, the subjacent arcuate fasciculus white matter tract, and Wernicke's area in the superior temporal gyrus. Extrasylvian sites that produce transcortical aphasia are present in surrounding cortices (*beyond dashed line*). (Modified from Mayeux R, Kandel ER. Disorders of language: the aphasias. In: Kandel ER, Schwartz JH, eds. *Principles of neural science,* 2nd ed. New York: Elsevier, 1985, with permission.)

(Comprehension of grammar is an important exception to this rule. Agrammatism is associated with damage to inferior frontal language regions.)

C. Repetition impairment

    1. Repetition of spoken language is linguistically and anatomically a distinct language function. For most patients, repetition impairment parallels other deficits in spoken language. Occasionally, however, relatively isolated disordered repetition is the dominant clinical feature (conduction aphasia). For other patients, repetition may be well-preserved despite severe deficits in spontaneous speech (transcortical aphasia). In rare instances, such patients have echolalia, a powerful, mandatory tendency to repeat all heard phrases.

    2. Anatomic correlate. Impaired repetition indicates damage within the core perisylvian language zone. Preserved repetition signals that these areas are intact.

D. Paraphasic errors. Paraphasia is substitution of incorrect words for intended words. Paraphasic errors are classified into three types.

    1. Literal or **phonemic** paraphasia occurs when only a part of the word is misspoken, as when "apple" becomes "tapple" or "apfle."

    2. Verbal or **global** paraphasia occurs when an entire incorrect word is substituted for the intended word, as when "apple" becomes "orange" or "bicycle." **Semantic** paraphasia occurs when the substituted word is from the same semantic field as the target word ("orange" for "apple"). Fluent output contaminated by many forms of verbal paraphasia is **jargon speech.**

    3. Neologistic paraphasia occurs when an entirely novel word not extant in the speaker's native lexicon is substituted for the intended word, as when "apple" becomes "brifun."

    4. Anatomic correlate. Paraphasic errors can occur with lesions anywhere within the language system and do not carry strong anatomic implications. To some extent, phonemic paraphasia is more common with lesions in the frontal language fields, and global paraphasia more common with lesions in temporoparietal areas.

E. **Word-finding difficulty (anomia)**

1. Retrieval of target words from the lexicon is almost always disturbed in aphasia. Patients may have frequent hesitations in spontaneous speech while they struggle with word finding.

2. **Circumlocution** occurs when patients "talk around" words they fail to retrieve, providing lengthy definitions or descriptions to convey the meanings of words they are unable to access.

3. **Anatomic correlate.** Word-finding difficulty occurs with lesions located throughout the language dominant hemisphere and possesses little localizing value.

F. **Reading and writing**

1. In most cases of aphasia, reading impairment (**alexia**) and writing impairment (**agraphia**) parallel oral language comprehension and production deficits. Occasionally, however, isolated reading impairment, writing impairment, or both can occur in the setting of fully preserved oral language function.

2. **Anatomic correlate.** The anatomy of reading and writing incorporates both the core perisylvian language zones and additional function-specific sites. Reading requires primary and higher-level visual processing in the occipital and inferior parietal lobes. Writing depends on visual stores in the inferior parietal lobe and graphomotor output regions in the frontal lobe.

IV. **Evaluation**

A. **History.** Abrupt onset of language difficulty suggests a cerebrovascular lesion. Subacute onset suggests tumor, abscess, or another more moderately progressive process. Slow onset suggests a degenerative disease, such as Alzheimer's or Pick's. Interviewing family members and other observers is crucial when the patient's language difficulty limits direct history taking.

B. **Physical examination**

1. **Elementary neurologic signs.** A detailed elementary neurologic examination allows identification of motor, sensory, or visual deficits that accompany the language disorder and aids neuroanatomic localization. Important "neighborhood" signs are the presence or absence of hemiparesis, homonymous hemianopia or quadrantanopia, and apraxia.

2. **Mental status examination.** It is important to assess the patient's wakefulness and attentional function, lest language errors resulting from inattentiveness be wrongly ascribed to intrinsic linguistic dysfunction. Nonverbal tests to evaluate memory, visuospatial, and executive functions should be used if severe language disturbance precludes routine verbal assessment.

3. **Language examination.** A careful language examination is critical in the evaluation of aphasia, profiling the patient's impaired and preserved language abilities, and allowing a syndromic, localizing diagnosis.

   a. **Spontaneous speech.** The patient's spontaneous verbal output in the course of conversation and in response to general questions should be judged for fluency versus nonfluency and presence or absence of paraphasia. It is important to ask open-ended questions, such as, Why are you in the hospital? or What do you do during a typical day at home? because patients may mask major language derangements with yes-or-no answers and other brief replies to more structured interrogatories.

   b. **Repetition.** The patient is asked to repeat complex sentences. If difficulty is evidenced, simpler verbal sequences from single-syllable words to multisyllabic words and short phrases are given to determine the level of impairment. At least one sentence rich in grammatical/functor words, such as "No ifs, ands, or buts," should be used to test for isolated or more pronounced difficulty in grammatical repetition, as may occur in Broca's and other forms of anterior aphasia.

   c. **Comprehension.** An initial judgment of auditory comprehension can be made in the course of obtaining the medical history and from spontaneous conversation. Tests that require no or minimal verbal responses are essential to evaluation of auditory comprehension for persons with severe disturbance of speech production and those with an endotracheal tube in place.

   (1) Commands. One simple bedside test is orally to instruct the patient to carry out one-step and multistep commands, such as Pick up a piece of paper, fold it in half, and place it on the table. Cautions to recall when interpreting results are that (1) apraxia and other motor deficits can cause impairment not related to comprehension deficit, and that (2) midline motor acts on command, such as closing and opening the eyes and standing up, draw on distinct anatomic systems and may be preserved, even in the setting of severe aphasic comprehension disturbance.

   (2) Yes/no responses. If the patient can reliably produce verbal or gestural yes/no responses, this output system can be used to assess auditory comprehension. Questions of graded difficulty should be used for precise gauging of the degree of comprehension disturbance. Queries should range from simple (Is your name Smith?) to complex (Do helicopters eat their young?).

   (3) Pointing. This simple motor response also allows precise mapping of comprehension impairment by means of questions of graded difficulty. The examiner should use both simple pointing commands (Point to the chair, nose, door) and more lexically and syntactically complex pointing commands (Point to the source of illumination in this room.).

d. Naming. Difficulty with naming is almost invariable in all the aphasia syndromes. Consequently, naming tasks are a sensitive, although not specific, means of testing for the presence or absence of aphasia.

   (1) Confrontation naming. The patient is asked to name objects, parts of objects, body parts, and colors pointed out by the examiner. Common, high-frequency words ("tie," "watch") and uncommon, low-frequency words ("knot" of the tie, "watchband") should be tested.

   (2) Word list generation. Another type of naming test is to ask the patient to generate a list of items in a category (animals, cars) or words beginning with a given letter (*F, A, S*). A normal response is to produce 12 or more words per letter in 1 minute.

e. Verbal automatism. Patients with profound disruptions of speech production should be requested to produce (1) overlearned verbal sequences, including the numbers from 1 to 10 and the days of the week. (2) overlearned verbal material, such as the pledge of allegiance, and (3) songs, such as "Happy Birthday to You." These utterances draw on subcortical and nondominant hemisphere areas and indicate residual capacities of impaired patients that may be capitalized on in rehabilitation.

f. Reading. Patients should be asked to read sentences aloud. Written sentences that are commands (Close your eyes) allow simultaneous testing of reading aloud and reading comprehension.

g. Writing. In order of difficulty, patients may be asked to write single letters, words, and short sentences. Obtaining a signature is insufficient, because this overlearned sequence may be retained when all other graphomotor function is lost.

C. Laboratory studies

   1. Computed tomography (CT). CT delineates most focal structural lesions affecting the language regions of the brain. CT findings may be normal in the first 24 hours after acute aphasia from new-onset ischemic stroke.

   2. Magnetic resonance imaging (MRI). MRI is somewhat more sensitive than CT at depicting morphologic abnormalities. MRI is the preferred study if readily available. Imaging in the sagittal, coronal, and axial planes allows precise mapping of lesions within known neural language regions.

V. Syndromic diagnosis. Distinctive features of a patient's language disturbance can be used to assign a syndromic diagnosis that has localizing value (Table 3.1). Eight classic

Table 3.1 Clinical features of aphasia syndromes

Syndrome	Language findings					Associated findings		
	Verbal output	Paraphasia	Comprehension	Repetition	Naming	Hemiparesis	Hemisensory loss	Visual field defect
Broca	Nonfluent	Rare, literal	Good	Poor	Poor	Common	Rare	Rare
Wernicke	Fluent	Frequent, mixed	Poor	Poor	Poor	Rare	Variable	± Quadrantanopia
Conduction	Fluent	Frequent, literal	Good	Poor	Poor	Rare	Common	± Hemianopia
Global	Nonfluent	Frequent, mixed	Poor	Poor	Poor	Common	Common	Hemianopia
Transcortical motor	Nonfluent	Rare	Good	Good	Poor	Occasional	Rare	Rare
Transcortical sensory	Fluent	Frequent, mixed	Poor	Good	Poor	Occasional	Common	± Hemianopia
Mixed transcortical	Nonfluent	Rare	Poor	Good	Poor	Common	Common	Hemianopia
Anomic	Fluent	Frequent	Good	Good	Poor	Rare	Rare	Rare
Striato-capsular	Nonfluent or fluent	Frequent	Good	Good	Poor	Common	Variable	Rare
Thalamic	Fluent	Frequent	Poor	Good	Poor	Rare	Rare	Rare

±, may or may not be present.

cortical aphasia syndromes are differentiated on the basis of fluency, comprehension, and repetition (Fig. 3.2). Approximately 60% of all aphasic patients have one of these symptom clusters. Most of the remaining patients with "atypical" aphasia are found to harbor subcortical lesions. It is important to consider the time after onset when these syndromes are used for clinicoanatomic correlation. Soon after an acute insult, deafferentation, edema, and other mechanisms of diaschisis produce exaggerated clinical deficits. Later, neuroplasticity-mediated recovery of function reduces clinical deficits. The aphasia syndromes have maximal localizing value 3 weeks to 3 months after onset.

A. **Perisylvian aphasias**
 1. **Broca's aphasia.** Patients with Broca's aphasia have (1) nonfluent, dysarthric, effortful speech, (2) similarly disordered repetition, and (3) relatively intact comprehension with mild difficulty in understanding syntax and relational grammar. Their verbal output is often telegraphic, containing substantive nouns and verbs but omitting small, connecting, functor words. Most patients have faciobrachial hemiparesis. Patients often exhibit frustration over their language deficits and are at elevated risk of depression.
   a. Lesions producing Broca's aphasia lie in the posterior portion of the inferior frontal gyrus (Broca's area) and extend to involve surrounding motor, premotor, and underlying white matter territories. Lesions restricted solely to Broca's area produce mild, transient aphasia and more persistent dysarthria.
   b. Broca's area is supplied by the superior division of the middle cerebral artery.
 2. **Wernicke's aphasia.** Patients with Wernicke's aphasia evince fluent, effortless, well-articulated output, almost always contaminated with paraphasia and neologisms. Repetition demonstrates parallel impairment with fluent but paraphasic output. The leading feature of Wernicke's aphasia is severe disturbance of auditory comprehension. Two types of behavioral responses to this comprehension deficit are observed. Most often in the acute phase, patients seem unaware of their inability to comprehend spoken language, calmly providing inappropriate and grossly paraphasic answers to observer inquiries. Less frequently, patients are irritable and paranoic, perhaps

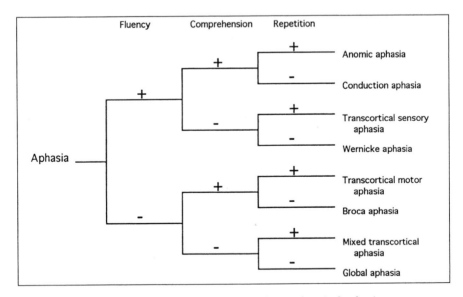

FIG. 3.2 Algorithm for diagnosis of the eight classic forms of cortical aphasia.

because of their inability to understand what others say. Superior homony-mous quadrantanopia is frequently present. However, the absence of more dramatic motor or sensory deficits and the fluid production of speech can mislead medical personnel into believing that the patient is confused or psy-chotic rather than aphasic and can delay diagnosis while metabolic or psy-chiatric disturbances are sought.

   a. The core of lesions engendering Wernicke's aphasia map to the posterior third of the superior temporal gyrus (Wernicke's area), an auditory asso-ciation area. Lesion size varies considerably, and damage often extends to the middle temporal gyrus and the inferior parietal lobe.

   b. Wernicke's area is supplied by the inferior division of the middle cere-bral artery.

3. Global aphasia. The most profound form of aphasia, called *global aphasia,* is characterized by drastically nonfluent output, severe disruption of com-prehension, and little repetitive ability. Spontaneous speech often is absent initially or is marked by production of a few stereotyped sounds. Patients neither read nor write. Hemiplegia is almost invariably present, and hemi-sensory loss and hemianopia are frequent.

   a. The typical insult involves the entire left perisylvian region, encom-passing Broca's area in the inferior frontal lobe, Wernicke's area in the posterior temporal lobe, and all the interposed parietofrontal cortices. In rare cases, separate, discrete lesions of Broca's area and Wernicke's area produce global aphasia without hemiparesis.

   b. The perisylvian region lies within the territory of the middle cerebral artery. Internal carotid and middle cerebral artery occlusions are the most common causes of global aphasia.

4. Conduction aphasia. The hallmark of conduction aphasia is a dispropor-tionate disruption of repetition. Comprehension of spoken language is rela-tively intact. Fluent spontaneous output often is marred by occasional hesitations and phonemic paraphasia but is not as disturbed as repetition. Naming also tends to show mild paraphasic contamination. Motor and sen-sory disturbances usually are absent or mild.

   a. Two neural loci tend to give rise to conduction aphasia: (1) the supra-marginal gyrus, sometimes with extension to the subinsular white mat-ter, and (2) the primary auditory cortex, insula, and subjacent white matter. The arcuate fasciculus, a subcortical white matter tract con-necting Wernicke's and Brodmann's areas, is often, but not invariably, involved.

   b. These regions are variably supplied by branches of the inferior or supe-rior divisions of the middle cerebral artery.

B. Extrasylvian aphasia. The extrasylvian aphasic syndromes share the clinical characteristic of preserved repetition and the anatomic trait of sparing of the core perisylvian language zone. They occur less commonly than perisylvian aphasia. Many arise from watershed infarcts, but they also can appear in con-junction with tumors, abscesses, hemorrhage, and other lesions.

   1. Transcortical motor aphasia is characterized by discrepant spontaneous speech and repetition. Spontaneous output is severely disrupted, nonfluent, and halting. In contrast, the ability to repeat sentences verbatim is pre-served, as is reading aloud. Comprehension is undisturbed. Naming may be mildly impaired.

   a. Transcortical motor aphasia results from damage at one of two foci: (1) the prefrontal cortices and subjacent white matter anterior or supe-rior to Broca's area, or (2) the supplementary motor area and cingulate gyrus. These lesions disconnect Broca's area from limbic areas and other sources of the drive to communicate.

   b. Lesions anterosuperior to Broca's area lie in the vascular border zone between the middle and anterior cerebral arteries. The supplementary motor area and cingulate gyrus regions are irrigated by the anterior cerebral artery.

2. **Transcortical sensory aphasia.** Patients with transcortical sensory aphasia have severely disturbed comprehension of spoken language but preserved repetition. Spontaneous speech is fluent, although often paraphasic. Echolalia—automatic repetition of overheard phrases—is common. Reading aloud can be fairly preserved, whereas reading comprehension is quite poor. Motor deficits are generally absent, but hemisensory deficits are uncommon.

   a. Lesions can occur over a wide distribution posterior and superior to the posterior perisylvian region, including the middle temporal gyrus, the angular gyrus, and underlying white matter. These insults disconnect Wernicke's area from multiple posterior association cortices, preventing retroactivation by aural word forms of the widely distributed neural representations that convey their meanings.

   b. The lesions generally lie within the vascular watershed between the posterior and middle cerebral arteries.

3. **Mixed transcortical aphasia.** This rare and remarkable condition is analogous to global aphasia, except for preserved ability to repeat. Spontaneous speech is minimal or absent. Patients are unable to comprehend spoken language, name, read, or write. Repetition of spoken language, however, is preserved. Patients often have echolalia. Mild hemiparesis and hemisensory loss affecting proximal greater than distal extremities may be observed.

   a. Lesions are an additive combination of those producing transcortical motor and sensory aphasia. Insults anterosuperior to Broca's area and posterosuperior to Wernicke's area cut off the perisylvian language zone from access to other cortices. **Isolation of the speech area** is a synonym for *mixed transcortical aphasia.*

   b. The lesions fall in the crescentic vascular border zone among the anterior, middle, and posterior cerebral arteries.

4. **Anomic aphasia.** Patients with anomic aphasia have difficulty retrieving verbal tags in spontaneous speech and confrontation naming. The remainder of language functions are relatively intact. Auditory comprehension, repetition, reading, and writing are normal. Spontaneous speech is preponderantly fluent, although interrupted by occasional hesitations for word-finding. In severe cases, output is lengthy but empty with recurrent circumlocution.

   a. A variety of lesions, including both dominant and nondominant hemisphere loci, can produce anomic aphasia. Particularly common sources are insults to (1) the dominant inferior parietal lobe and (2) the dominant anterior temporal cortices. The latter insults have been associated with **category-specific naming deficits,** in which naming in different semantic categories (e.g., living versus nonliving entities) is differentially impaired.

   b. The angular gyrus and anterior temporal cortices are supplied by different branches of the inferior division of the middle cerebral artery.

C. **Subcortical aphasia syndromes.** Focal lesions confined to subcortical structures strongly interconnected with language cortices produce aphasia. Delineation of the subcortical aphasia is a rapidly evolving and still unsettled enterprise, but two major profiles can be discerned.

1. **Striatocapsular aphasia.** The language deficit in striatocapsular aphasia resembles that in anomic or transcortical motor aphasia. Patients may or may not be fluent but are almost invariably have dysarthria. Mild to moderate anomia coexists with generally intact auditory comprehension, repetition, reading, and writing. Generation of complex syntactic sentences is impaired. Hemiparesis is common, hemisensory loss variable, and hemianopia infrequent. Lesions involve the dominant putamen, dorsolateral caudate, anterior limb of the internal capsule, and rostral periventricular white matter.

2. **Thalamic aphasia.** The language deficit in thalamic aphasia resembles that in transcortical sensory or mixed transcortical aphasia. Output can be nonfluent or relatively fluent, auditory comprehension is deficient, and rep-

etition is preserved. Impairment of naming, reading comprehension, and writing are present. Contralateral emotional facial paresis (diminished facial movement in expressing spontaneous emotions but preserved facial movements to command) and contralateral hypokinesia often are the only elementary neurologic deficits. Lesions are situated in the dominant anterolateral thalamus.

D. Additional classic syndromes. Strategically placed lesions can produce dissociated impairment of reading, writing, and oral language function. The following three have well-characterized localizing properties.

  1. Alexia without agraphia (pure alexia)

    a. Reading is severely impaired, whereas spontaneous speech, repetition, and auditory comprehension are normal. Writing is preserved, but dramatically, after a delay, patients are unable to read phrases they themselves have written. Recognition of words spelled aloud and traced on the palm is normal. Only words presented visually pose difficulty. Patients frequently have a slow, letter-by-letter reading strategy, painstakingly recognizing and stating aloud each letter in a word and then, from the spoken letters, string-determining the target word. Right homonymous hemianopia is common but not invariable. Disorders of color vision, including achromatopsia and color anomia, may be present.

    b. The most common neuroanatomic substrate comprises simultaneous lesions of the left occipital lobe and the splenium of the corpus callosum, depriving the angular gyrus region critical for word recognition of visual input from either the left or the right hemisphere. The smallest sufficient injury is a single lesion of the paraventricular white matter of the mesial occipitotemporal junction (the forceps major), interrupting interhemispheric and intrahemispheric visual tracks to the angular gyrus but sparing the corpus callosum and left occipital cortex.

  2. Alexia with agraphia

    a. Patients have loss of literacy—inability to read or write—but relatively well-preserved oral language function. Speech is fluent, although anomia often is present, and auditory comprehension and repetition are intact. Hemisensory deficits are frequent, and hemiparesis and hemivisual disturbances are variable. A full-fledged Gerstmann's syndrome, including dyscalculia, dysgraphia, left–right confusion, and finger agnosia, may be present.

    b. The underlying lesion involves the dominant inferior parietal lobule (angular and supramarginal gyri).

  3. Pure word deafness

    a. Patients resemble those with Wernicke's aphasia. Comprehension and repetition of spoken language are impaired, whereas speech is fluent. Unlike patients with Wernicke's aphasia, however, patients with pure word deafness rarely have paraphasia. More important, comprehension of written material is intact. Writing production also is normal. Although uncomprehending of word sounds, patients have intact hearing and generally is successful in identifying meaningful nonverbal sounds such as car horns or telephone rings.

    b. Two types of lesions underlie pure word deafness, both disconnecting Wernicke's area from input from primary auditory cortices. Some patients have bilateral superior temporal lesions. A roughly equal number have a single deep superior temporal lesion in the dominant hemisphere that blocks ipsilateral and crosses callosal auditory pathways.

E. Aprosodia. Meaning is conveyed not only through the propositional content of speech but also through prosody—the melody, rhythm, timbre, and inflection of the speaker. Prosody frequently is disturbed in nonfluent aphasia. However, patients may have normal propositional language yet have disturbances of the production, comprehension, or repetition of prosody. In general, the nondominant hemisphere plays a greater role in production and comprehension of emotional prosody than does the dominant hemisphere.

VI. Differential diagnosis. Acquired speech impairment can be caused by disruption of lower-order neural and muscular mechanisms for implementing sound production rather than disturbances of central processing of language. It is important to differentiate these nonaphasic speech impairments from genuine aphasia, because they differ in localizing importance and spectrum of etiologic factors.

    A. Dysarthria is abnormal articulation of spoken language.

        1. At least five types of nonaphasic dysarthria can be differentiated.

            a. Paretic dysarthria is caused by weakness of articulatory muscles. Soft, low-pitched, nasal voicing is characteristic. Causes include myopathy, neuromuscular junction disorders such as myasthenia gravis, and lower motor neuron disease.

            b. In **spastic dysarthria**, speech is typically strained, slow, and monotonic. Bilateral upper motor neuron lesions compromising the corticobulbar tracts are the cause.

            c. In **ataxic dysarthria,** jerky irregular speech rhythm and volume reflect lesions to the cerebellum or its connections. Multiple sclerosis is a common cause.

            d. Extrapyramidal dysarthria includes hypokinetic dysarthria, which occurs in parkinsonism, and choreic dysarthria, which occurs in Huntington's disease and other chorea syndromes.

            e. In **aphemia (cortical dysarthria),** small lesions within Broca's area or the dominant frontal oral motor cortex produce dysarticulation without disturbing core language function.

        2. Aphasic dysarthria—dysarticulation occurring as one manifestation of an aphasic language syndrome—is common with anterior aphasia such as Broca's syndrome. The nonaphasic forms of dysarthria can be differentiated from aphasic dysarthria by means of demonstration of preserved intrinsic language functions, including naming, comprehension, and reading. Intact writing is most telling and shows normal productive language capacity when a nonoral output channel is used.

    B. Mutism. Aphasia—disordered language—can be securely diagnosed only on the basis of exemplars of disturbed output (or comprehension). Patients with acute aphasia, especially Broca's or global aphasia, often are unable to speak for the first few hours or days. However, a wide variety of other insults can produce total cessation of verbal output (Table 3.2). The full differential diagnosis of mutism includes (1) psychiatric causes (schizophrenia, depression, catatonia, and psychogenic illness), (2) abulia/akinetic mutism (bilateral prefrontal, diencephalic, and midbrain lesions), (3) acute dominant supplementary motor area lesions, (4) pseudobulbar palsy, (5) locked-in syndrome from bilateral ventral pontine or midbrain lesions, (6) acute bilateral cerebellar lesions, (7) lower motor neuron lesions, and (8) laryngeal disorders.

    C. Thought disorders

        1. When an intact language apparatus is placed in service of an underlying thought disorder, bizarre utterances arise that superficially resemble the fluent aphasic output of patients with Wernicke's or conduction aphasia. Demographic features are helpful. For example, schizophrenia with psychotic speech of new onset tends to appear among persons in their 20s and 30s, whereas fluent aphasia clusters among older persons with vascular risk factors.

        2. Several features of the utterances differentiate thought-disordered from fluent aphasic speech.

            a. Paraphasia is common in aphasia but rare in schizophrenia.

            b. The neologisms of persons with aphasia are frequent and changing, whereas those of persons with schizophrenic are infrequent and consistent.

            c. Open-ended questions tend to prompt briefer responses from persons with aphasia than from those with schizophrenia.

            d. Bizarre and delusional themes appear only in schizophrenic discourse.

Table 3.2 Differential diagnosis of mutism

Psychiatric disorders	Pseudobulbar palsy
Schizophrenia	Abulia
Depression	Akinetic mutism
Catatonia	Locked-in syndrome
Psychogenic	Chronic vegetative state
Aphasic syndromes (acute period)	Cerebellar lesions (bilateral)
Global aphasia	Lower motor neuron lesions
Broca's aphasia	Guillain–Barré syndrome
Aphemia (acute period)	Laryngeal disorders
Dominant supplementary motor area lesion	

VII. Course

A. Some degree of spontaneous recovery of language function is invariable after static brain injury.

   1. An **initial accelerated period** of improved function occurs over the first few days or weeks after insult and is attributable to resolution of edema, ischemic penumbra, and other causes of dysfunction at a distance from the site of permanent injury.

   2. The **second, slower phase** of recovery reflects use of parallel circuits, retraining, and structural neural plasticity. The bulk of this functional recovery takes place in the first 3 months after injury, and some may continue as long as 1 year, rarely longer. Among the aphasia syndromes, the greatest recovery compared with baseline tends to occur in Broca's and conduction aphasia. **Anomic aphasia** is a common end stage into which other aphasia subtypes tend to evolve.

B. Factors favoring greater spontaneous improvement, as well as response to speech therapy, are young age, left-handedness or ambidexterity, higher education, smaller lesion size, no or few nonlanguage cognitive defects, absence of emotional difficulties such as depression and neglect, and strong family support. Patients with traumatic aphasia tend to recover more fully than do patients with ischemic lesions.

VIII. Referral

A. Neurologist. Most patients with aphasia need neurologic consultation. The neurology specialist confirms the presence of aphasia, clarifies the type, aids in etiologic diagnosis, and provides the patient and family with an informed prognosis.

   In selected cases, neurologists consider **pharmacotherapy** for aphasia. Results in small series of cases have suggested that noradrenergic and cholinergic agonists may increase neuroplasticity and facilitate recovery from aphasia when begun within 1 month of the onset of the deficit. Dopamine agonists such as bromocriptine have been used to improve output of speech among patients with speech initiation deficits, such as in transcortical motor aphasia. These uses, which have not been approved by the U.S. Food and Drug Administration, are the subject of active investigation.

B. Speech and language pathologist. All patients with aphasia need an evaluation by a speech and language pathologist.

   1. The speech therapist performs a formal diagnostic assessment, profiling the patient's language strengths and weaknesses with normed tests. A variety of standardized language assessment batteries, including the Boston Diagnostic Aphasia Examination, the Western Aphasia Battery, the Porch Index of Communicative Ability, and the Communication Abilities in Daily Living, can be drawn on to survey a patient's abilities. The therapist uses the results to design and implement an individualized program of aphasia therapy.

   2. Although controversy regarding the effectiveness of aphasia therapy persists, the preponderance of evidence suggests that systematic language rehabilitation programs improve patient outcome. Treatment is tailored to each individual's pattern of linguistic and cognitive competencies and deficits. It exploits spared brain systems to reestablish, circumvent, or compensate for lost language capacities. A variety of deficit-specific programs supplement general language stimulation. For nonfluency, treatments include (1) melodic intonation therapy, (2) sign language and other gestural communication training, and (3) communication boards. Syntax training may benefit agrammatism. Specific word-retrieval therapies have been developed for anomia and comprehension training programs for auditory comprehension deficits.

3. Speech therapy programs generally last for 2 to 3 months in 30 to 60 minute sessions conducted two to five times per week. Self- and family-administered home exercises provide additional stimulation. Computer-based training is expanding in scope and sophistication.

C. **Neuropsychologist.** Patients who have major nonlinguistic cognitive deficits in addition to aphasia and whose diagnosis is unclear need neuropsychological evaluation. Formal neuropsychological evaluation with tests that minimize language requirements allows detailed profiling of memory, visuospatial reasoning, executive function, praxis, and concept formation than can be obtained by means of bedside mental status examination. Findings can aid the physician in making a diagnosis by suggesting the pattern of neural system involvement and aid the speech pathologist in prescribing therapy by helping identify the extent to which different extralinguistic capacities can support various compensatory strategies.

D. **Patient support groups.** The National Aphasia Association (156 Fifth Avenue, Suite 707, New York, NY 10156, 1-800-922-4622, www.aphasia.org) is an excellent resource for patients and their families. The American Heart/Stroke Association and National Stroke Association also provide beneficial programs and information.

Recommended Readings

Alexander MP, Naeser MA, Palumbo C. Broca's area aphasias: aphasia after lesions involving the frontal operculum. *Neurology* 1990;40:353–362.

Benson DF. Aphasia. In: Heilman KM, Valenstein E, eds. *Clinical neuropsychology.* 3rd ed. New York: Oxford University Press, 1993:17–36.

Berthier ML. *Transcortical aphasias.* East Sussex, UK: Psychology Press, 1999.

Broca P. Remarks on the seat of the faculty of articulate speech, followed by the report of a case of aphemia (loss of speech). In: Rottenberg DA, Hochberg FH, eds. *Neurologic classics in modern translation.* New York: Hafner, 1977:136–149.

Cummings JL, Benson F, Hill MA, et al. Aphasia in dementia of the Alzheimer type. *Neurology* 1985;35:394–397.

Cummings JL, Benson DF, Houlihan JP, et al. Mutism: loss of neocortical and limbic vocalization. *J Nerv Ment Dis* 1983;17:255–259.

Damasio AR. Aphasia. *N Engl J Med* 1992;326:531–539.

Damasio AR. Category-related recognition defects as a clue to the neural substrates of knowledge. *Trends Neurosci* 1990;13:95–98.

Damasio H. Neuroanatomical correlates of the aphasias. In Sarno M, ed. *Acquired aphasia.* 3rd ed. New York: Academic Press, 1998:43–70.

Damasio H, Grabowski TJ, Tranel D, et al. A neural basis for lexical retrieval. *Nature* 1996; 380:499–505.

Devinsky O. *100 maxims in behavioral neurology.* London, UK: Edward Arnold, 1992.

Geschwind N. Disconnexion syndromes in animals and man. *Brain* 1965;88:237–294, 585–644.

Grodzinsky Y. The syntactic characterization of agrammatism. *Cognition* 1984;16:99–120.

Hanlon RE, Lux WE, Dromerick AW. Global aphasia without hemiparesis: language profiles and lesion distribution. *J Neurol Neurosurg Psychiatry* 1999;66:365–369.

Heiss WD, Kessler J, Theil A, et al. Differential capacity of left and right hemispheric areas for compensation of poststroke aphasia. *Ann Neurol* 1999;45:430–438.

Hughes JD, Jacobs DH, Heilman KM. Neuropharmacologic and linguistic neuroplasticity. *Brain Lang* 2000;71:96–101.

Kreisler A, Godefoy G, Delmaire C, et al. The anatomy of aphasia revisited. *Neurology* 2000; 54:1117–1123.

Mega MS, Alexander MP. Subcortical aphasia: the core profile of capsulostriatal infarction. *Neurology* 1994;44:1824–1829.
Mesulam MM. Primary progressive aphasia. *Ann Neurol* 2001;49:425–432.
Nadeau SE, Rothi LJG, Crosson B, eds. *Aphasia and language: theory to practice.* New York: Guilford Press, 2000.
Price CJ. The functional anatomy of word comprehension and production. *Trends Cogn Sci* 1998;2:281–288.
Robey RR. The efficacy of treatment for aphasic persons: a meta-analysis. *Brain Lang* 1994;47: 582–608.
Ross ED. The aprosodias: functional-anatomic organization of the affective components of language in the right hemisphere. *Arch Neurol* 1981;38:561–569.
Ross ED. Acute agitation and other behaviors associated with Wernicke aphasia and their possible neurological basis. *Neuropsychiatry Neuropsychol Behav Neurol* 1993;6:9–18.
Schiff HB, Alexander MP, Naeser MA, et al. Aphemia: clinical-anatomic correlation. *Arch Neurol* 1983;40:720–727.
Starkstein SE, Robinson RG. Depression following cerebrovascular lesions. *Semin Neurol* 1990;10:247–253.
Walker-Batson D, et al. Pharmacotherapy in the treatment of aphasia. In: Goldstein LB, ed. *Restorative neurology: advances in pharmacotherapy for recovery after stroke.* Armonk, NY: Futura, 1998.

4. APPROACH TO THE PATIENT WITH MEMORY IMPAIRMENT

Daniel Tranel
Natalie L. Denburg

The term **amnesia** refers to conditions in which patients lose, partly or completely, the ability to learn new information or to retrieve information acquired previously. Amnesia (also referred to here as *memory impairment* or *memory dysfunction*) is extremely common in neurologic diseases that affect the telencephalon or diencephalon and is surely the most frequent problem voiced by patients. In an outpatient setting, a substantial majority of patients have memory dysfunction. Varying degrees of amnesia also are common in inpatient populations.

Amnesia is a defining characteristic of some of the most frequently encountered neurologic diseases, including progressive dementia such as Alzheimer's disease. Reports of memory impairment must be taken seriously, because such reports frequently constitute one of the earliest manifestations of neurologic disease.

Accurate diagnosis and effective management of memory disorders are very important. A considerable clinical challenge is presented, however, by the facts that (1) the most frequent neurologic diseases affect elderly persons and (2) a certain degree of decline in memory is associated with normal aging. Hence it can be difficult to differentiate reports of memory problems that are more or less normal manifestations of aging from reports that signal the presence of neurologic disease. Memory problems also are common in nonneurologic conditions such as psychiatric disease, and this constitutes another reason for careful diagnosis. Such distinctions often require laboratory testing of the type that can be conducted by means of neuropsychological assessment procedures.

    I. Types of memory and memory systems in the brain. There are several fundamental distinctions between different types of memory and the different neural systems to which different types of memory are related (Table 4.1).
        A. Anterograde and retrograde memory
            1. Anterograde memory refers to the capacity to learn new information—that is, to acquire new facts, skills, and other types of knowledge. Anterograde memory is closely dependent on neural structures in the mesial temporal lobe, especially the hippocampus and interconnected structures, such as the amygdala, the entorhinal and perirhinal cortices, and other parts of the parahippocampal gyrus.
            2. Retrograde memory refers to the retrieval of information that was acquired previously—that is, retrieval of facts, skills, and other knowledge learned in the recent or remote past. This type of memory is related to nonmesial sectors of the temporal lobe, including the polar region (Brodmann's area 38), the inferotemporal region (including Brodmann's areas 20, 21, and 36), and the occipitotemporal region (including Brodmann's area 37 and the ventral parts of areas 18 and 19). Autobiographical memory, a special form of retrograde memory that refers to knowledge about one's own past, is linked primarily to the anterior part of the nonmesial temporal lobes, especially in the right hemisphere.
        B. Verbal and nonverbal memory. Knowledge can be divided into that which exists in **verbal** form, such as words (written or spoken) and names, and that which exists in **nonverbal** form, such as faces, geographic routes, and complex musical patterns. This distinction is important, because memory systems in the two hemispheres of the human brain are specialized differently for verbal and nonverbal material (Table 4.2). Specifically, systems in the left hemisphere are dedicated primarily to verbal material, and systems in the right hemisphere are dedicated primarily to nonverbal material. This arrangement parallels the general arrangement of the human brain, in which the left hemisphere is specialized for language, and the right hemisphere for visuospatial processing. This distinction applies to almost all right-handed persons and to approximately two thirds of left-handed persons (in the remaining minority of left-handers, the arrangement may be partially or completely reversed).

Table 4.1 Subdivisions of memory

Dichotomy	Characteristics
Retrograde	Retrieval of knowledge acquired previously, especially knowledge acquired before onset of brain injury
Anterograde	Learning of new knowledge, especially learning of knowledge after onset of brain injury
Verbal	Words, names, verbally coded facts; word-based material
Nonverbal	Faces, geographic routes, complex melodies; spatially based material
Declarative	Information that can be brought into consciousness, "declared," held in the "mind's eye"
Nondeclarative	Performance-based, motor output, habits and conditioning, automatic tendencies
Short-term	Ephemeral (30–45 sec), limited capacity (7 ± 2 words, numbers)
Long-term	Permanent, unlimited capacity

C. Declarative and nondeclarative memory
  1. **Declarative memory** (also known as **explicit memory**) refers to knowledge that can be "declared" and brought to mind for conscious inspection, such as facts, words, names, and individual faces that can be retrieved from memory, placed in the "mind's eye," and reported. The acquisition of declarative memories is intimately linked to the functioning of the hippocampus and other mesial temporal lobe structures.
  2. **Nondeclarative memory** (also known as **implicit memory**) refers to various forms of memory that cannot be declared or brought into the mind's eye. Examples include sensorimotor skill learning, autonomic conditioning, and certain types of habits. Skating and skiing, for example, rely on motor skills that constitute forms of nondeclarative memory. Nondeclarative memory requires participation of the neostriatum, cerebellum, and sensorimotor cortices. A remarkable dissociation between declarative and nondeclarative learning and memory has been repeatedly found among patients with amnesia (including those with Korsakoff's syndrome, bilateral mesial temporal lobe lesions, medial thalamic lesions, and Alzheimer's disease). Among such persons, sensorimotor skill learning and memory often is preserved, whereas declarative memory is profoundly impaired.
D. Short-term and long-term memory
  1. The term **short-term memory** is used to designate a time span of memory that covers from 0 to approximately 45 seconds, a brief period during which a limited amount of information can be held without rehearsal. Short-term memory (also known as **primary memory**) does not depend on the hip-

Table 4.2 Hemispheric specialization of memory systems

Left	Right
Verbal	Nonverbal
Words	Patterns
Names	Faces
Stories	Geographic routes
Lyrics	Complex melodies
Sequential, feature based	Holistic, gestalt based
Lexical retrieval	Unique personal knowledge

pocampus or other temporal lobe memory systems but is linked closely to cerebral mechanisms required for attention and concentration.

2. The term **long-term memory** refers to a large expanse of time that covers everything beyond short-term memory—that is, knowledge held for days, years, and even decades, in more or less permanent form. Long-term memory (also known as **secondary memory**) can be divided into **recent** (the past few weeks or months) and **remote** (years or decades ago). Unlike short-term memory, the capacity of long-term memory is enormous, and information can be retained in long-term memory almost indefinitely. The mesial temporal system, including the hippocampus, is required for acquisition of knowledge into long-term memory. Other systems in the temporal lobe and elsewhere are required for consolidation and retrieval of knowledge from long-term memory.

E. **Working memory** refers to a short time during which the brain can hold several pieces of information in an active register and perform operations on them. Working memory is akin to short-term memory but implies a somewhat longer duration (several minutes) and more focus on the **operational** features of the mental process rather than simply the acquisition of information. Working memory can be thought of as "on-line" processing and operating on knowledge that is being held in activated form. For example, consider the act of deciding to videotape a television program. One may consult a television listing for the relevant information about channel, time, and so forth. One then programs the video cassette recorder while holding in working memory the relevant information about the program as well as bringing into mind knowledge that is required for operating the recorder.

Working memory depends on the integrity of the frontal lobes. More specifically, many recent functional imaging studies have linked working memory to the dorsolateral prefrontal sector of the frontal lobes. A laterality effect also has been noted wherein verbal memory tasks depend on the left dorsolateral prefrontal sector while spatial working memory tasks depend on the right dorsolateral prefrontal sector. Interesting is that the ventromedial prefrontal region has not been found to be involved in working memory.

II. **Clinical manifestations.** Several frequent neurologic conditions damage memory-related neural systems and lead to various profiles and severities of amnesia (Table 4.3).

A. **Degenerative diseases**

1. **Cortical dementia**

a. **Alzheimer's disease.** The neuropathologic mechanism of Alzheimer's disease is characterized by two principal features—the neurofibrillary tangle and the neuritic plaque. Early in the course of Alzheimer's disease, the entorhinal cortex, which is a pivotal way station for input to and from the hippocampus, is disrupted by neurofibrillary tangles in cortical layers II and IV. The perforant pathway, which is the main route for entry into the hippocampal formation, is gradually and massively demyelinated. The hippocampus eventually is almost deafferentated from cortical input. Alzheimer's disease also breaks down the efferent linkage of the hip-

Table 4.3 Causes of and conditions associated with amnesia

Degenerative disease (e.g., Alzheimer's, Pick's, Parkinson's)
Head injury
Cerebrovascular accident (e.g., infarction, ruptured aneurysm)
Toxic conditions (e.g., alcoholism)
Anoxia, ischemia
Herpes simplex encephalitis
Surgical ablation
Neoplasm
Normal pressure hydrocephalus
Transient global amnesia
Functional amnesia

---

pocampus back to the cerebral cortex through destruction of the subiculum and entorhinal cortex. The hallmark behavioral sign of this destruction is amnesia—specifically, an anterograde (learning) defect that covers declarative knowledge but largely spares nondeclarative learning and retrieval. Early in the course of the disease, retrograde memory is relatively spared, but as the pathologic process extends to nonmesial temporal sectors, a defect in the retrograde compartment (retrieval impairment) appears and gradually worsens.

  b. **Pick's disease,** characterized by Pick bodies (cells containing degraded protein material), is an uncommon form of cortical dementia that often shows a striking predilection for one lobe of the brain, producing a state of circumscribed lobar atrophy. The disease often is concentrated in the frontal lobes, in which case personality alterations, rather than amnesia, are the most prominent manifestations. However, the disease can affect one or the other temporal lobe and produce signs of a material-specific learning and retrieval disorder (verbal or nonverbal amnesia).

  c. **Frontal lobe dementia** is another form of cortical dementia. It involves focal atrophy of the frontal lobes, which causes personality changes and other signs of executive dysfunction. This condition is similar to Pick's disease, except there is no predominance of Pick bodies.

  d. **Frontotemporal dementia** is characterized by symmetric atrophy of the frontal and temporal lobes. The earliest and most prominent cognitive symptoms involve personality and behavioral changes. Although reports of memory problems are common in frontotemporal dementia, they are never the sole or dominating feature. Severe amnesia is considered an exclusionary criterion. Memory functioning is described as selective (e.g., "she remembers what she wants to remember"). Knowledge regarding orientation and current autobiographical events remains largely preserved.

2. **Subcortical dementia**
  a. **Parkinson's disease.** With its pathologic mechanism focused in subcortical structures, Parkinson's disease influences memory in a manner different from that of cortical forms of dementia such as Alzheimer's and Pick's disease. Disorders of nondeclarative memory (e.g., acquisition and retrieval of motor skills) are more prominent, and there may be minimal or no impairment in learning of declarative material. Patients with Parkinson's disease often have more problems in **recall** of newly acquired knowledge than in **storage.** When cuing strategies are provided, the patients have normal levels of retention.

  b. **Huntington's disease.** Similar to Parkinson's disease, the pathologic mechanism of Huntington's disease is concentrated in subcortical structures. The amnesia of patients with Huntington's disease also resembles that of patients with Parkinson's disease. In particular there is disproportionate involvement of nondeclarative memory. Patients with Huntington's disease also tend to have disruption of **working memory** and have trouble holding information "on-line" and performing mental operations on it.

  c. **Progressive supranuclear palsy** is another primarily subcortical disease process that frequently produces problems with memory. In general, however, the amnesia of progressive supranuclear palsy is considerably less severe than that of Alzheimer's disease. Laboratory assessment often shows relatively mild defects in learning and retrieval despite the patient's reports of forgetfulness.

3. **Other degenerative conditions**
  a. **Dementia related to human immunodeficiency virus disease and acquired immunodeficiency syndrome (HIV/AIDS).** Persons with HIV infection and those with AIDS frequently have varying degrees of memory impairment, the severity being roughly proportional to the overall progression of the disease. Early in the course, memory defects

may be the sole signs of cognitive dysfunction. The problems center on acquisition of new material, particularly material of the declarative type. Memory defects in this disease appear to be attributable mainly to defective attention, concentration, and overall efficiency of cognitive functioning rather than to focal dysfunction of particular memory-related neural systems. One research approach in this area has been to identify variables predictive of the onset or severity of neuropsychological deficits. The goal is to develop immunologic or virologic indicators. Various investigators have found that the rate of percentage of CD4 lymphocyte cell loss is associated with and may represent a risk factor for cognitive dysfunction among persons with HIV/AIDS.

   b. **Multiple sclerosis.** Many patients with multiple sclerosis (MS) have varying degrees of amnesia, although the severity can wax and wane considerably in concert with other neurologic symptoms. Many patients with MS have no memory defects during some periods of the disease. When present, the memory impairment most commonly manifests as defective recall of newly learned information. Encoding and working memory are normal or near-normal. Patients with MS often benefit from cuing. The amnesia of MS usually affects declarative material of both verbal and nonverbal types; defects in nondeclarative memory are rare.

B. **Head injury** is a frequent cause of amnesia, especially among young men, who sustain most severe head injuries. Several distinct types of amnesia are associated with head injury.

   1. **Posttraumatic amnesia** refers to the period of time following head trauma during which patients do not acquire new information in a normal and continuous manner, despite being conscious and "awake." During this time, the patient may appear alert and attentive and may even deny having memory problems. It becomes apparent later that the patient was not forming ongoing records of new experiences. Information is simply not encoded, and no amount of cuing will uncover memories that would normally have been acquired during this period. The **duration** of posttraumatic amnesia is a reliable marker of the severity of head injury and constitutes one of the best predictors of outcome.

   2. **Retrograde amnesia.** Patients with head injuries often have retrograde amnesia—that is, defective recall of experiences that occurred immediately before the injury. Information from the time closest to the point of injury is most likely to be lost, and the farther back in time one goes, the less is the impairment. The extent of retrograde amnesia typically "shrinks" as the patient recovers, so that as time goes on, fewer and fewer retrograde memories are missing. Patients may be left with only a small island of amnesia for the few minutes or hours immediately before the trauma.

   3. **Learning defects (anterograde amnesia).** Moderate and severe head injuries often produce permanent damage to mesial temporal lobe structures, such as the hippocampus, with resultant defects in learning (anterograde amnesia). The impairment is centered on declarative knowledge; nondeclarative learning is rarely affected. The defect may be unequal for verbal and nonverbal material if there is asymmetry of the structural injury. Patients with head injury tend to be exquisitely sensitive to distraction, fatigue, the effects of alcohol, and other influences that produce suboptimal learning performance.

C. **Cerebrovascular disease**

   1. **Stroke** is a frequent cause of amnesia, and the nature and degree of memory disturbance are direct functions of which neural structures are damaged and to what extent. Amnesia is most likely to result from infarction that damages the mesial temporal region, the basal forebrain, or the medial diencephalon, especially the thalamus.

      a. **Mesial temporal lobe.** The parahippocampal gyrus and hippocampus proper can be damaged by infarction in territories supplied by branches of the middle cerebral or posterior cerebral arteries. (Strokes in the region of the anterolateral temporal lobe are decidedly uncommon.) Infarction of this type almost always is unilateral and almost always produces incomplete damage to mesial temporal memory structures; hence the profile is one of a partial material-specific (left–verbal, right–nonverbal) defect in anterograde memory for declarative knowledge.

   b. **Thalamus.** Damage to the thalamus can produce amnesia. The most severe memory impairment results from bilateral infarcts situated in the anterior part of the thalamus in the interpeduncular profundus territory. Unilateral lesions caused by lacunar infarction in anterior thalamic nuclei produce material-specific learning defects reminiscent of those observed with mesial temporal lobe lesions. Patients with thalamic damage, however, tend to have both anterograde and retrograde defects. In the retrograde compartment, there usually is a **temporal gradient** to the defect—that is, the farther back in time one goes, the less the severity of the amnesia.

 2. **Ruptured aneurysms.** Rupture of aneurysms located either in the anterior communicating artery or in the anterior cerebral artery almost invariably causes infarction in the region of the basal forebrain—a set of bilateral paramidline gray nuclei that includes the septal nuclei, the diagonal band of Broca, and the substantia innominata. The amnesia associated with basal forebrain damage has several distinctive features. Patients have an inability to link correctly various aspects of memory episodes (whens, wheres, whats, and whys). This problem affects both the anterograde and retrograde compartments. Confabulation is common among patients with basal forebrain amnesia. Cuing markedly improves recall and recognition of both anterograde and retrograde material.

 3. **Vascular dementia** (previously known as cerebrovascular dementia and multiinfarct dementia) refers to conditions in which repeated infarction produces widespread cognitive impairment, including amnesia. The term is used most commonly to denote multiple small strokes (lacunar strokes) in the arterioles that feed subcortical structures; hence the usual picture is "subcortical" dementia. The memory impairment in vascular dementia generally affects encoding of new material (anterograde amnesia), and nondeclarative learning also may be defective. Retrograde memory tends to be spared.

D. **Toxic conditions**
 1. **Alcoholism.** Chronic long-term alcohol abuse can produce permanent damage to certain diencephalic structures, particularly the mammillary bodies and dorsomedial thalamic nucleus, that has been linked to amnesic manifestations. This presentation is known as **alcoholic Korsakoff's syndrome** or **Wernicke–Korsakoff syndrome.** The amnesic profile in patients with Korsakoff's syndrome is characterized by (1) anterograde amnesia for both verbal and nonverbal material with defects in both encoding and retrieval, (2) retrograde amnesia with a strong temporal gradient— that is, progressively milder defects as one goes farther back in time, and (3) sparing of nondeclarative memory. Confabulation is characteristic of patients with Korsakoff's syndrome, especially in the early days following detoxification.

 2. **Other neurotoxins.** Amnesia can result from acute or chronic exposure to neurotoxins such as metals, especially lead and mercury, solvents and fuels, and pesticides. The relation between exposure to these substances and cognitive dysfunction is poorly understood. Conclusive scientific evidence for a specific cause-and-effect relation is almost nonexistent. Nonetheless, there is little doubt that memory impairment often does result from excessive exposure to these neurotoxins. The amnesia tends to manifest as a deficiency in new learning (anterograde amnesia) that covers various types of material, including verbal, nonverbal, and nondeclarative. Defects of concentration, attention, and overall cognitive efficiency are frequent contributing factors. In most cases, the memory impairment occurs in the setting of more widespread cognitive dysfunction.

E. Anoxia/ischemia. Cerebral anoxia or global ischemia, which frequently occurs in the setting of cardiopulmonary arrest, often leads to the selective destruction of cellular groups within the hippocampal formation. The extent of damage is linked fairly directly to the number of minutes of arrest. Brief periods of anoxia/ischemia can cause limited damage, and longer periods produce greater destruction. With a critical length of deprivation, the damage concentrates bilaterally in the CA1 ammonic fields of the hippocampus. The result is selective anterograde amnesia affecting declarative verbal and nonverbal material. The amnesia associated with anoxia/ischemia is reminiscent of the memory defect produced by early-stage Alzheimer's disease.

F. Herpes simplex encephalitis (HSE) causes a severe necrotic process in the cortical structures associated with the limbic system, some neocortical structures in the vicinity of the limbic system, and several subcortical limbic structures. The hippocampus, amygdala, and basal forebrain nuclei are frequent targets of HSE. The parahippocampal gyrus—particularly the entorhinal cortex in its anterior sector and the polar limbic cortex (area 38)—is frequently damaged. HSE also may destroy neocortices of the anterolateral and anteroinferior regions of the temporal lobe (areas 20, 21, anterior 22, and parts of 36 and 37). The destruction may be bilateral, although in recent years, with the advent of early diagnosis and treatment with acyclovir, circumscribed unilateral damage has become more common.

   The profile of amnesia caused by HSE is dictated by the nature of neural destruction. Damage confined to the mesial temporal region (hippocampus, amygdala, and entorhinal cortex) produce anterograde declarative memory impairment. If both sides are involved, both verbal and nonverbal material are affected. If the destruction is unilateral, a material-specific learning defect may appear—that is, only verbal (left-sided damage) or nonverbal (right-sided damage) material is covered by the amnesia.

   When HSE-related pathologic changes extend to nonmesial temporal structures in anterolateral and anteroinferior sectors, the amnesia involves progressively greater portions of the retrograde compartment. Patients are not able to retrieve memories from the past and are not able to learn new information. The retrograde defect can be quite severe if nonmesial temporal structures are extensively damaged. In the worst case, a patient can lose almost all capacity to remember declarative information from the past. Such a defect, coupled with the anterograde impairment, constitutes **global amnesia.**

G. Surgical ablation. Surgical management of intractable epilepsy, especially temporal lobectomy, can result in memory impairment, depending on the nature of the resection. Even if the lobectomy spares most of the hippocampus proper, the resection usually involves other anterior regions of the mesial temporal lobe, including the amygdala and entorhinal cortex, resulting in mild but significant memory defects. In the most common presentation, the patient has a material-specific learning defect after temporal lobectomy. In addition to being material specific (nonverbal if the resection is on the right, verbal if it is on the left), the amnesia affects only declarative knowledge. However, mild retrograde amnesia also can result if there is sufficient involvement of the anterolateral and anteroinferior temporal sectors. Other factors being equal, patients whose seizures began at an early age (e.g., before 5 years) are less affected by temporal lobectomy than are patients whose seizures began later (e.g., adolescence).

H. Neoplasm. Cerebral neoplasms can lead to amnesia, depending on their type and location. Impaired memory is a common symptom of brain tumors, especially those centered in the region of the third ventricle (in or near the thalamus) or in the region of the ventral frontal lobes (in or near the basal forebrain). The most common therapies for high-grade malignant brain tumors, including resection and radiation, often produce memory defects. Radiation necrosis, for example, can damage the lateral portions of the temporal lobes and lead to a focal retrograde amnesia (in which new learning is spared).

I. Normal pressure hydrocephalus is a partially reversible condition in which gait disturbance, incontinence, and dementia, especially memory impairment, compose a hallmark triad of presenting features. Early in the course, memory impairment can be minimal, but most patients with normal pressure hydrocephalus go on to have marked memory defects. The typical situation is anterograde amnesia for declarative material; however, problems with attention and concentration can exacerbate the amnesia and make the patient appear even more impaired than he or she actually is.

J. Transient global amnesia (TGA) is a short-lasting neurologic condition in which the patient has prominent impairment of memory in the setting of otherwise normal cognition and no other neurologic defect. The duration of TGA typically is approximately 6 or 7 hours, after which the condition spontaneously remits, and the patient returns to an entirely normal memory status. The cause of TGA is unknown, although psychological stress, vascular factors, and migraine have been proposed as causes. During the episode, the patient has severe impairment of anterograde memory for verbal and nonverbal material. Retrograde memory also is impaired, although to a lesser degree. After recovery, patients are unable to remember events that transpired during the TGA episode. Sometimes a short period of time immediately before the onset of TGA also is lost. Otherwise, there is no long-term consequence.

K. Functional amnesia. Amnesia can occur in the absence of any demonstrable brain injury, as a consequence of severe emotional trauma, hypnotic suggestion, or psychiatric illness. These presentations have been called *functional amnesia* to differentiate them from amnesia caused by "organic" factors, although at the molecular and cellular levels the mechanisms may not be distinguishable. A common form is **functional retrograde amnesia,** in which the patient loses most or all memory of the past (including self-identity), usually after a severe emotional or psychological trauma. Curiously, anterograde memory can be entirely normal, and the patient may even have "relearning" of the past. Spontaneous recovery is frequent, although most patients never are able to remember events that transpired during the episodes in which they had amnesia. Another interesting form is **posthypnotic amnesia,** the phenomenon whereby patients cannot remember events that transpired while they were under hypnosis (generally after being told by the hypnotist during the hypnosis that amnesia would ensue).

III. Evaluation

A. History

1. **Onset.** Through careful history taking, the clinician should determine as precisely as possible the timing of the **onset** of the problem. Memory defects that began years ago and have gradually worsened over time point to degenerative disease, and Alzheimer's is the most likely candidate. Reports of sudden memory impairment among younger patients, for whom psychological factors (e.g., severe stress and depression) can be identified as being temporally related to the problem, should raise the question of nonorganic etiologic factors.

2. **Course.** The history taking should document carefully the **course** of the concern. Progressive deterioration in memory signals a degenerative process. Memory defects after head injury or cerebral anoxia, by contrast, tend to resolve gradually, and reports to the contrary raise the question of other factors (e.g., psychological illness).

3. **Nature.** The clinician should explore the **nature** of the problem. With what types of information, and in what situations, is the patient having trouble? Patients often produce vague, poorly specified concerns (e.g., "My memory is bad," "I can't remember things," or "I'm forgetful"), and it is important to request specific examples to form an idea as to the actual nature of the problem. Patients tend to use the term "memory impairment" to cover a wide range of mental status abnormalities, and, again, elicitation of examples is informative. Patients who say they "can't remember" may actually have circumscribed impairment of word finding, proper name retrieval, or hearing or vision.

B. Bedside examination.
Memory assessment is covered to some extent by almost all bedside or screening mental status examinations, including such measures as the Mini-Mental State Examination, the Blessed Dementia Rating Scale, and

the Dementia Assessment Battery. If patients pass such examinations, do not report memory impairment, and are not described by spouses or caretakers as having memory difficulties, it is safe to assume that memory is normal. If any of these conditions is not met, a more complete evaluation of memory is warranted. Referral for neuropsychological assessment provides the most direct access to such evaluation. In bedside memory testing, there should be at least some coverage of the following aspects of memory and mental status.

1. **Learning.** Can the patient learn the examiner's name? Three words? Three objects?
2. **Working memory.** Backward spelling, serial subtraction, and the digit span backward subtest from the Wechsler Adult Intelligence Scale, third edition (WAIS-III) are good probes of working memory.
3. **Delayed recall.** It is important to ask for retrieval of newly acquired knowledge after a delay, for example, approximately 30 minutes. This may reveal a severe loss of information on the part of a patient who performed perfectly in an immediate recall procedure.
4. **Retrograde memory.** The patient should be asked to retrieve knowledge from the past. This should be corroborated by a spouse or other **collateral person,** because patients with memory defects may confabulate and otherwise mislead the examiner.
5. **Orientation.** The patient should be asked for information about time, place, and personal facts. Defects in orientation often are early clues to memory impairment.
6. **Attention.** Marked impairment of attention produces subsequent defects on most tests of memory. The diagnosis of amnesia, however, should be reserved for patients who have normal attention but still cannot perform normally on memory tests. Attentional impairment per se is a hallmark other abnormalities, not necessarily of an amnesic condition.

C. **Laboratory studies** of memory are conducted in the context of neuropsychological assessment, which provides precise, standardized quantification of various memory capacities. Examples of some widely used procedures are as follows.

1. **Anterograde memory** is assessed most conventional neuropsychological tests of memory, including the Wechsler Memory Scale, third edition (WMS-III). The WMS-III and other such instruments assess **learning of declarative knowledge,** and it should not be assumed that all aspects of memory are normal simply because the patient passes these procedures. For example, these tests do not measure nondeclarative memory, and they rarely provide adequate investigation of the retrograde compartment. Nonetheless, the WMS-III and related procedures provide sensitive, standardized means of quantifying many aspects of memory.
   a. **Verbal.** In addition to several verbal memory procedures that comprise part of the WMS-III (e.g., paragraph recall and paired-associate learning), there are several well-standardized list-learning procedures in which the patient attempts to learn and remember a list of words. The Rey Auditory-Verbal Learning Test, for example, requires the patient to learn a list of 15 words. Five successive trials are administered, and then a delayed recall procedure is performed after about 30 minutes. The patient's learning capacity, learning curve, and degree of forgetting can be determined.
   b. **Nonverbal memory tests** typically involve administration of various designs, such as geometric figures, that the patient must remember. The WMS-III includes one design-learning subtest. Another well-known test is the Benton Visual Retention Test, in which the patient is required to learn and reproduce various geometric figures. Face-learning procedures also provide good tests of nonverbal memory.
2. **Retrograde memory.** There are several standardized procedures for measuring retrograde memory, including the Remote Memory Battery, the Famous Events Test, and the Autobiographical Memory Questionnaire. These procedures probe recall and recognition of various historical facts,

famous events and persons, and autobiographical knowledge. Corroboration of retrograde memory, particularly with regard to autobiographical information, is extremely important; otherwise, even mild confabulation can completely mislead the clinician into underestimating the severity of retrograde memory defects.

3. **Nondeclarative memory.** A standard procedure for measuring nondeclarative learning is the rotor pursuit task, which requires the patient to hold a stylus in one hand and attempt to maintain contact between the stylus and a small metal target while the target is rotating on a platter. Successive trials are administered, and are followed by a delay trial. This procedure allows measurement of acquisition and retention of the motor skill. A normal result is to show steady improvement on this task, which is retained after a delay period.

4. **Working memory.** The digit span backward subtest from the WAIS-III provides a sensitive means of quantifying working memory. The Trail-making Test, which requires the patient to execute a psychomotor response while tracking dual lines of information, also is a good probe of working memory. Another commonly used procedure is the Paced Auditory Serial Addition Test, in which the patient must add numbers in an unusual format under increasingly demanding time constraints. Finally, two subtests from the WMS-III, Spatial Span and Letter-number Sequencing, together create a Working Memory Index. Spatial span is the visual–spatial analogue of the aforementioned auditory–verbal subtest, digit span. Rather than recalling numbers in forward and backward order, spatial span requires the examinee to replicate, forward and backward, an increasingly long series of visually presented spatial locations. In letter–number sequencing, the patient is read a combination of numbers and letters of varying lengths and is asked to repeat them by first stating the numbers in ascending order and then the letters in alphabetical order.

5. **Long-term memory,** which depends not only on the ability to acquire new information but also on the consolidation and storage of that information and its retrieval at a later time, is the real crux of memory. In a practical sense, it is not very helpful to have normal short-term memory if one cannot transfer the information into a more permanent storage area. Hence, delayed recall and recognition procedures, which yield information about the status of long-term memory, are very important in memory assessment.

IV. **Differential diagnosis.** Different causes of amnesia have different implications for diagnosis and management. The following common differential diagnoses are particularly challenging.

A. **Normal aging.** A seemingly minor but practically difficult challenge is to differentiate true memory impairment from the influences of normal aging. Aging produces certain declines in memory, which can be misinterpreted by patients and clinicians alike as signs of neurologic disease. Many elderly persons who report "forgetfulness" turn out to have peer-equivalent performances on all manner of standard memory tests, and the diagnosis of amnesia is not applicable. A considerable degree of "Alzheimer-phobia" has developed among elderly persons as the devastating consequences and widespread nature of Alzheimer's disease have gained increasing attention in the popular media. Patients may be quick to interpret any episode of memory failure as a sign of Alzheimer's disease, or they may adamantly deny memory dysfunction in the face of obvious real-world impairment. In both cases, careful quantification of the memory profile aids in the differential diagnosis.

B. **Psychiatric disease.** Many psychiatric diseases produce some degree of memory impairment. Accurate diagnosis is critical, because most memory defects caused by psychiatric disease are reversible, unlike most of amnesia that occurs in the setting of neurologic disease.

1. **Pseudodementia.** A condition that produces memory impairment and other cognitive defects resembling "dementia" but not caused by neurologic

disease is **pseudodementia.** Severe depression is the typical cause. Patients with pseudodementia often have memory impairment such as anterograde amnesia that is quite similar to that in the early stages of degenerative dementia. However, depressed patients respond to treatment with antidepressant medications and psychotherapy; when the affective disorder lifts, memory returns to normal.

    2. Depression is a common cause of memory impairment among all age groups. Distinguishing features, however, help differentiate amnesia due to depression from amnesia caused by neurologic disease. Depressed patients tend to have problems in concentration and attention, and they may have defects in working memory and other short-term memory tasks. Long-term memory is less affected, and retrograde memory is normal. Apathetic, "don't know" responses are common among depressed patients, whereas patients with a neurologic disorder more often give incorrect, off-target responses. Depressed patients also tend to describe their memory problems in great detail, whereas patients a neurologic disorder, such as those with suspected Alzheimer's dementia, generally discount memory problems. The history often is informative. In the evaluation of patients with depression, the clinician usually can find evidence of major stress, catastrophe, or other reasons for depression, and it is apparent that the onset of the memory problems coincided with the onset of the affective disorder.

  C. Side effects of medication. Many medications commonly prescribed for elderly persons produce adverse side effects on cognitive function, including memory. It is important to know what medications a patient has been taking and to account for the extent to which those medications may be causing memory impairment. The history often reveals that the onset of memory problems coincided with or soon followed the beginning of use of a particular medication. Memory defects caused by medication side effects also tend to be variable—for example, worse at certain times of the day. The main problems concern attention, concentration, and overall cognitive efficiency; memory defects are secondary.

V. Diagnostic approach. The diagnostic approach to a patient with amnesia should include any procedures necessary for establishing both the most likely **cause** and the precise **nature** of the memory impairment. The most commonly used procedures are as follows.

  A. Neurologic examination should establish whether a memory problems is present, the general degree of severity, and the history of the problem. It is not uncommon for patients with amnesia to underestimate or even deny the problem; information from a spouse or caretaker is a critical part of the history. Careful mental status testing can provide sufficient characterization of the amnesia profile.

  B. Neuroimaging procedures, including magnetic resonance imaging (MRI) and computed tomography (CT), almost always are helpful in diagnosing the cause of amnesia. Functional imaging, such as positron emission tomography (PET), may demonstrate abnormalities suggestive of Alzheimer's disease earlier in the natural course of the disease than may MRI, CT, or clinical assessment. However, PET procedures have for the most part not been standardized adequately for routine neurodiagnostic purposes. In the early stages of Alzheimer's disease, metabolic decrements usually are bilateral and focal and predominantly involve the parietal and temporal lobes.

  C. Neuropsychological assessment provides detailed quantification of the nature and extent of memory impairment. Such testing should be considered for almost all patients with amnesia, although there may be instances in which the mental-status-testing portion of the neurologic examination provides sufficient information. The cost of neuropsychological testing varies considerably from one clinical center to another, but it is almost always worth the investment.

VI. Criteria for diagnosis. The diagnosis of amnesia is appropriate whenever there are memory defects that exceed those expected given the patient's age and background. Some conditions, such as severe aphasia, make it difficult to assess memory in a meaningful way. Amnesia should not be diagnosed if the patient is in a severe confusional state, in which attentional impairment rather than memory dysfunction is the principal manifestation. Otherwise, amnesia can occur in isolation or coexist with almost any other form of impairment of mental status. It is customary to regard patients as having **amnesia** if there is considerable discrepancy between the level of intellectual function and one or more memory functions. There are many different subtypes of amnesia. Diagnosis of such subtype usually requires fine-grained quantification, such as that provided in a neuropsychological laboratory.

VII. Referral

A. **Neuropsychological** evaluation is appropriate for almost all patients with serious concerns about or manifestations of amnesia. The following situations that occur commonly in clinical practice particularly call for such a referral.

1. **Precise characterization of memory capacities.** For a patient who has sustained brain injury, neuropsychological assessment provides detailed information regarding the strengths and weaknesses of the patient's memory, which is useful in planning for placement, rehabilitation, and return to work. In most instances, memory assessment should be performed as early as possible in the recovery period. This evaluation provides a baseline to which recovery can be compared. Follow-up assessments assist in monitoring recovery, determining the effects of therapy, and making long-range decisions regarding educational and vocational rehabilitation.

2. **Monitoring the status of patients who have undergone medical or surgical intervention.** Serial neuropsychological assessment of memory is used to track the course of patients who are undergoing medical or surgical treatment of neurologic disease. Typical examples include drug treatment of patients with Parkinson's disease or a seizure disorder and surgical intervention for patients with normal pressure hydrocephalus or a brain tumor. Neuropsychological assessment provides a baseline memory profile with which changes can be compared and provides a sensitive means of monitoring changes in memory that occur in relation to particular treatment regimens.

3. **Differentiating "organic" from psychiatric disease.** Neuropsychological assessment can provide evidence crucial to the distinction between amnesic conditions that are primarily or exclusively "organic" and those that are primarily or exclusively "psychiatric." A common diagnostic dilemma faced by neurologists and psychiatrists is differentiating "true dementia" (e.g., cognitive impairment caused by Alzheimer's disease) and "pseudodementia" (e.g., cognitive impairment associated with depression).

4. **Medicolegal situations.** There has been a proliferation of cases in which "brain injury" and "memory impairment" are claimed as damages by plaintiffs who allegedly have sustained minor head injuries or have been exposed to toxic chemicals. In particular, there are many cases in which hard or objective signs of brain dysfunction (e.g., weakness, sensory loss, impaired balance) are absent, neuroimaging and electroencephalographic (EEG) findings are normal, and the entire case rests on claims of cognitive deficiencies, particularly memory dysfunction. Neuropsychological assessment is crucial to the evaluation of such claims.

5. **Conditions in which known or suspected neurologic disease is not detected with conventional neurodiagnostic procedures.** There are situations in which the findings of standard diagnostic procedures, including neurologic examination, neuroimaging, and EEG, are equivocal, even though the history indicates that brain disease and amnesia are likely. Examples include mild closed head injury, the early stages of degenerative dementia syndromes (e.g., Alzheimer's disease and Pick's disease), and early HIV-related dementia. Neuropsychological assessment in such cases provides the most sensitive means of evaluating memory.

6. **Monitoring changes in cognitive function over time.** A situation that warrants special mention is the evolution of changes in memory over time. In degenerative dementia in particular, equivocal findings in the initial diagnostic evaluation are not uncommon. In such cases, follow-up neuropsychological

evaluation can provide important confirming or disconfirming evidence regarding the status of the patient's memory.

B. Rehabilitation. Another common application of neuropsychological assessment is the case in which a patient undergoes cognitive rehabilitation for amnesia. Neuropsychological data collected at the initial assessment can help determine how to orient the rehabilitation effort. Subsequent examinations can be used to measure progress during therapy.

Acknowledgment

Supported by National Institute of Neurological Disorders and Stroke Program Project Grant NS 19632.

Recommended Readings

Adolphs R, Tranel D, Denburg NL. Impaired emotional declarative memory following unilateral amygdala damage. *Learn Mem* 2000;7:180–186.

Alexander MP. Mild traumatic brain injury: pathophysiology, natural history, and clinical management. *Neurology* 1995;45:1253–1260.

Bachevalier J, Meunier M. Cerebral ischemia: are the memory deficits associated with hippocampal memory loss? *Hippocampus* 1996;6:553–560.

Baddeley AD. Working memory. *Science* 1992;255:566–569.

Burke A, Heuter F, Reisberg D. Remembering emotional events. *Mem Cognit* 1992;20:277–290.

Butters N, Stuss DT. Diencephalic amnesia. In: Boller F, Grafman J, eds. *Handbook of neuropsychology.* Vol 3. Amsterdam: Elsevier, 1989:107–148.

Cabeza R, Nyberg L. Imaging cognition, II: an empirical review of 275 PET and fMRI studies. *J Cogn Neurosci* 2000;12:1–47.

Cohen NJ, Squire LR. Preserved learning and retention of pattern-analyzing skill in amnesia: dissociation of knowing how and knowing that. *Science* 1980;210:207–210.

Corkin S. Lasting consequences of bilateral medial temporal lobectomy: clinical course and experimental findings in H.M. *Semin Neurol* 1984;4:249–259.

Damasio AR. Time-locked multiregional retroactivation: a systems-level proposal for the neural substrates of recall and recognition. *Cognition* 1989;33:25–62.

Damasio AR, Eslinger PJ, Damasio H, et al. Multimodal amnesic syndrome following bilateral temporal and basal forebrain damage. *Arch Neurol* 1985;42:252–259.

Graff-Radford NR, et al. Diencephalic amnesia. In: Vallar G et al., eds. *Neuropsychological disorders associated with subcortical lesions.* New York: Oxford University Press, 1992:143–168.

Heindel WC, Salmon DP, Shults CW, et al. Neuropsychological evidence for multiple implicit memory systems: a comparison of Alzheimer's, Huntington's and Parkinson's disease patients. *J Neurosci* 1989;9:582–587.

Hyman BT, Kromer LJ, Van Hoesen GW. A direct demonstration of the perforant pathway terminal zone in Alzheimer's disease using the monoclonal antibody Alz-50. *Brain Res* 1988;450:392–397.

Kapur N. Focal retrograde amnesia in neurological disease: a critical review. *Cortex* 1993;29:217–234.

Kopelman MD. The neuropsychology of remote memory. In: Boller F, Grafman J, eds. *Handbook of neuropsychology.* Vol 8. Amsterdam: Elsevier, 1993:215–238.

Kroll NE, Markowitsch HJ, Knight RT, et al. Retrieval of old memories: the temporofrontal hypothesis. *Brain* 1997;120:1377–1399.

Lezak MD. Neuropsychological assessment, 3rd ed. New York: Oxford University Press, 1995.

Markowitsch HJ. Which brain regions are critically involved in the retrieval of old episodic memory? *Brain Res Rev* 1995;21:117–127.

McGaugh JL. Memory: a century of consolidation. *Science* 2000;287:248–251.

Milner B, Squire LR, Kandel ER. Cognitive neuroscience and the study of memory. *Neuron* 1998;20:445–468.

Poon L, ed. *Handbook for clinical memory assessment of older adults.* Washington, DC: American Psychological Association, 1986.

Scheinberg, P. The hidden costs of medicolegal abuses in Neurology. *Arch Neurol* 1994;51:650–652.

Squire LR. Memory and the hippocampus: a synthesis from findings with rats, monkeys, and humans. *Psychol Rev* 1992;99:195–231.

Stickgold R. Sleep: off-line memory reprocessing. *Trends Cogn Sci* 1999;2:484–492.

Thompson RF. The neurobiology of learning and memory. *Science* 1986;233:941–947.

Tranel D, Damasio AR. The covert learning of affective valence does not require structures in hippocampal system or amygdala. *J Cogn Neurosci* 1993;5:79–88.

Tranel D, Damasio AR. Neurobiological foundations of human memory. In: Baddeley AD, Wilson BA, Kopelman M, eds. *Handbook of memory disorders,* 2nd ed. New York: John Wiley and Sons Ltd., 2001 (*in press*).

Tranel D, Damasio AR, Damasio H, et al. Sensorimotor skill learning in amnesia: additional evidence for the neural basis of nondeclarative memory. *Learn Mem* 1994;1:165–179.

Tranel D, Damasio H, Damasio AR. Amnesia caused by herpes simplex encephalitis, infarctions in basal forebrain, and anoxia/ischemia. In: Boller F, Grafman J, eds. *Handbook of neuropsychology,* 2nd ed. Amsterdam: Elsevier Science, 2000:85–110.

Van Hoesen GW. The parahippocampal gyrus. *Trends Neurosci* 1982;5:345–350.

5. APPROACH TO THE COMATOSE PATIENT

Frank A. Rubino

Consciousness consists of wakefulness, self-awareness, and the capacity to formulate goal-directed behavior. **Awareness** is the content of consciousness and is the sum of cognitive and affective mental functions such as learning, memory, self-awareness, and adaptive behavior. All of these functions depend on the functional integrity of cerebral cortical neurons and associated subcortical nuclei. **Arousal** is closely linked to wakefulness and is an independent autonomic–vegetative function maintained by the ascending reticular activating formation, the intralaminar thalamic nuclei, and projections to the cerebral cortex. Awareness requires wakefulness, but mere arousal does not guarantee cognition. Arousal is composed of two components—tonic and phasic. **Tonic arousal** relates to fluctuations in the degree of wakefulness that occur on a diurnal basis, independent of sensory events and mediated by the caudal reticular formation. **Phasic arousal** involves rapid fluctuations in wakefulness in response to warning signals and unexpected stimuli and depends on the midbrain reticular formation, thalamic and hypothalamic nuclei, and mesial frontal structures (septum, anterior cingulate, and supplementary motor area). **Unconsciousness** implies global or total unawareness.

Coma is a state of consciousness in which there is lack of both wakefulness and awareness. Coma denotes unarousability, absence of sleep–wake cycles, and inability to react with the environment. Coma means advanced brain failure, and most causes of coma quickly and seriously threaten life or recovery of neurologic function. Causes must be promptly identified and managed. Diagnosis and treatment have to proceed concurrently.

Coma tends to occur in conjunction with acute or subacute brain lesions. Altered or reduced consciousness implies either diffuse bilateral impairment of cerebral hemispherical function, failure of the brainstem ascending reticular activating system, or both. However, even functional impairment can later cause structural pathologic changes, especially in the cortical neurons (diffuse cortical laminar necrosis). Mechanisms for the production of coma can be considered in two broad categories—structural and metabolic.

Diseases that produce coma fall into the following three categories:
1. **Supratentorial** lesions that also impair function of the opposite cerebral hemisphere, brainstem–diencephalic structures, or both.
2. **Infratentorial** lesions that directly impair the ascending reticular activating system.
3. **Metabolic (systemic)** disorders that diffusely impair cerebral hemispheric function and later brainstem–diencephalic structures.

Supratentorial and infratentorial structural lesions usually produce focal neurologic signs as well as pupillary and ocular motility abnormalities. Systemic causes of coma usually occur without focal neurologic signs or symmetric abnormalities (e.g., asterixis, myoclonus, or tremor).

    I. Etiology (Table 5.1)
        A. Supratentorial structural lesions
            1. **Unilateral cerebral hemisphere lesions** cause focal neurologic signs but not coma.
            2. **Bilateral hemisphere lesions** producing bilateral cerebral dysfunction can result in coma. These are usually extensive bilateral lesions, although left hemispheric strokes have been reported to affect consciousness more than have right-sided lesions.
            3. **Unilateral lesions** produce coma by secondarily encroaching on deep diencephalic structures so as to compress or damage physiologic systems that interact with both hemispheres. There may be central herniation with downward displacement of the diencephalon and midbrain through the tentorium cerebelli. There also may be uncal herniation with compression of the third cranial nerve or its nucleus (ipsilateral pupillary dilatation) and later compression of the midbrain.
            4. Typical lesions include **cerebral infarction; primary** or **secondary neoplasm; subdural, epidural,** or **intracerebral hemorrhage; abscess; focal encephalitis** (e.g., herpes simplex); **granuloma;** and **venous sinus thrombosis.**

Table 5.1 Causes of coma by approximate percentage

Cause	Percentage
Sedative drugs and toxins	40
Hypoxic–ischemic (cardiac arrest and anesthetic accidents)	25
Structural lesion	20
Other diffuse dysfunction (e.g., metabolic disturbances, systemic infection, systemic organ failure)	15

   B. Infratentorial structural lesions
      1. Lesions directly damage the deeper activating systems of the upper brainstem, hypothalamus, and thalamus, which normally activate both cerebral hemispheres.
      2. Typical lesions include **brainstem infarction** and **hemorrhage, intraaxial** and **extraaxial neoplasms, abscess,** and **granuloma.**
      3. One must consider lesions of the cerebellum that can secondarily compress the brainstem, especially infarction and hemorrhage. Posterior fossa lesions can cause upward herniation through the tentorium cerebelli or downward herniation through the foramen magnum.
         a. These lesions can necessitate emergency neurosurgical decompression.
         b. The lesions also can cause acute obstructive hydrocephalus.
   C. Primary neurologic diseases that produce **no mass effect** or necessarily produce focal neurologic signs
      1. Seizure disorders
         a. Postictal states
         b. Nonconvulsive status epilepticus
      2. Subarachnoid hemorrhage
      3. Disease of the leptomeninges
         a. Infection: meningitis and meningoencephalitis (viral, bacterial, or fungal)
         b. Neoplasia: carcinomatosis and lymphomatosis of the leptomeninges
         c. Inflammatory disease: sarcoidosis
   D. Diffuse disease and systemic disease (extracerebral causes)
      1. These disorders widely depress or interrupt the function of both the cerebral hemispheres and the brainstem.
      2. These disorders usually cause acute confusional states before causing stupor and coma.
      3. Causes
         a. Anoxic ischemic conditions
         b. Toxins
         c. Metabolic disturbances
         d. Systemic infections
         e. Electrolyte imbalance
         f. Systemic organ failure of any type
         g. Hyperthermia–hypothermia
II. Clinical manifestations
   A. Between the extreme states of consciousness and coma are a variety of **altered states of consciousness.**
      1. Various confusing terms have been used in the literature.
      2. The following terms have been defined.
         a. Drowsiness is a state of apparent sleep from which the patient can be aroused, often only briefly with an oral command.
         b. Stupor is a state in which the patient does not respond to oral commands but does respond to some degree to painful or noxious stimuli.
         c. Coma is unarousable unresponsiveness.
         d. Acute confusional state (delirium) is a fluctuating state of impairment of both arousal and awareness and has been termed an attentional disorder.

B. The Glasgow Coma Scale (Table 5.2)

  1. This scale may be a useful way to communicate the patient's clinical state to various medical personnel.
  2. Patients are considered to be in coma if they
     a. Do not open their eyes in response to verbal commands.
     b. Perform no better than weak flexion in response to pain.
     c. Utter only unrecognizable grunting in response to pain.

III. Evaluation

A. History

  1. In general, coma is likely to manifest in one of the following three ways:
     a. As the predictable progression of an underlying illness.
     b. As an unpredictable event in the case of a patient with a previously known disease.
     c. As a totally unexpected event.
  2. The history obtained from witnesses reviews
     a. The situation and the timing of the altered state of consciousness.
     b. Important previous medical and surgical illnesses.
     c. Previous psychological and neurologic conditions.
     d. Medications, including over-the-counter drugs.
     e. Social history, including use of tobacco, alcohol, and "recreational drugs."
     f. History of immediate or recent trauma (even minor trauma).
     g. Family members' thoughts or theories, which at times can give valuable clues.
     h. Important information obtained from other witnesses, such as ambulance personnel and police.

B. Physical examination

  1. **General physical examination.** A rapid, thorough physical examination can provide clues to the cause of stupor and coma.
     a. **Skin**
        (1) Careful examination can reveal signs of trauma, especially around the head and neck.

Table 5.2 The Glasgow Coma Scale

Circle the appropriate number and compute the total.

Eyes Open	
Never	1
To pain	2
To verbal stimuli	3
Spontaneously	4
Best Verbal Response	
No response	1
Incomprehensible sounds	2
Inappropriate words	3
Disoriented and converses	4
Oriented and converses	5
Best Motor Response	
No response	1
Extension (decerebrate rigidity)	2
Flexion abnormal (decorticate rigidity)	3
Flexion withdrawal	4
Localizes pain	5
Obeys	6
Total	3–15

Adapted from Teasdale G, Jennett B. Assessment of coma and impaired consciousness: a practical scale. *Lancet* 1974;2:81–84, with permission.

(2) There may be signs of liver disease, needle marks, and evidence of infection or embolic processes.

(3) Anemia, jaundice, or cyanosis can be identified.

(4) Exanthem may indicate a viral infection.

(5) Petechial rash is an indication of meningococcal infection.

(6) Hyperpigmentation suggests the possibility of Addison's disease.

(7) Bullous lesions can be seen with barbiturate intoxication.

b. **Temperature**

(1) Fever usually indicates infection, rarely a "central" cause.

(2) Hypothermia can be caused by exposure, intoxication with alcohol or barbiturates, peripheral circulatory failure, or, rarely, myxedema and Wernicke's encephalopathy.

c. **Breath**

(1) May smell like alcohol.

(2) May suggest the presence of hepatic disease (fetor hepaticus).

(3) May emit the uriniferous smell of uremia.

(4) May indicate ketoacidosis of diabetes.

d. **Blood pressure**

(1) Hypotension can indicate shock, septicemia, intoxication, myocardial infarction, or Addison's disease.

(2) Hypertension is a less helpful sign and can be the result of or the cause of lesions such as cerebral hemorrhage and infarction.

e. **Cardiovascular system**

(1) An important arrhythmia may be detected.

(2) Various valvular lesions may be detected.

f. **Abdomen**

(1) May reveal signs of trauma or rupture of viscera.

(2) May exhibit hepatomegaly or splenomegaly.

2. **Neurologic examination**

a. Rather than using vague and confusing terms, one should use everyday terms to describe the patient's responses to verbal, noxious, and painful stimuli.

(1) For noxious stimuli, vigorously rub the sternum with the knuckles.

(2) For painful stimuli, apply pressure with the fingers over the supraorbital nerve area or press the base of the fingernails or toenails with the rounded surface of a pen or pencil.

(3) Test pain with the gentle prick of a pin.

(4) Do not use maneuvers that can harm the patient, such as heavy pressure with a pin that draws blood or twisting the skin or nipples.

b. **Head and neck examination**

(1) Head and neck trauma often are associated with one another.

(2) If no history is available, the neck must be immobilized until fracture dislocation of the cervical spine has been ruled out.

(3) Check the neck for signs of meningeal irritation.

(4) Look for **Kernig's sign,** which is elicited by means of flexing the thigh of the recumbent patient to a right angle and attempting to extend the leg at the knee; this is accompanied by pain, spasm of hamstring, and limitation of extension.

(5) Look for **Brudzinski's neck sign,** in which passive flexion of the head on the chest is followed by flexion of both thighs and legs.

c. **State of consciousness**

(1) Describe the patient in everyday terms and describe any spontaneous movements, either normal or abnormal, and the patient's response to various stimuli.

(2) Terms such as *semicoma, lethargy,* and *obtundation* should be avoided.

(3) The **Glasgow Coma Scale** may be used. A score of 8 or less is considered standard for the diagnosis of coma.

d. Pupillary response

  (1) A patient cannot be in a coma resulting from a brainstem lesion without having impairment of pupillary function, ocular motility, or both.

  (2) The pupillary light reflex is resistant to metabolic dysfunction.

  (3) The presence or absence of the light reflex is the single most important physical sign for differentiating structural from metabolic coma.

  (4) A unilateral fixed, dilated pupil suggests brain herniation (uncal herniation) or a posterior communicating artery aneurysm (in a conscious patient, a unilateral fixed dilated pupil usually is benign).

  (5) Midbrain lesions result in midposition pupils that do not react to light.

  (6) Pontine lesions can result in small, pinpoint pupils.

  (7) Most drug intoxications cause pupils to be small but sluggishly reactive.

  (8) Atropine drugs can cause pupils to be large and unreactive.

  (9) Other agents that can cause pupils to be unreactive include barbiturates, succinylcholine, lidocaine, phenothiazines, methanol, and aminoglycoside antibiotics.

  (10) Hypothermia can fix the pupils.

  (11) Anoxia or ischemia, if severe, can lead to large, fixed pupils, which, if present more than several minutes after an acute anoxic insult, carry a poor prognosis.

  (12) Examination of the optic fundi may reveal evidence of papilledema, hemorrhage, emboli, or subhyaloid hemorrhage, which is indicative of subarachnoid hemorrhage.

e. Ocular motility

  (1) The pathway for ocular motility in the brainstem lies adjacent to the ascending reticular activating system in the paramedian pontine reticular formation, making ocular motility an important clinical sign of stupor and coma.

  (2) Asymmetric ocular motility accompanies structural more often than metabolic causes of coma.

  (3) If the brainstem is intact, the eyelids are closed and the eyes, slightly divergent, drift slowly from side to side (roving eye movements).

  (4) Roving eye movements indicate that coma is a result of cerebral hemisphere dysfunction.

  (5) If ocular motility is severely impaired but the pupillary reflex is more or less intact, the cause of the coma is metabolic and most likely attributable to abuse of drugs such as benzodiazepines, barbiturates, or alcohol.

  (6) Conjugate deviation of the eyes suggests the possibility of an ipsilateral cerebral hemispherical lesion or a contralateral brainstem lesion as the cause of the coma.

  (7) If there are no spontaneous eye movements, ocular motility can be tested by means of assessment of the oculocephalic reflex (doll's eye maneuver) and the oculovestibular reflex (caloric testing).

    (a) The oculocephalic reflex is tested by means of turning the patient's head from side to side. If the brainstem is intact, the eyes move fully and conjugately to the opposite side.

    (b) The oculovestibular reflex provides a stronger stimulus and is tested after the head of the bed is elevated 30 degrees and an intact tympanic membrane is observed; 50 to 200 mL of ice water is instilled into the external auditory canal, and after 5 minutes the opposite ear is tested.

      (i) The normal response of a conscious patient is development of nystagmus with the fast component away from the site of stimulation.

(ii) Nystagmus is not produced in response to the oculo-vestibular reflex in coma from any cause; thus the production of nystagmus indicates that the patient is conscious.

(iii) Tonic conjugate full movement of the eyes toward the stimulated side indicates that the brainstem is intact and that the coma is a result of cerebral hemisphere dysfunction.

(iv) A disconjugate response (internuclear ophthalmoplegia; INO) or no response indicates brainstem impairment, usually structural. However sedative drug intoxication and severe anoxic encephalopathy can result in INO.

(v) Conjugate deviation of the eyes to one side as a result of a supratentorial lesion usually can be overcome by the oculovestibular reflex; conversely, conjugate deviation of the eyes to one side as a result of an infratentorial lesion cannot be overcome by the oculovestibular reflex.

(vi) If a cerebral hemispherical lesion causes conjugate deviation of the eyes, unless the patient is having a seizure, the eyes "look toward the lesion," whereas with a brainstem lesion the eyes "look away from the lesion."

(vii) Drugs or conditions that can block the oculovestibular reflex include ototoxic drugs such as gentamicin; vestibulosuppressant drugs such as barbiturates and other sedative drugs, phenytoin, and tricyclic antidepressants; neuromuscular blockers such as succinylcholine; and preexisting vestibular disease.

(viii) Vertical gaze disturbances indicate brainstem disease.

(ix) Ocular bobbing consists of rapid downward eye movements followed by a slow drift back to the original position. Ocular bobbing usually is associated with absent horizontal eye movements and indicates extensive pontine structural damage.

f. Corneal reflex

(1) The corneal reflex has a high threshold in comatose patients and usually is retained until coma is very deep.

(2) If there is bilateral loss of the corneal reflex of a patient with light coma, one must consider drug-induced coma or a local anesthesia in both eyes.

(3) If there is unilateral impairment of the corneal reflex, one might consider a focal neurologic lesion that causes decreased sensation on the ipsilateral side or impairment of eye closure from weakness on the ipsilateral side.

(4) Although unilateral impairment of the corneal reflex suggests a structural lesion, one cannot differentiate a cerebral hemispheric lesion from a brainstem lesion.

g. Motor responses. In eliciting motor responses, one looks for symmetric and asymmetric responses.

(1) **Asymmetric responses** suggest a focal neurologic sign and thus a structural lesion in either the cerebral hemisphere or brainstem.

(2) **Symmetric responses** suggest a more diffuse process such as a metabolic encephalopathy.

(3) **Paratonia (gegenhalten)**

(a) This is a type of rigidity in which there is increased resistance in the opposite direction from which one passively moves a limb.

(b) This type of rigidity is common in elderly patients with altered states of consciousness from any cause and is prominent in the neck in all directions moved.

      (c) In metabolic coma, paratonia is seen symmetrically in the limbs and neck.

      (d) Paratonia of the limbs on one side and flaccidity of the limbs on the opposite side suggests hemiparesis involving the flaccid limbs and indicates the presence of a structural lesion in the cerebral hemisphere or brainstem causing focal neurologic signs.

(4) Movement of the limbs

      (a) The patient may move the limbs only on one side spontaneously or as a reaction to stimuli, suggesting a structural lesion in the cerebral hemisphere or brainstem.

      (b) Rarely is metabolic coma accompanied by hemiparesis.

      (c) If the patient does not move the limbs spontaneously or in response to stimuli, one can lift the patient's arms from the bed and flex the patient's legs at the knees and release the limbs one at a time. In light coma, if the cause is a diffuse one, the limbs fall slowly and symmetrically to the resting position; however, paretic limbs fall like "dead weights" and thus hemiparesis or monoparesis can be detected. **Symmetric** responses suggest a diffuse process; **asymmetric** responses suggest a focal, structural cause.

(5) Decorticate rigidity

      (a) Characterized by adduction of the arm at the shoulder with flexion at the elbow and pronation and flexion at the wrist with the leg extended at the hip and knee.

      (b) Usually indicates a structural lesion of the cerebral hemisphere or diencephalon with the decortication contralateral to the hemispherical lesion.

(6) Decerebrate rigidity

      (a) The arm is extended, adducted, and internally rotated (hyperpronated), and the leg is extended.

      (b) Supratentorial lesions causing downward herniation, upper brainstem structural lesions, and even severe metabolic disorders can give rise to decerebrate rigidity.

(7) Other movements

      (a) Partial simple motor (focal motor) seizures usually result from focal cerebral hemisphere lesions but occasionally are found in metabolic coma, such as nonketotic hyperosmolar coma.

      (b) In general, asymmetric motor findings speak against metabolic encephalopathy.

      (c) Abnormal movements such as tremors, asterixis, myoclonus, and generalized tonic–clonic seizures often are found in association with toxic–metabolic disorders; however, focal and multifocal motor seizures can accompany metabolic disorders such as nonketotic, hyperosmolar, and hyperglycemic states.

h. Respiratory patterns

    (1) The presence of abnormal respiratory patterns can be helpful in localizing the level of structural lesions in the central nervous system early in coma, but metabolic abnormalities can affect the respiratory centers of the brainstem and produce patterns resembling those found in neurologic diseases.

    (2) A normal breathing pattern suggests that the brainstem is intact.

    (3) Cheyne–Stokes respiration suggests the brainstem is intact. Although this breathing pattern can have neurologic causes, it usually is observed in conjunction with metabolic disturbances.

    (4) Deep, rapid hyperventilation in a comatose patient suggests pneumonia or rectification of metabolic acidosis.

    (5) Central neurogenic hyperventilation, however, can suggest a lesion in the midbrain or pons.

        (6) Apneustic breathing characterized by a deep inspiration followed by a pause suggests a lesion in the lower pons, but this breathing pattern is rare in humans.

        (7) Cluster breathing characterized by clusters of breaths in an irregular sequence suggests a lesion in the low pons or high medulla.

        (8) Ataxic breathing characterized by an irregular pattern of breathing with inspiratory gasps of diverse amplitude and length and periods of apnea suggests a lesion of the respiratory center in the medulla. This breathing pattern is probably the only reliable predictor of lesion site based on ventilatory pattern.

        (9) Yawning and sneezing suggest that the brainstem is intact, but coughing, swallowing, or hiccuping can occur in patients with severe brainstem failure.

C. Laboratory studies

1. Blood and urine screens for drugs and toxins
2. Complete blood cell count, urinalysis, blood chemistry, blood gases
3. Electrocardiography (ECG)
4. Neuroimaging studies—computed tomography (CT) or magnetic resonance imaging (MRI)
5. Lumbar puncture
6. Electroencephalography (EEG)

IV. Differential diagnosis (Table 5.3)

A. Brain death

1. Brain death is the **permanent cessation of all brain function.**
2. There is absence of function of both the cerebral cortex and the brainstem.
3. Patients are irreversibly comatose and apneic and have lost all brainstem reflexes and cranial nerve function.
4. Brain death is a clinical diagnosis.

B. Locked-in syndrome

1. Consciousness and cognition are retained.
2. Movement and communication are markedly impaired because of quadriplegia, inability to speak and swallow, and inability to move the eyes in a horizontal direction.
3. This syndrome usually results from lesions of the corticospinal and corticobulbar pathways, frequently in the base of the pons.
4. This syndrome also has been observed occasionally in patients with severe peripheral neuropathy (Guillain–Barré syndrome) or myasthenia gravis and after administration of neuromuscular blocking agents.
5. The patient usually communicates by means of eye blinks or vertical eye movements.
6. The syndrome also has been referred to as a de-efferented state.

C. Vegetative state

1. A state of wakefulness without detectable awareness.
2. There is preservation of vital vegetative functions such as heart rate and rhythm, respiration, and maintenance of blood pressure, but there is bowel and urinary bladder incontinence.

Table 5.3 Differential diagnosis of coma

Brain death
Locked-in syndrome
Vegetative state
Frontal lobe disease
Nonconvulsive status epilepticus
Transient unresponsiveness of the elderly (idiopathic recurring stupor)
Psychiatric disorder (catatonia, depression)
Neocortical death
Minimally conscious state

3. Patients remain unaware of self and environment.
4. Patients have sleep–wake cycles but no ascertainable cerebral cortical function; there is no evidence of language comprehension or expression.
5. This state has been referred to as a de-afferented state, and there is no evidence of sustained reproducible purposeful or voluntary behavioral response to visual auditory tactile, or noxious stimuli.
6. Patients are considered unconscious because although they are wakeful, they lack awareness.
7. Patients have extensive damage of the forebrain, especially the neocortex, with relative sparing of the brainstem.
8. The most common acute causes are head trauma and hypoxic ischemic encephalopathy.
9. This condition lasting 1 month is called the **persistent vegetative state.**

D. **Frontal lobe disease**
   1. Lesions are prefrontal and bilateral and include disorders such as hydrocephalus, subfrontal meningioma, bilateral frontal lobe tumors (primary or metastatic), intracerebral hemorrhage, cerebral trauma, and cerebral infarction in the distribution of both anterior cerebral arteries.
   2. Patients are described as **abulic.**
      a. Patients have long delays between stimulation—noxious, painful, or verbal—and reaction.
      b. A slowness or "viscosity" is applicable to verbal output and motor responsiveness.

E. **Nonconvulsive status epilepticus**
   1. **Complex partial status epilepticus**
      a. This is an important syndrome that is more common than is suspected.
      b. This condition takes one of two forms
         (1) A prolonged twilight state with partial responsiveness, impaired speech, and quasipurposeful automatism.
         (2) A series of complex seizures with staring, total unresponsiveness, speech arrest, and stereotyped automatism with a twilight state between seizures.
      c. There is often prolonged clouding of consciousness with cycling of ictal and postictal states.
   2. **Absence status epilepticus**
      a. Altered consciousness often is accompanied by mild clonic movements of the eyelids and hands with automatism of the face and hands.
      b. There are bilateral synchronous spike-wave discharges on an EEG.
      c. This is usually a disease of childhood.
      d. It can occur among adults as an acute confusional state.
         (1) Usually no apparent cause.
         (2) Sometimes occurs in association with diffuse insults such as metrizamide myelography or electroconvulsive therapy.
         (3) Also reported after benzodiazepine withdrawal.

F. **Transient unresponsiveness of the elderly** (idiopathic recurrent stupor)
   1. This condition usually occurs among elderly persons.
   2. There are one or more self-limited episodes of unresponsiveness unrelated to obvious structural, toxic, metabolic, convulsive, or psychiatric disorders.
   3. Flumazenil, a specific benzodiazepine receptor antagonist, can reverse the episode.

G. **Psychiatric disorders**
   1. **Pseudocoma** (hysterical coma)
      a. This relatively rare syndrome is a diagnosis of exclusion.
      b. Patient may hold eyes forcibly closed and resist eyelid opening or may keep eyes in a fixed stare interrupted by quick blinks.
      c. Pupils are of normal size, position and, reactivity (unless cycloplegic drugs have been used).
      d. Oculovestibular testing shows normal awake response.
      e. Patient may hyperventilate or breathe normally.

      f. EEG findings are normal.

      g. Harsh, painful stimulation is inappropriate; instead, one can stimulate the palpebral reflex or tickle the nose with a wisp of cotton.

    2. Severe vegetative depression

    3. Catatonia

      a. In the past, catatonia was considered a variety of schizophrenia.

      b. Catatonia now is considered to occur as a conversion reaction or a dissociative state.

H. Neocortical death

    1. This is an extreme form of the vegetative state and most often is the result of anoxic–ischemic injury.

    2. There may be normal brain stem function but no purposeful behavior.

    3. The EEG result is isoelectric.

    4. The pathologic process is diffuse cortical necrosis (laminar necrosis).

 I. Minimally conscious state

    1. A condition of severely altered consciousness in which minimal but definite behavior evidence of self or environmental awareness is demonstrated.

    2. Outcomes may be better than those of vegetative state.

V. Diagnostic approach

  A. Screening the blood and urine for drugs and toxins can yield valuable information.

    1. Sedative drugs and alcohol overdoses usually are nonlethal and carry a good prognosis as long as circulation and respiration are supported.

    2. However, drugs often depress brainstem function, and if drug overdose is not suspected, impairment of brainstem function can be misinterpreted as a poor prognostic sign.

  B. Complete blood cell count, urinalysis, blood chemistry including electrolytes, and blood gases all are performed to detect hepatic failure, renal failure, hyperglycemia, hypoglycemia, electrolyte disturbances, or acidosis.

  C. ECG is important in detecting various forms of cardiac arrhythmia.

  D. If a structural lesion is suspected in either of the cerebral hemispheres, the brainstem, or the cerebellum, neuroimaging is needed.

    1. CT of the head without contrast material is a good initial study because it can be performed quickly and can help identify acute intraparenchymal and subarachnoid hemorrhage better than can MRI.

    2. Plain CT of the head can help detect most structural lesions causing stupor and coma, including subarachnoid hemorrhage and subdural and epidural hematoma.

    3. MRI of the brain provides more information about lesions involving the temporal lobes, posterior fossa structures, and sellar and parasellar areas.

  E. Lumbar puncture with cerebrospinal fluid analysis is necessary in cases of suspected meningitis or meningoencephalitis as well as other lesions involving the leptomeninges.

  F. Electroencephalography

    1. The main role of EEG is detection of nonconvulsive status epilepticus.

    2. EEG also may be helpful in detecting feigned or psychological coma, in which cases it the EEG findings are normal.

    3. EEG also can help detect postictal states and show diffuse abnormalities with metabolic and toxic causes of coma. Some drugs and toxins also cause fast activity.

    4. *EEG should not be used as a screening tool* and is not needed in the emergency department unless nonconvulsive status epilepticus is suspected.

    5. Continuous EEG monitoring can be useful in an intensive care setting because EEG is tightly linked to cerebral metabolism, is sensitive to hypoxic and ischemic injury, provides dynamic information about reversible neuronal dysfunction and neuronal recovery, helps detects epileptic activity, and provides useful information about cerebral topography.

VI. Management

  A. One manages the patient initially with the **ABCs of resuscitation** (airway, breathing, circulation) of advanced cardiac life support or advanced trauma life support while evaluating the patient.

B. Any causes found are managed appropriately.

C. Nonspecific therapeutic endeavors can be performed to prevent permanent brain damage.

1. Assure an adequate airway for oxygenation.
2. Maintain circulation.
3. Manage increased intracranial pressure (unilateral dilated pupil) with hyperventilation (to a Pco_2 of 25 to 30 mm Hg) and intravenous (i.v.) mannitol (20% to 25% solution) 0.75 to 1 g/kg initially then 0.25 to 0.5 g/kg every 3 to 5 hours.

D. Manage any seizures that occur with i.v. benzodiazepine (diazepam, lorazepam), i.v. phosphenytoin, i.v or intramuscular phenobarbital, or i.v. valproate.

E. Manage any infections.

F. Restore electrolyte and acid–base balance.

G. Control body temperature.

H. Give 100 to 300 mg thiamine i.v.

I. Consider using a narcotic antagonist. Naloxone 0.8 to 2.0 mg i.v. should be given if narcotics are suspected.

J. Consider using a selective benzodiazepine antagonist.

1. Benzodiazepines are the drugs most commonly used for self-poisoning.
2. Flumazenil is a highly specific and competitive benzodiazepine antagonist.
   a. Flumazenil has a relative short half-life.
   b. The drug is given IV at a rate of 0.25 mg/min until a response is observed or until total of dose of 2.0 mg is reached.
   c. If the patient responds, there may be no need for further diagnostic studies.
   d. Because of the short half-life, repeated boluses or continuous infusions may be needed.
   e. Flumazenil must be given with caution to patients with mixed drug ingestion, especially if there has been an overdose of a tricyclic antidepressant, because the benzodiazepine may play a role in preventing tricyclic-induced convulsions.

K. 50% Dextrose

1. 50 mL of a 50% dextrose solution usually is recommended.
2. Results of some studies suggest that glucose administration worsens the neurologic and histologic outcome of cerebral ischemia.
   a. Some experts state that empiric administration of glucose should be avoided in the care of patients with acute stroke, cardiac arrest, or severe hypotension or during administration of cardiopulmonary resuscitation.
   b. A bedside finger-stick blood glucose estimation should be performed on patients with altered mental status.
   c. Administration of 50% dextrose should be reserved for patients in whom hypoglycemia is demonstrated.

VII. Prognosis

A. Patients who fit the criteria for brain death usually do not survive for more than a few days.

B. In patients in coma with preserved brainstem function, so-called cerebral death, the outcome is more difficult to predict. The condition of some of these patients may evolve into a persistent vegetative state.

C. If pupillary reflexes and ocular motility are absent after 6 hours of the onset of coma (especially with hypoxic–ischemic encephalopathy), the fatality rate is 95%.

1. At 24 hours, the absence of corneal, pupillary light, oculocephalic, and oculovestibular reflexes is not compatible with recovery to independence.
2. The most accurate prediction of outcome is obtained from the clinical examination.

D. "**Myoclonus status**" after cardiopulmonary arrest is a grave prognostic sign.

1. This is defined as spontaneous or stimulus-induced repetitive, irregular brief jerks involving the face, limbs, or both.
2. This indicates severe anoxic brain damage.

VIII. Referral. Patient in a coma should be referred to a **neurologist or neurosurgeon** in the following circumstances.

    A. There is structural cause in the cerebrum or brainstem.

    B. Seizures occur.

    C. The cause is obscure.

    D. Trauma is involved.

    E. There is involvement of the leptomeninges by a disease process (e.g., subarachnoid hemorrhage, meningoencephalitis, or neoplastic invasion).

    F. Brain death is suspected.

    G. Other states, such as locked-in syndrome or persistent vegetative state, are suspected.

Recommended Readings

Adams RD, Victor M. *Principles of neurology,* 5th ed. New York: McGraw-Hill, 1993.

Bates D. The management of medical coma. *J Neurol Neurosurg Psychiatry* 1993;56:589–598.

Browning RG, Olson DW, Stueven HA, et al. 50% dextrose: antidote or toxin? *Ann Emerg Med* 1990;19:683–687.

Feske SK. Coma and confusional states: emergency diagnosis and management. *Neurol Clin* 1998;16:237–256.

Giacino JT. Disorders of consciousness: differential diagnosis and neuropathologic features. *Semin Neurol* 1997;17:105–111.

Haimovic JC, Beresford HR. Transient unresponsiveness in the elderly. *Arch Neurol* 1992; 49:35–37.

Jordan KG. Continuous EEG monitoring in the neuroscience intensive care unit and emergency department. *J Clin Neurophysiol* 1999;16:14–39.

Mercer WN, Childs NL. Coma, vegetative state, and the minimally conscious state: diagnosis and management. *Neurologist* 1999;5:186–193.

O'Callahan W, Ranzi FP. Neurologic emergencies: stupor and coma. In: Stine RJ, Chudnofsky CR, eds. *A practical approach to emergency medicine.* 2nd ed. Boston: Little, Brown, 1994:803–848.

Plum F, Posner JB. *The diagnosis of stupor and coma.* 3rd ed. Philadelphia: Davis, 1980.

Samuels MA. The evaluation of comatose patients. *Hosp Pract* 1993;28:165–182.

Simon RP. Coma. In: Joynt RJ, Griggs RC, eds. *Clinical neurology.* Philadelphia: Lippincott Williams & Wilkins, 1998:1–38.

Teasdale G, Jennett B. Assessment of coma and impaired consciousness: a practical scale. *Lancet* 1974;2:81–84.

Tinuper P, Montagna P, Plazzi G, et al. Idiopathic recurring stupor. *Neurology* 1994;44:621–625.

Winkler E, Almog S, Kriger D, et al. Use of flumazenil in the diagnosis and treatment of patients with coma of unknown etiology. *Crit Care Med* 1993;21:538–542.

6. APPROACH TO THE PATIENT WITH SEIZURES

Vicenta Salanova

I. Introduction

A. Seizures result from the paroxysmal, hypersynchronous, abnormal activity of neurons in the cerebral cortex. Seizures are common symptoms and can be manifestations of toxic–metabolic abnormalities or of infection, can be secondary to a variety of disorders that affect neuronal function, or can be idiopathic with unknown cause.

1. **Nonrecurrent seizures**—e.g., toxic–metabolic, hypoxia.
2. **Recurrent seizures** or epilepsy—inherited, acquired, or structural cortical lesions

B. The **international classification of epileptic seizures** consists of two main categories—partial seizures and generalized seizures.

1. **Partial seizures** (focal) result from localized epileptogenic lesions, except in children with benign focal epilepsy, who have no structural lesions. Partial seizures are subdivided into
   a. **Simple partial seizures** if there is preservation of consciousness.
   b. **Complex partial seizures** if there is impairment of consciousness. A partial seizure typically begins as a simple partial seizure consisting of an aura reflecting the site of seizure origin (or ictal spread to the symptomatogenic area) and then evolves into a complex partial seizure. Both simple and complex partial seizures can evolve into secondarily generalized seizures.

2. **Generalized seizures** can be convulsive or nonconvulsive and are subdivided into absence (typical and atypical absences), myoclonic, clonic, tonic, tonic–clonic, and atonic seizures.

C. There is also an **international classification of epilepsy** and epilepsy syndromes. This classification takes into account the age at onset, possible etiologic factors, inheritance, findings at neurologic examination, prognosis, and seizure type (partial or generalized).

1. **Localization-related epilepsy**
   a. **Idiopathic** (benign childhood rolandic and occipital epilepsy)
   b. **Symptomatic,** which is acquired and based mainly on the anatomic localization.

2. **Generalized epilepsy and syndromes**
   a. **Idiopathic** with **age-related** onset (e.g., benign neonatal familial convulsions, childhood and juvenile absence epilepsy, juvenile myoclonic epilepsy, epilepsy with grand mal seizures on awakening)
   b. **Symptomatic** (e.g., infantile spasms, Lennox–Gastaut syndrome). The international classification includes two other categories: (1) epileptic syndromes with both focal and generalized seizures (e.g., acquired epileptic aphasia) and (2) special syndromes (e.g., febrile convulsions). This chapter reviews the etiology, clinical manifestations, evaluation, and differential diagnoses of some of these types of seizures with emphasis on patients with partial seizures.

II. Etiology

A. **Toxic–metabolic**

1. **Systemic illness.** Hypoglycemia, nonketotic hyperglycemia, hypoxia, hypocalcemia (in patients with or without a history of hypoparathyroidism), hyponatremia (inappropriate antidiuretic hormone syndrome and water intoxication), hypomagnesemia, uremia and hepatic failure, sickle-cell anemia, thrombotic thrombocytopenic purpura, Whipple's disease.

2. **Drugs and toxins.** Cocaine, amphetamines, phencyclidine, lidocaine, lead poisoning. Others can lower the seizure threshold and increase the risk of seizures usually among patients with other predisposing factors (tricyclics, theophylline, phenothiazine, penicillins).

3. **Withdrawal syndromes.** Alcohol, hypnotics

4. **Pyridoxine deficiency**

B. Acquired structural lesions
1. **Infection:** brain abscess, meningitis, encephalitis (e.g., herpes simplex encephalitis), postinfectious encephalomyelitis, cysticercosis, opportunistic infections in acquired immunodeficiency syndrome, neurosyphilis
2. **Vascular:** vasculitis (systemic lupus erythematosus, hypersensitivity, and infectious vasculitis), ischemic or hemorrhagic cerebrovascular disease, cerebral venous thrombosis, arteriovenous malformation, cavernous angioma
3. **Trauma:** usually penetrating, subdural hematoma
4. **Neoplasms** and other lesions: primary or metastatic tumors, hamartomas, cortical dysplasia
5. **Mesial temporal sclerosis:** usually postfebrile convulsions
6. **Other:** Alzheimer's disease, Creutzfeldt–Jakob disease, and in rare instances, multiple sclerosis

C. Familial
1. **Primary generalized epilepsy**
2. **Benign focal epilepsy of childhood**
3. **Febrile convulsions**
4. **Autosomal dominant nocturnal frontal lobe epilepsy**
5. **Familial temporal lobe epilepsy**

D. Other genetic syndromes associated with seizures (tuberous sclerosis, neurofibromatosis), disorders of amino acid, lipid, and protein metabolism (e.g., phenylketonuria, maple syrup urine disease, porphyria)

III. Clinical manifestations

A. Metabolic–toxic and hypoxic insults. Patients with seizures attributable to metabolic or toxic causes have generalized tonic–clonic seizures, but focal seizures and epilepsia partialis continua can occur with nonketotic hyperglycemia. Posthypoxic coma usually causes multifocal myoclonus; however, periodic lateralized epileptiform discharges (PLEDs) may be seen, at times associated with focal motor seizures.

B. Meningitis and encephalitis can cause either generalized or focal seizures with secondarily generalized seizures. Patients with herpes simplex encephalitis often have complex partial seizures typical of those of temporal lobe origin. The electroencephalogram (EEG) shows focal slowing in one or both temporal regions and periodic lateralized epileptiform discharges. Magnetic resonance imaging (MRI) shows hypodense lesions in one or both temporal lobes.

C. Partial seizures (functional–anatomic classification of epilepsy). Clinical features and EEG findings indicate focal origin.
1. **Temporal lobe seizures** are the most common partial seizures. In 30% of these patients, the seizures are refractory to medical treatment.
    a. **Signs and symptoms.** The findings at neurologic examination often are normal, except for memory disfunction, which can be seen in patients with bitemporal epilepsy. Most of these patients have an epigastric aura (nausea, an epigastric rising sensation, stomach upset, or even pain). Other aurae consist of fear, complex visual or auditory hallucinations, déjà vu, and olfactory and gustatory sensations. The clinical manifestations are stereotypical, and most patients have one seizure type. Most patients exhibit staring, unresponsiveness, and oroalimentary and gestural automatism. Some patients also have contralateral arm dystonic posturing. Ictal or postictal language difficulties also have lateralizing value. Ictal speech occurs in patients with seizures arising from the nondominant temporal lobe. Patients with seizures originating from the dominant temporal lobe may exhibit ictal and postictal dysphasia.
    b. **Etiologic factors and pathologic features.** Mesial temporal sclerosis is the most common pathologic finding. There is a strong association between mesial temporal sclerosis and prolonged complex febrile seizures in patients younger than 5 years of age. There usually is a silent interval between the occurrence of febrile seizures and the onset of mesial temporal lobe epilepsy, which often begins toward the end of the first decade of life or soon after. Other pathologic findings include tumors, such as

ganglioglioma, cortical dysplasia, and cavernous malformation. As many as 15% of patients with medically refractory temporal lobe epilepsy have evidence of a dual pathologic process. Mesial temporal sclerosis can occur with temporal lobe developmental lesions such as cortical dysplasia and subependymal heterotopia.

c. **EEG findings** include epileptiform discharges over the anterior temporal region and often polymorphic slowing. Thirty percent to 40% of these patients have bitemporal independent interictal epileptiform discharges, usually with predominance on the side of ictal onset.

d. **Imaging studies.** MRI volumetric studies usually show a smaller hippocampus and increased signal intensity on T2-weighted images that are indicative of hippocampal sclerosis. These changes can be seen in as many as 80% of patients with refractory temporal lobe epilepsy.

e. **Secondarily generalized** tonic–clonic seizures and convulsive status epilepticus can occur; nonconvulsive complex partial status epilepticus is rare.

f. Patients with temporal lobe seizures should be differentiated from patients with **familial temporal lobe epilepsy (FTLE)**. The first series described FTLE as a benign disorder with late age of onset, excellent outcome, and normal finding on the MRI of the head. A second report, however, showed that some cases of FTLE were refractory to medical treatment, requiring surgical treatment. The most recent report concluded that FTLE is a clinically heterogeneous syndrome. The authors found hippocampal atrophy in 57% of their patients, including those with a benign course or remission of seizures. They concluded that the findings indicated the presence of a strong genetic component in the development of mesial temporal sclerosis in the families studied.

2. **Focal motor seizures.** These seizures originate in the vicinity of the rolandic motor cortex. Consciousness is preserved.

a. **Signs and symptoms.** Examination may show contralateral mild hemiparesis or hyperreflexia. Seizures commonly begin with focal contralateral twitching of the face or hand and then spread to involve the rest of the extremity. When seizures originate in the nondominant hemisphere, patients usually are able to speak during the seizures. When seizures originate in the dominant hemisphere, patients may have ictal and postictal aphasia. Clonic eye movements, blinking, and conscious contraversion also may occur. Ictal focal motor manifestations, postictal hemiparesis, and postictal aphasia are contralateral to the side of seizure onset. Some patients have continuous focal motor activity (epilepsia partialis continua lasting weeks, months, or even years).

b. **Imaging studies.** Focal structural lesions are common.

c. **EEG** shows focal slowing and focal epileptiform discharges over the frontal lobe; however, some patients have no epileptiform discharges on scalp recordings or have bifrontal epileptiform abnormalities.

d. Patients with focal motor seizures have to be differentiated from patients with benign rolandic epilepsy with centrotemporal spikes, which begins between the ages of 3 and 13 years. These children have normal findings at neurologic examination and imaging studies. They have nocturnal generalized seizures and partial seizures beginning in the face with preservation of consciousness, at times with speech arrest. The EEG shows centrotemporal, high-amplitude, broad, sharp waves and slow discharges, with a horizontal dipole, occurring predominantly during sleep. The prognosis is excellent.

3. **Supplementary motor seizures** originate in the supplementary motor cortex, which is located in the mesial frontal lobe anterior to the primary motor leg area.

a. **Signs and symptoms.** Findings at examination usually are normal. Almost one half of these patients have a somatosensory aura consisting of tingling or numbness of the extremities, which can be contralateral or bilateral. These patients have unilateral or bilateral tonic posturing of the extremities at onset, vocalization, speech arrest, and laughter. Other manifestations include fencing posture, thrashing, kicking, and pelvic movements. Responsiveness is preserved unless the seizure evolves into a secondarily generalized tonic–clonic seizure. Supplementary motor seizures are common during sleep and are of short duration without postictal confusion or amnesia.

    b. Imaging studies. MRI of the head may show lesions in the supplementary motor area.

    c. The **EEG** may show epileptiform discharges over the vertex, but some patients may have no interictal epileptiform discharges on scalp recordings. Ictal recordings often are nonlateralized. A few patients may have no ictal EEG changes during scalp recordings.

4. Complex partial seizures of frontal lobe origin

    a. Signs and symptoms. The examination usually is normal. Patients may have a cephalic aura that is followed by staring or looking ahead, unconscious contraversion, and complex motor automatism such as bicycling, kicking, thrashing, running, and bouncing up and down. Vocalization and tonic posturing may occur toward the end of the seizure as manifestations of ictal spread to the supplementary motor area. Complex partial (nonconvulsive) status epilepticus, manifested by alteration of consciousness with automatic behavior often in a cyclical manner lasting hours to days, also may occur. Secondarily generalized tonic–clonic seizures and convulsive status epilepticus are believed to be more common in patients with frontal lobe seizures.

    b. Imaging studies. MRI may show lesions in the frontopolar, dorsolateral, orbitofrontal, and other frontal regions.

    c. The **EEG** may show focal slowing and interictal epileptiform discharges over one frontal lobe, lateralized to one hemisphere, or bilateral frontal epileptiform abnormalities.

    d. These patients with acquired frontal lobe epilepsy should be differentiated from those with **autosomal dominant nocturnal frontal lobe epilepsy (ADNFLE).** In ADNFLE, the seizures begin in childhood and usually persist through adult life. They occur in clusters during sleep and are characterized by vocalization, thrashing, hyperkinetic activity, or tonic stiffening. Patients have a normal findings at neurologic examination and on imaging studies. An ictal EEG may show bifrontal epileptiform discharges. The seizures usually respond to carbamazepine monotherapy. These seizures often are misdiagnosed as parasomnia or familial dyskinesia.

5. Occipital lobe seizures are rare, but they may be difficult to differentiate from seizures originating from the posterior temporal lobe. These patients have to be differentiated from patients with benign occipital epilepsy, the onset of which is in childhood and has similar symptoms but no occipital lesions. The age at onset of benign occipital epilepsy ranges from 15 months to 17 years (with a peak between 5 and 7 years), and more than one third of patients have family histories of epilepsy.

    a. Signs and symptoms. Occipital manifestations are common. Patients may have visual field defects, visual aurae consisting of elementary visual hallucinations described as colored flashing lights, or ictal blindness. Other manifestations include contralateral eye deviation, a sensation of eye movement, nystagmoid eye movements, and blinking. After the occipital manifestations, many patients have typical temporal lobe automatism as well as focal motor seizure activity resulting from ictal spread to the temporal and frontal lobes. Because of these different spread patterns, many patients have more than one type of seizure. Almost two thirds of patients have lateralizing clinical features, such as contralateral head deviation and visual field defects contralateral to the epileptogenic zone.

      b. Imaging studies. On CT scans and MR images, many patients have occipital lesions ipsilateral to the epileptogenic zone.

      c. The **EEG** may show focal slowing and epileptiform discharges over one occipital lobe. However, most often the EEG shows posterior temporal epileptiform discharges. Some patients have bilateral posterior temporal–occipital epileptiform abnormalities.

   6. Parietal lobe seizures are uncommon.

      a. Signs and symptoms. The examination may show contralateral impaired two-point discrimination, but more often the findings are normal. These patients have somatosensory aurae described as contralateral tingling or numbness and painful and thermal sensations. Other aurae consist of disturbances of body image, a sensation of movement in one extremity, or a feeling that one extremity is absent. Vertiginous sensations and visual illusions can occur, as can an aphasic aura. Some of these patients have seizures of multiple types as a result of ictal spread to the temporal and frontal lobes. Tonic posturing of extremities, focal motor clonic activity, head and eye deviations, and temporal lobe automatism are commonly observed.

      b. Imaging studies. MRI may show focal lesions in the parietal lobe.

      c. The **EEG** most often shows lateralized epileptiform discharges to one hemisphere rather than localized discharges.

D. Primary (idiopathic) generalized epilepsy. There is usually a family history of epilepsy. The first clinical manifestations indicate involvement of both cerebral hemispheres. This form of epilepsy can be **convulsive** or **nonconvulsive.**

   1. Childhood absence epilepsy begins between the ages of 4 and 8 years. The findings at neurologic examination are normal.

      a. Signs and symptoms. There is a brief loss of consciousness, usually lasting 10 seconds or less and almost always lasting less than 30 seconds. There is no aura or postictal confusion. Blinking, brief facial twitching, or other clonic component, decreased postural tone, and automatism such as swallowing, lip smacking, and fumbling with clothes are common. Forty percent to 50% of patients also may have tonic–clonic seizures.

      b. The **EEG** shows the typical generalized, bilaterally synchronous 3-Hz spike–wave epileptiform discharges. Hyperventilation for 3 to 5 minutes often provokes an absence seizure with typical generalized, bifrontally dominant, regular, synchronous 3-Hz spike–wave complexes with abrupt onset and termination. In some patients the epileptiform discharges may be maximum over the posterior head regions.

      c. The **prognosis** is favorable, and for many patients the seizures remit in adolescence. The prognosis is less favorable if tonic–clonic seizures occur.

      d. Absence status. Rare patients may have prolonged confusion that lasts hours or all day and is associated with continuous 3-Hz spike–wave discharges.

   2. Juvenile absence epilepsy is less common than childhood absence epilepsy.

      a. The **clinical manifestations** are similar, but seizures begin during puberty or later. The absences tend to occur on awakening and are not as frequent as those in the childhood form. Myoclonic seizures also may occur.

      b. The **EEG** may show generalized 3-Hz spike–wave discharges or higher-frequency (4 to 5 Hz) discharges.

      c. The **prognosis** is not as favorable as in the childhood form, and generalized tonic–clonic seizures are more frequent. Absence status also is more frequent than in the childhood form.

   3. Juvenile myoclonic epilepsy. Age at onset is in the second decade. The findings at neurologic examination are normal. The diagnosis often is missed because of failure to recognize the myoclonic jerks.

      a. Signs and symptoms. These patients have awakening myoclonic and generalized tonic–clonic seizures. Absence seizures occur in 15% of patients. During brief myoclonic jerks, consciousness is preserved. Myoclonic seizures may precede the onset of generalized tonic–clonic seizures by a few years, or they may have simultaneous onset. The generalized tonic–clonic seizures usually follow a series of myoclonic seizures. Seizures may be precipitated by sleep deprivation or alcohol intake.

   b. The **EEG** shows generalized polyspike and wave discharges in most patients. Some patients are photosensitive and have photoparoxysmal responses. During the myoclonic jerks, the EEG shows abrupt onset of high-amplitude polyspike and wave complexes lasting from 2 to 10 seconds.

   c. **Prognosis.** Although these patients have an excellent response to valproic acid, the electroclinical trait persists for life, and most patients need lifelong treatment.

4. **Generalized tonic–clonic seizures.** A patient with primary generalized tonic–clonic seizures usually has a family history of epilepsy. The findings at neurologic examination are normal. Age at onset usually is during puberty.

   a. **Signs and symptoms.** There is no aura. A few patients may have a prodrome (nervousness, irritability) hours before the seizure. The seizure begins with brief tonic flexion of the axial muscles and muscular contraction of the extremities followed by a longer period of tonic extension of the axial muscles. The mouth is closed, and this may lead to tongue biting. Apnea can occur as a result of contraction of the respiratory muscles. The arms are semiflexed, and the legs are extended. After the tonic phase, there is diffuse tremor, and then there is a clonic phase. Autonomic changes usually occur at the end of the tonic phase. Heart rate and blood pressure can more than double during the tonic phase. There is also increased bladder pressure.

   b. **Complications** during a prolonged tonic–clonic seizure may include tongue biting, dislocation of shoulders, vertebral compression fractures, aspiration pneumonia, and even sudden death. The mechanism of sudden death is unclear; several factors, such as apnea, pulmonary edema, and cardiac arrhythmias, may be involved.

   c. The **EEG** shows generalized 4- to 5-Hz spike–wave activity, or multiple spike–wave complexes. More irregular spike–wave discharges can occur. The likelihood of recording the epileptiform discharges increases if the EEG is obtained 1 to 5 days after a seizure. Some patients have a photoparoxysmal response with bisynchronous, generalized irregular spike and spike–wave discharges. EEG ictal changes show generalized low-voltage fast activity (recruiting rhythm) followed by high-amplitude generalized polyspike or polyspike and wave discharges. During the clonic phase, high-amplitude polyspike or polyspike and wave discharges alternate with low-amplitude slowing. Postictally, there is low-amplitude slowing.

   d. **Generalized tonic–clonic status epilepticus** begins with recurrent, brief tonic–clonic seizures without full recovery of consciousness or with a prolonged generalized tonic–clonic seizure lasting 30 minutes.

E. **Secondary (symptomatic) generalized epilepsy.** These patients have multifocal cortical abnormalities, including infantile spasms (West's syndrome) and Lennox-Gastaut syndrome.

   1. **West's syndrome.** The onset usually is between 3 and 6 months of age and always before 1 year. Some infants have no identifiable etiologic factors (cryptogenic subgroup). Symptomatic West's syndrome is more common and can result from trauma, infection, Down's syndrome, tuberous sclerosis, phenylketonuria, and other disorders. These infants have frequent infantile spasms, developmental delay, and a characteristic EEG pattern (hypsarrhythmia).

   2. **Lennox–Gastaut syndrome** is one of the most severe epileptic syndromes. These children usually have developmental delay, neurologic deficits, and seizures of multiple types, which are often medically refractory (drop attacks, atypical absence, myoclonic, tonic, and tonic–clonic seizures). The EEG shows generalized slow (<2.5 Hz) spike–wave discharges.

    a. Drop attacks represent atonic seizures and are characterized by sudden loss of tone, at times preceded by a generalized clonic jerk. There is head drop, and often the child collapses. The ictal EEG shows an electrodecremental response.

    b. Atypical absences usually last longer than typical absences and are commonly associated with motor findings and postictal confusion. They are more common during drowsiness and are not usually activated by hyperventilation. The EEG shows generalized slow spike–wave discharges and diffuse slowing of the background.

    c. Absence status is common. Patients come to medical attention with prolonged absences (spike–wave stupor), blinking, and at times facial twitching with continuous generalized spike–wave discharges.

    d. Tonic seizures are common in Lennox–Gastaut syndrome. The arms are elevated in a semiflexed position, and there is impairment of consciousness and autonomic changes.

IV. Evaluation

  A. History

    1. The following should be documented: **age at onset** and **frequency** of seizures, **family history** of epilepsy, psychosocial history, possible etiologic factors such as history of head trauma, difficult birth, febrile seizures, meningitis, or encephalitis. **Precipitating factors** include medical illnesses that can lead to metabolic abnormalities and exposure to drugs or toxins.

    2. The **presence and type of aura,** detailed description of the seizure by a family member, presence of automatism, ictal speech, dystonic or tonic posturing, postictal language difficulties, Todd's paralysis, or the presence of myoclonus can help to **differentiate focal from generalized seizures.**

    3. **Response to anticonvulsants** and possible side effects.

  B. Physical examination

    1. **Detailed examination,** including the skin, for signs of neurocutaneous lesions associated with seizures, such as neurofibromatosis, tuberous sclerosis, and Sturge–Weber syndrome. Cranial bruits may be present in patients with arteriovenous malformations, and cervical bruits in patients with seizures resulting from cerebrovascular disease.

    2. **Limb asymmetry** suggestive of injuries early in life. **Focal neurologic deficits,** such as subtle hemiparesis, hyperreflexia, decreased two-point discrimination, or visual field defects, may suggest the location of the epileptogenic lesion. **Memory deficits** can be elicited in some patients with bitemporal epilepsy.

  C. Laboratory studies include complete blood cell count; a Venereal Disease Research Laboratory test; measurement of erythrocyte sedimentation rate and blood levels of glucose, calcium, sodium, and magnesium; liver and renal function tests; drug and toxicology screening if indicated by the history or examination findings; and human immunodeficiency virus testing for patients with risk factors.

  D. Cerebrospinal fluid examination is performed if vasculitis or infection is suspected or if the serologic result is positive for syphilis.

  E. The **EEG** is essential to confirm the diagnosis of epilepsy and to characterize the seizure type. It usually shows focal slowing and epileptiform abnormalities in patients with partial seizures or generalized epileptiform discharges in those with generalized seizures. Seizures are rarely recorded on routine EEGs. The exception is absence seizures, which can be precipitated by hyperventilation. Metabolic encephalopathy associated with seizures usually have diffuse slowing or periodic patterns, such as triphasic waves, in patients with hepatic or renal failure.

    1. **Activation procedures,** such as photic stimulation, hyperventilation, and sleep, are performed.

    2. **Special electrodes.** Earlobe, anterior temporal, or zygomatic electrodes often are used. Nasopharyngeal electrodes are traumatic and produce arti-

facts, and they should not be used. Sphenoidal electrodes are reserved for patients undergoing presurgical evaluation.

    3. Video EEG recordings. In some patients with recurrent seizures and no interictal epileptiform discharges on serial EEGs, prolonged video EEG recording may be needed to confirm the diagnosis and to characterize the seizure type.

  F. Imaging studies. When the history, neurologic examination, EEG findings, and seizure type suggest partial seizures, the procedure of choice is **MRI of the head.** Although the CT of the head may be helpful, some patients with partial seizures have lesions that do not appear on CT scans, such as hamartoma, cortical dysplasia, low-grade glioma, or cavernous malformation.

V. The **differential diagnosis** includes many neurologic, psychiatric, and medical disorders. The most common are psychogenic seizures and syncopal episodes.

  A. Syncope is defined as a brief episode of loss of consciousness as a result of a transient decrease in cerebral blood flow. Episodes last a few seconds. Brief tonic–clonic movements and incontinence of urine and feces can occur (convulsive syncope). An EEG during the prodromal period (light-headedness) shows diffuse high-amplitude slowing, and when tonic or clonic activity occurs, the EEG result is isoelectric.

  B. Psychogenic seizures are suspected when a patient has seizures precipitated by stress when others are present, no response to anticonvulsants, seizures of long duration up to 15 or 30 minutes or even hours, side-to-side head movements, pelvic thrusting, arrhythmic jerking, bilateral motor activity with preservation of consciousness, bizarre and aggressive behavior, and crying. There is no postictal confusion after generalized tonic–clonic jerking. However, some of these symptoms (bizarre complex automatism, pelvic thrusting, bilateral motor activity) can occur among patients with complex partial seizures of frontal lobe origin and supplementary motor seizures.

  C. Panic attacks

  D. Cerebrovascular disorder: transient global amnesia

  E. Basilar artery migraine

  F. Sleep disorder: narcolepsy

  G. Movement disorder: myoclonus, choreoathetosis, familial paroxysmal dystonia

  H. Paroxysmal vertigo

  I. Toxic–metabolic disorder: alcohol withdrawal, hypoglycemia

  J. Daydreaming episodes

VI. Diagnostic approach

  A. The **history and examination** are central to determine the type of seizure (generalized or focal, psychogenic, related to syncope or metabolic causes, and so on), obtain descriptions of the aura (if present) and the seizure by a witness, and identify subtle neurologic deficits. It is helpful to ask a family member to mimic the seizure. After the initial evaluation, a presumptive etiologic diagnosis and a tentative seizure classification often are possible and should determine the extent of the evaluation.

  B. Laboratory evaluation should include serum electrolytes, baseline renal and hepatic function tests to rule out metabolic causes, drug screening, and other tests as indicated by the history and examination findings.

  C. If syncope is suspected, **electrocardiography** and **Holter monitoring** are performed as indicated by the history and examination findings. More extensive evaluation for cardiac causes of syncope may be needed.

  D. Sleep and awake EEGs are obtained with activation procedures (hyperventilation and photic stimulation) and special electrodes. An ambulatory EEG may be helpful in the evaluation of patients with suspected seizures or pseudoseizures or suspected convulsive episodes of syncope.

  E. Prolonged video EEG may be needed to confirm the diagnosis, characterize the seizure type, and exclude psychogenic seizures. Complex partial seizures of frontal lobe origin and supplementary motor seizures often are misdiagnosed as psychogenic seizures, and ictal recordings often are needed.

   F. Sleep studies (multiple sleep latency test and polysomnography) may be
      needed in the evaluation of some patients with suspected sleep disorders.
   G. MRI should be performed on patients with partial seizures and secondary
      (symptomatic) generalized epilepsy.
VII. Referral.
   A. For patients with recurrent seizures, an initial **neurologic consultation,**
      including an EEG to clarify the seizure type, allows the proper choice of anti-
      convulsants.
   B. When the diagnosis remains unclear after the initial evaluation or there is lack
      of response to anticonvulsants, the patient should be referred to a **comprehen-
      sive epilepsy center.** Evaluation at such centers includes prolonged video EEG
      with sphenoidal electrodes. It is important to emphasize that patients with
      poorly controlled epilepsy have a higher mortality rate than does the general
      population. Death usually is caused by accidents, status epilepticus, sudden
      unexplained death, cardiac arrhythmias, and suicide. However, when seizures
      are completely controlled after surgery, the mortality rate is not different from
      that of the age-matched general population.
      1. Because the treatment and prognosis are based on the seizure type and
         epileptic syndrome, **ictal recordings** are invaluable and allow the proper
         choice of anticonvulsants.
      2. Ictal recordings are the most effective way to diagnose psychogenic seizures,
         but patients with psychogenic seizures may also have epileptic seizures, and
         all the habitual seizure types should be recorded. To compound the prob-
         lem, some patients with supplementary motor seizures and other simple
         partial seizures may have no ictal EEG changes on scalp recordings, or the
         EEG activity may be obscured by muscle artifacts. Inpatient prolonged video
         EEG recordings with reduction of anticonvulsants may clarify the diagnosis
         by recording secondarily generalized seizures.
   C. Identification of surgical candidates. Approximately 30% of cases of com-
      plex partial seizures of temporal lobe origin are refractory to medical treatment,
      and many patients benefit from surgery. Prolonged video EEG, MRI with volu-
      metric studies, and tests of focal functional deficits (FDG-PET scans) are con-
      ducted at epilepsy centers to identify surgical candidates.
   D. Patients with medically refractory temporal lobe epilepsy are the largest group
      of patients undergoing epilepsy surgery, and 70% to 80% of these patients become
      seizure free after surgery. A longitudinal study of a large number of patients who
      underwent temporal resection showed the lasting benefits of epilepsy surgery.
      The best surgical outcome was observed among patients with small lesions such
      as cavernous malformation, followed by patients with mesial temporal sclerosis.
      Studies also have shown considerable improvement in the quality of life of
      patients who became seizure free after surgery.

Recommended Readings

Aicardi J. *Epilepsy in children.* International Review of Child Neurology Series. New York:
   Raven Press, 1994.
Andermann F, Robb JP. Absence status: a reappraisal following review of 38 patients.
   Epilepsia 1972;13:177–187.
Berkovic S, McIntosh A., Howell RA, et al. Familial temporal lobe epilepsy: a common dis-
   order identified in twins. *Ann Neurol* 1996;40:227–235.
Cendes F, Cook MJ, Watson C, et al. Frequency and characteristics of dual pathology in
   patients with lesional epilepsy. *Neurology* 1995;45:2058–2064.
Commission on Classification and Terminology of the International League Against Epilepsy.
   Proposal for classification of epilepsy and epileptic syndromes. *Epilepsia* 1985;26:268–278.
Engel J. *Seizures and epilepsy.* Contemporary Neurology Series. Philadelphia: FA Davis Co,
   1989.
French JA, Williamson PD, Thadani VM, et al. Characteristics of medial temporal lobe
   epilepsy, I: results of history and physical examination. *Ann Neurol* 1993;34:774–780.
Gloor P. Generalized epilepsy with spike and wave discharge: a reinterpretation of its elec-
   trographic and clinical manifestations. *Epilepsia* 1979;20:571–588.

Gloor P, Olivier A, Quesney LF, et al. The role of the limbic system in experiential phenomena of temporal lobe epilepsy. *Ann Neurol* 1982;12:129–144.

Holmes G. *Diagnosis and management of seizures in children.* Vol 30. Philadelphia: WB Saunders, 1987.

Kanner AM, Morris HH, Luders H, et al. Supplementary motor seizures mimicking pseudoseizures: some clinical differences. *Neurology* 1990;40:1404–1407.

Kobayashi E, Lopes-Cendes I, Guerreiro CAM, et al. Seizure outcome and hippocampal atrophy in familial mesial temporal lobe epilepsy. *Neurology* 2001;56:166–172.

Kotagal P, Lüders H, Morris HH, et al. Dystonic posturing in complex partial seizures of temporal lobe onset: a new lateralizing sign. *Neurology* 1989;39:196–201.

Lüders H, Lesser R, eds. *Epilepsy: electroclinical syndromes.* London: Springer-Verlag, 1987.

Markand O, Salanova V, Whelihan E, et al. Health-related quality of life outcome in medically refractory epilepsy treated with anterior temporal lobectomy. *Epilepsia* 2000;41:749–759.

Morris H 3rd, Dinner DS, Lüders H, et al. Supplementary motor seizures: clinical and electrographic findings. *Neurology* 1988;38:1075–1092.

Penfield W, Jasper H. Epilepsy and the functional anatomy of the human brain. Boston: Little, Brown, 1954.

Salanova V, Andermann F, Olivier A, et al. Occipital lobe epilepsy: electroclinical manifestations, electrocorticography, cortical stimulation and outcome in 42 patients treated between 1930 and 1991. *Brain* 1992;115:1655–1680.

Salanova V, Markand O, Worth R. Clinical chaacteristics and predictive factors in 98 patients with complex partial seizures treated with temporal resrection. *Arch Neurol* 1994;51:1008–1013.

Salanova V, Markand O, Worth R. Longitudinal follow-up in 145 patients with medically refractory temporal lobe epilepsy treated surgically between 1984 and 1995. *Epilepsia* 1999;40:1417–1423.

Salanova V, Morris HH, Van Ness P, et al. Frontal lobe seizures: electroclinical syndromes. *Epilepsia* 1995;36:16–24.

Scheffer I, Bhatia K, Lopez-Cendes I, et al. Autosomal dominant frontal lobe epilepsy misdiagnosed as sleep disorder. *Lancet* 1994;343:515–517.

Scheffer I., Bhatia K, Lopez-Cendes I, et al. Autosomal dominant frontal lobe epilepsy: a distinctive clinical disorder. *Brain* 1995;118;61–73.

Williamson PD, Boon PA, Thadani VM, et al. Parietal lobe epilepsy: diagnostic considerations and results of surgery. *Ann Neurol* 1992;31:193–201.

Williamson PD, French JA, Thadani VM, et al. Characteristics of medial temporal lobe epilepsy, II: interictal and ictal scalp electroencephalography, neuropsychological testing, neuroimaging, surgical results and pathology. *Ann Neurol* 1993;34:781–787.

Williamson PD, Spencer DD, Spencer SS, et al. Complex partial seizures of frontal lobe origin. *Ann Neurol* 1985;18:497–504.

Williamson PD, Thadani VM, Darcey TM, et al. Occipital lobe epilepsy: clinical characteristics, seizure spread patterns and results of surgery. *Ann Neurol* 1992;31:3–13.

Wyllie E, Lüders H, Morris HH, et al. The lateralizing significance of versive head and eye movements during epileptic seizures. *Neurology* 1986;36:606–611.

7. APPROACH TO THE PATIENT WITH SYNCOPE

Gary J. Martin
Martin J. Arron

Syncope can be defined as transient (less than 30 minutes) loss of consciousness accompanied by loss of postural control. Causes range from the relatively benign vasovagal syncope to life-threatening cardiac arrhythmia. This range is illustrated by several epidemiologic facts. Approximately one third of healthy young adults have had at least one episode of loss of consciousness. For the most of these persons, it is a relatively benign event. On the other hand, 5% of sudden cardiac death victims have had a recent history of syncope. The potential prognostic significance of the syncopal event makes it necessary to carefully evaluate each patient.

I. **Etiology**
   A. The major **mechanisms** of syncope include obstruction of cerebral blood flow, decreased cardiac output secondary to decreased heart rate or stroke volume, decreased peripheral vascular resistance, and insufficient blood constituents (oxygen, glucose). In the elderly, multiple mechanisms can contribute to the syncope. For example, postprandial fluid shifts can exacerbate mild preexisting orthostatic hypotension, sinus node dysfunction, and impaired autoregulation of cerebral blood flow.
   B. **Obstruction of cerebral blood flow** is a rare cause of true syncope. Most carotid artery distribution (anterior circulation) transient ischemic attacks (TIAs) cause unilateral visual impairment, weakness, or loss of sensation. Posterior circulation (vertebrobasilar artery distribution) TIAs generally manifest as diplopia, vertigo, ataxia, or "drop attacks," but not loss of consciousness. Rare patients with TIAs may have transient loss of consciousness, but isolated syncopal episodes without accompanying neurologic symptoms should not be ascribed to a TIA.
   C. **Generalized hypotension** can cause inadequate cerebral perfusion. This is the main mechanism of most episodes of syncope. The hypotension can be cardiogenic, due to rhythm disturbances such as bradycardia or tachyarrhythmia that reduce cardiac output, or secondary to valvular dysfunction resulting in outflow obstruction as in aortic stenosis or idiopathic hypertrophic subaortic stenosis. Probably the most common mechanism of hypotension is the loss of peripheral vascular tone. Vasovagal syncope is the most common disorder in this group. Drug toxicity and various disorders associated with orthostatic hypotension also can cause impaired peripheral vascular resistance.
   D. **Inadequate blood constituents such as severe hypoxemia** or **hypoglycemia** are associated with true loss of consciousness. Profound hypoglycemia often causes longer episodes of impaired consciousness and can induce coma, as opposed to the brief, transient loss of consciousness characteristic of syncope.
   E. Table 7.1 lists the common causes of syncope identified in a large number of prospective studies. The most common causes of syncope among patients arriving in emergency departments are vasovagal (vasodepressor) reactions, seizures, orthostatic hypotension, cardiac diseases such as dysrhythmia and outflow obstruction, situational syncope (postmicturition or posttussive), and hypoglycemia. Rarer causes include TIAs, migraine headaches, pulmonary embolism, and psychiatric disorders.
   Syncope of unknown origin is a legitimate diagnosis made after a careful history, physical examination, and selected laboratory tests have failed to elucidate a specific etiologic factor. This diagnosis is clinically useful because it is associated with a distinct prognosis that is considerably better than that of patients who have identifiable cardiac causes of syncope. Long-term follow-up studies have shown that the risk of sudden death among middle-aged and older patients with a defined cardiac cause of syncope is as high as 24% during the first year after the syncopal event. Patients with a history of cardiac or neurologic disease also have a significantly increased long-term mortality. Patients with syncope of unknown causation have a relatively low incidence of sudden death (0 to

Table 7.1 Causes of syncope

Cause	Percentage	Cause	Percentage
Vasovagal	36	Situational	4
Idiopathic	24	Psychogenic	3
Cardiac	13	Metabolic/drug	2
Neurologic	11	Miscellaneous	1
Orthostatic	4		

1363 pooled patients.

3%). Their risk is comparable with that of patients who, after further investigation, are given the diagnosis of a noncardiovascular cause of syncope.

II. Clinical manifestations. Table 7.2 lists associated signs and symptoms found among patients with syncope. These have been grouped into two categories. The first are fairly **nonspecific** symptoms associated with decreased cerebral perfusion regardless of the etiologic factor. The second category of signs and symptoms are those that are somewhat more suggestive of **specific** etiologic factors.

III. Evaluation

    A. History

        1. Information about the **prodromal period** is most helpful diagnostically. A useful technique is to ask the patient to "walk through" the sequence of events occurring just before the loss of consciousness.

            a. A patient's **activity and posture** before the episode should be noted. A supine position suggests cardiac dysrhythmia or seizure and makes a vasovagal reaction or syncope due to orthostatic hypotension unlikely. Syncope during physical exertion is a characteristic finding in aortic stenosis, whereas loss of consciousness after exercise indicates that idiopathic hypertrophic subaortic stenosis may be a causal factor. Loss of consciousness while urinating, coughing, or laughing is strongly suggestive of situational syncope. Episodes that follow the assumption of an upright posture, particularly if it occurs within 30 seconds to 2 minutes after standing implies that orthostatic hypotension is the inciting cause. The nadir in blood pressure following a meal in the elderly occurs within 15 to 90 minutes. Syncope occurring within this time suggests a postprandial induction or exacerbation of orthostatic hypotension. Episodes that follow neck extension, flexion, or rotation implicate carotid sinus hypersensitivity, whereas those taking place during a prolonged period of standing often are caused by vasovagal reactions.

            b. Specific symptoms experienced during the prodromal period are important predictors of the cause of the episode. Most symptoms are

Table 7.2 Syncope: Associated symptoms

Nonspecific	Specific
Paresthesia	Aura
Diaphoresis	Palpitations
Dizziness	Vertigo and ataxia
Lightheadedness	Anginal or pleuritic chest pain
Blurred or fading vision	Diplopia
Auditory impairment	Olfactory hallucinations
Tinnitus	Dyspnea
Nausea	Epigastric discomfort

nonspecific and merely reflect the presence of cerebral hypoperfusion. Examples include light-headedness, wooziness, nausea, a warm or flushed sensation, diaphoresis, paresthesia, and impaired visual acuity. Some of these symptoms are not unique to syncope and may also be felt just before a seizure. A classic but uncommon prodrome for a seizure disorder is a new smell or **olfactory hallucination. Epigastric distress** occurs with vasovagal syncope and inferior wall myocardial infarction. Although suggestive of pulmonary embolism, **dyspnea** also occurs with hyperventilation and other psychiatric disorders associated with syncope. **Facial pallor** suggests decreased cerebral blood flow from any cause (orthostatic hypotension, vasovagal reaction, arrhythmia) and helps rule out a seizure. In the latter instance, facial cyanosis during the ictus epilepticus or postictal facial plethora are more typical.

    c. The perceived **duration of the warning period** provides clinically relevant information. Very brief intervals (less than 10 seconds) are a characteristic of cardiac causes, micturition syncope, orthostatic hypotension, and seizure disorders. On the other hand, vasovagal syncope typically has a more sustained warning period lasting 1 or 2 minutes. This often can be elicited with careful questioning.

    d. Focal neurologic symptoms may indicate a TIA and can be present immediately before or after the loss of consciousness. Specific examples include vertigo, diplopia, ataxia, dysarthria, hemiparesis, and unilateral numbness. Posterior circulation TIAs usually manifest as a cluster of these symptoms.

    e. A variety of factors can trigger **vasovagal syncope** in predisposed persons. Emotionally charged situations such as anger, fear, and seeing blood can induce vasodepressor activity. Pregnant patients and those experiencing physical trauma, pain, fatigue, or sleep deprivation are at increased risk. Hot, enclosed, or crowded environments, particularly if the patient is standing for sustained periods, increase the likelihood of vasovagal syncope.

2. The **events during the syncopal period** are of great importance in defining a specific etiologic factor. A detailed history confirming the presence of a true transient episode of loss of consciousness and associated neuromuscular activity is extremely important.

    a. Given that patients are unconscious during most of this period, firsthand reports from **witnesses** are crucial. Clinicians should make sincere efforts to interview witnesses either in person or over the telephone.

    b. Although prolonged episodes of cerebral anoxia (more than 10 to 15 seconds) can induce brief involuntary motor activity, the presence of more sustained episodes of alternating **tonic and clonic** muscle action is strongly suggestive of a seizure. The same is true of the presence of facial cyanosis, tongue biting, and excessive salivation.

    c. Brief episodes of unconsciousness are more typical of most cardiovascular causes of syncope. Hypoglycemia can induce episodes of more sustained duration. Seizures also tend to have a more prolonged duration.

    d. Urinary **incontinence** is more frequent among patients with seizure, although it can accompany syncope of any cause. Fecal incontinence is more specific for seizures.

3. The events during the **immediately postsyncopal period** provide important clues to the cause of loss of consciousness. Patients may be unable to recount specific details regarding this period because they may have remained cognitively impaired for a large portion of this time. It is important to seek out and interview persons who may have witnessed the event.

    a. Prolonged duration of postictal confusion, **amnesia,** or lethargy implicates seizure or another primary central nervous system injury as the precipitating disorder.

    b. The presence of focal neurologic symptoms or signs point to an inciting neurologic event such as a seizure with residual functional deficit (Todd's paralysis) or ischemic injury.

      c. Facial **pallor** points to syncope, and facial **plethora** is more suggestive of seizure.

      d. Diffuse **muscle soreness** suggests seizure activity.

  4. Medical history

    a. Comorbid disorders

      (1) A variety of **cardiovascular disorders** are risk factors for syncope. Structural heart diseases such as coronary artery disease, congestive heart failure, hypertrophic obstructive cardiomyopathy, and valvular disorders predispose patients to syncope. Ventricular tachycardia, atrial fibrillation, and bradycardia are examples of dysrhythmias that may result in transient loss of consciousness. Chronic hypertension can induce left ventricular systolic and diastolic dysfunction, impair cerebrovascular autoregulation, and expose patients to hypotensive therapy.

      (2) A variety of **neurologic disorders** predispose patients to syncope or seizure. Primary or metastatic neoplasia and scars from previous trauma, ischemic injury, or infection provide foci for seizures. Peripheral or autonomic neuropathy induced by diabetes mellitus, alcohol abuse, vitamin B_{12} deficiency or other metabolic disorders can cause orthostatic hypotension. Preexisting cerebrovascular disease can make patients more susceptible to relatively minor reductions in cerebral perfusion. Various movement disorders, such as Parkinson's disease, are associated with a higher incidence of orthostatic hypotension and nonsyncopal falls.

      (3) Anxiety disorders and depression are examples of **psychiatric illnesses** that have been linked to syncope.

    b. A large number of **medications** can induce syncope. **Antihypertensive** drugs and **psychotropic** medications are the most risk prone. The former can impair cerebral perfusion by two primary mechanisms, either reducing cardiac output or lowering peripheral vascular resistance. Psychotropic medications can induce orthostatic hypotension and, in the case of the tricyclic antidepressants, predispose patients to a variety of cardiac rhythm disturbances.

    c. A brief **gynecologic history** should be elicited to identify risk factors for pregnancy, particularly in ectopic locations. Pregnant patients are at increased risk of syncope due to orthostatic hypotension and vasovagal reactions. Moreover, a ruptured ectopic pregnancy occasionally manifests with syncope. The recent occurrence of sexual intercourse without the use of contraception, the presence of amenorrhea, and any symptoms of pregnancy should be elicited.

B. Physical examination

  1. Vital signs should be accurately assessed. For accurate detection of the presence of orthostatic hypotension, the supine blood pressure should be obtained after prolonged recumbency and the standing blood pressure measured after the patient has been erect for a minimum of 2 minutes. Blood pressure readings in the sitting position are not accurate in the detection of postural hypotension. Orthostatic hypotension has been arbitrarily defined as present if the systolic arterial blood pressure decreases 20 mm Hg or the diastolic pressure 10 mm Hg after the patient moves from a supine to a standing posture.

  2. A detailed **cardiovascular examination** should be performed. Palpation of the carotid arteries may reveal pulsus tardus et parvus (delayed, low-volume carotid pulsation), which occurs with hemodynamically significant aortic stenosis, or pulsus bisferiens (equally intense, biphasic carotid pulsation), which is characteristic of idiopathic subaortic stenosis. The presence of a carotid bruit signifies a high likelihood of diffuse atherosclerotic vascular disease involving the cerebral, coronary, and peripheral vasculature.

    If continuous electrocardiographic (ECG) monitoring is used and cardiac resuscitation equipment is readily available, carotid massage can be performed to detect the presence of carotid sinus supersensitivity. Cardiac examination should be performed to detect evidence of rhythm abnormalities, murmurs suggestive of significant valvular heart disease, or parasternal heaves or gallops characteristic of left ventricular dysfunction. Evidence of a subclavian steal syndrome, such as a supraclavicular bruit or a diminished upper extremity arterial pulsation, should be sought.

3. A screening **neurologic examination** should be pursued to detect postictal cognitive impairment, the presence of focal neurologic defects indicative of either acute neurologic injury or a preexisting substrate for a seizure disorder, peripheral neuropathy that would predispose to orthostatic hypotension, or a movement disorder that would cause nonsyncopal falls.

4. A **digital rectal examination** should be performed to detect evidence of occult or overt gastrointestinal bleeding, such as melena or hematochezia.

C. **Laboratory studies**

1. **Electrocardiography**

   a. A resting **12-lead ECG** is the single most useful test for both prognosis and triage. This is true even though it provides enough information for a diagnosis in only 5% to 10% of cases. It is uncommon for the etiologic rhythm disturbance to be detected on an ECG tracing. However, research suggests that the presence of left axis deviation, left bundle branch block, or left ventricular hypertrophy points to an underlying cardiac cause. These generally are markers of the underlying substrate that can cause ventricular arrhythmia or bradyarrhythmia. Other, less common ECG findings are helpful. Signs of acute right heart strain ($S_1Q_3T_3$ or right bundle branch block pattern) suggest pulmonary embolism.

   b. More sophisticated forms of ECG monitoring frequently are helpful. **Ambulatory electrocardiography** is a moderately sensitive diagnostic tool. This test, however, has limited specificity because certain rhythm disturbances, such as brief pauses, premature atrial and ventricular contractions, and nonsustained ventricular tachycardia, can be detected even when they are not responsible for the syncopal episode. If symptoms occur during monitoring and no ECG abnormalities are detected, a rhythm disturbance is effectively excluded as an etiologic factor. Continuous ambulatory monitoring for more than 24 hours usually is unnecessary. Patient-activated or even subcutaneous loop recorders can be used for patients with recurrent but infrequent symptoms and a high pretest likelihood of a cardiac cause of syncope. Exercise ECG may be used in the uncommon instance when ischemically mediated rhythm disturbances are suspected.

   c. **Echocardiography** can be useful in evaluating ejection fraction and underlying heart disease when suspected clinically.

2. **Serum chemistry.** Determination of serum electrolyte concentrations has limited utility.

   a. If evaluated within an hour of the syncopal event, some patients have a depressed **bicarbonate** level. This can be a clue to a seizure disorder because the transient lactic acidosis generated during a convulsion can cause a lowering of the serum bicarbonate concentration. This generally normalizes within 1 hour.

   b. Elevated **prolactin** levels have been reported in some patients hours after generalized tonic–clonic seizures.

   c. The same is true for **creatine kinase** (CK) levels, although increased serum concentrations also can be caused by injury during a syncopal episode.

   d. Serum **glucose** levels are most valuable at the time of the event, particularly in evaluation of diabetic patients who have recently increased their insulin or oral hypoglycemic therapy or decreased their caloric intake.

3. **Complete blood count.** The main component that is occasionally helpful is the **hemoglobin** level. It is most useful when acute or subacute blood loss or severe anemia is suspected. In the former instances, clinically apparent bleeding usually is present.

4. **Arterial blood gas analysis** can be useful in evaluation of the occasional patient in whom pulmonary embolism is suspected because of the history, physical examination findings, or ECG results.
5. **Electrophysiologic studies.** This sophisticated assessment of the integrity of the cardiac conduction system is a reasonably accurate test. Its true sensitivity, specificity, and predictive values are unclear and often vary with the aggressiveness of the diagnostic protocol and the clinical suspicion of a dysrhythmia. The results are most often abnormal in patients with known heart disease or those with significant abnormalities on a routine ECG. These studies should be pursued when there is high clinical suspicion of life-threatening cardiac rhythm disturbances. They appear particularly useful in the evaluation of elderly persons with organic heart disease, recurrent symptoms, and abnormal findings on noninvasive evaluation.
6. **Tilt-table testing.** The utility of both passive and active tilt-table tests for the diagnosis of vasovagal syncope remains poorly defined. It is only a moderately sensitive and specific test. A positive result is reproducible only 70% of the time. Tilt-table testing also can be used to gauge the effectiveness of therapy. The limited reproducibility of the test and the variable natural history of unexplained syncope reduce its utility in the latter role.
7. **Carotid sinus massage.** Carotid sinus hypersensitivity, a rare cause of syncope, can be detected by means of monitoring changes in blood pressure and heart rate after 5 to 40 seconds of unilateral carotid artery massage. Responses are characterized as cardioinhibitory if asystole lasting 3 seconds or more develops; vasodepressor if systolic arterial blood pressure decreases 50 mm Hg or more without associated changes in heart rate or 30 mm Hg with associated syncope; and mixed when both cardioinhibitory and vasodepressor responses are present. Carotid sinus hypersensitivity occurs in a substantial minority of elderly patients, most of whom have no symptoms. This diagnosis should be made only when the history is strongly suggestive and an abnormal response to carotid sinus massage is elicited.
8. **Radiographic studies.** Routine computed tomography and magnetic resonance imaging of the head have low yields but may be useful in the evaluation of patients who have sustained major head trauma, have a newly diagnosed seizure disorder, or have focal deficits on the neurologic examination. Routine skull radiography, nuclear brain scans, and cerebral angiography are not useful screening tests for patients with syncope.

IV. Differential diagnosis. The differential diagnosis provided in Table 7.3 lists some clues for distinguishing seizure from syncope, as well as vasovagal syncope from cardiac syncope. This can be quite difficult in that patients frequently have unwitnessed events or witnesses are not available at the time of the physician's evaluation. It is also true that there is substantial overlap in the typical signs and symptoms of these disorders. For example, patients with decreased cerebral perfusion may have secondary brief (less than 10 seconds) seizure activity that can be mistaken for a primary seizure even by experienced observers. One of the main differentiating features is the prolonged duration of the postictal state after generalized tonic–clonic seizures. This may last 10 to 15 minutes as opposed to the relatively brief (less than 1 minute) confusional state that can follow syncope from cardiovascular causes.

V. Diagnostic approach
   A. History and physical examination initially provide the etiologic factor in one half to more than two thirds of diagnosed cases. Laboratory testing should be done selectively.
   B. A resting **ECG** should be obtained unless a benign, noncardiac cause of syncope is readily apparent. For patients in whom cardiac causes are suspected, up to 24 hours of ambulatory ECG monitoring is recommended. Loop recording devices are quite useful for selected patients with recurrent but infrequent (every few weeks) symptoms. For very infrequent recurrent syncope, a subcutaneous recording device can be quite helpful. For patients who have marked arrhythmia detected or patients with serious underlying heart disease and unexplained syncope, such as those with known myocardial infarction or left ventricular dysfunction, electrophysiologic studies often are recommended.

Table 7.3 Typical features of vasovagal syncope, cardiac syncope, and seizure

Feature	Vasovagal	Seizure	Cardiac
Onset	Subacute onset Prodromal weakness, nausea, diaphoresis, or visual changes	Sudden onset or brief aura Auditory hallucinations	Sudden onset Chest pain, dyspnea, palpitations, and other cardiac symptoms may be present
Typical milieu or precipitating factor	Fatigue Delayed meals Prolonged standing Crowded enclosed confines Pregnancy Pain or trauma Emotional situation	Spontaneous onset Triggered by flashing light or monotonous sensory stimulation	Often spontaneous onset During or after following exertion Known or suspected structural heart disease
Posture at time of onset	Standing or sitting	Standing, sitting, or supine	Standing, sitting, or supine
Appearance	Pallor Brief tonic–clonic motor activity possible Occasional urinary incontinence	Normal or cyanotic Stertorous respiration Stereotypic motor activity Transient loss of awareness Urinary and fecal incontinence common	Pallor Brief periods of tonic–clonic motor activity possible Urinary incontinence uncommon
Residual	Rapid recovery Reoccurrence with resumption of upright posture possible	Delayed recovery Postictal cognitive impairment Todd's paralysis	Rapid or briefly delayed recovery If prolonged hypoxia, evidence of central nervous system injury present Symptoms of cardiac dysfunction

C. Tilt-table testing can be helpful to patients with unexplained syncope, particularly when a cardiac cause is not suspected. However, therapy based on tilt-table testing itself is not especially reliable. This is because the test–retest reliability of tilt testing is not high and because many patients improve over time without therapy (or with placebo). Tilt-table testing should be reserved for patients with unexplained syncope who are older, have recurrent events, or have suffered serious injury with their episodes.

D. Computed tomography and magnetic resonance imaging are of little value in most evaluations for syncope unless a true seizure disorder or structural disease of the central nervous system is suspected.

VI. Referral. When a seizure disorder is suspected, **neurologic consultation** generally is appropriate. When a potentially life-threatening arrhythmia is strongly suspected or discovered, referral to a **cardiologist,** particularly one with advanced training in arrhythmia, is helpful. Referral to a **psychiatrist** may be indicated if the syncope is related to a psychiatric illness.

Recommended Readings

Benditt DG, Peterson M, Lurie KG, et al. Cardiac pacing for the prevention of recurrent vasovagal syncope. *Ann Intern Med* 1995;122:204–209.

Brignole M, Menozzi C, Gianfranchi L, et al. A controlled trial of acute and long-term medical therapy in tilt-induced neurally mediated syncope. *Am J Cardiol* 1992;70:339–342.

Day SC, Cook EF, Funkenstein J, et al. Evaluation and outcome of emergency room patients with transient loss of consciousness. *Am J Med* 1982;73:15–23.

Fenton AM, Hammill SC, Rea RF, et al. Vasovagal syncope. *Ann Intern Med* 2000;9:714–725.

Grubb BP, Kosinski D. Dysautonomic and reflex syncope syndromes. *Cardiol Clin* 1997;15: 257–268.

Grubb BP, Temesy-Armos P, Hahn H, et al. Utility of upright tilt-table testing in the evaluation and management of syncope of unknown origin. *Am J Med* 1991;90:6–10.

Hanlon JT, Linzer M, MacMillan JP, et al. Syncope and presyncope associated with probable adverse drug reactions. *Arch Intern Med* 1990;150:2309–2312.

Kapoor W, Peterson J, Karpf M. A rapid identification of low-risk patients with syncope: implications regarding hospitalization and cost. *Clin Res* 1986;34:823A.

Kapoor W, Peterson J, Wieand S, et al. Predictors of sudden death in patients with syncope. *Clin Res* 1985;33:255A.

Kapoor WN. Syncope. *N Engl J Med* 2000;25:1856–1862.

Kapoor WN, Karpf M, Wieand S, et al. A prospective evaluation of syncope in patients presenting to the emergency department. *N Engl J Med* 1983;309:197–204.

Krahn AD, Yee R, Klein GJ, et al. Syncope: experience with the implantable loop recorder. *ACC Curr J Rev* 1999;8:80–84.

Kroenke MK. Orthostatic hypotension. *West J Med* 1985;143:253–255.

Krol RB, Morady F, Flaker GC, et al. Electrophysiologic testing in patients with unexplained syncope: clinical and noninvasive predictors of outcome. *J Am Coll Cardiol* 1987;10:358–363.

Kuller L, Cooper M, Perper J. Epidemiology of sudden death. *Arch Intern Med* 1972;129:714.

Lipsitz LA, Wei JY, Rowe JW. Syncope in an elderly, institutionalized population: prevalence, incidence, and associated risks. *Q J Med* 1985;55:45–54.

Martin GJ, Adams SL, Martin HG, et al. Prospective evaluation of syncope in patients presenting to the emergency department. *Ann Emerg Med* 1984;13:499–504.

Middlekauff HR, Stevenson WG, Stevenson LW, et al. Syncope in advanced heart failure: high risk of sudden death regardless of origin of syncope. *J Am Coll Cardiol* 1993;21:110–116.

Murdoch BD. Loss of consciousness in healthy South African men: incidence, causes and relationship to EEG abnormality. *S Afr Med J* 1980;57:771–774.

Stumpf JL, Mitrzyk B. Management of orthostatic hypotension. *Am J Hosp Pharm* 1994;51: 648–660.

Thames MD, Alpert JS, Dalen JE. Syncope in patients with pulmonary embolism. *JAMA* 1977; 23:2509–2511.

Wayne HH. Syncope: physiological considerations and an analysis of the clinical characteristics in 510 patients. *Am J Med* 1961;30:418–438.

Zaidi A, Clough P, Cooper P, et al. Misdiagnosis of epilepsy: many seizure-like attacks have a cardiovascular cause. *J Am Coll Cardiol* 2000;36:181–184.

8. APPROACH TO THE PATIENT WITH GAIT DISTURBANCES AND RECURRENT FALLS

Rodger J. Elble

Gait disturbances and recurrent falls are caused by many neurologic, visual, vestibular, and musculoskeletal illnesses. These illnesses are common in all age groups and are particularly common among older persons. Impaired locomotion is a source of disability for approximately 15% of persons older than 65 years, rivaling dementia as the leading form of neurologic impairment. Each year, approximately 250,000 elderly Americans sustain hip fractures and 7,000 die as a result of falls, and the estimated annual expense of this problem is $7.2 billion. The number of hip fractures and the expense will double by the year 2040 because of an exponential increase in the number of older Americans.

  I. **Pathophysiology.** Successful locomotion requires the integrated control of posture and movement.
    A. **Postural control** is necessary for static and dynamic stability during stance and locomotion. Somatic, visual, and vestibular sensory information is used in complex feedback (reflex) pathways that enable the nervous system to respond to altered stability. These sensory inputs are also combined with experience to adjust the pattern of stance or locomotion in anticipation of threatened stability. This anticipatory or feedforward control of movement is critically important because reflex responses are too slow and inaccurate for normal locomotion. Altered sensorium and impaired cognition impede feedforward modifications of posture and movement.
    B. **Locomotion.** The basic locomotor rhythm emerges from spinal neuronal networks that interact directly with several brainstem nuclei and the cerebellum (Fig. 8.1).
      1. The **midbrain locomotor region** of the dorsolateral midbrain contains a heterogeneous group of neurons that connect with the basal ganglia and with raphe and reticular nuclei in the caudal pons and rostral medulla. The midbrain locomotor region and its connections play a critical role in the initiation of gait and control of posture.
      2. The **cerebellum** interacts with pontomedullary reticular nuclei, the red nucleus and the vestibular nuclei in the coordination of posture and rhythmic limb motion. The cerebellum receives input from the spinal locomotor network, from peripheral somatosensory, vestibular and visual pathways, and from cerebral cortex by way of the pontine, olivary and other brainstem nuclei. These connections enable the cerebellum to play a pivotal role in the feedback and feedforward control of posture and movement.
      3. The reticulospinal and vestibulospinal pathways in the **ventral spinal cord** are necessary for rudimentary control of the spinal networks. The corticospinal pathways are needed for flexible, adaptive control, and this "highest level control" is accomplished through rich cortical connections with the basal ganglia, thalamus, and cerebellum. Thus the nervous system can modify posture and locomotion as dictated by environmental constraints, body mechanics, and personal desires.
 II. **Etiology**
    A. **Gait disturbances.** A disturbance of locomotion can occur at any level of the neuraxis. Gait disturbances are caused by any disease affecting the frontal and parietal lobes, basal ganglia, thalamus, brainstem motor nuclei, cerebellum, spinal cord, peripheral nerves, eyes, labyrinth, and musculoskeletal system. The causes of locomotor impairment are myriad. The list in Table 8.1 is not exhaustive, and multiple coexistent etiologic factors are common, particularly among older persons. Neurologic disturbances commonly lead to secondary skeletal deformities, muscle deconditioning, and cardiopulmonary deconditioning, which cause further impairment of locomotion.
    B. **Causes of recurrent falls.** Environmental hazards and errors in judgment are responsible for 35% to 50% of falls in some studies, but underlying neurologic,

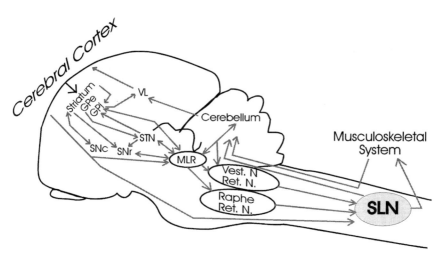

FIG. 8.1 Schematic of the principal neural pathways of locomotor control. *GPe* and *GPi,* globus pallidus externa and interna; *VL,* ventrolateral thalamus; *SNc* and *SNr,* substantia nigra pars compacta and reticulata; *STN,* subthalamus; *MLR,* midbrain locomotor region; *Vest. N.,* lateral vestibular nucleus; *Ret. N.,* pontomedullary reticular nuclei; *SLN,* spinal locomotor network (central pattern generator).

visual, or vestibular disease is present in most patients (Table 8.1). Most older persons who fall are impaired by previous stroke, Parkinson's disease, severe arthritis, orthostatic hypotension, dementia (confusion), poor vision, or vestibular disease. Medications are also a common contributing factor or primary cause.

III. Clinical manifestations. The examination of gait is useful in neurologic diagnosis and functional assessment. However, many patterns of abnormal walking provide only rough indications of the site of the pathologic process (Table 8.2) and must always be interpreted in the context of other neurologic signs. The parts of the nervous system involved in locomotion are widely distributed and highly integrated (Fig. 8.1), so lesions in one area can mimic damage to another. For example, damage to the frontal lobes, thalami, or cerebellum can produce similar ataxia of gait with poor balance and uncoordinated extremity motion.

   A. Features of normal walking. The gait cycle is defined as the time between successive heel–floor contacts with the same foot (Fig. 8.2). One gait cycle consists of two steps (one stride). From right heel–floor contact to left toe-off is a period of double-limb support, which lasts approximately 10% of the total gait cycle. This phase of the cycle is followed by the left swing phase, which is simultaneous with and equal to the right single-limb support phase. The time from left heel–floor contact to right toe-off constitutes the second of two double-limb support phases in a gait cycle and is followed by the right swing phase and left single-limb support phase.

      1. Stride length (length of two successive steps) and cadence (steps per minute) determine the velocity of walking (stride length × cadence ÷ 2). The magnitudes of arm swing, toe–floor clearance, and hip and knee rotations are proportional to stride length and velocity, whereas the percentage time in double-limb support increases with reductions in gait velocity.

      2. The total-body center of mass oscillates vertically at a frequency equal to the cadence and horizontally at one-half the cadence. During a gait cycle, the two maxima in vertical oscillation occur in the middle of right and left single-limb support, and the two minima occur in the middle of the two phases of double-limb support. The left- and right-most horizontal excursions of the center of gravity occur at the times of mid-left and -right single-limb support.

Table 8.1 Causes of gait disturbances

Vascular disease
   Stroke
   Binswanger's disease
   Collagen vascular disease
Visual and vestibular disturbances
Degenerative and hereditary movement disorders
   Basal ganglia (e.g., Parkinson's disease, progressive supranuclear palsy, multiple system
      atrophy, Huntington's disease)
   Hereditary ataxia
   Generalized dystonia (dystonia musculorum deformans, dopa-sensitive dystonia)
   Hereditary spastic paraparesis
   Amyotrophic lateral sclerosis
Cognitive disturbances
   Dementia (e.g., Alzheimer's disease, diffuse Lewy body dementia, normal pressure
      hydrocephalus)
   Depression
   Acute confusional state
Metabolic and toxic disorders
   Vitamin B_{12} or thiamine deficiency
   Thyroid disorder
   Ethanol
   Organic solvents
   Medications (neuroleptics, anticonvulsants, sedative–hypnotics, lithium,
      metoclopramide)
Skeletal disease
   Spinal and pelvic deformities
   Hip, knee, and ankle arthropathy
   Foot disorder (e.g., flatfoot, clubfoot)
Cervical spondylosis and other compressive myelopathies
Trauma
   Subacute and chronic subdural hematoma
   Posttraumatic positional vertigo
   Bilateral frontal lobe or brainstem contusions
   Spinal cord trauma and posttraumatic syringomyelia
Neoplasms
   Adults: frontal lobe (e.g., parasagittal), cerebellopontine angle, or spinal tumor
   Children: brainstem, cerebellar, or spinal tumor
   Carcinomatous meningitis causing hydrocephalus
   Paraneoplastic disease
Multiple sclerosis
   Spastic, hemiparetic, or ataxic gait
Acute cerebellar ataxia of childhood
Infectious disease
   Creutzfeldt–Jakob disease causing ataxia
   Fungal and tuberculous meningitis causing hydrocephalus
Neuromuscular (acquired and hereditary)
   Peripheral polyneuropathy
   Inflammatory myopathy
   Drug-induced myopathy
   Muscular dystrophy
   Congenital myopathy
   Muscular deconditioning
   Spinal muscular atrophy

Table 8.1 *(continued)*

Cerebral palsy
Spastic diplegia
Spastic quadriplegia
Spastic hemiparesis
Choreoathetosis
Ataxia (rare)

Congenital malformations
Cerebellar dysgenesis
Dandy–Walker syndrome ·
Arnold–Chiari malformation
Syringomyelia
Meningomyelocele
Aqueductal stenosis

These vertical and horizontal excursions of the center of mass are optimized in such a way that the center of mass (body) moves forward with the least amount of expended energy. Consequently, most gait disturbances increase expended energy.

B. Normal development of walking. Most children walk independently by 15 months, and a fairly mature pattern of lower limb movement is achieved 3 months after walking begins. Maturation of gait and balance probably continues throughout childhood, but most of this maturation is accomplished by 3 or 4 years of age. At this age, most children have lost their lordotic posture and are capable of walking on narrow beams and standing with feet together and eyes closed. Failure to walk by 18 months should be investigated systematically with regard to the following four systems.

1. **Sensory systems and postural control.** Somatosensory, visual, and vestibular reflexes are sufficient for stable stance and walking by 15 months. Even so, toddlers walk with a wide base and abducted arms to achieve adequate balance. Independent walking is delayed in blind children, only 50% walking by 24 months.

2. **Rhythmic pattern generation and extremity coordination.** Evidence of spinal rhythmic pattern generation reminiscent of walking is detectable at birth with the stepping reflex (infant stepping). By 9 to 12 months, subcortical and cerebellar control of the spinal pattern generator and postural control are sufficient for supported walking. Unassisted walking is initially accomplished with exaggerated hip flexion during the swing phase and initiation of the support phase with the toes or flat foot, instead of the heel.

3. **Musculoskeletal strength and development.** Muscle weakness, joint contractures, and maldevelopment of the limbs or spine can delay or prevent independent walking. These problems also can exist with central nervous system disease, such as cerebral palsy.

4. **Highest-level adaptive and motivational systems (see III.D.1.).** Frontal lobe and basal ganglia disease can impede postural control and locomotion in ways evident only during the testing of stance and gait. Children and adults with profound disturbances of stance and gait can have relatively normal findings at bedside examinations of strength, tone, coordination, and sensation. These patients often have impaired cognitive development.

C. Abnormal patterns of walking. Descriptions of abnormal gaits have generated a fairly large and redundant terminology, which is summarized in Table 8.2. The characteristics of an abnormal gait generally are a mixture of primary abnormalities (direct effects of the underlying pathologic condition), secondary musculoskeletal changes, and compensatory changes. All must be considered when deciphering a patient's gait.

(text continues on page 91)

Table 8.2 Clinical manifestations and abbreviated differential diagnosis of gait disturbances

Abnormal gait or sign	Related term	Site of pathologic lesion	Clinical condition
Cautious gait	Senile gait	Any part of the central or peripheral nervous system involved in locomotion and higher cortical function	Mild neurologic or musculoskeletal disease Sensory disturbance
Dysequilibrium	Frontal ataxia Frontal dysequilibrium Thalamic ataxia Subcortical dysequilibrium Cerebellar ataxia Sensory ataxia	Frontal lobes Ventrolateral thalamus Brainstem motor nuclei Midline cerebellum and fastigial nucleus Multiple involvement of peripheral visual, vestibular, and somato-sensory systems Spinal cord	Stroke Binswanger's disease NPH PSP MSA Hereditary ataxia Multiple sensory deficit Toxic–metabolic disorders
Start hesitation and freezing	Gait ignition failure Magnetic gait Frozen gait Akinetic gait Slipping clutch syndrome	Frontal lobes Basal ganglia Dorsolateral midbrain locomotor region	Binswanger's disease NPH Frontal lobe (parasagittal) mass Parkinson's disease PSP
Short, shuffling steps and en bloc turning with or without festination	Parkinsonian gait Lower-half parkinsonism Marche á petits pas Gait apraxia Magnetic gait	Basal ganglia Frontal lobes	Parkinson's disease Binswanger's disease PSP MSA (striatonigral degeneration)
Choreic gait	Hyperkinetic gait	Basal ganglia	Huntington's disease Sydenham's chorea Cerebral palsy Drug toxicity

Gait	Pattern	Site	Causes
Dystonic gait	—	Basal ganglia	Torsion dystonia Dopa-sensitive dystonia Cerebral palsy Drug toxicity
Hemiparetic gait	Hemiplegic gait Circumducting gait	Supraspinal pyramidal tract lesion	Stroke, tumor, abscess, trauma, demyelination, or other focal lesion
Spastic gait	Scissoring gait Paralegic gait	Thoracic or cervical spinal cord damage	Compressive and intrinsic spinal cord disease
Spastic diplegic gait	Crouch gait Scissoring gait	Bilateral perinatal frontal lobe damage	Cerebral palsy
Ataxic gait	Sensory ataxia Spinal ataxia Cerebellar ataxia Reeling, lurching gait	Peripheral nerves Dorsal spinal columns and spinocerebellar pathways Cerebellum Brainstem motor nuclei Spinal cord	Large-fiber sensory neuropathy Tabes dorsalis Pernicious anemia Hereditary ataxia PSP MSA (OPCA variant) Alcoholic cerebellar degeneration Drug toxicity
Toe walking	—	Bilateral pyramidal tract disease Hip girdle weakness Tight heel cords Ankle contractures	Cerebral palsy Duchenne muscular dystrophy Idiosyncratic
Myopathic gait	Lordotic-waddling gait Waddling gait	Hip girdle weakness	Acquired, congenital and hereditary myopathies
Steppage gait	Bilateral foot drop	Bilateral weakness of muscles innervated by the peroneal nerves	Hereditary or acquired distal motor polyneuropathy Bilateral peroneal neuropathy

continued

Table 8.2 (continued)

Abnormal gait or sign	Related term	Site of pathologic lesion	Clinical condition
Ataxic gait	Sensory ataxia Spinal ataxia Cerebellar ataxia Reeling, lurching gait	Peripheral nerves Dorsal spinal columns and spinocerebellar pathways Cerebellum Brainstem motor nuclei Spinal cord	Large-fiber sensory neuropathy Tabes dorsalis Pernicious anemia Hereditary ataxia PSP MSA (OPCA variant) Alcoholic cerebellar degeneration Drug toxicity
Antalgic gait	Hyperesthetic gait Limping gait	Foot, spine, pelvis, or lower extremity	Lumbar radiculopathy Skeletal pathologic lesion Foot deformity Tarsal tunnel syndrome Morton neuralgia
Hysterical gait	Psychiatric astasia–abasia	—	Somatoform disorder Affective disorder with conversion reaction Factitious disorder, malingering

NPH, normal pressure hydrocephalus; PSP, progressive supranuclear palsy; MSA, multisystem atrophy; OPCA, olivopontocerebellar atrophy.

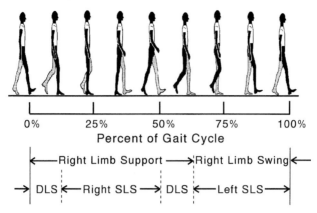

FIG. 8.2 Phases of the normal gait cycle, expressed as percentage of total stride. *DLS,* double limb support; *SLS,* single limb support.

1. **Cautious gait** is a slow, guarded, or restrained pattern of walking that resembles someone walking on a slippery surface or in a threatening environment. There is stooped posture, reduced arm swing, increased time with both feet on the floor (double-limb support), loss of the normal heel–toe sequence of foot–floor contact during stance phase, slightly widened base, and reduced hip and knee rotations, all of which are commensurate with the patient's reduced stride and gait velocity. This pattern of walking is a nonspecific compensatory response produced by most causes of impaired locomotion. The features of cautious gait frequently dominate the clinical signs and symptoms of patients with mild neurologic impairment and provide the clinician with little clue to the underlying pathologic process. **Senile gait** is a cautious gait in an older person.

2. **Dysequilibrium** is a disturbance of postural control and balance. Severe dysequilibrium produces a staggering, wide-based gait, particularly when the disturbance is acute. Mild or chronic dysequilibrium often is associated with a predominantly slow, cautious gait. Sudden or rapid movements (e.g., standing, turning, bending, and running) are avoided because they are most destabilizing. Dysequilibrium can result from damage at any level of the neuraxis (Fig. 8.1).

   a. **Sensory dysequilibrium** occurs when there is a loss or conflict among vestibular, somatosensory, and visual feedback caused by disturbances of primary sensory pathways. Disabling dysequilibrium generally does not persist unless at least two sensory modalities are impaired or unless there is concomitant impairment of the central nervous system. A cautious pattern of walking is typical among patients with isolated chronic peripheral visual, vestibular, or somatosensory deficits.

      (1) **Vestibular dysequilibrium** is associated with vertigo when the condition is acute.

      (2) **Somatosensory dysequilibrium** is most evident when the eyes are closed.

      (3) **Visual dysequilibrium** occurs when movement of the surroundings produces an illusion of body movement or when peripheral vision is reduced or distorted (e.g., with new glasses).

   b. **Dysequilibrium due to lesions in the central nervous system** can cause profound loss of balance despite normal sensory feedback.

      (1) **Frontal dysequilibrium.** Frontal lobe damage can cause profound dysequilibrium due to inappropriate postural synergies. Patients

lean the wrong direction in such a way that stability is impeded. For example, patients may lean backward when being helped from a chair, or they may lean away from the pivot foot when attempting to turn. Bilateral frontal damage is most disabling.

    (2) Subcortical dysequilibrium occurs with lesions in the basal ganglia, ventrolateral thalamus, or dorsolateral midbrain (midbrain locomotor region; Fig. 8.1). Patients tend to fall backward and to the side opposite the lesion. With ischemic lesions, the dysequilibrium is temporary unless the damage is bilateral. Progressive supranuclear palsy produces bilateral destruction of these sites, so early impairment of balance is common in this disorder.

    (3) Vestibulocerebellar dysequilibrium occurs with damage to the vestibulocerebellum and its brainstem connections. Patients tend to fall toward the side of the cerebellar lesion. Damage to the vestibular nucleus can produce a sensation that the environment is tilted and that the body is being pulled toward the side of the lesion.

3. **Start hesitation and freezing** are signs of akinesia. Patients move their extremities relatively normally while seated or recumbent, but their feet appear to stick to the floor while walking. Gait is often initiated with a few delayed, aborted, shuffling steps or is tricked into action by stepping over a self-imposed obstacle (e.g., the handle of an inverted cane) or by stepping onto a targeted spot on the floor. These tricks work best for patients with akinesia due to basal ganglia disease (e.g., Parkinson's disease and progressive supranuclear palsy). Environmental distractions and obstacles exacerbate start hesitation and elicit abrupt cessation of movement, called *freezing* (e.g., at a doorway).

4. **Short shuffling steps with en bloc turning** are common among patients with damage to the frontal lobes and basal ganglia. A greater reduction in arm swing than reduction in stride is characteristic of **Parkinson's disease**. Arm swing is increased in relation to the reduced stride of **lower-half parkinsonism**, which is exhibited by patients with multiple small infarcts and subcortical white matter degeneration in the basal ganglia and frontal lobes. **Festination of gait** can occur in which the patient's forward lean increases as walking proceeds, and the steps become increasingly short and rapid. Festination is more common in idiopathic Parkinson disease than in other causes of parkinsonism, and festination is commonly associated with start hesitation and freezing.

5. **Choreic gait** consists of extremity movements and postural shifts interrupted by sudden, variable flinging or dance-like movements (chorea) of the extremities and torso. Gait appears bizarre and hazardous. Huntington's disease is the most common etiologic factor. Suppression of chorea with neuroleptic medications (e.g., haloperidol) produces a disappointing improvement in gait when there are concomitant disturbances in postural control (subcortical dysequilibrium).

6. **Dystonic gait** is a variable pattern of walking in which extremity movements and postural shifts are interrupted by tonic (sometimes phasic) co-contractions of antagonistic muscles in the limbs or torso. The limbs, trunk, and neck may be contorted into bizarre postures that depend on the relative strengths of muscle contraction. Dystonia can be focal or generalized and can emerge during a particular phase of the gait cycle (e.g., the swing phase). In addition to the conditions listed in Table 8.2, dystonia occasionally complicates the shuffling gait of Parkinson's disease.

7. **Hemiparetic gait** varies with the magnitude and distribution of weakness and spasticity. Reduced arm swing with flexor or dangling arm posture occurs in combination with a hyperextended lower extremity. Reduced hip and knee flexion and tonic ankle plantar flexion make foot–floor clearance during the swing phase of gait impossible unless the patient leans away from the hemiparetic limb and swings the spastic lower extremity outward and forward (**circumduction**). The toes scuff the floor, and the swing phase

ends with the ball of the foot hitting the floor, instead of a normal heel strike. Patients with little spasticity and greater hip and knee mobility clear the floor during swing phase with increased hip flexion.

8. **Spastic (paraplegic) gait** varies with the magnitude and distribution of weakness and spasticity in the lower extremities and also varies with the degree of sensory loss (see **III.C.10.d.**). Movement of the upper extremities depends on the level of the spinal cord lesion. Upper extremity movement may be increased relative to lower extremity movement if the lesion is below the cervical cord. The upper extremities may dangle or exhibit flexor posturing in patients with high cervical lesions. Adduction or abduction of the upper extremities can occur. Relatively pure bilateral pyramidal tract dysfunction produces stiff, labored, scissoring movements of the hyperextended lower extremities, which are tightly adducted.

9. **Spastic diplegic gait** occurs among some patients with cerebral palsy and is caused by perinatal bilateral corticospinal tract damage. The knees and hips are excessively flexed during the gait cycle, and the tightly adducted hips cause the lower extremities to move in a scissoring, shuffling manner. The upper extremities and speech (pseudobulbar palsy) are usually much less affected than are the lower extremities, in contrast to bilateral hemiparesis and prominent pseudobulbar palsy in an adult. There is variable flexor posturing of the upper extremities and abduction of the arms.

10. **Ataxic gait**
    a. **Cerebellar ataxia** occurs among patients with damage to the cerebellum or to the areas of the brainstem, ventrolateral thalamus, and frontal lobes that interact with the cerebellum. Gait is wide based, erratic, and reeling. Upper and lower limb movements are uncoordinated, and there is considerable stride-to-stride variability. Abnormal postural sway during quiet stance is present with eyes open and closed. Damage to the midline cerebellum or fastigial nucleus produces a predominantly truncal disturbance, as in the rostral vermis degeneration of chronic alcoholism. Unilateral hemispheric lesions produce ipsilateral ataxia and falling toward the lesion.
    b. **Thalamic ataxia.** Lesions in the ventrolateral thalamus can produce ataxia of the contralateral extremities and a tendency to fall away from the lesion or backward (subcortical dysequilibrium).
    c. **Somatosensory ataxia** is exhibited by patients with large-fiber sensory polyneuropathy or posterior spinal column disease, with or without spinocerebellar tract damage. Somatosensory ataxia consists of wide-based, deliberate steps and postural dysequilibrium. Patients compensate for their loss of proprioception by watching their feet while walking. Postural sway is modest during quiet stance but increases markedly with eyes closed, because of the loss of proprioception (Romberg sign). Thus gait is more impaired in the dark or when vision is otherwise hindered. Somatosensory ataxia and steppage gait frequently coexist in patients with large-fiber sensorimotor polyneuropathy and in patients with degenerative disease that affects both the spinal cord and peripheral nerves (e.g., tabes dorsalis, vitamin B_{12} deficiency, Friedreich's ataxia, and hereditary dysmyelinating diseases).
    d. **Spinal ataxia.** Disease of the spinal cord can cause somatosensory ataxia by affecting the dorsal columns. Lesions in the anterior columns produce an uncoordinated, dysrhythmic gait owing to impairment of the vestibulospinal and reticulospinal tracts. Furthermore, the ventral spinocerebellar tract is positioned in the anterolateral surface of the cord and provides feedback from the spinal locomotor network to the cerebellum. Thus ataxia and dysequilibrium commonly coexist with spasticity in patients with spinal cord lesions and can dominate the clinical picture in some cases.

11. **Gait disturbances resulting from neuromuscular weakness**
    a. **Waddling gait** is produced by muscle weakness in the hip girdle or, less commonly, by bilateral hip dislocations. Gait is wide based and short

stepped. Increased lateral shoulder sway occurs during the stance phase in compensation for weakness of the gluteus medius muscle. Increased arm abduction also may occur. Associated weakness in the paraspinal muscles produces exaggerated lumbar lordosis.

b. **Steppage gait** is produced by distal symmetric motor polyneuropathy or bilateral peroneal neuropathy. Weakness of the ankle dorsiflexors interferes with foot–floor clearance during the swing phase of gait, so a compensatory increase in hip and knee flexion is necessary to raise the foot higher. Steps are high and short. The foot commonly slaps the floor at the end of swing phase. With polyneuropathy there is often coexistent weakness of ankle plantar flexion, which limits propulsion of the body at the end of the support phase.

12. **Antalgic gait.** Stance and gait are modified to reduce pain. Restricted (guarded) lower extremity and pelvic rotation occurs in locations dictated by the origin of pain. Limping is common.

13. **Hysterical gait.** Psychiatric gait disturbances are bizarre and variable. Patients frequently lean, lurch, and gyrate in a manner that requires good balance and coordination. Distracting the patient's attention or making the locomotor task more difficult tends to improve gait. For example, gait and stability increase when finger-to-nose testing is executed while the patient attempts to walk or stand. Gait also may improve when patients walk on their heels or toes. Tandem gait may initially seem impossible, but this task is frequently accomplished when attention is distracted with simultaneous performance of finger-to-nose testing, a difficult cognitive task (e.g., reciting the months of the year backward), or both. *Be careful when making this diagnosis.* Dystonic gaits, choreatic gaits, and the gait disturbances of multiple sclerosis can be so bizarre that an erroneous diagnosis of psychiatric disease is made.

D. **Systems classification of gait disorders.** The clinical lexicon in **III.C.** lends little to the systematic evaluation of impaired mobility. Many experts consequently have emphasized a systems approach to gait analysis and classification. Most systems classification schemes borrow heavily from the classic hierarchical view of motor control described by Nutt et al., which is not entirely correct but is clinically useful because it encourages the clinician to consider the entire neuraxis and neuromuscular system in deciphering a patient's gait. Thus gait disorders can be roughly classified as emerging from the highest, middle, or lowest levels of motor control.

1. **Highest-level gait disorders** are caused by pathologic processes in the cortical–basal ganglia–thalamocortical pathways. Highest-level gait disturbances therefore are common in all forms of parkinsonism and most dementing illnesses. Cortical–basal ganglia–thalamocortical circuits play an important role in selecting desired postures, movements, and behaviors while suppressing undesired postures, movements, and behaviors. Damage to these circuits impedes adaptation gait to varying environmental and emotional circumstances. Highest-level gait disturbances are particularly severe when both sides of the brain are affected. The characteristics of gait become increasingly bizarre and maladaptive as the underlying disease progresses. The gait disturbance often is most evident in complex, unfamiliar environments and during transitional movements from one steady-state posture or movement to another (e.g., starting, stopping, standing up, sitting down, and turning). Examination while the patient is seated or recumbent may provide little clue to the characteristics and severity of impaired walking.

a. **Clinical characteristics.** Highest-level gait disorders have one or more of the following characteristics.

(1) Absent or inappropriate corrective actions to postural perturbation. Patients "fall like a log" or make little attempt to rescue themselves. Corrective reactions may consist of inappropriate limb movement or postural reactions.

(2) Inappropriate or bizarre foot placement, postural synergy, and interaction with the environment (e.g., crossing the lower limbs while

walking or turning; leaning toward the pivot foot when turning or leaning backward when attempting to rise from a chair or bed).

(3) Variable performance, influenced greatly by the environment and emotion. This variability can baffle caregivers unaware of this phenomenon.

(4) Hesitation and freezing, often when seemingly insignificant environmental objects or thresholds are encountered (e.g., a doorway)

b. **Clinical subtypes.** Patients with cortical–basal ganglia–thalamocortical abnormalities can have relatively pure subcortical dysequilibrium, frontal dysequilibrium, or freezing gait (gait ignition failure), but most patients have signs of all three conditions (frontal gait disorder).

2. Lowest- and middle-level gait disorders differ from highest-level gait disorders in that they cause little or no change with alterations in environment, emotion, or cognition. The clinical characteristics of lowest- and middle-level gait disorders usually are predictable from the neurologic or musculoskeletal deficits revealed during an examination while the patient is seated or recumbent. These characteristics do not change considerably during transitional movements from one steady-state posture or movement to another. Compensatory changes in gait are not inappropriate or maladaptive, although they can be limited by the underlying neurologic or musculoskeletal deficit.

a. **Middle-level gait disorders** are caused by ascending or descending sensorimotor tract lesions, cerebellar ataxia, bradykinesia, hyperkinesia, and dystonia. Clinical subtypes are hemiparetic gait, spastic (paraplegic) gait, choreic gait, dystonic gait, spinal ataxia, and cerebellar ataxia.

b. **Lowest-level gait disorders** are caused by disease of the muscles, peripheral nerves, skeleton, peripheral vestibular system, and anterior visual pathway. Also included are the effects of secondary muscle deconditioning (type II atrophy), limb contracture, spinal ankylosis, and reduced pelvic mobility, which are common among older persons.

IV. **Evaluation**

A. **History** is critical in determining a specific cause and in identifying coexistent illnesses that can adversely affect the patient's performance (e.g., cardiopulmonary disease, arthritis, glaucoma, macular degeneration, painful feet).

1. **Functional disability** is largely determined with a careful history. The frequency and circumstances of falls and the ability to perform various activities of daily living (dressing, bathing, climbing stairs, and getting in and out of bed and chairs) are important measures of disability.

2. **Associated symptoms** such as rest tremor (Parkinson's disease), oscillopsia, and vertigo (vestibular or labyrinthine disease), urinary incontinence (frontal lobe lesions, hydrocephalus, myelopathy), dementia, numb clumsy hands (high cervical cord lesion causing loss of dexterity, fine touch, vibration sensation, and proprioception), dysarthria and dysphagia (supraspinal lesion), and muscle wasting (peripheral neuromuscular disease) are helpful in making a diagnosis.

B. **Physical examination** is essential because abnormal patterns of gait often provide only rough indications of the locus of the pathologic condition (Table 8.2). One must carefully search for more diagnostic or localizing neurologic signs (e.g., rest tremor, pyramidal tract signs) and general physical signs (cardiopulmonary disease, poor visual acuity, musculoskeletal disease). The examination of gait and station is performed with the intent of localizing the lesion and establishing the degree of disability (Table 8.3). Bedside measurements of gait velocity, average step length, and cadence over a 40-foot (12 m) walkway correlate well with all other valid measures of ambulatory ability.

C. **Laboratory studies** are useful mainly in corroborating the diagnosis derived from history and physical examination. A complete blood count and thyroid, renal, and liver function studies are performed in most cases. Measurement of vitamin B_{12} level is recommended in suspected subacute combined degeneration of the spinal cord and for elderly patients with a symmetric gait disturbance and cognitive or psychiatric symptoms. Radiologic studies are performed as needed: radiography of the hips, spine, and extremities; myelography; computed tomography

Table 8.3 Performance-oriented examination of locomotion

Static posture
  Curvature of spine
  Head position
  Pelvic tilt
  Flexion of knees and hips
  Stance base

Postural control and balance
  Romberg test
  Nudging or pulling on the upper torso
  Bending over
  Reaching while standing

Walking
  Sitting and rising from a chair
  Starting, stopping, and turning
  Coordination and amplitude of upper and lower limb movements
  Step length, width, rhythmicity, and symmetry; gait velocity
  Foot–floor clearance and contact
  Walking path
  Walking on heels and toes
  Tandem walking

---

or magnetic resonance imaging of the head and spine. Electromyography and nerve conduction studies are helpful when neuromuscular disease is suspected. Eye movement recordings can be helpful in identifying subtle abnormalities and in differentiating Parkinson's disease from other parkinsonian syndromes (e.g., progressive supranuclear palsy). Quantitative vestibular testing (electronystagmography) occasionally reveals vestibular dysfunction in patients with undiagnosed dysequilibrium. Quantitative posturography and quantitative motion analysis with computed photogrammetric methods do not have an established role in the evaluation of most patients.

  V. Differential diagnosis is particularly difficult for illnesses of older persons that produce a roughly symmetric gait disturbance with short, shuffling, hesitant steps (Table 8.4).

  VI. The **diagnostic approach** is to identify the primary cause of gait impairment and all contributing illnesses. Many contributing illnesses are easily overlooked in the evaluation of patients with neurologic gait disturbances: vitamin B_{12} deficiency, hypothyroidism, depression, foot disorder (e.g., flat feet, painful feet, clubfeet), muscle deconditioning, arthritic limbs, spinal deformities, cardiopulmonary disease, sleep apnea, orthostatic hypotension, visual impairment, benign positional vertigo, and medication use (e.g., sedative–hypnotics, antipsychotics, metoclopramide). These contributing illnesses are frequently more treatable than is the primary neurologic illness.

  VII. Criteria for diagnosis are well-established for most illnesses in Table 8.1. Many diagnoses are based largely or entirely on the findings of the history and physical examination. The diagnosis of **idiopathic normal pressure hydrocephalus** (NPH) in older persons is particularly difficult. The clinical triad of gait disturbance, urinary incontinence, and cognitive dysfunction is not specific and also occurs among patients with vascular dementia, chronic subdural hematoma, and degenerative dementia. In NPH, the cognitive dysfunction is a relatively mild and late component of the triad. Radiologic evidence of hydrocephalus is necessary but does not guarantee a beneficial response to ventriculoperitoneal shunting of cerebrospinal fluid (CSF). Improvement in gait after the removal of 30 to 40 mL of CSF by means of lumbar puncture supports the diagnosis but does not occur in all patients. Unfortunately, there is still no fully reliable method for predicting the response to CSF shunting. Improvement is achieved by approximately 50% of patients and sustained improvement by 30%. Complications occur in 20% of cases. Patients with an identifiable cause of hydrocephalus (e.g., aqueductal stenosis, Arnold–Chiari malformation, and previous meningitis or subarachnoid hemorrhage) are more likely to respond than are those with idiopathic hydrocephalus.

Table 8.4 Differentiating the neurologic causes of symmetric geriatric gait disturbances

Clinical feature	Parkinson's disease	Binswanger's disease	NPH	PSP	MSA	Cervical spondylosis
Reduced arm swing	++				+	
Asymmetric parkinsonism	++					
Rest tremor	++				+	
Facial masking	++			+	+	
Prominent response to levodopa	++					
Postural instability and falls during the first year of symptoms		+	+	++	+	+
Speech impairment during the first year of symptoms		+		++	++	
Stepwise progression		++				
Dementia		++	+	++		
Subcortical white matter degeneration and microinfarcts		++				
Urinary dysfunction		+	++		+	+
Definite improvement after removal of 30–40 mL cerebrospinal fluid by means of lumbar puncture			++			
Hydrocephalus (>5.5 cm span across frontal horns)			++			
Supranuclear downward gaze palsy				++		
Ataxia				+	++	
Symptomatic orthostatic hypotension					++	
Numb clumsy hands and Romberg sign						++
Spastic lower limb movement						++
Spondylotic cervical spine and cord compression						++

+, suggestive; ++, highly suggestive.
NPH, normal pressure hydrocephalus; PSP, progressive supranuclear palsy; MSA, multiple system atrophy.

VIII. Referral

    A. Neurologic consultation is recommended whenever the primary physician is uncertain or uncomfortable with the patient's diagnosis or treatment. A second opinion is advisable before performing shunting for a patient with presumed NPH and before operating on a patient with presumed cervical spondylosis. Drug-resistant parkinsonism is strong evidence against the diagnosis of idiopathic Parkinson's disease and is best managed by a specialist in movement disorders.

    B. Physical therapy and occupational therapy should be considered in most cases. An experienced occupational therapist, physical therapist, or visiting nurse can reduce falls and enhance mobility by performing a comprehensive safety evaluation of the patient's home. Handrails, raised toilet seats, adequate lighting, and rubber floor mats often are helpful. Elimination of electrical cords, clutter, and throw rugs throughout the home and repair of uneven floors and cracked sidewalks are additional considerations. Shoes with slippery soles or high heels should be avoided. Properly prescribed walking aids frequently are useful.

    C. Orthopedic and rheumatologic referrals should be considered when skeletal or foot abnormality impedes ambulation.

Recommended Readings

Baloh RW, Vinters HV. White matter lesions and disequilibrium in older people. *Arch Neurol* 1995;52:975–981.

Cummings SR, Rubin SM, Black D. The future of hip fractures in the United States. Numbers, costs and potential effects of postmenopausal estrogen. *Clin Orthop* 1990;252:163–166.

Elble RJ, Higgins C, Hughes L. The syndrome of senile gait. *J Neurol* 1991;239:71–75.

Gage JR. *Gait analysis in cerebral palsy.* New York: Cambridge University Press, 1991.

Garcia-Rill E. The basal ganglia and the locomotor regions. *Brain Res Rev* 1986;11:47–63.

Inman VT, Ralston HJ, Todd F. *Human walking.* Baltimore: Williams & Wilkins, 1981.

Lajoie Y, Teasdale N, Fleury M. Attentional demands for static and dynamic equilibrium. *Exp Brain Res* 1993;97:139–144.

Mori S. Integration of posture and locomotion in acute decerebrate cats and in awake, freely moving cats. *Prog Neurobiol* 1987;28:161–195.

Nutt JG, Marsden CD, Thompson PD. Human walking and higher-level gait disorders, particularly in the elderly. *Neurology* 1993;43:268–279.

Riley DE, Fogt N, Leigh RJ. The syndrome of "pure akinesia" and its relationship to progressive supranuclear palsy. *Neurology* 1994;44:1025–1029.

Smidt GL. Clinics in rehabilitation: gait in rehabilitation. New York: Churchill Livingstone, 1990.

Sudarsky L. Geriatrics: gait disorders in the elderly. *N Engl J Med* 1990;322:1441–1446.

Sutherland DH. *Gait disorders in childhood and adolescence.* Baltimore: Williams & Wilkins, 1984.

Tinetti M. Performance-oriented assessment of mobility problems in elderly patients. *J Am Geriatr Soc* 1986;34:119–126.

Tinetti ME, Speechley M. Prevention of falls among the elderly. *N Engl J Med* 1989;320:1055–1059.

Vanneste JA. Diagnosis and management of normal-pressure hydrocephalus. *J Neurol* 2000;247:5–14.

Wenning GK, Ebersbach G, Verny M, et al. Progression of falls in postmortem-confirmed parkinsonian syndromes. *Mov Disord* 1999;14:947–950.

Whitman GT, DiPatre PL, Lopez IA, et al. Neuropathology in older people with disequilibrium of unknown cause. *Neurology* 1999;53:375–382.

Woollacott MH, Assaiante C, Amblard B. Development of balance and gait control. In: Bronstein AM, Brandt T, Woollacott MH, eds. *Clinical disorders of balance, posture and gait.* London: Arnold, 1996:41–63.

9. APPROACH TO THE PATIENT WITH SLEEP DISORDERS

Mark Eric Dyken
Thoru Yamada

Sleep disorders are common and can lead to, exacerbate, or result from a variety of neurologic diseases. In the clinical setting, a few major issues create confusion when addressing a patient with a sleep disorder. The foundation of an accurate clinical diagnosis is the history. Physicians often fail to ask the basic questions concerning sleep that can aid in diagnosing many sleep disorders. To complicate matters, the field of sleep disorders medicine is in its relative infancy. Many sleep-related problems have only recently been identified, and as such the appropriate approach to certain specific disorders is not clear. In addition, the technologies used to define many sleep phenomena are constantly changing. As a result, the reliability, sensitivity, specificity, and validity of many diagnostic tools are still in question.

I. **General sleep**
   A. **History.** When patients have a pathologic process that occurs during sleep, they usually cannot recall significant elements of that process. Because of this, an attempt always should be made to elicit a sleep history from the person's bed partner, family members, or close associates. A 3-week sleep diary, begun before the initial clinic appointment, can be diagnostic in cases of poor sleep hygiene, irregular sleep–wake schedules, and circadian rhythm disorders (Fig. 9.1). Sleep disorders, almost by definition, are associated with **insomnia** (difficulty initiating or maintaining sleep). Subsequent sleep loss often leads to **excessive daytime sleepiness.** This is one of the most frequent and dangerous complications of almost any sleep disorder.
      1. **Questions.** What are the sleeping environment and the bedtime routine (what habits are associated with going to bed)? When is bedtime (regular or irregular)? What is the sleep latency (the amount of time it takes the patient to fall asleep "after the head hits the pillow")? What is the quality of sleep? Is it restful or restless and, if restless, why? How many arousals occur per night and for what reasons? What is the patient's final awakening time? Is assistance in waking necessary? How does the patient feel on waking? How many hours of sleep does the patient estimate are necessary for refreshment? Does the patient nap, and, if so, how often, how long, and how does the person feel after the nap (refreshed, unchanged, worse)? Does the patient experience excessive sleepiness or frank sleep attacks?
         a. Sleepiness can assist in rating the severity of any sleep disorder with the following set of operational **definitions:** mild—sleepiness that impairs social or occupational performance during activities that require little attention (reading or watching television); moderate—sleepiness that impairs social or occupational performance during activities that require some attention (meetings and concerts); and severe—sleepiness that impairs social or occupational performance during activities that require active attention (conversing or driving).
         b. A variety of **subjective measure scales** for sleepiness, such as the Stanford Sleepiness Scale, the Sleep–Wake Activity Inventory, and the Epworth Sleepiness Scale can routinely be used to help qualify, quantify, and follow problems with sleepiness (Fig. 9.2). Some chronically sleep-deprived persons underestimate their sleepiness as over time they lose the reference point from which to make comparisons—that is, they forget what it feels like to be fully rested. In such cases, excessive sleepiness can be suspected from reports such as memory loss, slow mentation, and amnestic periods associated with automatic behavior.
   B. **Examination.** The findings at physical examination often are normal, but in some instances, such as sleep-related breathing disorders, there often are associated signs that can include obesity, a small oropharynx, frank evidence of congestive heart failure (CHF), and even focal neurologic deficits. Sleepiness from any cause can lead to subtle neurocognitive deficits. Some nocturnal behavior

99

SLEEP DIARY

	Mon. a.m.	Tues. a.m.	Wed. a.m.	Thurs. a.m.	Fri. a.m.	Sat. a.m.	Sun. a.m.
1. What time did you go to bed last night?							
2. How many minutes did it take you to fall asleep?							
3. How many times did you wake up?							
4. How many total minutes did the awakenings keep you awake?							
5. What time did you wake up?							
6. What time did you get out of bed?							
Please use Wakefulness key below to answer the following questions:	Mon. p.m.	Tues. p.m.	Wed. p.m.	Thurs. p.m.	Fri. p.m.	Sat. p.m.	Sun. p.m.
1. How awake were you in the morning?							
2. How awake were you in the afternoon?							
3. How awake were you in the evening?							
4. Did you nap today? When and for how long?							

FIG. 9.1 Example of a typical week-at-a-glance sleep diary.

and movement disorders occur more frequently in association with neurodegenerative diseases (e.g., rapid eye movement [REM] sleep behavior disorder). Other findings unique to specific disorders are discussed in the appropriate sections.
II. **Investigative procedures**
   A. **Polysomnography (PSG)** is a combination of electroencephalography (EEG), electromyography (EMG), electrooculography, and a variety of other physiologic measures, such as oxygen saturation, heart rate, respiratory effort, airflow, and is often performed with simultaneous video monitoring. PSG allows differentiation of five sleep stages—non-REM (NREM) stages 1 through 4 and REM sleep—which can be associated with specific disorders (Table 9.1). The proven utility of technologic advances suggests that computer digitized polygraphic systems will offer data recording, scoring, and storage advantages that in many cases will replace traditional paper systems. The advent of compact, portable recording systems allows the evaluation of patients in medically unstable condition in the intensive care setting.
   B. **The multiple sleep latency test (MSLT)** allows quantification and qualification of sleepiness that results from the frequent arousals and microarousals associated with many sleep disorders. It is a cornerstone for the diagnosis of narcolepsy. The MSLT is a series of five 20-minute attempts at napping (during the patient's normal waking hours), which are separated by approximately 2-hour intervals. A mean sleep latency (the average time it takes the patient to fall

THE EPWORTH SLEEPINESS SCALE

Name: _____

Today's date: _____ Your age (years): _____

Your sex (male = M; female = F): _____

How likely are you to doze off or fall asleep in the following situations, in contrast to feeling just tired? This refers to your usual way of life in recent times. Even if you have not done some of these things recently try to work out how they would have affected you. Use the following scale to choose the *most appropriate number* for each situation:

    0 = would *never* doze
    1 = *slight* chance of dozing
    2 = *moderate* change of dozing
    3 = *high* chance of dozing

Situation	Chance of dozing
Sitting and reading	_____
Watching TV	_____
Sitting, inactive in a public place (e.g. a theater or a meeting)	_____
As a passenger in a car for an hour without a break	_____
Lying down to rest in the afternoon when circumstances permit	_____
Sitting and talking to someone	_____
Sitting quietly after a lunch without alcohol	_____
In a car, while stopped for a few minutes in the traffic	_____

Thank you for your cooperation

FIG. 9.2 The Epworth sleepiness scale. A score of 10 or greater suggests excessive daytime sleepiness. (From Johns MW. A new method for measuring daytime sleepiness: the Epworth sleepiness scale. *Sleep* 1991;14:540–545, with permission.)

asleep after the beginning of each individual nap period) less than 5 minutes indicates severe sleepiness, between 5 and 10 minutes suggest moderate sleepiness, and a latency greater than 10 minutes is not considered abnormal.

C. The **maintenance of wakefulness test** (MWT) is used to assesses the ability to remain awake in an environment conducive to sleep. Patients attempt to keep awake when placed in a warm, dark room, while lying in a semireclining position. The patient is monitored during five 20-minute sessions that are separated by 2-hour intervals. Each session ends if no sleep occurs for 20 minutes or after 10 minutes of sleep. The MWT is not a diagnostic test but is used primarily to document the effects of therapy.

Table 9.1 Classic polysomnographic findings associated with specific sleep disorders

Disorder	Finding
General insomnia	Increased sleep latency
	Increased stage 1 NREM sleep
	Reduced stage 3–4 NREM sleep
	Frequent arousals
	Increased sleep-stage shifts
	Increased time awake after sleep onset
	Reduced sleep efficiency
Insomnia in endogenous depression	Reduced REM latency
	Increased rapid eye movements in the first REM period
Sleep-related breathing disorder	Apnea, hypopnea
	Obstructive
	Mixed
	Respiratory effort–related arousals
	Central
	Hypoventilation
	±Snoring
	±Cardiac arrhythmia
PLM disorder, restless leg syndrome	PLMs often predominating in stage 2 NREM sleep
Rhythmic movement disorder	Head banging, body rocking, leg banging from drowsiness or early NREM sleep
REM behavior disorder	Violent behavior from REM sleep
	Elevated muscle tone in REM sleep
	PLMs and nonperiodic movements in REM or NREM sleep
Nocturnal paroxysmal dystonia	Dystonia from REM or NREM sleep
Sleep terrors, sleep walking	Sleep terrors or sleep walking from stage 3–4 NREM sleep
Circadian rhythm disorder	
ASPS	Early bedtime, early awakening time
DSPS	Late bedtime, late awakening time
ISWP	Irregular sleep periods
Narcolepsy	Short sleep latency, short REM latency
	MSLT with EDS with REM on two or more naps
Epilepsy	Increase in interictal discharge
	± Clinical seizure
Cluster headache and paroxysmal hemicrania	Headaches from REM
Fibromyositis	"Alpha–delta" sleep
	±PLMs

These classic polysomnographic findings may not necessarily be captured during an isolated study or observed in every patient. MSLT may or may not show evidence of EDS.

NREM, non–rapid eye movement; REM, rapid eye movement; ±, finding may or may not be present; PLM, periodic limb movement; ASPS, advanced sleep phase syndrome; DSPS, delayed sleep phase syndrome; ISWP, irregular sleep–wake pattern; MSLT, multiple sleep latency test; EDS, excessive daytime sleepiness.

D. Other tests. The use of extended PSG montages, which have extra channels, can allow more thorough assessment of variables such as the EEG (for nocturnal seizures) and EMG (for sleep-related movement and behavior disorders). Daytime provocative studies can be used to appropriately characterize phenomena such as cataplexy. Routine laboratory studies may be needed to rule out anemia, hypoxemia, infection, and metabolic and endocrinologic abnormalities. A Minnesota Multiphasic Personality Inventory (MMPI) with an interview by a neuropsychologist or psychiatrist familiar with sleep disorders can be helpful in cases in which an affective disorder is suspected. There is promise that for a number of intrinsic sleep disorders, such as narcolepsy, genetic testing may help to confirm the diagnosis.

III. Differential diagnosis. Sleep disorders can result from or be associated with a multitude of environmental, medical, and psychophysiologic factors. Often they simply result from poor sleep hygiene practices, but on occasion they exist without an obvious cause (idiopathic insomnia) or as subjective problems with no objective evidence of a sleep disturbance (sleep state misperception or malingering).

IV. Types of sleep disorders. This discussion uses terminology and outlines adapted from *The International Classification of Sleep Disorders: Diagnostic and Coding Manual* (ICSD).

   A. Insomnia resulting from psychological concomitants. Insomnia, the most common sleep problem, is only a symptom of many specific disorders. Difficulties with sleep are experienced by as much as 49% of the adult population in the United States. As many as 75% of cases result from specific problems with psychological associates, such as the intrinsic dyssomnia psychophysiologic insomnia, and from medical and psychiatric sleep disorders, which include depression, anxiety, and alcoholism.

   1. History. As many as 15% of patients with sleep problems have aspects of psychophysiologic, or conditioned, insomnia. These patients tend to respond to stress with somatized tension, which can occur in conjunction with learned sleep-preventing associations. An example is the person who sustains considerable psychological trauma (although in most cases no definite precipitating factor can be identified) and experiences acute insomnia secondary to affective concomitants. As affective issues are resolving, the person may negatively condition to the bedroom environment and sleep routine. Patients generally are overconcerned with their insomnia and deny psychological concomitants. Paradoxically, the sleep problems become worse as the persons tries harder to sleep and improve when the persons does not try to sleep. Often the persons sleeps much better in situations that differ from the routine sleep environment to which the somatized tension has been negatively conditioned, such as in the sleep laboratory.

   Because chronic insomnia can lead to depression, anxiety, and dependence on alcohol, drug, or medication, it is important to differentiate these secondary problems from primary disorders. In primary disorders, there usually is a history of major recurrent problems of mood, anxiety, or alcohol or drug abuse.

   2. PSG. Insomnia in general is associated with increased sleep latency, a relative increase in stage 1 NREM sleep, a relative decrease in stage 3 and 4 NREM sleep, an increased number of sleep-stage shifts, and an increase in wakefulness after sleep onset with a subsequent overall decrease in sleep efficiency. On occasion, a patient with psychophysiologic insomnia reports a much better night of sleep in the sleep laboratory setting than in the normal sleep environment with an unusually excellent sleep efficiency during PSG. Patients with depression often have early onset of the first REM sleep period with an increased frequency of rapid eye movements, whereas patients with secondary depression generally have normal first REM period latencies of approximately 90 minutes. Chronic alcoholism can cause a reduction in slow-wave sleep and total sleep time, which may improve only gradually after years of abstinence.

   3. MSLT. If sleep disruption is severe, pathologic sleepiness can occur, although in patients with anxiety disorders, there may be a normal or even increased sleep latency.

    4. Other tests. Psychological testing with the MMPI and the Beck depression and anxiety inventories may show repression, denial, somatization, depression, or anxiety. For patients with a history of alcohol abuse, liver function tests may be of value.

B. Sleep-related breathing disorders are problems that tend to occur more frequently among men and generally worsen with obesity and increasing age. The four major syndromes, defined by a combination of clinical and polysomnographic features, include obstructive sleep apnea–hypopnea syndrome (OSAHS), central sleep apnea–hypopnea syndrome (CSAHS), Cheyne–Stokes breathing syndrome (CSBS), and sleep hypoventilation syndrome (SHVS).

  1. General sleep-related breathing disorders assessment

    a. History. Patients often report excessive daytime sleepiness, short sleep latencies, restless or unrefreshing sleep, and extreme fatigue on awakening. Frequent reports of insomnia may be the result of arousals or microarousals associated with shortness of breath, choking, diaphoresis, palpitations, gastroesophageal reflux, nocturia, chest pain, and headache. The bed partner and family members may report loud snoring, gasping respirations, and frank apneic episodes. Sleep-related breathing disorders have been associated with chronic systemic hypertension, pulmonary hypertension, CHF, and stroke. When excessive daytime sleepiness is the major concern, the patient may actually have another or concomitant intrinsic sleep disorder (e.g., periodic limb movement disorder [PLMD] or narcolepsy) or an extrinsic disorder (e.g., inadequate sleep hygiene or alcohol- or drug-dependent sleep disorder). Because the ICSD contains more than 80 categories of sleep problems that can cause sleepiness, the history must be thorough.

    b. PSG. *The following descriptions pertain only to adults. Different PSG standards exist for children.* Obstructive events often are worse during REM sleep as a result of upper-airway hypotonia. In some cases, central apnea has a tendency to improve during REM sleep. Severity is determined by the **number of abnormal respiratory events,** the degree of associated **oxygen desaturation,** and the presence of associated **cardiac dysrhythmia.**

      (1) Apnea and hypopnea are generally considered events that occur for a minimum of 10 seconds with associated absent or markedly reduced airflow compared to the "baseline," oxygen desaturation of more than 3%, and arousals.

      (2) Apnea and hypopnea can be further classified as obstructive, central, or mixed. Obstruction is associated with persistent respiratory effort. During central events, respiratory effort is absent. Mixed apnea has an initial central component followed by obstruction.

      (3) One severity measure is the **apnea–hypopnea index** (AHI). Using the standard physiologic monitoring techniques available to most sleep laboratories, the AHI is considered by definition in the ICSD to be interchangeable with the **respiratory disturbance index** (RDI). The AHI represents the total number of episodes of apnea and hypopnea divided by the total sleep time. Although controversial, the following standards (based on convention, consensus, and an association between hypertension and higher AHIs) have been suggested: mild, 5 to 15 events per hour; moderate, 15 to 30 events per hour; and severe, more than 30 events per hour.

      (4) Another estimate of severity is the **lowest value of oxygen saturation** (SaO_2) during an event—90% or greater is considered normal; 80% to just less than 90%, mildly significant; 70% to just less than 80%, moderately severe; and less than 70% (or any event that appears to induce marked cardiac arrhythmia), severe. In addition, sustained oxygen desaturation greater than 10% compared with baseline and greater than 50% of total sleep time associated with an absolute oxygen saturation less than 85% also is considered significant.

(5) The sleep architecture with sleep-related breathing disorders often reveals an increase in stage 1 NREM sleep, a reduction in stage 3 and 4 NREM and REM sleep, and reduced sleep efficiency with frequent sleep-stage shifts and an increase in the total wake time after sleep onset.

c. MSLT. The MSLT should be performed 1½ to 3 hours after the completion of PSG. An MSLT should not be performed as an isolated test and should always immediately follow PSG. Disrupted sleep continuity associated with any sleep disorder can produce marked sleepiness.

d. Other tests. Most clinically performed PSG studies include the use of a variable combination of chest and abdomen airflow, snoring, and oxygen saturation monitoring devices. Becoming more commonplace, and considered essential by some, is the use of **capnography** for end-tidal CO_2 ($ETCO_2$) monitoring in patients with significant hypoventilation. In the future, we may see routine use of the devices considered the reference standards for PSG measurements in research. These include pneumotachometry, in which a tight-fitting mask is used to measure oronasal airflow for tidal volume measurements, and esophageal balloon pressure monitoring for detection of respiratory effort. In general, resting supine arterial blood gas measurement, complete blood cell count with differential, and liver, renal, and thyroid function tests are performed to screen for concomitant medical disorders that can induce, exacerbate, or result from sleep-related breathing disorders.

2. **OSAHS** is classically associated with repeated episodes of upper airway obstruction during sleep. It is common. In a random sample of persons 30 to 60 years of age, the prevalence was been reported to range from 9% to 24% for men and 4% to 9% for women. Upper airway obstruction is realized as a spectrum from incomplete (hypopnea) to complete (apnea) with persistent inspiratory effort. Hypopnea and mixed and obstructive apnea are believed to represent the same type of pathophysiologic event. These obstructions often result in oxygen desaturation, possible elevation in $PaCO_2$, and frequent arousals, which disrupt sleep continuity and lead to excessive daytime sleepiness.

This syndrome often occurs among sleepy, middle-aged, overweight men with insomnia who snore. Women are less commonly affected. This disorder also has been associated with systemic and pulmonary hypertension, nocturnal cardiac arrhythmia and angina, gastroesophageal reflux, nocturia, and an overall reduction in quality of life. Predisposing factors include familial tendencies, redundant pharyngeal tissue (e.g., adenotonsillar hypertrophy), craniofacial disorders (e.g., micrognathia, retrognathia, and nasal obstruction), endocrinopathy (e.g., acromegaly and hypothyroidism with myxedema), and neurologic disease. The overall severity of the disorder is determined by the most significant element of the evaluation (sleepiness, AHI, oxygen desaturation, or associated cardiac dysrhythmia).

a. History. The patient or bed partner often reports restless, unrefreshing sleep and sleep maintenance insomnia with arousals associated with gasping, choking, or heroic snoring, possibly exacerbated by fatigue, alcohol, weight gain, or the supine sleeping position. Snoring may force the person to sleep alone and may persist even when he or she is sitting. Although patients may not report daytime sleepiness, problems with fatigue, memory, and concentration are frequent. A family history of similar problems should be carefully sought.

b. Examination. The blood pressure, body mass index, and neck circumference should be documented, because hypertension and upper body adiposity may be predisposing factors for OSAHS. Oral and nasopharyngeal patency and abnormalities of the tonsils, adenoids, tongue, soft and hard palate, uvula, nasal septum, turbinates, and temporomandibular joint as well as fatty infiltration of soft tissues in the upper airways should be documented.

   c. **PSG.** Oximetry tracings often show a "sawtooth" pattern, which reflects recurrent obstruction with associated hypoxemia, and subsequent microarousals that lead to resaturation. Apneas and hypopnea generally last as long as 50 seconds and appear worse in the supine position and during REM sleep. It is not unusual to observe a microarousal within 3 seconds and the lowest level of associated oxygen desaturation within 30 seconds after an obstructive event has resolved. Tachycardiac and bradycardiac arrhythmias and asystolic periods may be documented to occur in direct relation to prolonged obstructive events.

   A mixture of hypopnea and mixed and obstructive apnea is routinely seen. Central apnea also may be appreciated. Limitations in the sensitivity and specificity of the commonly used monitoring techniques may lead not only to underscoring of obstruction but also on occasion to misscoring it as a central event. Medical decisions should be influenced by the overall clinical findings and by the most significant PSG phenomena.

   d. **Differential diagnosis.** Loud snoring and respiratory effort related arousals (RERA) and excessive daytime sleepiness might occur with no PSG evidence of OSAHS. Nevertheless, many experts believe that RERA (commonly referred to as *upper airway resistance syndrome*) are pathophysiologically similar to other obstructive events of OSAHS. Confident diagnosis of RERA requires an esophageal balloon recording that reveals episodes (10 seconds or greater duration) of increasingly negative pressure (corresponding to increased respiratory effort) that terminate with arousal that occurs in association with a return to baseline, resting esophageal pressure.

   e. **Other tests.** In general, results of routine laboratory studies are nonspecific. In severe cases, electrocardiography (ECG), chest radiography, and echocardiography may suggest pulmonary hypertension and right ventricular hypertrophy. Because OSAHS has been associated with multiple medical problems, an interdisciplinary approach with cephalometric evaluations of the upper airways, pulmonary function tests, and extensive cardiovascular and cerebrovascular assessments may be necessary.

3. **Idiopathic CSAHS.** This syndrome is a rare disorder of unknown causation characterized by repetitive episodes of sleep-related central apnea and hypopnea that occur without upper airway obstruction. These events are associated with oxygen desaturation, nocturnal arousals, and subsequent daytime problems. During normal sleep, there is a relative withdrawal of some of the waking stimulus to breathe. This is associated with a routine decrease in tidal volume and a mild increase in $PaCO_2$. Patients with CSAHS have an abnormal increased ventilatory response to this mild elevation in $PaCO_2$ and hyperventilate. The hyperpnea results in hypocarbia and subsequently transient cessation of breathing.

   a. **History and examination.** Patients often report excessive daytime sleepiness with sleep maintenance insomnia and frequent, vaguely described nocturnal arousals.

   b. **PSG.** During an event, there is a relative absence of airflow with a paucity of respiratory effort and no significant snoring or tachycardia or bradycardia. Associated oxygen desaturation is mild compared with OSAHS and SHVS. Central events tend to occur during the transition from wake to sleep, are less common in stage 2 NREM and REM sleep, and are rare in stage 3 and 4 NREM sleep. The central elements alternate with periods of hyperpnea. Episodes of hyperpnea are associated with frequent arousals. The sleep architecture shows an increased number of sleep-stage shifts with a relative increase in wake time after sleep onset and reduced sleep efficiency.

   c. **Differential diagnosis.** Patients with sleep-related, central-appearing respiratory abnormalities should be divided into two groups—those who are normocapnic or hypocapnic and those with hypercapnia (implying significant alveolar hypoventilation). When central events occur with hypercapnia, SHVS should be considered. Metabolic disorders, such as renal failure, CHF, and a variety or neurologic diseases can be associated with a Cheyne–Stokes respiratory pattern. CSAHS is not associated with the classic crescendo–decrescendo pattern. Alcohol and other central nervous system (CNS) depressants in and of themselves can cause cessation of respiratory effort. Finally, physiologic central apnea normally occurs with sleep-stage transitions and during phasic eye movements of REM sleep but are not associated with oxygen desaturation.

   d. Other tests. Arterial blood gas measurements obtained while the patient is awake and supine reveal a low to normal $Paco_2$ less than 45 mm Hg. Formal pulmonary function studies show an increased ventilatory response to carbon dioxide. Although high-altitude sleep apnea can result in central sleep apnea and a low to normal waking $Paco_2$, differentiation from CSAHS can usually be made with the history and the presence of a periodic breathing pattern with high-altitude sleep apnea.

4. **CSBS.** Severe CHF and in some cases neurologic dysfunction, classically stroke of brainstem medullary respiratory centers ("Ondine's curse"), can appear with PSG features that resemble those of central apnea–hypopnea. These appear with a cyclic, waxing and waning, fluctuating pattern of central apneic or hypopnic events that alternate with episodes of hyperpnea (Cheyne–Stokes respiratory pattern). Normally in adults the $Paco_2$ rises as high as 7 mm Hg in sleep. It is hypothesized that reduced cardiac function leads to a prolonged circulation time with a central delay in response to these fluctuating $Paco_2$ levels associated with sleep. The result is a Cheyne–Stokes breathing pattern. In most cases, a specific anatomic lesion to clearly explain this phenomenon cannot be discerned.

   a. History and examination. Many experts believe that to qualify for the diagnosis of CSBS in sleep, a patient must have severe CHF or cerebrovascular disease. These patients can appear with sleep maintenance insomnia. When the primary problem is severe, the Cheyne–Stokes respiratory pattern can be appreciated when the patient is awake. The examination should address peripheral signs, which can suggest underlying CHF and should include auscultation of the heart and chest for murmurs, gallops, rales, and rhonchi. There also should be a careful search for focal neurologic signs suggestive of brainstem injury.

   b. PSG. In general, there must at least three distinct periods of cyclical crescendo–decrescendo breathing, each lasting longer than 10 seconds. A significant disorder also is considered to exist when a single Cheyne–Stokes breathing period continues for 10 or more consecutive minutes. Severity can be reported as the proportion of the total sleep time spent in association with a Cheyne–Stokes breathing pattern. Cheyne–Stokes breathing is most frequent in NREM sleep. Respiratory frequency tends to parallel heart rate and blood pressure changes. Arousals are most frequent during the maximum of a hyperpneic period. The presence of Cheyne–Stokes breathing while awake is a greater predictive factor for mortality than is Cheyne–Stokes breathing isolated to sleep.

   c. Differential diagnosis. CSBS can coexist with OSAHS. The characteristic clinical features of CHF or cerebrovascular disease and crescendo–decrescendo breathing patterns differentiate CSBS from CSAHS. The clinical presentation and history help differentiate CSBS from high altitude–induced, sleep-related periodic breathing.

   d. Other tests. Measurement of $Paco_2$ while the patient is waking as well as supine often is low or low normal. Formal pulmonary function tests may reveal an increased ventilatory response to carbon dioxide. In addition to chest radiography, ECG, and measurement of cardiac enzymes, formal cardiac function studies can be considered because Cheyne–Stokes breathing is reported in as many as one half of all patients with CHF and a left ventricular ejection fraction less than 40%. Magnetic resonance imaging (MRI) of the brain and brainstem may be helpful when the history and examination findings suggest CNS injury.

5. **SHVS.** The most consistent finding in this disorder is a sleep-related increase in $Paco_2$ with subsequent hypoxemia. This is common in morbid

obesity (pickwickian syndrome) and in disorders that affect the mechanics of chest wall and lung function. This includes patients with chronic obstructive pulmonary disease and neuromuscular disorders that affect respiration. In the absence of the stereotypic concomitants, there may be an intrinsic dysfunction of medullary respiratory centers (central alveolar hypoventilation syndrome).

   a. **History.** Idiopathic hypoventilation appears in early adulthood and causes insomnia and sleepiness. Other forms of hypoventilation can occur at any age in association with obesity, chronic obstructive pulmonary disease, brainstem and cervical spinal injury, anterior horn cell disease, poliomyelitis, dysautonomia, muscular dystrophy, and diseases affecting the thorax and diaphragm. Patients may have erythrocytosis, cor pulmonale, or pulmonary hypertension secondary to severe, chronic hypoxemia.

   b. **Examination.** Body mass index should be calculated and a careful evaluation of the oral and nasopharynx and cardiovascular and cerebrovascular systems performed. A musculoskeletal visual survey should be performed for evidence of kyphoscoliosis. In some patients pretibial pitting edema may be the most obvious sign suggesting underlying cardiovascular insufficiency.

   c. **PSG.** Evidence of hypoxemia is often seen throughout the study as low baseline oxygen saturation, possibly apparent even in the supine waking state. Hypoventilation appears on oximetry tracings as prolonged (more than 1 minute) periods of reduced respiratory effort associated with sustained oxygen desaturation of more than 10%. This gradual desaturation can appear independently or with the superimposed classic "picket fence" pattern of OSAHS. Oxygen desaturation is generally worse in REM sleep. Because clinically significant SHVS can occur with only a few prolonged hypoventilatory events, the use of the RDI routinely leads to gross underestimation of the severity of this disorder. To address this issue, some experts recommend SHVS be considered severe when more than half of the total sleep time is spent with an oxygen saturation less than 85%. A "hypoventilation index" also can be calculated with the RDI if one considers each 3% oxygen saturation decrement of every hypoventilatory period a unique event. It can be difficult to differentiate hypoventilation from central apnea with routine PSG techniques. The use of capnography with $ETCO_2$ monitoring is becoming a more common method of addressing SHVS.

   d. **Other tests.** Arterial blood gas measurements should be obtained while the patient is awake and supine. In SHVS and chronic airflow limitation disorders, waking $PaCO_2$ often is greater than 45 mm Hg. During sleep, an increase in $PaCO_2$ of more than 10 mm Hg usually occurs. Early on, pulmonary function may be normal with the exception of a reduced respiratory response to hypercarbia and hypoxemia. Later there may be chronic elevation of hemoglobin level and hematocrit; the chest radiograph may reveal biventricular heart failure; ECG may indicate right ventricular hypertrophy, and pulmonary capillary wedge pressure may be elevated. Ruling out certain forms of endocrinopathy associated with weight gain, such as hypothyroidism, with thyroid function tests can be considered. When clinically indicated, as in evaluation for amyotrophic lateral sclerosis, MRI of the brain and brainstem or EMG and nerve conduction velocity studies may be helpful.

C. **Movement disorders**
   1. **PLMD and restless legs syndrome (RLS).** PLMD and RLS often occur concomitantly. Periodic limb movements (PLMs), often inappropriately referred to as *nocturnal myoclonus,* are sleep-related movements that primarily affect the lower extremities and can lead to insomnia and daytime sleepiness. Patients with RLS report dysesthesia and an uncontrollable need to move the legs that occurs on lying down to sleep or after sitting for a prolonged period. Although frequently observed in otherwise healthy middle-

aged and elderly adults, PLMD and RLS are associated with pregnancy, iron deficiency anemia, uremia, tricyclic antidepressant use or drug withdrawal, and a variety of CNS disorders. PLMD can be familial and has no sex predominance.

   a. History. It is essential that the bed partner be questioned, because the patient may be unaware of these movements. These movements increase with age and generally are not appreciated in patients younger than 30 years. With RLS, patients classically report minutes to hours of lower-extremity discomfort that is associated with rest, substantially improves with leg movement, and returns with rest.

   b. Examination. The findings at physical and neurologic examinations usually are normal.

   c. PSG. PLMs appear as elevated EMG activity from the tibialis anterior muscle, which persists for 0.5 to 5.0 seconds and coincides with episodes of repetitive, stereotypic extension of the large toe with ankle, knee, and hip flexion. Consecutive movements, with intermovement intervals of 4 to 90 seconds, occur primarily from stage 2 NREM sleep. The number of PLMs per hour (PLM index) is used to quantify severity: five or more movements per hour but fewer than 25 is considered mild; 25 or more but less than 50 is moderate; and 50 or more is severe. When PLMs are followed by an arousal, a PLM/arousal index of five or more movements per hour is significant, and more than 25 is considered severe.

   d. Differential diagnosis. Nonperiodic myoclonic movements associated with epilepsy and many neurodegenerative disorders should be considered. RLS-like problems may be associated with muscle overuse syndromes, nocturnal leg cramps, peripheral neuropathic dysesthesia, and rheumatologic pain disorders.

   e. Other tests. Routine laboratory analyses should include a complete blood count, iron and folate studies, measurement of serum glucose, and renal function tests. Drug screens, assessment of rheumatoid factor, and possibly a pregnancy test may be considered. If a neurologic lesion is suspected, MRI of the brain and brainstem or EMG and nerve conduction velocity studies may be helpful.

2. **Rhythmic movement disorder (RMD)** is a form of parasomnia that primarily affects children. The movements are sleep related, stereotypical, repetitive movements of the head, neck, or large muscle groups and often are associated with rhythmic vocalization that includes head banging (jactatio capitis nocturna), body rocking, and leg banging.

   a. History. Rhythmic body movements often begin in normal children between 8 and 18 months of age and rarely lead to injury. These movements generally resolve by 5 years of age, although persistence may be associated with stress, stimulus deprivation, or CNS lesions. Head banging is more common in boys. Both head banging and body rocking can occur in families. Family members generally are concerned about the noise and sometimes violent nature of these behaviors. Repeated, rhythmic striking of the head generally occurs in the supine position, whereas body rocking is associated with anteroposterior whole-body movements and can occur in many positions.

   b. PSG. Because RMD may not occur nightly, several consecutive study nights of infrared video analysis often are scheduled. Rhythmic movements generally occur with a frequency of 0.5 to 2 Hz during drowsiness and light sleep and can last from 15 minutes to 4 hours.

   c. Differential diagnosis. Seizures, night terrors, sleepwalking, and self-abusive and other psychogenic behaviors should be considered.

   d. Other tests. A baseline EEG (awake and sleeping) should be considered to rule out seizure. If the disorder is persistent, neuropsychiatric assessment may be appropriate.

3. **REM sleep behavior disorder (RBD).** This disorder is associated with violent behavior during sleep that reflects dream enactment. Events begin during REM ("dreaming" or "paralyzed") sleep and are followed, after

arousal, by reports of dream imagery compatible with the actions observed during the spell.

    a. History. This disorder generally appears, although not exclusively, in elderly men, often those with neurologic disease. The patients have histories of potentially harmful sleep-related body movements associated with dreaming. Patients frequently report sleep-related injuries, which include bruises, lacerations, dislocations, fractures, and subdural hemorrhage.

    b. PSG. Because major episodes may occur only once every 2 to 3 weeks, several consecutive study nights may be scheduled. During REM sleep, muscle tone generally is elevated and a variety of nonviolent movements, such as PLMs, can occur in REM and NREM sleep. Behavior appearing as dream enactment may be appreciated during REM sleep.

    c. Differential diagnosis. Violent behavior associated with dreams have been reported in association with posttraumatic stress disorder and sleep apnea, whereas elevated muscle tone in REM sleep may be observed with narcolepsy, drug use, and neurodegenerative disease. Excessive movements during sleep have been associated with some psychiatric disorders (dissociative states and nocturnal panic attacks).

    d. Other tests. RBD appears to result from dysfunction of the brainstem generators responsible for the atonia normally associated with REM sleep. This allows movement (dream enactment) during REM sleep, a state otherwise associated with essential paralysis. Although anatomic injury may not be appreciated with imaging studies, MRI of the brain and brainstem may be helpful in some cases. MSLT, drug screening, or neurocognitive and psychiatric testing may be considered for specific patients.

4. Nocturnal paroxysmal dystonia (NPD). NPD exists within a spectrum of disorders that includes paroxysmal arousals and episodic nocturnal wandering. The clinical characteristics, interictal EEG findings, and response to anticonvulsants suggest that NPD may actually be a complex-partial seizure disorder originating from the frontoorbital or mesial–temporal area. Much controversy continues to surround the true nature of this phenomenon, because the EEG findings generally are normal during a typical spell.

    a. History. NPD has an onset that ranges from infancy to late middle age and shows no sex preference. It is generally not considered a familial disorder. Episodes can persist for more than 20 years and have been associated with reports of daytime and nocturnal seizures. "Short-lasting" spells of NPD generally last 1 minute and can occur as many as 20 times nightly. The spells begin during sleep with several seconds of stereotypic dystonic, choreoathetotic, or opisthotonic posturing of the head, trunk, and extremities, which is often followed by semipurposeful, repetitive, violent movements. Patients may appear awake, although not necessarily fully conscious. After the spell, the patient is coherent and often goes back to sleep immediately. The episodes may be associated with partial amnesia, are not linked with dreamlike imagery, and are not associated with tongue biting or bowel or bladder incontinence.

    b. Examination. The findings at physical and neurologic examinations are generally normal.

    c. PSG. Onset of spells has been reported during stage 2 NREM sleep (occasionally following K-complexes, which are phenomena often associated with arousal), in stage 3 and 4 NREM sleep, and during transitions to REM sleep. The event persists during apparent arousal with a normal waking EEG pattern (although electroencephalographic evidence of epileptiform activity followed by generalized tonic–clonic activity has been reported).

    d. MSLT. Because frequent NPD can cause substantial sleep interruption, daytime sleepiness may be documented.

    e. Differential diagnosis. NPD can mimic sleep terrors, nightmares, somnambulism, RMD, or RBD and at times may suggest a conversion disorder or malingering. Atypical reports include a long-lasting form of NPD, which is associated with 2 to 50 minutes of dystonic or dyskinetic (choreoathetoid, ballistic) movements (familial Huntington's disease developed in one patient with this form of NPD 20 years after onset of NPD), and patients with characteristic movements precipitated during wakefulness.

    f. Other tests. Findings of brain imaging studies and interictal EEG generally are normal, although on occasion the interictal, sleep-deprived EEG shows focal slowing, paroxysmal bursts of φ activity, and generalized and focal epileptic discharges from the temporal lobes. Positron emission tomography has shown frontal and temporal hypometabolism.

  5. Sleep terrors (pavor nocturnus in children, pavor incubus in adults) and sleepwalking (somnambulism). These phenomena are closely related forms of parasomnia that can occur in a familial pattern, occur primarily among children, and begin in slow-wave (stage 3 and 4 NREM) sleep. The spells are associated with a general lack of responsiveness to the environment, with automatic actions, confusion, disorientation, and occasional injuries. After these events, from which the patient is generally unarousable, there usually is amnesia without dream recall. These disorders generally resolve by puberty, but when diagnosed in adults they can be associated with a psychopathologic condition.

    a. History. Sleep terrors tend to occur more often in boys, with an onset between 4 and 12 years and resolution by puberty. During the spell, the patient often appears glassy eyed and frightened, with tachycardia, tachypnea, diaphoresis, and inconsolable screaming and crying that can last from a few seconds to 20 minutes. Sleepwalking generally occurs at 4 to 8 years of age, often after sleep terrors have resolved. Patients walk in a confused manner and are subject to injury.

    b. Examination. The findings at physical and neurologic examinations generally are normal. Evidence of infection, fever, or drug use, any of which can exacerbate these forms of parasomnia, should be sought.

    c. PSG. Because these spells may not occur nightly, several consecutive nights of video PSG should be considered. Classically, an event follows a sudden arousal from stage 3 and 4 NREM sleep in the first third of the night. Partial arousals from stage 3 and 4 sleep are not uncommon. Often a spell cannot be captured, and the diagnosis is based primarily on the history.

    d. MSLT. One may be able to document sleepiness, because sleep deprivation can precipitate or exacerbate these disorders.

    e. Differential diagnosis. The differential diagnosis includes nightmares, seizures, RMD, RBD, psychogenic disorders, and malingering. Confusional arousal (arousal from sleep not associated with fear, walking, or hallucinations) also must be considered.

    f. Other tests. When the disorder is persistent, is associated with injury, or affects an adult, an MMPI and neuropsychological assessment may be important. Baseline EEG (awake and asleep) may be necessary to evaluate for seizures.

D. Circadian rhythm disorders (disorders of the timing of the sleep–wake pattern). These disorders occur when there are incongruities between the sleep–wake schedule demanded by society and the intrinsic sleep–wake pattern of the patient (determined in large part by the circadian pacemaker—the suprachiasmatic nuclei of the anterior hypothalamus). When not extrinsic or self-imposed ("jet lag" or shift work), these problems are believed to result from abnormal intrinsic physiologic responses to environmental time cues (*Zeitgebers*) such as sunlight (which exerts its effects through retinal–hypothalamic pathways). The patient's state of sleepiness or arousal subsequently is out of synchrony with that of the general population. The result is alternating sleepiness and insomnia when the patient tries to follow a normal schedule.

1. **History.** In many cases, the diagnosis can be made with a sleep log. By accurately documenting, for a period of 1 to 2 months, all bedtimes, final awakening times, and all nap times, a sleep log can help differentiate a circadian rhythm disorder from poor sleep hygiene. The log should be filled out during a vacation or "free" time so as to avoid societal constraints that prevent the patient from following his or her intrinsic sleep–wake pattern.
2. **PSG.** The PSG findings should corroborate the sleep log reports.
3. **MSLT.** In general, if patients are allowed to follow their intrinsic sleep–wake rhythm, there should be no evidence of sleepiness during normal waking hours.
4. **Differential diagnosis.** Poor sleep hygiene, drug use, affective problems, and a variety of disorders that can be detected with PSG and MSLT must be considered.
5. **Other tests.** Some sleep disorder centers can monitor hormonal rhythms (such as those of cortisol and melatonin) and 24-hour body temperature fluctuations, which can lose normal circadian fluctuations and amplitudes in circadian sleep disorders. Referral to such centers may be necessary.
6. **Other syndromes**
   a. **Advanced sleep-phase syndrome.** When free to follow their desired sleep–wake schedules, persons with this syndrome go to sleep very early in relation to the setting of the sun, arise very early in relation to sunrise, and do not report excessive sleepiness during their "normal" waking hours. This tendency increases with age and is generally addressed only if it impairs the quality of the patient's work, social, or family life.
      (1) **Sleep log.** The sleep log reveals a consistently early bedtime and early final awakening time with normal sleep continuity and total sleep time. Patients do not report excessive sleepiness unless they attempt to follow societal schedules.
      (2) **PSG/MSLT.** The ICSD suggests that the patient history be confirmed with consecutive sleep studies. All PSGs should show early evening sleep onset, with normal sleep latency and sleep architecture and early morning final awakening. MSLT should not reveal excessive sleepiness.
   b. **Delayed sleep-phase syndrome.** This disorder occurs primarily among adolescents. Patients report chronically late bedtimes with late final awakening times.
      (1) **Sleep log.** The sleep log confirms that the patient's problems are associated with normal sleep continuity and normal total sleep times. These patients do not report sleepiness unless they attempt to follow the normal societal sleep–wake schedule.
      (2) **PSG.** When the patient is allowed to follow his or her "normal" sleep pattern, PSG reveals a very late sleep onset and a late final awakening. The sleep latency usually is more than 30 minutes (this subsequently leads to relatively low sleep efficiency). Sleep continuity and architecture are otherwise normal.
   c. **Non-24-hour sleep–wake syndrome (hypernycthemeral syndrome).** Patients with this syndrome have an inability to synchronize (entrain) the physiologic desire for a sleep–wake schedule that is greater than 24 hours with a normal 24-hour day. Subsequently these patients continually "phase delay" and on a day-to-day basis show a progressive 1 to 2 hour delay of bedtime and final awakening times. When they attempt to keep regular sleep–wake schedules (with a fixed bedtime and final awakening time), they experience recurrent periods without sleep problems (when their intrinsic schedules match society's), which are then followed by the gradual onset of periods associated with sleep-onset insomnia, difficulty waking in the morning, and daytime sleepiness (when their intrinsic schedules are out of synchrony with society's).
      (1) **History.** Many of these patients are blind (from a variety of causes, including tumor of the optic chiasm). The disorder has been reported

in association with mental retardation and schizophrenia and only rarely in the normal population.

   (2) Sleep log. The sleep log reveals a day-to-day delay in bedtime and final awakening time.

   (3) Other tests. Imaging studies of the brain can be considered, because this disorder has been associated with suprasellar lesions.

   d. **Irregular sleep–wake pattern.** In this disorder there is no definitive sleep–wake rhythm. Patients subsequently have intermittent nocturnal insomnia and variable periods of daytime sleepiness, which generally result in three or more irregularly timed naps during a 24-hour period. The total sleep time during a 24-hour period is normal, but the timing of sleep is not predictable.

   (1) History and examination. This disorder is common among patients with severe congenital, developmental, and degenerative brain disorders.

   (2) PSG. Prolonged, continuous PSG for 24 to 72 hours shows irregular periods of sleep that vary from day to day. In patients with significant brain injury, the presence of diffuse slow-wave activity with a loss of normal sleep architecture is not unusual.

   (3) Other tests. Imaging studies of the brain should be considered.

E. **Sleep disorders associated with the CNS**

   1. **Narcolepsy** is generally considered a disorder of excessive sleepiness. Although some investigators believe a history of pathologic sleepiness and cataplexy is sufficient for diagnosis, narcolepsy may involve the classic full clinical tetrad of excessive sleepiness, cataplexy, sleep paralysis, and hypnagogic hallucinations.

   a. **History.** The onset generally is during puberty or young adulthood with symptoms of excessive sleepiness and sleep attacks. Sleep attacks can occur while the person is driving, engaged in active conversation, or eating. Brief 10 to 20 minute naps may refresh the patient for hours. Once the sleepiness stabilizes, it generally does not progress, but the other symptoms associated with narcolepsy may come and go. Cataplexy, often precipitated by strong emotion, involves attacks that range from brief sensations of weakness to essential paralysis. The spells are transient and do not produce cognitive impairment. Hypnagogic (at sleep onset) and hypnopompic (on awakening) hallucinations are generally frightening visual, auditory, or movement perceptions that essentially represent dreaming while awake. Sleep paralysis occurs during the transition from sleep to waking (or waking to sleep). The patient may experience brief paralysis (seconds to minutes) with the inability to speak. Other symptoms of narcolepsy can include insomnia, poor memory, depression, and automatic behaviors.

   b. **PSG.** REM sleep normally begins approximately 90 minutes after sleep onset. The REM latency of persons with narcolepsy can be less than 20 minutes. A short sleep latency and reduced sleep efficiency also may be appreciated.

   c. **MSLT** should show evidence of excessive sleepiness with two or more REM-onset sleep periods, although a variety of factors, including a noisy testing environment (hospitals in general), can produce false-negative results. For a 2-week period before the sleep studies, the patient should keep a diary, documenting good sleep hygiene and the avoidance of centrally active drugs. Both sleep deprivation and drug withdrawal can be associated with REM rebound, which can mimic narcolepsy electrophysiologically.

   d. **Genetic testing.** The major histocompatibility complex of chromosome 6 contains genetic markers for narcolepsy, the strongest being the human leukocyte antigen allele, HLA DQB1*0602. The presence of such markers correlates strongly with narcolepsy, but these markers have been associated with false-positive and false-negative results. Nevertheless, publications concerning the orexin (hypocretin) gene suggest that genetic testing will eventually be part of the routine approach to a quick and accurate diagnosis of narcolepsy.

   e. Differential diagnosis. Many sleep disorders can disrupt sleep continuity and produce sleepiness and an MSLT result suggesting narcolepsy. A thorough sleep history and an accurate sleep log, along with PSG and MSLT, generally prevent misdiagnosis in such cases. In addition, cataplectic-like events can occur in conjunction with sleep drunkenness, complex partial seizures, fugue states, and transient global amnesia.

     Idiopathic (CNS) hypersomnolence can be differentiated from narcolepsy by means of history and sleep studies. This is a lifelong disorder, beginning during adolescence or young adulthood, that is associated with continual sleepiness without cataplexy. Naps are long and unrefreshing, and drowsiness generally precedes sleep attacks. PSG reveals normal sleep, whereas MSLT confirms sleepiness. However, REM-onset sleep is not recorded with MSLT.

     The history usually differentiates narcolepsy from disorders of recurrent hypersomnolence, such as Kleine–Levin syndrome, which primarily affects adolescent boys. These patients suffer two to 12 sleep attacks per year, which last hours to days, that have been associated with hyperphagia and sexual inappropriateness.

2. Sleep-related epilepsy. For persons with epilepsy, focal interictal discharges and secondarily generalized tonic–clonic seizures during NREM sleep are not unusual. Sudden death during sleep is rare, but it has occurred in association with poor seizure control and nontherapeutic anticonvulsant levels. Seizure disorders associated with sleep (although not necessarily occurring exclusively in sleep) include juvenile myoclonic epilepsy (with seizures often occurring soon after awakening), electrical status epilepticus of sleep (primarily an EEG phenomenon that occurs during sleep and otherwise is not associated with clinical seizures), and Landau–Kleffner syndrome (acquired epileptic aphasia associated with mental deterioration).

   a. Diagnosis. Nocturnal seizures often can be diagnosed with the history and the baseline waking–sleeping EEG. If necessary, several consecutive nights of extended PSG and EEG monitoring may be helpful.

   b. Differential diagnosis. Other sleep disorders associated with sleep-related movements, such as obstructive sleep apnea (OSA), PLMD, RMD, RBD, and NPD, should be considered.

3. Sleep-related pain

   a. Headaches. Sleep studies often can lead to the diagnosis of, and assist in differentiating, primary sleep-related headaches (associated with specific sleep stages) and secondary sleep-related headaches that occur as a result of intrinsic sleep disorders such as OSA and epilepsy. Headaches that can be exacerbated by lying down or by sleep include those associated with cerebral edema, intracranial hypertension, and obstructive hydrocephalus. They often manifest with a crescendo time profile (generally over a period lasting as long as 3 months). The most frequent type of morning headache is associated with the hangover that results from alcohol use. The differential diagnosis includes headaches associated with systemic hypertension, depression, sinus inflammation, and sleep apnea. Postictal headaches associated with seizures can occur anytime throughout sleep, whereas headaches reported to occur just before sleep onset may represent the "exploding-head syndrome," a disorder associated with a sudden sensation of an explosion going off in the head.

      (1) Cluster headaches. Patients usually also experience daytime headaches (from one every other day to eight per day), although as many as 75% of the headaches may occur during REM sleep.

         (a) History. These headaches affect men far more frequently than they do women and tend to occur during periodic clusters lasting from 7 days to 1 year (generally 2 weeks to 3 months) and separated by at least 14 pain-free days. Patients wake with severe, unilateral eye and facial pain, often associated with tearing, conjunctival vasodilatation, rhinorrhea, nausea, vomiting, and occasionally Horner's syndrome. Episodes may last 15 to 180 minutes and can occur several times per night.

    (b) PSG. Typical headaches, associated with arousals from REM sleep, can be captured during extended PSG monitoring.

  (2) Paroxysmal hemicrania (REM sleep-locked headache). These headaches occur primarily among adult women and, like cluster headaches, are unilateral and associated with REM sleep, but they generally are briefer and occur more frequently than cluster headaches. These headaches can last from 2 to 45 minutes (usually 5 to 20 minutes) and occur day or night during waking or sleep, as many as 30 times during a 24-hour period. Therapeutically they respond with absolute effectiveness to indomethacin.

b. Fibrositis syndrome (fibromyalgia, fibromyositis) is a chronic disorder of diffuse musculoskeletal pain that often is worse at night and can lead to insomnia and sleepiness.

  (1) History. This disorder, when it first appears, generally affects young adults, women more than men, often after a febrile illness. The symptoms are diffuse myalgia and arthralgia, which can be exacerbated by climatologic changes and minimal trauma. The chronicity of the disorder can lead to psychological concomitants.

  (2) Examination. Diffuse tenderness, most prominent in the neck and shoulder muscles, can be appreciated with deep palpation. Specific areas to assess include the medial borders of the trapezius muscle and the scapula, the sternal border of the pectoralis major muscle and the second costochondral junction, the cervical and lumbar erector spinae muscles and intervertebral ligaments, the middle aspect and upper outer quadrant of the gluteus maximus muscle, the anterior superior iliac spine, the lateral portions of the elbows, and the medial aspects of the knees.

  (3) PSG may show α-δ sleep patterns, in which α EEG activity (the normal 8- to 12-Hz occipital activity observed in waking patients when their eyes are closed) appears in the slow waves of stage 3 and 4 NREM, or δ sleep. PLMs occasionally may be appreciated.

  (4) The **differential diagnosis** includes myopathy, polymyalgia rheumatica, arthritis, chronic fatigue syndrome, and primary affective disorders.

  (5) Other tests. Results of laboratory tests for inflammation, infection, and rheumatologic disorders and of radiographic studies should be normal. Associated affective disorders may necessitate neuropsychological evaluation.

4. Dysfunction of specific neurologic systems. In general, injury and trauma to the CNS can lead to sleep-related problems through diffuse effects that often involve the hypothalamus and brainstem.

  a. Large hemispheric strokes are associated with sleepiness and insomnia, which may be attributable to an inversion of the sleep–wake rhythm. Loss of sleep spindles and normal stage 2 NREM sleep architecture are associated with a poor prognosis.

  b. Diencephalic lesions involving the anterior hypothalamus and injuries to the preoptic area and the amygdala, as reported in conjunction with some forms of encephalitis, can result in insomnia. Lesions of the posterior hypothalamus can cause hypersomnia. Symptomatic narcolepsy and cataplexy can occur in association with several diseases involving the hypothalamic–upper brainstem area and the third ventricle, including craniopharyngioma, glioma, sarcoidosis, colloid cyst, pituitary adenoma, and mesencephalic glioma.

c. **Brainstem lesions** involving the mesencephalon and the rostral–central tegmentum (as in "top of the basilar syndrome") can produce sleepiness (possibly as a result of reticular activating system injury), gaze palsy, hallucinations, and unreactive, dilated pupils. Pontine lesions, often with involvement of the median raphe, resulting from vascular (medial tegmental pontine stroke), inflammatory (poliomyelitis), and degenerative (spinocerebellar degeneration) diseases, can produce indeterminate sleep patterns, with a paucity of normal sleep architecture, and insomnia. RBD has been reported with dorsopontomesencephalic lacunar infarction. Damage to tegmentoreticular tracts is hypothesized to produce disconnection of peri–locus ceruleus centers (generators of muscular atonia) from the medullary inhibitory center of Magoun and Rhines.

Bulbar poliomyelitis, lower brainstem stroke, spinal (high cervical) surgery, syringobulbia, encephalitis, striatonigral degeneration, Creutzfeldt–Jakob disease, and olivopontocerebellar degeneration are associated with central sleep apnea (CSA). Apnea can manifest as Ondine's curse, in which no spontaneous respiration occurs during sleep, necessitating continuous ventilatory support. Arnold–Chiari malformation can be associated with central and obstructive respiratory phenomena. Associated cranial nerve dysfunction can reduce the oropharyngeal opening as a result of jaw and tongue instability, phrenic nerve dysfunction, and atrophy of accessory respiratory muscles.

d. **Degenerative disorders**, including Parkinson's disease, Shy–Drager syndrome, progressive supranuclear palsy, olivopontocerebellar and spinocerebellar degeneration, fatal familial insomnia, Huntington's chorea, dyssynergia cerebellaris myoclonica of Ramsay Hunt, and many forms of dementia, have been associated with a variety of sleep disorders, including insomnia, indeterminate sleep, daytime sleepiness, nocturnal myoclonus, sleep apnea, and RBD. In some cases, sleep disorders may be related to psychological concomitants or medications. Dopaminergic agents improve sleep disturbances for some patients, but for others have an alerting effect, enhancing hallucinations and exacerbating nightmares.

e. **Myopathy** may predispose patients to sleep-related respiratory disorders by reducing tidal volume during REM sleep. Myasthenia gravis can lead to mixed, obstructive, and central apnea in REM sleep. Myotonic dystrophy (possibly attributable to dorsomedial thalamic dysfunction) has been associated with hypersomnia, although craniofacial characteristics and impaired upper airway and inspiratory muscle function can contribute to OSA, CSA, sleep-related alveolar hypoventilation, and sleepiness.

f. **Acquired autonomic neuropathy**, such as that associated with diabetes, can lead to irregular breathing patterns, a decrease in tidal volume in NREM sleep, and hypoventilation and apnea in REM sleep.

V. Referral to a sleep disorder center. Sleep disorders are common, and general practitioners see many patients with sleep-related problems. An accurate clinical diagnosis often can be made if a full sleep history is routinely incorporated into the general examination. On occasion, successful treatment of many sleep problems can be achieved by correcting poor sleep hygiene practices or addressing primary social, psychological, and medical concomitants when they exist. When sleep problems persist, greatly impair the patient's quality of life, or necessitate formal sleep studies for diagnosis or therapy (as in narcolepsy and sleep apnea), referral to a reputable sleep disorder center should be considered.

Recommended Readings
General

Browman CP, Gujavarty KS, Sampson MG, et al. REM sleep episodes during the maintenance of wakefulness test in patients with sleep apnea syndrome and patients with narcolepsy. *Sleep* 1983;6:23–28.

Carskadon MA, Dement WC, Mitler MM, et al. Guidelines for the multiple sleep latency test (MSLT): a standard measure of sleepiness. *Sleep* 1986;9:519–524.

Culebras A. The neurology of sleep. *Neurology* 1992;42[Suppl 6]:6–8.

Engleman HM, Martin SE, Deary IJ, et al. Effect of CPAP therapy on daytime function on patients with mild sleep apnoea/hypopnoea syndrome. *Thorax* 1997;52:114–119.

Kryger MH, Roth T, Dement WC. *Principles and practice of sleep medicine,* 3rd ed. Philadelphia: WB Saunders, 2000.

Rechtschaffen A, Kales A. *A manual of standardized terminology, techniques and scoring system for sleep stages of human subjects.* Bethesda, MD: National Institutes of Health, 1986.

Thorpy MJ, Diagnostic Classification Steering Committee. *The international classification of sleep disorders: diagnostic and coding manual.* Rochester, MN: American Sleep Disorders Association, 1997.

Young T, Blustein J, Finn L, et al. Sleep-disordered breathing and motor vehicle accidents in a population-based sample of employed adults. *Sleep* 1997;20:608–613.

Young T, Peppard P, Palta M, et al. Population-based study of sleep-disordered breathing as a risk factor for hypertension. *Arch Intern Med* 1997;157:1746–1752.

Insomnia Resulting from Psychological Concomitants

Hauri PJ. Consulting about insomnia: a method and some preliminary data. *Sleep* 1993; 16:344–350.

Morin CM. *Insomnia: psychological assessment and management.* New York: Guilford, 1993.

Sleep-induced Respiratory Impairment

American Academy of Sleep Medicine Task Force. Sleep-related breathing disorders in adults: recommendations for syndrome definition and measurement techniques in clinical research. *Sleep* 1999;22:667–689.

Deveraux MW, Keane JR, Davis RL. Automatic respiratory failure associated with infarction of the medulla: report of two cases with pathologic study of one. *Arch Neurol* 1973;29:46–52.

Dyken ME. Cerebrovascular disease and sleep apnea. In: Lenfant C, Bradley TD, Floras JS, eds. *Sleep apnea: implications in cardiovascular and cerebrovascular disease.* New York, NY: Marcel Dekker, 2000:285–306.

Dyken ME, Somers VK, Yamada T. Stroke, sleep apnea and autonomic instability. In: Togawa K, et al., eds. *Sleep apnea and rhonchopathy.* Basel: Karger, 1993:166–168.

Hung J, Whitford EG, Parsons RW, et al. Association of sleep apnoea with myocardial infarction in men. *Lancet* 1990;336:261–264.

Kales A, Bixler EO, Cadieux RJ, et al. Sleep apnoea in a hypertensive population. *Lancet* 1984;2:1005–1008.

Young T, Palta M, Dempsey J, et al. The occurrence of sleep-disordered breathing among middle-aged adults. *N Engl J Med* 1993;328:1230–1235.

Movement Disorders

Broughton RJ. NREM arousal parasomnias. In: Kryger MH, Roth T, Dement WC, eds. *Principles and practice of sleep medicine,* 3 ed. Philadelphia: WB Saunders, 2000:693–706.

Culebras A, Moore JT. Magnetic resonance findings in REM sleep behavior disorder. *Neurology* 1989;39:1519–1523.

Dyken ME, Rodnitzky R. Periodic, aperiodic and rhythmic motor disorders of sleep. *Neurology* 1992;42:68–74.

Dyken ME, Lin-Dyken DC, Seaba P, et al. Violent sleep related behavior leading to subdural hemorrhage: polysomnographically documented REM sleep behavior disorder with split-screen electroencephalographic-video analysis. *Arch Neurol* 1995;52:318–321.

Lugaresi E, Cirignotta F. Hypnogenic paroxysmal dystonia: epileptic seizure or a new syndrome? *Sleep* 1981;4:129–138.

Mahowald MW, Schenck CH. REM sleep parasomnias. In: Kryger MH, Roth T, Dement WC, eds. *Principles and practice of sleep medicine,* 3rd ed. Philadelphia: WB Saunders, 2000:724–741.

Salva MAQ, Guilleminault C. Olivopontocerebellar degeneration, abnormal sleep, and REM sleep without atonia. *Neurology* 1986;36:576–577.

Schenck CH, Milner DM, Hurwitz TD, et al. A polysomnographic and clinical report on sleep-related injury in 100 adult patients. *Am J Psychiatry* 1989;146:1166–1172.

Circadian Rhythm Disorders
Campbell SS, Kripke DF, Gillin JC, et al. Exposure to light in healthy elderly subjects and Alzheimer's patients. *Physiol Behav* 1988; 42:141–144.
Rosenthal NE, Joseph-Vanderpool JR, Levendosky AA, et al. Phase-shifting effects of bright morning light as treatment for delayed sleep phase syndrome. *Sleep* 1990;13:354–361.

Sleep Disorders Associated with the Central Nervous System
Dyken ME, Yamada T, Lin-Dyken DC, et al. Diagnosing narcolepsy through the simultaneous clinical and electrophysiologic analysis of cataplexy. *Arch Neurol* 1996;53:456–460.
Guilleminault C, Anagnos A. Narcolepsy. In: Kryger MH, Roth T, Dement WC, eds. *Principles and practice of sleep medicine,* 3rd ed. Philadelphia: WB Saunders, 2000:676–686.
Mouret J. Differences in sleep in patients with Parkinson's disease. *Electroencephalogr Clin Neurophysiol* 1975;38:653–657.
Niedermeyer E. Epileptic seizure disorders. In: Niedermeyer E, Lopes da Silva F, eds. *Electroencephalography: basic principles, clinical applications and related fields,* 2nd ed. Baltimore: Urban & Schwarzenberg, 1987:405–510.
Olesen J, Headache Classification Committee of the International Headache Society. Classification and diagnostic criteria for headache disorders, cranial neuralgias, and facial pain. *Cephalgia* 1988;8:1–96.
Plum F, Posner JB. *The diagnosis of stupor and coma,* 3rd ed. Philadelphia: FA Davis Co, 1980.
Yasuhara A, Yoshida H, Hatanaka T, et al. Epilepsy with continuous spike-waves during slow sleep and its treatment. *Epilepsia* 1991;32:59–62.

10. APPROACH TO THE PATIENT WITH VISUAL LOSS

James J. Corbett

When **visual loss** is a patient's primary problem, symptoms vary depending on whether one or both eyes are affected; whether the visual loss is abrupt in onset, gradual in onset, or suddenly discovered long after its onset; whether the visual loss is complete or partial; and whether the visual loss is manifested as visual hallucinations or illusions. The probable causes of visual loss are narrowed to a few possibilities on the basis of the symptoms, the patient's age and sex, and the presumed anatomic location of the lesion (Table 10.1).

Patients with primary visual problems usually seek the attention of an ophthalmologist or optometrist. Referral to a neurologist commonly occurs with computed tomographic (CT) scans or magnetic resonance (MR) images already in hand. If the problem appears to be a tumor, the patient more often is referred directly to a neurosurgeon. The pattern of referral and the tests performed before referral further decrease the number of probable diagnostic options.

The visual pathway consists of elements easily examined directly at the bedside, such as the pupils, the retina, and the optic disk, and those that are indirectly examined with subjective tests, such as the more posterior elements of the optic nerve, chiasm, optic tract, lateral geniculate body, geniculocalcarine tract, and visual cortex. Damage to visual association cortices, parietal and inferior temporal, produces symptoms with preservation of visual acuity and sometimes normal visual fields.

I. **Bedside or office clinical examination of the visual system**
   A. **Visual acuity.** Although it is best to examine visual acuity with a distance chart, the neurologist almost always examines visual acuity with a near card. This should be done with a handheld Snellen chart or a Jaeger print card. If a near card is being used, be sure that patients are using their reading glasses. Push patients to give you the very best acuity possible. Do not rush them. Do not start with the largest type; rather, ask patients to read the 20/25 line and then the 20/20 line. If this fails, gradually work your way up. Three fingers held up are the equivalent of the large *E* on the distance acuity chart, and a patient who can count fingers at 20 feet (6 m) has 20/200 acuity. Thus, counting fingers at 5 feet (1.5 m) would be equivalent to 20/800 acuity. Visual acuity should be normal in pure homonymous hemianopia or pure bitemporal hemianopia. Acquired visual acuity deficits not attributable to refractive error imply a central scotoma.
   B. **Confrontation visual fields** should be evaluated at a distance of 1 m from the patient. Ask the patient cover one eye with the palm of the hand and to look at your nose. Present your fingers (one, two, or five) rapidly in each quadrant. Slowness to respond in one quadrant or hemifield can be the earliest sign of a homonymous visual field defect. After rapid finger counting, present your hands, palms forward, first in the two upper quadrants and then in the two lower quadrants. Ask the patient to compare the palms for brightness and clarity. Finally, place one finger on your nose and one at a distance of 0.5 m from your nose in the nasal, temporal, superior, and inferior fields and ask which of the two fingers is brightest and clearest. This is a test for central scotoma. Holding one of your hands above and one below the horizontal meridian and having the patient compare the two for brightness and clarity helps identify the altitudinal defects that accompany retinal and disk disease.
   C. **Color vision testing.** A book of Ishihara's color plates can be used one eye at a time to test color acuity. Although these plates were designed for testing red–green color blindness, this test can be used as a rough indicator of color acuity, which is a macular function. Test one eye at a time, and use this test especially when looking for evidence of optic nerve damage.
   D. **Pupil tests.** The single most useful objective bedside test of visual function is the pupillary light response test. When there is damage to the ganglion cells or their axons in one eye, optic disk, or optic nerve, there is a less vigorous (less complete) response to a light shone in that eye than to a light shone in the unaffected or normal eye. Damage to both eyes shows a defect in the eye with the greatest amount of visual field loss. There is no describable entity such as bilateral afferent

119

Table 10.1 Causes of visual loss by anatomic location

Retina[a]	Optic disk[b]	Optic nerve[c]	Chiasm/tract[d]	Retrochiasmal[e]
Detachment	Ischemic optic neuropathy	Demyelination	Tumor	Tumor
Ischemia (embolic)	Arteritic	Tumor	Pituitary	Glioma
Infection	Nonarteritic	Meningioma	Glioma	Meningioma
Cytomegalovirus	Optic neuritis (papillitis)	Glioma	Craniopharyngioma	Metastasis
Histoplasmosis	Papilledema	Sarcoid	Mucocele (sphenoid)	Stroke
Toxoplasmosis	Glaucoma	Mucocele	Meningioma	Demyelination
Toxic	Pits/colobomas	Pituitary	Rathke's cleft cyst	Alzheimer's disease
Phenothiazine	Tumors	Tumor	Aneurysm	Creutzfeldt–Jakob
Ethambutol	Sarcoid	Craniopharyngioma	Trauma	disease (Heidenhain)
Degenerative	Degenerative	Rathke's cleft cyst	Demyelination	
Aging	Carcinoma-associated	Aneurysm	Vascular	
Macular degeneration	optic neuropathy	Thyroid ophthalmopathy	Toxic	
Retinitis pigmentosa		Inflammation		
Carcinoma-associated		Trauma (indirect		
retinopathy		traumatic optic		
		neuropathy)		

[a] Appearance of fundus or disk and mode of presentation are key. Visual fields helpful.

[b] Appearance of fundus or disk and mode of presentation are key. Visual fields helpful.

[c] Optic nerve function, appearance of disk, proptosis, and appearance of disk and retinal nerve fiber layer are key. Visual fields helpful.

[d] Visual function—acuity, fields, fundus examination, and visual complaints—are key.

[e] Associated general neurologic findings, visual fields, and computed tomographic or magnetic resonance imaging findings are key.

pupil defect. Swinging the light from eye to eye elicits a brisker reaction (a more complete response) to light in the unaffected eye and a less brisk reaction or dilation of the pupil in the affected eye. This is the **relative afferent pupillary defect** (RAPD). If one eye is blind, the reaction to light is gone completely—this is an amaurotic pupil. For details of the examination of the pupil for RAPD, refer to Chapter 11.

E. **Ophthalmoscopy.** The fundus examination is key in establishing the appearance of the optic disk—pallor, swelling, or anomalous appearance—and the appearance of the retina and macula. In chronically choked optic disks, the venous drainage is frequently diverted into collaterals known as **optociliary collateral vessels,** which drain the venous blood out through the vortex veins into the orbit rather than into the cavernous sinus.

F. **Visual evoked potentials (VEPs).** This test tends to be overused, but it can be valuable for two types of patients: (1) patients with a history suggestive of optic neuritis and with minimal or no residual signs, who frequently have an abnormally prolonged latency and (2) patients who are functionally blind, provided the patient is attentive. Uncooperative patients with functional visual loss can focus past the VEP screen, defocus or look around the screen, and alter VEP latency (implicit time). Thus a normal latency in this setting is useful, but an abnormal latency may be misleading.

G. **Formal visual field testing** consists of three types of tests.

1. The **tangent screen examination** is performed on a flat black screen located 1 m from the patient. It is especially helpful in that it allows the examiner to back the patient up to 2 or 3 m and use the tangent screen to look for tunnel vision or to magnify small central visual defects. This type of visual field is useful only for the inner 20 to 30 degrees of vision. This is the most common type of formal field testing performed in a neurologist's office, but today it is uncommon to encounter a neurologist who actually conducts such studies.

2. **Kinetic perimetry** is performed on a Goldmann perimeter with suprathreshold kinetic targets and is conducted in an ophthalmologist's office. This form of perimetry is being supplanted by the static or Humphrey perimeter (see **3.**).

3. The **static (Humphrey) perimeter** is used to test threshold static targets. This test is performed in an ophthalmologist's office.

II. **Acute transient monocular visual loss (TMVL)**

A. **Clinical features.** Acute TMVL is relatively common and occurs in a host of forms (Tables 10.2 and 10.3). First, before concluding that the patient has had a monocular event, explore the possibility that the "monocular" event was really binocular—that is, homonymous hemianopia. Patients with homonymous visual defects say that halves of objects are gone or that they cannot see well to one side. They may insist that when they close one eye and then the other, the visual loss is only unilateral, but frequently they are simply seeing what they think they should be seeing. In addition, monocular visual loss occasionally is reported as being sudden in onset when in reality it was suddenly and unexpectedly discovered when the normal eye was covered and the patient could not see well out of the affected eye. The most common important cause of true monocular visual loss is artery-to-artery or heart-to-artery embolism, but there are many causes of transient or permanent acute visual loss (Table 10.2).

B. **Approach to TMVL**

1. Be sure historically that the spells are in one eye and not homonymous.

2. Look for evidence of optic disk anomaly, swelling, or residues of retinal embolism (hemorrhage, soft exudate, embolic plugs of cholesterol, platelets, fibrin, or calcium).

3. Look for RAPD, visual field loss, and loss of visual acuity.

4. Look for proptosis (sign of intraorbital mass lesion) causing intermittent amaurosis as a result of vascular compression by eye movement.

5. Auscultate the heart and carotid arteries for murmurs and bruits.

6. Request the following **laboratory studies:**

   a. Complete blood cell count, including platelets

   b. Erythrocyte sedimentation rate

Table 10.2 Sources of transient monocular visual loss

Intraocular
  Recurrent hyphema (intraocular lens haptics)
  Glaucoma[a]
  Papilledema[a]
  Disk drusen[a]
  Congenital cavitary disk anomalies[a]
  Anterior ischemic optic neuropathy
    Arteritic
    Nonarteritic
  Choroidal insufficiency (ocular ischemia)
Intraorbital (intermittent vascular compression)
  Hemangioma
  Osteoma
  Meningioma
Intracranial
  Arteriovenous malformations
  Brain tumors
Embolic to retina (central or branch retinal artery occlusion)
  Intracranial aneurysm
  Cardiac
    Valvular debris
      Infective endocarditis
      Rheumatic valvular disease
      Bicuspid aortic valve
      Mitral valve prolapse
    Clot
      Atrial fibrillation
      Ventricular subendocardial ischemia
      Akinetic segment
      Ventricular aneurysm
      Right-to-left shunt
        Patent foramen ovale
        Atrial septal defect
        Atrial septal aneurysm
      Atrial myxoma
  Aortic atherosclerosis
  Carotid disease
    Dissection
    Atherosclerosis
    Fibromuscular dysplasia
  Fat embolism
    Pancreatitis
    Fractures
Hematologic
  Polycythemia
  Sickle cell disease
  Thrombocytosis
Hypotension
Demyelinating disease
  Uhthoff's phenomenon
Vasospasm
  Hypertensive crisis, especially among paraplegic or quadriplegic patients
  Migraine

[a] These causes usually last seconds and are known as transient visual obscurations. They are frequently binocular as well as monocular.

Table 10.3 Syndromes of transient visual loss

Name	Synonym	Duration	Pain	Characteristics
Amaurosis fugax	Transient monocular visual loss, transient monocular blindness	Seconds to hours, usually <5 min	Rare	Complete, altitudinal, or quadrantic loss; spots or constriction
Transient visual obscuration	Transient obnubilation	Seconds	No	Gray-, black-, or white-out of vision
Uthhoff's phenomenon	None, usually in an eye that has had optic neuritis	Minutes to 1 h	No	Precipitated by heat or exercise
Migraine aura	Fortification specters or spectra, teichopsia	5–45 min	Usually following the visual symptoms, but occasionally painless (so-called acephalgic migraine)	Zigzags, flashes, lights sparkles, heat wave, or water-on-window sensation

        c. C-reactive protein level

        d. For patients younger than 40 years, strongly consider evaluation for hypercoagulable states

            (1) Protein C

            (2) Protein S

            (3) Antithrombin III

            (4) Prothrombin time and partial thromboplastin time

            (5) Lupus anticoagulant

            (6) Antiphospholipid antibodies

            (7) Fibrinogen

    7. Perform transthoracic and transesophageal **echocardiography,** looking especially at the aortic arch and the atrial septum for evidence of patent foramen ovale, atrial septal defect, atrial septal aneurysm (>1.0 cm), and atrial myxoma.

    8. Perform carotid **Doppler** and transcranial Doppler ultrasonography.

    9. Consider cerebral angiography.

    10. Remember that emboli from the carotid arteries are only one cause of TMVL and that there can be more than one convincing potential cause of TMVL. It is always valuable to **refer** the patient with visual loss as a primary problem for examination by an ophthalmologist, who can measure intraocular pressure, perform a dilated indirect ophthalmoscopic examination, perform formal visual field tests, and obtain fundus photos. Most patients examined by neurologists have already been examined by an ophthalmologist or optometrist if the primary problem is visual.

III. Subacute monocular visual loss occurs in two age groups: 15 to 45 years, when it is usually painful, especially with eye movement, and older than 50 years, when it is usually stepwise and painless.

    A. Clinical syndromes

        1. Optic neuritis occurs in younger patients with monocular painful visual loss. Visual loss may follow the pain by a matter of days. Pain is worse with eye movement. The visual loss is characterized as a "skim, scum, blur, fog, or haze" or may be described as if there were a cloud in front of the eye. Vision may be characterized as dim, dark, or bright.

        Colors are dim, washed out, or gone entirely, and low-contrast images are lost. One third of patients have swollen optic disks. Patients occasionally describe phosphenes (spots and sparkles) with loud noise. Visual acuity may range from 20/20 to no light perception, but 20/50 to 20/200 is the rule. The visual field loss is monocular and usually central, altitudinal, or both. The prognosis for visual return within weeks is excellent.

        2. Anterior ischemic optic neuropathy (AION). An older patient with monocular subacute, occasionally stepwise visual loss that is painless has ischemia to the optic disk known as AION. This condition has two forms.

            a. Nonarteritic AION (NAION). The nonarteritic form of AION is believed to be in large part related to ischemia, a predisposing factor to which is an anatomically small scleral canal through which all of the axons of the optic nerve pass on their way to the chiasm and beyond. This small scleral canal causes the disk to be small, tightly packed, and a set-up for an ischemic cascade that can be abrupt and cataclysmic or gradual and stepwise (Fig. 10.1). NAION is painless and usually produces inferior altitudinal, inferior nasal quadrantic, or central scotomatous visual field defects. In 40% of patients, the second eye is affected within 2 years.

            b. Arteritic AION. The main difference between NAION and the arteritic form of AION is age. Arteritic AION is attributable to giant cell arteritis and is usually a disease of the elderly. The added features with suspected giant cell arteritis include headache and superimposed antecedent brief amaurotic attacks resulting from choroidal ischemia especially affecting the optic disk. Other symptoms include tenderness of the scalp, jaw claudication, aching pain in the shoulders and hips, weight loss, fever, and night sweats. Arteritic AION causes sudden severe

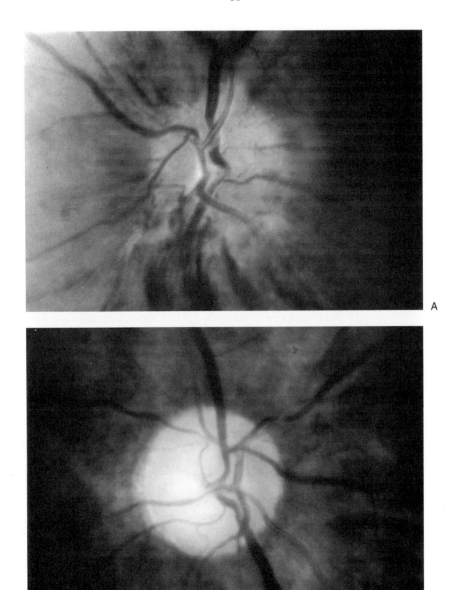

FIG. 10.1 Nonarteritic anterior ischemic optic neuropathy (NAION). **A:** Acute NAION in the right eye with swelling and hemorrhage. **B:** Previous atrophic NAION in the left eye. Marked temporal pallor and preserved tint of the nasal disk are evident. This combination of a swollen disk in one eye and a pallid disk in the fellow eye superficially resembles the rarely seen Foster Kennedy syndrome. Swelling of the disk in Foster Kennedy syndrome is caused by papilledema. In pseudo–Foster Kennedy syndrome the swelling is caused by anterior ischemic optic neuropathy and is associated with severe visual loss.

visual loss and is a diagnostic emergency. Visual acuity is 20/200 or less, and the visual field shows an altitudinal defect with a large central scotoma. There is an RAPD or in some cases an amaurotic (blind and unreactive) pupil. In addition to measurement of erythrocyte sedimentation rate and C-reactive protein, temporal artery biopsy should be performed.

A patient with suspected giant cell arteritis should be treated with 80 to 120 mg of prednisone per day. If there is already ischemic optic neuropathy, the dosage should be increased to 1 g/d methylprednisolone intravenously for 3 to 5 days. Treatment almost always relieves symptoms within 24 to 48 hours. If it does not, the diagnosis is in doubt. Relief of symptoms even with normal biopsy findings is strong evidence of giant cell arteritis. As with NAION, the disk is swollen, but it is usually pallid with a few small splinter hemorrhages (Fig. 10.2). Prognosis for return of vision is poor. The risk of involvement of the second eye, if left untreated, is high.

c. **Leber's optic neuropathy** is a syndrome of painless monocular visual loss over days, characteristically found among men in the teens to 20s (male-to-female ratio of 8:1). It is a disorder of mitochondrial DNA. The second eye is involved weeks to months after the first eye. The disk is slightly swollen and exhibits tortuous small telangiectatic vessels. After a few weeks, the nerve fiber layer becomes atrophic. This occurs first between the 7 and 11 o'clock positions in the right eye and between the 1 and 5 o'clock positions in the left eye. Later, both disks become diffusely pale. Visual loss ranges from acuity of 20/80 to 20/800 and central scotomas that can extend (break out) into the periphery of the visual field. The diagnosis is confirmed by means of examination of mitochondrial DNA to identify the appropriate mutations.

B. **Approach to permanent or long-lasting monocular visual loss**

1. Try to determine historically the pace of visual loss. Was it discovered when the unaffected eye was covered? Was there gradual and progressive visual dysfunction in that eye, or did the visual loss occur abruptly and the vision remain poor?

2. Look for evidence of optic disk swelling or pallor and for evidence of embolic material in the retina (Fig. 10.3).

3. Look for RAPD, perform confrontation visual field testing, and document visual acuity.

4. Decide whether this visual loss appears to have resulted from vascular embolic disease, in which case proceed as if the patient has TMVL—that is, look for a source of embolism (Fig. 10.4).

5. If the visual loss appears to be attributable to optic neuritis (pain on eye movement and subacute visual loss over a few days), proceed to MRI and lumbar puncture.

6. If it appears that the visual loss was actually more gradual in onset or has been present longer than recognized and there is evidence of optic disk pallor, perform CT and MRI to look for a compressive lesion from orbital apex to optic chiasm.

IV. **The syndrome of chronic progressive monocular visual loss** is characteristic of optic nerve compression. Visual acuity may well be normal early, but patients notice that something is not quite right. They report blurs or smudges and may repeatedly clean their glasses or have their refraction checked, resulting in one of the "handful of glasses" syndromes (Table 10.4). Visual loss usually is painless. If the optic nerve is being compressed by a mass in the orbit, there may be proptosis, limitation of ocular motility, and chemosis. If the optic nerve compression is in the optic canal or is intracranial, proptosis occurs only late.

Severe loss of visual acuity may occur rapidly, and visual field testing reveals a central scotoma that may break out (extend) into the periphery. Color vision is defective, and there is

(*text continues on page 129*)

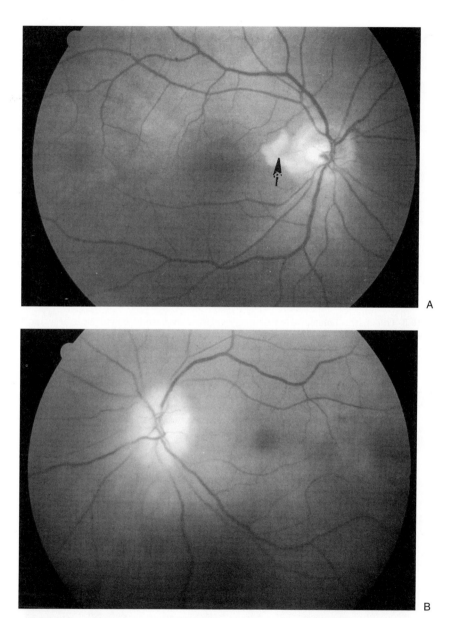

FIG. 10.2 Anterior ischemic optic neuropathy (arteritic). **A:** Disk infarction and a small "tail" of retinal infarction due to occlusion of the cilioretinal artery (CRA) caused by giant cell arteritis (GCA). Occlusion of cilioretinal arteries is almost pathognomonic of GCA (*arrow,* CRA and infarct). **B:** Fellow eye of same patient as in **A** with characteristic pallid swollen disk infarct due to GCA. This patient initially had episodes of transient monocular visual loss that could not be differentiated from embolic amaurosis.

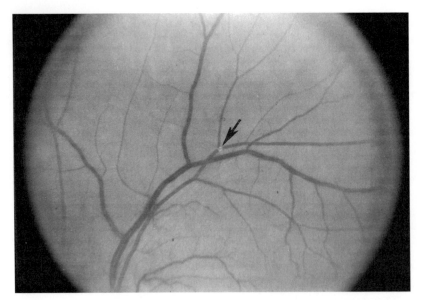

FIG. 10.3 This distal cholesterol embolus (*arrow*) is all that remains of an embolic event that caused total monocular visual loss lasting 15 minutes. Careful, dilated ophthalmoscopy may provide vital clues to the cause of such events.

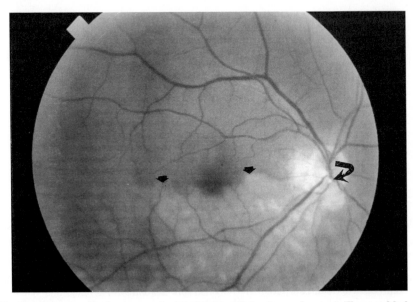

FIG. 10.4 Branch retinal artery occlusion due to embolus (*curved arrow*). The roughly horizontal superior margin of the arcuate nerve fiber layer infarct is marked by the *two smaller arrows*. The macula, which receives its blood supply, stands out as darker (redder) against the pale infarcted retina in a "hemi"-cherry-red macula.

Table 10.4 "Handful of glasses" syndromes

Early optic nerve compression
Bitemporal hemianopia with hemifield slide
Alexia without agraphia
Bilateral small occipital tip lesions
Eye-movement-induced myopia with convergence–retraction nystagmus

an RAPD (Marcus Gunn pupil) in the affected eye. Optic disk swelling, pallor, and atrophy or a mixture of pallor and swelling are common. Optociliary collateral shunt vessels appear on the disk and are evidence of chronic optic nerve compression occurring at the level of the disk with chronic papilledema, of end-stage glaucoma, or, most important, of retrobulbar strangulation of the optic nerve by meningioma, glioma, or sarcoidosis.

VEP testing in the early stages of optic nerve compression with normal or near-normal acuity reveals prolonged latency. After visual acuity has decreased, latency becomes strikingly prolonged, and the amplitude decreases. **Consultation with an ophthalmologist** is appropriate to rule out other treatable ocular causes of visual loss and to obtain formal visual fields and, when appropriate, photographs of the optic disks.

V. Abrupt binocular visual loss (Table 10.5) is rarely caused by bilateral optic disk disease such as ischemic optic neuropathy or optic neuritis. However, when this occurs, the typical patient announces that the vision in both eyes has acutely or subacutely been lost. On examination, one optic disk is pale and atrophic and the other is swollen. This "Foster Kennedy syndrome" is classically attributed to a frontal tumor causing monocular visual loss and optic atrophy in one eye and papilledema in the other eye. However, the most common cause of this ophthalmoscopic combination of atrophy and pallor and disk swelling is **pseudo–Foster**

Table 10.5 Causes of bilateral visual loss (excluding occipital lobe)

Ocular causes
    Anomalous disk[a]
    Papilledema[a]
    Disk drusen[a]
    Pseudo–Foster Kennedy syndrome (bilateral anterior ischemic optic neuropathy)
    Toxic
    Nutritional (tobacco–alcohol amblyopia)
    Medications: ethambutol, chloramphenicol, plaquenil, thioridazine
    Leber's optic neuropathy
Intracranial causes
    Chiasmal
    Tumor (craniopharyngioma, Rathke's cleft cyst, pituitary tumor, meningioma, and other
      rare tumors)
    Aneurysm
    Sphenoid mucocele
    Trauma (chiasmal tear)
    Pituitary apoplexy
    Demyelination
    Vascular (dolichoectatic anterior cerebral artery)
    Combined chiasmal and optic nerve disease caused by any of the above result in
      combinations of bitemporal and central visual loss
Optic tract
    Tumor—same as chiasm
    Demyelination
    Trauma

[a] These causes result in transient visual obscurations, which may be bilateral.

Kennedy syndrome of bilateral sequential anterior ischemic optic neuropathy in a patient who did not notice visual loss in the first eye. The loss of vision in the only properly seeing eye suddenly plunges the patient into unexpected bilateral visual loss.

Transient visual obscuration found among patients with papilledema, drusen of the disk, and other conditions (Tables 10.2 and 10.3) causes transient bouts of binocular dimming or blindness precipitated by a Valsalva maneuver or postural changes. Examination of the fundus should identify any of the congenitally anomalous or swollen disks.

Longer-lasting binocular visual disturbances of rather rapid onset occasionally affect patients with migraine who have basilar migraine. This is a historical diagnosis; laboratory examination is helpful only in ruling out other conditions.

Abrupt binocular visual loss occurs on rare occasions after radiographic procedures. The use of metrizamide for myelography or for intracranial positive contrast studies occasionally can result in bilateral blindness from a toxic–metabolic cause (cortical hypoglycemia). Posterior fossa angiography and coronary angiography also are occasionally attended by what appears to be a toxic reaction to contrast associated with vasospasm.

VI. **Binocular visual loss as a result of chiasmal damage** is found in the pure form, in which there is no damage to optic nerves or optic tracts.
A. **Clinical features**
1. **Bitemporal visual loss.** If the lesion is coming from below (typically pituitary adenoma), the visual loss is superior bitemporal. If the compression is from above (typically an aneurysm of the anterior cerebral artery or craniopharyngioma), the visual field defect is inferior bitemporal. Complete, macula-splitting, bitemporal defects usually are attributable to tumors or traumatic chiasmal tears.

   The visual problems of patients with bitemporal visual loss are not losses of peripheral vision but rather symptoms caused by instability of the two nasal visual fields abutting the midline. These symptoms consist of intermittent and brief doubling of objects, loss of objects, and strange visual effects as a result of vertical sliding of the two hemifields that cause the right halves of images to slip vertically in relation to the left halves. These symptoms are known collectively as the **hemifield slide phenomenon** and are another cause of handful of glasses syndrome (Table 10.4). Because patients with visual symptoms see eye doctors first and rarely articulate the nature of the visual dysfunction adequately, they are commonly provided with new refractions.
2. **Junctional syndrome.** If the chiasmal compression is far anterior, one optic nerve may be compressed at the junction with the chiasm. This produces symptomatic optic nerve compression (see **IV.**) and asymptomatic superior temporal quadrantic visual loss in the other eye. This is caused by damage to a loop of fibers from the inferior nasal part of the contralateral eye that loops into the optic nerve at its junction with the chiasm **(Wilbrand's knee).** Thus a visual field combination of central loss in one eye and a superior temporal defect in the other eye is known as a **junctional syndrome.**
3. **Pituitary apoplexy.** Abrupt onset of unilateral or bilateral visual loss, usually with ocular motility disturbances resulting from paresis of cranial nerves III, IV, and VI and associated with headache, agitation, fever, stiff neck, and blood in the cerebrospinal fluid, occurs with hemorrhage into a pituitary tumor either spontaneously or from emboli following carotid endarterectomy or cardiac surgery. Diagnosis must be suspected and is confirmed with MRI or CT, but patient agitation frequently makes these studies less than optimal for interpretation. Although pituitary apoplexy rarely causes purely visual loss and usually involves ocular motility disturbance, it should be high on the list of causes of sudden onset of bilateral visual loss.
4. **Combination of central and bitemporal visual loss.** Both optic nerves may be gradually compressed by large lesions that also compress the chiasm. This causes both central visual loss and a bitemporal visual field defect. Unless the bitemporal field loss is complete, it is rare for the amount of field loss to be the same in both eyes. Thus the eye with the greatest visual field loss has an RAPD.

B. Clinical approach to subacute or chronic binocular visual loss

1. Look for symptoms in the history that are consistent with hemifield slide and determine which eye seemed to be more affected.

2. Perform confrontation visual field testing to look for bitemporal and central visual field losses. Perform visual acuity tests to look for evidence of optic nerve disease. Perform ophthalmoscopy to look for evidence of optic disk swelling or pallor.

3. Obtain CT scans or MR images to look especially at the suprasellar space, the pituitary fossa, and the sphenoid sinus.

4. Evaluate the fundus. Fundus findings in chiasmal compression depend on the nature of the lesion and whether there is an associated increase in intracranial pressure. Papilledema rarely is found with pituitary adenoma unless the tumor has caused hydrocephalus, and even then optic atrophy may preclude disk swelling. For reasons that are not clear, disk swelling is fairly common in patients with craniopharyngioma, as is severe optic atrophy.

VII. Bilateral visual loss resulting from homonymous hemianopia can be caused by lesions in the optic tract, geniculate nucleus, geniculocalcarine tract, or occipital cortex.

A. Localization of lesions. If hemianopia is complete and splits fixation and there are no other symptoms or signs, the lesion is in either the optic tract or the occipital cortex. Lesions between the optic tract and visual cortex rarely produce complete hemianopia without causing other problems such as hemiparesis, hemisensory loss, aphasia, or neglect. Most cases of hemianopia are incomplete, and location, density, and congruity (superimposability of one field on the other) help to determine the location of the lesion in the neuraxis. With CT and MRI, however, these lesions are rarely a mystery, and homonymous and visual field defects caused by tumors, strokes, and arteriovenous malformations are easily accounted for with these techniques. Occipital lobe damage produces pure visual loss if damage is confined to the calcarine cortex. Total loss of calcarine cortex on one side produces complete homonymous hemianopia, which is rare. More commonly, the macular area is "spared" to some extent because so much of the visual cortex subserves the inner 20 degrees of vision. Conversely, small infarcts in the cortex that represents the inner 20 degrees of the visual field can cause small but disturbing visual field loss that may not be found at Goldmann or Humphrey perimetry and is best identified with a tangent screen. These patients complain bitterly of visual loss that cannot be corrected with glasses (Table 10.3) and frequently go from one eye doctor to another without having the occipital lobe damage detected.

B. Migraine aura. Far and away the most common cause of repeated homonymous visual loss is the visual aura (visual hallucination) of migraine. This is frequently mistaken for visual loss in one eye. The characteristic features of this visual event are movement and "buildup" of the visual loss usually beginning in the center and moving over minutes to the periphery of the visual field. The hallucinations consist of zigzag lines—silvery, colored, bright white, and black—that pulsate, turn, swirl, or glimmer. Although most patients characterize this as a "circle" or "horseshoe" shape to one side, some patients describe a visual image that is central in both eyes "as if a flashbulb just went off" or an arc of shimmering, flashing zigzags in both the right and left fields "like a rainbow." The next most common description is a "heat wave" sensation or the image of water running down a window. These visual events usually last 5 to 45 minutes and are followed by a headache. The headache is usually unilateral but may be generalized and need not be severe or long lasting. Some patients have only the visual aura and no headache—the so-called **acephalgic migraine.**

C. Visual seizures. Metastatic brain tumor, primary glioma, and arteriovenous malformation can cause primary visual seizures with no secondary generalization. These seizures produce sparkles, flashes, and colors, but unlike migraine, they produce no characteristic buildup and progression of the visual event from center to periphery. CT and MRI rapidly depict these conditions, and electroencephalography shows epileptiform activity.

D. **Degenerative diseases.** The common causes of homonymous hemianopsia either are benign and leave no trace (migraine) or produce lesions in the brain that can be detected with CT or MRI (stroke or tumor). Creutzfeldt–Jakob disease may manifest as homonymous hemianopia (the so-called Heidenhain variety); focal Alzheimer's disease also can manifest as homonymous hemianopia. Neither of these conditions has specific CT or MRI findings. Progressive multifocal leukoencephalopathy, a condition much more common among immuncompromised patients, often manifests as dense homonymous hemianopia and large, demyelinating plaques detected in the white matter by means of MRI. This condition characteristically spares the U fibers and the cortex.

VIII. **Syndromes of visual disturbances resulting from higher cognitive dysfunction,** although sometimes caused by tumors, primary or metastatic, are mostly attributable to strokes and are particularly common after cardiac surgical procedures. They frequently go unrecognized.

A. **Alexia without agraphia.** This syndrome is caused by damage to the connections between the primary visual cortices and the angular gyrus. It is the result of either a lesion in the left splenial outflow and the connections of the left occipital lobe to the angular gyrus or of a combination of left occipital infarction and a lesion of the splenium of the corpus callosum. Patients frequently appear with a history of many visits to eye doctors for new glasses because of their inability to read.

B. **Balint's syndrome,** which is caused by bilateral damage to the watershed between the middle and the posterior cerebral circulation, consists of visual disorientation, spasm of fixation (apraxia of gaze), optic ataxia or ataxia of visually guided hand movements, and simultanagnosia (loss of panoramic vision). Patients do not deny their visual troubles but usually suffer in silence unable to verbalize satisfactorily what is wrong. They are not agitated and do not have aphasia or dementia.

C. **Bilateral inferior temporal lobe syndrome.** Damage to the inferior temporal lobe bilaterally in the region of area V4 of the fusiform gyrus causes one or both of the following syndromes: **prosopagnosia** (the inability to recognize faces) and **central achromatopsia** (central color vision loss).

1. **Prosopagnosia** manifests as either sudden bilateral visual disturbance or previous damage to the inferior temporal lobe (which may or may not have been recognized) and a second lesion in the other inferior temporal lobe. Occasional patients have only one lesion, usually in the left hemisphere. They report being unable to recognize faces, but they also have trouble picking out their own cars from other cars and their own dogs from other dogs. In short, although they can identify classes of objects, they have trouble singling out specific items from the general class or group without other clues. Differentiating features of a person's voice or the way a person walks become the cues to identifying people. These patients commonly report that colors are washed out and that whites (linens, snow) look dirty or brownish. They may have homonymous superior quadrantic visual field disturbances or may have no visual field loss.

2. **Central achromatopsia.** Patients with central achromatopsia may also have prosopagnosia or a unilateral defect in color vision known as *central hemiachromatopsia.* Color loss can be profound or consist simply of the desaturation and dirtying of color described by patients with prosopagnosia.

D. **Anton's syndrome** consists of visual loss produced by bilateral damage to the occipital and parietal lobes and the denial of blindness. Patients confabulate elaborately in response to questions about their visual environment.

E. **Approach to patients with homonymous visual field defects**

1. Obtain the best corrected visual acuity.
2. Perform confrontation visual field testing to determine the completeness and the location of the visual field defect.
3. Perform a fundus examination to confirm that disease of the retina or disk is not responsible for the visual loss.
4. Obtain a CT scan or preferably MR images.
5. Refer the patient to an ophthalmologist for formal visual field testing.
6. Perform a neuropsychological evaluation of patients with higher cortical defects.

IX. Functional visual loss. Patients with functional visual loss claim either total or partial loss in one or both eyes. Whatever the motivation or underlying problem, it is possible to uncover functional monocular visual loss simply by looking for an RAPD. In the absence of an RAPD, severe (or even moderate), neurologically significant visual loss does not occur. Patients with functional binocular blindness can be uncovered in one of two ways. Use of an optokinetic target (tape or drum) usually is sufficient, but some patients are able to "look through" these targets. A foolproof method to test for one "blind" eye or bilateral "blindness" is the use of a mirror held in front of the patient's face and tilted up, down, and from side to side. This maneuver produces an irresistible sensation of environmental movement, and the patient's eyes move in an orienting response. Such eye movement proves that the patient can see at least partially.

The most difficult problem is that of the patient who appears with moderate functional visual loss that is equal in both eyes (e.g., 20/50 OU). An RAPD is of no help, and the acuity is too good to make the mirror or optokinetic target useful. In this setting and in the setting of other functional visual loss, referral to an ophthalmologist to ensure that there is no underlying serious ocular disorder is in order. Remember that it is possible for patients voluntarily to alter VEP latency and wave form; thus an abnormal VEP is not helpful. A normal VEP is helpful. Accurate color identification suggests that the central vision is better than the patient claims. Before pronouncing a patient's visual loss functional, be sure to use a pinhole to "refract" or to send the patient for an ophthalmologic refraction.

A. Approach to the patient with functional visual loss

1. Document every visual test performed and the patient's response. This includes how the patient entered the examining room, found the chair and sat down, and regarded the examiner as well as how vigorously testing was resisted.

2. The greater the resistance and complaints about the test, the more likely it is that the patient is a deliberate malingerer. A more naive patient with functional loss gladly cooperates with the examination regardless of the obvious contradictions in performance behavior.

3. Confronting the patient with accusations of malingering is fruitless and counterproductive. Gentle suggestion that vision is better than the patient thinks it is and that the patient's vision is likely to improve reassures almost all but hard-core malingerers.

4. Radiographic or electrophysiologic studies should be performed and the results interpreted for the patient to ensure that no nagging doubts remain. The patient should be told that no disease of the central or peripheral nervous system has been identified.

5. *Do not give drops or pills or refer the patient to a psychiatrist.* Prescriptions for medication give double messages (i.e., "nothing is wrong, but take this medication"), and psychiatric referrals for functional problems do not produce useful results. Simple reassurance is the key.

B. General rules for referral of patients who report visual loss

1. If the patient has seen several eyecare specialists (optometrists or ophthalmologists) and continues to report visual loss, consider the syndromes in Table 10.4.

2. Interpret imaging studies with the visual pathways in mind. If the visual loss is monocular, look at the orbit and intracranial optic nerve. If the visual loss is bitemporal, look at the chiasm and perichiasmal structures.

3. Enlist an ophthalmologist for visual examination if the patient has not yet seen one. Ask that visual field testing be done and for an interpretation of the findings. If the optic disk looks abnormal or the fundus appears abnormal, have photographs taken. As physicians, we obtain chest radiographs for lung disease, and we should obtain fundus photographs for eye disease. Remember that the ophthalmologist can put corneal, lenticular, and visible vitreous and retinal diseases into perspective in regard to visual loss.

4. If a tumor or stroke is causing visual loss, referral to a neurologist is appropriate. If the problem is pituitary apoplexy, it is an emergency. Refer the patient immediately to a neurosurgeon.

Recommended Readings

Aldrich MS, Alessi AG, Beck RW, et al. Cortical blindness: etiology, diagnosis and prognosis. *Ann Neurol* 1987;21: 149–158.

Barton JJS, Corbett JJ. Neuro-ophthalmologic vascular emergencies in the elderly. *Clin Geriatr Med* 1991;7:525–548.

Bernstein EF, ed. *Amaurosis fugax.* New York: Springer-Verlag, 1987.

Brown G, Tasman W. *Congenital anomalies of the optic disc.* New York: Grune & Stratton, 1983.

Bruno A, Corbett JJ, Biller J, et al. Transient monocular visual loss patterns and underlying vascular abnormalities: a prospective study of 100 consecutive patients. *Stroke* 1990;21:34–39.

Carr RE, Siegel IM. *Electrodiagnostic testing of the visual system: a clinical guide.* Philadelphia: FA Davis Co, 1990.

Damasio A, Yamada T, Damasio H, et al. Central achromatopsia: behavioral, anatomic and physiologic aspects. *Neurology* 1980;30:1064–1071.

Frisén L. The neurology of visual acuity. *Brain* 1980;103:639–670.

Ghanchi FD, Dutton GN. Current concepts in giant cell (temporal) arteritis. *Surv Ophthalmol* 1997;42:99–123.

Grant M. *Toxicology of the eye,* 3rd ed. Springfield, IL: Charles C Thomas Publisher, 1986.

Hayreh SS, Podhajsky PA, Zimmerman B. Ocular manifestations of giant cell arteritis. *Am J Ophthalmol* 1998;125:509–520.

Hughes B. Indirect injury to the optic nerves and chiasm. *Bull Johns Hopkins Hosp* 1963;111:98–126.

Hupp SL. Syndromes of the optic chiasm. In: Tusa RJ, Newman SA, eds. *Neuro-ophthalmological disorders: diagnostic workup and management.* New York: Marcel Dekker, 1995: 65–75.

Hupp SL, Kline LB, Corbett JJ. Visual disturbances of migraine. *Surv Ophthalmol* 1989; 33:221–236.

Kathol RG, Cox TA, Corbett JJ, et al. Functional visual loss: follow up of 42 cases. *Arch Ophthalmol* 1983;101:729–735.

Lessell S. Indirect optic nerve trauma. *Arch Ophthalmol* 1989;107:382–386.

Rizzo M. The role of striate cortex: evidence from human brain lesion studies. In: Peters A, Rockland K, eds. *Cerebral cortex.* Vol 10. New York: Plenum, 1994:504–540.

Rizzo M, Nawrat M. Human visual cortex and its disorders. *Curr Opin Ophthalmol* 1993; 4:30–37.

Thompson HS. Functional visual loss. *Am J Ophthalmol* 1985;100:209–213.

Thompson HS, Corbett JJ. Swinging flashlight test. *Neurology* 1989;39:154–156.

Trobe JD, Acosta PC, Krischer JP, et al. Confrontation visual field techniques in the detection of anterior visual pathway lesions. *Ann Neurol* 1981;10:28–34.

Wray SH. Amaurosis fugax. In: Tusa RJ, Newman SA, eds. *Neuro-ophthalmological disorders: diagnostic workup and management.* New York: Marcel Dekker, 1995:3–26.

11. APPROACH TO THE PATIENT WITH ABNORMAL PUPILS

Aki Kawasaki

The **pupillary light reflex** is composed of an afferent and an efferent limb. The **afferent limb** begins with the retinal ganglion cells, which transmit light (visual) and pupillary impulses through fibers of the optic nerve, chiasm, and tract. At the distal end of the optic tract, homonymous sets of light and pupillary impulses separate from each other to reach different synaptic sites: light (visual) impulses to the lateral geniculate nucleus and pupillary impulses to the pretectal nucleus. Each pretectal nucleus in the dorsal midbrain continues the afferent relay by sending pupillary impulses to both the ipsilateral and contralateral Edinger–Westphal nucleus of the oculomotor nuclear complex. The Edinger–Westphal nucleus begins the **efferent limb** of the pupillary light reflex and transmits pupillomotor impulses through the parasympathetic fibers of the oculomotor nerve. After synapsing in the ciliary ganglion of the orbit, the short ciliary nerves complete the efferent neural connection to the pupilloconstrictor muscle of the iris. Pupil size and reactivity are equal as long as the output signals from the Edinger–Westphal nuclei are equal.

Proper equipment for pupillary examination includes a millimeter ruler, a bright handheld light source (a nonhalogen penlight is not bright enough), a darkened room, 4% or 10% cocaine hydrochloride eyedrops, and 1% pilocarpine eyedrops. Be sure to ask the patient whether any ophthalmic medications have been used in the past 24 hours.

    I. Pupillary examination. *Objective:* To recognize abnormal pupils and then differentiate afferent and efferent pupillary defects.

        A. Hippus. An awake patient sitting quietly in room light has spontaneous oscillations of pupil size. This phenomenon is known as *hippus,* and it reflects spontaneous fluctuation in the tone and activity of the parasympathetic and sympathetic nervous systems. Supranuclear stimuli such as a startle or pain activate the sympathetic system and inhibit the parasympathetic system, thus dilating the pupils. Conversely, drowsiness causes progressive miosis.

        B. Pupil size. Average pupil diameter is greatest (7.0 to 7.5 mm) during the teenage years and then gradually decreases with increasing age. Have the patient fixate a distant target in dim room light and record the pupil size. Anisocoria of 0.4 mm or more is clinically visible. If any asymmetry of size exists, carefully note whether the anisocoria is greater in darkness or under bright lights. (To measure anisocoria in darkness, turn off the room light and hold a handlight at the level of the patient's chin, illuminating the eyes just enough to view and measure the pupils.)

           1. Normal pupils are sometimes slightly unequal in size, but seldom by more than 1.0 mm, and the difference can increase a small amount in darkness (see **III.B.1**).

           2. Significant anisocoria (greater than 1.0 mm) indicates an efferent pupillomotor problem (see **III.**).

           3. Subtle Horner's syndrome can be missed because there may be very little anisocoria under regular room light conditions. Anisocoria is easier to detect in darkness (see **IV.A.1**).

        C. Pupillary light reaction

           1. Direct light response. Have the patient fixate on a distant target in a dark room. Shine a bright focal light directly onto one pupil for 3 seconds and record the amplitude and velocity of constriction. Do this for each pupil two or three times for a mental "average."

           2. Consensual pupillary response. Sometimes it is important to view the consensual pupillary response, the reaction of one pupil while shining a light onto the other pupil. The consensual response is not routinely checked; it is difficult to see because the consensual pupil is not illuminated. If a pupil consistently has poor or sluggish direct light reaction, check its consensual reaction (shine a light in the other pupil while observing this pupil). If this pupil also has a poor and sluggish consensual reaction, there is an efferent defect, either in the parasympathetic pupilloconstrictor pathway or in the iris sphincter muscle itself. In the resting state, anisocoria that is more apparent under bright lights also is typically present.

Simply noting that a pupil is "sluggish" to direct light stimulation is not enough information to differentiate an afferent from an efferent pupillary defect.

   a. A pupil with an efferent defect does not react well to any afferent stimulation—direct light, consensual light, or near effort—unless there is aberrant regeneration of damaged axons.

   b. A pupil with injury to its afferent limb of the pupillary light reflex (relative afferent pupillary defect; RAPD) reacts poorly only to direct light stimulation. It is capable of a normal brisk constriction if given another stimulus such as a consensual light or near effort.

   c. An afferent defect (RAPD) is not a cause of anisocoria.

D. Alternating light test. This is the standard clinical technique for identifying asymmetry of afferent input between the two eyes. This asymmetry is referred to as *RAPD*, sometimes called *Marcus Gunn pupil*. The patient usually reports poor vision in the eye with an RAPD.

   1. Have the patient fixate a distant target in a dark room. Shine a bright focal light directly onto one pupil for 3 seconds, then quickly swing the light onto the other pupil for 3 seconds. Repeat this for four or five alternations of light stimulation. Watch only the illuminated pupil (direct light response). The normal response is symmetric pupillary constriction followed by equal redilation in both eyes.

   2. In an eye with a **large RAPD,** the pupil of the bad eye constricts poorly compared with the opposite pupil during an alternating light test (comparison of the direct pupillary light responses). Because the pupil of the bad eye is constricting normally to consensual light stimulation—that is, shining the light into the good eye—then this pupil seems to dilate when the light is quickly alternated back onto it. In other words, the bad eye "sees" less light as compared with the good eye.

   3. A **small-to-moderate RAPD** is a bit more difficult to detect than is a large defect. The bad eye generates a good pupillary constriction to direct light but on close inspection, it is a less vigorous response compared with that of the pupil of the good eye. The pupil of the bad eye may also "escape," that is, redilate, sooner after the initial constriction.

      a. Neutral density filters can be used to "titrate" the pupil responses to a balance point and quantitate the RAPD. Place progressively darker neutral density filters over the good eye and repeat the alternating light test until the pupil responses are equal.

      b. If only one pupil is working properly, compare its direct light response to its consensual light response. The reactions should be equal if the afferent functions of both eyes are intact.

II. Afferent pupillary defect. The presence of an RAPD is a sensitive indicator of unilateral or asymmetric injury to the afferent limb of the pupillary light reflex. If an RAPD is found, it needs to be investigated. In general, the size of the RAPD (asymmetry of afferent pupillary impulses) correlates with the asymmetry of visual field loss. It also tends to vary with the location of the lesion within the afferent pathway (Fig. 11.1).

   A. Ocular and retinal lesions

      1. Large unilateral retinal lesions such as central retinal artery occlusion or trauma produce a clear RAPD. Visual acuity is generally poor. Findings of a careful dilated funduscopic examination usually provide enough information for diagnosis, so an ophthalmology consultation is important.

      2. Cataracts, corneal opacities, and vitreous lesions do not cause an RAPD, even when the visual loss is severe.

   B. Optic nerve lesions. Damage to the optic nerve almost always produces an RAPD, and a visual field defect is almost invariably detected at formal perimetry testing. Loss of acuity is variable. The optic disk can appear normal or swollen in the acute phase of injury but later has pallor. Examples of optic nerve disorders include optic neuritis, ischemic optic neuropathy, hereditary optic neuro-

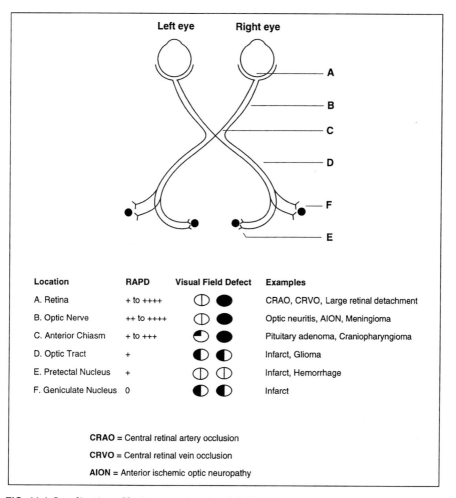

FIG. 11.1 Localization of lesions causing visual field defects and relative afferent pupillary defect (RAPD). *Plus signs* (+) represent grading of RAPD. Visual fields are represented as right-eye visual field on the right side and left-eye visual field on the left.

pathy, compressive lesions, exposure to toxins, trauma, and cellular infiltration (see Chapter 10).

1. The largest RAPDs occur in association with unilateral optic nerve disorders.
2. "Resolved" optic neuritis can result in optic disk pallor and a residual RAPD despite functional recovery to normal visual acuity and normal visual field.
3. The extent of damage in bilateral optic nerve disorders is rarely symmetric. Therefore, an RAPD is found on the side with greater damage. Look carefully.

C. Optic chiasm
1. Compressive lesions of the optic chiasm can produce asymmetric visual loss and therefore an RAPD. A junctional scotoma commonly is found.
2. Truly symmetric bitemporal hemianopsia is not associated with an RAPD because the injury to the visual and pupillary pathways is symmetric.

   D. Optic tract lesions. Anatomically, there are slightly more optic nerve fibers
      that decussate at the chiasm than do not. Therefore, a complete optic tract lesion
      can produce a small RAPD in the contralateral eye. Consider an optic tract lesion
      in any patient with complete homonymous hemianopsia and an afferent defect
      (RAPD) in the eye with the temporal field loss.
   E. Pretectal nucleus
      1. The pretectal nucleus in the dorsal midbrain is the final synaptic site of
         pupillary impulses coming from the optic tract through the brachium of the
         superior colliculus. Visual impulses, however, have separated to the lateral
         geniculate nucleus. Therefore, a unilateral dorsal midbrain lesion such as
         stroke or tumor that involves the pretectal nucleus on one side can produce
         a small contralateral RAPD and no visual loss.
      2. RAPDs arising from optic tract or midbrain lesions are small usually and
         are fairly rare.
III. Efferent pupillary defect. The differential diagnosis of anisocoria is either a structural (mechanical) defect of the iris muscles or a neural efferent (parasympathetic or sympathetic) pupillary defect (Fig. 11.2). Physiologic anisocoria and pharmacologically manipulated
pupils are two nonpathologic conditions that must always be considered in the differential
diagnosis.
   A. Structural iris damage: "ophthalmologic" anisocoria. The iris contains two
      muscles that modulate pupil size and shape—the circular sphincter and the
      radial dilator. Therefore, structural iris defects can distort the size and shape of
      the pupil as well as its constriction and dilation responses, even though the neural
      afferent and efferent pathways are intact. If iris mechanics are suspect, first
      examine the iris muscles under a slit-lamp because this might avoid unnecessary
      ancillary tests.
      1. **History.** Inquire about any previous ocular infection, inflammation, trauma,
         or surgical procedures.
      2. **Examination.** Some iris defects, such as iris coloboma and iridectomy, are
         visually apparent, whereas others, such as synechiae (adhesions) and small

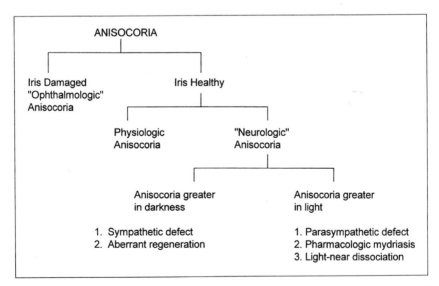

FIG. 11.2 Differential diagnosis of anisocoria. Sometimes it is difficult to say whether the
anisocoria becomes worse in dark or light. In this circumstance, a detailed history and other
examination findings may provide clues.

sphincter tears, require slit-lamp biomicroscopy. Marked irregularity of the pupillary margin, unusual distortions of pupillary shape, and differences in iris color are clues that iris damage may be present. A dusting of iris pigment may be observed in a ring on the lens of a patient who has had a blow to the eye.

B. Structurally intact iris. If the iris appears healthy, the next important determination is whether the anisocoria is physiologic.

   1. Physiologic anisocoria

      a. This disorder has been called *benign* or *essential anisocoria* and *simple central anisocoria.*

      b. Incidence. Approximately 20% of the healthy population have pupillary inequality of 0.4 mm or more in dim lighting.

      c. Clinical characteristics

         (1) Physiologic anisocoria usually is a difference in pupil diameter of 0.4 to 1.0 mm.

         (2) Physiologic anisocoria is slightly greater in darkness than in bright light. Patients often notice anisocoria "disappears" in the sunlight.

         (3) Physiologic anisocoria can vary in amplitude (even within a few minutes).

         (4) Physiologic anisocoria can even "reverse" sides—that is, the larger pupil can be on one side at first but on the other side later.

         (5) Pupillary constriction to light and near stimulation is normal in both eyes.

         (6) Pupillary dilation to darkness is normal.

      d. Work-up: none. Physiologic anisocoria can be confused with Horner's syndrome because both conditions cause greater, more apparent anisocoria in darkness (Fig. 11.3). Look for other clinical evidence of oculosympathetic damage (see **IV.A.1.**).

   2. "Neurologic" anisocoria is discussed in **IV.** The discussion concerns a healthy iris when physiologic anisocoria has been ruled out. The guidelines in **IV.** are not applicable to bilateral or mixed sympathetic or parasympathetic pupil defects.

IV. Neurologic anisocoria. (Read **III.** first.) Two iris muscles regulate pupil size. The sphincter (pupilloconstrictor) is innervated by the parasympathetic system, and the dilator (pupillodilator) is innervated by the sympathetic system. Determine whether anisocoria is greater in darkness (dilation problem in the eye with the smaller pupil) or in bright light (constriction problem in the eye with the larger pupil).

  A. Anisocoria greater in darkness

    1. Horner's syndrome (oculosympathetic defect)

      a. Clinical characteristics

         (1) Ptosis. There is upper lid ptosis and "upside-down" lower lid ptosis (elevation of the lower lid). Together they create the impression

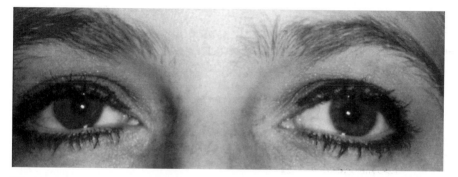

FIG. 11.3 Patient with a physiologic anisocoria.

of enophthalmos but do not constitute true enophthalmos. The upper-lid ptosis of Horner's syndrome is generally mild. Especially in older patients, it can be inapparent if the opposite eyelid is dehiscent or droopy from age-related skin changes.

- (2) **Smaller pupil.** The anisocoria usually is not marked in room light but is more apparent in darkness. Remember that the anisocoria stems from a failure of the smaller pupil to dilate (Fig. 11.4).
- (3) **Dilation lag.** When the lights are first turned off, a normal pupil dilates promptly, but the smaller Horner's pupil initially dilates more slowly—that is, it "lags." Illuminate the patient's face from below with a flashlight. Turn off the room lights and watch the anisocoria slowly change. The anisocoria is barely visible in bright light, then maximally visible at 5 seconds of darkness, and then smaller again after 15 to 20 seconds of darkness as the Horner's pupil finally dilates. (Drowsiness causes miosis and obscures dilation lag. Arouse the patient before testing for dilation lag.)
- (4) **Ipsilateral facial anhidrosis.** This finding is not present with postganglionic sympathetic lesions (see **IV.A.1.c.**).
- (5) **Heterochromia iridis** (different iris color) accompanies congenital Horner's syndrome.

b. **Pharmacologic testing: cocaine test.** Cocaine inhibits presynaptic reuptake of released norepinephrine at the postganglionic neuromuscular synapse. When the entire oculosympathetic pathway is intact, cocaine normally dilates the pupils. (Inform the patient that the urine will test positive for cocaine for the next 48 to 72 hours.)

- (1) Do not touch the corneas or use eyedrops before the cocaine test— that is, do not check corneal reflexes or intraocular pressure. Contact lenses should not be worn 24 hours before the test.
- (2) Place 2 drops (1 minute apart) of 4% to 10% cocaine hydrochloride ophthalmic solution in each eye. Wait 40 to 60 minutes.
- (3) A normal pupil will dilate. A Horner's pupil will not dilate. Postcocaine anisocoria of 1.0 mm or greater is considered confirmation of the diagnosis.

c. **Anatomy of the oculosympathetic pathway**

- (1) The central oculosympathetic neuron originates in the posterolateral hypothalamus and descends in the lateral brainstem to the spinal cord.
- (2) The preganglionic neuron originates in the lateral horn of the spinal cord at C8–T2, the ciliospinal center of Budge–Waller. Its fibers skirt the apex of the lung and under the subclavian artery before ascending in the anterior neck.
- (3) The postganglionic neuron originates in the superior cervical ganglion, and its pupillary fibers are intimately associated with the

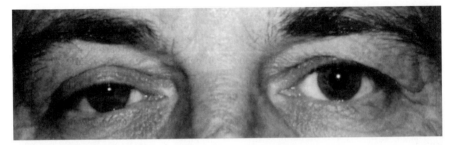

FIG. 11.4 Patient with Horner's syndrome of the right eye. Note the anisocoria, which is clearly visible in dim room light. Upper and lower lid ptosis of the right eye create a false impression of enophthalmos.

internal carotid artery through the neck, base of the skull, and cavernous sinus. (The vasomotor sympathetic fibers travel separately with the external carotid artery.) In the orbit, the oculosympathetic fibers are carried in the long ciliary nerves.

  d. Etiology of Horner's syndrome. In general, central Horner's syndrome is stroke related. Preganglionic lesions can be neoplastic, and postganglionic lesions are mostly benign (Table 11.1). Painful postganglionic Horner's syndrome should be evaluated for internal carotid artery dissection.

  e. Work-up for Horner's syndrome

    (1) Clinical localization

        (a) Central Horner's syndrome usually is accompanied by other symptoms or signs of brainstem dysfunction (e.g., Wallenberg's syndrome). There is also anhidrosis throughout the ipsilateral face, neck, and body.

        (b) Preganglionic Horner's syndrome causes ipsilateral anhidrosis of the face only. Weakness and wasting of the ipsilateral hand muscles suggest injury to the C8–T2 spinal rootlets or brachial plexus. If there is also pain in the supraclavicular fossa, an apical lung tumor can be suspected. Inquire about any past surgical procedures on or trauma to the neck or chest, such as use of central catheters, thyroidectomy, or history of physical assault or choking.

        (c) Horner's syndrome in a patient with vascular headaches usually is postganglionic in origin. There is no clinically appreciable facial anhidrosis. Sudden pain in the jaw, ear, throat, or peritonsillar area is characteristic of carotid dissection. Painful postganglionic Horner's syndrome with ipsilateral trigeminal dysfunction (dysesthesia, numbness) is called **Raeder's paratrigeminal syndrome** and has been associated with a variety of lesions in the parasellar–cavernous sinus region.

    (2) Pharmacologic localization: 1% hydroxyamphetamine. Hydroxyamphetamine testing helps differentiate central or preganglionic Horner's syndrome from a postganglionic Horner's syndrome. Hydroxyamphetamine releases stored catecholamines from the postganglionic fiber terminal if the postganglionic fiber is intact. Therefore, the pupil of the eye with a postganglionic oculosympathetic defect does not dilate with administration of hydroxyamphetamine.

        (a) Central or preganglionic Horner's syndrome. If no brainstem symptoms or signs exist, obtain computed tomographic scans or magnetic resonance (MR) images of the neck and chest. If the findings are normal, obtain cranial MR images. If brainstem signs are present, cranial MR imaging is indicated first.

        (b) Postganglionic Horner's syndrome requires head and neck MR imaging. Angiography can be considered if carotid dissection is a diagnostic differential. Cluster headaches can cause postganglionic Horner's pupil in as many as 22% of cases. If the history is typical of cluster headache and other neurologic deficits are absent, radiologic studies are not necessary.

2. Aberrant regeneration of the oculomotor nerve

  a. Pathophysiology. When a structural lesion compresses or transects the oculomotor (third cranial) nerve, the fibers innervating the extraocular muscles can sprout misguided collaterals that aberrantly innervate the iris sphincter. Primary ischemic injury such as diabetic third nerve palsy essentially never causes aberrant regeneration.

Table 11.1 Causes of injury to the oculosympathetic pathway (Horner's syndrome)

Central	Preganglionic	Postganglionic
Hypothalamus	Cervicothoracic cord, spinal roots	Superior cervical ganglion
Infarct	Trauma	Iatrogenic (surgical removal, tonsillectomy)
Tumor	Intramedullary or paravertebral tumor	Trauma
Brainstem	Syrinx	Internal carotid artery
Ischemia	AVM	Dissection
Hemorrhage	Spondylosis	Trauma
Tumor	Epidural anesthesia	Thrombosis
Demyelination (MS)	Lower brachial plexus	Tumor
Cervical cord	Birth trauma	Migraine, cluster headache
Trauma	Acquired trauma	Base of skull, carotid canal
Tumor	Pulmonary apex, under subclavian artery	Tumor (e.g., nasopharyngeal carcinoma, lymphoma)
Syrinx	Vascular anomalies (e.g., subclavian aneurysm,	Trauma
AVM	aortic tortuosity)	Middle ear
	Pancoast (apical lung) tumor	Tumor (e.g., cholesteatoma)
	Cervical rib	Infection
	Iatrogenic (e.g., chest tube)	Cavernous sinus
	Infection (e.g., apical tuberculosis)	Tumor (meningioma, pituitary adenoma)
	Anterior neck	Inflammation (Tolosa–Hunt syndrome)
	Iatrogenic (thyroid surgery, neck dissection, catheter)	Cavernous carotid aneurysm
	Trauma	Thrombosis
	Tumor (lymphoma, breast metastasis)	Fistula

Of all outpatient cases of Horner's syndrome, 3% to 13% have a central cause. Of all outpatient cases of Horner's syndrome, 41% have a preganglionic cause, and of these, 50% are neoplastic. Many cases of benign postganglionic Horner's syndrome are associated with pain. Every infant or child with congenital Horner's syndrome needs evaluation for mediastinal neuroblastoma.
MS, multiple sclerosis; AVM, arteriovenous malformation.

b. Clinical characteristics

(1) **Aberrantly regenerated fibers cause simultaneous unilateral pupilloconstriction** during attempted adduction, supraduction, or infraduction of the globe.

(2) **Miosis.** The aberrantly innervated pupil is typically smaller than the normal pupil, and because it does not dilate well, the anisocoria is more apparent in darkness.

(3) **Reversed anisocoria.** Although aberrantly innervated, the original parasympathetic innervation to the iris sphincter has been disrupted by the structural lesion, and the oculomotor nerve has been damaged. Therefore, that pupil has poor constriction to light. In some cases, the aberrantly innervated pupil is the smaller pupil in darkness and yet is also the larger pupil under bright light.

3. Physiologic anisocoria. See III.B.1.

B. Anisocoria greater in bright light

1. Oculomotor (third cranial) nerve palsy

a. Clinical characteristics

(1) **Ptosis.** Upper-lid ptosis usually is present but can be absent, slight, or complete. Lower-lid ptosis is not present.

(2) **Larger pupil.** Anisocoria is more apparent under bright light. The pupil is rarely "blown"—completely nonreactive—in a noncomatose patient with acute third nerve palsy.

(3) **Ophthalmoplegia.** The patient reports diplopia resulting from limitation of adduction, supraduction, and infraduction.

b. Anatomy of the oculoparasympathetic pathway

(1) **Oculomotor nerve.** The preganglionic neuron originates in the Edinger–Westphal subnuclei in the dorsal midbrain. Its fibers exit at the interpeduncular fossa and then enter the cavernous sinus. At the anterior cavernous sinus–superior orbital fissure, the oculomotor nerve divides into a superior division, which innervates the levator palpebrae and superior rectus muscles and an inferior division that contains fibers for accommodation, pupilloconstriction, and the inferior rectus, medial rectus, and inferior oblique muscles.

(2) **Short ciliary nerves.** The postganglionic neuron originates in the ciliary ganglion of the orbit. The ciliary ganglion is mesial to the lateral rectus muscle, approximately 1 cm behind the globe. Its fibers are the short ciliary nerves that serve both accommodation and pupilloconstriction.

c. Etiology of oculomotor nerve palsy. See Table 11.2 and Chapter 12.

d. Work-up. Any painful oculomotor nerve palsy with pupillary involvement warrants **emergency angiography** to look for an expanding or ruptured posterior communicating artery aneurysm. Remember that early compression by an aneurysm can cause partial oculomotor palsy and no initial pupil dysfunction.

2. Tonic pupil (Adie's pupil). The site of injury for a tonic pupil is the ciliary ganglion cell bodies or their postganglionic parasympathetic fibers carried in the short ciliary nerves. A tonic pupil is the most common neurologic cause of a dilated unreactive pupil in an otherwise healthy patient.

a. Symptoms include anisocoria, photophobia, and blurred near vision.

b. Clinical characteristics

(1) **Larger pupil.** A fresh tonic pupil is very large but becomes smaller over several months.

(2) **Poor light reaction.** Pupillary constriction to light stimulation is minimal and segmental when present but can be completely absent.

(3) **Light-near dissociation (LND).** Pupillary constriction to near stimulation is delayed in onset and slow in velocity. The pupil remains tonically constricted; thus it is called "tonic." The amplitude of the near reaction exceeds the amplitude of the light constriction, which is why there is LND.

Table 11.2   Causes of injury to the oculoparasympathetic pathway resulting in a large, poorly reactive pupil.

Preganglionic (oculomotor nerve)	Postganglionic: "tonic pupil" (ciliary ganglion or short ciliary nerve)
Brainstem (midbrain)—"fascicular" Ischemia Hemorrhage Tumor Arteriovenous malformation	Intraorbital Viral ganglionitis Trauma Ocular surgery Tumor
Interpeduncular fossa, subarachnoid space Basal aneurysm	Systemic peripheral neuropathy Hereditary (e.g., Charcot–Marie– Tooth disease, Riley–Day syndrome)
Basal infection (granulomatous meningitis, fungal meningitis) Intraneural ischemia—"vasculopathic" (e.g., diabetes, hypertension)	Acquired (diabetes, alcohol, toxins, amyloid, vasculitis) Idiopathic (Adie) tonic pupil
Cavernous sinus, superior orbital fissure Tumor (e.g., meningioma, pituitary adenoma) Inflammation (Tolosa–Hunt syndrome) Cavernous carotid aneurysm Thrombosis Fistula	

Brainstem "fascicular" oculomotor nerve palsy occasionally occurs as an isolated finding but is more commonly associated with other neurologic deficits (i.e., Weber's, Benedikt's, Claude's, and Nothnagel's syndromes). Vasculopathic oculomotor nerve palsy tends to spare the pupil. Compressive lesions typically involve the pupil.

    (4) Pupillary redilation after near constriction is slow owing to the tonic constriction. Thus it also has "tonic" redilation.

    (5) Accommodation paresis. Accommodation is lost acutely but may gradually improve.

    (6) Segmental palsy of the iris sphincter necessitates slit-lamp examination. On near effort, the innervated areas of sphincter draw up like a pulled purse string, but the denervated areas flatten out. A tonic pupil is the larger pupil in light because it reacts to light poorly, but because it also dilates tonically, it can be the smaller pupil in darkness (see **IV.A.2.**).

c. Pharmacologic testing: 0.1% pilocarpine

    (1) Dilute regular strength 1% pilocarpine to a 1:10 weak strength ophthalmic solution (0.1%) with saline solution.

    (2) Place 2 drops (1 minute apart) in each eye. Wait 25 to 30 minutes.

    (3) Weak (0.1%) pilocarpine generally does not affect the normal pupil sphincter but induces constriction of the suspected tonic pupil because of cholinergic denervation supersensitivity of the sphincter. (The diagnostic utility of weak pilocarpine testing is based on the assumption that there is one tonic pupil and one normal pupil for comparison.)

d. Pathophysiology

    (1) Acute denervation. Injury to the ciliary ganglion or short ciliary nerves denervates the ciliary muscle and its sphincter; thus accommodation and pupilloconstriction are acutely abolished.

    (2) Aberrant reinnervation. Neurons originally destined for the ciliary muscle for accommodation regrow and correctly reinnervate the ciliary muscle but in addition sprout collaterals to aberrantly reinnervate the iris sphincter. Accommodation improves and tonic pupilloconstriction accompanies accommodation (near effort).

    e. Etiology. See Table 11.2. The most common tonic pupil is idiopathic and unilateral, typically affects women between the ages of 20 and 40 years, and may be associated with generalized hyporeflexia (Adie's syndrome), segmental anhidrosis (Ross' syndrome) or both.

    f. An isolated tonic pupil does not require imaging studies.

  3. Pharmacologic mydriasis

    a. Mydriatic ophthalmic agents include atropine, scopolamine, homatropine, cyclopentolate, tropicamide, phenylephrine, cocaine, and hydroxyamphetamine.

    b. The pupil is maximally dilated and nonresponsive to light or near stimulation.

    c. Other ocular or neurologic findings are absent. There is no history of recent ocular trauma.

    d. Instillation of regular strength 1% pilocarpine does not produce constriction in a pharmacologically dilated pupil. A pupil dilated as a result of a parasympathetic defect (third nerve palsy or tonic pupil) promptly constricts with administration of regular strength 1% pilocarpine.

  4. LND. The amplitude of pupilloconstriction to a light stimulus typically is greater than that to a near stimulus. Never test the near response with a bright light, because the two stimuli summate and create the false impression of LND. LND occurs under the following two circumstances.

    a. The light response limb of the reflex is defective (reduced), but the near response is spared (normal). This circumstance arises with any isolated lesion to the afferent pupillary pathway. It is said that the most common cause of LND is optic neuropathy.

    b. The light response and the near response are defective, but only the near response is restored (aberrant regeneration). The classic example is tonic (Adie's) pupil.

    c. Examples of LND

      (1) Midbrain LND (sylvian aqueduct syndrome, dorsal midbrain syndrome). Both pupils are typically midsize with LND. Associated motility dysfunction includes bilateral lid retraction, supranuclear vertical gaze palsy, and convergence–retraction nystagmus.

      (2) Argyll Robertson pupils. Both pupils are typically small and irregular in shape with an impaired light response, brisk near response, and poor dilation in darkness. Visual function is intact. These pupils originally were described as a sign of central nervous system syphilis.

      (3) Bilateral LND. Bilateral old Adie's pupils and diffuse peripheral neuropathy such as diabetes can cause bilaterally small pupils that have LND. Any bilateral LND warrants serologic testing for syphilis.

  V. Referral. Any diagnostic dilemma regarding the afferent or efferent pathways of the pupil should be referred to a neuroophthalmologist.

Recommended Readings

Corbett JJ, Thompson HS. Pupillary function and dysfunction. In: Asbury AK, McKhann GM, McDonald WI, eds. *Diseases of the nervous system: clinical neurobiology.* Philadelphia: WB Saunders, 1992:490–500.

Cox TA, Thompson HS, Corbett JJ. Relative afferent pupillary defects in optic neuritis. *Am J Ophthalmol* 1981;92:685–690.

Cremer SA, Thompson HS, Digre KB, et al. Hydroxyamphetamine mydriasis in Horner's syndrome. *Am J Ophthalmol* 1990;110:71–76.

Czarnecki JSC, Thompson HS. The iris sphincter in aberrant regeneration of the third nerve. *Arch Ophthalmol* 1978;96:1606–1610.

Digre KB, Smoker WR, Johnston P, et al. Selective MR imaging approach for evaluation of patients with Horner's syndrome. *AJNR Am J Neuroradiol* 1992;13:223–227.

Grimson BS, Thompson HS. Horner's syndrome: overall view of 120 cases. In: Thompson HS, ed. *Topics in neuro-ophthalmology.* Baltimore: Williams & Wilkins, 1979:151–156.

Kardon RH, Denison CE, Brown CK, et al. Critical evaluation of the cocaine test in the diagnosis of Horner's syndrome. *Arch Ophthalmol* 1990;108:384–387.

Lam BL, Thompson HS, Corbett JJ. The prevalence of simple anisocoria. *Am J Ophthalmol* 1987;104:69–73.

Loewenfeld IE. The Argyll Robertson pupil, 1869–1969: a critical survey of the literature. *Surv Ophthalmol* 1969;14:199–299.

Loewenfeld IE. "Simple, central" anisocoria: a common condition, seldom recognized. *Trans Am Acad Ophthalmol Otolaryngol* 1977;83:832–839.

Loewenfeld IE, Thompson HS. The tonic pupil: a re-evaluation. *Am J Ophthalmol* 1967;63: 46–87.

Loewenfeld IE, Thompson HS. Mechanism of tonic pupil. *Ann Neurol* 1981;10:275–276.

Maloney WF, Younge BR, Moyer NJ. Evaluation of the causes and accuracy of pharmacologic localization in Horner's syndrome. *Am J Ophthalmol* 1980;90:394–402.

Thompson HS. The pupil. In: Hart WM Jr, ed. *Adler's physiology of the eye: clinical application,* 9th ed. St. Louis: Mosby, 1992:412–441.

Thompson HS, Corbett JJ. Swinging flashlight test [Letter]. *Neurology* 1989;39:154–156.

Thompson HS, Corbett JJ, Cox TA. How to measure the relative afferent pupillary defect. *Surv Ophthalmol* 1981;26:39–42.

Thompson HS, Kardon RH. Pretectal pupillary defects [Editorial comment]. *J Clin Neuro-ophthalmol* 1991;11:173–174.

Thompson HS, Kardon RH. *Clinical importance of pupillary inequality.* Focal points: clinical modules for ophthalmologists. Vol. 10. San Francisco: American Academy of Ophthalmology, 1992:1–12.

Thompson HS, Miller NR. Disorders of pupillary function, accommodation and lacrimation. In: Miller NR, Newman NJ, eds. *Walsh and Hoyt's clinical neuro-ophthalmology.* 5th edition. Baltimore: Williams & Wilkins, 1998:961–1040.

Thompson HS, Newsome DA, Loewenfeld IE. The fixed dilated pupil: sudden iridoplegia or mydriatic drops? A simple diagnostic test. *Arch Ophthalmol* 1971;86:21–27.

12. APPROACH TO THE PATIENT WITH DIPLOPIA

Robert D. Yee

Strabismus is a misalignment of the eyes that can cause **binocular diplopia,** or double vision. In binocular diplopia, both images are clear, and covering either eye abolishes the diplopia. Abnormalities of the cornea and lens, such as astigmatism and cataract, create **monocular diplopia.** Double vision persists when the normal eye is covered. The primary image is clear, and the secondary image is blurred. However, diplopia disappears when the abnormal eye is occluded. Disorders of the extraocular muscles, orbit, cranial nerves, and brainstem cause binocular diplopia. The physical examination reveals the location of the lesion, and the history usually indicates its cause. The work-up and management of diplopia usually allow time for observation, except when the etiologic factor may be an intracranial aneurysm. An aneurysm can cause sudden pain, diplopia, third nerve palsy with dilated pupil and abnormal pupillary reactions, or sixth nerve palsy. Because of the risk of severe morbidity and mortality with rupture of the aneurysm, magnetic resonance imaging (MRI), magnetic resonance angiography (MRA), helical computed tomography (CT), or perhaps cerebral angiography should be performed immediately. Other causes of diplopia also demand urgent evaluation. Phycomycosis of the orbit, cavernous sinus thrombosis, pituitary apoplexy, and ischemia of the extraocular muscles or cranial nerves from giant cell arteritis cause sudden pain, diplopia, and ophthalmoplegia and must be evaluated immediately.

I. **Etiology and clinical manifestations**
   A. **Extraocular muscles.** Table 12.1 describes the patterns of eye findings that establish the anatomic locations of lesions causing ophthalmoplegia. Table 12.2 lists the common and potentially serious causes of diplopia arranged according to anatomic location. Diseases that affect the extraocular muscles (EOMs) directly (ocular myopathy) include myasthenia gravis, chronic progressive external ophthalmoplegia, muscular dystrophy, myositis, and Graves' ophthalmopathy. Ocular myopathy usually does not limit extraocular movements in patterns suggesting cranial nerve palsy. However, when they do, the presence of ptosis (drooping of the upper eyelid), weakness of the orbicularis oculi muscles (inability to keep the eyelids shut), and retraction or edema of the eyelids can indicate that myopathy exists.
      1. **Myasthenia gravis** causes ptosis and diplopia that vary throughout the day (worse in the evening) and from day to day. Asymmetric ptosis and weakness of eyelid closure (orbicularis oculi) are usually present. EOM weakness is asymmetric and produces a pattern that can mimic cranial nerve palsy or internuclear ophthalmoplegia (limitation of adduction). Pupillary reactions always are normal. Voluntary eye movements (saccades) made by affected muscles can have normally high velocity despite limited amplitude.
      2. Chronic progressive external ophthalmoplegia (CPEO) is associated with mitochondrial disorders and manifests as progressive, bilateral ptosis over years. Patients with CPEO usually do not report diplopia because ptosis occludes one eye, the characteristically symmetric EOM weakness does not cause misalignment of the eyes, or the image of one eye is suppressed by the brain. As in myasthenia gravis, the orbicularis oculi muscles are weak. Because weakness usually is symmetric among the EOMs of each eye and between the two eyes, CPEO usually does not mimic cranial nerve palsy. As in myasthenia gravis, however, the medial rectus muscles often are most affected, and a pattern of pseudointernuclear ophthalmoplegia results. Saccades are very slow. CPEO and atypical retinitis pigmentosa compose **Kearns–Sayre syndrome.** Cardiac conduction defects can develop in this syndrome. **Oculopharyngeal dystrophy** and **myotonic dystrophy** are autosomal dominant forms of muscular dystrophy that cause ophthalmoplegia. **Abetalipoproteinemia (Bassen–Kornzweig syndrome)** also produces atypical retinitis pigmentosa and CPEO.
      3. Myositis is a form of idiopathic inflammatory pseudotumor of the orbit in which the EOMs are infiltrated by chronic inflammatory cells. Impaired contraction of muscle fibers and restriction limit eye movements. Severe pain usually accompanies the gradual or sudden onset of diplopia. The conjunctiva

Table 12.1 Patterns at anatomic locations

Extraocular muscles
  Individual muscles (usually not cranial
    nerve pattern)
  Pseudocranial nerve palsy
  Pseudo–internuclear ophthalmoplegia
  Ptosis
  Facial muscle paresis
Orbit
  Individual muscles
  Cranial nerve palsy
  Proptosis
  Periocular edema and inflammation
  Visual loss (orbital apex syndrome)
  Infraorbital nerve sensory loss
Cranial nerve palsy
  Third nerve palsy
    Exotropia and hypotropia
    Limited adduction (medial rectus),
      supraduction (superior rectus),
      infraduction (inferior rectus), supra-
      duction in adduction (inferior
      oblique)
    Pupillary dilation, diminished
      constriction to light and near reflex
    Decreased accommodation (ciliary
      muscles)
  Fourth nerve palsy
    Hypertropia and excyclotorsion
    Deviation increases in contralateral
      horizontal gaze, downgaze, and head
      tilt to ipsilateral shoulder
    Limited infraduction in adduction

Sixth nerve palsy
  Esotropia
  Limited abduction
**Cavernous sinus, superior orbital
fissure**
  Single or multiple nerve palsy
  Complete or partial pupil-sparing third
    nerve palsy
  Horner's syndrome (sixth nerve palsy)
  Facial sensory loss (first and second
    divisions of fifth nerve)
  Decreased orbital venous return (dilated
    retinal veins)
Brainstem
  Oculomotor nucleus
    Ipsilateral third nerve palsy
    Bilateral limited supraduction
    Bilateral ptosis
  Trochlear nucleus
    Contralateral fourth nerve palsy
  Abducens nucleus
    Ipsilateral horizontal gaze palsy
  Fascicles
  Internuclear ophthalmoplegia
    Ipsilateral limited adduction
    Slow saccades by ipsilateral medial
      rectus
    Abducting nystagmus in contralateral
      gaze
  Skew deviation

and lids may be injected and edematous, and pressure on the globes may be painful. Myositis can be associated with systemic vasculitis and granulomatous disorders.

4. In **Graves' ophthalmopathy,** lymphocytes, plasma cells, and edema distend the EOMs and orbital fat, causing restriction. Supraduction and abduction are typically impaired. Upper eyelid retraction, periocular edema, conjunctival injection, and proptosis often occur in both eyes. The ophthalmopathy usually follows the onset of hyperthyroidism and often occurs after iatrogenic hypothyroidism is present. However, some patients with Graves' disease have ophthalmopathy before hyperthyroidism or have normal results of thyroid function tests (euthyroid Graves' disease).

5. On rare occasions, **metastatic tumors** and **lymphoma** infiltrate the EOMs and occasionally **giant cell arteritis** cause ischemia of the EOMs. Acute **botulism** causes dilated, areflexic pupils and ophthalmoplegia by blocking transmission at cholinergic synapses.

B. **Orbit.** Masses in the orbit displace the globe, mechanically interfere with the EOMs, and cause cranial nerve palsy. **Mass lesions** include orbital inflammatory pseudotumor, lymphoma, primary tumors (cavernous hemangioma, rhabdomyosarcoma, and lacrimal gland neoplasms), metastatic tumors (adenocarcinoma, leukemia, and neuroblastoma), vascular lesions (venous varix and arteriovenous malformation), and lesions of the paranasal sinuses. Most orbital disorders produce proptosis.

Table 12.2 Location and causes of ophthalmoplegia

Extraocular muscles
  Myasthenia gravis
  Chronic progressive external ophthalmo-
    plegia
  Muscular dystrophy (oculopharyngeal
    dystrophy, myotonic dystrophy)
  Myositis (idiopathic inflammatory
    pseudotumor of orbit)
  Graves' ophthalmopathy
  Metastatic tumor, lymphoma
  Botulism
Orbit
  Idiopathic inflammatory pseudotumor of
    orbit
  Primary neoplasm
  Metastatic neoplasm
  Vascular malformation
  Paranasal sinus mucocele
  Orbital cellulitis (bacterial infections,
    phycomycosis)
  Orbital wall fractures
Cranial nerves
  Microvascular occlusion (diabetes melli-
    tus, hypertension, arteriosclerosis,
    migraine)
  Intracranial aneurysm
  Trauma
  Inflammation
	Infection (Gradenigo's syndrome, menin-
	    gitis, herpes zoster)
	  Neoplasm (parasellar, meninges, clivus)
	  Transtentorial herniation
	  Increased intracranial pressure
	  Subarachnoid hemorrhage
	  Congenital
	**Cavernous sinus, superior orbital
	  fissure**
	  Tumor (meningioma, hemangioma,
	    pituitary neoplasm, parasellar tumor,
	    metastatic tumor)
	  Intracavernous aneurysm
	  Cavernous sinus thrombosis
	  Carotid–cavernous fistula
	  Tolosa–Hunt syndrome
	  Herpes zoster
	Brainstem
	  Demyelination (multiple sclerosis,
	    postviral)
	  Ischemia
	  Hemorrhage
	  Trauma
	  Infection (encephalitis, AIDS)
	  Tumors
	  Vascular malformation
	  Congenital hypoplasia

1. The rapidity of onset and progression depend on the behavior of the mass lesions. For example, cavernous hemangioma causes gradual, painless, forward displacement of the eye over many years. Diplopia develops late in the clinical course. A **venous varix** manifests as intermittent proptosis and diplopia precipitated by a Valsalva maneuver. **Mucoceles** of the frontal and ethmoid sinuses gradually displace the eye downward and laterally but can cause sudden pain and diplopia with infection (pyomucocele).

2. Inflammation, infection, and neoplasms at the orbital apex impair eye movements (nerve palsy or mechanical restriction) and damage the optic nerve. **Phycomycosis** in patients with metabolic acidosis (e.g., diabetic ketoacidosis) extends from the nasopharynx, oropharynx, and paranasal sinuses into the orbit and causes a fulminant orbital apex syndrome.

3. A blow to the face might cause an **orbital wall fracture**. In blowout fractures of the orbital floor, entrapment of the inferior rectus muscle and other tissues in the fracture restricts supraduction. Damage to the infraorbital nerve causes numbness below the eye. The medial rectus muscle can be caught in a medial wall fracture, and the result can be limitation of abduction.

C. **Cranial nerves.** Microvascular occlusion, aneurysms, tumors, trauma, inflammation, infection, and increased intracranial pressure cause acquired cranial nerve palsy.

   1. The pattern of **third nerve palsy** includes ptosis, pupillary dilation, decreased pupil reactions to light and in the near reflex, and limitation of adduction (medial rectus muscle), supraduction (superior rectus and inferior oblique muscles), and infraduction (inferior rectus muscle) (Fig. 12.1). The affected eye is deviated laterally (exotropia) and downward (hypotropia).

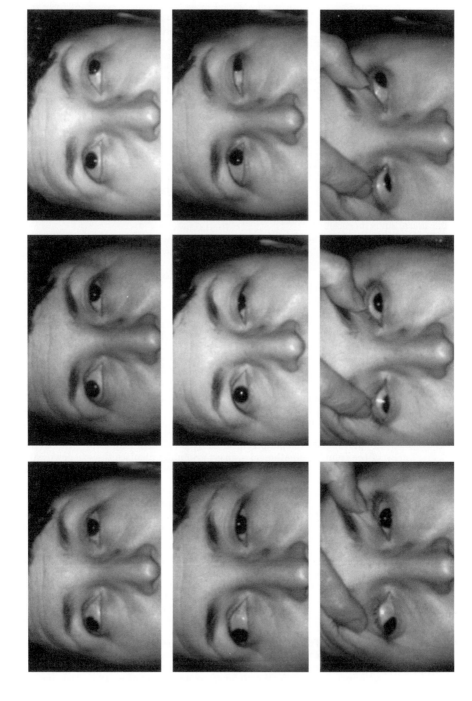

2. Fourth nerve palsy causes limitation of infraduction while the eye is adducted (superior oblique muscle). The affected eye is deviated upward (hypertropia), and the 12 o'clock position of the cornea is rotated laterally relative to the vertical meridian (excyclotorsion). The patient reports vertical and torsional diplopia.

3. The pattern of a **sixth nerve palsy** includes impaired abduction (lateral rectus muscle) and nasal deviation of the eye (esotropia) (Fig. 12.2).

4. The most common etiologic factor in older adults is microvascular occlusion causing ischemia of the peripheral cranial nerves. The common associated systemic diseases are **diabetes mellitus, hypertension, arteriosclerosis,** and **migraine.** Diplopia occurs suddenly and is often accompanied by retrobulbar pain. In third nerve palsy, pupillary size and reactions are normal or nearly normal (pupil sparing). Spontaneous improvement occurs in a few weeks, and complete resolution occurs in almost all patients within 6 months.

5. Intracranial aneurysms cause third and sixth nerve palsy. The onset can be abrupt or gradual, and moderate or severe pain often exists. In third nerve palsy, the pupil is dilated and the pupillary contractions to light and near are diminished. Pain may accompany cranial nerve palsy caused by tumors (sellar and parasellar neoplasms). Diplopia usually begins slowly and gradually increases.

6. Head trauma can produce sudden diplopia and is the most frequent cause of fourth nerve palsy.

7. Aberrant regeneration after traumatic third nerve palsy results in pupillary miosis, lid elevation, or both on attempted adduction or infraduction or on adduction on attempted up or down gaze. Oculomotor synkinesis occurs a few months after trauma or compression by aneurysms or tumors. The upper eyelid elevates or the pupil constricts, or both occur when the eye adducts or infraducts. Regenerated axons that originally innervated the medial rectus or inferior rectus muscles reach the eyelid levator muscle or the iris sphincter muscle. If aberrant regeneration is found without a history of acute oculomotor paralysis, a slowly growing, parasellar neoplasm, such as meningioma of the cavernous sinus, should be suspected.

8. Inflammatory disorders, such as sarcoidosis or postviral encephalitis, can produce cranial nerve palsy. The diplopia and pain respond quickly to systemic corticosteroids.

9. Increased intracranial pressure produces bilateral papilledema and unilateral or bilateral sixth nerve palsy. Fourth nerve palsy occurs occasionally, and third nerve palsy rarely.

10. Inflammatory, infectious, and neoplastic disorders of the **meninges** and head **trauma** with shearing forces can damage single or several cranial nerves. Severe mastoiditis causes sixth nerve palsy associated with ipsilateral facial pain and facial palsy (Gradenigo's syndrome).

11. **Guillain–Barré syndrome** and its variant, **Fisher's syndrome** (ophthalmoplegia, ataxia, and areflexia), can cause cranial nerve palsy.

12. **Transtentorial herniation** or an intracranial aneurysm can compress the third cranial nerve, initially producing pupillary dilation and later causing EOM paresis as it progresses. Compression lesions that cause only pupillary dilation are rare.

13. **Congenital cranial nerve palsy** is less common than acquired palsy. Patients with congenital third nerve palsy usually have miotic pupils with abnormal reflexes. The miosis results from aberrant regeneration. Congenital

---

FIG. 12.1 Third nerve palsy of the left eye. Evident are ptosis of left upper lid, extropia of left eye **(center),** and limitation of left medial rectus **(center right),** superior rectus **(top left),** inferior oblique **(top right),** and inferior rectus **(bottom right)** muscles.

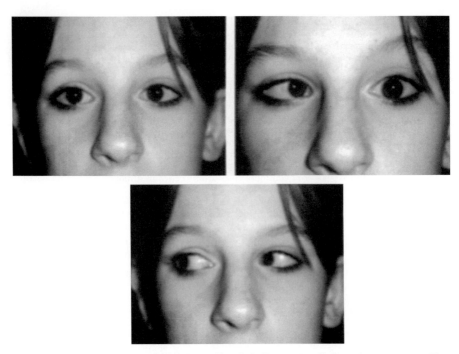

FIG. 12.2 Sixth nerve palsy of the left eye. **Top left.** Esotropia of left eye in center gaze. **Top right.** Greater esotropia in left gaze due to limitation of left lateral rectus. **Bottom.** No esotropia in right gaze.

sixth nerve palsy usually is associated with other neurologic or systemic malformations, such as **Möbius' syndrome** (bilateral sixth and seventh nerve palsy). In **Duane's retraction syndrome,** sixth nerve palsy is associated with narrowing of the ipsilateral palpebral fissure and retraction of the paretic eye backward into the orbit when the paretic eye adducts.

D. **Cavernous sinus.** Because nerves in the cav rnous sinus continue into the adjacent superior orbital fissure, syndromes of both structures are similar. Lesions in the cavernous sinus, such as tumors, aneurysms, and **carotid-cavernous fistulas,** produce single or multiple cranial nerve palsy.

1. Granulomatous inflammation at the superior orbital fissure or in the cavernous sinus in **Tolosa–Hunt syndrome** also causes multiple cranial nerve palsy and severe pain. The pain and diplopia improve with treatment with systemic corticosteroids. However, ophthalmoplegia caused by aneurysms and tumors can produce the same findings that respond partially to corticosteroids.

2. The third, fourth, sixth, and fifth cranial nerves (sensory divisions 1 and 2) and the postganglionic sympathetic axons to the eye and eyelids traverse the cavernous sinus. Sensory loss in the face and **Horner's syndrome** (sympathetic axons travel with the sixth nerve in the posterior part of cavernous sinus) can accompany diplopia.

3. In third nerve palsy, the pupils are totally or partially spared and are normal in size or only slightly dilated. Simultaneous damage to postganglionic sympathetic axons to the iris dilator muscle prevents greater pupillary dilation. Lesions of the cavernous sinus often cause dilation of the retinal veins by obstructing venous flow from the eye and orbit into the cavernous sinus.

4. **Meningioma** is the most common primary tumors in adults. **Pituitary tumors** can extend into an adjacent cavernous sinus. Hemorrhagic infarction of a pituitary adenoma produces severe pain, obtundation, bilateral cranial nerve palsy, and bilateral blindness (**pituitary apoplexy**).

5. **Cavernous sinus thrombosis** from bacterial infection extending from the orbit (orbital cellulitis) into the cavernous sinus causes unilateral or bilateral cranial nerve palsy, severe pain, and dilation of retinal veins. *It is a medical emergency.*

6. **Intracavernous carotid aneurysms** cause cranial nerve palsy, often with pain. The risk of rupture is less than that with other intracranial aneurysms because the intracavernous aneurysm is supported by the surrounding venous sinus.

7. **Traumatic and spontaneous carotid cavernous fistulas** cause unilateral or bilateral cranial nerve palsy, periocular edema, and dilation (arterialization) of conjunctival veins arranged radially around the corneas (caput medusa sign).

E. **Brainstem.** Brainstem lesions cause diplopia from nuclear and fascicular cranial nerve palsy, internuclear ophthalmoplegia, and skew deviation. Common causes are **demyelination** (multiple sclerosis and postviral) and ischemia (hypertension, diabetes mellitus, arteriosclerosis, and vasculitis).

1. Unilateral lesions of the **oculomotor nucleus** cause ipsilateral paresis of the EOMs innervated by the third cranial nerve, bilateral ptosis, and bilateral superior rectus paresis. The ipsilateral superior rectus subnucleus projects to the contralateral superior rectus. The crossing fibers from the contralateral subnucleus to the ipsilateral superior rectus also are interrupted by the nuclear lesion. Patients have bilateral ptosis because the levator superioris palpebrae subnucleus that innervates both lid levators is located in the midline.

2. The **trochlear nucleus** innervates the contralateral superior oblique muscle. Head trauma and hydrocephalus can produce bilateral fourth nerve palsy by damaging the fascicles decussating in the anterior medullary velum.

3. Lesions of the **abducens nucleus** cause ipsilateral horizontal gaze palsy. The nucleus contains motor neurons of the ipsilateral lateral rectus and interneurons that decussate and project through the contralateral medial longitudinal fasciculus to the contralateral medial rectus subnucleus.

4. **Fascicular lesions** or **nuclear lesions** of each cranial nerve usually damage adjacent structures in the brainstem. The syndromes that result include Nothnagel's syndrome (third nerve palsy and contralateral cerebellar ataxia), Benedikt's syndrome (third nerve palsy and contralateral tremor), Weber's syndrome (third nerve palsy and contralateral hemiparesis), Foville's syndrome (ipsilateral horizontal gaze palsy or sixth nerve palsy, facial palsy, facial analgesia, loss of taste, Horner's syndrome, deafness, and contralateral hemiplegia), Raymond Cestan syndrome (sixth nerve palsy and contralateral hemiplegia), and Millard–Gubler syndrome (ipsilateral sixth nerve palsy, facial palsy, and contralateral hemiplegia).

5. Damage to the medial longitudinal fasciculus produces **internuclear ophthalmoplegia** (INO). INO is characterized by paresis of the ipsilateral medial rectus muscle, slowing of saccades generated by the medial rectus, overshooting of abducting saccades (contralateral lateral rectus), and dissociated nystagmus in contralateral gaze (nystagmus in abducting eye larger than in adducting eye). Patients report diplopia in contralateral gaze. Upbeat nystagmus and skew deviation often are present. Demyelination is the most common cause of bilateral INO; ischemia is the most common cause of unilateral INO.

6. **Skew deviation** is vertical misalignment of the eyes that is not a result of a third or fourth nerve palsy. It is usually caused by lesions of the brainstem or cerebellum.

II. **Evaluation**

A. **History.** The type of onset (gradual or sudden); the presence, type, and location of pain; and the progression over time (increasing, decreasing, stable, or variable) should be discerned. The history should establish the direction of the diplopia (vertical, horizontal, oblique, or torsional) and whether closure of either eye abolishes diplopia (binocular diplopia versus monocular diplopia). Other ocular symptoms (ptosis, pupillary dilation, visual loss, periocular edema, injection, ptosis, and proptosis), neurologic symptoms, and the existence of systemic diseases are important.

B. Physical examination. The general physical examination and neurologic examination include a search for a compensatory head position (face turn in third and sixth nerve palsy and head tilt in fourth nerve palsy), facial palsy, and sensory loss in the face (fifth cranial nerve). The ocular examination includes assessment of visual acuity and confrontation visual fields and a search for signs of ptosis or retraction of the eyelids, periocular inflammation, proptosis, and anisocoria. Table 12.3 lists the eye tests used to evaluate ophthalmoplegia.

1. Covering each eye differentiates **monocular diplopia** from **binocular diplopia** (see **III.**).

2. The **cover test** helps detect tropia, which is misalignment of the eyes when both eyes are opened and binocular vision is possible. While the patient fixates a small target straight ahead, cover one eye with an occluder and watch the other eye. If that eye makes a refixation movement, it was not aligned on the target. If the eye moves nasally, it was misaligned temporally, and the patient has an exotropia. Temporal refixation signifies esotropia, downward movement indicates hypertropia, and upward movement reveals hypotropia. If the eye does not refixate, remove the occluder and pause momentarily to allow binocular vision to be reestablished. Then cover the second eye and look for refixation of the first eye.

   a. Third nerve palsy produces exotropia and hypotropia of the paretic eye. Sixth nerve palsy causes esotropia of the affected eye. Fourth nerve palsy produces hypertropia and excyclotorsion of the paretic eye.

   b. Tropia is commonly caused by **nonparalytic strabismus** beginning in childhood. The image from the deviated eye is suppressed, and there is no diplopia. Patients do not have ophthalmoplegia, and there is no limitation of eye movement. The cover test can be repeated in eccentric horizontal and vertical gaze. In nonparalytic strabismus, the amount of tropia does not change.

   c. In **paralytic strabismus,** tropia increases when the eyes gaze in the direction of action of the paretic muscle in which the muscle is maximally active, and it decreases in the opposite direction of gaze in which the paretic muscle is relaxed.

   d. Patients often have a habitual face turn that moves the eyes away from the field of action of the paretic muscle and minimizes tropia and diplopia. For example, a patient with right sixth nerve palsy turns the face to the right, placing the eyes in left gaze. The right sixth nerve palsy produces esotropia of the right eye in center gaze. The esotropia increases in right

Table 12.3 Eye tests for ophthalmoplegia

Monocular occlusion (monocular versus binocular diplopia)
Cover test for tropia (primary gaze, eccentric gaze)
Alternate cover test for phoria
Hirschberg corneal reflex test for tropia
Duction
Oculocephalic maneuver
Saccades
Eyelid position and movement
Pupil size and reflexes
Proptosis and periocular signs
Facial sensation, corneal reflex

---

gaze and decreases in left gaze. Patients with fourth nerve palsy often tilt the head toward the shoulder opposite the side of the paretic superior oblique muscle to decrease hypertropia and cyclotorsional diplopia.

    e. The **Park's three-step test** is used to detect the pattern of fourth nerve palsy.

        (1) In center gaze, the hypertropic eye is the paretic eye. For example, right fourth nerve palsy produces right hypertropia.

        (2) Hypertropia increases when the patient looks to the opposite side. For example, right hypertropia is greater when the patient looks to the left than to the right.

        (3) Hypertropia increases when the patient tilts the head to the same side. For example, right hypertropia is larger when the head tilts toward the right shoulder than when it tilts toward the left shoulder.

3. If the cover test reveals no tropia, test for phoria with the **alternate cover test**. Phoria is misalignment of the eyes when binocular vision is absent. While the patient looks at the target straight ahead, cover one eye with the occluder and move the occluder quickly to cover the other eye so that there is no opportunity for binocular vision to be established. Move the occluder alternately between the eyes. If the eyes make refixation movements when they are uncovered, they were misaligned when occluded. Nasal movement confirms exophoria (each eye was deviated temporally under cover); temporal movement, esophoria; and vertical refixation movement, hyperphoria. Phoria does not cause diplopia because the eyes are aligned when both eyes are opened simultaneously. However, under certain conditions, such as fatigue or generalized central nervous system depression, phoria can "break down" and become tropia, which causes diplopia.

4. When a patient cannot fixate a small target (poor vision or cooperation), the **Hirschberg corneal reflex test** can be used to detect a tropia. Position a penlight in front of the eyes so that the bright corneal reflex is centered in the pupil of one eye. If the reflex in the other eye is also in the center of the pupil, the eyes are aligned. If it is displaced temporally, the eye is deviated nasally (esotropia). Nasal displacement signifies exotropia, upward displacement hypotropia, and downward deviation hypertropia.

5. The **duction** (range of motion) of the EOMs should be tested. While the first eye is occluded, the second eye follows the examiner's target, such as a pen point held in front of the patient. The examiner moves the target horizontally and vertically into the primary fields of action of the EOMs. The maximum range of motion from center gaze is normally 45 to 50 degrees. The examiner should try to estimate the range of motion—for example, one-third the maximum is 15 degrees, one-half is 30 degrees, and full movement is 45 degrees. This measurement reflects the severity of EOM palsy. The examiner covers the second eye and measures the duction of the first eye. Duction should be tested with monocular viewing, because binocular viewing can give a false impression of limited duction when nonparalytic strabismus is present. For example, if a patient has nonparalytic left esotropia and fixates the target with the right eye, in left gaze the left eye will not be fully abducted, giving the impression that weakness of the left lateral rectus muscle exists.

6. The **oculocephalic maneuver** (doll's eye test) is used to evaluate duction when the patient is unconscious. The examiner rapidly thrusts the patient's head horizontally and vertically. The vestibuloocular reflex rotates the eyes in the opposite direction. This maneuver can also help identify supranuclear gaze palsy in an alert patient. For example, patients with Parinaud's syndrome and a supranuclear palsy of upgaze cannot voluntarily look up, but thrusting of the head down rotates the eyes upward. Forced closure of the eyelids normally causes the eyes to supraduct (Bell's phenomenon). A patient with supranuclear palsy of upgaze can still have a normal Bell's phenomenon.

7. Saccades are rapid, conjugate, voluntary eye movements between objects. The examiner holds small targets (e.g., the fingertips) 30 degrees to the patient's right and 30 degrees to the left, or 30 degrees up and 30 degrees down, and commands the patient to look back and forth between the targets. Normal saccades have a high velocity (as high as 800 degrees per second) and are accurate.

   a. Most forms of ophthalmoplegia, such as cranial nerve palsy, internuclear ophthalmoplegia, and CPEO, cause slowing of saccades. When the paretic eye makes a saccade into the field of action of the weak muscle, the examiner detects that the eye reaches the target after the normal eye. The examiner can watch one eye and notice that the paretic eye has slow saccades into the field of the weak muscle and normal saccades into the opposite field. Slowing of saccades is a more sensitive sign of most forms of ophthalmoplegias than is limitation of duction.

   b. Many patients with myasthenia gravis can make small saccades with normal velocity despite limited duction. Saccades in restrictive orbitopathy, such as Graves' ophthalmopathy and orbital blowout fracture, can have normal velocity until they are made into the field of restriction.

8. The examiner should measure **lid position.** The margins of the upper eyelids usually intersect the edges of the corneas at the 10 and 2 o'clock positions. A higher position can signify pathologic lid retraction in Graves' ophthalmopathy or Parinaud's syndrome. A lower position can indicate ptosis.

   a. When asymmetric lid positions are present, the difference should be measured with a ruler. The examiner measures the actions of the lid levators (levator palpebrae superioris muscles) by measuring the excursion of the upper eyelid margin from extreme downgaze to extreme upgaze. The normal excursion is approximately 15 mm. In ptosis due to paresis of the lid levator, the excursion is decreased.

   b. Myasthenia gravis causes fatigue of the lid levator. The examiner uses fingers of one hand to press against the eyebrows to prevent brow lift and holds a target above the patient for 30 seconds. As the patient maintains upward gaze, the examiner watches for gradual descent of the upper lids. Myasthenia gravis can cause Cogan's lid twitch sign. The patient looks from downgaze to center gaze. The upper eyelid momentarily overshoots the normal lid position.

9. The examiner observes **pupillary size** and **reflexes.** The patient fixates a small distant target in a well-lit room. A difference in pupillary diameter between the eyes (anisocoria) of 1 mm can be normal.

   a. If the examiner finds small anisocoria (1 to 2 mm), the upper lid is 1 to 2 mm lower in the miotic eye, and the lower lid in the same eye is 1 mm higher, Horner's syndrome might be present. The examiner should measure the pupillary diameters in a dark room. In Horner's syndrome, anisocoria increases in the dark. Administration of topical cocaine can confirm the presence of Horner's syndrome. Topical hydroxyamphetamine can identify damage to the third-order neuron in the sympathetic pathway to the iris dilator muscle.

   b. In third nerve palsy, parasympathetic innervation to the iris sphincter muscle can be interrupted or spared (pupil sparing). If it is interrupted, the pupil is dilated, and pupillary constriction to direct stimulation by light and in the near reflex (focusing on a near target) is decreased or absent. While the patient fixates a distant target, the examiner shines a bright penlight beam into each eye and compares the speeds and amplitudes of the pupillary constrictions of the two eyes. If the parasympathetic innervation is partially interrupted (partial pupil sparing), the pupil is slightly dilated and its reactions are decreased, but still present.

10. The examiner looks for **proptosis** and **periocular signs.**

   a. Narrow palpebral fissures (openings between upper and lower lids) give the appearance of enophthalmos (recession of the eye into the orbit), and wide palpebral fissures make the eye look proptotic (bulging out of the orbit). To confirm the presence of enophthalmos or exophthalmos, the examiner stands behind the patient, looks over the patient's brows, and

compares the positions of the two corneas relative to themselves and to the superior orbital rims.
   b. A mass in the orbit increases resistance in the orbit. The examiner gently pushes against the closed eyelids and judges the resistance to retrodisplacement of each eye. The orbit with a mass lesion causing proptosis seems stiffer.
   c. The examiner also should look for lid edema and conjunctival injection.
   d. Perception of light touch and pin prick in the three sensory divisions of the trigeminal nerve and the corneal flex to light touch should be tested.
C. **Laboratory studies.** The probable locations and causes of ophthalmoplegia dictate which laboratory tests should be performed.
   1. **Blood tests**
      a. The work-up of **myopathy** and **orbital disorders** includes acetylcholine receptor antibody titers and antistriated muscle antibody titers for myasthenia gravis and triiodothyronine, thyroxine, and thyroid-stimulating hormone levels for Graves' ophthalmopathy. If myasthenia gravis affects only or primarily the extraocular muscles (ocular myasthenia gravis), acetylcholine receptor titers are elevated in only approximately 50% of patients. There is no direct correlation between thyroid hormone levels and the activity of Graves' ophthalmopathy. However, abnormal hormone levels indicate abnormal thyroid function, which can corroborate the ocular diagnosis, and hormone testing is important for the patient's general health.
      b. The work-up of **isolated cranial nerve palsy** should include tests for diabetes mellitus and vasculitis. Because a cranial nerve palsy can be the initial sign of type II diabetes, fasting blood sugar and a serum hemoglobin A_{1c} level should be measured. Complete blood cell count, antinuclear antibody titer, anti-DNA titer, and Westergren erythrocyte sedimentation rate can help identify vasculitis, such as systemic lupus erythematosus and giant cell arteritis. The work-up of **brainstem lesions** includes the tests for vasculitis. If ischemia is a possible cause in a young adult, the lupus anticoagulant syndrome, hyperhomocysteinemia, and other forms of coagulopathy can be considered and appropriate tests performed.
   2. **Cerebrospinal fluid.** A lumbar puncture should be performed to evaluate the cerebrospinal fluid in cranial nerve palsy if the examiner suspects that increased intracranial pressure is causing cranial nerve palsy or that inflammatory, infectious, or neoplastic diseases are producing cranial nerve palsy or brainstem disorders. The opening pressure must be recorded. CT or MRI should be performed before lumbar puncture if increased intracranial pressure is suspected.
   3. CT and MRI. Neuroradiologic studies are indicated in the evaluation of some forms of myopathy, orbital disorders, cranial nerve palsy, and brainstem disorders. CT usually is satisfactory in studying disorders of the EOMs and orbits. The examiner should request direct coronal and axial views of the orbits and paranasal sinuses with intravenous administration of contrast material or request spiral CT. Patients with obvious Graves' ophthalmopathy do not need CT unless visual loss from optic nerve compression occurs. MRI usually is better than CT in imaging the orbital apex, superior orbital fissure, cavernous sinus, sella, and sphenoid bone. The examiner should request coronal and axial views of the orbits and sellar area with and without injection of gadolinium and with fat-suppression techniques. MRI of the posterior fossa should be used to evaluate brainstem disorders.
   4. Other tests
      a. If myasthenia gravis is a likely cause of diplopia and ophthalmoplegia, the examiner should perform an antiacetylcholinesterase test. **Edrophonium** (Tensilon; ICN Pharmaceuticals, Costa Mesa, CA, U.S.A.) should be used for adults and older children. **Neostigmine** (Prostigmin; ICN Pharmaceuticals) is used for young children and other patients whose ability to cooperate is limited. The examiner must measure ptosis,

tropia, or limitation of duction before and after drug administration. For the edrophonium test, a short intravenous line (e.g., butterfly) is placed in a hand or arm vein and is kept opened and flushed with a 10- or 20-mL syringe of saline solution. In adults, 0.4 mg of atropine (1 mL of a 0.4 mg/mL solution) is given to block some of the systemic side effects of edrophonium. Saline solution flushes the intravenous line after each drug injection. The examiner injects small amounts of edrophonium (10 mg/mL) with a 1-mL tuberculin syringe. Aliquots of 1, 3, 3, and 3 mg are given serially to reduce systemic side effects. After each aliquot, the examiner measures the eye findings over the next 2 minutes. If definite improvement occurs, the next aliquot is not injected. An alternative is to inject 0.04 mg/kg of neostigmine intramuscularly (up to the adult dose of 1.5 mg) and measure the eye signs 30 minutes later. Whereas the effects of edrophonium persist for only several minutes, those of neostigmine can last as long as 1 hour.

    b. Patients with CPEO should undergo **electrocardiography** to detect cardiac myopathy (conduction defect) caused by the mitochondrial cytopathy and **blood tests** for mitochondrial DNA mutations.

III. Differential diagnosis. The aforedescribed disorders produce misalignment of the eyes and **binocular diplopia.** Covering either eye abolishes the diplopia. In **monocular diplopia**, the eyes are not misaligned. One eye usually has an abnormality of the ocular media and produces multiple images. When the abnormal eye is covered, diplopia disappears. Covering the abnormal eye does not abolish the diplopia. Uncorrected refractive errors, such as astigmatism, irregularities of the corneal surface, corneal opacities, and cataracts, are the most common causes of monocular diplopia. When the patient views with the abnormal eye, one image usually is clear and the second image is blurred (ghost image). Refraction or viewing through a pinhole usually abolishes monocular diplopia. In rare cases, lesions in the parietoccipital cortex cause monocular diplopia.

IV. Referral. If a patient persistently reports diplopia, tropia is detected, or a limitation of duction is found, the patient should be referred to a neurologist, ophthalmologist, or neuroophthalmologist. These specialists can confirm the findings, suggest the differential diagnosis, recommend laboratory tests, and help treat the patient. Treatment can include temporary patching of one eye, eyeglasses with prisms, or EOM surgery. Most cases of diplopia and ophthalmoplegia do not necessitate urgent referral. However, when patients are likely to have diseases that can quickly cause severe morbidity or mortality, the referral, work-up, and treatment must proceed rapidly. The sections that follow describe the initial management of patients with cranial nerve palsy (intracranial aneurysm), orbital apex syndrome (phycomycosis), cavernous sinus thrombosis (bacterial orbital cellulitis), pituitary apoplexy (pituitary adenoma), and ischemic myopathy (giant cell arteritis) as examples of why urgent referrals may be needed.

    A. Cranial nerve palsy

        1. Compression by an **aneurysm** at the junction of the posterior communicating artery and internal carotid artery is an infrequent, but important, cause of third nerve palsy because of the risk of spontaneous rupture and high risk of severe morbidity and mortality if a rupture occurs. Aneurysms of the posterior inferior cerebellar artery, basilar artery, and intracavernous carotid artery less frequently cause sixth nerve palsy. Intracavernous aneurysms are less likely to rupture because the venous structures and dura of the cavernous sinus surround them. Aneurysms rarely produce fourth nerve palsy.

        2. Ischemia of the subarachnoid or intracavernous portions of the cranial nerves is the most common cause of isolated cranial nerve palsy in adults (microvascular cranial nerve palsy). Patients usually have a history of diabetes mellitus, hypertension, arteriosclerosis, or migraine. Obstruction of small blood vessels supplying the peripheral nerve produces sudden diplopia and ophthalmoplegia that are often accompanied by pain behind the affected eye. Improvement in diplopia and ophthalmoplegia occurs within the following 4 to 6 weeks, and recovery is complete within 6 months for most patients.

        3. Microvascular third nerve palsy usually spares pupillary reactions. If the extraocular muscles innervated by the third nerve are severely affected but pupillary size and reactions to light and near are normal (**pupil-sparing third nerve palsy**), the most likely cause is ischemia, and an aneurysm is unlikely. After the initial examination and the screening laboratory tests mentioned earlier, the examiner reevaluates the patient in 2 weeks if diabetes mellitus, hypertension, arteriosclerosis, or migraine is present. If there is no history of these systemic diseases, the patient should return in 1 week to be examined for signs of pupillary involvement or progression of paresis. The paretic eye can be patched to avoid diplopia. In microvascular cranial nerve palsy, signs of improvement should be observed within 4 to 6 weeks after the onset. The examiner must measure tropia, duction, and lid findings at the initial examination so that improvement can be detected in follow-up visits.

4. If the pupil becomes affected, EOM paresis increases, improvement does not occur within 4 to 6 weeks, or full recovery does not occur within 6 months, MRI of the orbits, sella, and posterior fossa with and without gadolinium as well as MRA (or spiral CT) should be performed to seek other causes.

5. If the extraocular muscles are severely paretic, the pupil is mildly dilated, and pupillary reactions are slightly decreased (**partial pupil-sparing third nerve palsy**), microvascular third nerve palsy is probably present and aneurysmal compression is still unlikely. The patient can be followed as described in **4.** Compression of the third nerve in the cavernous sinus, as by meningioma of the cavernous sinus, often produces this type of third nerve palsy, but in this case the palsy usually does not show spontaneous improvement.

6. If the pupil is widely dilated and pupillary reactions are absent (**non-pupil-sparing third nerve palsy**), a microvascular cause is unlikely. Compression by an aneurysm or tumor, inflammation, or infiltration often is the cause. Diabetes mellitus occasionally causes non-pupil-sparing third nerve palsy, but aneurysmal compression is the most common cause. The examiner immediately should request MRI of the orbits, sella, and posterior fossa with and without gadolinium and MRA or spiral CT of the intracranial arteries. These studies can depict intracranial aneurysms with diameters of 5 mm or greater. The most common site of an aneurysm causing third nerve palsy is the junction of the posterior communicating artery and the internal carotid artery. *MRA and spiral cannot exclude smaller aneurysms.* Although small aneurysms are less likely to rupture than are larger ones, cerebral angiography is still the standard study and should be performed if the MRA or spiral CT findings are normal. The examiner should perform lumbar puncture if the results of neuroimaging studies are normal.

7. Pupil sparing when the third nerve EOMs are only mildly paretic or when some third nerve EOMs are not affected is not as reassuring that there is a microvascular etiology as is pupil sparing with severe EOM paresis. Compressive lesions in the subarachnoid space and cavernous sinus, including aneurysms and tumors, can produce pupil-sparing third nerve palsy. However, the EOM paresis usually is partial. In this instance, both MRI and MRA, or spiral CT, should be performed. If the results are normal, the patient is reevaluated in 1 month.

8. Patients with multiple cranial nerve palsies need MRI with and without gadolinium enhancement to find lesions at the orbital apex, superior orbital fissure, cavernous sinus, sella, meninges, and brainstem.

B. **Phycomycosis of the orbit.** Phycomycetes, such as *Mucor* organisms, cause opportunistic infections of the oronasopharynx and paranasal sinuses in patients with metabolic acidosis. Diabetic ketoacidosis is a frequent predisposing disorder. The infection rapidly spreads to the orbits, producing a painful orbital apex syndrome with ophthalmoplegia and loss of vision. The examiner should look for black, necrotic lesions of the mouth and nose; immediately obtain a CT scan of the orbits and paranasal sinuses; and request consultations to control the acidosis, begin administration of antimicrobial medications, and obtain biopsy specimens. Prompt reversal of acidosis, intravenous administration of amphotericin

B, lavage of infected tissues with amphotericin B, and excision of necrotic tissue can achieve recovery without extensive débridement of infected tissues.

C. **Cavernous sinus thrombosis.** Bacterial infection of the cavernous sinus causes abrupt, painful, bilateral cranial nerve palsy. Several cranial nerves to both eyes are affected because the cavernous sinuses are connected. The retinal veins are dilated because venous return from the orbits into the cavernous sinuses is obstructed. Cavernous sinus thrombosis usually occurs after orbital cellulitis has been present. Orbital cellulitis usually follows trauma to the eyelids or orbits and is rarely caused by hematogenous spread of bacteria. The examiner should immediately obtain CT scans of the orbits, paranasal sinuses, and cavernous sinuses and request consultations for drainage of an abscess, culturing of infected tissues, and institution of systemic antibiotics.

D. **Pituitary apoplexy.** Hemorrhagic infarction of a pituitary tumor causes sudden, severe pain, bilateral ophthalmoplegia, binocular loss of vision, and prostration from pituitary insufficiency. Cranial nerves in both cavernous sinuses and both intracranial optic nerves are damaged. The retinal blood vessels are dilated. The examiner should immediately begin therapy for pituitary insufficiency and obtain MR images or CT scans of the sella and cavernous sinuses. Urgent transsphenoidal decompression of the sella may salvage vision and cranial nerve function.

E. **Ischemic myopathy** and **cranial nerve palsy from giant cell arteritis.** Giant cell arteritis (temporal arteritis) produces characteristic systemic symptoms in the elderly. These symptoms include headache, enlarged and tender temporal arteries, scalp tenderness, jaw claudication, myalgia of limb muscles, fatigue, weight loss, and fever. Infarction of the short posterior ciliary arteries that supply the optic disks causes sudden, severe visual loss and pale swelling of the optic disk of one eye (anterior ischemic optic neuropathy). In rare instances, giant cell arteritis produces sudden ophthalmoplegia and diplopia by obstructing branches of the ophthalmic artery to the EOMs or ischemia of the cranial nerves.

   If a patient with sudden ophthalmoplegia has systemic symptoms suggestive of giant cell arteritis, the examiner should immediately obtain a Westergren sedimentation rate and C-reactive protein level. The sedimentation rate normally increases with age. Dividing a man's age (in years) by 2 approximates the upper limit of the normal sedimentation rate (mm/h) for that patient. For women, the patient's age plus 10 is divided by 2. Giant cell arteritis and other systemic inflammatory disorders also increase C-reactive protein level. If the sedimentation rate and C-reactive protein level are abnormally high, the patient immediately should begin taking 100 mg of prednisone a day, and a temporal artery biopsy should be performed in the next several days. The examiner obtains the laboratory tests and begins treatment immediately to avoid permanent visual loss from anterior ischemic optic neuropathy (infarction of the optic disk from occlusion of branches of the posterior ciliary arteries).

Recommended Readings

Biller J, Shapiro R, Evans LS, et al. Oculomotor nuclear complex infarction: clinical and radiological correlation. *Arch Neurol* 1984;41:985–987.

De Keizer RJW. Spontaneous carotid–cavernous fistulas. *Neuroophthalmology* 1981;2:35.

DiNubile MJ. Septic thrombosis of the cavernous sinuses. *Arch Neurol* 1988;45:567.

Feldon SE, Weiner JM. Clinical significance of extraocular muscle volumes in Graves' ophthalmopathy: a quantitative computed tomographic study. *Arch Ophthalmol* 1982;100:1266.

Forteza G, Burgeno M. Rhinocerebral mucormycosis: presentation of two cases and review of the literature. *J Craniomaxillofac Surg* 1988;16:80.

Gerbitz KD, Obermaier-Kusser B, Zierz S, et al. Mitochondrial myopathies: divergences of genetic deletions, biochemical defects and the clinical syndromes. *J Neurol* 1990;237:5–10.

Goldberg RT. Ocular muscle paresis and cranial arteritis: an unusual case. *Ann Ophthalmol* 1983;15:240.

Harley RD. Paralytic strabismus in children: etiologic incidence and management of third, fourth, and sixth nerve palsies. *Ophthalmology* 1980;86:24.

Hirst LW, Miller NR, Johnson RT. Monocular polyopia. *Arch Neurol* 1983;40:756.

Hunt WE, Brighton RP. The Tolosa–Hunt syndrome: a problem in differential diagnosis. *Acta Neurochir Suppl (Wien)* 1988;42:248.

Kline LB. The Tolosa–Hunt syndrome. *Surv Ophthalmol* 1982;27:79.

Kushner BJ. Errors in the three-step test in the diagnosis of vertical strabismus. *Ophthalmology* 1989;96:447.

Leigh RJ, Zee DS. The neurology of eye movements, 2nd ed. Philadelphia: FA Davis Co, 1991.

McKhann GM. Guillain–Barré syndrome: clinical and therapeutic observations. *Ann Neurol* 1990;27[Suppl]:S13.

Meienberg O, Buttner-Ennerver JA, Kraus-Ruppert R. Unilateral paralysis of conjugate gaze due to lesion of the abducens nucleus. *Neuroophthalmology* 1981;2:47.

Meienberg O, Ryffel E. Supranuclear eye movement disorders in Fisher's syndrome of ophthalmoplegia, ataxia, and areflexia. *Arch Neurol* 1983;40:402.

Miller NR, Newman NJ. *Walsh and Hoyt's clinical neuro-ophthalmology,* 5th ed. Vol 1. Baltimore: Williams & Wilkins, 1998.

Newman NJ. Third-, fourth-, and sixth-nerve lesions and the cavernous sinus. In: Albert DM, Jacobiec FA, eds. *Principles and practice of ophthalmology clinical practice.* Vol 4. Philadelphia: WB Saunders, 1994:2444.

Palestine AG, Younge BR, Piepgras DG. Visual prognosis in carotid–cavernous fistula. *Arch Ophthalmol* 1981;99:1600.

Richards BW, Jones FR, Younge BR. Causes and prognosis in 4,278 cases of paralysis of the oculomotor, trochlear, and abducens cranial nerves. *Am J Ophthalmol* 1992;113:489.

Sibony PA, Lessell S, Gittinger JW. Acquired oculomotor synkinesis. *Rev Surv Ophthalmol* 1984;28:382.

Soliven BC. Sero-negative myasthenia gravis. *Neurology* 1988;38:514.

Soni SR. Aneurysms of the posterior communicating artery and oculomotor paresis. *J Neurol Neurosurg Psychiatry* 1974;37:475.

Striph GG, Burde RM. Abducens nerve palsy and Horner's syndrome revisited. *J Clin Neuroophthalmol* 1988;8:13.

Terranova W, Palumbo JN, Breman JG. Ocular findings in botulism type B. *JAMA* 1979; 241:475.

Trobe JD. Isolated pupil-sparing third nerve palsy. *Ophthalmology* 1985;92:58.

Trobe JD, Glaser JS, Post JD. Meningiomas and aneurysms of the cavernous sinus: neuro-ophthalmologic features. *Arch Ophthalmol* 1978;96:457.

Wakai S, Fukushima T, Teramoto A, et al. Pituitary apoplexy: its incidence and clinical significance. *J Neurosurg* 1981;55:187–193.

Yee RD, Cogan DG, Zee DS, et al. Rapid eye movements in myasthenia gravis, II: electrooculographic analysis. *Arch Ophthalmol* 1976;94:1465–1472.

Yee RD, Whitcup SM, Williams IM, et al. Saccadic eye movements in myasthenia gravis. *Ophthalmology* 1987;94:219–225.

Younge BR, Sutula F. Analysis of trochlear nerve palsies: diagnosis, etiology, and treatment. *Mayo Clin Proc* 1977;52:11.

13. APPROACH TO THE PATIENT WITH FACIAL NUMBNESS

Betsy B. Love
Marianna R. Beattie

I. Introduction

A. Definition of facial numbness. Isolated facial numbness often is descriptive of impairment of sensation of the face as a result of dysfunction of the trigeminal system or central trigeminal pathways. Patients may report unilateral or bilateral facial numbness, paresthesia (a spontaneous abnormal sensation), or dysesthesia (an unpleasant abnormal sensation produced by normal stimuli). There may be associated symptoms of altered sensation of the mucous membranes of the nose, mouth, gums, palate, or teeth. Facial numbness may be a part of a syndrome involving other cranial nerves, in addition to the trigeminal nerve. Trigeminal nerve dysfunction associated with pain is discussed in Chapter 14.

B. Types. The types of facial numbness discussed in this chapter include conditions that may present with isolated facial numbness, including lesions of the trigeminal nerve branches (e.g., trauma, tumor, connective tissue diseases), the gasserian ganglion or root (e.g., infection, tumors, nontumorous masses), and the central trigeminal pathways (e.g., stroke, tumor, vascular anomalies). Facial numbness is an uncommon, but not rare, condition. A patient with facial numbness may see a dentist, primary physician, neurologist, or otolaryngologist. The typical clinical scenario is gradual onset of numbness in one or more regions of the face, usually unilaterally. Because the presence of facial numbness can indicate a serious underlying condition, each patient with this symptom needs a thorough evaluation.

C. Facial numbness as a symptom of a life-threatening disorder. Facial numbness can represent not only a serious underlying condition that needs to be evaluated expeditiously but also, in some rare instances, a medical condition that must to be dealt with as an emergency. In rare instances, facial numbness is the presenting sign of internal carotid artery dissection, carotid aneurysm, intracranial hemorrhage, or intracranial or nasopharyngeal tumor. However, in most instances, associated features point to one of these serious etiologic conditions. If there are features suggestive of carotid artery dissection or intracranial aneurysm, **emergency computed tomography (CT) of the brain and a cerebral arteriography** are warranted. Magnetic resonance imaging (MRI) of the head with contrast medium is indicated if there is suspicion of an intracranial tumor. Brain CT without contrast material is indicated if intracranial hemorrhage is a concern. An otolaryngology consultation should be obtained if symptoms suggest a nasopharyngeal tumor.

II. Etiology.
A brief review of the trigeminal pathways is necessary for an understanding of the location of dysfunction with facial numbness.

A. Neuroanatomy of the trigeminal nerve

1. The trigeminal nerve (cranial nerve V) is a mixed sensory and motor nerve.

   a. The sensory portion of the nerve is the largest portion, transmitting sensation from areas of the face, oral cavity, and nasal passages.

   b. There are three divisions of the **sensory portion** of the trigeminal nerve (Fig. 13.1).

      (1) **Ophthalmic (V1).** The ophthalmic division provides cutaneous supply to the forehead and anterior scalp to approximately the vertex, parts of the nose and the upper eyelid, and the upper half of the cornea. Branches of this division to the facial structures are the nasociliary, infratrochlear, supratrochlear, lacrimal, and supraorbital nerves.

      (2) **Maxillary (V2).** The maxillary division provides cutaneous supply to portions of the nose, upper lip, cheek, lower half of the cornea, upper gums and teeth, palate, and nasal mucosa. Branches of this division are the zygomaticofacial, zygomaticotemporal, and infraorbital nerves.

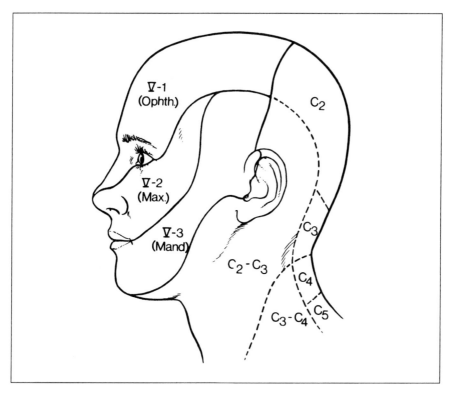

FIG. 13.1 Regions of the face supplied by the three sensory divisions of the trigeminal nerve (V-1, V-2, V-3). (From Sears ES, Franklin GM. Diseases of the cranial nerves. In: Rosenberg RN, ed. *Neurology*. New York: Grune & Stratton, 1980, with permission.)

> **(3) Mandibular (V3).** The mandibular division provides cutaneous supply to the lower lip, chin, portions of the jaw, ear, and mouth, lower gums and teeth, and the anterior two thirds of the tongue. Branches of this division are the auriculotemporal, buccal, and mental nerves. The combined nerve trunk of the mandibular division and the motor portion gives rise to the inferior alveolar nerves and the lingual nerves.
>
> **c.** The **motor portion** of the trigeminal nerve is a smaller division that travels with V3. It provides motor function to the muscles of mastication and the tensor tympani. This portion is not discussed further. However, it is important to examine the patient for dysfunction of the motor portion of the nerve.
>
> **2.** The three sensory divisions (V1, V2, and V3) enter the cranial cavity through the superior orbital fissure, foramen rotundum, and foramen ovale, respectively, to unite in the gasserian or semilunar ganglion, which lies at the apex of the petrous bones.
>
> **3.** Second-order sensory neurons enter the pons at the sensory root.

B. Localization of the lesion with facial numbness (Table 13.1). Facial numbness usually is unilateral and can be partial or total. Bilateral numbness can be associated with brainstem involvement, leptomeningeal disease, or systemic diseases, or it can be idiopathic. There are some generalizations that help localize the lesion.

Table 13.1 Types of numbness associated with lesions in different areas of the trigeminal sensory system

Location of lesion	Area of facial sensory loss
Ophthalmic (V1) division	Forehead, scalp, nose (except inferolateral), upper eyelid, upper half of cornea
Maxillary (V2) division	Lateral nose, upper lip, cheek, lower half of cornea, upper gums, palate, mucosa of lower nasal cavity
Mandibular (V3) division	Lower lip, lower jaw, chin, tympanic membrane, auditory meatus, upper ear, floor of mouth, lower gums and teeth, anterior two thirds of tongue
Proximal to gasserian ganglion	Entire face and all structures listed above
Brainstem	Onionskin sensory loss

1. Lesions of the divisions of cranial nerve V have distinct areas of sensory loss (Fig. 13.1).
2. Lesions proximal to the gasserian ganglion cause cutaneous numbness of the entire face and the anterior scalp (Fig. 13.2).
3. Lesions of the brainstem can produce an onionskin distribution of sensory loss (Fig. 13.3).
4. Lesions of cranial nerve V typically spare the angle of the jaw, which is supplied by C2 and C3 (Fig. 13.1).

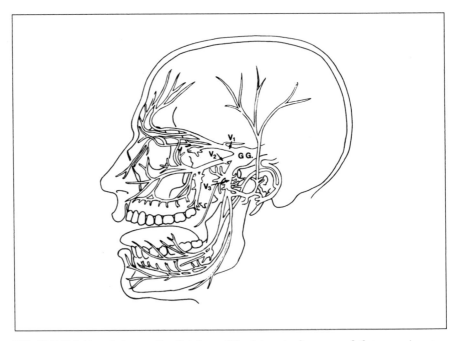

FIG. 13.2 Relations between the divisions of the trigeminal nerve and the gasserian ganglion (*GG.*).

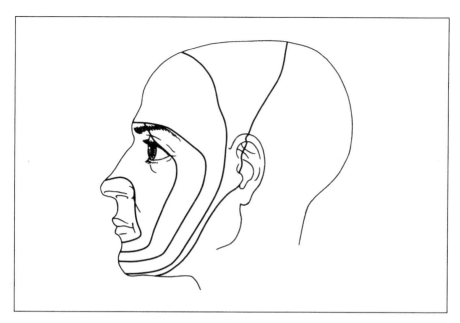

FIG. 13.3 Onionskin sensory loss resulting from brainstem lesions.

C. **Causes of facial numbness** (Table 13.2). There are many causes of facial numbness. The different causes are discussed according to the known or presumed site of involvement of the trigeminal pathway.
   1. **Lesions peripheral to the gasserian ganglion** (V1, V2, and V3)
      a. **Trauma.** Injury to the peripheral branches of the trigeminal nerve can occur with head or facial trauma, dental trauma or surgery, or any surgical procedure on the face (e.g., otorhinolaryngologic or dermatologic surgery).
         (1) **Head or facial injury.** The most frequently affected nerves are the superficial branches, including the supraorbital (branch of V1), supratrochlear (branch of V1), and infraorbital (branch of V2) nerves. The sensory loss is temporally related to the injury. Nerve regeneration can be accompanied by facial pain. The supraorbital branch can be damaged by blunt injury or as a result of a fracture of the upper margin of the orbit. The infraorbital nerve can be injured with closed head injuries or maxillary fractures. The entire ophthalmic division (V1) can be damaged in fractures through the foramen ovale. Transverse basilar skull fractures can injure the gasserian ganglion, resulting in anesthesia of the entire face and weakness of the masticatory muscles.
         (2) **Dental trauma.** Facial numbness can occur after tooth extraction. The inferior alveolar or lingual nerve can be damaged, and the result is transient anesthesia. Direct nerve injury also can occur as a result of needle trauma during dental anesthesia. In patients with severe mandibular bone resorption, denture use can cause pressure on the mental nerve, resulting in chin numbness.
         (3) **Facial surgery.** Any surgical procedure involving the face can lead to trigeminal nerve injury. Facial numbness has been described as a postoperative complication of microvascular decompression for trigeminal neuralgia due to trauma to the trigeminal root.

Table 13.2 Causes of facial numbness[a]

Lesions peripheral to the gasserian ganglion
Trauma (accidental, dental, surgical)
Infection (leprosy, herpes zoster)
Systemic diseases (sickle cell anemia, diabetes, diffuse connective tissue disease)
Tumor
Inflammatory
Drugs or toxins (stilbamidine, cocaine, others)
Idiopathic trigeminal sensory neuropathy
Lesions of the gasserian ganglion root
Infection (syphilis, tuberculosis, herpes zoster)
Tumor
Nontumorous mass lesions (aneurysm, hydrocephalus)
Sarcoidosis
Arachnoiditis
Amyloid
Drug (trichloroethylene)
Lesions of the central trigeminal pathways
Stroke
Tumor
Syringobulbia
Demyelinating disease
Vascular anomaly

[a]Presumed site of pathologic change.
Modified from Hagen NA, Stevens JC, Michet CJ Jr. Trigeminal sensory neuropathy associated with connective tissue disease. *Neurology* 1990;40:891–896.

    b. Infection
        (1) Leprosy. Worldwide, lepromatous leprosy is the most common cause of facial numbness. There can be facial hypalgesia and resultant accidental mutilation of the face.
        (2) Herpes zoster. Although the herpes zoster virus resides in the gasserian ganglion, evidence of active infection usually involves a division of the trigeminal nerve. The most commonly affected division is the ophthalmic division.
    c. Systemic disease
        (1) Sickle cell anemia. Numbness of the chin and lower lip resulting from mental neuropathy with sickle cell crisis has been described.
        (2) Diabetes. Facial numbness has been reported with diabetes and can accompany other forms of sensory neuropathy.
        (3) Diffuse connective tissue disease. The presence of facial numbness with a connective tissue disorder is rare. It has been associated with scleroderma, Sjögren's syndrome, mixed connective tissue disease, systemic lupus erythematosus, rheumatoid arthritis, and dermatomyositis.
    d. Tumors. Regional spread of a tumor along the trigeminal nerve can occur. Disease (most commonly of the lung and breast) metastasizing to the lower jaw can affect the inferior alveolar or mental nerve and cause numbness of the chin and lower lip. Cheek or malar numbness has been described with local spread of tumors along V2 or with leptomeningeal involvement with tumors. Nasopharyngeal tumors (squamous cell carcinoma is most common) arise most frequently in the roof of the pharynx. They can encroach on the trigeminal nerve, producing facial numbness. Associated features can include excessive lacrimation, facial pain, proptosis, hearing loss, and Horner's syndrome.

     e. Inflammatory lesions. Paranasal sinusitis can affect some branches of the trigeminal nerve.

     f. Drugs and toxins

       (1) Stilbamidine is an agent that has been used to treat leishmaniasis and multiple myeloma. Unilateral or bilateral facial numbness and anesthesia have been reported after treatment.

       (2) Cocaine abuse by the nasal route is a cause of facial numbness in the territory of the maxillary division (V2). Usually there is associated traumatic and ischemic necrosis of the nasal mucosa.

       (3) Other drugs. Many drugs can cause facial paresthesia. Circumoral paresthesia has been reported with labetalol, and mandibular neuropathy has been reported with allopurinol.

     g. Vascular disorders. In rare instances, carotid artery dissection can produce facial numbness.

     h. Idiopathic trigeminal sensory neuropathy. This diagnosis is one of exclusion after serious causes have been ruled out (see **III.**).

  2. Lesions of the gasserian ganglion or root

     a. Infection of the gasserian ganglion can occur with syphilis, tuberculosis, and herpes zoster.

     b. Tumor. Various tumors can affect the gasserian ganglion or root. Tumors that arise in the ganglion (ganglioneuroma or gangliocytoma) tend to have early, associated pain. Tumors that arise primarily in the root (neurinoma or neurofibroma) tend to have predominant sensory loss without pain. Tumors that can compress or invade the ganglion or root include acoustic neuroma, meningioma, schwannoma, cholesteatoma, pituitary adenoma, chordoma, nasopharyngeal carcinoma, and metastatic lesions.

     c. Nontumorous mass lesions (aneurysm, hydrocephalus)

     d. Sarcoidosis

     e. Arachnoiditis

     f. Amyloid. In rare instances, the gasserian ganglion or root can be the solitary site of amyloid deposits.

     g. Drug. Trichloroethylene is an industrial solvent that has been associated with facial numbness.

  3. Lesions of the central trigeminal pathways

     a. Stroke. Infarction in the lateral tegmentum of the medulla (Wallenberg's syndrome) can produce ipsilateral facial numbness along with other cranial nerve deficits and long tract signs. In rare instances, lateral pontine hemorrhage causes isolated facial numbness, perhaps as a result of involvement of the main sensory nucleus of the trigeminal nerve.

     b. Tumor. Tumors of the pons or medulla can affect the sensory nucleus of cranial nerve V, but there are usually other signs, including long tract and cranial nerve findings.

     c. Syringobulbia. This central cavitation of the medulla or pons can be associated with facial numbness.

     d. Demyelinating disease. Facial numbness is the initial symptom in 2% to 3% of patients with multiple sclerosis.

     e. Vascular anomalies. Isolated facial numbness very rarely results from a posterior fossa aneurysm or other vascular malformation.

III. Clinical manifestations

  A. Trigeminal sensory neuropathy. The literature is rather unclear in its definition of *trigeminal sensory neuropathy* (TSN). TSN has been used to describe different populations of patients with facial numbness. Blau et al. in 1969 described a population of patients with TSN who had self-limited facial paresthesia that in one half of the cases resolved in several months. There were no associated neurologic deficits. At neurologic examination, the corneal response was intact and the only finding was a subjective decrease in light touch and pinprick over the involved trigeminal distribution. Only 10% of these patients had identifiable causes of TSN, and 10% went on to have trigeminal neuralgia. In contrast to this population, with a seemingly benign course, Horowitz in 1974 found that 88% of a population with facial numbness had an identifiable, usually serious condition. This population almost always had other neurologic deficits (cranial nerve or ataxia). It may be concluded that these two studies involved quite different populations.

TSN is best defined as a general term for facial numbness of which there are many different causes, as previously discussed. Any area of the face can be involved. **Idiopathic TSN** is used to describe purely sensory impairment of unknown causation in a territory of the trigeminal nerve (usually V2 or V3) on one or both sides of the face. It can be associated with pain, paresthesia, or dysfunction of taste. Because the data currently available do not allow one to differentiate consistently between facial numbness that is benign and facial numbness that is attributable to a serious condition, idiopathic TSN remains a diagnosis of exclusion after an appropriate, thorough evaluation. Available data do indicate that the presence of associated neurologic signs and deficits usually points to a more ominous process.

B. Numb chin and numb cheek syndromes

    1. Numb chin syndrome is an uncommon forms of facial neuropathy. However, the occurrence of this syndrome is notable, because numb chin syndrome rarely is caused by benign lesions and often is a symptom of more ominous processes such as involvement of the mental or inferior alveolar nerves (branches of V3) by systemic cancer.

        a. Any tumor metastasizing to the jaw can produce this syndrome, but malignant tumors of the breast, lung, and lymphoreticular system are found most commonly. Numb chin syndrome also can be caused by metastasis to the proximal mandibular root at the base of the skull or by leptomeningeal involvement with malignant tumors such as lymphoma.

        b. Most patients already have a known diagnosis of cancer. However, mental neuropathy can be the initial symptom of malignant disease or it can herald tumor recurrence or progression.

        c. The **clinical presentation** involves ipsilateral numbness or anesthesia of the skin and mucosa of the lower lip and chin that extends to the midline. There is usually no associated pain, but there can be lip swelling and ulcerations from biting of the numb lip.

        d. The **evaluation** of patients with numb chin syndrome should include radiographs of the mandible with particular attention to the mental foramen, radiographs of the basal skull, MRI of the brain with contrast enhancement, and if there is concern of leptomeningeal infiltration, cerebrospinal fluid analysis.

        e. Although a numb chin is a seemingly benign problem, it should be thoroughly evaluated because of its clinical importance as a possible sign of malignant disease.

    2. Numb cheek syndrome. Numbness over the malar region can have implications similar to those of numb chin syndrome. Squamous or basal cell carcinoma of the face can spread along the trigeminal nerve. Such tumors also can spread from regional nerves to the skull base and into the intracranial space. Numbness of the anterior gums and teeth suggests a more peripheral lesion, whereas both anterior and posterior gum and teeth involvement suggests leptomeningeal disease.

IV. Evaluation

    A. History. It is important to obtain as much detailed information as possible about the patient's facial numbness. The points that should be addressed include the following:

        1. Sites of numbness, including whether the numbness is unilateral or bilateral.

        2. Duration of numbness

        3. Quality of numbness

        4. Associated features (pain, altered taste, and nasal, dental, and cerebrovascular symptoms)

5. History of **trauma** (accidental, dental, or surgical)

6. History of **malignant disease**

7. **Medications** used currently and in the past

B. Physical examination

1. General physical examination. A thorough, complete examination is necessary to evaluate for a potential cause of the facial numbness. Particular attention must be paid to evaluating for an underlying malignant lesion (including nasopharyngeal tumor), a dental problem, or an underlying rheumatologic condition. Although many different areas need to be assessed, the following areas are especially important.

    a. Head and neck. Inspection of the nose, mouth, and teeth and palpation for adenopathy are important.

    b. Vascular disorders. Bilateral blood pressure should be checked to evaluate for vascular disease. Auscultation for carotid or vertebral bruits should be performed. If there is suspicion of an intracranial aneurysm, listen for cranial bruits.

    c. Breast

    d. Pulmonary

    e. Lymphatic

    f. Rheumatologic

    g. Skin

2. Neurologic examination. A thorough neurologic examination is necessary. It is particularly important to evaluate all of the functions of the trigeminal nerve and to evaluate for evidence of dysfunction of other cranial nerves.

    a. Clinical evaluation of the trigeminal nerve

        (1) Sensory evaluation. Touch, pain, and temperature are tested in the distribution of the three divisions. Each division is tested individually and compared with the opposite side. The sensation in the nasal and oral mucosa, the anterior two thirds of the tongue, and the anterior portion of the ear (tragus and anterior helix) should be assessed.

        (2) Motor evaluation. The motor functions of the trigeminal nerve are assessed by means of testing the muscles of mastication. By having a patient clench the jaw, the strength of the masseters and temporalis can be tested bilaterally. Weakness is evidenced by absent or reduced contraction of the muscles on the side of the lesion. The lateral pterygoids are tested by having the patient move the jaw from side to side against the resistance of the examiner's hand. The jaw deviates toward the paralyzed side on opening the mouth because of contraction of the intact contralateral lateral pterygoid muscle. It cannot be deviated to the opposite, nonparalyzed side. Finally, the patient should be asked to protrude the jaw. Any evidence of atrophy or fasciculation is noted.

        (3) Reflex evaluation

            (a) Corneal reflex. This reflex is assessed by means of touching a wisp of a sterile cotton-tipped applicator to the edge of the cornea (not the sclera) bilaterally. The afferent portion of the reflex is carried by V1 (upper cornea) and V2 (lower cornea), and the efferent portion is carried by cranial nerve VII, both ipsilaterally and contralaterally. Lesions of the trigeminal nerve may cause a diminished or absent response both ipsilaterally and contralaterally.

            (b) Orbicularis oculi reflex (blink reflex). This reflex is assessed by means of tapping the glabella or supraorbital ridge. This elicits an early ipsilateral blink followed by bilateral blinking.

            (c) Sternutatory reflex. This reflex is assessed by means of checking light touch sensation of the lateral nasal mucosa with a cotton-tipped applicator. The appropriate response is immediate withdrawal from the irritating stimulus. This reflex may be diminished or absent in lesions of the maxillary division (V2).

(d) **Masseter reflex or jaw jerk.** This reflex is assessed by means of tapping the slightly opened lower jaw. Lesions of the trigeminal nerve may result in a hypoactive ipsilateral jerk, whereas bilateral supranuclear lesions may result in a hyperactive response.

b. **The rest of the neurologic examination**
   (1) **Speech.** Dysarthria may be present with profound facial, tongue, or oral sensory deficits.
   (2) **Cranial nerves.** Careful attention should be paid to associated abnormalities of cranial nerves, especially II, III, IV, VI, VII, and VIII.
   (3) **Motor and muscle stretch reflexes**
   (4) **Sensory loss.** It is important to evaluate for evidence of other regions of sensory loss, especially generalized sensory neuropathy.
   (5) **Coordination.** Coordination can be impaired by a process such as a tumor in the cerebellopontine angle.
   (6) **Gait and station**

C. **Laboratory studies**
   1. **Biochemical tests** include complete blood cell count with differential, complete chemistry profile including liver function tests and glucose level, and erythrocyte sedimentation rate. In certain situations, a Venereal Disease Research Laboratory test, antinuclear antibody determination, rheumatoid factor, extractable nuclear antigen antibodies, or an angiotensin-converting enzyme level may be necessary. Skin scraping or biopsy is necessary when leprosy is a consideration.
   2. **A purified protein derivative test** should be done if there is suspicion of tuberculosis.
   3. A **chest radiograph** should be obtained to evaluate for a malignancy pulmonary disease or tuberculosis.
   4. **Skull and sinus radiography.** A radiograph if the mandible is indicated if there is a numb chin.
   5. **Lumbar puncture** is essential if there is suspicion of infection or a malignant tumor of the leptomeninges.
   6. A **blink reflex** may be elicited electrophysiologically by means of electrical stimulation of the supraorbital nerve. It can be helpful in detecting subtle central or peripheral lesions of the trigeminal nerve.
   7. **Brain imaging.** All patients with facial numbness MRI of the brain. MRI is more sensitive than CT as a detector of lesions of the trigeminal nerve and of posterior fossa abnormalities such as acoustic neuroma. Suspicion of acoustic neuroma may necessitate special cuts through the acoustic canals with administration of contrast medium. Suspicion of an intracranial tumor may necessitate administration of contrast material. CT with and without contrast enhancement may be indicated if MRI is not available or if there are contraindications to MRI.

V. **Differential diagnosis.** Specific locations of lesion causing facial numbness are detailed in Table 13.1.
   A. Tumor
   B. Infection
   C. Trauma
   D. Connective tissue disease
   E. Drug or toxin
   F. Nontumor mass lesion
   G. Vascular disorder
   H. Demyelinating disorder
   I. Other systemic or rare disease
   J. Idiopathic disorder

Table 13.3 Tests used in the evaluation of facial numbness and the relative cost

Test	Cost
Complete blood cell count with differential	$
Chemistry profile	$
Erythrocyte sedimentation rate	$
Venereal Disease Research Laboratory test	$
Antinuclear antibodies	$
Rheumatoid factor	$
Extractable nuclear antigen antibodies	$$
Angiotensin-converting enzyme	$
Purified protein derivative	$
Chest radiograph	$$
Skull radiograph	$$
Sinus radiograph	$$
Lumbar puncture	$$
Blink reflex	$$
Brain computed tomography	$$$
Brain magnetic resonance imaging	$$$$

$, relatively inexpensive; $$, moderately expensive; $$$, expensive; $$$$, very expensive.

VI. Diagnostic approach

A. The first step is to define clinically whether the deficit involves a division or divisions of the trigeminal nerve, the gasserian ganglion or root, or the central trigeminal pathways. Detecting involvement of other cranial nerves or signs of associated diseases can help to limit the number of diagnostic possibilities.

B. Appropriate tests are performed depending on the results of the examination. Unless there is an obvious history of trauma, the following tests should be performed: complete blood cell count with differential, chemistry profile, erythrocyte sedimentation rate, chest radiography, and brain MRI. For selected patients, other tests are indicated, such as Venereal Disease Research Laboratory test, antinuclear antibody determination, extractable nuclear antigen antibodies determination, angiotensin-converting enzyme measurement, purified protein derivative test, blink reflex, lumbar puncture, skull radiography, sinus radiography, and brain CT. The tests that may be indicated, and their relative costs, are listed in Table 13.3.

VII. Referral.
Because the range of possible underlying diseases that can cause facial numbness is so wide, it is often necessary to use a teamwork approach to this problem. A **neurologist,** who should be most familiar with localization of lesions of the trigeminal nerve, should be consulted initially. It is often necessary to consult an **otolaryngologist** to evaluate for the presence of a nasopharyngeal tumor, acoustic neuroma, or sinusitis. A **dentist** or an **oral surgeon** may be needed to assist in ruling out a dental cause of facial numbness. In selected instances, a **rheumatologist** may be needed if there is evidence of associated connective tissue disease.

Recommended Readings
Ashworth B, Tait GBW. Trigeminal neuropathy in connective tissue disease. *Neurology* 1971; 21:609.

Blau JN, Harris M, Kennett S. Trigeminal sensory neuropathy. *N Engl J Med* 1969;281: 873–876.

Brazis PW, Masdeu JC, Biller J. The localization of lesions affecting cranial nerve V. In: Brazis PW, Masdeu JC, Biller J, eds. *Localization in clinical neurology,* 3rd ed. Boston: Little, Brown, 1996:251.

Bruyn RPM, Boogerd W. The numb chin. *Clin Neurol Neurosurg* 1991;93:187.

Burt RK, Sharfman WH, Karp BI, et al. Mental neuropathy (numb chin syndrome): a harbinger of tumor progression or relapse. *Cancer* 1992;70:877–881.

Francis KR, Williams DP, Troost BT. Facial numbness and dysesthesias: new features of carotid artery dissection. *Arch Neurol* 1987;44:345–346.

Gibbin KP, Griffith IP. Idiopathic sensory trigeminal neuropathy. *J Laryngol Otol* 1978;92:915.

Goldstein NP, Gibilisco JA, Rushton JG, et al. Trigeminal neuropathy and neuritis: a study of etiology with emphasis on dental causes. *JAMA* 1963;184:458–462.

Goor C, Ongerboer De Visser BW. Jaw and blink reflexes in trigeminal nerve lesions: an electrodiagnostic study. *Neurology* 1976;26:95.

Greenberg HS, Deck MD, Vikram B, et al. Metastasis to the base of the skull: clinical findings in 43 patients. *Neurology* 1981;31:530–537.

Hagen NA, Stevens JC, Michet CJ. Trigeminal sensory neuropathy associated with connective tissue disease. *Neurology* 1990;40:891–896.

Holtzman RNN, Zablozki V, Yang WC, et al. Lateral pontine tegmental hemorrhage presenting as isolated trigeminal sensory neuropathy. *Neurology* 1987;37:704–706.

Horowitz SH. Isolated facial numbness: clinical significance and relation to trigeminal neuropathy. *Ann Intern Med* 1974;80:49.

Kuntzer T, Bogousslavsky J, Rilliet B, et al. Herald facial numbness. *Eur Neurol* 1992;32:297–301.

Lecky BR, Hughes RA, Murray NM, et al. Trigeminal sensory neuropathy: a study of 22 cases. *Brain* 1987;110:1463–1485.

Massey EW, Moore J, Schold SC Jr, et al. Mental neuropathy from systemic cancer. *Neurology* 1981;31:1277–1281.

Searles RP, Mladinich EK, Messner RP, et al. Isolated trigeminal sensory neuropathy: early manifestation of mixed connective tissue disease. *Neurology* 1978;28:1286.

Sears ES, Franklin GM. Diseases of the cranial nerves. In: Rosenberg RN, ed. *Neurology*. New York: Grune & Stratton, 1980.

Thrush DC, Small M. How benign a symptom is facial numbness? *Lancet* 1970;2:851.

14. APPROACH TO THE PATIENT WITH FACIAL PAIN

Julius M. Goodman

A careful work-up usually reveals the source of most **facial pain,** but some patients with severe facial pain have normal results of physical examinations and diagnostic tests. It is important for the primary care physician to realize that some of these patients may have pain of neurologic or psychological origin. Sometimes such pain is erroneously attributed to disorders of the paranasal sinuses, teeth, or jaw and leads to a series of therapeutic misadventures by surgical and dental specialists with interest in facial pain. This chapter reviews an approach to patients with **trigeminal and glossopharyngeal neuralgia, cluster headache, herpetic and postherpetic neuralgia,** and a variety of other conditions that can be associated with facial pain. Some patients with chronic facial pain of unknown causation may have **atypical facial pain** syndrome, which is thought to be of psychological origin. Long-term treatment and guidance of these distraught patients may become the responsibilities of the primary care physician.

I. **Trigeminal neuralgia** (tic douloureux or tic) is the most common paroxysmal pain disorder of the face and one of the most painful afflictions known.
A. **Etiology.** The exact mechanism of trigeminal neuralgia has not been definitely established. Some cases have been associated with structural lesions (symptomatic trigeminal neuralgia), but in most patients ordinary imaging studies do not reveal a cause (idiopathic trigeminal neuralgia).
1. **Symptomatic.** Approximately 1% to 2% of patients with trigeminal neuralgia have a posterior fossa lesion in the area of the ipsilateral trigeminal nerve: tumor (epidermoid, acoustic schwannoma, or meningioma), vascular malformation, or anomaly or tumor of the skull. At times, there is a mass on the side opposite the pain or even in the supratentorial area. In such cases, it has been postulated that secondary distortion of the brainstem is responsible. More likely is that some of these remote lesions are incidental and not related to trigeminal neuralgia. Approximately 2% of patients with multiple sclerosis may have trigeminal neuralgia, usually secondary to an area of demyelination near the root entry zone of the trigeminal nerve in the pons. When a young person comes to medical attention with trigeminal neuralgia, it is important to rule out occult multiple sclerosis or a structural lesion.
2. **Idiopathic.** Most patients with trigeminal neuralgia have no discernible lesions. Some neurosurgeons believe that most but not all patients may have compression of the trigeminal nerve root near its exit from the pons by a normal or ectatic artery or a vein. Refinements in magnetic resonance imaging (MRI) have made noninvasive visualization of some of these vessels possible (see **I.D.**). It has been postulated that vascular pulsations cause an area of demyelination on the trigeminal root with resulting ephaptic (nonsynaptic) transmission or "short circuit" from thickly myelinated sensory fibers to thinly myelinated pain fibers.
B. **Symptoms.** Most patients with trigeminal neuralgia are older than 50 years. Women are affected somewhat more frequently than are men. Trigeminal neuralgia is characterized by intermittent paroxysms of severe, brief (seconds), lancinating, "shocklike" pain. Patients often use phrases such as "a bolt of lightning" or "an electric shock" when describing the pain. The pain of trigeminal neuralgia can occur spontaneously or be brought on by talking, eating, brushing the teeth, washing, or lightly touching the face. Some patients refuse to go outdoors, fearing that a breeze will precipitate pain.
1. Most patients have a **trigger zone,** which is a localized area of skin or mucous membrane that is highly sensitive. When this area is touched lightly, a paroxysm of pain can be triggered. The first attack of trigeminal neuralgia can be so spectacular that the patient recalls it vividly, even after many years. Trigeminal neuralgia is sometimes mistakenly attributed to dental disease, and many patients undergo tooth extractions or root canals to no avail.

2. Tic pain usually involves a single trigeminal division or two adjacent divisions simultaneously but rarely all three; the first (ophthalmic) division is least involved. Pain never crosses the midline. In 4% of patients, symptoms may become bilateral, but simultaneous bilateral pain is extremely rare. Patients with multiple sclerosis are more prone to eventual bilateral involvement. This fact must be kept in mind when ablative surgical lesions are contemplated.

3. Spontaneous remission of trigeminal neuralgia pain may last for months or years, especially at the outset. After many years, trigeminal neuralgia pain tends to change to a more constant discomfort with fewer attacks of lancinating pain, thus making diagnosis more difficult. When seeing a patient at a late stage for the first time, it is helpful to ask for a description of the pain experienced at onset.

C. **Signs.** Characteristically the findings at neurologic examination are normal, and the diagnosis is suspected from the history. The patient may refuse to speak for fear of setting off a paroxysm of pain. A startle reaction to spontaneous trigeminal neuralgia pain helps confirm the diagnosis when observed by the examiner. If the patient allows it, the examiner can lightly touch a trigger area and cause a very brief sudden flinch or wince, during which the patient may draw a hand up toward the face. A member of the patient's family may be able to describe these quick jerks that occur with pain. During the neurologic examination, signs and symptoms of tumor or multiple sclerosis should be sought. The presence of **objective or subjective facial sensory loss, facial weakness, decreased hearing, or ataxia** should raise suspicion of a **structural lesion.**

D. **Diagnosis.** There is no laboratory test for trigeminal neuralgia. The key to diagnosis is an accurate history. A dramatic response to carbamazepine is reassuring, because most patients with trigeminal neuralgia have an initial response. Other types of facial pain are not relieved in this manner. Imaging studies to rule out a structural lesion are not essential in the treatment of elderly patients with normal neurologic findings, but most clinicians consider MRI part of the workup. MRI is strongly advised for patients younger than 60 years, for all those with abnormal neurologic findings or in whom multiple sclerosis is suspected, and when a surgical procedure is contemplated. MRI with and without contrast enhancement is preferred over computed tomography because MRI is superior in visualizing intraaxial and extraaxial lesions in the posterior fossa. If treatment by microvascular decompression is being considered, some surgeons may be influenced by several newer MRI protocols that can depict small vessels close to the trigeminal nerve as it exits the brainstem. Conventional angiography and electrophysiologic studies are not helpful.

E. **Treatment**
   1. **Medical**
      a. Initially almost all patients with trigeminal neuralgia respond to the anticonvulsant **carbamazepine.** An unequivocal response can be used as a diagnostic test for trigeminal neuralgia. Because carbamazepine stimulates its own metabolism in the liver by means of autoinduction, administration must begin with a low dose (100 mg twice a day) followed by gradual escalation to avoid unpleasant side effects. The dose of carbamazepine required to control symptoms varies from 200 to 1,200 mg per day. The medication should be titrated to the lowest dose that relieves pain with a minimum of drug-related symptoms. Measurement of carbamazepine blood levels is not helpful. Extended release tablets are available and may provide smoother control for some patients. Dizziness, unsteadiness, and drowsiness are the most common **adverse reactions** on initiation of therapy. Older patients often report disturbed mentation and forgetfulness. Because of potential serious **drug interactions,** patients taking carbamazepine must be cautioned to check with their physician any time they receive a new medication. The most common offenders are propoxyphene, cimetidine, erythromycin, and verapamil, all of which can cause extremely high carbamazepine blood levels.

Carbamazepine frequently causes mild leukopenia and slightly abnormal results of liver function tests, which are not ordinarily a justification for stopping the medication. A rare patient may have serious bone marrow or liver failure.

b. Oxcarbazepine, a newer medication, is as effective as carbamazepine and has lesser liver, hematopoietic, and skin reactions but causes a greater incidence of acute hyponatremia. A practitioner should carefully review the pharmacologic properties of carbamazepine and related drugs before prescribing them (see Chapter 39).

c. Other medications, which are less effective, that can be used alone or in combination with carbamazepine are phenytoin, gabapentin, baclofen, clonazepam, and lamotrigine.

2. **Surgical.** Approximately 50% of patients who obtain initial relief with medication eventually need surgical therapy for trigeminal neuralgia, either for persistent or recurrent pain or for medication intolerance. A few specialists unfamiliar with surgical therapy are reluctant to refer patients for operation and continue futile treatment with a wide variety of drugs, resulting in very unhappy patients. There is no perfect operation for trigeminal neuralgia, but a variety of contemporary procedures can afford sustained relief. Age, general health, patient preference, willingness to accept risk and the risk of side effects, and the experience and bias of the surgeon are all factors in selecting a procedure. The following are currently the most popular operations for trigeminal neuralgia.

a. Microvascular decompression in the posterior fossa usually is reserved for patients younger than 65 years but is occasionally offered to older patients in excellent health. This is the only procedure that addresses what many surgeons believe is the most common cause of trigeminal neuralgia. The operation is performed through a small opening in the skull just medial to the mastoid. With the use of a surgical microscope, the trigeminal nerve is identified as it exits the brainstem. If there is nerve compression or indentation by a vessel, a small surgical sponge is placed between the nerve and the offending vessel. In the occasional patient in whom no such vessel can be identified, a small incision into the nerve or manual compression of the nerve usually is performed. Approximately 80% of patients obtain long-lasting pain relief without considerable facial sensory loss. Although it is a major neurosurgical procedure, **experienced neurosurgeons** usually can perform microvascular decompression with minimal morbidity.

b. Percutaneous procedures that partially injure the trigeminal root as it exits the posterior fossa to enter the middle fossa can be performed on outpatients and often afford immediate pain relief with minimal risk. However, the patient must be willing to accept a variable amount of permanent facial sensory loss, which occasionally can be quite bothersome. To avoid unpleasant sensory symptoms, an attempt is made to make the sensory loss minimal, although a lesser degree of nerve injury increases the failure and recurrence rates and the need for repeat surgery. The production of profound anesthesia can lead to a central deafferentation pain syndrome (anesthesia dolorosa), for which there is no good treatment and which can be more disabling than trigeminal neuralgia. When the pain involves the first trigeminal division, great care must be taken to avoid corneal anesthesia.

All percutaneous procedures are performed with a needle that enters the cheek approximately 3 cm lateral to the mouth. The needle passes between the mandible and maxilla into the foramen ovale, through which the mandibular division and motor root of the trigeminal nerve exit the skull. A heat lesion by a radiofrequency current (**radiofrequency rhizotomy**), a pressure lesion by a balloon catheter (**balloon microcompression**), or a chemical lesion by injection of glycerol (**glycerol rhizotomy**) are options and to a large extent depend on the surgeon's preference and experience. These percutaneous procedures can be used to treat patients with trigeminal neuralgia and multiple sclerosis. Aged, infirm, seriously ill, malnourished, and demented patients seem to tolerate percutaneous procedures well.

c. **Gamma knife radiosurgery** has recently been used to cause partial radiation injury to the trigeminal nerve as it exits the pons. Radiosurgery is becoming quite popular in the management of trigeminal neuralgia, because it is entirely noninvasive, outpatient, and painless. A single dose of highly focused gamma rays converges on the trigeminal root with minimal effect on the adjacent brain stem. Complete pain relief can be obtained in 50% to 70% of patients and partial relief in some of the others. Delayed mild sensory loss occurs in 10% of patients. A major disadvantage is a latent period of 2 weeks to 2 months from the time of treatment to onset of effective relief. Consequently, the operation is not ideal for patients incapacitated by medically nonresponsive excruciating pain and those who are unable to eat. The optimal radiation dose and technique are still being determined. However, when gamma knife therapy is successful, it is so elegant that some surgeons are recommending that it be the first line of surgical treatment and that it even be offered earlier to patients without pain who are not happy with medical management. Multiple sclerosis patients with trigeminal neuralgia may respond to this treatment. A distinct advantage for them is sparing of the motor root and minimal if any sensory loss, because patients with multiple sclerosis may eventually need a procedure on the opposite side.

d. **Warning.** *These surgical procedures are only for patients with trigeminal neuralgia. When performed for other types of facial pain, including those in which the etiologic factor may be obscure, facial pain can be made worse.*

II. Glossopharyngeal neuralgia is characterized by paroxysmal lancinating pain similar to that of trigeminal neuralgia but centered on the tonsil and ear. Pain can be triggered by swallowing, yawning, or food contact on the pharynx. Glossopharyngeal neuralgia is rare in comparison with trigeminal neuralgia. **It can be associated with neoplasms involving the skull base.** The diagnosis is made by history. Patients should have an otolaryngology consultation to look for an occult neoplasm. Anesthetizing the pharynx with topical anesthesia can aid in the diagnosis if it temporarily halts lancinating pain triggered by touch or swallowing. A rare manifestation of glossopharyngeal neuralgia is episodes of **bradycardia** or **asystole** secondary to increased reflex sensitivity in the distribution of the ninth and tenth cranial nerves. Glossopharyngeal neuralgia is less responsive than is trigeminal neuralgia to anticonvulsants. Microvascular decompression of the glossopharyngeal nerve or sectioning of the glossopharyngeal nerve and the upper two rootlets of the vagus nerve are the preferred surgical options.

III. Herpes zoster virus neuralgia has no relation to trigeminal neuralgia in regard to etiology, symptoms, or management. Herpes zoster usually involves the thoracic dermatomes, but the ophthalmic division (V1) of the trigeminal nerve is affected approximately 10% to 20% of the time, resulting in facial pain. Zoster infection results from reactivation of latent varicella-zoster virus in the gasserian (trigeminal) sensory ganglion. Elderly patients with declining immune systems and patients with diseases that compromise immunity are most susceptible. An acute painful disorder and a chronic pain syndrome are associated with herpes zoster of the face. Acute **herpes zoster ophthalmicus** is a term that includes the preeruptive phase, painful skin lesions, and persistent discomfort for 1 month. Chronic **postherpetic neuralgia** (PHN) refers to a central pain syndrome that develops in some patients after the acute phase.

A. **Herpes zoster ophthalmicus** in the preeruptive phase is difficult to recognize and can be confused with other types of facial neuralgia and cranial arteritis until the characteristic herpetic rash appears. There may be burning or lancinating pain in the ophthalmic distribution associated with nausea, malaise, and mild fever. Clusters of skin vesicles (shingles) usually appear within 4 days of the onset of pain, but sometimes the appearance of skin lesions may be delayed for many days. In rare instances, there is pain and no development of skin lesions. If the diagnosis is suspected, it can be confirmed by the presence of increasing herpes zoster virus antibody titers. The virus also can involve the globe, leading to ocular pain and visual loss. In the acute phase, the level of protein in the spinal fluid may be elevated, and pleocytosis may be present.

B. **PHN** involving the ophthalmic division is a type of central pain and is not caused by stimulation of pain nerve endings by damaged tissue, as in acute infection. Severe pain during the acute phase and age older than 80 years seem to make a patient more prone to development of PHN. The pain is incapacitating for the patient and extremely frustrating for the physician attempting to manage it.

   1. **Symptoms** of PHN begin approximately 4 weeks after the cutaneous phase has subsided at the site of the herpetic eruption. PHN pain is described as "burning" or "ice burning," which differs from shingles pain. Tactile allodynia can be caused by a nonnoxious stimulus such as hair brushing or wind. The pain of PHN should not be confused with the shock-like pain of trigeminal neuralgia, which can also be triggered by similar stimuli. A moist cloth over the skin may afford some relief. Sleep usually is not disturbed. Emotional stress can aggravate symptoms and cause depression, as in other types of central pain.

   2. **Signs.** Residual skin scarring of herpes zoster ophthalmicus may be evident. Careful sensory testing in the involved areas may reveal deficits in response to light touch, pinprick, hot and cold, and two-point discrimination.

IV. **Cluster headache** (migrainous neuralgia) is a paroxysmal, recurring disorder of unknown causation that is characterized by episodes of intense, strictly unilateral facial pain lasting approximately 30 minutes to 2 hours. The pain tends to occur once or several times daily over a period of weeks to months and followed by spontaneous remission lasting months to years.

A. **Symptoms.** Periocular pain is characteristic, but the cheek and forehead can be involved. The pain is as excruciating as trigeminal neuralgia but is of longer duration. Pain occasionally may be lancinating, but the existence of a trigger area is rare. Unlike trigeminal neuralgia, cluster headaches frequently awaken a patient from sleep. Unlike migraine, (1) the disorder is more common among men, (2) onset in childhood is unusual, (3) a family history of migraine is not as common, (4) the patient usually is hyperactive during an attack, whereas a persons with migraine prefers a quiet, dark room, (5) auras do not occur, and (6) nausea and vomiting are not characteristic.

B. **Signs.** During an attack there may be ipsilateral flushing of the face, conjunctival injection, and nasal stuffiness. The findings of neurologic examination are normal during an attack except for occasional partial Horner's syndrome that manifests as slight ptosis and miosis. **Horner's syndrome associated with any other type of facial pain is ominous and deserves a detailed search for a structural lesion.**

C. **Variants**

   1. **Cluster–tic syndrome.** A rare patient with cluster headache may also have symptoms of trigeminal neuralgia. The pain is always on the same side and division and can be provoked by similar stimuli, suggesting that this is a separate entity and not the coexistence of the two disorders. The success rate of medical or surgical therapy is not well established.

   2. **Cluster–migraine.** Migraine headaches occur among 1% to 3% of patients with cluster headaches and vice versa.

   3. **Paroxysmal hemicrania.** In this rare condition, pain and signs are similar to those of cluster headache, but each episode is shorter in duration with as many as eight paroxysms in 24 hours. It occurs somewhat more commonly among women than among men. Recognition of this disorder is important, because symptoms often, but not always, respond rapidly and specifically to indomethacin.

   4. **Posttraumatic cluster headaches.** Clusterlike headaches have occurred after facial trauma. The mechanism is not known, and these headaches are more resistant to abortive and prophylactic treatment.

V. Atypical facial pain. Physicians often use this term to describe facial pain for which no organic cause can be found and that does not meet the criteria for established facial pain syndromes. However, atypical facial pain should be regarded as a diagnosis in its own right and not as a wastebasket term when chronic facial pain cannot be explained.

   A. Signs and symptoms. The typical patient is a middle-aged woman with continuous deep facial pain that is poorly localized and not in the anatomic distribution of one of the trigeminal branches. Initially the pain is unilateral, but in one third of cases, bilateral symptoms eventually occur. The patient may have difficulty describing the pain and use terms such as "pulling," "aching," "tearing," and "drawing." The pain intensity may fluctuate, but discomfort is always present. Activities and weather may aggravate the pain but not to the extent observed with trigeminal neuralgia. Many of these patients are prone to exaggeration. They may claim that facial pain is ruining their lives, but when examined they do not appear very sick. Mood swings and irritability are common. Insomnia is a frequent symptom, but pain does not ordinarily awaken the patient. The typical patient has already seen a variety of medical specialists and may have undergone numerous diagnostic studies with normal results, unsuccessful anesthetic blocks, and failed surgical procedures. These patients characteristically look forward to additional operations, hoping that eventually someone will find the cause of and a cure for their discomfort. Patients often carry lists of drugs that have failed to alleviate their suffering or to which they are allergic. *Beware that patients with typical trigeminal neuralgia, after many years of suffering, may have continuous pain that can be difficult to differentiate from atypical facial pain. A careful history of the initial pain is important.*

   B. Etiology. Approximately one half of patients with atypical facial pain attribute the onset to trauma or a dental procedure. Most authorities believe that the disorder is primarily psychological. The diagnosis must not be made until other causes of facial pain are ruled out.

VI. Other causes of facial pain.

   A. Paranasal sinus disease. Acute sinusitis usually is clinically evident; chronic sinusitis is rarely a cause of facial pain. However, isolated sphenoid sinusitis can be an obscure cause of headache and pain referred to the face. Remember that thickened mucous membranes and paranasal cysts are commonly seen on routine imaging studies of patients who have no symptoms.

   B. Temporomandibular joint (TMJ) disorders are frequently implicated as a cause of chronic facial pain. The disorder should be considered when there is mechanical pain on jaw movement, restriction of mouth opening, localized trauma, and abnormal imaging studies. However, the diagnosis of TMJ disorder is controversial and difficult and is often made inappropriately. It is important for the primary care physician to keep this in mind when monitoring the evaluation and treatment of patients thought to have TMJ disorder.

   1. Many patients have dental malocclusion but no TMJ symptoms.

   2. Many persons without symptoms have abnormal findings at TMJ imaging studies and arthrography that include arthritis and TMJ meniscus disorders.

   3. The incidence of TMJ disorder decreases with age, which would be unusual if degenerative disease of the TMJ were the cause of pain.

   4. Joint tenderness, teeth grinding, and electromyographic abnormalities occur with equal frequency among patients considered to have TMJ disorders and among controls.

   Multiple opinions and prolonged conservative treatment should be considered before a patient is advised to proceed with a TMJ procedure. Although oral appliances are widely prescribed by dentists, valid evidence that supports the efficacy of these devices is lacking.

   C. Toothache is an easily recognized cause of acute facial pain, but when bad teeth coexist with a neurologic disorder such as trigeminal neuralgia, dentists may perform extractions before the neuralgia is recognized. Moreover, some dentists believe that small cavities in the jaw, apparently occurring after tooth extraction but not visible on radiographs, can cause chronic oral pain. If the pain is relieved with a block, curettage of the mandible usually is recommended. However, these procedures are not often successful in relieving chronic facial pain. **Phantom tooth pain** is a recently recognized type of deafferentation pain syndrome that occurs in a small percentage of patients after tooth extraction or endodontic treatment. The cause is thought to be similar to pain that occurs after amputation of other parts of the body.

D. **Temporal arteritis** may be present in an elderly person with pain in the distribution of the external carotid artery. Pain with chewing, tenderness and thickening over the branches of the superficial temporal arteries, acute visual loss, occasional redness or ulceration of the skin of the forehead, and systemic symptoms may be present. The erythrocyte sedimentation rate is almost always elevated (see Chapter 10).

E. **Cranial nerve disorders** may manifest as pain before the appearance of neurologic signs that make the cause obvious.

   1. **Optic neuritis** or **retrobulbar neuritis** can cause retroorbital pain that precedes visual loss by hours or days. An early abnormal afferent pupillary reflex should be sought.

   2. **Ischemia** or **infarction** of the oculomotor or other cranial nerves can be associated with pain so severe that the neurologic deficit is overshadowed, as in early diabetic oculomotor palsy.

F. **Ocular pain**

   1. **Acute glaucoma** as a cause of pain in the eye and adjacent face usually is obvious by virtue of clouding of the cornea and other changes in the globe. However, subacute glaucoma can manifest as eye pain and physical findings that may not be readily evident to an inexperienced examiner.

   2. **Refractive errors** and squint should **not** ordinarily be considered causes of unexplained facial pain.

G. **Thalamic pain** is a central pain syndrome that develops in rare instances after thalamic infarction. Painful dysesthesia may be limited to the contralateral face. Sensory loss usually is present but may be difficult to elicit. Good-quality MR images should show the thalamic infarct.

H. **Anesthesia dolorosa** is a dreaded form of central pain that can occur after any of the various surgical procedures for trigeminal neuralgia that cause a variable amount of sensory loss. After the ablative procedure, a constant and very unpleasant feeling is noticed in an area of skin or mucous membrane with diminished sensation. Surgeons attempt to minimize the level of anesthesia produced to lessen the likelihood of anesthesia dolorosa.

   1. **Symptoms** usually begin weeks to months after the procedure. The patient describes the unpleasant sensation as burning or stinging. A feeling of crawling and itching can occur around the mouth or eye. An irrepressible urge to scratch the anesthetic area results in skin erosion or abrasion. Insomnia from night pain is common.

   2. **Management** with medication or operation is difficult.

I. **Cancer** can be an indolent cause of facial pain. Even though a patient with chronic facial pain may have seen numerous physicians, each new consultant as well as the patient's own physician must periodically repeat a complete history and examination and review previous imaging studies. If symptoms change or do not respond to treatment, additional imaging studies should be considered. **The presence of any of the following should raise the possibility of a serious structural lesion:** a subjective or objective sensory deficit in the trigeminal distribution, hearing loss, serous otitis, chronic nasal obstruction, enlarged cervical lymph nodes, weakness or atrophy of the muscles of mastication, cranial nerve palsy, diplopia, proptosis, lid edema, subjective or objective bruits, or Horner's syndrome.

VII. **Referral**

A. When a **structural lesion** is found or a **neoplasm** is suspected, referral should be made to the appropriate specialist for evaluation.

B. **Trigeminal neuralgia** should be evaluated by a neurologist or neurosurgeon if the diagnosis is in doubt or if there are abnormal neurologic signs, symptoms, or imaging findings. Neurosurgical consultation should not be delayed if there is failure to respond to medication, a relapse, or medication intolerance. If a surgical procedure is contemplated, the primary physician should be aware of the percutaneous, radiosurgical, and open operations available, because certain centers and surgeons may be biased toward a particular procedure. Dental operations, such as extraction and root canal, do not relieve trigeminal neuralgia, and *alcohol blocks by dentists must be discouraged*.

C. **Glossopharyngeal neuralgia** is rare and difficult to diagnose. A neurologist or neurosurgeon should be involved. Because malignant disease can be associated with this condition, the patient should also be examined by an otolaryngologist.

D. **Cluster headache** and its variants should be referred to a neurologist if there is doubt about the diagnosis or if there is failure to respond to the usual medications.

E. **Herpes zoster ophthalmicus** and **postherpetic neuralgia** involving the face do not ordinarily require neurologic referral once the diagnosis has been established. Many specialists have experience with these disorders, including ophthalmologists, dermatologists, oncologists, and infectious disease physicians. The primary care physician, however, should follow the patient's case. As "last resort" management of postherpetic neuralgia, a sympathetic or overzealous surgeon may recommend an ablative procedure used for trigeminal neuralgia or another serious operation. Most interventions should be avoided, because they do not relieve postherpetic pain and can make the patient's condition worse.

F. **Atypical facial pain** is notoriously difficult to manage. A neurologist or a neurosurgeon with an interest in facial pain may be helpful in establishing the diagnosis and suggesting medication. The advice of other consultants, such as otolaryngologists, ophthalmologists, neuroradiologists, and oral surgeons may be needed to exclude occult disorders that can cause facial pain and to assure the patient that there is no structural lesion or malignant tumor. However, **the generalist should screen and protect the patient against futile nerve blocks and dental or surgical operations done on the "hope" that they might relieve the patient's pain.** Surgical procedures, often advised by an out-of-town consultant as acts of desperation, are fraught with hazard because they often aggravate an already bad situation. Referral to a psychotherapist who lacks special interest and expertise with atypical facial pain usually is another disappointing experience for the patient. Support and a compassionate relationship between the patient and the primary physician are important.

Recommended Readings

Brown JA, Gouda JJ. Percutaneous balloon compression of the trigeminal nerve. *Neurosurg Clin N Am* 1997;8:53–62.

Burchiel K, Slavin KV. On the natural history of trigeminal neuralgia. *Neurosurgery* 2000;46:152–155.

Ferrante L, Artico M, Nardacci B, et al. Glossopharyngeal neuralgia with cardiac syncope. *Neurosurgery* 1995;36: 58–63.

Jannetta PJ. Outcome after microvascular decompression for typical trigeminal neuralgia, hemifacial spasm, tinnitus, disabling positional vertigo, and glossopharyngeal neuralgia. *Clinical Neurosurgery* 1997;44:331–383.

Maesawa S, Salame C, Flickinger, et al. Clinical outcomes after stereotactic radiosurgery for idiopathic trigeminal neuralgia. *J Neurosurgery* 2001;94:14–20.

Marbach JJ. Medically unexplained chronic orofacial pain, temporomandibular pain and dysfunction syndrome, orofacial phantom pain, burning mouth syndrome, and trigeminal neuralgia. *Med Clin North Am* 1999;83:691–710.

Rovit R, et al., eds. *Trigeminal neuralgia*. Baltimore: Williams & Wilkins, 1990.

Taha JM, Tew JM. Treatment of trigeminal neuralgia by percutaneous radiofrequency rhizotomy. *Neurosurg Clin North Am* 1997;8:31–39.

Tekkok IH, Brown JA. The neurosurgical management of trigeminal neuralgia. *Neurosurg Q* 1997;6:89–107.

Young RF, Vermulen S, Posewitz A. Gamma knife radiosurgery for the treatment of trigeminal neuralgia. *Stereotact Funct Neurosurg* 1998;70[Suppl 1]:192–199.

15. APPROACH TO THE PATIENT WITH FACIAL WEAKNESS

Askiel Bruno
Engin Y. Yilmaz

Facial weakness is a common neurologic problem that can be caused by a large number of diverse disorders. The diagnosis needs to be established rapidly to minimize neurologic damage and prevent recurrence. A systematic approach to localization of lesions and differential diagnosis optimizes patient care.

  I. Etiology. Table 15.1 summarizes the causes of facial weakness. The innervation of the facial muscles starts in the precentral gyrus of the cerebral motor cortex. The region controlling the facial muscles is located most laterally and inferiorly near the sylvian fissure. Above this region is the cortical region for hand movement, then the region for arm movement, and finally, on the medial surface, in the interhemispheric fissure, the region for leg movement. The middle cerebral artery supplies blood flow to the lateral portion of the cerebral motor cortex controlling face and arm movement. The anterior cerebral artery supplies blood flow to the medial portion of the cerebral motor cortex controlling leg movement. From the motor cortex, the axons pass through the centrum semiovale and converge in the internal capsule. Within the internal capsule, the motor fibers to the face are located at the genu, the fibers to the arm are located posteriorly to the facial fibers, and the fibers to the leg are posterior to the arm fibers. The motor fibers continue down through the cerebral peduncles in the midbrain, where the facial fibers are most medial, the arm fibers are lateral to them, and the leg fibers are most lateral. The motor fibers then continue down to the lower pons, where some innervate the parts of the ipsilateral and contralateral facial nuclei that control the upper facial muscles (frontalis and orbicularis oculi). Other fibers cross in the lower pons and upper medulla oblongata to innervate the part of the contralateral facial nucleus that controls the lower facial muscles. From the facial nucleus, the fibers exit the pons ventrally, travel through the subarachnoid space, the temporal bone, the parotid gland, and the subcutaneous facial region to the muscles of facial expression. The differential diagnosis of facial weakness depends on which segment of this pathway is affected.

  II. Clinical manifestations. Facial weakness usually is apparent at rest and becomes obvious during testing. It is important to determine whether **an upper or a lower motor neuron lesion** is the cause of facial weakness. This distinction can be easily made at examination (Fig. 15.1; see **III.B.**). Drooping of one side of the face with flattening of the nasolabial fold is observed at rest. With lower motor neuron type weakness, flattening of the forehead wrinkles and palpebral fissure widening also may be apparent. The eye may be red and dry as a result of impaired blinking or decreased lacrimation. Speech usually is slurred.

  Taste may be impaired if a lesion of the facial nerve is proximal to the chorda tympani nerve branch within the temporal bone. This branch carries taste sensation from the ipsilateral anterior two thirds of the tongue. Sounds may be exaggerated (hyperacusis) if a lesion of the facial nerve is proximal to the stapedius nerve branch in the temporal bone. This branch supplies the ipsilateral stapedius muscle to dampen loud sounds.

  III. Evaluation

  A. History. The most useful facts to be obtained from the medical history are the rate of onset of the weakness, whether there are any other neurologic symptoms, and what preexisting medical problems might possibly be causing the facial weakness.

   1. Sudden or rapid **onset** (within hours) of nontraumatic facial weakness suggests a vascular cause such as stroke or peripheral ischemic neuropathy if the weakness is unilateral and Guillain–Barré syndrome if the weakness is bilateral. Facial weakness progressing over days or weeks is most likely idiopathic (Bell's palsy) or the result of infection or a tumor.

   2. The status of eye closure on the affected side and the presence or absence of other **neurologic symptoms** helps localize the lesion. Inability to close the eye suggests a lower motor neuron lesion, and preservation of eye closure suggests an upper motor neuron (brain) lesion. Presence of central nervous system symptoms such as hemiparesis, hemisensory loss, or hemineglect, in

Table 15.1 Causes of facial weakness

Upper Motor Neuron Causes
  Stroke: 80–85% ischemic, 15–20% hemorrhagic
  Brain tumor: metastatic or primary, hemispheric or brainstem
  Brain abscess
Lower Motor Neuron Causes
  Bell's palsy (idiopathic)
  Guillain–Barré syndrome (may be associated with human immunodeficiency virus
    infection)
  Direct facial nerve infection: herpesviruses
  Vasculitis
  Neurosarcoidosis, Behçet's syndrome, polyarteritis nodosa, Sjögren's syndrome,
    syphilis
  Meningitis: common bacteria (pneumococci, meningococci, *Haemophilus influenzae*),
    Mycobacterium tuberculosis, Lyme borreliosis, syphilis, fungus
  Meningeal carcinomatosis
  Temporal bone fracture
  Temporal bone tumor: metastatic, invasive meningioma
  Middle ear infection: common organisms, *Pseudomonas aeruginosa*
  Middle ear tumor
  Parotid gland tumor or infection
  Facial laceration
  Intracranial carotid artery dissection
  Drug effect (chemotherapeutic agents)
  Aftermath of insertion of cochlear implant
Disorders Affecting the Neuromuscular Junction
  Myasthenia gravis
  Botulism
Disorders Affecting the Facial Muscles
  Muscular dystrophy
  Myopathy

---

addition to facial weakness, suggests a brain lesion. The presence of lower
motor neuron symptoms, such as sensory disturbances in distal lower extremities or muscle atrophy, suggests a neuropathy.

3. Certain **medical conditions** are predisposing factors for facial weakness.
   Increasing age, tobacco smoking, diabetes mellitus, and hypertension
   increase the risk of ischemic stroke and of ischemic peripheral neuropathy.
   Ear and parotid gland infections increase the risk of facial nerve damage.
   Head trauma with basal skull fracture can cause facial nerve compression or
   laceration within the temporal bone. Malignant tumors are predisposing factors for metastatic facial nerve infiltration and carcinomatous meningitis.

B. The **physical examination** confirms the suspicion from clinical history and
   uncovers additional useful findings.

1. Upper motor neuron facial weakness can be differentiated from lower motor
   neuron weakness rapidly and reliably at examination (Fig. 15.1).

   a. **Upper motor neuron facial weakness** is caused by contralateral
      brain lesions above the level of the upper medulla oblongata. Only the
      lower facial muscles are affected. The appearance of the forehead and
      the width of the palpebral fissure are normal. Eyebrow elevation, forehead wrinkling, and eye closure are intact. The nasolabial fold is flattened, the corner of the mouth is lowered, and smiling and grinning are
      impaired. Speech usually is slurred, and when the cheeks are puffed
      with air, the air escapes between the lips on the weak side. The corneal
      reflex is intact because the lesion is above this reflex arc. Emotional

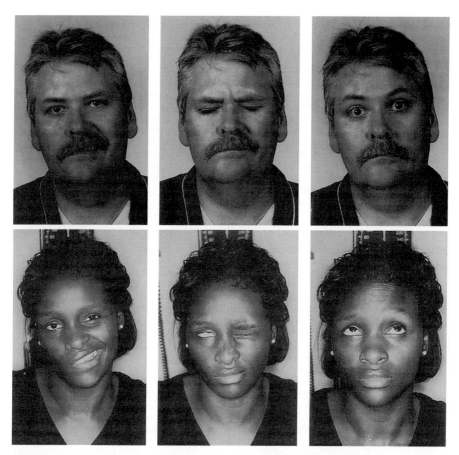

FIG. 15.1 Right facial weakness resulting from left cerebral infarction **(top)** and from Bell's palsy **(bottom).** At rest, neither patient had obvious facial weakness (*not shown*). Voluntary smiling produces obvious facial asymmetry with a similar appearance of the facial weakness in both patients **(left).** Eye closure **(center)** and eyebrow elevation **(right)** are impaired only in the patient with lower motor neuron facial weakness. The upward eye deviation during eye closure **(bottom center)** is the normal Bell's phenomenon.

facial movements, such as smiling, usually are intact despite weakness of voluntary facial movements.
   (1) The upper facial muscles are spared by unilateral upper motor neuron lesions because the portion of the facial nerve nucleus that controls the upper facial muscles receives bilateral cerebral innervation (see **I.**). Therefore a unilateral cerebral lesion impairs only the lower facial muscles. In patients with upper motor neuron weakness of voluntary facial movements, emotional movements usually are intact.
   (2) Emotional facial movements are intact when voluntary facial movements are not because facial innervation for voluntary movements comes from the pyramidal motor cortex, whereas facial innervation for emotional facial expressions comes from extrapyramidal cerebral regions.

        b. Lower motor neuron facial weakness is caused by lesions affecting the facial nerve nucleus, its fibers within the lower pons, or the peripheral portion of the facial nerve. The facial nucleus and nerve contain all the nerve fibers that innervate the ipsilateral facial muscles. Therefore a lesion in the facial nucleus or nerve impairs all the ipsilateral facial muscles. In addition to lower facial weakness, forehead creases are flattened, the palpebral fissure is widened, and the patient is unable to raise the eyebrow, wrinkle the forehead, or close the eye tightly. Emotional movements are impaired. The corneal reflex is impaired because the lesion affects the efferent part of this reflex arc.

        c. The distinction between upper and lower motor neuron facial weakness made at examination is very reliable if made during acute weakness. However, after partial recovery has occurred, lower motor neuron facial weakness can resemble upper motor neuron weakness.

    2. The rest of the neurologic examination is important as a means of looking for **other focal deficits** that help localize the lesion or lesions and suggest the best differential diagnosis. The presence of multiple cranial neuropathy suggests basilar meningitis or vasculitis. Hemiparesis on the same side as the facial weakness suggests a hemispheric brain lesion contralateral to the weakness. Hemisensory loss on the side opposite the lower motor neuron facial weakness, or gaze palsy on the same side as the facial weakness, suggests a pontine lesion on the side of the facial weakness (see **V.B.4.**).

    3. Examination of the ear for a patient with facial weakness is important. Infections and tumors of the tympanic cavity can be detected with an otoscope and can account for facial nerve damage. The facial nerve passes near the tympanic cavity in the temporal bone. Vesicles on the external ear suggest varicella-zoster neuronitis (Ramsay Hunt syndrome). Parotitis and parotid tumors also can cause peripheral facial palsy.

C. Laboratory studies

    1. Magnetic resonance imaging (MRI) is indicated when a brain lesion is suspected. Overall, it is a more sensitive brain imaging test than is computed tomography (CT), especially in the posterior fossa, where CT is limited by bone artifacts.

    2. CT is superior to MRI in depicting basal skull fractures. When an acute stroke is suspected, CT is preferred as the initial neuroimaging study to differentiate hemorrhage from ischemia.

    3. Lumbar puncture should be done when there is an indication of meningitis or vasculitis, such as fever, headache, nuchal rigidity, or systemic signs of vasculitis.

    4. Electrodiagnostic studies such as electroneurography are used to prognosticate recovery but are not needed to make the diagnosis.

    5. Tears and saliva can be tested with **polymerase chain reaction** for viral DNA.

IV. Differential diagnosis

  A. Guillain–Barré syndrome is a serious acute neurologic disorder involving multiple peripheral nerves. Sometimes facial weakness is the predominant initial finding. In that situation, the facial weakness is bilateral. Weakness in other muscles and loss of muscle stretch reflexes are always part of this syndrome. The most dreaded acute complications are respiratory insufficiency resulting from neurogenic respiratory muscle weakness and autonomic instability resulting from autonomic neuropathy. Prompt diagnosis is essential for optimal management.

  B. Acute stroke can manifest as predominantly facial weakness. Other deficits, such as hemiparesis or hemisensory loss, usually are present. Upper motor neuron facial weakness develops suddenly or over minutes to a few hours.

  C. Meningitis manifests as headache, fever, and nuchal rigidity. The infection or inflammation can damage the facial nerve where it passes through the subarachnoid space and the meninges to enter the temporal bone. Cerebrospinal fluid analysis is needed to differentiate infectious (bacterial or fungal) meningitis from carcinomatous meningitis caused by metastatic infiltration of the meninges.

D. **Otitis media** manifests as ear pain and inflammation in the tympanic cavity. Because it passes close to the tympanic cavity, the facial nerve can become damaged by otitis media.

E. **Brain tumor or abscess** can manifest as upper motor neuron facial weakness as the predominant finding. Infiltrating pontine tumors, such as glioma or lymphoma, or a cerebellopontine angle tumor, can manifest as lower motor neuron facial weakness as the predominant finding. The weakness progresses over days to months, and often there is headache or fever.

F. **Bell's palsy** is diagnosed when there is peripheral facial nerve palsy (lower motor neuron facial weakness) without other neurologic deficits and without an apparent cause. Serologic and pathologic evidence suggests that a large proportion of apparently idiopathic cases of facial neuropathy may be caused by neuronitis resulting from a herpesvirus, such as varicella-zoster or human herpes virus 6. In a patient with vascular risk factors, ischemic facial neuropathy is a likely etiologic factor.

V. **Diagnostic approach.** First determine whether the facial weakness is of the upper or lower motor neuron type (Fig. 15.1). Second, determine the rate of onset of facial weakness and whether there are other associated symptoms. Third, determine whether there are other neurologic deficits and whether they represent a central or a peripheral lesion. Fourth, localize the problem to a single lesion if possible or to multiple lesions. Fifth, generate a differential diagnosis list based on the localization of the lesion and rate of onset of the facial weakness (Fig. 15.2). Sixth, request the diagnostic tests needed to confirm or exclude the serious or treatable conditions in the differential diagnosis list.

A. **Upper motor neuron facial weakness** indicates a brain lesion. Sudden onset of weakness suggests a stroke, and weakness progressing over days or weeks suggests a brain tumor or an abscess. If an acute stroke is suspected, cranial CT should be performed without contrast material. With the scans, differentiation of ischemic and hemorrhagic stroke is easy and reliable. If another brain lesion is suspected, MRI should be performed, usually with contrast material, to differentiate the various possible causes.

B. **Lower motor neuron facial weakness** indicates involvement of the facial nerve.

1. **Isolated unilateral lower motor neuron facial weakness** without other neurologic deficits is most likely idiopathic (Bell's palsy) or ischemic and the result of small-vessel disease. If the patient has no vascular risk factors, such as hypertension, smoking, diabetes mellitus, or advanced age, the most likely diagnosis is Bell's palsy. Polymerase chain reaction testing of tears and saliva has been used to detect herpes virus DNA in patients with Bell's palsy. If the patient has vascular risk factors, the diagnosis of ischemic facial neuropathy is likely.

2. **Bilateral facial weakness.**

   a. **Rapid onset** of bilateral facial weakness should alert the physician to the possibility of Guillain–Barré syndrome, neurosarcoidosis, or other types of vasculitis causing multiple cranial neuropathy (Table 15.1). With Guillain-Barré syndrome, there is progressive weakness over hours to days, other muscles usually are weak, including the respiratory muscles and extremities, and the muscle stretch reflexes are always absent or depressed.

   b. **Slow-onset or long-standing** bilateral facial weakness should alert the physician to the possibility of muscular dystrophy, such as facioscapulohumeral muscular dystrophy, of myasthenia gravis, or of congenital hypoplasia of the facial nuclei (Möbius' syndrome). In muscular dystrophy and in myasthenia gravis, other muscles always are involved. In facioscapulohumeral muscular dystrophy, there is bilateral proximal upper extremity weakness. In myasthenia gravis, there is usually weakness in the ocular muscles, neck muscles, pharynx, or proximal limbs, and the weakness is intermittent throughout the day. In Möbius' syndrome, there also may be hypoplasia of the abducens (cranial nerve VI) nucleus and other brainstem nuclei.

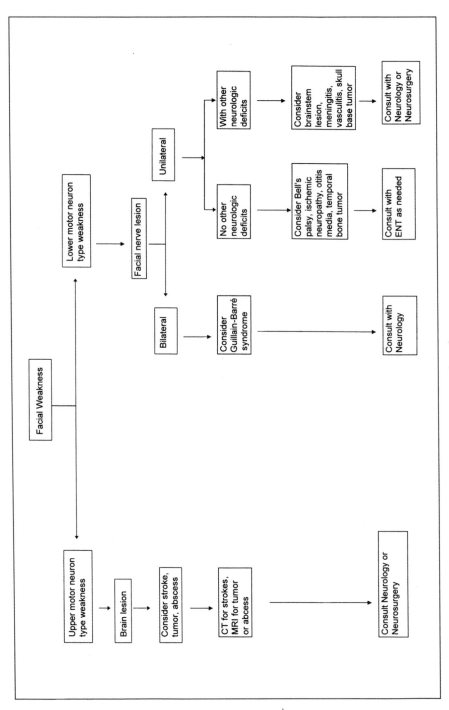

FIG. 15.2 Diagnostic algorithm for evaluation of patients with facial weakness.

3. Multiple cranial nerve deficits. If multiple cranial nerve deficits are associated with facial weakness, infectious and carcinomatous basilar meningitis, vasculitis, and basilar skull tumor should be considered. Any of these problems is likely to cause headache, fever, nuchal rigidity, and elevated erythrocyte sedimentation rate. However, these findings are nonspecific. The presence of an extracranial malignant lesion suggests possible carcinomatous meningitis. The presence of collagen vascular disease suggests possible vasculitis. MRI should be performed to rule out a skull base tumor. If a lesion is detected, gadolinium-enhanced MRI should be performed to determine the enhancement pattern. Tumor excision or biopsy usually is needed for definitive diagnosis. If the MRI findings are normal, lumbar puncture should be performed to look for meningitis. The spinal fluid should be stained and inspected for bacteria, fungi, and malignant cells. It also should be cultured for bacteria and fungi. Bacterial stains and cultures always should include mycobacteria. Cerebrospinal fluid protein, glucose, and cell count abnormalities are important indicators of disease, but they are not reliable for differentiation among the various disorders in question.

4. Brainstem lesions. The facial nerve and nucleus can be involved by lesions within the pons. Because of the proximity of other structures in the pons to the facial nucleus and nerve, additional neurologic deficits help establish the correct diagnosis. The facial nerve fibers wrap around the abducens nucleus (cranial nerve VI), which is located dorsally to the facial nucleus. A lesion in the abducens nucleus produces lateral gaze palsy on the side of the lesion. The spinal trigeminal nucleus and tract are lateral to the facial nucleus. A lesion in the trigeminal tract or nucleus produces pain and temperature sensory loss on the same side of the face. The trigeminothalamic and spinothalamic tracts are ventral to the facial nucleus. A lesion in the trigeminothalamic tract produces pain and temperature sensory loss on the face on the side opposite the lesion. A lesion in the spinothalamic tract produces pain and temperature sensory loss on the body below the neck on the side opposite the lesion. Cerebellar fibers from above and from below travel to the cerebellum through the pons. A lesion involving these fibers produces ipsilateral dysmetria of the arm, leg, or both. Large pontine lesions can involve the ventrally located corticospinal tract and cause hemiparesis on the other side of the body. The so-called "crossed signs"—cranial nerve deficit contralateral to hemiparesis or hemisensory loss—can be explained by a single lesion only in the brainstem.

VI. Referral

A. None. When the findings of the history and physical examination are consistent with Bell's palsy or ischemic facial neuropathy, referral may not be necessary. Slow spontaneous improvement is expected.

B. Neurologist. Consultation with a neurologist is indicated when there is suspicion of acute stroke, Guillain–Barré syndrome, meningitis, or vasculitis.

C. An **ear, nose, and throat specialist** should be consulted when unusual otitis media or tumor in the tympanic cavity or parotid gland is suspected.

D. A **neurosurgeon** should be consulted when a tumor or abscess is found.

Recommended Readings

Adour KK. Diagnosis and management of facial paralysis. *N Engl J Med* 1982;307:348–351.

Bateman DE. Facial palsy. *Br J Hosp Med* 1992;47:430–431.

Brazis PW, Masdeu JC, Biller J. The localization of lesions affecting cranial nerve VII. In: *Localization in clinical neurology,* 3rd ed. Boston: Little, Brown, 1996:271–292.

Engstrom M, Thuomas KA, Naeser P, et al. Facial nerve enhancement in Bell's palsy demonstrated by different gadolinium-enhanced magnetic resonance imaging techniques. *Arch Otolaryngol Head Neck Surg* 1993;119:221–225.

Finestone AJ, Byers K. Acute facial paralysis: Is it a stroke or something else? *Geriatrics* 1994;49:50–52.

Furuta Y, Takasu T, Sato KC, et al. Latent herpes simplex virus type 1 in human geniculate ganglia. *Acta Neuropathol (Berl)* 1992;84:39–44.

Keane JR. Bilateral seventh nerve palsy: analysis of 43 cases and review of the literature. *Neurology* 1994;44:1198–1202.

Morgan M, Nathwani D. Facial palsy and infections: the unfolding story. *Clin Infect Dis* 1992;14:263–271.

Murr AH, Benecke JE Jr. Association of facial paralysis with HIV positivity. *Am J Otolaryngol* 1991; 12:450–451.

Olsen KD. Facial nerve paralysis: general evaluation, Bell's palsy. *Postgrad Med* 1984;75:219–225.

Olsen KD. Facial nerve paralysis: all that palsies is not Bell's. *Postgrad Med* 1984;76:95–105.

Pitkäranta A, Piiparinen H, Mannonen L, et al. Detection of human herpesvirus 6 and varicella-zoster virus in tear fluid of patients with Bell's palsy by PCR. *J Clin Microbiol* 2000;38:2753–2755.

Terao S, Miura N, Takeda A, et al. Course and distribution of facial corticobulbar tract fibers in the lower brain stem. *J Neurol Neurosurg Psychiatry* 2000;69:262–265.

Walling AD. Bell's palsy in pregnancy and the puerperium. *J Fam Pract* 1993;36:559–563.

16. APPROACH TO THE PATIENT WITH DIZZINESS AND VERTIGO

Timothy C. Hain
Mohammad Kaleem Uddin

Dizziness and **vertigo** are common symptoms. Approximately 2.5% of all primary care visits are for dizziness, and approximately 1% are for vertigo. Dizziness and vertigo have diverse causes. For this reason, a broad-based approach to a patient with dizziness is necessary. At times, life-threatening medical problems such as cardiac arrhythmia must be differentiated from the more common inner ear disease and dizziness with a source that cannot be localized.

    I. Etiology. Vertigo can be categorized into four types: otologic, central, medical, and unlocalized (Table 16.1). The largest category, unlocalized vertigo, includes approximately 50% of patients with vertigo.

        A. Otologic vertigo is caused by dysfunction of the inner ear. It accounts for approximately one third of all patients with vertigo. Table 16.1 lists entities that account for approximately 95% of all cases of otologic vertigo.

            1. Benign paroxysmal positional vertigo (BPPV) is the most common single type of otologic vertigo, accounting for approximately 20% of cases of vertigo of all causes and 50% of all otologic cases. BPPV manifests as brief vertigo provoked by changes in the orientation of the head to gravity. BPPV is caused by loose debris within the posterior canal of the inner ear.

            2. Vestibular neuritis manifests as vertigo, nausea, ataxia, and nystagmus. It is attributed to viral infection of the vestibular nerve. Labyrinthitis manifests as the same symptom complex combined with tinnitus, hearing loss, or both. Vestibular neuritis and labyrinthitis together account for approximately 15% of all cases of otologic vertigo.

            3. Ménière's disease manifests as intermittent vertigo accompanied by hearing problems (see **IV.A.3.**). It is attributed to dilation and periodic rupture of the endolymphatic compartment of the inner ear. Ménière's disease accounts for approximately 15% of cases of otologic vertigo.

            4. Bilateral vestibular paresis manifests as oscillopsia and ataxia, usually caused by loss of vestibular hair cells. The typical history includes therapy for several weeks with an intravenous or intraperitoneal ototoxic antibiotic (gentamicin is the most commonly encountered). Much more rarely, bilateral vestibular paresis can be due to autoimmune disorders such as Cogan's syndrome—in this situation, vestibular paresis usually is accompanied by bilateral hearing loss. Bilateral vestibular loss is uncommon.

            5. Perilymphatic fistula (PLF) and superior canal dehiscence syndrome (SCD) manifest as pressure sensitivity, vertigo induced by sound (the Tullio phenomenon), or ataxia provoked by activity. In PLF, a rupture has occurred between the fluid-filled inner ear and the air-filled middle ear. Barotrauma, such as from scuba diving, is the common mechanism. Ear surgery for otosclerosis or cholesteatoma also is a well-known cause of PLF. Spontaneous PLF is uncommon. In SCD, bone over the superior semicircular canal is absent. SCD is thought to be due to congenital idiosyncrasy in bone thickness over the superior canal that is exacerbated by trauma.

            6. Tumors compressing the eighth cranial nerve manifest as asymmetric hearing combined with mild ataxia. Eighth nerve tumors are uncommon in the population with vertigo but are more common among persons with unilateral hearing impairment.

        B. Central vertigo is caused by dysfunction of central structures that process sensory input from the inner ear. Central vertigo accounts for 2% to 23% of vertigo diagnoses, depending on the specialty setting in which patients are seen. In most instances, central vertigo is caused by vascular disorders such as stroke, transient ischemic attack (TIA), and vertebrobasilar migraine. Table 16.1 lists entities accounting for only approximately 60% of central vertigo diagnoses; the others are individual unusual conditions (e.g., spinocerebellar degeneration).

Table 16.1 Causes of vertigo

Otologic Vertigo	Medical Vertigo
Benign paroxysmal positional vertigo	Postural hypotension
Vestibular neuritis and labyrinthitis	Arrhythmia
Ménière's disease	Hypoglycemia and diabetes
Bilateral vestibular paresis or loss	Medication effect
Perilymph fistula and superior canal dehiscence	Viral syndrome
Tumors compressing the eighth cranial nerve	**Unlocalized Vertigo Syndromes**
	Unknown
Central Vertigo	Anxiety and panic
Stroke and transient ischemic attack	Posttraumatic vertigo
Vertebrobasilar migraine	Hyperventilation
Seizure	Malingering
Multiple sclerosis	
Arnold–Chiari malformation	

1. **Stroke** and **TIA** involving the brainstem or cerebellum cause approximately one third of all cases of central dizziness. Pure vertigo can occasionally be the only symptom preceding a posterior fossa stroke, and there are no reliable means of differentiating a TIA affecting the vestibular nucleus from another process affecting the vestibular nerve or end organ.
2. **Vertebrobasilar migraine** ordinarily manifests as vertigo and headache, but it can also manifest as isolated vertigo. Migraine causes approximately 15% of cases of central vertigo. Migraine is particularly common among women in their thirties.
3. **Seizures** manifest as vertigo combined with motor symptoms or confusion, or more frequently as quick spins. Approximately 5% of cases of central vertigo are caused by seizures. Dizziness is a common symptom among persons with known epilepsy.
4. **Multiple sclerosis (MS)** combines vertigo with other central signs, such as cerebellar dysfunction. MS is an uncommon source of vertigo, although many patients suspect it as a cause of symptoms. In the care of persons with known MS, it is important not to attribute vertigo to MS without considering common peripheral causes that may be coincident, such as BPPV. MRI assists in the diagnosis. Approximately 2% of cases of central vertigo are caused by MS.
5. **Arnold–Chiari malformation** is a hindbrain malformation wherein the cerebellar tonsils herniate 5 mm or more below the foramen magnum. Patients report vertigo, ataxia, and posterior headaches and often have downbeat nystagmus. As with PLF, symptoms can be precipitated by straining or coughing. MRI of the posterior fossa establishes the diagnosis. Approximately 1% of cases of central vertigo are caused by Arnold–Chiari malformation.
6. **Cervical vertigo** is a controversial syndrome. The diagnosis is most often made after a whiplash injury in which the findings usually include vertigo, tinnitus, and neck pain. Examination usually reveals a nonspecific symptom complex including neck movement limited by pain and reports of nausea or vertigo on neck positioning. Generally, no nystagmus is found even with video-recording methods, and there are no definitive clinical or laboratory tests for cervical vertigo. Rare patients also have been reported in whom vertigo can be traced to compression of a vertebral artery after neck rotation. Because of the lack of clarity in the diagnosis of cervical vertigo, the prevalence is unknown.
C. **Medical vertigo** is caused by altered blood pressure, decreased blood sugar, or metabolic derangements associated with medication or systemic infection. Medical vertigo is largely encountered in the emergency department, where it accounts

for approximately 33% of all cases of dizziness. Medical vertigo is unusual in subspecialty settings (2% to 5%). Table 16.1 lists nearly all causes of dizziness reported in studies of vertigo as it is encountered in emergency departments.

1. **Postural hypotension** manifests as giddiness, light-headedness, or syncope. Dizziness occurs only while the patient is upright.

2. **Cardiac arrhythmia** manifests as syncope or drop attacks. Like those of postural hypotension, symptoms are characteristically present only when patients are upright.

3. **Hypoglycemia** and **metabolic derangements** associated with diabetes manifest as giddiness or light-headedness. Hypoglycemia often is accompanied by autonomic symptoms resembling a panic attack, such as palpitations, sweating, tremor, or pallor. Together they account for approximately 5% of the cases of dizziness in general medical settings.

4. **Medication effect** or **substance abuse** usually manifests as giddiness or light-headedness but also can manifest as true vertigo. These diagnoses account for approximately 16% of cases of dizziness seen in the emergency setting but are rare outside the emergency department. Medications commonly encountered include antihypertensive agents, especially α_1-adrenergic blockers such as terazosin (Hytrin; Abbott Laboratories, Abbott Park, IL, U.S.A.), calcium channel blockers with strong vasodilating effects such as nifedipine (Procardia; Pfizer, New York, NY, U.S.A.), and sedatives. Certain common benzodiazepines, such as alprazolam (Xanax; Pharmacia & Upjohn, Kalamazoo, MI, U.S.A.), cause dizziness as part of the withdrawal syndrome. Vestibular suppressant medications, such as meclizine (Antivert; Pfizer) and scopolamine (Transderm Scop; Novartis Consumer Health, Summit, NJ, U.S.A.), can cause dizziness through direct effects on central vestibular pathways.

5. **Viral syndromes** not involving the ear are the reported cause of dizziness in 4% to 40% of all cases seen in the emergency department. Such syndromes include, for example, gastroenteritis and influenza-like illnesses.

D. **Unlocalized vertigo** includes symptoms attributed to psychiatric disorders, symptoms are attributed to events without further definition (such as head trauma), and vertigo and dizziness of unknown origin. Common variants of unlocalized vertigo include psychogenic vertigo, hyperventilation syndrome, posttraumatic vertigo, and nonspecific dizziness. Approximately 50% of all patients with dizziness or vertigo fall into this category.

1. **Unknown (nonspecific dizziness).** Diagnostic procedures are insensitive, and in dizziness evaluations it is usual that a large population of patients have no detectable abnormalities at careful clinical examination and thorough testing. Some authors wrongly consider these patients to have *psychogenic vertigo*.

2. **Psychogenic.** Patients with anxiety disorders, panic disorder, and posttraumatic stress disorder may report dizziness, ataxia, and autonomic symptoms. This is a common presentation. It is often impossible to determine whether anxiety is the sole cause or a reaction. In somatization disorder, symptoms may be present without anxiety.

3. Patients with **posttraumatic vertigo** report vertigo after head injuries but have no findings at examination or vestibular testing. BPPV is excluded by a negative Dix–Hallpike maneuver. Posttraumatic vertigo is common.

4. Patients with **hyperventilation syndrome** have vertigo resulting from hyperventilation and have no other findings. Most authors report that hyperventilation syndrome is uncommon.

5. **Multisensory dysequilibrium of the elderly.** Most elderly persons have age-related multisensory impairment. Like the diagnosis of psychogenic vertigo, this diagnosis often is used in situations in which the examination findings are otherwise normal.

6. **Malingering.** Because vertigo can be intermittent and disabling and frequently follows head injury, vertigo may be claimed in an attempt to obtain compensation. Malingering is common only among patients who are being compensated for illness.

II. Clinical manifestations

A. Primary symptoms. The primary symptoms listed in Table 16.2 are mainly the result of a disturbed sensorium.

   1. **Vertigo** denotes a sensation of rotation—either of the person or of the world. Vertigo can be horizontal, vertical, or rotatory (around the front–back axis). It is also described as visual "blurring" or "jumping." **Horizontal** vertigo is the most common type, usually resulting from dysfunction of the inner ear. When vertigo is associated with nystagmus, patients most commonly report movement of the visual scene opposite the direction of the slow phase. **Vertical** vertigo is rarer. When transient, vertical vertigo usually is caused by BPPV. When constant, it is usually of central origin and accompanied by downbeat or upbeat nystagmus. **Rotatory** vertigo is the least frequent. When transient, rotatory vertigo usually is caused by BPPV. When chronic, it is always central and usually is accompanied by rotatory nystagmus.

   2. **Impulsion** denotes a sensation of translation, usually described as brief sensations of being pushed or tilted. Variants include rocking, floating, and perceived changes in the directions of up and down. Impulsion indicates dysfunction of the otolithic apparatus of the inner ear or central processing of otolithic signals.

   3. **Oscillopsia** is illusory movement of the world evoked by head movement. Patients with bilateral vestibular loss are unable to see when their heads are in motion because of oscillopsia. Patients with unilateral vestibular loss often say that "the world doesn't keep up" when they rapidly rotate their heads laterally to the side of the bad ear.

   4. **Ataxia,** unsteadiness of gait, is nearly universal among patients with otologic or central vertigo and is variably observed among patients with medical and unlocalized vertigo.

   5. **Hearing symptoms.** Vertigo often is accompanied by tinnitus, hearing reduction or distortion, and aural fullness.

B. Secondary symptoms include nausea, autonomic symptoms, fatigue, headache, and visual sensitivity. These symptoms accompany vertigo in varying amounts according to individual susceptibility. Although most secondary symptoms are self-explanatory, **visual sensitivity,** also known as the "grocery store syndrome," is not encountered frequently in other contexts. Patients describe dizziness related to the types of patterned visual stimulation that occur when one views grocery store aisles, drives past picket fences or through bridges, or views large screen movies. Grocery store syndrome is a nonspecific common late symptom among patients with vertigo and presumably reflects a visual–vestibular mismatch.

C. Giddiness and lightheadedness. These terms have no precise meanings in common usage. They are rarely used by patients with documented inner ear dysfunction but are frequently used by patients with vertigo related to medical problems (e.g., postural hypotension or hypoglycemia).

Table 16.2 Symptoms in patients with dizziness and vertigo

Primary Symptoms	Pallor, bradycardia
Vertigo	Fatigue
Impulsion and rocking	Headache
Oscillopsia	Visual sensitivity
Ataxia	**Nonspecific Symptoms**
Hearing symptoms	Giddiness
Secondary Symptoms	Lightheadedness
Nausea, emesis, diarrhea	

III. Evaluation

  A. History. Because the numerous potential causes of vertigo cut across four sub-specialty areas, the history must either be all-encompassing or follow a heuristic technique whereby questions are dynamically selected as the interview progresses. The following represents the all-encompassing approach.

    1. Definition. Does the patient report vertigo (spinning), a secondary symptom (e.g., nausea), a nonspecific symptom (giddiness or light-headedness), or something entirely different (e.g., confusion)?

    2. Timing. Are symptoms constant or are they episodic? If episodic, how long do they last?

    3. Triggering or exacerbating factors are listed in Table 16.3. All patients should be queried regarding these factors, either by going through them one by one or by using an interview heuristic whereby one attempts to rule in or rule out a symptom complex (see **IV.**).

    4. Otologic history. Ask about hearing loss, tinnitus, and fullness. Positive answers are indications for an audiogram. Ask about the type of tinnitus— "roaring" tinnitus suggests Ménière's disease.

    5. Medication history. Numerous medications can induce vertigo, including ototoxins (especially gentamicin), anticonvulsants, antihypertensives, and sedatives. All current medications as well as previous exposure to ototoxins should be considered sources of vertigo.

    6. Family history. Has anyone in the immediate family had similar symptoms? Is there a family history of migraine, seizures, Ménière's disease, or early-onset hearing loss?

    7. The **review of systems** should explore psychiatric problems (anxiety, depression, and panic), vascular risk factors, cancer, autoimmune disease, neurologic problems (migraine, stroke, TIA, seizures, and MS), otologic surgery, and general medical history (especially thyroid dysfunction, diabetes, Lyme disease, or syphilis).

    8. Previous studies relevant to dizziness (see **III.C.**) should be reviewed.

  B. Physical examination. The physical examination of a patient with vertigo is outlined in Table 16.4. It is ordered in such a way that procedures can be added on the basis of previous results. Because a full examination may be quite long, it is most practical to expand or contract the examination dynamically. As an exception to the following procedure, *if there is a history of positional vertigo, it is best to go immediately to the Dix–Hallpike test* (see **III.B.5.b.**).

    1. General examination. Blood pressure and pulse are measured with the patient standing. Arrhythmia is noted, if present. If the standing blood

Table 16.3 Triggering or exacerbating factors

Changes in position of the head or body
Standing up
Rapid head movements
Walking in a dark room
Loud noises
Coughing, blowing the nose, sneezing, straining, or laughing
Underwater diving, riding in elevators, airplane travel
Exercise
Later time in the day
Shopping malls, narrow or wide-open spaces, grocery stores, escalators
  (visual sensitivity complex)
Foods, not eating, salt, monosodium glutamate
Alcohol
Menstrual period
Boat or car travel
Anxiety or stress

Table 16.4 Examination procedures for dizziness and vertigo

Procedures	Triggers for additions
General Examination	
Orthostasis assessment	
Arrhythmia evaluation	
Test for carotid sinus hyperreactivity	Syncope
Balance Assessment	
Observation of gait	
Eyes-closed tandem Romberg test	
Pulsion and retropulsion	Parkinsonian gait
Otologic Examination	
Hearing	
Tympanic membranes	
Neurologic Examination	
Cranial nerves	
Long tract signs	
Cerebellar	
Position sense testing	Fails Romberg test
Nystagmus Assessment	
Spontaneous nystagmus	
Dix–Hallpike positional test	
Head-shake test	Normal examination findings so far
Fistula test	Pressure sensitivity
Hyperventilation test	Normal examination findings so far
Vestibuloocular Reflex Gain Assessment	
Dynamic illegible "E" test	Fails Romberg test
Ophthalmoscope test	Fails "E" test

Procedures in *italics* are always performed; procedures not in italics are performed only for certain symptom complexes.

pressure is low (110/70 mm Hg or lower), check blood pressure with the patient lying flat. The heart and the carotid and subclavian arteries are auscultated. In patients with potential syncope, who are younger than 70 years, 10 seconds of carotid sinus massage may be undertaken. This is done with the patient in the sitting position, first on one side and then on the other, to see whether symptoms are reproduced.

2. **Balance** is assessed by means of observation of gait (apraxic, antalgic, ataxic, bizarre, normal, or parkinsonian) and the eyes-closed tandem Romberg test. The tandem Romberg test is extremely useful. Low normal performance consists of the ability to stand heel-to-toe with eyes closed for 6 seconds. Young adults should be able to perform this test for 30 seconds, but performance declines with age.

It is helpful to develop a judgment about how much ataxia is appropriate for a given degree of ear injury. Patients with **bilateral vestibular loss** have moderate ataxia—they make heavy use of vision and are unsteady when their eyes are closed (with a narrow base). No patient with bilateral loss can stand in the eyes-closed tandem Romberg test for 6 seconds. Patients with an additional superimposed position sense deficit are unsteady with eyes open (with a narrow base). Patients with **chronic unilateral vestibular loss** have very little ataxia, and they usually have normal results of the eyes-closed tandem Romberg test. The need to gauge ataxia does not come up in evaluations of patients with recent unilateral vestibular imbalance, because these patients have prominent nystagmus. Patients with **cerebellar disorders,** such as alcoholic cerebellar degeneration, have greater ataxia than is appropriate for the degree of nystagmus or vestibular paresis. Patients who are malingering also typically emphasize imbalance, which is the disabling aspect of their symptoms.

In head injury or when there is another reason to suspect a central nervous system (CNS) origin of imbalance, also test basal ganglia function (pulsion–retropulsion tests).

3. **Otologic examination.** A brief screening test is adequate for hearing. The examiner rubs a thumb and first finger together at arm's length from one of the patient's ears. Persons with normal hearing can perceive this sound at an arm's length. If the sound is not perceived, the source is brought in closer and closer until it is heard, and the distance is recorded. This simple test helps identify high-tone hearing loss—for example, most elderly persons are able to hear when the examiner's hand is approximately 6 inches (15 cm) away on either side. The tympanic membranes should be inspected for wax, perforation, otitis, discoloration, and mass lesions. Wax always should be removed before more sophisticated diagnostic procedures are performed.

4. **Neurologic examination.** An abbreviated neurologic examination is adequate. The cranial nerve examination includes ophthalmoscopy, extraocular movements (range, saccadic accuracy and velocity, and pursuit), and facial movement. It usually is convenient to check the vestibuloocular reflex (VOR) and nystagmus with the ophthalmoscope at this point (see **III.B.5.a.** and **III.B.6.b.**). The motor examination includes tests for reflexes, Babinski sign, and gross assessment of power. The cerebellar examination includes finger-to-nose testing and rapid alternating movement testing. Sensory examination of position sense is done when ataxia is present.

5. **Nystagmus** (involuntary movement of the eyes) indicates an inner ear, brain, or ocular muscle disorder.

   a. **Spontaneous nystagmus** is best assessed with Frenzel goggles, which are illuminated, magnifying goggles worn by the patient. The goggles are placed on the patient, and the eyes are observed for spontaneous nystagmus for 10 seconds. The typical nystagmus produced by inner ear dysfunction is primary position jerk nystagmus—the eyes slowly deviate off center, and then there is a rapid jerk, which brings them back to the center position. Most nystagmus of other patterns (e.g., sinusoidal, gaze-evoked, and saccadic) is of central origin.

   If Frenzel goggles are not available, similar information about nystagmus can be obtained from the ophthalmoscopic examination. One simply monitors movement of the back of the eye. As the back of the eye moves opposite to the front of the eye, for horizontal and vertical movement, one must remember to invert the direction of the nystagmus when making notes. Fixation can be removed by covering the opposite eye. Nystagmus deriving from the inner ear is increased by removal of fixation.

   b. **Dix–Hallpike positional test** (Fig. 16.1). The Frenzel goggles are temporarily removed, and the patient is repositioned on the examination table so that when the patient lies flat, the head extends over the end of the table. If Frenzel goggles are available, they are replaced on the patient, but ordinarily they are not necessary. The patient is then moved rapidly to the head-hanging position. If no dizziness or nystagmus is appreciated after 20 seconds, the patient is sat back up. The head is then repositioned 45 degrees right, and the patient is brought down to the head-right supine position. After another 20 seconds, the patient is sat up again, and the procedure is repeated to the left (head-left position). One hopes to see a burst of nystagmus provoked by either the head-right or the head-left position. The nystagmus of classic BPPV beats upward and also has a rotatory component, such that the top part of the eye beats toward the down ear. The nystagmus typically has a latency of 2 to 5 seconds, lasts 5 to 60 seconds, and is followed by downbeat nystagmus when the patient is sat up. There is also a lateral canal variant of BPPV in which the eyes beat horizontally toward the ear that is down.

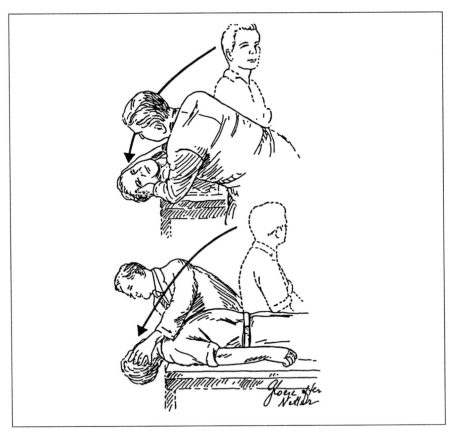

FIG. 16.1 Dix–Hallpike positional test. To precipitate the characteristic nystagmus of benign paroxysmal positional vertigo, the patient is rapidly brought into a head position that makes the posterior canal vertical and also brings it through a large angular displacement. (From Bahloh RW, Honrubia V. *Clinical neurophysiology of the vestibular system,* 2nd ed. Philadelphia: FA Davis Co, 1990:124, with permission.)

     c. Head-shake test and **neck vibration test.** If there is no spontaneous nystagmus or positional nystagmus and if Frenzel goggles are unavailable, the head-shake test may be performed. The patient's eyes are closed, and the head is moved in the horizontal plane, back and forth, for 20 cycles. One aims for 45-degree excursion of the head to either side and a frequency of 2 cycles per second. Nystagmus lasting 5 seconds or more is an indication of an organic disorder of the ear or CNS and supports the need for further investigation.

     A newer test that is even more helpful than the head-shaking test is the vibration test. A video Frenzel goggle system is necessary. The eyes are observed in complete darkness while vibration is applied to the sternocleidomastoid muscle for 10 seconds, first on one side and then on the other. Strong, direction-fixed nystagmus indicates a compensated peripheral vestibular lesion. The nystagmus beats away from the lesion.

    d. The **fistula test** is performed if the history shows a pressure sensitivity symptom complex (see **IV.**). Three or four pulses of pressure are delivered to each external ear canal in turn while the patient watches an eye chart or is observed for nystagmus with Frenzel goggles or a similar device. A positive test result consists of dizziness, nystagmus, or apparent movement of the eye chart correlated with pressure. Movement of the eye with pressure is sometimes called *Hennebert's sign.*

    e. The **hyperventilation test** is performed if so far the examination findings have been entirely normal. The patient takes 30 deep, hard breaths. Immediately after hyperventilation, the eyes are inspected for nystagmus with the Frenzel goggles and the patient is asked whether the procedure has reproduced the symptoms. A positive test result without nystagmus suggests the diagnosis of hyperventilation syndrome. Nystagmus induced by hyperventilation suggests a tumor of the eighth cranial nerve or MS.

  6. Assessment of VOR gain. The following maneuvers are aimed at documenting bilateral vestibular loss. They need not be done unless the patient has failed the eyes-closed tandem Romberg test.

    a. The **dynamic illegible "E" test.** With an eye chart at a distance of at least 10 feet (3 m), visual acuity is recorded with the head still. Then the examiner gently moves the patient's head horizontally at approximately 1 Hz, ±30 degrees, and visual acuity is again recorded. Patients with normal vestibular function drop from zero to two lines of acuity with head movement. Patients with partial to complete bilateral loss of vestibular function drop from three to seven lines of acuity. Patients with complete bilateral loss usually drop seven lines of acuity.

    b. The **ophthalmoscope test** is done to obtain objective corroboration when the result of the illegible "E" test is positive. The examiner focuses on the optic disk and then gently moves the head as described in **a.** If the disk moves with the head, this confirms that the VOR gain is abnormal. This test is less sensitive than is the illegible "E" test.

C. Laboratory studies. Table 16.5 lists laboratory procedures commonly used for evaluation of patients with vertigo and dizziness as well as the indications for the tests. For efficiency and cost containment, procedures should be selected according to specific symptom complexes and should be done sequentially. Algorithms are discussed in **IV.** and **V.**

  1. Audiologic testing is not needed for every patient with dizziness but may be appropriate when there are hearing problems. If the diagnosis is uncertain, audiometry is recommended even for patients who have no hearing abnormalities,

    a. Audiogram. The audiogram is used to measure hearing. Abnormalities suggest otologic vertigo. Audiograms often include a battery of procedures such as tympanometry and acoustic reflex testing. When cost containment is important, the two latter procedures may be contingent on reduced hearing.

    b. The **brainstem auditory evoked response** (BAER) test is used to assess the auditory nerve and brainstem pathways. Because BAERs are of little use for patients who have no high-frequency hearing, audiometry is recommended before BAER testing. Abnormal BAERs are indications for MRI of the posterior fossa (T1-weighted sequences with contrast material). For cost efficiency, BAER testing need not be performed if MRI is planned.

    c. Electrocochleography (ECOG) is a variant of the BAER test in which electrodes are positioned in the external ear canal. Like BAER, ECOG requires reasonable high-frequency hearing. Abnormal ECOG findings suggest Ménière's disease.

    d. Miscellaneous tests. The MLR, or middle latency response, is a central variant of the BAER test. Otoacoustic emission tests are used to measure sound generated by the ear itself. At present, neither of these recently developed tests has found a place in the usual diagnostic process.

Table 16.5 Laboratory procedures for dizziness and vertigo

Test	Indication
Audiologic Tests	
Audiogram	Vertigo, hearing symptoms
BAER	Asymmetric hearing loss
Electrocochleography	Secondary test for Ménière's disease and
Middle latency response	perilymphatic fistula
Otoacoustic emissions	
Vestibular Tests	
ENG	Vertigo
Rotatory chair test	Bilateral loss, secondary to confirm ENG
Fistula test	Pressure sensitivity
Posturography	Malingering
Blood Tests	
Fluorescent treponemal antibody absorption test	Vertigo with hearing symptoms
Glycohemoglobin	Hydrops symptom complex
Antinuclear antibody	Hydrops symptom complex
Thyroid-stimulating hormone	Hydrops symptom complex
Lyme borreliosis titer	Vertigo in person from endemic area
Radiologic Tests	
MR imaging of head	Central vertigo, abnormal BAER
MR angiography, vertebrobasilar	Transient ischemic attack
Computed tomography of temporal bone	Pressure sensitivity or Tullio's sign, mastoiditis, congenital abnormality, substantial head trauma
Other Tests	
Electroencephalography	Quick spins, head trauma
Ambulatory event monitoring (Holter monitoring)	Cardiogenic syncope
Tilt-table test	

BAER, brainstem auditory evoked response; ENG, electronystagmography; MR, magnetic resonance.

2. **Vestibular testing** is not needed for every patient with dizziness. The primary study—electronystagmography (ENG)—is helpful when there is no clear diagnosis after the history has been obtained and the examination performed.
   a. **ENG** is a battery of procedures used to identify vestibular asymmetry (such as that caused by vestibular neuritis) and to document spontaneous or positional nystagmus (such as that caused by BPPV). ENG is an intrinsically inaccurate test, and an abnormal result that does not fit the clinical picture should be confirmed with rotatory chair testing.
   b. **Rotatory chair testing** is used to measure the vestibular function of both inner ears together. Rotatory testing is highly sensitive and specific for bilateral loss of vestibular function. In unilateral loss, it is sensitive but not specific. Also, it does not help identify the side of the lesion.
   c. **Fistula testing** involves recording of nystagmus induced by pressure in the external ear canal. Its sensitivity to PLF is only 50%.
   d. **Posturography** is an instrumented Romberg test. Except to document malingering, posturography has no diagnostic value.
3. **Blood tests** are triggered by specific symptom complexes (see **IV.**), and no "routine" set is obtained for every patient with dizziness. In particular, a chemistry panel, complete blood cell count, glucose tolerance test, and allergy tests need not be routinely ordered.

   4. Radiologic investigations. Skull radiographs, cervical spinal radiographs, CT of the head, and CT of the sinuses are not recommended routinely in the evaluation of vertigo.
   a. MRI of the head is performed to evaluate the structural integrity of the brainstem, cerebellum, periventricular white matter, and eighth nerve complexes. T1-weighted MRI with contrast enhancement is the most useful variant. MRI is not routinely needed to evaluate vertigo without accompanying neurologic findings. Although MRI may show enhancement of the vestibular nerve in vestibular neuritis, it seems unreasonable to use this expensive modality to document the existence of a self-limited condition.
   b. CT of the temporal bone provides higher resolution of ear structures than does MRI and is better for evaluating lesions involving bone.
   5. Other tests
   a. Electroencephalography (EEG) is used to diagnose seizures. Because EEG is insensitive, several studies may be needed.
   b. Ambulatory event monitoring, or Holter monitoring, is used to detect arrhythmia or sinus arrest.
   c. Tilt table testing sometimes is advocated for diagnosis of syncope. However, because of a lack of data establishing a link between tilt table test abnormalities and successful treatment outcome, the appropriate role of the tilt table test in the evaluation of dizziness is unclear.
   IV. Differential diagnosis. We now discuss symptom complexes, their differential diagnosis, and algorithms used to narrow the differential. This approach can be time-consuming and is intended for use by an examiner who has approximately an hour to make an evaluation. Table 16.6 enumerates five specific symptom complexes. When a patient's findings do not fit into a complex in Table 16.6, one can fall back to grouping the findings by duration of symptoms only, as in Table 16.7.

Table 16.6 Specific symptom complexes

Positional Vertigo (Bed Spins)
  Benign paroxysmal positional vertigo (95%)
  Central vertigo
  Vestibular neuritis
  Postural hypotension
Headaches and Vertigo
  Vertebrobasilar migraine
  Posttraumatic vertigo
  Arnold–Chiari malformation
  Unlocalized Vertigo
Hydrops Symptom Complex (Fluctuating Hearing, Vertigo, Tinnitus, Fullness)
  Ménière's disease
  Perilymphatic fistula
  Posttraumatic hydrops
  Syphilis
Pressure Sensitivity Symptom Complex
  Perilymphatic fistula
  Ménière's disease
  Superior canal dehiscence
  Arnold–Chiari malformation
  Stapes malformation or prosthesis
Medicolegal Situations
  Malingering and disability evaluations

Table 16.7 Typical duration of selected conditions causing dizziness

---

1–3 Seconds (Quick Spins)
Epilepsy
Vestibular nerve irritation
Ménière's disease variants
BPPV variants
Less Than 1 Minute
BPPV
Arrhythmia
Ménière's disease variants
Minutes to Hours
Transient ischemic attack
Ménière's disease
Panic attacks, situational anxiety, hyperventilation
Orthostasis
Hours to Days
Ménière's disease
Vertebrobasilar migraine
Two Weeks or More
Vestibular neuritis and labyrinthitis
Central vertigo with structural lesion
Anxiety
Malingering
Bilateral vestibular paresis or loss
Multisensory dysequilibrium of the elderly
Drug intoxication

BPPV, benign paroxysmal positional vertigo.

A. Approach based on specific symptom complexes
    1. Bed spins and positional syndromes. Patients report a brief burst of rotatory vertigo when getting into or out of bed or on rolling over from one side to the other. This symptom strongly suggests the diagnosis of BPPV.
        a. BPPV. If typical nystagmus is observed in Dix–Hallpike positional testing, no other diagnoses need be considered. Because approximately 95% of all positional nystagmus is caused by BPPV, even in cases in which atypical positional nystagmus is observed, it usually is most efficient to try one of the currently available treatments before considering other diagnoses. MRI of the head is indicated when atypical BPPV is refractory to treatment.
        b. Central disorders. Strong positional nystagmus can accompany brainstem and cerebellar disorders (e.g., medulloblastoma and Arnold–Chiari malformation). MRI is indicated when positional nystagmus is combined with abnormal findings at neurologic examination or when atypical BPPV is refractory to treatment.
        c. Vestibular neuritis. Weak horizontal positional nystagmus may be found with peripheral vestibulopathy. ENG and an audiogram are indicated.
        d. Postural hypotension manifests as dizziness on getting out of bed but never occurs in bed. It is diagnosed when there is a symptomatic decrease in blood pressure or an increase in pulse rate between the supine and standing positions. A decrease of 20 mm Hg mercury is significant.
    2. Headaches and vertigo
        a. Migraine. One large group of patients are women in their thirties with perimenstrual exacerbations. Food triggers, motion sickness, and a pos-

itive family history are frequent associations. There is a weak association between BPPV and migraine. The diagnosis of migraine associated
vertigo should prompt consideration of BPPV. Empirical trials of antimigraine medication (verapamil or a β-blocker) may be the only way to
make this diagnosis.

   b. **Posttraumatic vertigo.** Audiometry, ENG, CT of the head, and EEG
      are indicated.
   c. **Arnold–Chiari malformation.** The headache is posterior, and there
      are downbeat nystagmus and ataxia. The diagnosis is obtained by means
      of sagittal T1-weighted MRI.
   d. **Unlocalized vertigo.** Audiometry and ENG are indicated for the ver-
      tigo component. The headache component (e.g., tension, migraine, sinus)
      is considered separately.
3. **Hydrops.** Patients report spells of vertigo, roaring tinnitus, and transient
   hearing loss, each preceded by aural fullness. Audiometry should be performed for all patients, as should fluorescent treponemal antibody absorption
   (FTA), erythrocyte sedimentation rate, and thyroid-stimulating hormone
   blood tests.
   a. **Ménière's disease.** The usual duration of vertigo is 2 hours, but it can
      vary from seconds to weeks. Audiometry is crucial to document the fluc-
      tuating low-tone sensorineural hearing loss (Fig. 16.2). The diagnosis of
      Ménière's disease is highly probable when a typical history is obtained
      and when fluctuating hearing is documented. ECOG may be performed
      in difficult cases in an attempt to "rule in" the diagnosis. Approximately
      10% of all cases of bilateral Ménière's disease are autoimmune. Thyroid
      disease is frequent among patients with Ménière's disease.
   b. **PLF.** Fistula occasionally manifests as hydrops rather than the pres-
      sure sensitivity symptom complex (see **IV.A.4.**). The only clue may be a
      history of barotrauma. Fistula testing is indicated.
   c. **Posttraumatic hydrops** is a variant of the Ménière's disease symptom
      complex that appears after a strong blow to the ear with presumed
      bleeding into the inner ear.

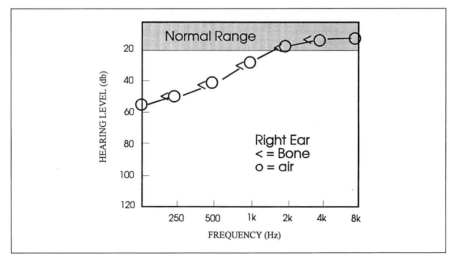

FIG. 16.2 Low-tone hearing loss. Unilateral low-frequency sensorineural pattern hearing
loss often is observed in early Ménière's disease.

d. Syphilis. Hearing loss is bilateral. Diagnosis is by means of FTA antibody absorbent (FTA-ABS) testing.

4. **Pressure sensitivity.** Patients report dizziness or ataxia evoked by nose blowing, high-speed elevators, cleaning of the ear with a cotton swab, straining as at stool, after the landing of an airplane, or after diving. In addition to pressure sensitivity, patients report vertigo induced by loud noises (Tullio's phenomenon) and by exercise. Patients often are extremely motion intolerant and visually sensitive. Audiometry and the fistula test are indicated.

   a. PLF is the main source of pressure sensitivity. Most patients have a history of barotrauma. Audiometry and the fistula test are indicated. ECOG may be used as a secondary test if audiometry and the fistula test fail to establish the side of injury.

   b. Ménière's disease. Mild pressure sensitivity occurs in approximately one third of patients with Ménière's disease. See **IV.A.3.** for a differential diagnosis.

   c. SCD syndrome. Vertigo and nystagmus can be provoked by loud noise or pressure. This syndrome is caused by dehiscence of bone overlying the superior semicircular canal. Diagnosis is made by means of high-resolution CT of the temporal bone.

   d. Arnold–Chiari malformation and **platybasia.** Vertigo is correlated with straining but not with pressure in the external ear canal. The downbeat nystagmus and abnormal MRI findings of Arnold–Chiari malformation also separate it from the other entities.

   e. Stapes malformation. Remarkable pressure sensitivity with torsional movement of the eye occurs among patients with congenital malformations of the stapes footplate and also among patients in whom stapes prostheses (for otosclerosis) of excessive length have been inserted. High-resolution CT of the temporal bone is indicated in this situation, if there has been no stapes surgery.

5. **Medicolegal situations.** The possibility of malingering often arises in disability evaluations, worker's compensation cases, and legal situations in which patients may be compensated for having vertigo. These patients usually present no objective evidence at physical examination or testing. Often they resist examination by closing their eyes at inappropriate times or refusing to perform key positional maneuvers. Their problems often cannot be resolved into one of the symptom complexes discussed earlier (see **I.D.6.**). Objective testing (audiometry, ENG, or an MRI of the head) is nearly always appropriate. Posturography also may be helpful. This test can trick a malingering patient by presenting a series of protocols that gradually become more and more difficult. A malingerer trying to fail a posturography test frequently performs equally poorly on the easy and difficult subtests, producing a nonphysiologic pattern.

B. **Approach based on timing only.** These categories, as documented in Table 16.7, are less useful for diagnosis than those based on symptom complexes, but they can be used when a patient's condition does not fall into any category. As such, these categories form a clinical "fall back" strategy.

1. **Quick spins** are brief spells (1 to 3 seconds) of true vertigo unaccompanied by secondary symptoms. EEG and BAER testing should be performed. A trial of carbamazepine may be helpful.

   a. Epilepsy. Spells often are very frequent (20 per day), and there is often a history of head injury. Cognitive impairment is frequent.

   b. Microvascular compression syndrome. Frequent spells are possible. There also may be hearing symptoms such as a "sizzling" tinnitus. The BAER may be abnormal. Magnetic resonance angiography (MRA) occasionally depicts a vertebral or basilar artery compressing the brainstem. If the EEG findings are normal, a good response to carbamazepine suggests the diagnosis.

   c. Ménière's disease variants. Frequency of spells is daily at most. Hearing often is affected. For diagnosis, see **IV.A.3.**

    d. BPPV variants. Spells are of no more than daily frequency. The presumption is that otoconial debris is caught on a canal wall and suddenly slips down. Diagnosis is achieved with the Dix–Hallpike maneuver. It may take several visits to obtain a positive result.

2. Less than 1 minute. These are mainly postural syndromes.

    a. Classic BPPV. If there is positional vertigo, this diagnosis is easy. However, poor "historians" may omit to mention that they have adopted sleeping strategies (e.g., two pillows) to avoid bed spin. BPPV also can be triggered by unusual head positions such as looking up at a top shelf. Diagnosis is achieved with the Dix–Hallpike maneuver.

    b. Cardiac arrhythmia. The clues usually are that vertigo spells occur only while the persons is standing and that light-headedness is a more prominent symptom than is spinning. Ambulatory event monitoring is the best method of documenting this problem. Holter monitoring can be used in contexts in which event monitoring is not available.

    c. Ménière's disease variants. See **IV.B.1.c.**

3. Minutes to hours

    a. TIA. Spells of pure vertigo lasting 2 to 30 minutes and of abrupt onset and ending in a patient with vascular risk factors are diagnosed as TIA until proved otherwise. Suspicion is reduced if there is a positional trigger. MRA of the vertebrobasilar circulation is the single most useful test.

    b. Ménière's disease. A typical Ménière's attack lasts 2 hours. If there are hearing symptoms, see **IV.A.3.** If not, be cautious about proposing this diagnosis. Sometimes the term *vestibular Ménière's disease* is used to denote episodic vertigo having the typical timing of classic Ménière's disease but without any ear symptomatology. It is unclear whether this entity exists, and there is no method of confirming this diagnosis.

    c. Panic attacks, situational anxiety, and **hyperventilation** can produce symptoms of this duration (minutes to hours). The patients ordinarily have no symptoms during the examination. A detailed history is the most useful diagnostic test. If hyperventilation reproduces symptoms in patients without other findings, the diagnosis is hyperventilation syndrome. If hyperventilation also induces nystagmus, MRI is indicated.

    d. Cardiac arrhythmia and orthostasis

4. Hours to days

    a. Ménière's disease

    b. Vertebrobasilar migraine. Migraine is so common in the general population that even unusual variants, such as manifestation solely as a vertiginous aura, are common. Diagnosis is suggested by age (twenties and thirties), sex (usually female), positive family history, and attacks provoked by the usual migraine triggers.

5. Two weeks or more

    a. Vestibular neuritis. The diagnosis is made by combining a long duration with spontaneous nystagmus or an abnormal ENG result. ENG may document nystagmus or significant vestibular paresis (a conservative criterion is paresis of 40% or more). After 2 months of vertigo, central vertigo becomes more likely and MRI is indicated. For labyrinthitis, the diagnosis is made by combining the vestibular neuritis pattern with hearing symptoms. Audiometry, a serum FTA test, erythrocyte sedimentation rate, and fasting glucose measurement are indicated.

    b. Central vertigo with a fixed structural CNS lesion. This diagnosis should be considered when neurologic symptoms or signs accompany vertigo. Central vertigo can last indefinitely. For example, the combination of peripheral vestibular loss with a cerebellar lesion can occur after acoustic neuroma surgery. Nevertheless, acoustic neuroma is an extremely uncommon source of peripheral or central vertigo because of its rarity compared with disorders such as BPPV. MRI is the most effective method of diagnosis of central vertigo. There are no examination maneuvers that can reliably separate peripheral vertigo (such as that caused by vestibular neuritis) from central vertigo that lacks any "central signs."

   c. **Anxiety.** With this duration of symptoms (2 weeks or more), patients may experiencing vertigo during the office visit. If a patient is describing vertigo, but no spontaneous nystagmus is evident under Frenzel goggles, one can reasonably conclude that the vertigo is functional in origin. Patients with anxiety typically report that nearly every trigger factor in Table 16.4 exacerbates the symptoms. Interesting is that whereas most patients with inner ear problems report that stress makes their symptoms worse, patients with anxiety frequently are sensitive about this diagnosis and perversely claim that everything except stress triggers vertigo. A positive response to a trial of a benzodiazepine such as lorazepam supports this diagnosis but does not establish it, because many organic vestibular disorders also respond well to these medications.

   d. **Malingering.** Malingerers persist in reporting symptoms as long as necessary to accomplish the purpose of obtaining favorable court settlements or disability rulings. Posturography may be helpful.

   e. **Bilateral vestibular paresis or loss.** All patients with these disorders fail the dynamic illegible "E" test and the eyes-closed tandem Romberg test. The ataxia is worse in the dark. At audiometry, usually only high-frequency hearing is affected. Rotatory chair testing is the best way to confirm this diagnostic impression.

   f. **Multisensory dysequilibrium of the elderly** is essentially unlocalized vertigo in an elderly patient. If the diagnosis is accurate, this usually is a permanent condition.

   g. **Drug intoxication.** The diagnosis depends on withdrawal of medications.

V. Diagnostic approach

  A. Obtain the history and perform the examination as outlined in **II.** and **III.**

  B. Approximately 20% to 40% of cases are diagnosed immediately at examination.

    1. BPPV with Dix–Hallpike maneuver (15% to 20% of population with vertigo)

    2. Orthostatic hypotension, arrhythmia, and carotid sinus hypersensitivity (2% to 5%)

    3. Bilateral vestibular paresis or loss on dynamic illegible "E" test (5%)

    4. Fistula at fistula test (0 to 5%)

    5. Acute vestibular neuritis through spontaneous nystagmus (2% to 5%)

  C. For the other patients, proceed as follows.

    1. If the patient's findings fits into a symptom complex category, follow the procedures in **IV.A.**

    2. If patient's findings do not fit into a symptom complex, follow the procedures in **IV.B.**

     a. If the symptoms are intermittent, follow the procedures in **IV.B.1.–3.**

     b. Otherwise, if symptoms are constant, proceed as follows.

      (1) If the duration has been less than 2 weeks, treat symptomatically or simply reassure and have patient return if symptoms persist for more than 2 weeks.

      (2) If the duration has been more than 2 weeks, follow the procedures in **IV.B.**

VI. Referrals

  A. Otology

    1. Cerumen disimpaction and microscopic examination. Ear wax can be safely removed with an examining microscope, a standard piece of otologic equipment.

    2. Progressive or acute hearing loss has potential medicolegal ramifications, and otologic consultation should be obtained.

    3. A **perforated tympanic membrane** or a **mass** in the canal or behind the tympanic membrane may necessitate referral for closure of the perforation or surgical management of the tumor.

    4. Mastoiditis and **chronic otitis media** are commonly managed with a combination of surgery, cleaning, antibiotics, and antiseptics that requires otologic supervision.

    5. Surgical management of acoustic neuroma, Ménière's disease, fistula, and cholesteatoma.

B. Internal medicine

    1. Cardiac or blood pressure problems

    2. Management of diabetes or thyroid dysfunction

C. Psychiatry

    1. Undiagnosed conditions (after thorough evaluation)

    2. Anxiety or panic

    3. Malingering

Recommended Readings

Brandt T. *Vertigo: its multisensory syndromes.* London: Springer-Verlag, 1991.

Drachman D, Hart CW. An approach to the dizzy patient. *Neurology* 1972;22:323–334.

Fife TD, Tusa RJ, Furman JM, et al. Assessment: vestibular testing techniques in adults and children. *Neurology* 2000;55;1431–1441.

Fisher CM. Vertigo in cerebrovascular disease. *Arch Otolaryngol* 1967;85:85–90.

Herr RD, Zun L, Mathews JJ. A directed approach to the dizzy patient. *Ann Emerg Med* 1989;18:664–672.

Kroenke K, Lucas CA, Rosenberg ML, et al. Causes of persistent dizziness. *Ann Intern Med* 1992;117:898–904.

Macrae D. The neurologic aspects of vertigo: analysis of 400 cases. *California Med* 1960;92: 255–259.

Madlon-Kay DJ. Evaluation and outcome of the dizzy patient. *J Fam Pract* 1985;21:109–113.

Nedzelski JM, Barber HO, McIlmoyl L. Diagnoses in a dizziness unit. *J Otolaryngol* 1986;15: 101–104.

Sloane PD. Dizziness in primary care: results from the national ambulatory medical care survey. *J Fam Pract* 1989;29:33–38.

17. APPROACH TO THE PATIENT WITH HEARING LOSS

Richard T. Miyamoto
Michael K. Wynne

Hearing loss is the most prevalent physical ailment in the United States, affecting approximately one in 10 persons. It produces substantial communication problems and can be the presenting symptom of serious underlying medical disorders. A detailed medical and audiologic evaluation is required to establish a specific etiologic factor and management plan.

    I. Etiology. There are various and complex causes of hearing loss. In many cases, particularly among children, the cause of the hearing loss may remain unknown or idiopathic even after an extensive medical and audiologic work-up.
        A. Despite the diversity of the patients and their presenting symptoms, the causes of hearing loss can be classified as **hereditary** or **adventitious,** although there is not a clear distinction between the two. For example, there is a genetic disposition for certain populations to be more susceptible to noise-induced hearing loss.
        B. The **onset** of hearing loss serves as a useful indicator when describing the cause. Hearing loss is considered **congenital** when the it was caused before birth, **perinatal** when the hearing loss occurs during the birthing process, and **postnatal** when the onset of the hearing loss occurs after birth.
        C. Nonorganic hearing losses are not uncommon and can be found among young children or patients with previously confirmed organic hearing loss.
    II. Anatomy and physiology of the auditory system. The auditory system is divided into four anatomical regions: (1) the external ear, (2) the middle ear, (3) the inner ear, and (4) the central auditory pathway.
        A. The **external ear,** consisting of the pinna and the external auditory canal, collects and directs sound to the tympanic membrane. Because of its physical dimensions, the external ear provides an important resonance boost between 2,000 and 5,000 Hz, a frequency range that contributes to the perception of speech.
        B. The **middle ear** consists of the tympanic membrane, three ossicles (malleus, incus, and stapes), two middle ear muscles (tensor tympani and stapedius), and the ligaments that suspend the ossicles in the middle ear cavity. The middle ear structures transmit acoustic energy from the external environment to the inner ear and serve as a mechanical transformer recovering energy that would otherwise be lost as sound is transmitted from a gaseous medium (air) to a liquid medium (endolymph).
        Two middle ear mechanisms restore most, but not all, of the sound pressure lost in the energy transfer. Most of the mechanical gain results from a concentration of the energy collected by the relatively large tympanic membrane on the small oval window. The areal ratio between the tympanic membrane and the oval window recovers approximately 23 dB of the 30 dB lost. An additional 2 or 3 dB is gained as a result of a lever action that occurs because the handle of the malleus is slightly longer than the long process of the incus.
        C. Inner ear. The inner ear is divided into the **vestibular portion** consisting of three semicircular canals as well as the utricle and saccule and the **auditory portion** consisting of the cochlea. The semicircular canals provide information regarding angular acceleration, and the utricle and saccule provide information regarding gravitational or linear acceleration. The vestibular system, coupled with the visual and proprioceptive systems, functions as the body's balance mechanism. The cochlea is the end organ of hearing. The cochlea is a fluid-filled cavity divided by the cochlear partition into three cavities—the scala vestibuli, the scala media, and the scale tympani. With stapes displacement, a traveling wave moves up the cochlear partition and displaces the basilar membrane. This displacement results in a shearing action of the stereocilia at the top of the one set of inner hair cells and the three sets of outer hairs cells. The inner hair cells are considered sensory cells, and the outer hair cells are considered motor cells. When the stereocilia of the inner hair cell are sheared toward the basal body of

the cell (the human cochlear hair cell has no kinocilium but rather a basal body located at the base of the "U" or "W" pattern of the stereocilia), the inner hair cell depolarizes and discharges neurotransmitters at its base and into the synaptic space with the afferent fibers of the eighth cranial nerve. Because of the stiffness and mass characteristics of the cochlear partition, the traveling wave envelope reaches its peak at a given location along the cochlear partition, and then the displacement is heavily damped. This location corresponds to a specific frequency region equivalent to the frequency of the auditory stimulus. Thus the inner ear acts as a low-pass filter with high-frequency sounds encoded at the basal region of the cochlea and low-frequency sounds encoded at the apical region of the cochlea. This tonotopic arrangement is maintained throughout the central auditory system.

    D. Central auditory system. The central auditory system consists of the auditory portion of the eighth cranial nerve, the cochlear nucleus, the intermediate stria or trapezoid body, the superior olivary complex, the lateral lemniscus, the inferior colliculus, the medial geniculate body of the thalamus, and finally the auditory cortex. The level of neural complexity increases exponentially with each higher order neuron or central auditory nucleus.

III. Medical evaluation. Evaluation of the auditory system is accomplished by means of obtaining a detailed history and performing a physical examination and audiologic studies. In selected cases, radiologic imaging is indicated.

    A. History. The otologic history includes inquiry into symptoms of ear disease, including hearing loss, ear pain (otalgia), discharge from the ear (otorrhea), tinnitus or other head noises, and vertigo or dizziness. If any of these symptoms is present, a detailed characterization is performed. The clinical significance of hearing loss is related to the time and acuity of onset, severity, and the tendency to fluctuate or progress. The deleterious effects of hearing loss are particularly great when the onset occurs before the development of spoken language (prelingually).

    B. Physical examination

        1. The **otologic examination** begins with inspection of the pinna and palpation of periauricular structures, including the periauricular and parotid lymph nodes.

        2. Otoscopic examination of the external ear canal and tympanic membranes is performed to identify abnormalities of these structures. Pneumatic otoscopy is helpful in assessing the mobility of the tympanic membrane and is particularly useful in identifying subtle middle ear effusion.

        3. A complete **head and neck examination** is performed, including a cranial nerve screen and cerebellar testing.

        4. Tuning fork tests are an important part of the otologic functional examination for hearing acuity. They are particularly useful in differentiation between conductive and sensorineural hearing loss. The most useful tuning forks are those with vibrating frequencies of 512 and 1,024 cycles per second. The two most commonly used tuning fork tests are the **Weber test** and the **Rinne test.**

            a. The **Weber test** is performed by placing the stem of the tuning fork on the midline plane of the skull. The patient is asked to identify the location of the auditory percept within the head. The signal lateralizes to the ear with conductive hearing loss provided normal hearing is present in the opposite ear. This occurs because the ambient room noise present in the usual testing situation tends to mask the normal ear, but the poorer ear with a conductive loss does not hear such noise and better hears bone-conducted sound. If a sensorineural loss is present in one ear and the opposite ear is normal, the fork is heard louder in the better ear.

            b. The **Rinne test** is performed by alternately placing a ringing tuning fork opposite one external auditory meatus and firmly on the adjacent mastoid bone. The loudness of the tuning fork in these two locations is compared. The normal ear hears a tuning fork about twice as long with air conduction as with bone conduction. Conductive hearing loss reverses this ratio, and sound is heard longer with bone conduction than with air conduction. Patients with sensorineural hearing loss hear better by means of air conduction than by means of bone conduction, although hearing is reduced with both air and bone conduction.

IV. Hearing. The audiologic evaluation characterizes the type, severity, and configuration of a hearing loss. Loss of hearing can be either partial or total. It can affect the low, middle, or high frequencies in any combination. The acuity of onset and the tendency to fluctuate or progress in severity influence the negative impact of hearing loss.

    A. Range of hearing. Although the human ear is sensitive to frequencies between 20 and 20,000 Hz, the frequency range from 300 to 3,000 Hz is most important for understanding speech.

        1. During an audiologic evaluation, pure-tone thresholds are routinely obtained for frequencies at octave intervals between 250 and 8,000 Hz. This approximates a range from middle C (262 Hz) to just under one octave above the highest note on a piano (5,274 Hz).

        2. The range of sound pressure to which the human ear responds is immense. Infinitesimal movement of the hair cells produces a just audible sound, yet a trillion-fold increase is still tolerable.

        3. The large range of numbers needed to describe audible sound pressure is best represented by a logarithmic ratio comparing a sound to a standard reference sound. This is called the **decibel.** The decibel is defined in relation to the physical reference of sound, or **sound pressure level (SPL),** to the average threshold of normal hearing for young adults, or **hearing level (HL),** or to a patient's own threshold for the sound stimulus, or **sensation level (SL).**

        4. Speech sounds vary in their acoustic characteristics. Vowels tend to have most of their energy in the low to middle frequencies and are produced at relatively higher intensities than consonants. Thus vowels carry the power of speech. Consonants tend to contain higher frequency information and have low power. Much of the actual understanding of speech depends on the correct perception of consonants. Consequently, speech may not be audible for patients with hearing loss across the entire frequency range. Patients with hearing loss in the higher frequencies may hear speech but not understand it.

    B. Audiogram. A graphic representation of pure-tone responses is provided by the audiogram presented in Fig. 17.1. **Frequency** (pitch) is represented on the horizontal axis and **intensity** (loudness) is presented on the vertical axis. The 0 dB HL line represents the average threshold level for a group of normal-hearing young adults with no history of otologic disease or noise exposure. Conversational speech at a distance of 1 m has an intensity level of approximately 50 to 60 dB HL. Most persons with normal hearing or sensorineural hearing loss would find speech uncomfortably loud at about 80 to 90 dB HL.

V. Hearing loss. Hearing loss is broadly classified into two types—conductive and sensorineural. Each type has a wide variety of pathologic causes. Table 17.1 presents a summary of the diagnostic and audiologic findings associated with various types of hearing loss.

    A. Conductive hearing loss occurs when sound cannot efficiently reach the cochlea. The blockage may be due to abnormalities of the ear canal, the tympanic membrane, or the middle ear ossicles, including the footplate of the stapes.

        1. Hearing loss due to **obstruction of the external auditory canal** can result from impacted cerumen, foreign bodies in the canal, and swelling of the canal during infection. **Cerumen impaction** is the most common cause of conductive hearing loss. Cerumen is normally secreted by glands in the outer one third of the ear canal to protect the ear canal skin from moisture. It is normally carried to the outside by the canal skin as it migrates from the tympanic membrane to the external auditory meatus. Another cause is **congenital atresia** of the external auditory canal, in which the canal does not develop.

        2. Conductive hearing loss may result from **damage to the tympanic membrane or middle ear** as a result of trauma or infection. Perforation of the tympanic membrane and ossicular discontinuity are surgically correctable.

(*text continues on page 214*)

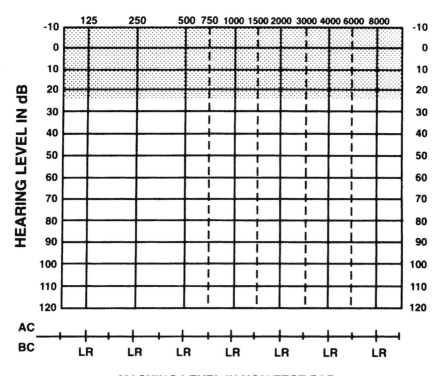

FIG. 17.1 Audiogram and audiometric symbols.

Table 17.1 Summary of types of hearing loss with general diagnostic and audiologic patterns

Type of lesion	General diagnostic and audiologic pattern	Tuning fork	Speech audiometry	Tympanogram	Acoustic reflexes	Recruitment/ adaptation
Conductive	Unilateral or bilateral hearing loss Rising or flat audiometric configuration Bone conduction thresholds: normal Maximum conductive loss cannot exceed 60–70 dB Paracusis willisii: "I hear better in a noisy place" If speech is presented at a sufficient intensity, discrimination is excellent No loudness tolerance difficulties Often can be treated medically Can be transient or fluctuating Examples: cerumen impaction, otitis media, otosclerosis, TM perforation	Weber: to ear with greatest conductive loss Rinne: negative, bone is better than air Bing: no occlusion effect	SRT: consistent with pure-tone average Discrimination: excellent Normal dynamic range	Jerger type B: fluid in middle ear space Jerger type C: retracted TM Jerger type A or A_s: otosclerosis or ossicular fixation Jerger type A_D: tympano-sclerosis or ossicular discontinuity	Absent	None seen
Sensorineural	Unilateral or bilateral hearing loss ranging from mild to profound in severity Flat or falling audiometric configuration—may have notch if noise induced or rising in Ménière's disease No air–bone gap; bone conduction thresholds are poorer than normal limits Speech discrimination is variable, depending on severity, configuration, and cause of hearing loss	Weber: to ear with best cochlear reserve Rinne: positive, air is better than bone Bing: occlusion effect	SRT: consistent with pure-tone average Discrimination: excellent to minimal Reduced dynamic range	Jerger type A: normal TM compliance at normal pressure	Present but can vary as a function of severity of hearing loss	Partial or complete recruitment No adaptation

Type	Characteristics	Speech audiometry	Tympanometry	Acoustic reflex
	Abnormal growth of loudness and reduced dynamic range Otoacoustic emissions are generally absent BSER has normal latencies for high intensity clicks, recruitment Tinnitus is common, ranging from high-pitched ringing to low-frequency roar to unusual head noises Some patients experience vertigo Occasionally can be managed medically Can be assisted with hearing aids, cochlear implants, assistive listening devices, and speechreading Examples: presbycusis, noise-induced hearing loss, Ménière's disease, ototoxicity, congenital loss			
Mixed	Combination of the conductive and sensorineural hearing losses described above Marked air–bone gaps with bone conduction thresholds poorer than normal Conductive component may respond to medical treatment, still requires amplification or other aural rehabilitation strategies	Weber: to ear with greatest conductive loss Rinne: negative, bone is better than air Bing: no occlusion effect SRT: consistent with pure-tone average Discrimination: excellent to minimal Dynamic range may be reduced	Absent Jerger type B: fluid in middle ear space Jerger type C: retracted TM Jerger type A or A_s: otosclerosis or ossicular fixation Jerger type A_D: Tympano-sclerosis or ossicular discontinuity	None seen owing to the overriding conductive component

(continued)

Table 17.1 (Continued)

Type of lesion	General diagnostic and audiologic pattern	Tuning fork	Speech audiometry	Tympanogram	Acoustic reflexes	Recruitment/ adaptation
Neural	Usually unilateral or asymmetric hearing loss, ranging from normal hearing to profound loss Characterized by asymmetric configuration No air–bone gap Speech discrimination generally poorer in the affected ear Abnormal adaptation Otoacoustic emissions may be present or absent BSER shows prolonged latency between waves I and V or between ears Vertigo and tinnitus common Often managed surgically, trying to preserve hearing when possible Example: acoustic neuroma	Weber: to ear with best cochlear reserve Rinne: positive, air is better than bone Bing: occlusion effect	SRT: consistent with or poorer than pure-tone average Discrimination: poor to minimal in affected ear Reduced dynamic range	Jerger type A: normal TM compliance at normal pressure	Elevated or absent Abnormally rapid decay	Can have partial or complete recruitment Abnormal adaptation is common

| Central | Audiogram is generally normal but can show any other type of hearing loss
Characterized by difficulties processing speech in the presence of noise
Often diagnosed by abnormally poor scores on specialized speech tests
Otoacoustic emissions usually are normal but can have unusual contralateral suppression characteristics
BSER is normal, but middle and late evoked potentials and event-related potentials may be abnormal
Generally poor academic and reading performance | Normal | SRT: consistent with pure-tone average
Discrimination: excellent in quiet, reduced in noise or if signal is distorted
Normal dynamic range | Jerger type A: normal TM compliance at normal pressure | Generally present at normal levels | None seen |

TM, tympanic membrane; SRT, speech recognition threshold; BSER, brainstem evoked response

3. **Otitis media with effusion** is the most common cause of conductive hearing loss among children. This condition can be associated with adenoid hypertrophy. The middle ear effusion may necessitate treatment with myringotomy and tube placement.

4. **Otosclerosis** is the most common cause of conductive hearing loss among persons between the ages of 15 and 50 years. Otosclerotic bone progressively fixes the stapes in the oval window. This condition can be successfully managed with stapedectomy.

B. **Sensorineural hearing loss.** Sensorineural hearing loss results from lesions central to the footplate of the stapes that involve the cochlea or cochlear division of the eighth cranial nerve. When the site of lesion is **within the cochlea,** the hearing loss is considered **sensory** (end organ). When the site of lesion is **within the neural pathways,** the hearing loss is **neural or retrocochlear.** In sensorineural hearing losses, both air- and bone-conduction thresholds are outside the normal range of hearing sensitivity.

1. Sensorineural hearing loss may be hereditary; at least 100 genetic syndromes that involve hearing loss have been identified. It has been estimated that 50% of childhood sensorineural hearing loss is due to **genetic factors.** Genetic forms of hearing loss may be congenital or delayed in onset, unilateral or bilateral, and progressive or nonprogressive.

2. **Infection.** A number of viruses, including cytomegalovirus, rubella, and herpes simplex, have been implicated as etiologic agents in congenital and acquired hearing loss. Congenital syphilis and bacterial meningitis are contemporary causes of deafness despite of greatly improved treatment modalities.

3. **Other common causes** of sensorineural hearing loss are noise exposure, metabolic and systemic changes in the auditory system, ototoxic medications, aging (presbycusis), and head trauma. In patients with unilateral progressive sensorineural hearing loss, acoustic neuroma must be suspected. Bilateral acoustic neuroma is the hallmark of neurofibromatosis type 2 and must be suspected when a patient has a positive family history (autosomal dominant inheritance).

C. **Mixed hearing loss.** Mixed hearing loss exists when both conductive and sensorineural hearing losses occur in the same ear. The lesions are additive, resulting in marked air–bone gaps with the bone-conduction thresholds falling outside the normal range of hearing sensitivity.

D. **Auditory neuropathy.** Some patients have normal peripheral ears up to and including the outer hair cells but have hearing difficulties. These hearing difficulties can range from normal hearing sensitivity to tones but considerably reduced speech discrimination to the complete absence of a response to any auditory stimulus. These patients typically have normal immittance results and normal otoacoustic emissions, yet they have anomalies in evoked potentials, particularly in the auditory brainstem response, and in the behavioral response under earphones or in the sound field. These patients are said to have auditory neuropathy. Although the causes of auditory neuropathy are unclear, it does appear that the pathologic process affects the inner hair cell or the auditory processing abilities of the brainstem. Because of the possible dead regions in the cochlea or neural involvement, these patients do not respond typically to some of the traditional treatment protocols.

E. **Central auditory processing disorder.** Patients with this type of disorder do not perceive and use acoustic information because the central auditory system is incapable of appropriately processing the signals transduced by the cochlea. Patients with central auditory processing disorders can be taught compensation strategies to improve their ability to comprehend speech. Many adults with sensorineural hearing losses also may have a concomitant central auditory processing disorder, which confounds the evaluation and management of the sensorineural hearing loss.

F. **Degree of hearing loss.** Although a percentage of hearing handicap can be determined for medicolegal purposes as presented in Table 17.2, the degree of hearing loss cannot be completely defined as a percentage because the effects of

Table 17.2 Calculation of hearing handicap as a percentage

1. Obtain air-conduction thresholds in dB HL for both ears.
2. Calculate the average of the thresholds obtained for 500, 1,000, 2,000, and 3,000 Hz for each ear.
3. If the average exceeds 25 dB (low fence), subtract 25 and multiply the remainder by 1.5% up to a maximum of 100% which is reached at 92 dB (high fence). This score represents percentage monaural impairment.
4. If the monaural percentage figure is the same for both ears, that figure expresses the percentage handicap. If the percentage monaural impairments are not the same, multiply the smaller percentage (better ear) by 5, add this figure to the larger percentage (poorer ear), and divide the sum by 6 to compute the total hearing handicap.

the loss depend on the type, severity, and configuration of the hearing loss. Table 17.3 presents the range and effects of the various degrees of hearing loss, particularly as the degrees affect educational outcomes for children. Table 17.4 presents some of the common hearing loss configurations.

Findings reported in the literature suggest that cochlear hearing loss is associated with complete destruction of the inner hair cells along a certain area of the cochlear partition that results in a dead region of the cochlea. That is, no transduction occurs in that region of the cochlea. If there is no retrocochlear or neural involvement, the data suggest that a sensory hearing loss between 20 and 65 dB HL (and possibly 50 dB HL in the low frequencies) may be due to "pure" outer hair cell dysfunction or a combination of outer and inner hair cell dysfunction. When the thresholds exceed 65 dB HL (and possibly 50 dB HL in the low frequencies), the sensory hearing loss is likely due to a combination of outer and inner hair cell dysfunction. When the thresholds exceed 90 dB HL (or 75 to 80 dB HL in the low frequencies), the hearing loss is likely associated with a dead region of the cochlea. Signals that have most of their information within the frequency boundaries of these dead regions do not have clear pitch percepts or intelligibility. Amplifying signals to stimulate the dead regions of the cochlea may not only result in poor perception but also may further reduce the perception of other signals that fall outside these dead regions.

VI. **Audiologic evaluation**
   A. **Screening for hearing loss.** Because hearing is critical for speech and oral language development in children, early identification of hearing loss is a primary concern for health care professionals and educators. The recent **Joint Committee on Infant Hearing 2000 Position Statement and Guidelines** endorse universal hearing screening of newborn infants and provides specific guidelines for hearing screening of newborns and infants. It also recommends that hearing screenings be conducted through the first 3 years of life if the child is at risk of development of postnatal hearing loss. The position paper identifies indicators associated with sensorineural and conductive hearing loss that can be used to ascertain which infants should undergo hearing screening (Table 17.5).
   B. **Pure-tone threshold audiometry.** The thresholds obtained during pure-tone threshold audiometry are the faintest intensity level at which a pure-tone stimulus can be detected by the patient. Thresholds are generally obtained for air-conduction stimuli presented through earphones or in a sound field and for bone-conduction stimuli presented with a vibrator placed on the mastoid or forehead.

   For adults and compliant older children, pure-tone testing simply requires a behavioral response to pure-tone stimulation. For infants older than 5 months, **visual reinforcement audiometry** can be used to obtain thresholds and to obtain information about other auditory functions. In this testing, infants are reinforced with illuminated, animated toys when they demonstrate a head turn
(*text continues on page 218*)

Table 17.3 Degree and possible effects of hearing loss

Range of hearing loss	Severity	Possible effects	Possible educational needs
–10–15 dB HL	Normal	None	None
16–25 dB HL	Slight	The child may have difficulties hearing faint speech, especially in difficult listening situations. The child may be unaware of subtle conversational cues, which can cause some inappropriate behavior. The child may be more fatigued owing to increased listening effort.	The child benefits from preferential seating and possibly from routine medical or audiologic monitoring. The child may benefit from mild-gain hearing assistance technologies. The child may need speech–language services.
26–40 dB HL	Mild	At 30 dB, a child can miss 25%–40% of the speech signal. In difficult listening environments, up to 50% of the primary speech signal may be missed. The child may not attend to speech and becomes easily fatigued owing to increased listening effort.	The child benefits from amplification and hearing assistance technologies. The child may need additional educational services to address any deficits in speech–language skills and in academic performance. Teacher in-service training is strongly recommended.
41–55 dB HL	Moderate	The child likely understands conversational speech only at a close distance, in a clear and distinct manner, and in a favorable listening situation. The hearing loss likely has some effect on speech and language skills as well as academic performance.	Amplification and hearing assistance technology are essential in the classroom. The child likely benefits from additional educational services to address any deficits in speech–language skills and in academic performance. Teacher in-service training is strongly recommended.

56–70 dB HL	Moderate to severe	Without amplification, conversational speech is very difficult to hear. The child has some delayed or disordered speech and language skills. Needing to constantly wear hearing aids, the child is perceived as a special learner.	Full-time amplification is required, and hearing assistance technologies are essential in the classroom. The child likely needs additional educational services to address any deficits in speech–language skills and in academic performance. Teacher in-service training is necessary.
71–90 dB HL	Severe	Without amplification, speech must be very loud if it is to be heard. Even when aided, the child may have great difficulty hearing and understanding speech. The child has some delayed or disordered speech and language skills. Needing to constantly wear hearing aids, the child is perceived as a special learner.	In addition to the communication and educational needs above, the child may need to use a sign language system as part of the overall communication program.
>90 dB HL	Profound	Even when aided with conventional hearing aids, speech is very difficult to understand. In many cases, the child may only be aware of sound and not appropriately perceive it. The child likely relies on visual cues to communicate effectively.	In addition to the communication strategies for less severe hearing losses, the child may need cochlear implants or tactile aids to perceive the acoustic cues of speech. Some families may choose a bilingual, bicultural approach to language development.

Table 17.4 Configurations (slopes) of hearing loss

Flat	Approximately equal hearing loss for all frequencies, <15 dB variation across frequencies.
Gradual sloping	Progressively greater hearing loss for higher frequencies at a slope of 5–10 dB per octave.
Sloping	Progressively greater hearing loss for higher frequencies at a slope of 15–20 dB per octave.
Precipitous sloping	Progressively greater hearing loss for higher frequencies at a slope of >20 dB per octave.
Rising	Progressively better hearing loss for higher frequencies.
Notch	Precipitously sloping hearing loss reaching a peak with some precipitous rise to better hearing in the higher frequencies above the center frequency. At least a 15-dB drop and recovery must occur within two octaves before the hearing loss is considered to have a notch.
"Cookie bite"	Greater loss in the middle frequency with at least 20 dB better hearing in the lower and higher frequencies.

response away from midline and toward the reinforcer. Visual reinforcement audiometry is a successful means to measure the hearing status of older infants and young toddlers. **Play audiometry** typically is used to assess the hearing of preschool children. In this technique, play activities are used as operant reinforcers for a child's response to auditory signals. If an older infant or a child does not condition with visual reinforcement audiometry or play audiometry, electrophysiologic testing may be needed.

C. **Speech audiometry.** Speech signals can be used to assess hearing sensitivity and the processing capabilities of the auditory system. Speech must first be audible to be understood. However, even when speech is audible, various physiologic and environmental factors can reduce the intelligibility of the speech signal so that the patient can have difficulties understanding speech despite hearing it. Two tests are used to measure these two parameters—speech threshold tests and speech recognition or discrimination tests.

1. **Speech threshold tests.** When testing for hearing sensitivity, a speech recognition threshold (SRT) or a speech awareness threshold (SAT) is obtained for each ear individually or for both ears in the sound field. The SRT is obtained at the lowest intensity level at which the patient can repeat the spondee words (two-syllable words with equal stress on each syllable) 50% of the time. The SAT is the lowest intensity level at which the patient gives any consistent behavioral response to the presentation of speech stimuli. Both the SRT and the SAT are used to provide a valid estimate of hearing sensitivity and to verify the accuracy and reliability of the pure-tone thresholds when they are available. The SRT and pure-tone average of the thresholds obtained at 500, 1,000, and 2,000 Hz should be within ±7 dB of one another. If a discrepancy exists, the examiner should doubt the validity or accuracy of the patient's thresholds.

2. **Speech discrimination.** Word recognition or speech discrimination testing determines how well a patient can "understand" speech when the stimuli are above threshold. Speech recognition or discrimination scores depend on the type, severity, and configuration of the hearing loss and on the type of pathologic condition of the ear. The scores depend on a number of stimulus and response characteristics. The patient's attending and cognitive skills also can influence the results, particularly in examinations of children and elderly persons.

Although several pathologic conditions can markedly decrease speech recognition or discrimination scores, a rollover phenomenon in which the

Table 17.5 Indicators associated with sensorineural or conductive hearing loss from the Joint Committee on Infant Hearing 2000 position statement and guidelines

For use with neonates (birth–28 d) when universal screening is not available
   Illness or condition requiring admission of 48 hours or more to a neonatal intensive care unit
   Stigmata or other findings associated with a syndrome known to include sensorineural or conductive hearing loss
   Family history of permanent childhood sensorineural hearing loss
   Craniofacial anomalies, including those with morphologic abnormalities of the pinna and ear canal
   In utero infection such as cytomegalovirus, herpes, toxoplasmosis, or rubella
For use with infants (29 d–3 y) when certain health conditions develop that necessitate rescreening
   Parent or caregiver concern regarding hearing, speech, language, or developmental delay
   Family history of permanent childhood hearing loss
   Characteristics or other findings associated with a syndrome known to include sensorineural or conductive hearing loss
   Postnatal infection associated with sensorineural hearing loss, including bacterial meningitis
   In utero infection such as cytomegalovirus, herpes, rubella, syphilis, and toxoplasmosis
   Neonatal indicators, specifically hyperbilirubinemia at a serum level necessitating exchange transfusion, persistent pulmonary hypertension of the newborn associated with mechanical ventilation, and conditions necessitating use of extracorporeal membrane oxygenation
   Syndromes associated with progressive hearing loss, such as neurofibromatosis, osteoporosis, and Usher's syndrome
   Neurodegenerative disorders, such as Hunter syndrome, or sensory motor neuropathy, such as Friedreich's ataxia or Charcot–Marie–Tooth disease
   Head trauma
   Recurrent or persistent otitis media with effusion for at least 3 mo

scores first increase and then dramatically decrease with increasing presentation levels is characteristic of retrocochlear lesions. Patients who have excellent word recognition scores at or near their threshold for speech often have a nonorganic component to their results. Children and adults with central auditory processing disorders show markedly reduced scores when the speech signals are altered in frequency content or when the speech is presented in background noise but at a favorable message-to-competition ratio.

VII. **Physiologic measures of audition.** Whenever possible, behavioral measures of hearing should be used to assess the status of the auditory system. These measures provide a more specific description of the auditory stimuli that elicit a response from a patient and how the patient perceives and responds to the stimuli. Owing to many variables that can affect the validity and reliability of these measures, particularly when testing the hearing of infants and young children, physiologic techniques can be used assess the integrity of the auditory system. In some instances, the results provide excellent estimates of hearing sensitivity.

   A. **Immittance audiometry** consists of measuring the impedance of the tympanic membrane for the transmission of a tone or the amount of sound reflected back from the tympanic membrane.

      1. **Tympanometry** is sensitive to disorders of the middle ear that affect the tympanic membrane, middle ear space, and ossicular chain. It is particularly useful in documenting the presence of middle ear effusion, ossicular discontinuity, and ossicular fixation. However, it lacks specificity for infants younger than 6 months because of the high compliance of their external ear canal walls. Figure 17.2 illustrates typical results obtained during tympanometry.

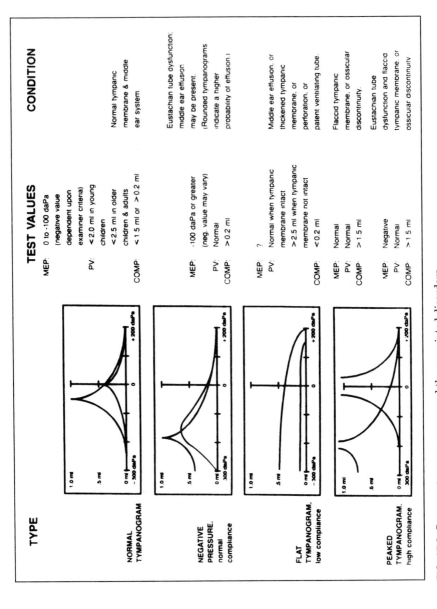

FIG. 17.2 Common tympanograms and the associated disorders.

2. **Acoustic reflex.** When an ear with normal hearing is exposed to an intense auditory signal, the stapedius muscle contracts and then changes the orientation of the stapes footplate to the oval window to produce additional impedance to the flow of energy to the inner ear. This acoustic reflex occurs bilaterally regardless of which ear is stimulated, if the system is functioning normally. The presence or absence of the reflex and the intensity levels at which the reflex is obtained provide information useful in identifying lesions within the auditory system up to the level of the superior olivary complex. In the case of lesions of the eighth cranial nerve, the decay of the acoustic reflex occurs rapidly, indicating abnormal adaptation of the neural response.

B. **Brainstem evoked response (BSER) audiometry** consists of measuring the electrical potentials generated by the neurons within the eighth cranial nerve and lower auditory brainstem to rapid-onset, short-duration acoustic signals such as a click stimulus. Because these signals are low level and are often buried in noise, signal averaging techniques are used to record the electrical response of the auditory system.

1. An example of normal BSER results obtained from an adult patient is presented in Fig. 17.3. The response is judged by the presence of positive wavelets occurring within a certain latency range. The latency, amplitude, and morphologic features of the responses depend on the patient's age, the stimulus characteristics, and the recording parameters. Persons with normal peripheral ear and lower auditory brainstem system integrity have a response to clicks at intensities as low as 5 dB normal HL (nHL). Under most stimulus conditions, the response is sensitive to the hearing status between 2,000 and 4,000 Hz. Although different methods of evoked potential testing can be used to estimate hearing sensitivity outside this frequency range, the testing is difficult and the results have less reliability.

2. The test parameters and interpretation criteria for BSER depend on the nature of the questions asked by the clinicians. Because the amplitude measures are highly variable and more susceptible to artifacts, clinicians typically use latency measures to assess integrity of the system. When screening

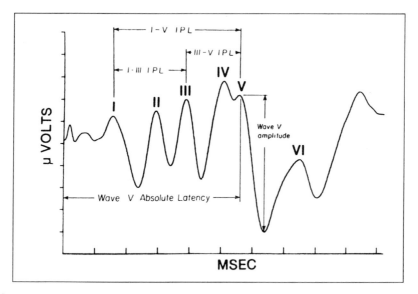

FIG. 17.3 Normal brainstem evoked response obtained from a young adult.

for hearing loss, the clinician examines the waveform for the presence of distinctive peaks, particularly in wave V, as the intensity of the stimulus changes and compares any measurable latency with the normative values available for the type of patient. In the differential diagnosis of retrocochlear lesions, a prolonged wave I–V latency difference becomes the most sensitive indicator of this condition, although other prolonged values for interpeak latency and interaural latency differences can be enough information for a diagnosis. Absolute latencies values tend to provide the least information for diagnosis of retrocochlear lesions. Knowledge of the hearing sensitivity between 2,000 and 4,000 Hz in each ear is critical for appropriate interpretation of BSER results during differential diagnosis.

  3. BSERs can be obtained without intentional responses from patients, and frequency is used to assess the integrity of the auditory system in populations such as infants. Although the click-evoked BSER can appear as early as the 25th week of gestation and is typically present at the 27th week of gestation, there are developmental changes in the response until approximately 2 years of age. The decrease in the absolute latency of the response is the most salient change during this maturational period. Therefore, interpretation of the BSER to identify hearing loss depends on age-appropriate norms. Still, if wave V of the BSER is present in a test ear at 35 dB nHL, it is likely that the infant has normal hearing sensitivity between 2,000 and 4,000 Hz in the test ear. An example of normal results from BSER screening of an infant is presented in Fig. 17.4. Clinicians must resist the urge to "peak pick" when judging a BSER waveform with either poor morphologic characteristics or low-amplitude wavelets.

C. **Otoacoustic emission** testing is a relatively new means of detecting hearing loss. The cochlea generates a low-intensity acoustic echo in response to an auditory stimulus in persons with normal hearing. Hearing losses due to cochlear or middle ear lesions can be readily identified with otoacoustic emissions; however, these measurements generally do not define the severity of the hearing loss. There are two classes of otoacoustic emissions—spontaneous otoacoustic emissions and evoked otoacoustic emissions. Evoked otoacoustic emissions can be further divided according to the type of stimulus used during measurement: **stimulus frequency emissions, transient evoked otoacoustic emissions**

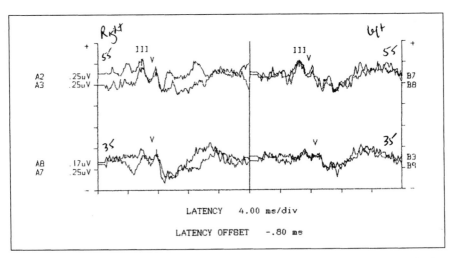

FIG. 17.4 Normal series of brainstem evoked responses obtained from an infant during screening for hearing loss.

(TEOAEs), and **distortion product otoacoustic emissions (DPOAEs).** TEOAEs and DPOAEs tend to be preferred for clinical measurement owing to the equipment difficulties encountered when trying to obtain stimulus frequency emissions. Results of recent studies have suggested that otoacoustic emissions may be an effective means of identifying hearing loss among infants and young children.

1. Figure 17.5 illustrates a TEOAE of a school-age child whose hearing was evaluated as a baseline measure of auditory sensitivity before administration of ototoxic medication and radiation to manage an intracranial tumor. A variety of scoring protocols have been suggested to describe the clinical outcome of TEOAEs.

2. Figure 17.6 illustrates a DPgram (DPOAE amplitude plotted as a function of the frequency of the F_2 stimulus across a number of frequencies from 500 to 8,000 Hz) of a school-age child with normal hearing. DPOAEs represent distortions of the two primary stimuli and are relatively easy to detect because they occur at frequencies different from the stimulus frequencies. The most robust distortion typically occurs at a frequency of $2F_1 - F_2$, which is known as the cubic difference tone. The DPOAE response is observed at a level that is between 50 and 60 dB below the level of the primary stimuli and only occurs when the primary stimuli fall within a region of the cochlea that responds normally to auditory stimulation.

VIII. Management and referral lists. When any hearing loss is suspected or identified, the patient should be referred for otologic examination and audiologic evaluation to determine the appropriate means of treatment. For conductive hearing loss, medical management is the primary course of treatment. The nature and outcome of medical management are determined to a great extent by the type and severity of the pathologic condition present. Although many patients with sensorineural hearing loss require medical treatment and follow-up care, the primary course of management of this type of hearing loss is amplification, whether through hearing aids, cochlear implants, or assistive listening devices.

A. **Amplification.** Hearing aids differ in design, size, amount of amplification, ease of handling, volume control, and availability of special features. But they do have similar components, which include a microphone to pick up sound, amplifier

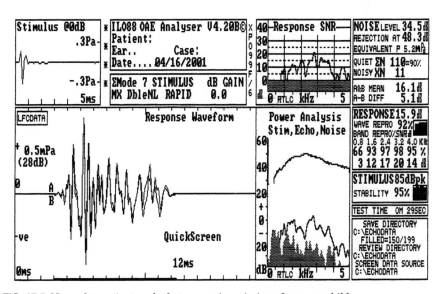

FIG. 17.5 Normal transient evoked otoacoustic emission of a young child.

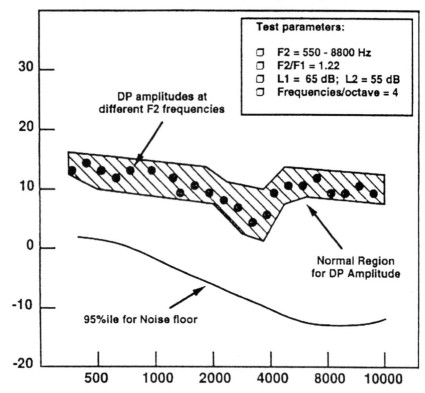

FIG. 17.6 DPgram (distortion-product otoacoustic emissions) of a child with normal hearing sensitivity.

circuitry to make the sound louder, a receiver to deliver the amplified sound into the ear, and batteries to power the electronic parts.

   1. **Hearing aid styles.** Although there are more than four basic styles, most hearing aids fall into one of four categories. The completely-in-the-canal (CIC) hearing aid is the smallest and most cosmetically appealing style. It also is the most expensive. This hearing aid requires some form of automatic signal processing because it is difficult to manipulate controls with its small size and its location deep inside the ear canal of the user. The next two styles, the in-the-canal (ITC) and in-the-ear (ITE) hearing aids are the most common dispensed in the United States. They offer some cosmetic value to the user owing to the small size, but they still sit outside the ear canal and allow manipulation of various controls on the hearing aid. The last style is the behind-the-ear (BTE) hearing aid. This hearing aid rests behind the ear and requires an earmold to direct the flow of sound into the ear and enhance sound quality. This style is often chosen for young children for safety and growth reasons.

   2. **Hearing aid circuitry.** Hearing aids also are differentiated according to technology or circuitry.

      a. **Conventional analog** hearing aids are designed with a particular frequency response based on the audiogram. The hearing aid has a series of potentiometers that the dispenser can adjust to approximate the values of amplification needed by the user. Although this technology is the least expensive and can be appropriate for many users, it is hampered by limitations in the analog circuitry.

   b. Analog programmable hearing aids contain a microchip that allows the aid to have settings programmed for different listening environments, such as quiet conversation in the home, noisy situations as in a restaurant, or large areas such as a theater. The dispenser uses a computer to program the hearing aid for different listening situations depending on the degree and configuration of the hearing loss and the growth of loudness for sounds in particular frequency bands or channels. Advantages of these hearing aids are that they can be programmed to meet specific targets for the user, they generally are more flexible and have a longer life span, and many of them come with a multiple memory option or directional microphones or both for changing the response to different listening environments.

   c. Digital programmable hearing aids have all of the advantages of analog programmable hearing aids, but the dispenser also uses digital signal processing to change the characteristics of the signal to maximize its frequency and intensity characteristics to meet the individual user's needs at any given moment in time. These hearing aids, although the most flexible, are often the most expensive.

 3. **Cochlear implants** are a set of amplification devices used to fit children and adults who have severe and profound hearing loss. Although the external processor is similar to that of a digital hearing aid, the internal components of the cochlear implant stimulate the neural cells of the eighth cranial nerve directly and therefore bypass any mechanisms of the peripheral ear, which may not even be functional owing to the severity of the hearing loss and the dead regions within the cochlea. Cochlear implants have been found a successful alternative to providing auditory input to persons who would not benefit from hearing aids.

 4. **Assistive listening devices** are specialized listening systems that may or may not interface with hearing aids and cochlear implants. These devices are designed to augment communication function by improving the signal-to-noise ratio during listening activities. The type of assistive listening device usually is designated by the type of transmission properties the device uses such as frequency modulation (FM) systems, infrared systems, loop (wire inductance) systems, and hard-wired systems. These devices are particularly effective for listening in large-group situations such as in classrooms, churches, or public meetings. They are also effective in bridging the gap between many audio devices, such as televisions and radios, with the user's hearing aids.

B. Referral: The following organizations can assist the reader in locating patient education materials and appropriate otologic and audiologic service providers in their geographic areas:

American Academy of Otolaryngology—Head and Neck Surgery
1 Prince St.
Alexandria, VA 22314
(703) 836-4444
(703) 683-3100 fax
E-mail: entinfo@aol.com
www.entnet.org
American Speech-Language-Hearing Association
10801 Rockville Pike
Rockville, MD 20852
(301) 897-5700
(301) 571-0457 fax
www.asha.org
professional.asha.org

American Academy of Audiology
1735 N. Lynn St., Suite 950
Arlington, VA 22209-2022
(800) 222-2336
(703) 790-8631 fax
E-mail: mail@audiology.org
www.audiology.org

Recommended Readings

Allen JB, Neely ST. Micromechanical models of the cochlea. *Physics Today* 1992;45:40–47.
American Speech-Language-Hearing Association. Report on audiologic screening. *Am J Audiol* 1995;4:24–40.
Bess FH, Humes LE. *Audiology: the fundamentals,* 2nd ed. Baltimore: Williams & Wilkins, 1994.
Canalis RF, Lambert PR. *The ear: comprehensive otology.* Philadelphia: Lippincott Williams & Wilkins, 2000.
Deconde-Johnson C, Benson PV, Seaton JB. *Educational audiology handbook.* San Diego: Singular Publishing Group, 1997.
Diefendorf AO, Reitz PS, Wagner-Escobar M, et al. Pediatric assessment: TIPS (testing–interpreting–promoting–securing) for early amplification. In: Bess FH, Gravel JS, Tharp AM, eds. *Amplification for children with auditory deficits.* Nashville: Bill Wilkerson Center Press, 1997:123–143.
Hall JW III, Mueller HG III. *Audiologist's desk reference, volume I: diagnostic audiology: principles, procedures and practices.* San Diego: Singular Publishing Group, 1997.
Hall JW III, Baer JE, Byrn A, et al. Audiologic assessment and management of central auditory processing disorder (CAPD). *Semin Hear* 1993;14:254–263.
Joint Committee on Infant. Year 2000 position statement: principles and guidelines for early hearing detection and intervention programs. *Am J Audiol* 2000;9:9–29.
Miyamoto RT, Kirk KI. Cochlear implants. In: Baily BJ, ed. *Head and neck surgery—otolaryngology,* 3rd ed. Philadelphia: Lippincott Williams & Wilkins, 2001.
Miyamoto RT, Kirk KI, Svirsky MA, et al. Longitudinal communication skill acquisition in pediatric cochlear implant recipients. *Adv Otorhinolaryngol* 2000;57:212–214.
Miyamoto RT, Robbins AM, Kirk KI, et al. Aural rehabilitation. In: Hughes GB, Peñsak ML, eds. *Clinical otology,* 2nd ed. New York: Thieme Medical Publishers, 1997:395–405.
Moore BCJ. Dead regions in the cochlea: diagnosis, perceptual consequences, and implications for the fitting of hearing aids. *Trends Amplif* 2001;5:1–34.
Muller HG III, Hall JW III. *Audiologist's desk reference, volume II: audiologic management, rehabilitation, and terminology.* San Diego: Singular Publishing Group, 1998.
Northern JL, Roush, J. Diagnostic audiology. In: English GM, ed. *Otolaryngology.* Philadelphia: JB Lippincott, 1994:1014–1032.
Norton SJ, Gorga MP, Widen JE, et al. Identification of neonatal hearing impairment: evaluation of transient evoked otoacoustic emission, distortion product otoacoustic emission, and auditory brainstem response test performance. *Ear Hear* 2000;21:508–528.
Nozza RJ, Bluestone CD, Kardatzke D, et al. Towards the validation of aural acoustic immittance measures for diagnosis of middle ear effusion in children. *Ear Hear* 1992;13:442–453.
Pender DJ. *Practical otology.* Philadelphia: JB Lippincott Co, 1992.
Pickles JO. *An introduction to the physiology of hearing,* 2 ed. New York: Academic Press, 1988.
Roeser RJ, Valente M, Hosford-Dunn H. *Audiology diagnosis.* New York: Thieme Medical Publishers, 2000.
Ruenes R. *Otologic radiology with clinical correlations.* New York: Macmillan, 1986.
Schuknecht HF. *Pathology of the ear,* 2 ed. Philadelphia: Lea & Febiger, 1993.
Valente M, Hosford-Dunn H, Roeser RJ. *Audiology treatment.* New York: Thieme Medical Publishers, 2000.
Wynne MK, Diefendorf AO, Wagner-Escobar M, et al. Hearing care for children: never too early. *J Dev Learn Disabil* 1997;1:219–276.
Yost WA. *Fundamentals of hearing: an introduction,* 3rd ed. San Diego: Academic Press, 1994.

18. APPROACH TO THE PATIENT WITH DYSPHAGIA

Jeri A. Logemann

    I. Dysphagia: difficulty swallowing. Dysphagia is common after sudden-onset neurologic damage such as stroke, head injury, or spinal cord injury. Oropharyngeal swallowing problems also are common among patients with degenerative neurologic disease such as motor neuron disease, including amyotrophic lateral sclerosis and postpolio syndrome, myasthenia gravis, multiple sclerosis, and Parkinson's disease. Dysphagia can be the first symptom of neurologic disease. It is critical to identify the presence of a swallowing problem early, define the exact nature of the physiologic or anatomic problem, and institute appropriate compensatory or therapeutic procedures to prevent costly medical complications (see **B. 4.**).
    A. Symptoms of oropharyngeal dysphagia
        1. Coughing at meals
        2. Struggling to eat
        3. Taking longer to eat
        4. Chronic excessive secretions including tracheal secretions, chronic bronchitis, asthma
        5. Weight loss of unexplained origin
        6. Pneumonia, especially recurrent
        7. Gurgling voice quality, especially during or after meals
        8. Recurrent fevers or increased secretions within 1 to $1\frac{1}{2}$ hours after meals
        9. Elimination of some consistencies of foods from the diet
      10. Difficulty managing own saliva
      11. Patient report of difficulty swallowing
    B. Effects of dysphagia on health and the health care system
        1. Aspiration pneumonia. A positive correlation has been found between the aspiration observed during a modified barium swallow (MBS) examination and the development of pneumonia within the next 6 months.
        2. Malnutrition
        3. Dehydration
        4. Increased costs of health care, including hospitalization for aspiration pneumonia and other expensive medical complications, nonoral feeding, and nursing care, if dysphagia is not managed properly.
    C. Prevention: reason for evaluation and management of oropharyngeal dysphagia. In patients with neurologic damage or disease, dysphagia cannot be prevented, but the expensive medical complications that result from swallowing disorders can be prevented with appropriate assessment and treatment.
        1. Prevent expensive medical complications. Aspiration pneumonia alone is a substantial cost to the healthcare system. In the midwest, an average hospital stay for aspiration pneumonia costs $18,000 to $20,000 in 1995 dollars.
        2. Facilitate the patient's return to safe and efficient oral intake. Nonoral feeding requires greater nursing care and often specially prepared feedings, both of which are more expensive than oral feeding.
    II. Normal swallowing. At all ages, normal swallowing is safe and efficient, moving food or liquid from the mouth, through the pharynx and into the cervical esophagus in 2 seconds or less, and through the esophagus in an additional 8 to 20 seconds.
    A. Swallowing stages
        1. Oral preparatory stage (variable duration). The oral preparatory stage includes chewing and other oral manipulations, which reduce food to a consistency appropriate for swallowing and provide taste and pleasure of eating. It does not depend on good dentition. Lip closure, circular and rotary action of the tongue, normal facial tone, and rotary jaw action are included in this stage of swallowing. Circular tongue action and fine motor control of the tongue are most important, because tongue action controls food in the mouth.
        2. Oral stage (approximately 1 second). The tongue is responsible for propelling food through the oral cavity and for providing sensory input that contributes to triggering the pharyngeal stage of swallow.

   3. **Pharyngeal triggering (0.5 second or less).** Pharyngeal triggering involves sensory input from the oral cavity to the cortex and brainstem. The input is recognized as a swallow stimulus in the nucleus tractus solitarius in the brainstem. This sensory information is passed to the nucleus ambiguous, which triggers the pharyngeal motor response.
   4. **Pharyngeal stage (less than 1 second).** The pharyngeal stage involves closure of the airway to prevent entrance of food into the airway (aspiration), opening of the upper esophageal sphincter to allow food to pass into the esophagus, and pressure applied to the bolus by the tongue and pharyngeal walls to clear food efficiently into the esophagus.
   5. **Esophageal stage (8 to 20 seconds).** The esophageal phase involves sequential contraction of the esophageal muscle fibers from top to bottom. The contraction propels the bolus ahead of the contractile wave into the stomach. This phase also involves relaxation of the lower esophageal sphincter to allow the bolus to pass into the stomach.
B. **Neuromuscular components of the normal swallow**
   1. **Lip closure** is maintained from the time food is placed in the mouth until the pharyngeal swallow is completed. If lip closure cannot be maintained, the nasal airway may not be patent.
   2. **Lingual control.** Oral tongue action is required in oral preparation, because the tongue controls the food in the mouth during chewing. The tongue also forms the food into a ball or bolus in preparation for the swallow, subdividing the food in the mouth if necessary, to ensure the appropriate size bolus for swallowing. The oral portion of the tongue then propels the food through the oral cavity and into the pharynx.
   3. **Rotary, lateral jaw motion.** Jaw action crushes the food, which is placed on the biting surfaces of the teeth by the tongue.
   4. **Velar or soft palate elevation and closure of the velopharyngeal port** prevents food from entering the nasal cavity.
   5. **Posterior motion of the base of the tongue** generates pharyngeal pressure on the bolus, as does sequential contraction down the pharyngeal wall.
   6. **Airway closure** prevents aspiration. Airway closure begins at the true vocal folds, proceeds to the level of the airway entrance, that is, the false vocal folds, arytenoids, and base of the epiglottis, and ends as the epiglottis is folded over the airway. The most critical level of airway closure is at the entrance, that is, the arytenoid cartilage and the base of epiglottis and false vocal folds. This level of closure prevents food from entering the airway.
   7. **Opening of the upper esophageal sphincter** involves a complex set of actions including (1) relaxation of the cricopharyngeal muscular portion of the valve, which does not open the sphincter, (2) laryngeal upward and forward motion, which opens the sphincter by carrying the anterior wall of the sphincter, the cricoid cartilage, away from the pharyngeal wall, and (3) arrival of the bolus under pressure, which increases the width of the opening of the upper sphincter.
   8. **Esophageal peristalsis** begins when the tail of the bolus enters the esophagus and follows the bolus through the esophagus.
C. **Systematic changes in oropharyngeal swallow with changes in volume and viscosity of the incoming food and voluntary control.** Not all swallows are alike. The physiologic mechanism of normal oropharyngeal swallowing changes systematically as the volume and viscosity of the food being swallowed increase. A great deal of voluntary control also can be exerted over the oropharyngeal swallow. These systematic changes help to explain why patients have more difficulty with one type of food than another. The swallows are different for different foods.
   1. **As bolus volume increases,** the duration of the oral and pharyngeal stages of the swallow increases. The duration of airway closure and cricopharyngeal opening increase systematically.
   2. **Greater viscosity** of food increases the width of cricopharyngeal opening.
   3. **Volitional control** also changes the characteristics of the oropharyngeal swallow.

     a. Breath-holding can extend the duration of airway closure at the vocal folds or at the entrance to the airway. This is often done in anticipation of swallowing a large volume of liquid, as from a cup.

     b. Volitional control can open the upper esophageal sphincter and prolong the duration of upper esophageal sphincter opening.

     c. Volitional control can extend the duration and extent of laryngeal elevation.

     d. Increasing effort during swallow increases oropharyngeal pressure. Voluntary changes can occur spontaneously as patients "work" to swallow, or patients can be taught these movements as compensation for swallowing problems.

D. Effects of normal aging

1. Oral transit time slows 0.5 to 1.0 seconds with increasing age, probably because older adults hold the bolus on the anterior floor of the mouth and must pick it up with their tongue to begin the swallow.

2. Slightly slower shift from the oral to pharyngeal stage occurs in persons older than 60 years, probably because of slower neural processing.

3. After 80 years of age, the range of motion of pharyngeal structures decreases; that is, there is less muscle reserve and less flexibility in the swallow. This is particularly true of men.

4. After 60 years of age, esophageal peristalsis becomes less efficient.

5. Healthy elderly persons do not aspirate more often than do young persons. Elderly patients (older than 80 years) who become generally weak and sick have a weak swallow because of reduced muscular reserve. This can cause aspiration.

E. Efficiency and safety

1. Normal swallows are efficient, moving food quickly through the mouth and pharynx and into the esophagus in less than 2 seconds.

2. Only occasional aspiration occurs, usually when the mechanism is stressed or when eating and talking are attempted at the same time.

3. Efficiency and safety do not change substantially with age.

III. Swallowing disorders can occur in any stage of swallow and involve one or more of the neuromuscular actions or sensory inputs described earlier as involved in the swallow.

A. Swallowing disorders can be **anatomic** or **physiologic** in nature.

B. Effective management of swallowing disorders requires identification of the specific anatomic or physiologic abnormalities in each patient's swallow, such as reduced laryngeal elevation, poor airway closure, or reduced tongue base movement.

C. Aspiration and inefficient swallowing causing oral or pharyngeal residue are symptoms of swallowing disorders. They are not disorders. These symptoms disappear when the patient's swallowing function returns to normal.

IV. Definitive assessment of the oropharyngeal swallow: modified barium swallow

A. The MBS is performed by a speech–language pathologist and a radiologist. This radiographic (videofluorographic) study is used to examine the anatomic and physiologic features of the oral and pharyngeal stages of swallowing. These areas must be examined separately from the esophagus, which is anatomically and physiologically distinct from the oral cavity and pharynx and requires a different technique for assessment (**barium swallow**). MBS assessment is used to examine the ability of the pharynx to manage small to large volumes and thin to thick viscosities of food. An esophageal assessment requires presentation of a large amount of liquid to distend the esophagus, which as a collapsed muscular tube cannot be examined adequately unless distended.

1. **Purpose**

     a. Define the physiologic mechanism of the oral and pharyngeal phase of swallowing in relation to patient's swallowing symptoms.

     b. Define physiologic characteristics of the swallow that are symptomatic of neurologic disease.

    c. Examine the effectiveness of management strategies designed to assist patients in continuing to eat safely by mouth or to begin eating safely by mouth.

    d. Define a treatment plan to rehabilitate oropharyngeal swallow function and to eliminate symptoms of dysphagia, including aspiration, and thereby prevent the development of aspiration pneumonia.

    e. Define the safest and most efficiently swallowed diet (food consistency).

  2. Procedure. The procedure of the MBS is designed to minimize the risk of aspiration by presenting calibrated small to large amounts of liquid, pudding, and masticated material as tolerated by the patient.

    a. The patient seated upright initially and examined in the lateral plane to define the speed, efficiency, and safety (aspiration) of the swallow.

    b. Liquids are given in 1-mL, 3-mL, 5-mL, and 10-mL cups. The patient drinks the liquid in 2 swallows each to observe the "dose response" of the pharynx and to define the optimal volume for each patient.

    c. If and when the patient aspirates or has a highly inefficient swallow, various treatment strategies are provided and the effects observed radiographically, including

      (1) Posture changes

      (2) Increased sensory input

      (3) Therapeutic procedures (requires normal cognition)

      (4) Increased bolus viscosity. Nectar or honey-thickened liquids as needed if thin liquids are aspirated and no other strategy is effective.

    d. Pudding (1 to 2 mL) and a small bite of cookie are given (2 swallows each) as tolerated by patient.

    e. The patient is turned and examined in the anteroposterior plane to define symmetry of the swallow.

    f. The report contains (1) a description of the oral and pharyngeal anatomic features and swallow function causing the patient's dysphagia symptoms, (2) identification of the types and amounts of foods safely swallowed, (3) a statement about whether or not partial or full nonoral feeding is needed, and (4) a statement regarding the effectiveness of and need for compensatory strategies or swallow therapy.

  3. Reevaluation. To ensure patient safety, the oropharyngeal swallow may have to be reevaluated when the patient appears ready to move to oral intake.

B. Barium swallow is performed to examine the esophageal stage of swallowing, particularly the anatomic configuration of the esophagus and any anatomic abnormalities, such as strictures or tumors. Because this assessment requires the patient to swallow large volumes of liquid, it should be completed after oropharyngeal assessment (MBS) to be sure the patient can tolerate the larger volumes.

  1. Used to assess esophageal anatomy and peristaltic action

  2. Misses reflux disease 60% to 80% of the time

V. Screening tests for oropharyngeal dysphagia. The results of these tests are not definitive and tend to over-identify patients as at risk of swallowing disorders in the pharyngeal stage of swallowing.

A. A bedside or clinical examination usually is performed by a speech–language pathologist. A bedside or clinical, noninstrumental assessment of swallowing cannot reliably define swallowing function or the presence of dysphagia symptoms, such as aspiration.

  1. Complete medical history including history of the swallowing problem

  2. Complete oromotor test of lip, jaw, tongue, pharyngeal, and laryngeal function

  3. Trial swallows with small amounts of food are observed

B. The **3-oz water test** involves giving the patient 3 oz (90 mL) of water to swallow continuously.

  1. If patient coughs or has difficulty, referral for MBS should be made.

  2. This test *can be dangerous if the patient aspirates a large amount of liquid.*

  3. The result does not show the physiologic characteristics of the patient's swallow, so treatment cannot be planned.

VI. Screening test for risk of pneumonia after stroke: the laryngeal cough reflex test

   A. The patient inhales a mixture of tartaric acid and water from a nebulizer with nose blocked.

   B. An immediate strong cough by a patient who has had a stroke indicates good airway protection.

   C. No cough indicates poor or no airway protection.

   D. The result does not provide information on the anatomic or physiologic characteristics of the swallow.

   E. The test is valid only for stroke patients.

VII. Referrals for further testing

   A. Computed tomography or **magnetic resonance imaging** to localize the lesion. A small lesion causing dysphagia may not be identified with these procedures, however.

   B. Other instrumental assessments of the oropharyngeal swallow, such as endoscopy, are limited in depicting a swallow and providing information about the swallow. None of these procedures is as useful as MBS (see **IV.A.**).

      1. Endoscopy, usually is performed by an otolaryngologist or speech–language pathologist, is used to examine the pharynx from above before and after but not during a swallow.

      2. Ultrasonography depicts the oral stages of swallowing but not the pharynx. Ultrasonography usually is performed by a speech–language pathologist.

      3. Manometry provides information about the pressures generated in the pharynx during a swallow and about relaxation of the cricopharyngeal muscle if done concurrently with MBS. Manometry usually is performed by a gastroenterologist.

   C. Neurologic evaluation. Some patients with swallowing problems and no known medical diagnosis need in-depth neurologic testing before an accurate diagnosis can be made.

   D. A **gastroenterology** consultation may be needed in the diagnosis of esophageal aspects of the swallowing disorder.

   E. An **otolaryngology** consultation may be helpful if voice changes are present.

   F. A **speech–language pathology** consultation may be helpful in defining voice, speech, and swallowing disorders that indicate neurologic disease.

VIII. Patients with known neurologic damage or disease with swallowing problems

   A. Progressive neurologic disease. Dysphagia is frequent in progressive neurologic disease at some point in the patient's deterioration. Many neurologic diseases that can manifest as swallowing difficulties include Parkinson's disease, motor neuron disease, postpolio syndrome, myasthenia gravis, multiple sclerosis, Guillain–Barré syndrome, and stroke.

      1. Parkinson's disease

         a. Swallowing problems may come early or later in the disease progression.

         b. The patient may aspirate silently; that us, there is no cough.

         c. The symptoms are those of a swallowing disorder

            (1) The patient may slow down while eating because of characteristic (pathognomonic) rocking, rolling tongue motion.

            (2) The patient may swallow two or three times with each bite of food because the swallow is not efficient and there is residue in the pharynx.

            (3) Increased chest secretions occur—"bronchitis" with chronic cough—that are actually signs of chronic aspiration.

            (4) The patient has a gurgling voice quality because residual food remains at the top of the airway.

         d. Referrals

            (1) MBS

            (2) Swallowing therapy as indicated by results of MBS

         e. Progression is slow. The condition may worsen very slowly over 10 years, 20 years, or more.

    f. Parkinson medications may alleviate the swallowing disorder for some patients.

    g. Swallow therapy is moderately successful.

2. Amyotrophic lateral sclerosis

    a. A swallowing or speech disorder may be first symptom. The disorder usually affects the oral stage of swallowing first with a reduction in tongue strength and fine control so that chewing is increasingly difficult.

    b. Symptoms of swallowing disorders

        (1) Diet change. The patient eliminates foods from the diet that require chewing; thicker foods require more muscle effort to swallow.

        (2) Weight loss

        (3) Coughing usually occurs during swallowing of liquids, which are not controlled well by the tongue and splash into the pharynx and into the open airway.

        (4) There may be **slight aspiration.**

    c. Referrals. MBS at regular intervals (3 to 4 months) for patients with brainstem involvement to define the best eating strategies. Direct exercise fatigues muscles.

    d. Progression

        (1) Often rapid among patients with predominantly brainstem involvement. Patient may be advised to stop eating and accept gastrostomy when within $1\frac{1}{2}$ to 2 years of diagnosis because of chronic aspiration.

        (2) Very slow among patients with predominantly spinal involvement. May be 10 to 15 years before dysphagia is severe enough to cause weight loss or chronic aspiration.

3. Postpolio syndrome

    a. Onset. Dysphagia may begin as patients reach their forties or fifties, particularly patients with a history of bulbar polio.

    b. The patient may have **reduced awareness** of the swallow problem.

    c. Symptoms of a swallowing disorder

        (1) Feeling of food left in throat, particularly thicker, heavier foods, which require increased muscle activity to swallow.

        (2) Fatigue as meal progresses.

    d. Referrals. MBS is indicated to define optimum eating strategies. Often the problem is unilateral weakness in the pharynx, and head rotation toward the damaged side of the pharynx during eating facilitates improved clearance of food. Direct exercise fatigues the mechanism.

    e. Progression is slow, worsening over years.

4. Myasthenia gravis

    a. A swallowing or speech disorder may be the first symptom.

    b. Symptoms may include

        (1) Fatigue in selected muscles of mouth or pharynx as eating progresses. May become severe enough so that no swallowing is possible.

        (2) Increasing nasality, hoarseness, imprecision in speech sounds as patient continues to talk.

    c. Referrals. MBS to define involved musculature and extent of fatigue.

    d. Progression. Slow worsening of symptoms. Medication may greatly improve swallowing.

5. Multiple sclerosis

    a. Swallowing problem may be first symptom, but is more likely to occur as disease progresses. Patient often is unaware of the swallowing problem.

    b. Wide range of swallowing disorders as various parts of the nervous system are affected.

    c. Symptoms may include

        (1) Difficulty swallowing liquids with coughing because of pharyngeal swallow delay.

        (2) Feeling of food "stuck in the throat" because of reduced strength of tongue base and pharyngeal wall movement.

     d. Responds well to **swallowing therapy**

     e. Referrals

       (1) MBS

       (2) Swallowing therapy, if indicated by results of MBS

B. Sudden-onset neurologic disorders. Stroke, head injury, and spinal cord injury can cause dysphagia from which a patient can recover with appropriate management. The focus of management should be early radiographic assessment (MBS) with swallowing therapy to prevent medical complications. The more medical problems and complications a patient sustains, the longer is recovery.

  1. Stroke. Single or multiple strokes can cause swallowing problems.

    a. A **single infarct** in the cortex, subcortical region, or brainstem can cause swallowing problems that are worse within the first week after the stroke. By 3 weeks after the stroke, patients usually have functional swallowing unless they are taking medications that affect swallowing or have additional medical complications that slow swallowing recovery.

    b. Brainstem stroke poses the greatest risk of dysphagia. Some patients who have had a brainstem stroke, particularly those with lateral medullary syndrome, need intensive swallowing therapy.

    c. Patients who have had **multiple strokes** often have more severe swallowing problems and need more rehabilitation than do other patients who have had strokes but usually do recover to full oral intake.

    d. Referrals

      (1) MBS when the patient is alert and awake (3 to 4 days after the stroke) to determine the need for nonoral feeding and swallowing therapy. Repeat study 3 weeks after the stroke to determine progress and discontinue nonoral feeding if no longer needed.

      (2) Swallowing therapy, if indicated by the results of MBS.

  2. Head injury. Approximately one third of patients with head injury have swallowing problems. Dysphagia can result from the neurologic injury, from other injuries to the head or neck, such as laryngeal fractures, and from acute care procedures, such as long-term intubation. Neuromuscular damage usually is present in both the oral and pharyngeal phases of swallowing.

    a. Referrals

      (1) MBS

      (2) Swallowing therapy, if indicated by results of MBS

    b. Most patients regain oral intake with therapy. Some patients with severe head injury need maintenance therapy from a caregiver to maintain safe and adequate oral intake.

  3. Cervical spinal cord injury. Patients with injuries to the cervical spinal cord who undergo anterior spinal fusion are at greatest risk of dysphagia. The pharyngeal phase of swallowing usually is impaired.

    a. Referrals

      (1) MBS

      (2) Swallowing therapy

    b. Most often swallowing problems are in the pharyngeal phase of the swallow.

    c. With swallowing therapy, most patients recover. The length of time in recovery depends on the extent of physical damage and the number of medical complications sustained.

IX. Patients who report swallowing disorders (dysphagia) but have no medical diagnosis

  A. Most often these patients have a progressive neurologic disease, have had a stroke, or have a brain tumor. Rarely does the dysphagia indicate head or neck cancer. Rarely is dysphagia a psychogenic problem. Anatomic or physiologic disorders should be ruled out first, before a psychogenic cause is considered.

  B. Testing

    1. A complete medical and swallowing **history** should be taken, including

      a. Pattern of difficulty

        (1) Fatigue at the end of a meal, which can indicate myasthenia gravis.

(2) Foods the patient finds difficult.
(3) Gradual or sudden onset. Gradual onset usually indicates neurologic disease. Sudden onset can indicate a stroke.
  b. **Family history** of any swallowing problem
2. **Symptoms.** Asking the patient to describe the symptoms is helpful.
  a. Food remains in mouth—indicates oral stage problem.
  b. Food hesitates at top of neck—may indicate difficulty triggering pharyngeal stage.
  c. Food remains in throat—may indicate pharyngeal stage problems.
  d. Feeling of pressure at the base of the neck or feeling that food remains at base of neck—usually indicates an esophageal stage problem.
  e. Pressure, feeling of food caught in chest—usually indicates esophageal stage problem.
3. **Other motor signs**
  a. **Gait changes**
  b. **Tremor** in the tongue, jaw, pharynx, or larynx at rest may indicate Parkinson's disease.
  c. **Speech or voice changes.** Many patients with neurologic disease may have speech or voice changes and swallowing problems.
  X. Summary. Early MBS assessment by a speech–language pathologist can reduce the medical complications of dysphagia and thereby reduce costs to the health care system. One hospitalization for aspiration pneumonia can equal the cost of MBS and follow-up swallowing therapy for three to five patients for 3 months. Careful and aggressive management of dysphagia can save the health care system substantial costs in hospitalization and other medical services.

Recommended Readings

Buchholz D. Clinically probable brainstem stroke presenting primarily as dysphagia and nonvisualized by MRI. *Dysphagia* 1993;8: 235–238.

DePippo KL, Holas MA, Reding MJ. Validation of the 3 oz water swallow test for aspiration following stroke. *Arch Neurol* 1992;49:1259–1261.

Dodds WJ, Logemann JA, Stewart ET. Radiological assessment of abnormal oral and pharyngeal phases of swallowing. *AJR Am J Roentgenol* 1990;154:965–974.

Ergun GA, Miskovitz PF. Aging and the esophagus: common pathologic conditions and their effect upon swallowing in the geriatric population. *Dysphagia* 1992;7:58–63.

Horner J, Massey EW, Riski JE, et al. Aspiration following stroke: clinical correlates and outcomes. *Neurology* 1988;38:1359–1362.

Jacob P, Kahrilas P, Logemann J, et al. Upper esophageal sphincter opening and modulation during swallowing. *Gastroenterology* 1989;97:1469–1478.

Kahrilas PJ, Logemann JA, Lin S, et al. Pharyngeal clearance during swallow: a combined manometric and videofluoroscopic study. *Gastroenterology* 1992;103:128–136.

Kasprisin AT, Clumeck A, Nino-Murcia M. The efficacy of rehabilitative management of dysphagia. *Dysphagia* 1989;4:48–52.

Langmore SE, Schatz K, Olsen N. Fiberoptic endoscopic examination of swallowing safety: a new procedure. *Dysphagia* 1988;2:216–219.

Lazarus C, Logemann JA. Swallowing disorders in closed head trauma patients. *Arch Phys Med Rehabil* 1987;68:79–87.

Lazarus CL, Logemann JA, Rademaker AW, et al. Effects of bolus volume, viscosity and repeated swallows in normals and stroke patients. *Arch Phys Med Rehabil* 1993;74: 1066–1070.

Logemann J, Kahrilas P, Kobara M, et al. The benefit of head rotation on pharyngoesophageal dysphagia. *Arch Phys Med Rehabil* 1989;70:767–771.

Logemann JA, ed. Swallowing disorders & rehabilitation. *J Head Trauma Rehabil* 1989;4:1–92.

Logemann JA. Head and neck diseases in the elderly: effects of aging on the swallowing mechanism. *Otolaryngol Clin North Am* 1990;23:1045–1056.

Logemann JA. The dysphagia diagnostic procedure as a treatment efficacy trial. *Clin Commun Disord* 1993;3:1–10.

Logemann JA. *A manual for videofluoroscopic evaluation of swallowing,* 2nd ed. Austin, TX: Pro-Ed, 1993.

Logemann JA. *Evaluation and treatment of swallowing disorders,* 2nd ed. Austin, TX: Pro-Ed, 1998.

Logemann JA, Kahrilas PJ. Relearning to swallow post CVA: application of maneuvers and indirect biofeedback—a case study. *Neurology* 1990;40:1136–1138.

Logemann JA, Kahrilas PJ, Cheng J, et al. Closure mechanisms of the laryngeal vestibule during swallowing. *Am J Physiol* 1992;262:G338–344.

Logemann JA, Pauloski BR, Rademaker AW, et al. Temporal and biomechanical characteristics of oropharyngeal swallow in younger and older men. *J Speech Hear Res* 2000;43:1264–1274.

Martin BJ, Corlew M, Wood H, et al. The association of swallowing dysfunction and aspiration pneumonia. *Dysphagia* 1994;9:1–6.

Martin-Harris B, Logemann JA, McMahon S, et al. Clinical utility of the modified barium swallow. *Dysphagia* 2000;15:136–141.

Rasley A, Logemann JA, Kahrilas PJ, et al. Prevention of barium aspiration during videofluoroscopic swallowing studies: value of change in posture. *AJR Am J Roentgenol* 1993;160:1005–1009.

Robbins J, Levine R. Swallowing after unilateral stroke of the cerebral cortex: preliminary experience. *Dysphagia* 1988;3:11–17.

Robbins J, Logemann J, Kirschner H. Swallowing and speech production in Parkinson's disease. *Ann Neurol* 1986;19:283–287.

Robbins JA, Hamilton JW, Lof GL, et al. Oropharyngeal swallowing in normal adults of different ages. *Gastroenterology* 1992;103:823–829.

Schmidt J, Holas M, Halvorson K, et al. Videofluoroscopic evidence of aspiration predicts pneumonia and death but not dehydration following stroke. *Dysphagia* 1994;9:7–11.

Splaingard M, Hutchins B, Sulton D, et al. Aspiration in rehabilitation patients: videofluoroscopy vs. bedside clinical assessment. *Arch Phys Med Rehabil* 1988;69:637–640.

Tracy JF, Logemann JA, Kahrilas PJ, et al. Preliminary observations on the effects of age on oropharyngeal deglutition. *Dysphagia* 1989;4:90–94.

Veis SL, Logemann JA. Swallowing disorders in persons with cerebrovascular accident. *Arch Phys Med Rehabil* 1985;65:372–375.

19. APPROACH TO THE PATIENT WITH DYSARTHRIA

Marian P. LaMonte
M. Cara Erskine
Barbara E. Thomas

Communication disorders are common in neurologic practice and are the result of congenital, developmental, and acquired abnormalities. **Dysarthria** is a collective name for a group of motor speech disorders that result from focal, multifocal, or diffuse damage to the central or peripheral nervous system, or both. Dysarthria is classified according to descriptive categories that have been correlated with specific lesion sites and neuropathologic conditions. Production of speech occurs through the interaction of five systems: (1) respiration, (2) phonation, (3) resonance, (4) articulation, and (5) prosody. Examination of each system facilitates not only the diagnosis of a specific type of dysarthria but also neuroanatomic localization and, ultimately, the appropriate therapeutic intervention.

    I. Etiology. Neurologic conditions that produce dysarthria are numerous and diverse. Dysarthric symptoms also may remain stable, resolve, or progress, depending on the cause. Most patients with dysarthria have preceding substantial neurologic symptoms or accompanying neurologic signs that assist in diagnosis of the type of dysarthria. Lesions along the neuroaxis that produce motor dysfunction of any of the five speech systems produce a type of dysarthric speech. The lesions can be unilateral or bilateral and localize to the cortex, subcortex, brainstem, cranial nerves, or upper cervical nerves.

    II. Clinical manifestations of particular types of dysarthria are the result of nervous system damage to particular components of the speech system, and the effects manifest as patterns of dysfunctional speech. Table 19.1 presents a classification of dysarthria. The dysfunctional patterns are classified descriptively. An understanding of the normal components of the speech system followed by identification of specific system abnormalities and the common causes clarifies the resulting clinical manifestations.

    A. Normal speech systems

        1. Respiration

            a. Anatomic components include the **lungs, chest wall, diaphragm,** and **abdominal muscles.**

            b. Physiologically, respiration provides the air source and subglottal pressure necessary to force a constant column of air through the larynx and vocal folds.

            c. Respiration depends on intact connections from medullary centers to respiratory muscles.

        2. Phonation

            a. The anatomic unit is the **larynx.**

            b. Physiologic changes in the vocal fold length, elevation, opposition, and vibratory pattern as well as changes in the relations between cartilage movement and muscle tension bring about vocalization.

            c. Each person has a unique fundamental frequency as a controlled stream of air passes through the vocal folds. Pitch is a function of fundamental frequency changes produced by changing the length and tension of the vocal folds.

        3. Resonance

            a. The anatomic units are the **oropharynx** and the **nasopharynx,** but contributions are made by all the components of the respiratory outflow tract.

            b. Physiologically, the supraglottic space, also referred to as the **vocal tract,** provides a chamber in which various harmonics of the fundamental frequency are resonated to produce more complex sounds.

            c. Specific consonants rely on specific intact functions. An example is the contrast between /m/ and /b/ in "Mamie" (nasal resonance) and "baby" (oral resonance).

        4. Articulation

            a. Anatomic components include the **lips, teeth, cheeks, tongue, soft palate,** and **mandible.**

Table 19.1 Mayo clinic classification of dysarthria

Dysarthria type	Neurologic condition	Location of lesion	Most distinctive speech deviation
Flaccid	Bulbar palsy	Lower motor neuron	Marked hypernasality, often with nasal air emission; continuous breathiness; audible inspiration
Spastic	Pseudobulbar palsy	Upper motor neuron	Very imprecise articulation; slow rate; low pitch; harsh strained or strangled voice
Ataxic	Cerebellar ataxia	Cerebellum	Excess stress and monostress; phoneme and interval prolongation; dysrhythmia of speech and syllable repetition; slow rate; some excess loudness variation
Hypokinetic	Parkinsonism	Extrapyramidal system	Monopitch, monoloudness, reduced overall loudness; variable rate; short rushes of speech; some inappropriate silences
Hyperkinetic 1. Quick	Chorea	Extrapyramidal system	Highly variable pattern of imprecise articulation; episodes of hypernasality; sudden variations in loudness
	Myoclonus		Rhythmic hypernasality; rhythmic phonatory interruption
	Gilles de la Tourette's syndrome		Sudden ticlike grunts, barks, coprolalia
2. Slow	Athetosis	Extrapyramidal system	No distinct deviation
	Dyskinesias	Extrapyramidal system	No distinct deviation
	Dystonia	Extrapyramidal system	Prolongations of phonemes, intervals, unsteady rate, loudness
3. Tremors	Organic voice tremor	Extrapyramidal system	Rhythmic alterations in pitch, loudness, voice stoppages
Mixed	Amyotrophic lateral sclerosis	Multiple motor systems	Grossly defective articulation; extremely slow, laborious rate; marked hypernasality; severe harshness, strained or strangled voice; nearly complete disruption of prosody
	Wilson's disease		Reduced stress; monopitch; monoloudness; similar to hypokinetic dysarthria except no short rushes of speech
	Multiple sclerosis		Impaired control of loudness; harshness

Adapted from Johns DF, ed. *Clinical management of neurogenic communicative disorders,* 2nd ed. Boston: Little, Brown, 1985, with permission.

      b. Changes in the size and shape of the oral cavity in conjunction with the positions of the lips, teeth, and tongue, produce **phonemes**—distinctive units of speech sound.

      c. Vowel sounds are made with the vocal tract remaining in a relatively open position. Consonants are formed by a range of vocal tract constriction.

  5. Prosody

      a. Neurologic control of the speech system that produces prosody is diverse. Brain control and programming of speech are organized as for other movements.

      b. Integration of the functions of the premotor and motor cortex, the pyramidal and extrapyramidal systems, the cerebellum, afferent sensory nerves, and peripheral nerves results in control of the sequencing, timing, and rate of speech production.

      c. With alterations in pitch, intonation, stress, rhythm, and rate, different meanings and emphases are conveyed.

B. Abnormalities in speech systems

  1. Abnormalities in respiration result from hypofunction, hyperfunction, or mixed (incoordinated) function.

      a. Hypofunction is associated with decreased vital capacity, expiratory volumes, and expiratory force.

        (1) Diseases include obstructive and restrictive pulmonary diseases; chest wall restriction (e.g., kyphoscoliosis); nerve (mononeuropathy or polyneuropathy), neuromuscular junction, and muscle diseases; and intrathoracic and intraabdominal masses.

        (2) The results are quick fall-offs in pitch and loudness, loss of strength of all plosive consonants, shortened speech phrasing, and interruption by frequent wheezing and inspiratory stridor.

      b. Hyperfunction is related to upper motor neuron dysfunction, both pyramidal and extrapyramidal. It is associated with spasticity.

        (1) Constant hyperfunction is associated with spasticity and results from asynchrony between respiratory muscles. This condition is observed in pseudobulbar palsy and cerebral palsy and is characterized by choppy and explosive speech.

        (2) Mixed function or incoordination accompanies the hyperkinetic movement disorders of chorea and dystonia, wherein sudden changes in muscle tone result in abrupt stops and breaks in inspiration and expiration and lead to unwanted pauses and changes in pitch and loudness. Patients with this type of disorder speak in short phrases.

  2. Abnormalities in phonation. Abnormalities that produce faulty approximation of vocal folds (nerve, muscle, or joint injuries) or variation in vocal mass (tumors, nodules, inflammation, or edema) result in the following three types of abnormal phonatory patterns.

      a. Hypofunction results from impaired adduction of the vocal folds. Excessive escape of air through a patent glottis leads to loss of clear tonal musical sound. Instead, a breathy quality is heard. This condition can result from laryngeal nerve injury, tumor, surgical procedure, or recent extubation.

      b. Hyperfunction is the result of overadduction of the vocal folds and results in increased pitch and evidence of a strained or strangled quality resulting from the greater effort to produce a voice. This condition accompanies pseudobulbar palsy, dystonia, and cerebellar disease.

      c. Mixed phonation combines pathologic elements of both hypofunction and hyperfunction and imparts both a breathy and a harsh or hoarse character to the voice. Mixed phonation occurs in association with structural lesions of the vocal folds, such as tumors, polyps, and inflammation.

  3. Abnormalities in resonance. Defects in the shape of the vocal tract above the level of the larynx result in two types of resonance changes—variations in nasality, which are discussed here, and variations in articulation, which are discussed in **II.B.4.**

a. **Hypernasality** is associated with velopharyngeal incompetence, or weakness of the soft palate. There is excess escape of air into the nasal cavity. During speaking, there also may be nasal emission.

b. **Hyponasality** results from obstruction within the velopharyngeal opening or within the nostrils. Airflow is dissipated through the mouth during speaking.

   (1) For example, the nasal consonants /m/ as in "met" and /n/ as in "net" resemble their nonnasal counterparts /b/ as in "bet" and /d/ as in "debt."

   (2) Vowel sounds also are altered in hyponasal speech, producing an overall dull or muffled sound.

4. **Abnormalities in articulation** can result from hypofunction (weakness, decreased range of motion, slowness of movement), hyperfunction (increased tone), or incoordination among the anatomic components of articulation. Articulation disorders may be perceived as being generalized or specific.

   a. **Generalized articulation disorders** involve articulatory problems affecting all or most phonemes and occur with either central nervous system or systemic disease.

   b. **Specific articulatory disorders** involve problems affecting specific groups of phonemes and are associated with a local structural pathologic process or damage to one or more nerves.

   c. **Errors**

      (1) The types of errors that occur during articulation include omission, distortion, substitution, and addition of phonemes.

      (2) Misarticulation can be secondary to neurologic damage but also can be secondary to structural abnormalities of the articulators.

      (3) Common articulation errors among children are considered developmental and are not classified as dysarthria. True dysarthria can occur in childhood (e.g., cerebral palsy, posttraumatic brain injury) and, as in adulthood, results from disordered muscular control over speech mechanisms.

5. **Abnormalities in prosody** involve miscoordination of respiratory, phonatory, and articulatory components of speech that results in errors in rhythm and rate, stress, or intonation of speech.

   a. **Rhythm and rate** errors involve excessive speed, slowness, or inconsistency of articulation time, pause time, and the ratio between the two.

   b. **Stress errors** can occur within a word (e.g., re*cord, re*cord) or within a phrase or sentence (e.g., *Lee* wrote the book; Lee *wrote* the book), and can change the meaning of the utterance.

   c. **Intonation errors** can change meanings of sentences (e.g., You're going home. You're going home?)

   d. **Disordered prosody** is typically associated with ataxic dysarthria, hypokinetic dysarthria, and right hemispheric aprosodic dysarthria. Persons with the last disorder also may have deficits in comprehension of prosodic features in others' speech.

III. **Evaluation**

A. **History**

1. **Onset.** When did the patient or family first notice the change in speech? Were there preexisting developmental misarticulation problems?

2. **Tempo.** Did the speech change come on suddenly or gradually? Has it resolved, stabilized, or progressed since it was first noticed? Has it fluctuated in severity? Have there been periods of normal speech among periods of abnormality?

3. **Coexisting neurologic symptoms,** especially those related to the upper or lower motor system of the brain or to the cranial or cervical nerves.

4. **Previous neurologic diagnoses** and previous treatment.

5. **Medication history** and nonprescription drug use.

B. **Physical examination**

1. There are three steps in the physical examination.

   Step 1. Obtain adequate samples of both spontaneous and tested speech.

Step 2. Interpret the speech samples by focusing on each system and determining whether it is normal or abnormal and, if it is abnormal, the nature of the abnormality. Include a physical examination of the oral cavity, the oropharynx, the nasopharynx, and chest wall movement.

Step 3. Categorize the pattern of abnormalities found in the previous steps and compare it with known patterns resulting in clinical diagnoses of dysarthria (Table 19.1).

2. **Specific system testing**

   a. **Respiration.** Test fatigability by having the patient count to 20 during one breath. Note pitch fall-off, loudness, length of speech phrasing, choppiness, or explosiveness during attentive listening.

   b. **Phonation.** Have the patient phonate a constant vowel sound /ah/ as clearly and for as long as possible. Other phonemes, such as /ee/, place greater stress on the vocal folds, and the examiner should listen for variations in quality, duration, pitch, steadiness, and loudness. To assess true vocal fold efficiency, compare the times that the patient can sustain the /s/ and /z/ phonemes. Normal function makes it possible to sustain phonation of these two consonants for equal lengths of time. If /z/ is sustained for a markedly shorter period, inefficient use of the true vocal folds is indicated. Have the patient give a crisp cough to see if the abnormality clears. Refer the patient to an otolaryngologist for laryngoscopic visualization if abnormalities are noted.

   c. **Resonance** is evaluated by having the patient selectively pronounce words that emphasize nasal and plosive phonemes. Watch the soft palate at rest and during the phonation of /ah/. Have the patient sustain phonation as long as possible. Watch for fatigue. Another measure of nasality is taken by having the patient sustain /ee/ while the examiner alternately occludes and releases the nares; the sound should remain basically unchanged if resonance is normal.

   d. **Articulation.** During attentive listening, note whether the abnormality is general (mispronunciation of all or most phonemes) or specific (mispronunciation of only certain phonemes). Have the patient pronounce each of the following syllables repeatedly: "puh," "tuh," and "kuh." "Puh" is specific for bilabial function, "tuh" is specific for lingual–alveolar function, and "kuh" is specific for lingual–palatal function. Then have the patient rapidly alternate among the three syllables to bring out dysdiadochokinesia. An alternative is to use an expression that has more contextual meaning to assess misarticulation, such as "buttercup" or "pattycake." Inspection and palpation of intraoral structures are performed to search for abnormal coloration, clefts, malocclusion, missing teeth, and masses.

   e. **Prosody.** In careful listening to spontaneous speech, note rate, timing, spacing, melody, and stress. Have the patient imitate varied stress and intonation patterns using a common phrase such as "How are you?"

   f. Test **hearing** by recognition of words whispered into each ear or with a tuning fork.

C. **Laboratory studies**

   1. **Brain or cervical neuroimaging** is indicated in acute or subacute instances and in cases of progressive or chronic disorders when treatable illness is possible.

   2. **Electromyography** is used to diagnose specific peripheral nerve injury or focal dystonia, polyneuropathy, myopathy, bulbar palsy, motor neuron disease, or myasthenia gravis.

   3. **Certain blood tests** may be specific to the diagnostic possibilities producing dysarthria.

IV. **Differential diagnosis.** As with the classification of dysarthria, differential diagnosis can be approached in several different ways. If a general neurologic diagnosis and neuroanatomic localization are arrived at before speech testing, a relatively accurate diagnosis of the type of dysarthria can be made with attentive listening during conversation with the patient. As an alternative, if the neurologic diagnosis or neuroanatomic localization is elusive, careful application of the steps used to characterize the type of dysarthria may narrow the diagnostic search. Table 19.1 summarizes the type of dysarthria, neuroanatomic localization, differential diagnosis for dysarthria type, and the most prominent features during testing.

A. **Respiration.** The differential diagnosis of respiratory problems falls mainly into two categories—primary pulmonary disease and neurologic disease. Patients with pulmonary disease have diminished breath support, phrase length, and voice quality, but other characteristics most often are normal. Primary neurologic disorders characterized by respiratory system abnormalities include injury or dysfunction of the intercostal nerves, phrenic nerve, sympathetic plexus, spinal cord, brainstem, or vagus nerve; myopathic processes; and neuromuscular junction disorders. Although the act of respiration is affected by different processes depending on the diagnosis, the outcome is similar. Problems are caused by the inability of the system to maintain consistent subglottic airflow. Common diseases include

   1. **Myopathic disorders**
      a. Acute myopathy syndrome
      b. Hypokalemic periodic paralysis
      c. Periodic paralysis
   2. **Disorders of the neuromuscular junction**
      a. Persistent neuromuscular blockade
      b. Myasthenia gravis
      c. Hypermagnesemia
   3. **Peripheral nerve disorders**
      a. Critical illness polyneuropathy
      b. Guillain–Barré syndrome
      c. Acute intermittent porphyria
      d. Phrenic and intercostal nerve lesions from trauma or tumor infiltration
      e. Intoxication
   4. **Anterior horn cell disease**
   5. **Spinal cord disorder**

B. **Phonation** depends on the integrity of the vagus nerve and specifically its branches.

   1. The **recurrent laryngeal nerve** innervates the true vocal folds.
      a. **Lesions.** A unilateral lesion produces vocal fold paralysis in the abducted position. The result is a flaccid dysphonia, which is characterized by breathiness, lowered pitch, and possibly diplophonic sound caused by vibration of the vocal folds at two separate frequencies. In rare instances, unilateral lesions of the vagus nerve or recurrent laryngeal nerve can result in a normal voice, because the normal vocal fold may adduct across the midline to approximate the weaker vocal fold. Bilateral lesions result in vocal folds in the paramedian position with severe compromise of the airway, and speech may be dysphonic or aphonic. There may be a forced quality to the voice, which may result in monostress and monopitch.
      b. **Common causes** include accidental injury during open heart surgery, especially to the left recurrent laryngeal nerve as it passes around the aorta; trauma as from gunshot or knife wounds; tumor infiltration; and viral infection.
   2. The superior laryngeal nerve innervates the cricothyroid muscle. Bilateral damage results in loss of pitch control. The voice is slightly hoarse and fatigues quickly.
   3. An intramedullary or extramedullary lesion at the brainstem level affecting the main trunk of the vagus nerve produces unilateral or bilateral true vocal fold paralysis in the abducted position and causes considerable glottic air escape and a breathy voice quality combined with hypernasality.
   4. Paradoxical vocal cord motion occurs when the expiratory and inspiratory phases are out of synchrony with vocal fold abduction. Speech and biofeedback therapy are important interventions.

C. Resonance. Normal resonance depends on the integrity of the oropharynx, nasopharynx, nares, and oral cavity.

1. The **pharyngeal branch of the vagus nerve** innervates the soft palate. Lesions produce unilateral or bilateral weakness of the soft palate and incompetence of the velopharyngeal seal during speech and swallowing. Speech is hypernasal owing to escape of air through the nares.
2. Lesions of the trigeminal nerve or its mandibular branch produce flaccidity of the floor of the mouth due to loss of innervation of the mylohyoid and anterior digastric muscles.
3. Obstruction along the nasal passage by a mass or by edema results in excess escape of air through the mouth and gives the speech a hyponasal quality.

D. Articulation. Disordered articulation results from dysfunction of **cranial nerves VII and XII** (predominantly XII) but also, although less commonly, the **trigeminal nerve** that serves to open and close the jaw. Normal function of the muscles of facial expression and tongue are required for accurate production of phonemes.

1. The facial nerve provides innervation for motor manipulation of the mouth and lips. Paralysis produces problems with bilabial (e.g., /b/ as in baby) and labiodental (e.g., /f/ as in father) phonemes. Common causes of facial nerve lesions include idiopathic conditions (Bell's palsy), tumor within the temporal bone, Ramsay Hunt syndrome, mass lesions such as acoustic neuroma, aneurysm, Lyme disease, sarcoidosis, Guillain–Barré syndrome, trauma, and both supranuclear and pontine lesions.
2. Involvement can be unilateral or bilateral, resulting in lingual errors. One common type is a lisp, in which a /th/ may be substituted for /s/, /t/, /d/, /ch/, or /j/.
3. Dental malocclusion, dental absence, and structural deformity of the tongue can contribute to articulation errors.

E. Prosody. Aprosody or dysprosody can be the result of a lesion anywhere along the motor speech neuroaxis but is most prominently associated with hemispheric brain disease.

V. Diagnostic approach

A. Perform the three-step physical examination outlined in **III.B.1.**
B. Initiate a therapeutic plan based on system dysfunction and dysarthria type.

VI. Referrals

A. **Otolaryngology** consultation may be necessary for evaluation of the larynx and pharynx, especially if hypernasality is of recent onset, to rule out structural lesions and hearing problems. If a patient has been extubated for longer than 7 days and vocal quality remains impaired or not improving, referral may be indicated for nasopharyngeal laryngoscopy.
B. **Speech and language pathology** consultation is necessary to aid in diagnosis of speech and swallowing problems and to provide and administer a therapeutic plan.

Acknowledgment
The authors acknowledge Dr. Jeffrey Metter's outstanding contribution to the understanding of dysarthria by basing this chapter on his diagnostic approach.

Recommended Readings
Adams RD, Victor M, Ropper AH. Disorders of speech and language. In: Adams RD, Victor M, Ropper AH, eds. *Principles of neurology,* 6th ed. New York: McGraw–Hill, 1997: 472–493.

Barry WR, ed. *Clinical dysarthria.* San Diego: College Hill, 1983.

Brazis PW, Masdeu JC, Biller J. The localization of lesions affecting cranial nerve XII. In: *Localization in clinical neurology,* 3rd ed. Boston: Little, Brown, 1996:335–342.

Brookshire RH. *An introduction to neurogenic communication disorders,* 4th ed. St. Louis: Mosby, 1992.

Chapey R, ed. *Language intervention strategies in adult aphasia,* 2nd ed. Baltimore: Williams & Wilkins, 1986.

Costello J. *Speech disorders in adults.* San Diego: College Hill, 1985.

Critchley EMR. *Language and speech disorders: a neurophysiological approach.* Hillsdale, NJ: CNS Clinical Neuroscience, 1987.

Darby JK, ed. *Speech and language evaluation in neurology: adult disorders.* Orlando, FL: Grune & Stratton, 1985.

Duus P. *Topical diagnosis in neurology,* 2nd ed. New York: Thieme Medical Publishers, 1989.

Eldridge M. *A history of the treatment of speech disorders.* London: Livingstone, 1968.

Groher ME. *Dysphagia: diagnosis and management,* 2nd ed. Boston: Butterworth–Heinemann, 1992.

Hartman DE, Abbs JH. Dysarthria associated with focal unilateral upper motor neuron lesion. *Eur J Disord Commun* 1992;27:187–196.

Hird K, Krisner K. Dysprosody following acquired neurogenic impairment. *Brain Lang* 1993; 45:46–60.

Ichikawa K, Kageyama Y. Clinical anatomic study of pure dysarthria. *Stroke* 1991;22:809–812.

Johns DF. *Clinical management of neurogenic communicative disorders,* 2nd ed. Boston: College Hill, 1985.

Johnson JA, Pring PR. Speech therapy in Parkinson disease: a review on further data. *Br J Disord Commun* 1990;25:183–194.

Lass NJ, et al. *Handbook of speech, language pathology, and audiology.* Philadelphia: BC Decker, 1988.

Love RJ, Webb WG. *Neurology for the speech-language pathologist,* 2nd ed. Boston: Butterworth–Heinemann, 1992.

Matas M. Psychogenic voice disorders: literature review and case report. *Can J Psychiatry* 1991;36:363–365.

Mayo Clinic and Mayo Foundation for Medical Education and Research Members. Language and motor speech. In: Ahlskog JE, Atunson AE, Anger RG, ed. *Clinical examinations in neurology,* 6th ed. St. Louis: Mosby, 1991:46–84.

Metter J. *Speech disorders: clinical evaluation and diagnosis.* Dana Point, CA: PMA, 1985.

Moore CA, Yorkston KM, Beukelman DR, eds. *Dysarthria and apraxia of speech: perspective on management.* Baltimore: PH Brooks, 1991.

Nation JE, Aram DM. *Diagnosis of speech and language disorders,* 2nd ed. San Diego: College Hill, 1984.

Singh S, Lynch J. *Diagnostic procedures in hearing, language, and speech.* Baltimore: University Park, 1978.

Swigert NB. *The source for dysarthria.* East Moline, IL: LinguiSystems, 1997.

Yorkston KM, Buekelman DR, Bell KR. *Clinical management of dysarthric speakers.* Boston: College Hill, 1988.

20. APPROACH TO THE PATIENT WITH ACUTE HEADACHE

David L. Gordon

Acute headache is one of the most common reasons for visits to emergency departments. **Primary headache**, such as migraine and cluster, is a condition in which headache is a primary manifestation, and no underlying disease process is present. **Secondary headache** is a condition in which headache is a secondary manifestation of an underlying disease process. Most patients with acute headache have primary headache, particularly migraine. Performing an expensive battery of tests on all patients with acute headache is neither cost-effective nor appropriate. However, failure to perform diagnostic tests for certain patients with acute headache will result in failure to detect life-threatening, yet treatable, causes. The challenge to the clinician in the emergency setting is not to be lulled to sleep by the frequent migraine attacks and to remain vigilant for the other disease causes of acute headache.

Migraine is so common that many patients with a secondary headache have a history of migraine, making diagnosis in the acute setting quite difficult. Certain clues in the history and examination should lead to performance of a diagnostic evaluation in search of the cause of secondary headache. The primary goals of the clinician treating a patient with acute headache are threefold: (1) diagnose the cause of headache, (2) provide emergency therapy, and (3) provide the patient with a means of long-term care. These goals apply for patients with primary or secondary headache. Primary headaches are chronic conditions that manifest as multiple acute attacks. Secondary headaches generally are caused by diseases that necessitate both urgent and prolonged care. This chapter deals with the diagnosis of acute headache. The diagnosis of chronic headache and therapy for conditions that cause headache are dealt with elsewhere in Chapter 21.

I. **Pathophysiology.** The description of a headache alone is not a reliable predictor of whether a headache is primary or secondary. For example, hemicranial throbbing pain is not always a feature of migraine and can be a feature of intracranial disease. This suggests that primary and secondary headaches have common pathophysiologic mechanisms. Although current understanding of the cause of head pain is not complete, a plausible explanation of the pathophysiologic mechanism of headache that emphasizes the common final pathway of primary and secondary headaches is depicted in Fig. 20.1. The schema provides an explanation for the "migrainous" characteristics of some secondary headaches. Older theories regarding the vascular origin of migraine and the muscle-contraction cause of tension headache are not likely to be true.

II. **History**

    A. A **history of headaches** is perhaps the most important historical information needed to determine whether a diagnostic evaluation is necessary. A history of similar headaches for many years suggests a primary headache disorder. If, on the other hand, this is the **first** headache of the patient's life, if this is the **worst** headache that the patient has had, if the headache is **different** in character from past headaches, or if the pain is **persistent** despite the use of measures that relieved previous headaches, then a secondary headache is much more likely (Table 20.1). If the patient has had similar headaches for only a few months, weeks, or days, then the possibility of secondary headache increases, and further investigation is warranted. Although it is common for the character of primary headache disorders to change throughout a lifetime, if the current headache differs from previous headaches, the clinician is obligated to investigate.

    B. **Age at onset** of primary headache disorders is generally childhood to young adulthood. An age at onset older than 50 years is particularly suggestive of secondary headache.

    C. **Activity at onset of headache** may suggest cause of headache. Although migraine can be precipitated or exacerbated by Valsalva maneuver, changes in position, or head trauma, the presence of any of these features on history should raise the suspicion of secondary headache.

        1. A **Valsalva maneuver,** such as occurs with lifting, straining, or squatting, may precipitate aneurysmal rupture and resultant subarachnoid hemorrhage. Headache during coitus can occur as a result of aneurysmal rupture

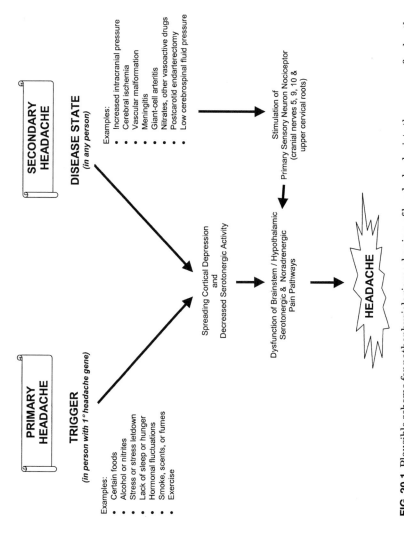

FIG. 20.1 Plausible schema for pathophysiologic mechanism of headache depicts the common final pathway of primary and secondary headaches.

Table 20.1 Clinical features suggestive of secondary headache

---

Headache Features
First headache
Worst headache
Different headache
Persistent headache
Exacerbation by head position
Onset
   With Valsalva maneuver
   With head trauma
   After 50 years of age
Associated Features
Focal neurologic signs (abnormal examination findings)
Change in consciousness
Fever
Seizure
Nuchal rigidity
Papilledema
Preretinal or retinal hemorrhage
History of
   Bleeding diathesis
   Hypercoagulable state
   Cancer
   Risk factor for human immunodeficiency virus infection or acquired immunodeficiency
     syndrome

---

or as a result of coital migraine. The first time a person experiences coital headache, he or she needs a complete evaluation to rule out aneurysmal subarachnoid hemorrhage.

2. **Changes in position** exacerbate several types of headache. Headaches worse in the supine position suggest sinusitis, cerebral venous thrombosis, or an intracranial mass. Improvement in the supine position and worsening with sitting or standing are characteristic of low-pressure headaches. Headaches that occur only in a particular head position may be caused by a mobile intracranial tumor, such as third ventricle colloid cyst, that intermittently obstructs the ventricles and thereby increases intracranial pressure.

3. Although **head trauma** can be a trigger for migraine, subdural hematoma must be ruled out before this diagnosis is possible.

4. **Exercise** can precipitate migraine headache.

D. The **characteristics of a headache** are most helpful in determining whether the current headache is different from previous headaches experienced by the patient. Certain characteristics are suggestive of but not pathognomonic for certain causes of headache.

1. **Severity** of pain is important in that any patient who says he or she has "the worst headache of my life" need an urgent and complete evaluation, with subarachnoid hemorrhage highest in the differential diagnosis. Both primary headaches and secondary headaches, however, can manifest as very severe or very mild pain.

2. The **time frame** of onset of pain is more discriminating. Sudden onset of a headache suggests a sudden increase in intracranial pressure, as occurs with subarachnoid hemorrhage. Mass lesions such as tumors, abscesses, and subacute or chronic subdural hematoma usually manifest gradually over days to months. Gradual onset of headache over minutes to hours is consistent with migraine. The headache of giant cell arteritis tends to be subacute to chronic in presentation.

   3. **Duration** of primary headaches is variable, although they typically last hours to days. Headaches that persist for longer periods despite treatment are worrisome because they suggest underlying cranial pathologic conditions.
   4. **Location** of headache and radiation of pain are nonspecific. Many posterior lesions cause frontal headache. Both primary and secondary headaches can be unilateral or bilateral. The pain of both migraine headaches and secondary headaches can radiate.
   5. **Quality** of headache is nondiscriminating. Despite the traditional teaching that migraines must be pounding or throbbing, they are just as often pressure like, squeezing, sharp, stabbing, or dull. Cluster headaches typically are described as boring, sharp, or lancinating, but so might the headaches associated with other pathologic processes.
   6. **Associated symptoms** of the headache can offer important clues to the cause of headache (Table 20.1).
      a. **Nausea and vomiting** are common features of migraine, but their presence in a person with new or sudden headache is worrisome because they suggest increased intracranial pressure or a posterior fossa lesion.
      b. **Photophobia and phonophobia** can be part of migraine or a meningeal process such as subarachnoid hemorrhage or meningitis.
      c. **Neck stiffness** is typical of a meningeal process.
      d. **Change in consciousness** is rare in a patient with primary headache; its presence should alert the clinician to more serious causes of headache.
      e. **Focal neurologic symptoms** (e.g., aphasia, visual symptoms, vertigo, ataxia, hemiparesis, or hemisensory deficit) can occur suddenly in association with headache in patients with stroke, seizure, subdural hematoma, and migraine. In this case, migraine is a diagnosis of exclusion, and the clinician is obliged to investigate for underlying disease. Transient ischemic attacks (TIAs) typically last 5 to 20 minutes. Stroke and subdural hematoma symptoms persist. The Todd's paralysis of partial seizures and the aura of migraine often last hours. The focal symptoms of ischemia or hemorrhage typically are static, whereas the focal symptoms of migraine typically travel over minutes to hours—for example, numbness that begins in the fingertips and progresses to involve the entire arm and perhaps the ipsilateral face or leg. Partial seizures can result in symptoms that travel over seconds. Binocular visual symptoms can be migrainous or due to occipital pathologic conditions. Headache in a person older than 50 years with monocular blurred vision and a swollen optic disk suggests the anterior ischemic optic neuropathy of giant cell arteritis. Certain visual symptoms are classic for migraine, such as scintillating scotomata (blind areas surrounded by sparkling zigzag lines), photopsia (unformed flashes of color), and fortification spectra (slowly enlarging, sparkling, serrated arcs).
      f. **Fever, diaphoresis, chills, or rigors** are worrisome because they suggest infection. Fever of any cause or generalized infection can cause headache, but if headache, neck stiffness, or decreased consciousness is a prominent symptom, meningitis is highest in the differential diagnosis.
   E. **Family history of headache** is important yet extremely difficult to obtain in the emergency setting of acute headache. Patients may be distracted by their pain and nausea and may have cognitive dysfunction as a feature of the headache (whether primary or secondary). Even if the patient is coherent or an accompanying relative is available, it is common for persons not to be aware of their family history of headache. Migraines tend to be most prominent in early adulthood, when children are too young to realize their parent has headaches, and the patient no longer lives under the same roof with parents or siblings. In addition, rationalization of relatives regarding the cause of the headache (e.g., "sinus" or "tension") usually is believed by the patient, making it difficult to obtain a family history of "migraine."
III. Physical examination may reveal signs of a disease that causes secondary headache. A detailed neurologic examination is particularly important; any subtle abnormality should be enough to stimulate a diagnostic evaluation (Table 20.1).

A. General examination

    1. Vital signs. Fever suggests an infectious cause of headache. The presence of arterial hypertension in a patient with headache is common and is not necessarily causative. Hypertension occurs as a result of migraine attacks, cerebral ischemia, and intracranial hemorrhage. In certain cases, especially when it comes on abruptly and reaches extreme levels, hypertension may be a primary cause of headache.

    2. General appearance. Cachexia may be present among patients with chronic diseases such as cancer, acquired immunodeficiency syndrome (AIDS), tuberculosis, and sarcoidosis. Headache due to tumor, abscess, granuloma, or meningitis may be the presenting symptom among such patients.

    3. Head. Evidence of cranial trauma includes face and scalp abrasions and contusions and the signs of skull fracture—depressed section of skull, Battle's sign (postauricular ecchymosis that occurs with basilar skull fracture), raccoon sign (periorbital ecchymosis), hemotympanum, cerebrospinal fluid (CSF) otorrhea, and CSF rhinorrhea. Skull tenderness to palpation can occur as a result of subdural hematoma. Poor dentition or dental abscesses may result in intracranial abscess. Tenderness to palpation over the mastoid process, frontal sinus, or maxillary sinus may suggest infection of these structures. Migraine, however, frequently results in external carotid territory vasodilatation with resultant sinus "fullness," "pressure," and tenderness. The presence of purulent discharge from the sinuses is more helpful in diagnosing sinusitis. Otoscopic examination may reveal ear infection as well as hemotympanum and otorrhea. Temporal tenderness or diminished temporal artery pulses in a person older than 50 years are consistent with giant cell (temporal) arteritis. Auscultation of the skull may reveal cranial bruits that occur as a result of arteriovenous malformation (AVM).

    4. Neck. Meningeal signs include nuchal rigidity (neck stiffness in the anteroposterior direction), Kernig's sign (inability to extend the knee after passive hip flexion in the supine position), and Brudzinski's sign (involuntary hip flexion after passive flexion of the neck in the supine position) and imply the presence of meningitis or subarachnoid hemorrhage. Evidence of neck trauma includes pain on lateral neck movement and neck immobility.

    5. Skin. A petechial rash over the axillae, wrists, and ankles is consistent with meningitis due to meningococcus. Skin examination may reveal bruising suggestive of a bleeding diathesis, splinter hemorrhages of the distal digits suggestive of cardioembolism, or lesions suggestive of a neurocutaneous disorder such as neurofibromatosis, tuberous sclerosis, or cutaneous angiomatosis; these conditions are associated with intracranial lesions that may cause headache. Melanoma suggests the possibility of cerebral metastasis causing headache. Lesions of Kaposi's sarcoma are consistent with AIDS, which is associated with several intracranial diseases that cause headache.

    6. Lymph nodes. Lymphadenopathy occurs among patients with cancer, AIDS, chronic infections, or chronic inflammatory diseases. The possible presence of any of these conditions should stimulate evaluation for a cause of secondary headache.

B. Neurologic examination. The neurologic findings are normal in patients with primary headache. A change in consciousness or focal deficit raises the possibility of secondary headache. The funduscopic examination may reveal papilledema (swollen disk with normal visual acuity) in patients with increased intracranial pressure, anterior ischemic optic neuropathy (swollen disk with decreased visual acuity or relative afferent pupillary defect) in patients with giant cell arteritis, or preretinal hemorrhage in patients with intracranial hemorrhage. Headache in association with either partial third nerve palsy or complete but pupil-sparing third nerve palsy is worrisome because it suggests posterior communicating artery aneurysm. A patient with these findings needs urgent four-vessel cerebral arteriography. The combination of proptosis, oculomotor findings, and headache suggests disease in the orbit, superior orbital fissure, or cavernous sinus; evaluation should be urgent. Acute glaucoma can manifest as headache, especially periorbitally. An injected conjunctiva and a hard globe are consistent with the diagnosis. Horner's syndrome (miosis, subtle upper- and lower-lid ptosis, and anhydrosis) can occur in isolation ipsilateral to a carotid dissection.

IV. Laboratory studies are necessary in the evaluation of any patient believed to have a secondary headache (Fig. 20.2). There are no laboratories that identify primary headache.

  A. Blood evaluation
    1. **Complete blood cell count.** Leukocytosis is consistent with infection, and marked leukocytosis is found in leukemia, which can cause headache through carcinomatous meningitis or cerebral venous occlusion. Leukopenia is found in AIDS. Anemia can occur in patients with cancer or giant cell arteritis. It also can be associated with a low-flow state that precipitates cerebral venous thrombosis. Essential thrombocythemia is a hypercoagulable state that can cause arterial or venous occlusions in the brain with resultant headache.
    2. **Chemistries.** Renal failure can be associated with headache. Both renal function and liver enzyme abnormalities have implications regarding past drug use and options for future medical management. In general, however, abnormalities in serum chemistries may provide clues to a generalized, underlying disease process that can cause headache.
    3. **Erythrocyte sedimentation rate (ESR)** and **C-reactive protein (CRP)** are the initial tests to perform if giant cell arteritis is suspected. Moderate elevations in ESR (up to 50 mm/h) are common among healthy elderly patients. Both ESR and CRP are nonspecific; elevations can be present in patients with infection, inflammatory disease, or cancer. Still, marked elevations of ESR or any elevation of CRP in a patient older than 50 years with new-onset headache should prompt administration of high-dose steroids and temporal artery biopsy.
    4. **Prothrombin time (PT)** and **partial thromboplastin time (PTT)** may provide evidence of a bleeding diathesis that results in intracranial hemorrhage and headache.
    5. **Thyroid function tests.** Thyroid disease can cause headache by serving as a trigger in a migraine patient or can cause headache by other mechanisms.
    6. **Hypercoagulable profile** is indicated for patients with suspected cerebral venous thrombosis and for patients younger than 50 years with suspected ischemic stroke or TIA (new-onset headache with transient neurologic deficit). In addition to CBC, PT, and PTT, the minimal evaluation should include fibrinogen, protein C, protein S (total and free), antithrombin III, lupus anticoagulant, anticardiolipin antibodies (IgG and IgM), and activated protein C resistance. If the platelet count is abnormal, platelet function studies should be performed.
    7. **Arterial blood gas.** Hypoxia can cause headache; arterial blood gas measurement should be performed if clinically indicated.
    8. **Drug screen.** Use of sympathomimetic drugs such as cocaine and amphetamines can be associated with intracranial hemorrhage or cerebral ischemia and resultant headache. Salicylate toxicity can result in diffuse cerebral edema with headache worsening. The use of excessive analgesics, whether over-the-counter or narcotic, can cause chronic analgesic rebound headache and interfere with acute headache management.
  B. Urine evaluation may reveal nephrotic syndrome (which can be associated with a hypercoagulable state and resultant cerebral venous thrombosis), infection (organisms and white blood cells), evidence of peripheral embolization (red blood cell casts), or use of illicit or analgesic drugs.
  C. Radiography. A chest radiograph may reveal hilar adenopathy or pulmonary lesions that provide clues regarding the identity of intracranial lesions that cause headache. Radiographs of the cervical spine may reveal evidence of neck trauma.
  D. Computed tomography (CT) is the preferred initial cerebral imaging study because of its sensitivity in the detection of acute blood. Noncontrast scanning is mandatory because both contrast material and blood present because of acute bleeding are white (hyperdense) on CT scans. If only a contrast scan is obtained,

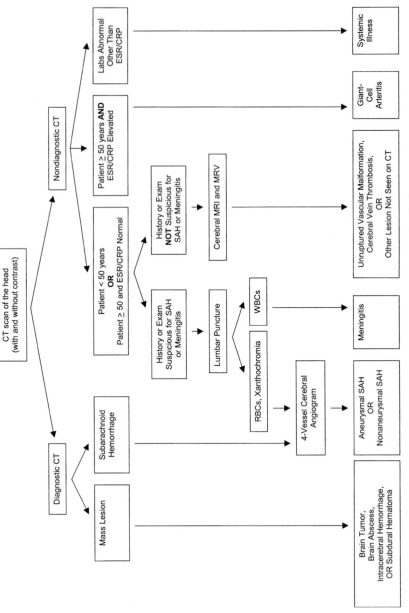

FIG. 20.2 Diagnostic algorithm for a patient with suspected acute secondary headache.

there may be confusion about whether a lesion is hemorrhage or an enhancing mass. With time, blood becomes increasingly dark on CT scans. Consequently, subacute (2 to 14 days) subdural hematoma is isodense with parenchyma on CT scans and may be difficult to detect. Magnetic resonance imaging (MRI) is better in the detection of subacute bleeding. The odds of detecting subarachnoid hemorrhage with CT decreases with time from onset of symptoms. Within a few days, a large percentage of CT scans are normal. Even in the acute phase, at least 5% of patients with subarachnoid hemorrhage have normal CT scans. For any patient with suspected subarachnoid hemorrhage, if the CT findings are normal, the clinician is obliged to perform lumbar puncture. Once noncontrast CT is performed, if a mass lesion is suspected, a contrast scan should be obtained. Mass lesions such as tumors and abscesses disrupt the blood–brain barrier and cause seepage of contrast medium around or in the lesion. A mass lesion can be isodense with parenchyma on noncontrast CT scans and therefore difficult to detect. Contrast scanning greatly increases the chance of detecting such a lesion. Patients with known allergic reactions to iodine-based contrast agents should be pretreated with steroids. CT contrast material is nephrotoxic and generally should not be used in examinations of patients with renal failure.

E. **MRI** is a secondary cerebral imaging procedure in the evaluation of acute headache owing to its inability to depict blood present because of acute bleeding. It is better than CT, however, in the detection of subacute bleeding and is especially useful in examinations of patients with suspected subacute subdural hematoma. MRI also is superior to CT and even angiography in the detection of vascular malformation. Any patient with suspected unruptured AVM as a cause of headache needs MRI. MRI is superior to CT in the detection of parenchymal lesions and the visualization of the posterior fossa and inferior temporal lobes. Unlike CT, MRI provides information regarding blood flow in cerebral vessels. MRI is the procedure of choice in examinations of patients with suspected cerebral venous thrombosis. It depicts both parenchymal and venous abnormalities and leads to a correct diagnosis of this condition approximately 75% of the time. MRI contrast material—gadolinium—is not iodine based, is not nephrotoxic, and generally does not cause allergic reactions.

F. **Magnetic resonance angiography (MRA)** is indicated in evaluation of patients with suspected cerebral venous thrombosis who do not undergo conventional angiography. MRA offers a noninvasive way of evaluating the cerebral vessels. Contrast medium is not necessary. MRA, however, is performed with complex technology and can mislead the clinician if not performed and interpreted properly. MRA entails gradient recall echo technology. Vessels with abnormal flow are not depicted, slow flow can mimic occlusion, and subacute thrombus can mimic normal flow. Selective **MR venography (MRV)** is performed by means of saturating arterial inflow. Acquisition of images should be perpendicular to flow to avoid in-plane flow artifact. Two-dimensional time-of-flight images are preferred for venography, although additional phase-contrast images may be necessary for clarification.

G. **Lumbar puncture (LP)**
   1. **Indications.** LP for CSF analysis is indicated if one suspects acute or chronic meningitis, subarachnoid hemorrhage, pseudotumor cerebri, or low-CSF-pressure headache.
   2. **Timing in relation to CT.** It is preferable to perform CT before LP. If CT shows significant mass effect such as shift across the midline, obliterated basilar cisterns, or a compressed fourth ventricle, LP should be avoided to avoid precipitating uncal or central herniation of brain tissue through the foramen magnum. If CT shows subarachnoid hemorrhage, LP is not necessary. If bacterial meningitis is suspected, antibiotics should be started on the way to CT and LP performed after normal CT findings are obtained. If CT is to be delayed for hours and one suspects bacterial meningitis, it is necessary to perform LP and treat the patient with appropriate antibiotics without CT. The prognosis among patients with meningitis is heavily influenced by promptness of treatment.

3. **CSF analysis.** Opening pressure is most important in patients with suspected pseudotumor cerebri (generally more than 250 mm Hg) or low-CSF-pressure headaches. If subarachnoid hemorrhage is suspected, one should obtain cell counts in the first and last tubes of CSF and test for xanthochromia. Knowing that the number of red blood cells does not change significantly between the two tubes helps to confirm the diagnosis and avoids the common dilemma of determining whether or not a bloody tap is "traumatic." Xanthochromia is the yellowish color of CSF supernatant that occurs because of either the presence of hemoglobin breakdown products or a very high protein concentration. If the patient arrives for treatment days after a subarachnoid hemorrhage, there may be no red blood cells in the CSF, but xanthochromia due to hemoglobin breakdown persists for up to 2 weeks. Samples for culture of bacteria, fungus, and tuberculosis should be sent. Polymerase chain reaction is a sensitive means of determining the presence of infection. A Venereal Disease Research Laboratory test and cryptococcal antigen assessment should be performed as well. If cancer is suspected, at least 10 mL of fluid should be sent for cytologic analysis.

H. **Cerebral angiography** should be performed urgently for any patient with evidence of subarachnoid hemorrhage at CT or LP. A four-vessel arteriogram is mandatory because predictions of aneurysm location based on CT findings are not always accurate, and many patients have multiple aneurysms. Delayed venous-phase images are the standard for the evaluation of cerebral venous thrombosis, which can cause subarachnoid bleeding.

I. **Electroencephalography** is indicated if seizures are being considered, as in evaluation of a patient with headache and associated loss of consciousness. Headaches often occur in association with seizures. Partial seizures can result in transient neurologic deficits and can be difficult to differentiate from migraine with aura and TIA.

V. Differential diagnosis
A. Primary headache
1. Migraine

a. **Definition.** Migraine is a genetic condition in which a person has a predisposition to episodic headaches, gastrointestinal dysfunction, or neurologic dysfunction. Contrary to popular belief, severe headache need not be a feature of migraine. The International Headache Society definition of migraine is quite specific for the purpose of research but probably is too limiting in clinical practice. Migraine is inherited in an autosomal dominant manner and generally is not life threatening; that is, it is inherited in the same way brown eyes are inherited. It stands to reason that approximately two thirds of all persons have migraine. There is convincing evidence that intermittent **tension-type headache** is a form of migraine rather than a separate entity.

b. **Triggers.** A migraine attack occurs when an external stimulus, or trigger, affects a person with the genetic predisposition to migraine. Examples of triggers include hormonal change, stress, stress letdown, certain foods, alcohol, smoke, certain scents, fumes, exercise, fatigue, lack of sleep, hunger, and head trauma. Women suffer more migraine attacks than do men because they are more frequently exposed to a trigger (estrogen level fluctuations of menstruation, pregnancy, oral contraceptives, and menopause), but they do not possess the gene more often than do men.

c. **Phases.** There are four main phases of migraine—prodrome, aura, headache, and postdrome. Not all phases need be present in any one migraine attack.

(1) The **prodrome** occurs hours to days before the headache and consists of mood changes (irritability, depression) or food cravings. Although chocolate, nuts, and bananas often are thought to be migraine triggers, it more likely that patients crave these foods as part of the migraine prodrome.

(2) The **aura** can be visual, sensory, motor, or reflective of brainstem (e.g., vertigo, diplopia) or cerebral cortex (e.g., aphasia) involvement. The symptoms are typically traveling in nature, such as moving or pulsating spots in the vision or numbness that starts in part of one extremity and travels over several minutes to hours to involve the entire extremity or other extremities. The traveling nature of the symptoms reflects the spreading wave of cortical depression that occurs during migraine. The visual symptoms can be any shape (spots, circles, wavy or zigzag lines), any color (clear, silver, black, white, or brightly colored), and hemianopic or present throughout the visual field and typically move (traveling across vision, floating, pulsating, heat wave sensation). An aura may the only symptom of a migraine attack (aura without headache, acephalgic migraine), may occur before, during, or after the headache (headache with aura, classic migraine), or may not be present at all (headache without aura, common migraine).

(3) The **headache** quality is not as helpful in diagnosis as is generally believed. Although the headache can be severe, throbbing, and hemicranial, it need not have any of these characteristics. Migraine headaches frequently are mild, squeezing or dull in nature or are bilateral. The onset of headache typically is gradual over minutes to hours, and the duration typically is several hours to a few days. The headache may be associated with nausea, vomiting, photophobia, phonophobia, or difficulty concentrating. Gastrointestinal symptoms such as abdominal cramping, flatulence, and diarrhea may predominate during this phase (so-called abdominal migraine). The abdominal symptoms often resolve soon after diarrhea occurs. Transient dysautonomia often occurs during this phase and results in blood pressure changes.

(4) The **postdrome** is marked by malaise for several hours after the headache. Mood changes, impaired concentration, and scalp or muscle tenderness also may be present. Sleep often helps migraine attacks, and patients tend to crave rest in a dark, quiet room.

   d. **Difficulties in migraine diagnosis.** Migraine is a purely historical diagnosis. Aided by folklore and advertising for over-the-counter medications, patients tend to believe their recurrent headaches are due to "sinus," "tension," or "regular headache." Consequently, obtaining a history of "migraine" often is difficult. It may be beneficial to educate the patient regarding migraine before obtaining a history. If there is any doubt in the clinician's mind regarding the diagnosis of migraine, a diagnostic evaluation is necessary to rule out other causes of headache.

  2. **Cluster headache** is much less common than migraine. It occurs primarily among men and manifests as severe, stabbing, periorbital pain with associated ipsilateral tearing, injected conjunctiva, nasal congestion, and rhinorrhea. Alcohol often precipitates attacks. The attacks occur most frequently at night, last 30 minutes to 3 hours, and can occur several times per day. Unlike patients with migraine, patients with cluster headaches prefer to pace and keep active during the attacks. The term *cluster* refers to the seasonal occurrence of multiple episodes over weeks to months with intermittent periods of remission. There are episodic and chronic forms.

B. Secondary headache

  1. **Subarachnoid hemorrhage (SAH)** is the most important consideration in evaluation of patients with a first or worst headache, yet it is frequently missed: 25% of patients with SAH are initially treated for another condition. Most patients with SAH have headache as the initial symptom. The headache is unilateral in 30% of patients, and findings at neurologic examination may be normal. Many patients (estimates range from 20% to 95%) have a milder sentinel headache that precedes the cataclysmic event. The clinician should consider the sentinel headache of SAH in evaluation of patients with

mild, yet different headaches. CT usually provides enough information for a diagnosis, but if SAH is suspected clinically and CT findings are normal, LP is mandatory. One should examine the CSF as described in **IV.G.** Once SAH is diagnosed with CT or LP, urgent four-vessel angiography is required to identify aneurysms amenable to surgical clipping.

2. **Meningitis**, particularly bacterial and viral meningitis, often manifests as acute headache. Fever, neck stiffness, confusion, decreased consciousness, and cranial neuropathy may be present. Bacterial meningitis is fatal if the patient is not treated. Administration of broad-spectrum antibiotics should be started as soon as there is clinical suspicion—before CT and LP are performed. If one suspects bacterial meningitis, CSF analysis is mandatory. If CT can be performed within minutes, one should perform CT before LP to rule out mass effect. **IV.G.** describes steps to take if CT cannot be performed immediately. Antibiotic therapy can be adjusted once culture results are known.

   Aseptic meningitis and the chronic meningitis also can manifest as acute, persistent headache. Cranial neuropathy is more common, and neck stiffness is less common in chronic meningitis. Conditions associated with chronic meningitis include syphilis, fungal infection (especially with cryptococcus), tuberculosis, sarcoidosis, Lyme disease, cancer, and lymphoma. Any patient with AIDS who has a headache and normal findings at contrast CT of the brain needs LP in search of cryptococcal meningitis. Patients with suspected carcinomatous or lymphomatous meningitis, may need several LPs for cytologic analysis of CSF before the diagnosis is confirmed.

3. **Subdural hematoma** occurs as a result of the tearing of bridging veins. When acute, it presents as a rapidly progressive neurologic deficit, but headache may be the only symptom of subacute or chronic subdural hematoma. Although subdural hematoma typically is caused by closed head trauma, in many cases a history of trauma is absent, especially in older patients. CT usually provides enough information for the diagnosis, but blood from subacute bleeding (2 days to 2 weeks) is isodense with brain parenchyma on CT scans, making it difficult to detect. MRI, although inferior to CT in the detection of acutely bleeding, is superior in the detection of subacute bleeding. **Epidural hematoma** caused by rupture of a meningeal artery and usually associated with skull fracture usually manifests as rapidly progressive neurologic deficit and decreased consciousness, rather than as headache. The classic sequence is head trauma, brief loss of consciousness, lucid interval, and rapid progression to coma.

4. **Intracerebral hemorrhage** manifests as focal neurologic findings and usually a change in consciousness or cognition. Estimates of headache incidence with intracerebral hemorrhage vary depending on the size and location of the hemorrhage. Among patients who are able to communicate, headache is more common with larger sites of hemorrhage and hemorrhage in the cerebellum and cortex (lobar hemorrhage). The classic description of cerebellar hemorrhage is acute posterior headache with nausea, vomiting, and inability to stand. CT provides enough information for the diagnosis, and emergency surgery may be life saving.

5. **Ischemic stroke and TIA** always manifest as a focal neurologic deficit. Headache occurs in 15% to 20% of patients with acute cerebral ischemia. The presence of headache with acute cerebral ischemia suggests at least temporary ischemia of the large artery territory, even if only a subcortical, "lacunar" infarct is seen on CT scans or MR images (not all small-artery "occlusions" are caused by small-artery "disease"). Despite traditional teaching, it is unclear whether headaches are more common in association with cardioembolic rather than atherosclerotic stroke. CT findings often are normal in the first 24 to 48 hours of ischemic stroke. Stroke should be the first thought when a patient has an acute focal neurologic deficit with headache. Patients with acute focal brain or brainstem dysfunction, headache, and normal CT findings or CT scans that show focal hypodensity need a thorough evaluation for a cause of ischemic stroke or TIA. The evaluation should

include assessment of cerebral arteries and the heart for a source of embolism and, in certain circumstances, assessment of the aorta and blood (hypercoagulability or vasculitis profile).

6. **Cervicocephalic arterial dissection** is often—but not always—associated with trauma. When trauma is the cause, symptoms may be delayed for several minutes to hours. Headache, facial pain, or neck pain may be the only symptom. Carotid dissection usually results in ipsilateral, steady, nonthrobbing headache and ipsilateral Horner's syndrome. Pain in the throat and focal cerebral ischemia also are prominent. Vertebrobasilar dissection causes occipital headache or neck pain and may be associated with neck manipulation or whiplash injury. Definitive diagnosis of arterial dissection requires MRI or cerebral angiography. MRI cross-sections of the artery typically show a circle of increased signal intensity (subintimal blood) surrounding a small area of low signal intensity (normal flow in a narrowed lumen). At cerebral arteriography, the classic finding is a tapered narrowing or occlusion.

7. **Giant cell arteritis** is almost exclusively a disease of persons older than 50 years and is much more prevalent among those older than 60 years. It should be considered when any person older than 50 years has a persistent or new headache. The term "temporal arteritis" is misleading because this condition often affects the short posterior choroidal arteries of the eye and branches of the external carotid artery other than the temporal artery. It also can affect the cerebral and coronary arteries. Possible associated symptoms include visual loss (arteritic anterior ischemic optic neuropathy), temporal tenderness, weight loss, malaise, fever, chills, polymyalgia rheumatica (pain without tenderness in the shoulders, neck, and hips), and jaw claudication. Anemia, leukocytosis, and elevated liver enzyme levels may be present. CRP elevation is more sensitive and more specific than is ESR elevation. Definitive diagnosis is made by means of temporal artery biopsy. Administration of steroids should be started as soon as serologic results are known. Treatment does not affect biopsy results for at least 2 weeks. Because of the frequent presence of skip lesions, long segments of artery should be obtained, and bilateral biopsy may be necessary.

8. **Cerebral venous thrombosis** is likely more common than previously thought and often goes unrecognized. It is a condition that occurs as a consequence of a predisposing disease. Diffuse headache due to increased intracranial pressure may be the only symptom. Other common symptoms include seizure, focal neurologic deficit, and change in consciousness. Predisposing conditions fall into one of three categories—hypercoagulable state, low-flow state, and vessel wall abnormality. Primary hypercoagulable states include deficiencies in the naturally occurring anticoagulants, lupus anticoagulant, and anticardiolipin antibodies (see **IV.A.6.**). A personal or family history of clotting episodes (deep venous thrombosis, pulmonary embolism, stroke, myocardial infarction, or several miscarriages) suggests a primary hypercoagulable state. Secondary hypercoagulable states include those associated with late pregnancy, the puerperium, and cancer. Low-flow states include dehydration, anemia, congestive heart failure, sickle-cell disease, and compression of cerebral sinus by tumor. Vessel-wall abnormalities can be caused by trauma, infection, cancer, or inflammation. Because the cerebral sinuses lie in the midline, lesions often are bilateral and parasagittal. Venous edema, infarction, or hemorrhage can occur; edema and infarct cannot be differentiated at cerebral imaging. CT findings often are suggestive but are not enough to make a diagnosis. MRI and MRV are the diagnostic studies of choice. One also can make the diagnosis with conventional cerebral angiography and delayed venous images. Cerebral venous thrombosis should be considered in the evaluation of any patient with a "pseudotumor" syndrome, especially men and thin women (see **V.B.9.**), any patient with headache and a history consistent with hypercoagulable state, and any patient with headache and bilateral "infarcts" or hemorrhages on cerebral images.

9. **Idiopathic intracranial hypertension (pseudotumor cerebri)** occurs mainly among young women who are obese. The diagnosis is based on the clinical findings of headache and papilledema, normal findings at cerebral imaging, and elevated opening CSF pressure (more than 250 mm Hg) at LP. Brain tumor and cerebral venous thrombosis in particular must be ruled out. Papilledema need not be present for diagnosis. The serious sequela of idiopathic intracranial hypertension is blindness due to chronic papilledema. Several drugs can cause intracranial hypertension, mimicking the idiopathic condition; these include tetracycline, aminoglycosides, and vitamin A. The syndrome of intracranial hypertension in a patient taking oral contraceptives should stimulate investigation for cerebral venous thrombosis, because oral contraceptives can exacerbate or cause a hypercoagulable state.

10. **Unruptured AVM** can cause migraine-like headaches. If an apparent migraineur always has hemicranial headaches on the same side, and there is no known family history of migraine (realizing the pitfalls of family headache history), one should use MRI to rule out unruptured AVM. It is likely that ischemia or rapid changes in cerebral blood flow incite spreading cortical depression and a migraine-like attack.

11. **Post–carotid endarterectomy** headaches occur in approximately 40% of patients undergoing the procedure. The headache usually develops several hours to days after endarterectomy, is ipsilateral to the side of the operation, and resembles a migraine. Patients with a history of migraine may have a typical attack. The presence of associated focal neurologic symptoms is concerning to patient and physician alike, but usually the headache lasts only a few hours and the neurologic symptoms resolve without sequelae. Nausea often is present. As is the case with AVM, the rapid change in cerebral blood flow may incite spreading cortical depression and migraine-like phenomena. Seizures and intracerebral hemorrhage also can occur after endarterectomy and should be included in the differential diagnosis.

12. **Bell's palsy,** idiopathic or herpetic mononeuropathy of cranial nerve VII, often is associated with retroauricular pain. Pain may be the first symptom and may be severe enough to be the patient's chief symptom, rather than the ipsilateral facial weakness involving the forehead, eye closure, and lips.

13. **Cerebral tumors and abscesses** usually manifest similarly as gradually progressive headache over weeks to months. They also may be associated with gradually progressive neurologic deficit. Both primary brain tumors and metastatic lesions can occur acutely if associated with hemorrhage or seizure. Abscesses generally do not hemorrhage, but they frequently cause seizures and can be associated with fever and other signs of sepsis. Any patient with a known history of cancer and new headache should be evaluated for cerebral metastasis. Colloid cysts may manifest as positional headaches, as in **II.C.2.**

14. **Dental abscesses** usually manifest as oral or jaw pain, but if the patient is not treated, these abscesses may cause more diffuse headache.

15. **Sinusitis** is a much less common cause of acute headache than is generally imagined. A sensation of nasal congestion is common in migraine owing to vasodilatation in the external carotid territory; this can even cause clear nasal drainage or mild nose bleed. Surgery for sinusitis should not be undertaken to manage the headache alone, because for most patients, the headache associated with sinus congestion is due to migraine. The diagnosis of sinusitis is more likely if the headache is associated with fever, purulent nasal discharge, cranial sinuses that are exquisitely tender to palpation, and increased densities in the sinuses on CT scans.

16. **Trigeminal neuralgia** usually is described as a sharp or burning pain rather than an ache and most commonly occurs unilaterally in the maxillary distribution of the trigeminal nerve, that is, over the cheek. It can occur sporadically or represent a symptom of multiple sclerosis (see Chapter 40).

17. **Low-CSF-pressure headache** can occur when CSF pressure is abnormally low, as occurs after LP (post-LP headache) or after nerve root sleeve

trauma and subsequent CSF leak. Symptoms typically resolve in the supine position and recur when the patient is upright.

18. **Acute glaucoma** often manifests as periorbital headache. Pupillary changes, conjunctival injection, lens clouding, and a globe hard to palpation are typical. Elevated intraocular pressure confirms the diagnosis.

19. **Arterial hypertension** most often occurs as a result of rather than as a cause of headache. Migraine and stroke both cause arterial blood pressure to increase. Headache can occur, however, when there is marked, acute in crease in blood pressure due to pheochromocytoma or ingestion of certain drugs, such as cocaine, amphetamines, phenylpropanolamine, and monoamine oxidase inhibitors. Such patients often are confused ("encephalopathic"), and papilledema may be present.

VI. Diagnostic approach. The diagnosis of primary headache conditions is based on a supportive detailed history and normal findings at neurologic examination. If the clinician has any suspicion at all that the patient may be having a secondary headache, a series of diagnostic tests is indicated to determine the cause of headache. Many of the conditions that cause secondary headache are fatal or disabling if the patient is left untreated. Fortunately, in many cases the conditions can be managed. Figure 20.2 depicts a diagnostic algorithm for patients with suspected acute secondary headache. If a patient has any one of the clinical features suggestive of secondary headache, the diagnostic evaluation should be undertaken, beginning with laboratories and noncontrast CT.

VII. Referral

A. **Primary headache.** Migraine, cluster, "tension-type," and analgesic rebound headaches are chronic conditions that manifest acutely. The proper management of primary headache conditions requires long-term care. Once the acute-care clinician diagnoses primary headache and offers emergency treatment, he or she is obligated to counsel the patient regarding the importance of long-term care and to refer the patient to a neurologist or generalist for definitive treatment. Increased patient education leads to improved patient care and lower health care costs by not spending emergency department resources on patients with recurrent headache.

B. **Secondary headache.** After initial diagnosis and emergency management, the definitive treatment of patients with secondary headache usually requires admission to the hospital and referral to a specialist. A neurosurgeon should be intimately involved with all aspects of care of patients with subarachnoid hemorrhage, subdural hematoma, or epidural hematoma. Patients with intracranial masses need immediate referral to a neurologist and often a neurosurgeon as well. If the mass turns out to be a tumor, referral to a neurooncologist may be necessary. If the mass is an abscess, referral to a specialist in infectious diseases is appropriate. Most patients with sinusitis and headache are best cared for by a generalist or infectious disease expert. Referral to an otolaryngologist is appropriate if surgery is deemed necessary. Patients with suspected giant cell arteritis should be treated with high-dose steroids by the acute-care clinician and then referred immediately to both a physician for long-term therapy with steroids (usually a neurologist or rheumatologist) and a surgeon for temporal artery biopsy (usually an ophthalmologist or neurosurgeon). One should not wait for the biopsy before beginning treatment with steroids. Patients with cerebral venous thrombosis need immediate referral to a neurologist or primary care physician for anticoagulation and hypercoagulability evaluation. These patients also should be treated in the acute setting by an ophthalmologist who follows visual fields carefully and performs optic nerve sheath fenestration if necessary.

Recommended Readings

Clinch CR. Evaluation of acute headaches in adults. *Am Fam Physician* 2001;63:685–692.

Diamond ML. Emergency department management of the acute headache. *Clin Cornerstone* 1999;1:45–54.

Ducharme J, Beveridge RC, Lee JS, et al. Emergency management of migraine: is the headache really over? *Acad Emerg Med* 1998;5:899–905.

Edmeads JG. Headache as a symptom of organic diseases. *Curr Opin Neurol* 1995;8:233–236.

Evans RW. Diagnostic testing for the evaluation of headaches. *Neurol Clin* 1996;14:1–26.

Goadsby PJ. Current concepts of the pathophysiology of migraine. *Neurol Clin* 1997;15:27–42.

Gordon DL. Cerebral venous thrombosis. In: Biller J, Mathews KD, Love BB, eds. *Stroke in children and young adults*. Boston: Butterworth–Heinemann, 1994:165–190.

Koudstaal P, van Gijn J, Kappelle J. Headache in transient or permanent cerebral ischemia. *Stroke* 1991;22:754–759.

Kurita H, Ueki K, Shin M, et al. Headaches in patients with radiosurgically treated occipital arteriovenous malformations. *J Neurosurg* 2000;93:224–228.

Lewis DW, Qureshi F. Acute headaches in children and adolescents presenting to the emergency department. *Headache* 2000; 40:200–203.

Mathew NT. Cluster headache. *Neurology* 1992;42[Suppl 2]:22–31.

May A, Goadsby PJ. The trigeminal system in humans: pathophysiologic implications for primary headache syndromes of the neural influences on the cerebral circulation. *J Cereb Blood Flow Metab* 1999;19:115–127.

Moskowitz MA. Basic mechanisms in vascular headache. *Neurol Clin* 1990;8:801–815.

Moskowitz MA. Neurogenic inflammation in the pathophysiology and treatment of migraine. *Neurology* 1993;43[suppl 3]:S16–S20.

Olesen J, Tfelt-Hansen P, Welch KMA, eds. *The headaches*. New York: Raven Press, 1993.

Rapoport AM, Silberstein SD. Emergency treatment of headache. *Neurology* 1992;42[suppl 2]:43–44.

Raskin NH. *Headache,* 2nd ed. New York: Churchill Livingstone, 1988.

Ries S, Steinke W, Neff W, et al. Ischemia-induced migraine from paradoxical cardioembolic stroke. *Eur Neurol* 1996;36:76–78.

Saper JR, Silberstein SD, Gordon CD, et al. *Handbook of headache management*. Baltimore: Williams & Wilkins, 1993.

Shuper A, Packer RJ, Vezina LG, et al. "Complicated migraine-like episodes" in children following cranial irradiation and chemotherapy. *Neurology* 1995; 45:1837–1840.

Silberstein SD. Advances in understanding the pathophysiology of headache. *Neurology* 1992;42[Suppl 2]:6–10.

21. APPROACH TO THE PATIENT WITH CHRONIC AND RECURRENT HEADACHE

David S. Lefkowitz

I. Primary headache disorders. Most chronic and recurrent headaches represent a benign recurrent headache syndrome. Migraine, tension-type headache, cluster headache, and chronic daily headache represent the overwhelming majority of headaches encountered in primary care. Chronic daily headache is common in referral-based practices specializing in headache. A revised classification of headache was published by the International Headache Society (IHS) in 1988. The classification scheme is phenomenologic and is based on symptoms and signs. The system in the *International Classification of Diseases of the World Health Organization* (ICD-10) published in 1997 is almost identical. The characteristics of various forms of primary benign recurrent headache are described herein and are summarized in Table 21.1.

   A. Migraine. Migraine is no longer referred to as "migraine headache of the vascular type" in the IHS system to reflect the growing consensus that migraine is a neurogenic disorder and that observed vascular changes are secondary phenomena.

   1. The following **clinical characteristics** of migraine are outlined in the IHS classification system.

      a. The duration of headache is 4 to 72 hours.

      b. The quality of headache fulfills at least two of the following criteria: unilaterality, pulsatility, moderate to severe intensity, and aggravation by routine physical activity.

      c. At least one of the following associated features is present: nausea or vomiting, photophobia, and phonophobia.

      d. Migraine, like other benign headache syndromes, is a diagnosis of exclusion without evidence of organic disease.

      e. A history of stereotypy is sought. There should be at least five such episodes if there is no aura, at least two if an aura is present.

   2. Migraine may be associated with **focal neurologic symptoms and signs.** A distinction is made between migraine with aura, in which neurologic features are present (formerly classic migraine) and migraine without aura (formerly common migraine). A spreading wave of cortical depolarization analogous to spreading depression of Leão may be an important mechanism in migraine with aura.

      a. By definition, the **aura** should meet at least three of the following criteria:

         (1) It consists of one or more fully reversible symptoms of focal cerebral or brainstem dysfunction.

         (2) One aura symptom develops gradually over more than 4 minutes. If two or more symptoms occur, they do so in succession.

         (3) No aura symptom lasts more than 60 minutes, or proportionately longer if there is more than one.

         (4) Headache follows within 1 hour of the aura, precedes the aura, or occurs simultaneously with it. An aura need not begin before the headache.

      b. Typical migraine auras include homonymous visual disturbance, unilateral paresthesia or numbness, unilateral weakness, aphasia, or unclassifiable speech disturbance. Sensory auras typically have a cheirooral distribution, and there may be a "march" from one body part to another.

      c. Migraine with prolonged aura (formerly referred to as complicated migraine) may be diagnosed if at least one aura symptom persists for more than 1 hour but less than 7 days and neuroimaging studies remain normal.

      d. Migrainous infarction is classified as a complication of migraine. It occurs when symptoms of the aura do not completely resolve within 7 days and there is evidence of infarction on imaging studies.

      e. Migraine aura without headache (previously referred to as migraine equivalent) occurs when the aura is not followed by a headache.

Table 21.1 Characteristics of benign recurrent headache disorders

Characteristic	Migraine	Tension-type headache	Cluster	Chronic daily headache
Age at onset	10–30 y	Any age	Middle age	3rd–4th decade
Sex	F > M	F > M	M > F	F > M
Duration	4–72 h	30 min–7 d	15–180 min	Constant or nearly constant
Frequency	Variable	Occasional to daily	At least daily for weeks to months	Daily or constant
Time of day	Any time	Later in day	Nocturnal	Constant
Quality	Pulsatile	Dull, aching, bandlike	Severe, boring	Variable
Location	Retroorbital, temporal, hemicranial or holocephalic	Bilateral, temporal or occipitonuchal	Unilateral, retroorbital	Variable
Associated symptoms	Nausea, vomiting, photophobia, phonophobia with or without neurologic accompaniments	Other symptoms rare, associated with stress in episodic form	Ipsilateral autonomic symptoms	Migraine history, analgesic abuse and psycho-pathologic condition common

3. Migraine often is associated with specific endogenous or environmental triggers, including ingestion of tyramine-containing foods, use of alcohol, changes in sleep pattern, and emotional stress. There also is a relation with hormonal factors. Migraine is more common among women than among men after the age of menarche. For most women, migraine is more frequent or severe at or around menses, and the headaches often are relieved after menopause.

B. **Tension-type headache** was previously referred to as "tension" or "muscle contraction headache" but the term has been changed in the IHS system because of evidence that muscle tension is not the underlying mechanism of pain.

  1. **Clinical characteristics** of tension-type headache include the following features:

    a. Headache duration is 30 minutes to 7 days.

    b. Pain conforms to at least two of the following: pressing or tightening in quality, nonpulsatile, mild to moderately intense, bilateral, not aggravated by routine physical activity.

    c. There should be no nausea or vomiting, although anorexia does occur. Photophobia or phonophobia may occur but not simultaneously.

    d. There is no evidence of organic disease.

  2. There may or may not be tenderness or increased electromyographic activity of pericranial muscles.

  3. Tension-type headache is episodic when there are fewer than 15 headache days per month or 180 days per year for at least 6 months and chronic when headache frequency exceeds these limits.

  4. There should be a history of 10 similar headaches.

C. Differentiating migraine from episodic tension-type headache.
   1. Benign recurrent headache. It has been postulated that migraine and tension-type headache are different phenotypic expressions of a common abnormality of serotoninergic nociceptive mechanisms referred to as *benign recurrent headache.* As frequency increases, headache severity and the association with autonomic and neurologic symptoms decreases.
   2. For some patients, it may be difficult to differentiate migraine without aura from episodic tension-type headache because both can be bilateral, nonthrobbing, moderately severe, and associated with anorexia, photophobia, or phonophobia without violating IHS criteria.
   3. Multiple headache types may exist in the same patient. IHS criteria do not recognize the existence of combined or mixed headaches that have properties of both migraine and tension-type headache.
D. Cluster headache. The clinical manifestations of cluster headache are quite characteristic, and the disorder is readily diagnosed from the history and physical examination findings.
   1. A diagnosis can be made with IHS criteria when there have been five or more attacks with the following features:
      a. Severe unilateral supraorbital or temporal pain lasting 15 to 180 minutes. The pain is usually described as boring in quality.
      b. Patients invariably have at least one ipsilateral autonomic sign, including conjunctival injection, eyelid edema, lacrimation, nasal congestion or rhinorrhea, forehead and facial sweating, miosis, or ptosis secondary to oculosympathetic paresis.
      c. Attacks occur from once every other day to eight times a day. There is a tendency for attacks to occur at the same time each day or to awaken the patient from sleep, usually in the early morning when the patient enters rapid eye movement sleep.
   2. The **typical episodic pattern,** for which this entity is named, consists of periods of headache lasting 1 week to 1 year separated by remissions of at least 2 weeks. When recurrent headaches persist for at least 1 year without interruption or if remission lasts less than 2 weeks, the disorder is referred to as **chronic cluster headache.** A chronic pattern may develop in patients who have had typical episodic cluster headache, in which case it is known as **secondary chronic cluster.**
E. Variants of cluster headache
   1. Chronic paroxysmal hemicrania is now classified as a variant of cluster headache. This is an unusual disorder that mainly affects women with multiple, brief, unilateral, cluster-like headaches occurring daily and absolute response to indomethacin.
   2. Raeder's paratrigeminal neuralgia. Raeder originally described five patients with a parasellar syndrome of neuralgic pain in the trigeminal distribution, oculosympathetic paresis, and dysfunction of the trigeminal and several other cranial nerves. The term *Raeder's syndrome* has come to be applied to a different syndrome of nonneuralgic head pain and oculosympathetic paresis without other cranial nerve palsies. This latter syndrome usually represents a variant of cluster headache.
   3. Cluster headache variant is an entity consisting of multiple daily atypical cluster headaches, a constant background vascular headache, multiple sharp jabs, and response to indomethacin.
   4. Lower-half headache refers to several arcane syndromes, referred to variously as *Sluder's neuralgia, sphenopalatine neuralgia, vidian neuralgia,* and *greater superficial petrosal neuralgia,* which manifest as facial pain and ipsilateral nasal congestion or rhinorrhea. These syndromes probably represent cluster headache.
F. Chronic daily headache.
   1. Chronic daily headache is defined as a primary headache disorder in which headaches occur at least 15 days per month.
   2. The IHS classification is of limited value in this area. Most cases of chronic daily headache are classified according to IHS criteria as chronic tension-type

headache, although most evolve from migraine and represent transformed migraine. Many patients with chronic tension-type headache have acute exacerbations of headache fulfilling IHS criteria for migraine. Chronic daily headache without antecedent migraine or tension-type headache has been referred to as *new daily persistent headache.*

   3. **Analgesic rebound headache.** Rebound or withdrawal headache related to overuse of narcotics, butalbital-containing analgesics, ergotamine, or over the counter pain medications frequently is a factor in chronic daily headache. These patients have a rhythmic cycle of headache and medication use. The patient awakens with early morning headache resulting from medication withdrawal, and the headache is relieved only by the next dose of medication. Patients may begin to use analgesics in anticipation of pain. Other symptoms of medication withdrawal include irritability, asthenia, and insomnia.
   4. **Hemicrania continua** is a type of chronic daily headache that is unilateral, moderately severe, and usually associated with autonomic signs similar to those of cluster headache and responsive to indomethacin.
G. **Idiopathic stabbing headache** sometimes is referred to descriptively as *jabs and jots* or *ice pick pains.* It frequently occurs in association with other primary headache syndromes such as migraine or cluster headache. The clinical pattern is distinctive, and the diagnostic criteria are as follows:
   1. Pain is localized to the head, mainly to the distribution of the ophthalmic division of the trigeminal nerve.
   2. The pain is stabbing in quality, lasts for a fraction of a second, and may occur singly or in series.
   3. Headache recurs at irregular intervals of hours to days.
   4. There are no structural changes at the site of the pain or in the distribution of the affected nerve.
II. **Secondary headache disorders.** Headache frequently is a symptom of disorders of the nervous system.
   A. **Tumor.** Head pain among patients with brain tumors arises from traction or pressure on pain-sensitive intracranial structures or from production of increased intracranial pressure. There is nothing pathognomonic about headache among patients with brain tumor, but there are some general rules.
   1. In most cases, headache is described as dull, aching, or pressure-like and resembles tension-type headache in quality. The headache is intermittent and moderate to severe in most patients. Worsening with bending or a Valsalva maneuver is not unusual. Headache from brain tumor rarely mimics migraine.
   2. A "typical" history of severe headache worse in the morning and associated with nausea or vomiting is relatively rare, as is a history of postural, cough, or exertional headache.
   3. Unilateral headache usually is on the side of the lesion. Bilateral headache usually is due to increased intracranial pressure or either midline or bilateral tumor.
   4. Supratentorial tumors generally produce frontal or bifrontal headache, which is relatively mild.
   5. The headache of infratentorial tumor is generally localized to the occiput.
   6. Increased intracranial pressure produces severe headache in the frontal area, vertex, or neck with nausea and vomiting.
   7. Involvement of the dura or skull may produce localized pain.
   B. **Cerebrovascular disease**
   1. **Intracranial hemorrhage.** Headache, nausea, and vomiting are more commonly associated with intracranial hemorrhage than with ischemic stroke. In some patients, recurrent subarachnoid hemorrhage may resemble migraine. Patients with aneurysmal subarachnoid hemorrhage often have a warning leak or sentinel headache several days to months before substantial hemorrhage occurs.
   2. **Unruptured aneurysms.** It is controversial how often unruptured aneurysms cause recurrent headache. In some patients, sudden onset of an intense

headache referred to as **thunderclap headache** simulates subarachnoid hemorrhage but actually represents a benign syndrome that may be a variant of migraine. Day and Raskin described a patient with recurrent thunderclap headache who proved to have an unruptured internal carotid artery aneurysm. The headaches ceased after surgical correction of the aneurysm. They hypothesized that stretching of the aneurysm wall accounted for the headaches. Thunderclap headache also may be associated with angiographic evidence of segmental narrowing or spasm.

3. **Arteriovenous malformation.** Chronic headache occurs in approximately 15% of patients with arteriovenous malformation. These headaches may be clinically indistinguishable from migraine. This relation may be coincidental because migraine is common in the general population and because arteriovenous malformation is rare in large series of patients with migraine who undergo imaging studies.

4. **Cerebral ischemia.** Headache occurs in 30% to 40% of patients with cerebral infarction and 25% to 40% of those with transient ischemia. It is usually nonthrobbing, ipsilateral to the infarct, and self-limited.

5. **Sinovenous thrombosis.** Occlusion of a major dural sinus frequently produces a syndrome of headache and papilledema indistinguishable from pseudotumor cerebri. Sinovenous occlusion should be suspected whenever acute or subacute neurologic dysfunction manifests as altered consciousness, focal deficits, seizures, or evidence of increased intracranial pressure.

6. In patients with chronic or recurrent headache associated with stroke, the following differential diagnoses should be considered:

   a. **Cervicocephalic dissection.** An ipsilateral throbbing or steady headache, with or without neck or jaw pain, frequently accompanies carotid dissections. Dissection may produce fixed or reversible neurologic deficits. Oculosympathetic paresis, visual scintillations, and dysgeusia are also clues to this diagnosis. Dissections may be overlooked when they occur without a previous history of trauma or after relatively trivial injuries.

   b. **Migrainous stroke and late-life migraine accompaniments.** When headache recurs in association with focal neurologic deficit, it may be challenging to distinguish between migrainous accompaniments and atherosclerotic cerebrovascular disease, especially in elderly patients. There need not be a history of preexisting migraine, and headache does not have to be a prominent feature of the individual episodes. Fisher suggested the following criteria for late-life migraine accompaniments.

      (1) Scintillations or other typical visual displays which may expand or "build up" after onset.

      (2) A sensory "march" from one body part to another or spread to the opposite side of the body.

      (3) Progression from one accompaniment to another without delay.

      (4) Episodes may be stereotyped, which should be less common with embolism.

      (5) Headache is frequently associated with the episode.

      (6) The attacks occur in characteristic flurries during mid- or late life and have a benign course.

      (7) Other causes of focal deficit, including atherosclerosis, should be excluded.

C. **Headaches resulting from disorders of intracranial pressure**

   1. **Pseudotumor cerebri or benign intracranial hypertension (BIH)**

      a. The primary features of this disorder are headache and visual disturbance (enlargement of the blind spot, visual obscurations, and progressive visual loss) resulting from elevated intracranial pressure. There may also be pulsatile tinnitus, dizziness, and nausea.

      b. BIH occurs most often in women. It is frequently associated with obesity and menstrual irregularities.

      c. Physical findings are limited to papilledema and nonlocalizing abducens nerve palsies. Papilledema may be unilateral, asymmetric, or absent.

     d. Cerebrospinal fluid (CSF) is acellular with elevated pressure, and the protein content may be low.

     e. Imaging may reveal slitlike ventricles or an empty sella, but no mass lesion. In some patients with BIH, imaging studies may reveal thrombosis of the superior sagittal or lateral sinuses. Sinovenous occlusion associated with ear infection has been referred to by the misnomer "otitic hydrocephalus."

     f. Most cases are idiopathic. BIH may be due to vitamin A intoxication, steroid withdrawal, hypoparathyroidism, systemic lupus erythematosus, or medications (tetracycline, nalidixic acid).

     g. BIH without papilledema should be considered in the differential of chronic daily headache.

  2. Hydrocephalus.

     a. Headache is not usually a feature of communicating hydrocephalus.

     b. Headache is common with obstructive hydrocephalus. It is usually occipital and may be associated with neck pain or stiffness, vomiting, or visual abnormalities. The headache may be present on awakening and more severe in the morning. Obstructive hydrocephalus resulting from intraventricular tumors may cause positional headache and life-threatening increases in intracranial pressure.

D. Pheochromocytoma. Approximately 10% of patients with pheochromocytoma present with headache and paroxysmal hypertension. The headache is usually bifrontal, severe, and throbbing. It may be exacerbated by coughing, bending, straining, or lying flat.

E. Inflammatory disorders

  1. Giant cell arteritis is rare before age 50 but increases in incidence with advancing age. Headache is almost invariably present. It is often localized to the temple and is sharp, throbbing, or boring in quality. There may be constitutional symptoms, joint complaints, or jaw claudication. Blindness is the most feared complication and results from ischemic optic neuropathy. Diplopia may arise from ischemia of oculomotor nerves or extraocular muscles.

  2. Physical findings include a tender, nodular, nonpulsatile, thickened superficial temporal artery.

  3. Diagnosis. The Westergren erythrocyte sedimentation rate is elevated in approximately 85% of patients. Other common laboratory abnormalities include elevated C-reactive protein, thrombocytosis, and anemia. Definitive diagnosis rests on the use of superficial temporal artery biopsy, but the biopsy may be negative because of patchy involvement (skip lesions).

  4. Systemic lupus erythematosus (SLE)

     a. Migrainous headaches, often associated with focal neurologic auras, occur frequently in patients with systemic lupus. Visual scintillations have been reported anecdotally as the presenting symptom of lupus. In a case-controlled prospective study of patients with SLE, there was a higher incidence of migraine, a higher percentage of migraine with aura, and later age of onset of migraine than in controls. There was also a tendency for headaches to parallel the activity of the lupus and sometimes to respond to steroids or immunosuppressive therapy.

     b. There is no proven association of antiphospholipid antibodies with migraine in SLE patients or with neurologic deficits in migraine patients who do not have lupus.

F. Post-traumatic headache

  1. Postconcussion syndrome is a distinct clinical entity following relatively minor head injuries that is manifested by recurrent headache, memory disturbances, irritability, difficulty concentrating, dizziness, and depressive symptoms. There is still controversy surrounding the etiology of the syndrome and how much of the symptomatology may be related to psychological factors or "compensation neurosis." Symptoms resolve within 6 months in most patients.

  2. Chronic subdural hematoma may present with headache, seizures or focal neurologic deficits.

3. **Intracranial hypotension.** The typical history includes postural headache with or without nausea and dizziness, which is worsened or initiated by assumption of the upright position and relieved by recumbency. The diagnosis is obvious when there is a history of a preceding lumbar puncture (LP).

    a. Postlumbar puncture headache may occasionally be protracted or complicate the evaluation of patients with chronic or recurrent headaches resulting from other causes. Demographic features associated with post lumbar puncture headache are youth, female gender, and lower body mass index (BMI). Technical aspects affecting the risk of post lumbar puncture headache include needle diameter, use of cutting (Quincke) needles and orientation of the bevel but not the duration of recumbency after the procedure or hydration.

    b. CSF hypotension may occur without a history of diagnostic LP as a result of CSF leakage following head trauma, Valsalva maneuver, or nerve-root avulsion.

    c. The diagnosis may be confirmed by low CSF pressure on repeat lumbar puncture. MR imaging demonstrates diffuse dural enhancement, descent of the cerebellar tonsils and subdural fluid collections.

4. **Occipital neuralgia.** The occipital nerve may be traumatized directly or compressed by spasm of the trapezius or semispinalis capitis muscle. There is usually a lancinating, neuralgic component to the pain, a Tinel's sign with percussion over the occipital condyle and decreased sensation over the ipsilateral occipital scalp.

5. **Post-traumatic migraine and tension-type headaches.** In some patients, head trauma may precipitate headaches identical in quality to migraine or tension-type headache or aggravate pre-existing ones. Post-traumatic cluster headache has also been reported. In some patients, headache is associated with scarring at the site of a scalp laceration and is relieved by infiltration of a local anesthetic.

6. **Post-traumatic dysautonomic cephalalgia.** Vijayan and Dreyfus described this syndrome in 1975. Throbbing headaches associated with nausea, photophobia, and signs of ipsilateral sympathetic overactivity such as sweating and mydriasis occur as delayed sequelae of penetrating neck injuries that damage the sympathetic fibers in the carotid sheath. This disorder should not be confused with cluster headache, which it superficially resembles.

G. **Temporomandibular joint (TMJ) dysfunction** is believed to be a myofascial syndrome related to dental malocclusion or bruxism. It may cause recurrent preauricular or temporal pain radiating into the neck. The pain is typically aggravated by chewing and is frequently worse in the morning. Physical findings include lateral jaw deviation and crepitus of the joint on opening the mouth and tenderness or spasm of the masticatory muscles.

H. **Trigeminal neuralgia** is often mentioned in the differential diagnosis of cluster headache, although typical trigeminal neuralgia is rarely confused with other entities. Onset usually occurs late in life except when it is a manifestation of multiple sclerosis.

    1. The IHS defines trigeminal neuralgia as follows.

        a. Paroxysmal attacks of facial or frontal pain lasting a few seconds to less than one minute.

        b. The attacks have at least four of the following characteristics.

            (1) Distribution along one or more divisions of the trigeminal nerve.

            (2) Sudden, intense, sharp, superficial, stabbing or burning quality.

            (3) Severe intensity.

            (4) Precipitation by stimulation of trigger areas or by daily activities such as eating, talking, washing the face, or cleaning the teeth.

            (5) The patient is asymptomatic between the paroxysms.

        c. Absence of neurologic deficit.

        d. Attacks are stereotyped.

    2. Most cases result from microvascular compression of the trigeminal nerve, but secondary causes include cerebellopontine angle tumors or vascular malformations.

III. Evaluation

    A. History. The history is the most important factor in the accurate diagnosis of headache. It is usually helpful to ask the patient to describe a typical headache from its onset. It is important to remember that as many as 30% to 40% of headache patients have more than one headache type and an accurate description should be obtained for each. Because the head does not exist in isolation, disorders of other organ systems may cause or modify headache. Therefore, the physician must inquire about general symptoms and signs of (CNS) dysfunction and conduct a detailed review of the medical history. The headache history should specifically include questions regarding the following areas.

        1. Age of onset. Onset of most benign headache syndromes occurs early in life, usually between childhood and the third decade, although tension-type headache may begin at any time. Late onset may suggest a more serious condition.

        2. Localization of pain. The location of headache may help in determining its etiology. Migraine is frequently unilateral, alternates sides, and involves the temple or retro-orbital area. Tension-type headache is usually bilateral, frontal, or occipital, and radiates into the neck and shoulders. Brief attacks of strictly unilateral orbital pain suggest cluster headache or chronic paroxysmal hemicrania. Dental, ocular, and sinus disorders often produce frontal pain. The site of headache may be of localizing value in patients with mass lesions, as discussed above (see section **II.A**).

        3. Temporal pattern. Headache syndromes may have characteristic patterns of headache duration and frequency. In general, longer-lasting headaches tend to be benign, particularly when headache is constant over more than several months without change in character or development of new signs. Headache resulting from meningitis may be constant, but not usually over a prolonged duration. Benign headache syndromes typically produce episodic headache. For instance, migraine usually lasts several hours and occurs several times a month. Cluster headache has a characteristic periodicity. Acute tension-type headache is usually brief and associated with emotional stress, but in its chronic form, tension-type headache becomes more frequent, prolonged, or constant and loses its association with psychosocial stressors. The mode of onset may also be helpful. Does the headache begin gradually or start suddenly? Sudden onset of headache is of greater concern because it may indicate intraparenchymal or subarachnoid hemorrhage.

        4. Quality and severity of pain. These are often very difficult for patients to verbalize. There is a tendency for the headache patient to describe severity when asked about the quality of pain. It may be necessary for the interviewer to provide the patient with some pain characteristics from which to choose. Migraine and headache associated with fever are usually throbbing and pulsatile, for instance. Tension-type headache is usually described as dull and nagging, tight and constricting, or bandlike. Tumor and meningitis typically produce a steady, aching pain. Severity of pain can be ranked on a scale of 1 to 10. An indirect indicator of severity is interference with work and social activities.

        5. Prodromal and associated symptoms. Symptoms that precede or coincide with headache onset may be valuable clues to the nature of the underlying headache. The patient with migraine may have mood or behavioral changes for several days prior to headache. Visual scintillations and fortification spectra are typical migraine prodromes, but visual symptoms may also be associated with carotid dissections and occipital arteriovenous malformations. Ipsilateral autonomic features are almost always present in cluster headache, the paroxysmal hemicranias, hemicrania continua, and short lasting unilateral neuralgiform headache with conjunctival injection and tearing (SUNCT).

        6. Precipitating factors. Provoking factors may suggest the diagnosis. Examples include precipitation of an attack of trigeminal neuralgia by cutaneous stimulation or of migraine by ingestion of certain foods or alcohol, stressful life events, glare, hypoglycemia, or sleep deprivation. Chewing may produce pain in patients with temporomandibular joint dysfunction or giant cell arteritis. Identification of precipitants may also provide information that will be helpful in treatment.

   7. Sleep onset. Migraine, hypertension, and cluster headache may awaken patients from sleep. Tension-type headache does so only rarely.

   8. Relieving or exacerbating factors. Patients with migraine typically report exacerbation of pain by movement, bending, straining, and coughing and relief with lying flat, avoiding bright light, sometimes by pressure over the superficial temporal artery or after vomiting. Post lumbar puncture headache is characteristically modified by postural factors.

   9. Family history. About 20% to 60% of patients with migraine report at least one affected family member. However, 6% of men and 18% of women report migraine, and thus it is not unusual for the family history to be positive for migraine in patients with other types of headaches.

B. Physical examination. Vital signs should be checked for fever and hypertension. In addition to a thorough general and neurologic examination, certain areas require special attention.

   1. Inspection, palpation, and percussion of the skull should be performed to check for signs of trauma, including areas of localized tenderness or scarring. There may be tenderness at the site of a skull neoplasm. Percussion over the site of a tumor or subdural hematoma may also produce pain. In children, head circumference should always be measured.

   2. Assessment of the ears, tympanic membranes, and mastoids may reveal evidence of otitis or mastoiditis.

   3. Evaluation of the temporomandibular joints. The temporomandibular joint and masticatory muscles may be tender to palpation, or there may be crepitus when the patient opens and closes the mouth. This can be felt externally or with the examiner's fingers in the external auditory canals. The jaw should also be observed for lateral deviation when the mouth is opened. When temporomandibular joint dysfunction results from muscle spasm, the joint is tender to direct palpation but not to palpation through the ear canal.

   4. Palpation of glandular and lymphatic tissues. Examination of the soft tissues of the neck may reveal evidence of infection or malignancy of the head and neck, sarcoidosis, or Behçet's syndrome.

   5. Inspection of the teeth and oropharynx. In some patients, headache may be referred from dental disease, although headache rarely occurs without concomitant tooth pain. Percussion of the teeth and inspection for caries and periodontal disease may reveal a dental origin of pain. Percussion of the maxillary teeth may also hint at maxillary sinusitis, which can arise from dental root infection.

   6. Assessment of the nose and paranasal sinuses. The nasal mucosa should be examined for polyps, septal deviation, and secretions. The maxillary and frontal sinuses may be palpated or percussed for tenderness. The sinuses can also be transilluminated with a flashlight in a darkened room. The ethmoid and sphenoid sinuses can not be adequately evaluated by bedside techniques.

   7. Assessment of the eyes. Ocular causes of headache are uncommon. Patients frequently consult an ophthalmologist or optometrist before seeking a neurologic opinion for chronic headache but eye strain and refractive errors rarely prove to be responsible. Examination of the eyes may, nevertheless, provide valuable data including papilledema or abducens palsy resulting from increased intracranial pressure, optic disk pallor from a compressive lesion, or ischemic optic neuropathy associated with giant cell arteritis. Acute glaucoma may sometimes present primarily with head pain.

   8. Assessment of the extracranial vasculature is especially important in cases of suspected giant cell or temporal arteritis, in which the superficial temporal artery may be tender, nodular, and nonpulsatile. Bruits may result from arterial stenosis or increased venous outflow in patients with arteriovenous malformations. Increased collateral flow may be a source of headache when there is extracranial vascular disease. In patients with migraine, compression of the superficial temporal artery may temporarily relieve the pain.

   9. **Palpation of the scalp and neck musculature and neck mobility.** Tenderness of the pericranial muscles and limited or painful range of motion of the neck may suggest tension-type headache or spinal pathology. Spinal disease may cause headache referred to the frontal area. Resistance to passive anteroposterior neck movement, and Kernig's and Brudzinski's signs, are indications of meningeal irritation due to CNS infection or subarachnoid bleeding.

   10. A **low hairline** may be a clue to craniovertebral junction abnormalities such as a Chiari malformation, basilar impression, or basilar invagination.

IV. **Indicators of structural disease.** Recurrent attacks of acute recurrent headache are usually migraine. Chronic nonprogressive headache usually represents analgesic overuse, benign intracranial hypertension, or chronic tension-type headache. Features that suggest structural disorders are as follows:

   A. **Altered consciousness or behavior.** Although loss of consciousness during headache may result from vasovagal syncope or as a manifestation of basilar migraine, in most cases it is a sign of increased intracranial pressure, seizure activity, or ischemia. Sudden headache with altered consciousness may represent subarachnoid hemorrhage. Changes in cognitive function may also accompany destructive lesions.

   B. **Neurologic deficit developing simultaneously with or following the onset of headache.** In general, the neurologic symptoms associated with migraine arise prior to the onset of headache, although this is not necessary by definition. For the other benign headache disorders except cluster headache, nonspecific subjective neurologic symptoms occur more often than objective signs of neurologic dysfunction. When a neurologic deficit develops at or after onset of headache, differential considerations include tumor, stroke, and abscess.

   C. **Headache associated with fever or meningeal signs** should always suggest infections such as encephalitis, meningitis, subdural empyema, or abscess. Recurrent meningitis may occur in patients with anatomic defects, after splenectomy, or immune compromise. Noninfectious causes of recurrent meningitis include craniopharyngiomas, dermoid cysts, sarcoidosis, Behçet's syndrome, and the Vogt-Koyanagi-Harada syndrome. Recurrent aseptic meningitis associated with large mononuclear endothelial cells is referred to as Mollaret's meningitis. It has been associated with Herpes simplex infection. Tuberculous and fungal meningitides are likely to present chronically. Subarachnoid hemorrhage may also produce meningismus and low-grade fever. Fever and headache may accompany sinusitis or dental abscess, but the physician should keep in mind the possibility of intracranial complications of extracranial infections of the head and neck, including sinovenous thrombosis and brain abscess.

   D. **Headache occurring exclusively on one side over time.** Side-locked headache has traditionally been described as a warning sign of structural disease, particularly vascular abnormalities. In reality, many benign headache syndromes, such as migraine, cluster headache, and atypical facial pain, may consistently affect one side of the head.

   E. **Onset after age 50.** Benign headache syndromes generally begin early in life.

   F. **Change in character or response to treatment of preexisting headache.** There is no reason why a patient with chronic recurrent headache cannot develop a second disorder. Therefore, the clinician should carefully approach the patient in whom a change in the pattern or quality of long-standing headaches occurs or in whom a progressive increase in frequency or severity of headache occurs over several months, particularly when presenting with sudden onset of the "worst headache of [his/her] life."

   G. **Vomiting preceding headache by days to weeks.** Vomiting, with or without preceding nausea, may be a sign of increased intracranial pressure resulting from tumor, hydrocephalus, or chronic infection.

H. Headache associated with paroxysmal hypertension. In addition to headache, pheochromocytomas cause tachycardia, tremor, nausea, or diaphoresis. In a small minority of patients, the tumor is located in the bladder and symptoms follow urination.

 I. Associated endocrine changes. The association of subacute or chronic headache with signs of secondary hypothyroidism, galactorrhea, hypo- or hypercortisolism, or other evidence of pituitary dysfunction raises suspicions of a sellar lesion such as a pituitary adenoma. Hypopituitarism may also occur with craniopharyngiomas.

 J. Headache precipitated by rapid changes in head position or head movement. Rapid changes in head position may produce pain when there is an intracranial mass. Intraventricular lesions such as colloid cysts of the third ventricle may cause obstructive hydrocephalus with a change in posture.

K. Headache initiated by Valsalva's maneuver or associated with exercise or sexual activity. Although migraine is often exacerbated by Valsalva's maneuver, the onset of headache with Valsalva's maneuver may have ominous significance. About 10% of patients with exertional or cough headache have an underlying structural abnormality such as a craniocervical junction abnormality, posterior fossa mass or pituitary tumor. These patients should always have MRI scans. Some patients with exertional headache have a benign disorder that is usually considered a form of migraine. The headaches are often self-limited and respond to indomethacin. Coital headache is usually bilateral, throbbing, and intense. It is more common in men than in women and usually occurs just prior to orgasm. The major differential diagnosis is subarachnoid hemorrhage.

 L. Headache not conforming to known functional headache patterns.

V. Laboratory studies. In many patients a diagnosis can be made on clinical grounds alone and treatment can be initiated without any further testing. Headache is rarely the sole symptom of serious nervous system disorders. Patients with any of the historical factors discussed in the preceding section or with fever, focal signs, changes in cognition or consciousness, or stiff neck on examination should be evaluated more extensively.

A. Blood work. Occasionally, routine blood work may provide evidence of infection, anemia, or electrolyte or hormonal abnormalities that are related to headache. Erythrocyte sedimentation rate (ESR) should be checked in all elderly patients with headache due to the possibility of giant cell arteritis. When the ESR is not elevated, other acute phase reactants such as C-reactive protein, haptoglobin, or the platelet count may be increased.

B. Imaging. Imaging studies are indicated when the clinical pattern suggests the presence of a secondary cause of headache.

   1. Uninfused CT is the procedure of choice for diagnosis of intracranial hemorrhage. Sagittal MRI readily demonstrates Chiari malformations. MRI with MR venography is preferable to CT for imaging dural sinus or vein occlusions. Tumors are also seen better with MR. Catheter angiography remains the definitive modality for imaging intracranial aneurysms but advances in technology may permit the use of magnetic resonance or CT angiography (MRA or CTA) as screening techniques in selected patients.

   2. Imaging studies in patients presenting with chronic, recurrent headaches are of limited value unless there is something unusual in the history or abnormal on examination. In a prospective consecutive series of 350 patients studied with CT for headache, 2% had clinically significant abnormalities, including metastatic tumor, epidural abscess, chronic subdural hematoma, and hydrocephalus. Another 7% of the patients had clinically insignificant CT abnormalities. Of those patients with abnormal examinations, 10% had clinically significant CT abnormalities compared with 11% if there was either an unusual history or an abnormal examination and none if both the history and the physical were normal.

   3. In patients with a history consistent with migraine, the yield of imaging studies is exceptionally low. Frishberg reviewed retrospective and prospective CT or MRI studies of patients with headaches and normal examinations and found that of 897 patients with histories compatible with migraine, only 0.4% had abnormal imaging studies. Of 1825 patients whose headaches were not migrainous, 2.4% had positive scans. He concluded that in patients with a history of migraine, imaging studies were unnecessary unless there was a history of a seizure, a change in headache pattern, or a focal neurologic sign on examination. For patients with "nonspecific" headaches, the role of imaging was not clear. This study is the basis for the American Academy of Neurology's guidelines on imaging in nonacute headache.

C. **Lumbar puncture (LP)** has a role in the diagnosis of certain headache syndromes.

   1. **Exclusion of subarachnoid hemorrhage.** CT is very sensitive to the presence of subarachnoid blood but still misses about 5% to 10% of acute subarachnoid hemorrhages. In these patients, the presence of CSF blood or xanthochromia may be diagnostic.

   2. **Diagnosis of CNS infection.** In patients with suspected encephalitis or meningitis, LP may indicate the presence of CSF pleocytosis. Patients should have an imaging procedure prior to undergoing LP except when bacterial meningitis is strongly suspected, in which case LP should be done immediately to prevent a potentially life-threatening delay in institution of antibiotic therapy.

   3. **Confirmation of elevated CSF pressure in BIH.** For the patient with chronic headache and signs of increased intracranial pressure, such as papilledema or small ventricles, especially in young obese women, benign intracranial hypertension should always be included in the differential diagnosis. When imaging studies exclude a mass lesion, LP should be performed to confirm an elevation of CSF pressure.

   4. **Cisternal taps.** Cisternal puncture may increase the likelihood of diagnosing fungal or tuberculous meningitis, which may primarily affect basal meninges.

D. **Electroencephalography.** EEG is not recommended for routine evaluation of patients with headache, unless associated symptoms suggest a seizure.

E. **Biopsy** of pathologic material is indicated under certain circumstances.

   1. **Diagnosis of giant cell arteritis.** Temporal artery biopsy is still the gold standard for diagnosing cranial arteritis. A specimen of adequate length is imperative because of the tendency of this disorder to affect the temporal artery at irregular intervals. The risk of blindness in untreated patients is sufficient to warrant initiation of steroids as soon as the diagnosis of cranial arteritis is contemplated. The incidence of positive biopsy results falls dramatically after even short trials of steroids, so moving to biopsy rapidly is recommended. There is a modest increase in diagnostic yield by biopsying the contralateral temporal artery if the initial biopsy specimen is negative in patients with signs and symptoms of giant cell arteritis. Biopsy may be of value in diagnosing other arteritides, such as polyarteritis nodosa, which may involve the temporal artery. The practice of preoperative angiography to select the site of biopsy is rarely of benefit because of confusion with arteriosclerotic changes, which commonly occur in this age group.

   2. **Meningeal biopsy.** In patients with chronic meningitis, meningeal biopsy may help establish diagnoses such as granulomatous angiitis, sarcoidosis, or meningeal carcinomatosis.

Recommended Readings

Allison MC, Gallagher PJ. Temporal artery biopsy and corticosteroid treatment. *Ann Rheum Dis* 1984;43:416–417.

Boyev LR, Miller NR, Green WR. Efficacy of unilateral versus bilateral temporal artery biopsies for the diagnosis of giant cell arteritis. *Am J Ophthalmol* 1999;128:211–1215.

Brightbill TC, Goodwin RS, Ford RG. Magnetic resonance imaging of intracranial hypotension syndrome with pathological correlation. *Headache* 2000;40:292–299.

Day JW, Raskin NH. Thunderclap headache: symptom of unruptured cerebral aneurysm. *Lancet* 1986;2:1247–1248.

Evans RW, Armon C, Frohman EM, et al. Assessment: prevention of post–lumbar puncture headaches—report of the Therapeutics and Technology Assessment Subcommittee of the American Academy of Neurology. *Neurology* 2000;55:909–914.

Fisher CM. Late-life migraine accompaniments as a cause of unexplained transient ischemic attacks. *Can J Neurol Sci* 1980;7:9–17.

Forsyth PA, Posner JB. Headaches in patients with brain tumors: a study of 111 patients. *Neurology* 1993;43:1678–1683.

Frishberg BM. The utility of neuroimaging in the evaluation of headache in patients with normal neurologic examinations. *Neurology* 1994; 44:1191–1197.

Gorelick PB, Hier DB, Caplan LR, et al. Headache in acute cerebrovascular disease. *Neurology* 1986;36:1445–1450.

Headache Classification Committee of the International Headache Society. Classification and diagnostic criteria for headache disorders, cranial neuralgias and facial pain. *Cephalalgia* 1988;8[Suppl 7]:1–96.

ICD-10 guide for headaches: guide to the classification, diagnosis and assessment of headaches in accordance with the tenth revision of the international classification of diseases and related health problems and its application to neurology. *Cephalalgia* 1997;17[Suppl. 19]: 1–82.

Kuntz KM, Kokmen E, Stevens JC, et al. Post–lumbar puncture headaches: experience in 501 consecutive procedures. *Neurology* 1992;42:1884–1887.

Marcelis J, Silberstein SD. Idiopathic intracranial hypertension without papilledema. *Arch Neurol* 1991;48:392–399.

Mathew NT, Ravishankar K, Sanin LC. Coexistence of migraine and idiopathic intracranial hypertension without papilledema. *Neurology* 1996;46:1226–1230.

Medina JL, Diamond S. Cluster headache variant: spectrum of a new headache syndrome. *Arch Neurol* 1981;38:705–709.

Mitchell C, Osborn RE, Grosskreutz SR. Computed tomography in the headache patient: is routine evaluation really necessary? *Headache* 1993;33:82–86.

Pless M, Rizzo JF 3rd, Lamkin JC, et al. Concordance of bilateral temporal artery biopsy in giant cell arteritis. *J Neuroophthalmol* 2000;20:216–218.

Quality Standards Subcommittee of the American Academy of Neurology. Practice parameter: the electroencephalogram in the evaluation of headache. *Neurology* 1995;45:1411–1413.

Quality Standards Subcommittee of the American Academy of Neurology. Practice parameter: the utility of neuroimaging in the evaluation of headache in patients with normal neurologic examinations [Summary statement]. *Neurology* 1994;44:1353–1354.

Silberstein SD, Lipton RB, Sliwinski M. Classification of daily and near-daily headaches: proposed revision to the IHS criteria. *Headache* 1994;34:1–7.

Vijayan N, Dreyfus PM. Posttraumatic cephalalgia. *Arch Neurol* 1975;32:649–652.

Vijayan N, Watson C. Pericarotid syndrome. *Headache* 1978;18:244–254.

22. APPROACH TO THE PATIENT WITH NECK PAIN WITH OR WITHOUT ASSOCIATED ARM PAIN

Scott A. Shapiro

I. **Traumatic neck pain without arm pain**
   A. Trauma to the neck secondary to a motor vehicle accident, work-related injury or athletic injury is a common cause of musculoskeletal neck pain. For most patients, posttraumatic neck pain is a self-limited problem that is not serious.
   B. **Etiology.** Straining of anteroposterior cervical muscles and tendons is the mechanism of pain for most posttraumatic neck pain syndromes. The most common cause in clinical practice is vehicular accidents with hyperextension and flexion of the neck (whiplash). Altercations, athletic injuries, especially football, and lifting and tugging work injuries also occur.
   C. **Evaluation**
      1. **History and physical examination.** The primary symptoms are posttraumatic neck pain and neck stiffness. The paracervical muscles are tender with limitation of motion, spinous process point tenderness may be present, and there may be associated interscapular pain and headache. Patchy arm numbness occasionally is reported, but the findings of neurologic examination of the upper extremities are normal for most patients.
      2. **Radiographs**
         a. **Plain radiographs** rule out most fractures and ligamentous instability. Among persons younger than 40 years, the most common finding is loss of the lordotic curve from muscle spasm. Among those older than 40 years, radiographs often show degenerative changes, such as narrowed disk spaces and osteophyte (bone spur) formation. The accident is not the cause of these radiographic changes, but certainly these changes can predispose the patient to more pain than does a normal spine.
         b. **Computed tomography (CT) and magnetic resonance imaging (MRI).** In the modern era, any clinical or radiographic evidence of acute fracture, subluxation (instability), or spinal cord injury necessitates a thorough evaluation, including plain radiographs with five cervical views (anteroposterior, lateral, right and left oblique, and open mouth odontoid), CT, consultation with a spine specialist and, more often than not, MRI.
   D. **Referrals**
      1. **First 2 to 3 weeks (medicate and wait)**
         a. **Soft collar.** Posttraumatic neck pain usually subsides on its own over a week or two. A narrow soft cervical collar can be helpful in taking the weight of the head off the neck and transferring it to the shoulders. The collar should not be so wide that it forces that patient into hyperextension, which is uncomfortable.
         b. **Medication.** An over-the-counter nonsteroidal antiinflammatory drug (NSAID; ibuprofen) with or without acetaminophen is the ideal analgesic. Other analgesics such as propoxyphene, codeine, or codeine analogues are acceptable, but no schedule III narcotics, such as oxycodone, meperidine, or morphine should be used. Muscle relaxants such as methocarbamol (Robaxin; A.H. Robins, Richmond, VA, U.S.A.) 500 mg by mouth every 6 to 8 hours, cyclobenzaprine (Flexeril; ALZA, Mountain View, CA, U.S.A.) 10 mg by mouth three times a day, or chlorzoxazone (Parafon Forte; McNeil, Spring House, PA, U.S.A.) 500 mg by mouth every 6 to 8 hours can help. Benzodiazepines should not be used because of the abuse potential. For a patient whose stomach is sensitive to nonsteroidal medications, an evening dose of an histamine-2 (H_2) receptor blocker such as cimetidine 300 to 600 mg by mouth can help prevent gastritis.
         c. **Time off from work.** Patients who do almost all their work at a desk who have mild to moderate neck pain can work, and most ambitious people are able to function. Heavy laborers may benefit from light duty or

1 to 2 weeks off work. Beware of patients who exhibit symptom magnification and functional overlay for purposes of secondary gain (worker's compensation and litigation). They have the tendency to abuse time off work. In these scenarios, early referral to a physical medicine and rehabilitation specialist who can scientifically assess for malingering can be helpful.

    2. Weeks 3 to 6 if pain still present

        a. Physical therapy. If the neck pain does not subside after 2 weeks, physical therapy—heat, ultrasound, massage and transcutaneous electrical nerve stimulation (TENS)—is reasonable.

        b. Pain clinic. Trigger point injections of anesthetics or steroids can be helpful but are probably best scheduled after evaluation by a spine specialist.

    3. After 6 to 8 weeks. When neck pain persists after 6 to 8 weeks despite rest and therapy, and the pain remains severe enough to interfere with work or recreation, the next diagnostic test should be cervical MRI to evaluate the cervical disks. The results usually are normal or show mild cervical disk dehydration with disk bulging. Neck pain from cervical disk dehydration can best be managed with cervical traction. Minor cervical disk bulging with chronic pain with normal neurologic findings is rarely sufficient indication for surgery. At this point, it is best to obtain the opinion of a neurosurgeon.

II. Nontraumatic neck pain of arthritic origin

  A. Neck pain from degenerative arthritis of the neck is of epidemic proportion (60% to 80%) in the elderly population.

  B. Etiology. Degenerative arthritis of the cervical spine occasionally manifests as early as the third decade of life but is much more common with increasing age. Disk dehydration and disk space narrowing with osteophyte formation are a process that occurs naturally with age. Facet arthritis also occurs. Small nerve fibers innervating the disk and facet can be involved, and neck pain ensues. Dural impingement by osteophytes also can produce neck pain, especially with extension or lateral gaze.

  C. Evaluation

    1. History and physical examination. Nontraumatic neck pain among persons older than 40 years is most often caused by cervical degenerative arthritis. The pain is gradual in onset and initially intermittent and then becomes constant. There can be associated occipital headache and interscapular pain. Motion, especially extension or lateral gaze, can aggravate the pain.

    2. Radiographs show narrowing of disk spaces with bone spur formation. At least 70% of the population older than 65 years has significant changes of degenerative arthritis. Regardless of how bad the radiographs look, if the patient has normal neurologic findings, MRI or surgery is not absolutely indicated.

  D. Referrals

    1. Medication. An over-the-counter NSAID (ibuprofen with or without acetaminophen) is the ideal analgesic. Other analgesics such as propoxyphene, codeine, or codeine analogues are acceptable, but no schedule III narcotics should be used. Muscle relaxants such as methocarbamol 500 mg by mouth every 6 to 8 hours, cyclobenzaprine 10 mg by mouth three times a day, or chloroxazone 500 mg by mouth every 6 to 8 hours can help. Benzodiazepines should not be used because of the abuse potential. For patients whose stomach is sensitive to nonsteroidal medication, an evening dose of an H_2 receptor blocker such as cimetidine 300 to 600 mg by mouth can help prevent gastritis.

    2. Physical therapy. Heat, ultrasound, massage, and TENS unit therapy can help.

    3. Pain clinic. Trigger point injections can help.

    4. Alternative therapies. Although chiropractors can help many people, we cannot advocate manipulation of the neck when obvious bone spurs exist. Neurologic catastrophes and lawsuits have occurred. Patients can seek chiropractic care at their own risk. Magnets have become popular in relieving arthritic problems with some scientific credence. Oral glucosamine also has been shown somewhat effective against arthritis, although the effect on cervical spondylosis remains to be determined.

5. **Spine specialists.** For most patients with neck pain and no arm pain, surgery is not indicated. The removal of large osteophytes ventral to the spinal cord can improve severe neck pain, occipital headache, and range of motion. Only an experienced spinal surgeon should make this decision based on a CT and MRI findings and repeated physical examinations over a period of time.

III. **Neck pain with arm pain (radiculopathy) from soft cervical disk bulging and herniation**

A. **Etiology.** Among persons older than 50 years, the most common cause is a single level soft cervical disk. The concept of a soft cervical disk means either an eccentric disk bulge or a free fragment herniation compressing a root. A disk consists of inner water-laden mucoid nuclear material and an outer fibrous annulus. The annulus can fissure, allowing the nucleus either to bulge or to herniate out. There is no osteophyte involved in the compression. The posterior longitudinal ligament extends beneath the entire spinal cord, protecting the cord from disk herniation, so disk herniation primarily projects laterally into the foramen, compressing the nerve only. In rare cases, sufficient force, as in trauma, can lead to large disk herniation and cause acute myelopathy.

B. **Anatomy.** A disk is named by the bordering vertebral bodies. Thus, the disk between vertebral bodies C5 and C6 is the C5-6 disk. The nerve root corresponding to a given vertebral body exits above the pedicle of that body. Thus the C5-6 disk compresses the C6 nerve root.

C. **Evaluation**

1. **History.** The classic story is intermittent neck pain followed by severe neck pain and arm pain. Rarely is this condition traumatic in origin. The pain radiates down the shoulder and into the arm. Some dermatomal patterns of radiation can help discern the level of herniation. Patients may report various combinations of suboccipital headache, interscapular pain, numbness, tingling, and weakness. The pain often awakens the patient from sleep.

2. **Physical examination**

a. **Neck examination.** There is posterior tenderness, especially tenderness at the spinous process near the level of involvement and paracervical tenderness. Painful limitation of motion with extension and lateral gaze to the side of arm pain is classic.

b. **Arm examination**

(1) **C5 radiculopathy (C4-5 disk herniation)** manifests as pain and numbness radiating to the shoulder and weakness of the deltoid muscle (shoulder abduction). Simultaneous testing of both deltoid muscles by means of compression on the outstretched upper arms helps detect minor weakness (Table 22.1). There is no true reflex to test.

(2) **C6 radiculopathy (C5-6 disk herniation).** C5-6 disk herniation is the second most common cervical disk herniation. Pain and numbness radiate across the top of the neck and along the biceps to the lateral aspect of the forearm and dorsal thumb and index finger. Numbness usually is more distal. A weak biceps, a reduced biceps reflex, and weak wrist extension are observed.

(3) **C7 radiculopathy (C6-7 disk herniation)** is the most common disk herniation. Pain radiates across the top of the neck, across the triceps, and down the posterolateral forearm to the middle finger. Numbness again is more distal. A weak triceps and reduced triceps reflex are observed.

(4) **C8 radiculopathy (C7-T1 disk herniation)** is uncommon. Pain and numbness radiate across the neck and down the arm to the small finger and ring finger. Wrist flexion and the intrinsic muscles of the hand are weak.

3. **Radiographic evaluation**

a. **Plain radiographs** provide little help. They may show slight narrowing of the disk space involved and loss of lordosis.

Table 22.1 Motor strength classification (0–5 scale)

0 = No movement
1 = Flicker of movement
2 = Able to move but not against gravity
3 = Able to move against gravity but offers no resistance
4 = Offers resistance but able to overcome or easy fatigue
5 = Normal

        b. MRI without contrast material is the study of choice for demonstrating soft cervical disk herniation (Fig. 22.1).

    4. Electromyography (EMG) and nerve conduction velocity studies. EMG for single-level disk herniation with radiculopathy is not absolutely necessary. EMG can help when other disorders, such as amyotrophic lateral sclerosis, carpal tunnel syndrome, and brachial plexopathy, have to be ruled out.

  D. Referrals

    1. Physical therapy. After diagnosis by means of MRI, a patient with a motor strength rating of 4/5 or more (Table 22.1) can be referred for cervical traction, heat, ultrasound, massage, and a soft collar. Cervical traction initially should be provided by a physical therapist. Inform the therapist that if traction is tolerated, the patient is to be instructed in home cervical traction at 10 pounds (4.5 kg) for 30 minutes every night. Approximately 60% to 80% of cases of soft disk herniation improve to the point of resolution of the radiculopathy with traction alone within 4 to 6 weeks. Not every patient can tolerate traction.

    2. Medication. A trial of 4 mg self-weaning methylprednisolone (Solu-Medrol; Pharmacia & Upjohn, Kalamazoo, MI, U.S.A.) dose pack can be used with some success early in treatment before nonsteroidal agents are given. An over-the-counter NSAID (ibuprofen with or without acetaminophen) is the ideal analgesic. Other analgesics such as propoxyphene, codeine, or codeine analogues are acceptable, but no schedule III narcotics should be used. Muscle relaxants such as methocarbamol 500 mg by mouth every 6 to 8 hours,

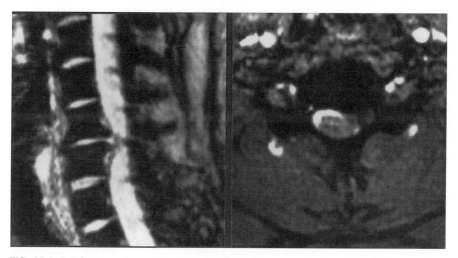

FIG. 22.1 Axial magnetic resonance image shows large eccentric cervical disk herniation compressing the spinal cord and nerve root.

cyclobenzaprine 10 mg by mouth three times a day, or chloroxazone 500 mg by mouth every 6 to 8 hours can help. Benzodiazepines should not be used because of the abuse potential. For patients whose stomach is sensitive to nonsteroidal medication, an evening dose of an H_2 receptor blocker such as cimetidine 300 to 600 mg by mouth can help prevent gastritis.

3. **Time off from work.** Desk workers with mild to moderate neck or arm pain can work, and most ambitious people are able to function. Heavy laborers may benefit from light duty or 1 to 4 weeks off work. Beware of patients who exhibit symptom magnification and functional overlay for purposes of secondary gain (worker's compensation and litigation). They have the tendency to abuse time off work. In these scenarios, early referral to a physical medicine and rehabilitation specialist who can scientifically assess for malingering may be helpful.

4. **Spine specialist.** For any patient with 3/5 strength or worse, immediate referral to a spine surgeon is indicated. The longer a root is compressed with severe weakness, the less likely it is that strength will return to normal. If strength remains 4/5 or better but pain persists after 3 to 6 weeks of traction, referral to a spine surgeon is indicated. A well-trained spine surgeon should be able to relieve arm pain and weakness for 90% to 95% of patients with soft cervical disk herniation.

IV. **Neck pain with arm pain from bone spurs (hard disk, cervical spondylosis)**
   A. **The combination of neck pain and arm pain in cervical spondylosis is of epidemic proportions in the elderly population.**
   B. **Etiology.** Disk dehydration and narrowing lead to bone spur formation at the margins of the vertebral body. The spurs can project into the foramen or canal, compressing the nerve root or the spinal cord, or both. Facet arthritis with resultant hypertrophy and ligamentous hypertrophy also narrow the spinal canal and neural foramina. With progressive age, more than one disk space usually is involved. The center of the process usually extends from C4 to C7.
   C. **Evaluation**
      1. **History.** This condition occurs primarily in patients older than patients with soft cervical disk herniation, although the two groups overlap. Approximately 90% of patients have gradual onset of neck pain with progression to neck and arm pain. The pain radiates down the shoulder and into the arm. Some dermatomal patterns of radiation can help discern the level of root compression. Suboccipital headache, interscapular pain, numbness, tingling, and weakness also may be present in varying degree.

      The pain often awakens the patient up from sleep. Approximately 10% of patients have asymptomatic degenerative arthritis. Then neck pain and arm pain often are precipitated by hyperextension–flexion injuries from trauma (motor vehicle accidents). A large percentage have multiple disk spaces involved, making it more difficult to determine which level or levels caused the radiculopathy.

      2. **Physical examination**
         a. **Neck examination.** There is posterior tenderness, especially tenderness at the spinous process near the level of involvement and paracervical tenderness. Painful limitation of motion with extension and lateral gaze to the side of arm pain are classic.
         b. **Arm examination (Table 22.1)**
            (1) **C5 radiculopathy (C4-5 disk degeneration)** manifests as pain and numbness radiating to the shoulder along with a weak deltoid muscle (shoulder abduction). Simultaneous testing of both deltoid muscles by means of compression on the outstretched upper arms detects minor weakness. There is no true reflex to test.
            (2) **C6 radiculopathy (C5-6 disk degeneration).** The C5-6 level is the second most common level for disk disease with spurring. Pain and numbness radiate across the top of the neck and along the biceps to the lateral aspect of the forearm and dorsal thumb and index finger. Numbness usually is more distal. A weak biceps, a reduced biceps reflex, and weak wrist extension are observed.

(3) **C7 radiculopathy (C6-7 disk degeneration).** The C6-7 level is the most common level for disk space involvement. Pain radiates across the top of the neck, across the triceps, then down the posterolateral forearm to the middle finger. Numbness is again more distal. A weak triceps and a reduced triceps reflex are observed.

(4) **C8 radiculopathy (C7-T1 disk degeneration)** is uncommon. Pain and numbness radiate across the neck and down the arm to the small finger and ring finger. Wrist flexion, and the intrinsic muscles of the hand, especially those for finger extension, are weak.

  c. **Leg examination (Table 22.2).** Gait usually is normal even in the face of considerable radiographic evidence of spinal cord compression. Myelopathy occasionally is present. Early on, gait is normal in the face of increased muscle stretch reflexes and a Babinski sign. With more severe and prolonged compression, one can observe spastic gait with bowel and bladder problems. In the most severe cases, the patient needs a cane or a walker. Rarely is the condition allowed to progress to wheel chair dependency.

3. **Radiographs**
  a. **Plain radiographs** show disk-space narrowing with osteophyte (bone spur) formation. Oblique radiographs can show neuroforaminal narrowing.
  b. **MRI (Fig. 22.2)** is excellent for showing nerve-root compression and cord compression from bone spurs. It does not provide as much detail about bone anatomy as does CT.
  c. **CT (Fig. 22.3)** shows better bone detail than does MRI but is not as good at showing the neural structures. The two studies together are ideal for this group of patients, but this is not cost-effective, so MRI is the first choice.

4. **EMG and nerve conduction velocity studies.** EMG can be helpful in discerning which roots are most involved in patients with multilevel spondylosis.

D. **Referrals**

1. **Medication.** Initially an over-the counter or prescription NSAID with or without acetaminophen is ideal. An evening dose of an H_2 receptor blocker such as cimetidine can prevent the gastritis associated with NSAIDs. Analgesics such as propoxyphene, codeine, or codeine analogues are acceptable. Muscle relaxants such as methocarbamol can help in some instances. Schedule III narcotics and benzodiazepines are ill advised because of the chronic nature of the disorder. However, abuse of these medications is less likely among the elderly, and thus one may be more willing to prescribe them for elderly patients.

2. **Soft cervical collar**

3. **Physical therapy.** Heat, ultrasound, massage, traction, and TENS can reduce the symptoms. Approximately 20% of cases of radiculopathy (arm pain, strength) can be relieved with medicine and therapy alone for many

Table 22.2 Nurick classification

Grade	Characteristic
1	Signs of spinal cord disease but normal gait
2	Slight gait abnormality not preventing full-time employment
3	Gait abnormality severe enough to prevent employment or housework; still able to walk independently
4	Requires a walker or someone else's help to walk
5	Uses a wheelchair full time

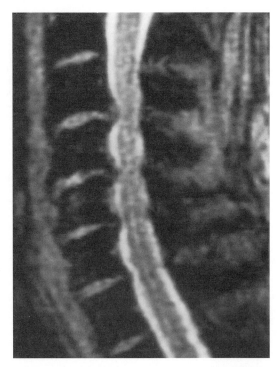

FIG. 22.2 Sagittal magnetic resonance image of cervical spondylosis shows involvement of multiple levels.

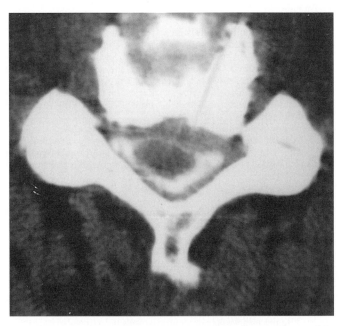

FIG. 22.3 Axial computed tomographic scan of a patient with cervical spondylotic radiculo-myelopathy shows cervical spondylosis with canal and foraminal stenosis.

years. Most patients have some pain with persistent mild weakness (if any weakness is present). Rarely does myelopathy develop in this group of patients.

4. **Spine specialist.** Surgery for cervical spondylotic radiculopathy is almost always elective. Results of surgery are much better for single-level disease than for multilevel disease, especially for neck pain. Arm motor strength of 3/5 or worse and any evidence of myelopathy is an indication for immediate referral to a spine surgeon. The anterior approach is superior to the posterior approach if bone spurs project under the entire spinal cord. Surgery relieves radiculopathy in 90% to 95% of cases of both single-level disease and multilevel disease, but neck pain improves for only 70% to 75% of patients with multilevel disease. Complete relief of radicular pain occurs in approximately 60% to 80% of cases. There is no age cutoff for surgery as long as the patient is in reasonable medical condition. The elderly tolerate surgery well with minimal morbidity. If myelopathy is present with gait abnormality and aggressive decompression is performed, an improvement of one grade on the Nurick scale (Table 22.2) can be expected for 70% to 80% of patients. Duration of symptoms is important for patients with gait problems. Thus early referral is indicated.

V. **Neck pain with or without arm pain due to metastatic cancer of the cervical spine**

A. As patients live longer with various malignant diseases, the number of patients with spinal metastases also increases. Tumors that most commonly involve the spine are lung cancer, breast cancer, prostate cancer, lymphoma, and multiple myeloma. As many as 20% of these tumors develop symptomatic spinal involvement. In approximately 10% of patients, metastatic spinal involvement is the mode of presentation with no known primary tumor.

B. **Evaluation**

1. **History and physical examination.** Both primary and metastatic tumors of the spine initially manifest as pain that is often worse at night. The pain continues to worsen over a very short period, and then neurologic symptoms such as radiculopathy and myelopathy develop fairly quickly. It is best to make the diagnosis when neurologic symptoms are minimal.

2. **Radiographs**

a. **Plain radiographs** can show destruction of the vertebral bodies and pedicles (Fig. 22.4). Pathologic compression fractures and lytic pedicles are common. The sensitivity of plain radiographs is approximately 60%.

b. **Bone scans** are sensitive—approaching 100%—in showing spinal metastases, including asymptomatic areas with no destruction.

c. **MRI** is ideal for delineating canal involvement, cord compression, and surgical feasibility.

C. **Referrals**

1. **Radiation therapy.** Diffuse disease involving large amounts of the spine is managed primarily with steroids and radiation therapy. Radiation usually is reserved for the symptomatic areas only. Dexamethasone 2 to 20 mg by mouth every 6 hours can be quite helpful in improving pain and neurologic symptoms.

2. **Surgery.** Early referral to a spine surgeon is warranted after diagnosis regardless of the findings at neurologic examination. If surgery is indicated, it is often best to perform the operation before radiation therapy, because this reduces the wound complication rate. In the face of a cervical myelopathy resulting from diffuse canal involvement and cord compression, laminectomy can be performed. Patients with lung cancer do very poorly, and it is difficult to justify scientifically surgery for metastatic lung cancer. The results with other tumors are better, but a good rule is that 30% to 50% of all tumors are relieved by means of laminectomy with a 10% mortality rate. Isolated vertebral body disease can be resected from an anterior approach—especially for breast cancer, prostate cancer, lymphoma and renal cell cancer—with excellent long-term results.

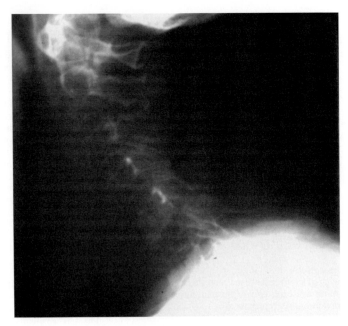

FIG. 22.4 Lateral radiograph shows lytic destruction of the C6 vertebral body.

VI. **Miscellaneous neck pain with/without arm pain**
  A. **Rheumatoid arthritis**
     1. **Etiology.** Rheumatoid arthritis can affect the C1-2 articulation and lead to erosion of the odontoid process and transverse atlantal ligament, which leads to C1-2 instability and cord compression from the developing panus.
     2. **Evaluation**
        a. **History and physical examination.** Severe neck pain usually is followed by arm pain and a progressive myelopathy.
        b. **Imaging.** Plain radiographs and MRI are best for showing erosion of the odontoid process with subsequent instability (Fig. 22.5).
     3. **Referrals and therapy.** Place a soft collar and refer the patient immediately to a spine surgeon. Posterior C1-2 fusion with transarticular screws is ideal for the problem. Anterior transoral odontoidectomy occasionally is needed. These treatments are not without risk and must be individualized.
  B. **Discitis and osteomyelitis**
     1. Bacterial discitis and osteomyelitis is extremely uncommon in the cervical spine, and fever may not be present.
     2. **Evaluation**
        a. **History and physical examination.** There may be a history of skin infection, urinary tract infection, or pulmonary infection. Iatrogenic diskitis or osteomyelitis complicating cervical spine surgery is known to occur. Perhaps the most common cause in urban settings is a history of intravenous drug abuse. Progressive neck pain with rapidly progressive myelopathy is the usual presentation.
        b. **Imaging.** Plain radiographs show disk-space collapse with erosion of the bordering vertebral bodies. MRI shows epidural spinal cord compression from kyphosis or epidural abscess.
     3. **Referrals.** The patient should be immediately referred to either a spine specialist or an infectious disease specialist. An immediate radiology-directed

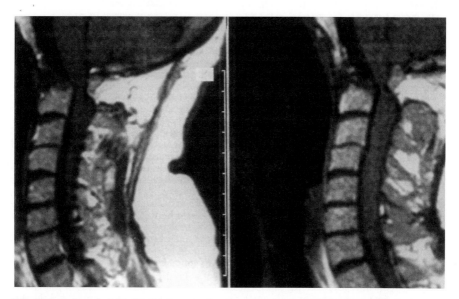

FIG. 22.5 *Left and right:* Sagittal magnetic resonance images of a patient with rheumatoid arthritis show destruction of the dens with compression of the medulla and spinal cord at the craniocervical junction.

needle biopsy with culture or open biopsy with culture and administration of intravenous bactericidal antibiotics for at least 6 weeks are indicated. Surgical débridement and decompression are performed for severe kyphosis and neurologic problems.

Recommended Readings
Adams R, Victor M, eds. *Principles of neurology.* New York: McGraw-Hill, 1993
Bracken M, Shephard M, Collins W, et al. Methylprednisolone or naloxone treatment after acute spinal cord injury: 1 year follow up data—results of the second national acute spinal cord injury study. *J Neurosurg* 1992;76:23–31.
DePalma, A, Rothman R, Levitt, et al. The natural history of severe cervical disc degeneration. *Acta Orthop Scand* 1972;43:392–339.
Melhem E. MR imaging of the cervical spine and spinal cord. *Magn Reson Imaging Clin N Am* 2000;8:435–650.
Modic M, Masaryk T, Ross J, eds. *Magnetic resonance imaging of the spine.* Chicago: Year Book, 1989.
Pellicci P, Ranawat C, Tsairis P, et al. A prospective study of the progression of rheumatoid arthritis of the cervical spine. *J Bone Joint Surg Am* 1981;63:342–350.
Rothman R, Simeone F, eds. *The spine.* Philadelphia: WB Saunders, 1992.
Shapiro S. Banked fibula: locking cervical plate following anterior cervical discectomy. *J Neurosurg* 1996;84:161–165.
Shapiro S. Spinal instrumentation with a low complication rate. *Surg Neurol* 1997;48:566–574.
Wilkins R, Rengachary S, eds. *Neurosurgery.* New York: McGraw–Hill, 1996.
Wong D, Fornasier V, MacNab I. Spinal metastases: the obvious, the occult and the imposters. *Spine* 1990;15:1–4.

23. APPROACH TO THE PATIENT WITH LOW BACK PAIN, LUMBOSACRAL RADICULOPATHY, AND LUMBAR STENOSIS

Paul B. Nelson

I. **Introduction**
   A. **Acute low back pain.** Back pain is extremely common. Most adults can remember at least one episode of back pain sometime in their lives. Approximately 50% of working adults have back pain at least 1 day per year. Back pain has become one of the most expensive health care problems and has become a leading cause of disability among persons younger than 45 years. The estimated annual cost of medical care of patients with low back pain is more than 8 billion dollars.
   B. **Lumbar disk disease with sciatica.** Patients with back and leg pain (sciatica) most likely have nerve-root compression secondary to rupture of a lumbar disk. Although it occurs occasionally in the pediatric and geriatric age groups, ruptured disk generally occurs in the third to fifth decades of life. Approximately 90% of cases of rupture of lumbar disks occur between L4-5 and L5-S1; 5% occur at L3-4. The incidence of disk rupture is the same among men and women.
   C. **Lumbar spinal stenosis** is any type of narrowing of the spinal canal, lateral recess, or intervertebral foramina secondary to congenital causes, disk degeneration, bony hypertrophy, ligamentous hypertrophy, or spondylolisthesis. Because it is caused primarily by degenerative change, the disease seldom occurs before the fifth decade of life. The mean age of patients undergoing operative procedures for lumbar stenosis is the sixth decade, although it sometimes occurs in the seventh and eighth decades. Lumbar stenosis is most commonly observed at L4-5 and L3-4.

II. **Etiology**
   A. **Acute low back pain.** Only about one half of patients with low back pain have associated injuries. With the disorder being so common and so often unassociated with injury, back pain must be considered a normal part of aging. Degenerative changes in the spine begin by the end of the second decade of life and are extremely common by the fifth decade.
   A small percentage of patients have structural abnormalities that account for low back pain. Spondylolisthesis, which is a forward slipping of one vertebral body over another, is caused by defects in the pars interarticularis (spondylolysis) in the younger age group and by degenerative changes in the older age group. Lumbar scoliosis, which is a lateral deformity of the spine, usually is caused by degenerative disease. Primary or metastatic bone tumors or infections of the disk or epidural space are much less common causes of back pain.
   B. **Lumbar disk disease with sciatica.** A lumbar disk acts as an articulation between the vertebrae and as a cushion. It is composed of a cartilaginous end plate and an outer annulus that surrounds the nucleus. Degenerative changes begin in the disk by the late twenties and are common by the fourth decade. Alterations in the lumbar disk from age alone and major or minor trauma can cause an intervertebral disk to rupture. The disk most commonly ruptures in a posterolateral direction. Disk extrusions and some protrusions can cause nerve-root or, less frequently, cauda equina compression.
   C. **Lumbar spinal stenosis.** Except in patients born with short pedicles, spinal stenosis is secondary to degenerative changes and many years of repetitive trauma. With age, the disk loses its water content and stops functioning as a cushion. There is increased stress on the bony vertebrae, the ligaments, and the facets. There is increased mobility of the vertebral bodies, ballooning of the disk, and hypertrophy of the ligaments. All these changes can cause narrowing of the lumbar canal. Absolute spinal stenosis is defined as a midsagittal diameter of 10 mm or less. A normal lumbar canal is 15 to 25 mm in diameter.

III. **Clinical manifestations and evaluation**
   A. **History**
      1. **Acute low back pain.** The history interview must determine whether there is associated injury. It must also determine whether there are any "red

flags" that suggest more serious causes of the back disorder (Table 23.1). Symptoms and histories that should alert the physician that there may be a disorder more serious than regular mechanical low back pain include night pain, fever, severe back spasms, leg pain, leg weakness, leg numbness, bladder or bowel dysfunction, major trauma, minor trauma in a patient with osteoporosis, weight loss, lethargy, back pain in a child, history of previous bacterial infection, history of carcinoma, history of intravenous drug use, and a worker's compensation or legal claim.

2. **Lumbar disk disease with sciatica.** A patient with sciatica usually has a history of back pain for several days before the development of leg pain. In L4-5 and L5-S1 disk disease, the back pain actually may be somewhat relieved as the patient goes on to have burning discomfort in the buttocks and unilateral pain in the posterolateral aspects of both the upper and lower leg. There may also be numbness or tingling in a portion of the foot or toes. The less common L3-4 disk disease can cause pain in the groin and anterior aspects of the thigh and upper leg. The history occasionally is one of severe sciatic pain from the onset. Bilateral leg pain and bladder or bowel dysfunction suggest large midline disk extrusion.

3. **Lumbar spinal stenosis.** In spinal stenosis, the history is more important than the examination. The patient typically reports back and leg discomfort, numbness, or heaviness with standing or walking. Symptoms improve with rest or forward bending. The leg symptoms usually are asymmetric. Occasional patients have true sciatica.

B. **Physical examination**
1. **Acute low back pain.** Examination of a patient with acute low back pain should begin with inspection and palpation of the low back. Paravertebral muscle spasms may be present. In most cases of mechanical back pain, straight-leg-raise testing causes back pain only. Straight-leg-raise testing that causes back and leg pain and neurologic findings that reveal neurologic deficits in the lower extremities suggest root or cauda equina compression. The neurologic examination should include walking on the heels and toes, squatting, and individual testing of the foot and toe dorsiflexors, the quadriceps, and the iliopsoas muscles. The general examination should include palpation of the abdomen, to rule out an abdominal aortic aneurysm, and a rectal examination.
2. **Lumbar disk disease with sciatica.** The patient walks in a slow, deliberate manner with slight forward tilt of the trunk. Paravertebral muscle tightness can cause decreased range of motion of the back, and asymmetric

Table 23.1 "Red flags" that suggest serious causes of low back pain

Symptoms, history	Possible diagnosis
Night pain	Tumor
Fever, history of recent bacterial infection or intravenous drug use, severe back spasms	Diskitis and epidural abscess
Leg pain	Nerve-root compression
Bilateral tower extremity weakness or numbness, bladder or bowel dysfunction, compression	Cauda equina or conus
Major trauma	Fracture, dislocation
Minor trauma in a patient with osteoporosis	Compression fracture
History of carcinoma	Metastatic disease
Systemic symptoms such as fever, weight loss	Multiple myeloma
Back pain in a child	Tumor, tethered cord
Worker's compensation or legal claim	Secondary gain

muscle tightness can cause associated scoliosis. The patient prefers to stand or lie rather than sit. The best position usually is lying on the unaffected side with the affected leg slightly bent at the knee and hip. The pain frequently is worsened by a Valsalva maneuver.

    a. Straight-leg-raise testing is important in the diagnosis of lumbar disk disease. The patient is in a supine position with the knee extended and the ankle plantar flexed. The examiner raises the leg slowly. Normally, the leg can be raised to 90 degrees without discomfort or with slight tightness in the hamstring. When the nerve root is compressed by a ruptured disk, the straight leg raise is limited and causes back and leg pain. It worsens with dorsiflexion of the foot. In most cases, the result of the straight-leg-raise test is positive only on the side of the disk rupture. If lifting the leg without symptoms causes pain in the leg with symptoms, one must consider disk rupture in the axilla of the nerve root.

    b. Motor testing is directed at the nerve roots most commonly affected. Compression of the L5 nerve root can cause foot and great toe dorsiflexion weakness (tibialis anterior and extensor hallucis longus). When the compression is severe, the patient may have foot drop. Compression of the S1 nerve root can cause plantar flexion weakness. This is difficult to detect at the bedside and is best tested by having the patient do toe raises one leg at a time. Weakness at L4 can cause quadriceps weakness. The patient may have the sensation that the leg is giving way. Disease of the L3-4 disk decreases the knee reflex, and disease of the L5-S1 disk decreases the ankle reflex.

    c. Sensory loss resulting from a disk rupture seldom occurs in a dermatomal pattern. Rupture of the L5-S1 disk can cause relative hypalgesia in the lateral aspect of the foot and little toe. Rupture of the L4-5 disk can cause relative hypalgesia in the dorsum of the foot and great toe. Rupture of the L3-4 disk can cause sensory loss in the anterior thigh and shin.

   3. Lumbar spinal stenosis. Findings at neurologic examination of the lower extremities may be relatively unremarkable at rest. One occasionally may find evidence of mild nerve-root dysfunction such as L5 numbness and weakness.

IV. Differential diagnosis

A. Acute low back pain with and without sciatica

    1. Lumbosacral sprain
    2. Degenerative arthritis
    3. Fracture
    4. Metastatic disease
    5. Primary bone tumor
    6. Diskitis
    7. Epidural abscess
    8. Ankylosing spondylitis
    9. Paget's disease
    10. Tethered spinal cord
    11. Spondylolisthesis
    12. Conversion reaction

B. Lumbar spinal stenosis

    1. Peripheral vascular disease. Arterial vascular insufficiency can cause leg discomfort during walking but is relieved by simply stopping rather than bending forward or sitting.

    2. Degenerative hip disease can cause limitation of standing and walking. The pain usually comes on with any type of weight bearing. Examination reveals a decreased range of motion of the hip, and hip rotation may exacerbate the discomfort. The pain associated with degenerative hip disease is most likely to be located in the proximal hip, thigh, and knee.

V. Diagnostic approach

A. Acute low back pain.
In the absence of red flags that suggest a more serious disorder, most testing should be delayed for 4 weeks. If the patient does not

respond to conservative treatment in 4 weeks, however, the following studies may be considered.
   1. Lumbosacral radiographs of the spine
   2. Magnetic resonance imaging (MRI)
   3. Computed tomography (CT) scan if MRI is not available or if the patient is claustrophobic. CT should include L3-4, L4-5, and L5-S1.
   4. Lumbosacral myelography and postmyelography CT seldom are needed unless it is impossible to perform MRI.
   5. Laboratory tests include complete blood cell count with differential and erythrocyte sedimentation rate.
   6. A bone scan can be done, especially if there is a history of carcinoma.
   B. **Lumbar disk disease with sciatica.** Few tests are needed in the first 4 weeks if the signs and symptoms are mild to moderate. Severe sciatica and sciatica associated with marked neurologic deficits and weakness of bladder and bowel movements should be evaluated earlier. The presence of a disk rupture on an imaging study does not necessarily imply nerve-root dysfunction. Approximately 75% of adult patients with symptoms have disk bulges or protrusions. Most severe sciatica is associated with disk extrusion.
   1. Plain lumbosacral radiographs of the spine should be performed.
   2. MRI is the procedure of choice for evaluating a lumbar disk rupture. L5-S1 disk extrusion causing severe right Sl nerve-root compression is shown in Fig. 23.1.

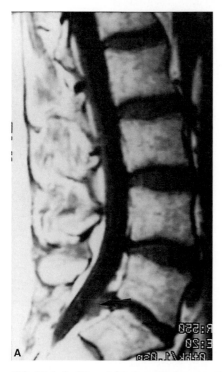
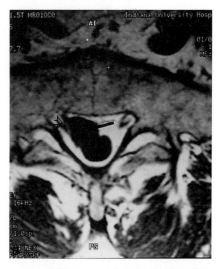

FIG. 23.1 A: T1-weighted sagittal magnetic resonance (MR) image shows a lumbar disk extrusion at L5-S1 that has gone down the lumbosacral canal (*arrow*). **B:** T2-weighted axial MR image shows a large, extruded L5-S1 disk fragment (*solid arrow*) compressing the right S1 nerve root (*open arrow*).

      3. CT may be used if the patient is unable to tolerate MRI.
      4. Myelography and postmyelography CT can be used occasionally if MRI and CT do not provide enough information for a diagnosis.
      5. Electromyography and nerve conduction velocity studies may be helpful if the signs and symptoms do not correlate well with the MRI or CT findings and if one suspects a peripheral nerve problem.
    C. Lumbar spinal stenosis. Unless the symptoms are severe, testing may not be done in the early stages of spinal stenosis. A patient who seeks medical therapy for spinal stenosis usually has a walking tolerance of less than 1 to 2 blocks and a standing tolerance of 20 minutes or less.
      1. Plain radiographs of the lumbosacral spine are indicated to assess the degree of degenerative change and bone density. Flexion–extension lateral views are needed to detect degenerative spondylolisthesis (Fig. 23.2). Degenerative spondylolisthesis frequently is associated with spinal stenosis.
      2. MRI is the best study for evaluating the number of levels involved and the severity of the spinal stenosis. Fig. 23.3. is an MR image that shows severe stenosis at L4-5.

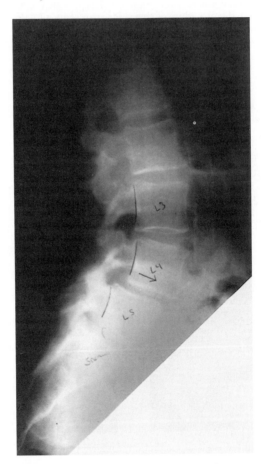

FIG. 23.2 Lateral plain radiograph of the lumbosacral spine shows spondylolisthesis of L4 on L5.

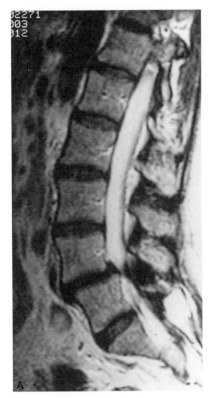
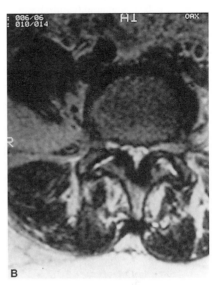

FIG. 23.3 A: T2-weighted sagittal magnetic resonance (MR) image shows segmental stenosis at L4-5. **B:** Axial T2-weighted MR image shows severe stenosis at L4-5. There is marked facet and ligamentous hypertrophy.

3. **CT** can be used if MRI is not available, but CT does not show the complete lumbar spine and has poorer resolution.
4. A **bone scan** should be obtained if there is a history of malignant disease.
5. **Radiographs of the hip** are needed if there is decreased range of motion of the hip or pain with rotation of the hip.
6. **Laboratory tests.** Complete blood cell count and differential and erythrocyte sedimentation rate should be obtained and possibly serum and urine protein electrophoresis performed if there are systemic symptoms. A prostatic specific antigen (PSA) assay should be performed for male patients older than 50 years.
7. **Arterial Doppler ultrasonography** should be performed if the patient has diminished or absent peripheral pulses.

VI. **Treatment**
   A. **Acute low back pain.** Approximately 90% of patients with acute low back pain recover within 1 month. Treatment is as follows.
   1. Restriction of patient activities as tolerated
   2. Acetaminophen
   3. Nonsteroidal antiinflammatory drugs (cyclooxygenase-2 inhibitors)
   4. Opioids, but for no longer than 2 weeks
   5. Short course of steroids (3 to 5 days)

      6. Muscle relaxants
      7. Heat
      8. Limit lifting to 20 pounds (9 kg) for moderate to severe back pain. Activity restrictions at work should seldom be extended beyond 3 months.
  B. Lumbar disk disease with sciatica. The initial management of sciatica is similar to that of acute low back pain. At least one half of patients with sciatica improve within 1 month.
      1. Two to 4 days of rest with gradual return to normal activities
      2. Acetaminophen
      3. Nonsteroidal antiinflammatory drugs (cyclooxygenase-2 inhibitors)
      4. Short course of opioids (no more than 2 weeks)
      5. Short course of steroids (3 to 5 days)
      6. Muscle relaxants
      7. Heat
      8. Limit lifting to 20 pounds (9 kg). Try to keep work-related activity restrictions to no more than 3 months.
  C. Lumbar spinal stenosis
      1. Conservative therapy requires that patients be taught to live within the limits of their walking and standing tolerances. They need to realize that they should get off their feet, if possible, when symptoms occur. Patient with severe limitation of walking may benefit from the use of license plates for persons with disabilities. Patients with degenerative spondylolisthesis may benefit from lumbosacral support. Flexion exercises should be considered.
      2. Surgical treatment should be considered only if the patient's condition is medically stable and the patient can no longer live with his or her degree of spinal claudication. Patients with true sciatica that does not respond to conservative therapy also can be considered for surgery. Surgical procedures that can be considered include lumbar laminectomy, lateral recess decompression, and spinal fusion. Seldom is surgery for spinal stenosis necessary in the first 3 months of symptoms. In most cases, the patient has symptoms for 12 to 18 months.
VII. Surgical referral
  A. Severe and disabling sciatica
  B. Neurologic deficits such as foot drop or bladder and bowel disturbance
  C. Poor response to at least 4 weeks of conservative therapy
  D. Other red flags (Table 23.1)

Recommended Readings

Clinical Practice Guidelines, Acute Low Back Problems in Adults: Assessment and Treatment. US Department of Health and Human Services, AHCPR publication no. 95-0643. December 1994.

Frymoyer JW. *The adult spine: principles and practice.* New York: Raven Press, 1991.

Jensen MC, Brant-Zawadzki MN, Obuchowski N, et al. Magnetic resonance imaging of the lumbar spine in people without back pain. *N Engl J Med* 1994;331:69–73.

Malmivaara A. The treatment of low back pain—bed rest, exercise, or ordinary activity? *N Engl J Med* 1995;332:351–355.

Mixter WJ, Barr JS. Rupture of the intervertebral disc with involvement of the spinal canal. *N Engl J Med* 1934;211:210–215.

Rockman RH, Simeone FA. *The spine.* Philadelphia: WB Saunders, 1992.

24. APPROACH TO THE PATIENT WITH UPPER EXTREMITY PAIN AND PARESTHESIAS AND ENTRAPMENT NEUROPATHIES

Mark A. Ross

Upper extremity (UE) pain and paresthesia are common in clinical practice. The conditions causing these symptoms often are reversible peripheral nervous system (PNS) or musculoskeletal (MSK) disorders. Common PNS disorders causing these symptoms include cervical radiculopathy, brachial plexopathy, and entrapment syndromes of individual peripheral nerves (mononeuropathy). In addition to pain and paresthesia, symptoms can include muscle weakness and atrophy. The location of symptoms and signs reflect the anatomy of the PNS. Thus knowledge of PNS anatomy is fundamental for diagnosis. Because symptoms and physical findings of several PNS disorders overlap, electrodiagnostic studies (EDS) are commonly used to clarify a specific diagnosis. Determination of the specific cause of UE problems is possible through the integration of clinical history, physical findings, and results of diagnostic studies.

I. **Differential diagnosis and causes of UE pain.** See Table 24.1.
II. **Evaluation**
   A. **History**
      1. **Symptoms.** The patient's description of symptoms should be obtained. Clarification of symptoms often is necessary because patients may misuse terms, such as saying "weakness" to describe numbness. The examiner should inquire about symptoms in the unaffected UE and legs to address the possibility of a generalized process.
         a. **Sensory symptoms**
            (1) **Pain.** Descriptions of pain are never pathognomonic of specific disorders. Tingling or radiating pain suggests a peripheral nerve, plexus, or root disorder, whereas dull, aching, nonradiating pain is typical of MSK disorders. Exceptions to this generalization occur frequently. Acute onset of excruciating pain in the shoulder or arm is common with idiopathic brachial plexopathy. Pain radiating from the neck to the arm or hand suggests radiculopathy. The location of pain often suggests the root involved, such as lateral arm (C5), lateral forearm or thumb (C6), middle finger (C7), or medial aspect of hand and forearm (C8). Pain localized to the shoulder can result from MSK disorders such as bicipital tendinitis, rotator cuff injury, and adhesive capsulitis, or from PNS disorders such as C5 radiculopathy, brachial plexopathy, and entrapment of the suprascapular or dorsal scapular nerves. Pain radiating distant from the site of the pathologic process may belie the location. For example, carpal tunnel syndrome (CTS) occasionally manifests as forearm or shoulder pain. Forearm pain can occur with C6 radiculopathy, plexopathy, or entrapment of nerves in the forearm. Pain involving specific digits can help narrow diagnostic considerations. Involvement of the thumb, index finger, or middle finger, or some combination thereof, suggests median mononeuropathy, a disorder of the upper or middle component of the brachial plexus, or C6 or C7 radiculopathy. Pain involving the ring and little fingers suggests ulnar mononeuropathy, a lower plexus disorder, or C8-T1 radiculopathy. Digital pain also can result from local MSK disorders, such as arthritis. Bizarre descriptions of pain are typical of psychological or functional disorders.
            (2) **Paresthesia and sensory loss.** Paresthesia is a spontaneous sensation originating from nerve fibers. Patients may describe it as "tingling" or "pins and needles." Sensory loss refers to the absence of normal sensation, which patients may describe as "numbness" or "like Novocain." Paresthesia and sensory loss can occur together or independently, and either suggests PNS disease is more likely than

Table 24.1 Differential diagnosis and causes of upper extremity pain

Disorder	Common cause
Peripheral Nervous System	
Radiculopathy	Root compression (disk, bone), trauma
Brachial plexopathy	Idiopathic conditions, trauma, tumor, radiation, compression (thoracic outlet syndrome)
Mononeuropathy	
Suprascapular n.	Trauma, IBP
Dorsal scapular n.	Trauma, IBP
Long thoracic n.	Trauma, IBP
Musculocutaneous n.	Trauma, IBP
Median n.	
Anterior interosseous n.	Compression, trauma
Pronator teres syndrome	Compression, trauma
Carpal tunnel syndrome	Compression
Ulnar n.	
Cubital tunnel syndrome	Compression, trauma
Guyon's canal	Compression, trauma
Radial n.	
Spiral groove	Compression, trauma
Posterior interosseous	Compression, trauma
Superficial radial	Compression, trauma
Musculoskeletal System	
Rotator cuff injury	Overuse, trauma
Biceps tendinitis	Overuse, trauma
Adhesive capsulitis	Immobility, shoulder weakness
Lateral epicondylitis	Overuse, trauma

IBP, idiopathic brachial plexopathy; n, nerve.

a MSK disorder. The distribution of paresthesia or sensory loss has localizing value similar to that described earlier for pain. However, in many cases of mononeuropathy or radiculopathy, paresthesia, sensory loss, and pain do not conform precisely to the known anatomic distribution of the affected nerve or nerve root. For example, a patient with a median mononeuropathy resulting from CTS may state that the entire hand is numb. Thus failure of sensory symptoms to localize precisely to a specific nerve or nerve-root distribution should not exclude the possibility of these disorders. The differential diagnosis of paresthesia and sensory loss has to include central nervous system (CNS) disease, especially when pain is absent.

    b. **Motor symptoms.** Patients who report weakness should be asked to describe specific activities that cause difficulty. Problems with fine motor skills, such as buttoning buttons, indicate distal muscle weakness and suggest involvement of the C8 or T1 roots, lower plexus, or nerves supplying hand muscles (median or ulnar nerves). Difficulty with arm and shoulder movements indicates proximal muscle weakness, suggesting involvement of the C5 or C6 roots, upper plexus, or nerves supplying proximal muscles (e.g., long thoracic, suprascapular, or axillary nerves). Patients with pain or sensory loss may misconstrue impaired motor performance as weakness. This possibility can be clarified during the examination or by asking the patient to state which factor chiefly limits his or her performance. CNS disorders can produce weakness of either the proximal or distal muscles.

2. **Onset and precipitating factors.** The history should address the patient's activity at or just before the onset of symptoms and whether or not physical activity exacerbates the symptoms.

   a. **Physical activity.** Some physical activities can be predisposing factors for the development of specific PNS disorders. Heavy lifting can cause cervical disk herniation and resultant radiculopathy. Head turning often exacerbates pain or paresthesia associated with radiculopathy. Arm abduction or shoulder rotation exacerbates the pain of MSK shoulder disorders and the pain associated with brachial plexopathy. Repetitive flexion and extension movements of the elbow or sustained elbow flexion can be predisposing factors for ulnar mononeuropathy at the elbow (cubital tunnel syndrome). Repetitive flexion and extension movements at the wrist or fingers can be predisposing factors for median mononeuropathy within the carpal tunnel (CTS). Repetitive pronation and supination can lead to hypertrophy of the pronator teres muscle and median nerve entrapment in the forearm (pronator teres syndrome). The radial nerve can be compressed in the axillary region by improper use of a crutch or in the arm when pressure is applied by a tourniquet, a hard surface, or the body's weight. Radial nerve compression in the arm is especially likely to occur when the patient's level of consciousness is reduced by anesthesia, sedatives, or alcohol intoxication. Handcuffs or other tight-fitting objects at the wrist, such as watchbands or bracelets, can injure the median, ulnar, or superficial radial sensory nerves. The history should review the patient's occupation, hobbies, and recent changes in physical activity. Sporting activities, playing musical instruments, gardening, and knitting are examples of physical activities that can contribute to development of compressive nerve injuries.

   b. **Trauma** often causes UE pain and sensorimotor problems. Even remote trauma can have a bearing on UE pain or sensorimotor symptoms. Examples include entrapment of a nerve by the callus of a healing fracture and development of a central cavity in the spinal cord (syringomyelia).

      (1) **Motor vehicle accident (MVA).** The severe trauma of an MVA can cause various PNS disorders, including vertebral fracture with direct spinal cord injury, nerve-root avulsion, radiculopathy, brachial plexus injury, peripheral nerve injury, or late development of syringomyelia. Arm traction or stretching the arm and neck in opposite directions can cause cervical root avulsion or stretch injury to the brachial plexus. An MVA can cause more than one PNS disorder, such as cervical nerve-root avulsion and concomitant peripheral nerve injury. After an MVA, attention to multiple life-threatening injuries or casting for multiple limb fractures can preclude detection of PNS disorders until late in the course of recovery.

      (2) **Fractures and dislocations** can cause specific nerve injuries. Shoulder dislocation or fracture of the humerus can injure the axillary nerve. Fracture of the clavicle can injure components of the brachial plexus. Fracture of the humerus is a predisposing factor for radial nerve injury in the spiral groove, whereas fracture or dislocation of the radius can injure the posterior interosseous branch of the radial nerve. Fracture of the elbow is a predisposing factor for ulnar mononeuropathy, which may not manifest until years after the trauma, hence the name "tardy ulnar palsy." A wrist fracture can cause either median or ulnar mononeuropathy.

      (3) **Laceration.** When UE pain or sensorimotor symptoms begin after a skin laceration or puncture wound, direct injury to a nerve has to be considered. Exploration is needed to determine whether the nerve requires repair.

   c. **Physiologic compression sites.** The median and ulnar nerves have sites where the anatomic relations between the nerve and normal ligamentous and bony structures make the nerve vulnerable to physical compression. The site of common compression injury is the wrist for the median nerve (carpal tunnel) and the elbow for the ulnar nerve (cubital tunnel). At these locations, the nerves are particularly susceptible to compression injury, hence the term **physiologic compression sites.** A patient with UE sensorimotor symptoms and no clear predisposing factors is likely to have an abnormality of one of these nerves.

    d. Systemic illness can be a predisposing factor for development of PNS disorders that manifest as UE sensorimotor symptoms. A complete list of systemic illnesses with PNS complications exceeds the scope of this chapter, but the following are common examples.

        (1) Endocrine disorders. Patients with diabetic polyneuropathy are more vulnerable to development of mononeuropathy at physiologic compression sites. Patients with hypothyroidism are prone to development of CTS.

        (2) Rheumatologic disorders. Several rheumatologic disorders predispose to UE nerve or nerve-root injury. Rheumatoid arthritis can cause degenerative disease of the spine that leads to cervical radiculopathy. Patients with rheumatoid arthritis also are susceptible to CTS and posterior interosseous neuropathy. Systemic vasculitis can involve individual peripheral nerves in either the UE or the lower extremity. Abrupt onset of mononeuropathy occasionally is the manifestation of systemic vasculitis. Primary amyloidosis and some hereditary forms are associated with CTS.

        (3) Renal failure and dialysis. Patients undergoing long-term hemodialysis are particularly likely to have CTS owing to deposition of amyloid material (β_2-microglobulin) within the carpal tunnel. Placement of arteriovenous fistulas for hemodialysis access can be associated with development of median or ulnar neuropathy and, less often, severe distal ischemic injury to all UE nerves, known as **ischemic monomelic neuropathy.** Diabetic patients seem particularly prone to this severe UE nerve injury.

        (4) Malignant disease. A patient with a history of cancer, particularly of the breast or lung, who has UE sensorimotor problems needs to be evaluated for metastasis to the brachial plexus. Patients who have undergone radiation therapy to the brachial plexus region may have radiation-induced brachial plexopathy, which can begin many years after radiation therapy.

  3. Other history. The medical history interview should include inquiries about symptoms of depression and a review of the social situation for factors that may influence the symptoms. Specific questions should be asked regarding employment, accidents, work injuries, and possible litigation. Evidence of CNS disease should be sought, which may include seizures, disturbed consciousness, personality change, or problems with cognition, language, or vision.

B. Physical examination

  1. Motor examination

    a. Muscle inspection. Muscles are inspected for evidence of atrophy and spontaneous muscle contractions. Muscle atrophy is present when reduction of the normal muscle bulk or contour is revealed by visual inspection or direct measurement of limb circumference. Atrophy of specific muscles helps localize the disorder. For example, atrophy of the thenar eminence alone suggests a disorder of the median nerve or the deep terminal branch of the ulnar nerve. Atrophy of the thenar and hypothenar areas and the interossei muscles should raise considerations of combined median and ulnar mononeuropathy, lower trunk brachial plexopathy, C8-T1 radiculopathy, or C8-T1 spinal cord disease. Winging or elevation of one scapula when the arms are extended forward suggests long thoracic nerve mononeuropathy. Inspection of muscles also involves a careful search for fine muscle twitches visible through the skin, called **fasciculations.** These twitches can occur as isolated symptoms or findings in healthy persons. When present in conjunction with muscle weakness and atrophy, fasciculations are a sign of disease. The examination should include inspection for fasciculations in all four limbs, as well as in the back and abdomen. Fasciculations occur most commonly with anterior horn cell diseases, such as amyotrophic lateral sclerosis, but also can occur with diseases affecting the motor root, plexus, or peripheral nerve.

   b. **Muscle strength ratings.** Muscle strength is assessed by means of manual muscle testing. The Medical Research Council strength rating scale is used (Table 22.1). Muscle strength ratings are made for proximal and distal muscles in all four limbs, which can reveal weakness of which the patient was not aware. Muscles that should be tested bilaterally in the UE include muscles for arm abduction (deltoid and supraspinatus), arm external rotation (infraspinatus), elbow flexion (biceps), elbow extension (triceps), wrist flexion (flexor carpi radialis and flexor carpi ulnaris), wrist extension (extensor carpi radialis), finger flexion (flexor digitorum superficialis and flexor digitorum profundus), finger extension (extensor digitorum communis), finger spreading (interossei), thumb abduction (abductor pollicis brevis), and grip strength.

   Patients with MSK disorders and patients with depression, psychological disturbances, or malingering can exhibit a type of weakness known as **breakaway weakness,** in which incomplete effort gives the appearance of weakness. Features suggesting breakaway weakness include reports of pain during testing, reasonable initial strength that diminishes, variability in motor performance on serial examinations, improved strength with encouragement, and absence of other objective signs of motor impairment. When patients exhibit breakaway weakness as a result of a psychological disturbance or malingering, they often make facial expressions or contortions of the tested limb that imply great effort is being made.

   c. **Muscle tone** is assessed by means of observing how easily the patient's limbs can be passively moved while the patient is asked to relax the limb tested. Tone is rated according to the Ashworth scale, in which normal tone is assigned a value of 1, and values 2 to 5 represent increasing degrees of abnormal stiffness. Muscle tone should be normal with all of the common PNS disorders that cause UE pain and sensorimotor symptoms. Increased muscle tone should raise the question of a CNS disorder. When increased muscle tone occurs with UE weakness and atrophy, a compressive lesion of the cervical spine or amyotrophic lateral sclerosis must be considered.

2. **Reflexes** are tested bilaterally in all four limbs, including the brachioradialis (C5-6), biceps (C5-6), triceps (C7-8), quadriceps (L2-4), and soleus (S1) tendons. Reflexes are rated as normal, decreased, or increased. Marked reflex asymmetry suggests abnormality of the nervous system. Radiculopathy involving a cervical root typically depresses the corresponding UE reflex on the affected side. Brachial plexopathy decreases reflexes corresponding to the part of the plexus involved. Radiculopathy of the C8 or T1 root or lower trunk brachial plexopathy can produce normal UE reflexes. Mononeuropathy of the UE does not usually influence the UE reflexes unless the nerve involved supplies the muscle tested in the reflex arc. For example, musculocutaneous nerve mononeuropathy can reduce the biceps reflex. Reflexes are preserved in MSK disorders and increased in CNS disorders.

3. **Sensory examination.** The sensory examination involves testing of light touch, pain (pinprick), vibration, and joint position sensations in the UE and lower extremity. Particular attention is paid to cutaneous areas where there are sensory problems.

4. **Maneuvers.** Several maneuvers can aid in the evaluation of UE sensorimotor problems.

    a. Tinel's sign, originally used for assessment of regenerating nerve fibers, is commonly used as an indication of paresthesia radiating in the cutaneous distribution of the nerve. It is elicited by means of mild tapping over the nerve. Tinel's sign may be observed in association with regenerating nerve fibers, neuroma, or focal demyelinating nerve lesions and even in healthy persons. Tinel's sign is easier to elicit from a diseased nerve than from a normal nerve, and thus it can help to localize an abnormal nerve. By means of tapping over the median nerve on the volar surface of the wrist, Tinel's sign is commonly used to assess for CTS.

    b. In **Phalen's maneuver,** the wrist is flexed for up to 1 minute in an attempt to induce numbness or tingling in the median nerve distribution. A positive Phalen's maneuver is supportive evidence of CTS.

    c. In **Adson's maneuver,** the arm is moved into an abducted and extended position, and the radial pulse is assessed. Although loss of the radial pulse with this maneuver is alleged to indicate compression of the subclavian artery by a cervical rib or hypertrophied or tight scalenus muscles, it is not a useful test, because it is subjective and can cause healthy persons to lose their radial pulse.

C. Laboratory studies

    1. Electrodiagnostic studies consist of nerve conduction velocity (NCV) studies and electromyography (EMG). These tests allow objective and quantitative assessment of individual peripheral nerves and muscles. They can substantiate a clinically suspected diagnosis or reveal unsuspected abnormalities. With rare exceptions, all patients with symptoms of UE pain and sensorimotor symptoms should undergo EDS as part of the initial diagnostic evaluation. When performed in the first few days after onset of nerve injury, EDS do not reveal as many abnormalities as when performed 7 to 10 days later. However, performing EDS soon after injury can document preexisting abnormalities that can be important for complicated diagnostic cases or when medicolegal issues occur. EDS are discussed in detail in Chapter 33.

    2. Radiologic studies

        a. Plain radiographs. After trauma with neck or UE injury, radiographs of the cervical spine or plain bone radiographs are necessary to evaluate for fractures. When cervical radiculopathy is suspected, cervical spinal radiographs may reveal narrowing of specific neural foramina. Cervical spinal radiographs also can be useful in detecting a cervical rib, which should be investigated when clinical and EDS evidence suggests neurogenic thoracic outlet syndrome (TOS). Patients with brachial plexopathy need chest radiographs to evaluate for malignant disease. If clinical evidence suggests Pancoast's syndrome, chest radiographs in the apical view should be included to search for an apical tumor. Plain radiographs can be also useful in evaluation of MSK disorders if they show evidence of degenerative arthritis or calcifications within tendons.

        b. Magnetic resonance imaging (MRI). Radiologic evaluation of cervical radiculopathy is most often accomplished by means of MRI. Myelography combined with computed tomography also can be used. MRI of the brachial plexus often is used to search for evidence of tumor as the cause of brachial plexopathy.

        c. Laboratory studies for investigation of systemic illnesses are performed for patients with UE sensorimotor problems, depending on individual circumstances. Tests that can be useful include complete blood cell count with differential, chemistry panel, blood sugar, erythrocyte sedimentation rate, antinuclear antibody, urinalysis, serum immunofixation electrophoresis, thyroid function, and spinal fluid tests.

D. Unexplained symptoms. Patients reporting UE pain or sensorimotor symptoms sometimes have no objective evidence of a PNS disorder after thorough evaluation. For such patients, possible explanations for symptoms include CNS disease, depression, psychological factors, or malingering. The symptoms and signs of CNS and PNS disease can overlap, particularly for slowly progressive conditions, such as brain tumor or multiple sclerosis. Evidence suggesting CNS disease includes painless weakness or sensory disturbance, upper motor neuron signs, altered consciousness or personality, or problems with cognition, language, or vision. Patients with depression can have unexplained UE pain or sensorimotor symptoms. Some patients with unexplained UE symptoms may not have frank depression but have unhappiness or conflict in the psychosocial realm, which manifests as symptoms of neurologic dysfunction. Often such patients cannot recognize or accept the relation between their symptoms and their psychological state. Others have onset of symptoms after accidents or injuries, and either the process of litigation or the power of suggestion from inquisitive physicians distorts the usual concept of wellness and perpetuates the symptoms. Patients with unexplained symptoms need neurologic consultation and may need to be observed for an extended period.

III. Diagnostic approach. Briefly, the history is used to form initial hypotheses about the cause of the symptoms, and these hypotheses are tested during the physical examination. Knowledge of PNS anatomy is essential for interpreting UE sensorimotor symptoms and signs. In almost all cases, EDS are performed to help localize a suspected PNS disorder or to exclude a PNS disorder. When a PNS disorder is present, EDS help determine the severity and type of pathologic process. Additional diagnostic assessments can include radiologic studies or laboratory tests, depending on individual patient circumstances.

IV. Selected disorders and criteria for diagnosis

    A. Peripheral nervous system disorders

        1. Mononeuropathy

            a. Median nerve

                (1) Carpal tunnel syndrome

                    (a) Anatomy and etiology. CTS is an extremely common disorder caused by compression of the median nerve at the wrist within the unyielding space known as the carpal tunnel. Many disorders compromise this space and result in median nerve compression. The most common cause is flexor tenosynovitis, which can be associated with excessive physical use of the hands. Patients with primary carpal stenosis—a narrow carpal tunnel—can be especially prone to CTS. Other local factors causing CTS include vascular lesions, abnormal tendons, ganglion cyst, tumoral calcinosis, pseudoarthrosis, and infection. Systemic illnesses associated with CTS include endocrine disorders, such as hyperparathyroidism, acromegaly, and hypothyroidism, and rheumatologic disorders, such as rheumatoid arthritis, systemic lupus erythematosus, polymyalgia rheumatica, temporal arteritis, scleroderma, and gout. Other conditions predisposing to CTS include diabetic and other forms of polyneuropathy, chronic hemodialysis, shunts for hemodialysis, and pregnancy.

                    (b) The **clinical features** of CTS include numbness or tingling involving one or more of the first four digits (thumb through ring finger), although occasionally the entire hand is involved. There can be pain in the fingers or wrist, and at times in the forearm or shoulder. Patients often report being awakened at night by these symptoms, and physical activity involving use of the hands can exacerbate the symptoms. Patients may observe weakness and atrophy of the thenar muscle. Physical examination reveals decreased sensation in the volar aspect of the first four digits. Because the median nerve innervation frequently supplies only the lateral half of the ring finger, sparing of sensation on the medial half of the ring finger is a helpful sign. Advanced cases show weakness and atrophy of the abductor pollicis brevis. Tinel's and Phalen's signs may be present.

(c) The **diagnosis** of CTS is established with the clinical history, physical findings, and EDS results. The EDS findings vary with the severity of the disorder. In mild cases, the amplitude of the median compound muscle action potential (CMAP) and sensory nerve action potential (SNAP) are normal, and the latency values of the median SNAP and CMAP from the wrist are increased, with focal slowing of median NCV across the wrist. Slowing of NCV in proximal median nerve segments should not exclude the diagnosis of CTS. In some cases, there can be conduction block at the wrist level. In more advanced cases, the median CMAP and SNAP amplitude values decline, and fibrillation potentials may be found in the abductor pollicis brevis muscle but not in other muscles, including median-innervated forearm muscles. The EDS results for the ulnar nerve in the same hand are normal.

(2) **Pronator teres syndrome**

  (a) **Anatomy and etiology.** *Pronator teres syndrome* refers to presumed compression of the median nerve in the forearm where it passes between the two heads of the pronator teres muscle. This disorder is uncommon and usually is related to an occupation that involves repetitive pronation of the forearm. Such activity or hypertrophy of the pronator teres muscle can compress the median nerve. A fibrous band from pronator teres to flexor digitorum superficialis and local trauma are other potential causes.

  (b) **Clinical features.** The predominant symptom is pain in the volar forearm. Weakness of the abductor pollicis brevis and median distribution sensory problems usually are not present but occasionally occur. The pronator teres muscle itself remains strong. Examination may show tenderness in the region of the pronator teres muscle, and there may be a Tinel's sign over the pronator muscle.

  (c) The **diagnosis** is established primarily with the clinical features. Results of EDS often are normal, but occasionally slow median NCV can be observed in the forearm segment.

(3) **Anterior interosseous syndrome**

  (a) **Anatomy and etiology.** This relatively uncommon median nerve disorder involves compression of the anterior interosseous branch of the median nerve in the forearm, usually by a fibrous band from the pronator teres or the flexor digitorum superficialis muscle. Other forearm anomalies or forearm trauma can also cause the disorder. The anterior interosseous nerve (AIN) is a purely motor nerve that supplies the flexor pollicis longus (FPL), flexor digitorum I and II, and pronator quadratus muscles.

  (b) The **clinical features** include forearm or elbow pain combined with weakness of flexion of the distal phalanx of the thumb (FPL) and the index and middle fingers (flexor digitorum), or weakness of some of these functions. Patients notice inability to pinch the thumb and index finger together but generally do not report weakness of pronation, because the major muscle involved with pronation, the pronator teres, is unaffected.

  (c) The **diagnosis** is established with the clinical features and EDS results. The results of median nerve conduction studies (NCS) are normal, because the AIN does not contribute to the muscle assessed for median NCS, and median sensory fibers do not travel in the AIN. EMG shows fibrillation potentials confined to one or more of the aforementioned muscles supplied by the AIN. When the AIN causes weakness confined to the FPL, EMG is extremely helpful for differentiating a partial AIN syndrome from rupture of the FPL tendon.

b. Ulnar nerve

    (1) Cubital tunnel syndrome

        (a) Anatomy and etiology. The most common cause of entrapment of the ulnar nerve in the elbow region is compression in the cubital tunnel. The floor of the tunnel is formed by the medial ligament of the elbow, and the roof is the aponeurosis of the flexor carpi ulnaris muscle. The ulnar nerve runs through this space, and then underneath the flexor carpi ulnaris muscle. Remote elbow trauma, with or without fracture, is a predisposing factor for later development of entrapment neuropathy in the elbow region (tardy ulnar palsy). However, many patients have ulnar neuropathy due to compression in the cubital tunnel without antecedent trauma. Repetitive movement at the elbow or prolonged flexion of the elbow can be predisposing factors.

        (b) The **clinical features** include sensory problems in the ulnar division of the hand (fifth digit and medial half of the fourth) and the ulnar-innervated portion of the hand and wrist. Sensory problems include decreased sensation, paresthesia, and pain. Pain can involve the medial forearm and elbow. Weakness involves the interossei, abductor digiti minimi, adductor pollicis, and flexor pollicis brevis muscles. When weakness is chronic, atrophy may be present, and a clawhand deformity can develop. Most often, the flexor carpi ulnaris muscle remains strong. A diagnosis of ulnar neuropathy requires normal strength in the C8-T1 muscles innervated by the median and radial nerves.

        (c) The **diagnosis** is established with the characteristic history and physical findings and with the EDS results. Ulnar neuropathy at the elbow can show reduction of the ulnar CMAP and SNAP. There may be evidence of conduction block in motor fibers that can be localized to the elbow region. Ulnar NCV can be focally slow across the elbow. EMG reveals fibrillation potentials or abnormal motor unit potentials (MUPs), or both, in ulnar-innervated hand muscles. Usually the flexor carpi ulnaris muscle does not show fibrillation potentials, although it may do so if its motor branch also is compressed.

    (2) Compression at the wrist (Guyon's canal)

        (a) Anatomy and etiology. Guyon's canal is a fibroosseous tunnel connecting the pisiform and hamate wrist bones through which the ulnar nerve travels. As it emerges from Guyon's canal, the ulnar nerve divides into a deep terminal branch, which is purely motor and supplies all of the ulnar-innervated hand muscles, and a superficial terminal branch, which supplies sensation to the medial distal half of the palm and the palmar surfaces of the fourth and fifth digits. Sensation to the medial proximal half of the palm is supplied by the palmar cutaneous branch of the ulnar nerve, which arises in the midforearm and does not pass through Guyon's canal. Sensation to the medial dorsal half of the hand is supplied by the dorsal cutaneous branch of the ulnar nerve, which arises above the wrist and also does not pass through Guyon's canal. Predisposing factors for ulnar neuropathy at the wrist include chronic compression, which occurs among cyclists, and local trauma, such as wrist fracture.

        (b) The **clinical features** vary depending on the precise level of abnormality. Compression of the entire ulnar nerve within

Guyon's canal or of the two branches as they leave the canal causes weakness of all ulnar-innervated hand muscles and sensory loss in the superficial terminal branch distribution. Sensation of the dorsal medial hand and the proximal half of the medial palm is spared because sensation is supplied by other branches. Compression of the deep terminal motor branch can occur in isolation either before or after it supplies the hypothenar muscles, producing ulnar-innervated hand muscle weakness with no sensory loss. Finally, compression of only the superficial terminal branch causes sensory loss in its palmar distribution with normal hand strength.

(c) The **diagnosis** is established with clinical examination and EDS. The EDS findings vary depending on which of the ulnar nerve branches is involved. If the superficial terminal sensory branch is involved, NCS show a reduced or absent SNAP recorded from the fifth digit, but the SNAP from the dorsal ulnar cutaneous nerve remains normal. If the abnormality involves the deep terminal branch, ulnar CMAP amplitude can be reduced, and there can be fibrillation potentials or abnormal MUPs in ulnar-innervated hand muscles.

c. Radial nerve

(1) Axilla or spiral groove compression

(a) **Anatomy and etiology.** The radial nerve can be compressed against the humerus by external pressure in the axilla or the spiral groove. Compression in the axilla can be caused by improper use of crutches. Compression in the spiral groove is likely to occur when someone falls asleep with the arm hanging over a chair or with a partner's head against the arm, and the effects of alcohol or sedatives prevent paresthesia from arousing the person to move the arm. The term *Saturday night palsy* has been used for such a radial nerve palsy. A similar outcome can result from use of an arm tourniquet during surgery. The radial nerve can also be injured in the spiral groove by blunt trauma, by fractures of the humerus, and in rare instances by vigorous arm exercise.

(b) The **clinical features** are weakness of radial-innervated muscles and sensory loss on the dorsal aspects of the hand, thumb, and index and middle fingers. Radial-innervated muscles include the triceps, brachioradialis, supinator, and the wrist and finger extensors. The triceps is affected by axillary compression but is spared by spiral groove compression. Weakness of wrist extensors causes wrist drop. Inability to stabilize the wrist and fingers as a result of radial-innervated extensor weakness frequently creates the false impression that ulnar-innervated hand muscles are weak.

(c) The **diagnosis** of radial mononeuropathy is confirmed with clinical features and EDS results that verify abnormalities confined to the radial nerve distribution. Nerve conduction studies show a reduced-amplitude radial CMAP and reduced or absent SNAP. The presence or absence of fibrillation potentials in the triceps muscle helps to localize the compression site (axilla or spiral groove).

(2) Posterior interosseous nerve (PIN)

(a) **Anatomy and etiology.** The PIN is the purely motor termination of the radial nerve in the forearm. The PIN supplies the supinator muscle and the wrist and finger extensors. Entrapment of the PIN is relatively uncommon. When it does occur, it is usually at the level of the supinator muscle. Predisposing factors include vigorous use of the arm, fracture of the head of the radius, and other local trauma. Hypertrophied synovia of the elbow joint in patients with rheumatoid arthritis can compress the PIN.

(b) The **clinical features** are weakness of the wrist and finger extensors. Some patients have pain in the elbow or dorsal forearm. There are no sensory abnormalities apart from pain, because the posterior interosseous nerve is purely motor.

(c) The **diagnosis** is established with the clinical features and EDS results. NCS show a reduced-amplitude radial CMAP and normal radial SNAP. EMG shows fibrillation potentials and abnormal MUPs in the radial-innervated muscles.

(3) The superficial sensory branch

(a) Anatomy and etiology. The superficial sensory branch of the radial nerve arises in the vicinity of the elbow and supplies sensation to the dorsolateral hand and the dorsal aspects of the first three digits. It can be injured at the wrist level by local trauma or compression from tight objects around the wrist, such as watchbands or handcuffs.

(b) The **clinical features** are purely sensory—paresthesia and sensory loss in the radial sensory distribution.

(c) The **diagnosis** is made with the history, physical findings, and NCS evidence of a reduced or absent superficial radial SNAP.

d. Axillary nerve

(1) Anatomy and etiology. The posterior cord of the brachial plexus divides into the radial and axillary nerves. The axillary nerve travels below the shoulder joint and gives off a branch innervating the teres minor muscle, which is an external rotator of the arm. The axillary nerve then courses behind and lateral to the humerus before dividing into anterior and posterior branches, which supply corresponding portions of the deltoid muscle. The posterior branch gives off a cutaneous nerve that supplies the skin over the lateral aspect of the deltoid muscle. The axillary nerve can be injured by shoulder dislocation or fracture of the humerus. It occasionally may be the only nerve affected by idiopathic brachial plexopathy (see **IV.A.2.a.**).

(2) Clinical features. The main clinical manifestation is impaired shoulder abduction resulting from weakness of the deltoid. The supraspinatus muscle initiates arm abduction, so patients may retain limited arm abduction ability. Weakness of the teres minor muscle can be difficult to demonstrate at physical examination because of normal infraspinatus muscle function. Sensory loss can be demonstrated over the lateral portion of the deltoid muscle.

(3) The **diagnosis** is confirmed with the finding of weakness limited to the deltoid muscle and EMG abnormalities restricted to the deltoid and teres minor muscles. Axillary NCS with surface recording from the deltoid muscle may show delay or reduced amplitude of the axillary nerve CMAP.

e. Musculocutaneous nerve

(1) Anatomy and etiology. The musculocutaneous nerve arises from the lateral cord of the brachial plexus and supplies the coracobrachialis, biceps, and brachialis muscles. It continues in the forearm as the purely sensory lateral antebrachial cutaneous nerve. Mononeuropathy of the musculocutaneous nerve is uncommon, but it can occur with shoulder dislocation, direct trauma or compression, or sudden extension of the forearm.

(2) The **clinical features** include impaired arm flexion resulting from weakness of the biceps and other musculocutaneous-innervated muscles. The biceps reflex may be normal or reduced, depending on the severity of the biceps weakness. Sensory loss is present over the lateral forearm.

(3) **Diagnosis.** The clinical features of musculocutaneous neuropathy closely parallel those of C5 radiculopathy. The diagnosis is established with the clinical features and EDS results that differentiate C5 radiculopathy from musculocutaneous nerve mononeuropathy. The lateral antebrachial SNAP is reduced or absent in musculocutaneous neuropathy but normal in C5 radiculopathy. EMG shows involvement of only the aforementioned muscles supplied by the musculocutaneous nerve.

f. **Long thoracic nerve**

(1) **Anatomy and etiology.** The long thoracic nerve is a purely motor nerve arising from the ventral rami of the C5, C6, and C7 spinal nerves. It courses along with other brachial plexus components underneath the clavicle then travels down the chest wall anterolaterally to supply the serratus anterior muscle. This large muscle fixes the scapula to the chest wall and provides general stability for the shoulder during arm movement. Injury to the long thoracic nerve can occur with trauma or with vigorous physical activity involving shoulder girdle movement. Long thoracic neuropathy can be caused by idiopathic brachial plexopathy.

(2) The **clinical features** of long thoracic mononeuropathy include pain and weakness in the shoulder. Patients have difficulty abducting the arm or raising it above the head. Winging of the scapula is demonstrated by having the patient extend the arms forward and push against a wall. The scapula elevates from the chest wall because the weak serratus muscle cannot hold it.

(3) The **diagnosis** is established with the clinical features and EMG that shows fibrillation potentials involving only the serratus anterior muscle. Long thoracic nerve NCS are technically difficult, and other NCS results are normal.

g. **Suprascapular nerve**

(1) **Anatomy and etiology.** The suprascapular nerve is a purely motor nerve arising from the upper trunk of the brachial plexus and passing through the suprascapular notch on the upper border of the scapula to supply the supraspinatus and infraspinatus muscles. The suprascapular nerve is most often injured by trauma in which there is excessive forward flexion of the shoulder. It can be involved in idiopathic brachial plexopathy.

(2) The **clinical features** are pain in the posterior shoulder and weakness of the supraspinatus and infraspinatus muscles. The supraspinatus initiates arm abduction, whereas the infraspinatus externally rotates the arm.

(3) The **diagnosis** is established with the clinical history, physical findings, and EDS results. Results of routine NCS are normal, but motor NCS with recording from the supraspinatus muscle can show reduced amplitude or prolonged latency relative to the unaffected side. EMG shows abnormalities confined to the supraspinatus and infraspinatus muscles on the affected side.

h. **Dorsal scapular nerve (DSN)**

(1) **Anatomy and etiology.** The DSN is a purely motor nerve arising from the upper trunk of the brachial plexus and passing through the scalenus medius muscle to supply the rhomboid and levator scapulae muscles. Injury to the DSN is relatively uncommon.

(2) The **clinical features** include pain in the scapular region and weakness of the rhomboid and levator scapulae muscles.

(3) The **diagnosis** is established with the clinical features and EMG results showing fibrillation potentials restricted to the muscles supplied by the DSN. There is no satisfactory NCS for the DSN.

2. **Brachial plexopathy**
   a. **Idiopathic brachial plexopathy**
      (1) **Anatomy and etiology.** Idiopathic brachial plexopathy, also known as *Parsonage–Turner syndrome* or *neuralgic amyotrophy,* is an uncommon condition believed to represent an immune-mediated neuropathy affecting various portions of the brachial plexus. An antecedent event such as an upper respiratory infection or immunization is present in approximately one half of cases.
      (2) The main **clinical features** are abrupt onset of severe pain in the shoulder and proximal arm followed at a variable interval (hours to weeks) by shoulder and arm muscle weakness. The pain is exacerbated by movement of the arm, shoulder, or neck, which can give the false impression of an MSK disorder. Any combination of muscles innervated by nerves arising from the brachial plexus can be involved, but there is a predilection for proximal muscles. Muscles supplied by the axillary, suprascapular, long thoracic, radial, musculocutaneous, and anterior interosseous nerves are commonly involved, but other nerves can be affected. Involvement can be extensive or restricted to a single nerve, and asymmetric bilateral involvement occurs in one third of patients. Sensory loss or paresthesia may be present, but these features are relatively minor (Fig. 24.1).
      (3) The **diagnosis** is established with the characteristic clinical history, physical findings, and results of EDS. Patients with this disorder typically seek evaluation and management of the severe pain early in the course. If EDS are performed early, abnormalities of MUP recruitment can be found, but the results may be otherwise normal. If EDS are repeated 7 to 10 days after weakness begins, NCS show evidence of axonal injury, the distribution varying according to the specific nerves involved. EMG shows fibrillation potentials in clinically weak muscles, and often in muscles that were not judged weak by physical examination. For this reason, EMG is essential for determining the extent of injury.
   b. **Neurogenic thoracic outlet syndrome**
      (1) **Anatomy and etiology.** "True" neurogenic TOS is a rare disorder in which the lower trunk of the brachial plexus is compressed by an elongated transverse process of C7, a rudimentary cervical rib, or a fibrous band running from either of these to the first rib.
      (2) The **clinical features** are weakness and wasting of the intrinsic hand muscles, most markedly affecting the abductor pollicis brevis muscle; pain involving the medial forearm or hand; and sensory loss involving the fourth and fifth fingers and the medial hand and distal forearm.
      (3) The **diagnosis** is established with the clinical features and characteristic results of EDS. Radiographic evidence of an elongated C7 transverse process or a rudimentary cervical rib is helpful but not mandatory for diagnosis, because the structural problem may be a fibrous band that may be fond only at surgical exploration. The nerve conduction findings of neurogenic TOS are the combination of severely reduced or absent median CMAP, normal median SNAP, reduced or absent ulnar SNAP, and mildly reduced or normal ulnar CMAP. EMG shows fibrillation potentials in muscles innervated by the lower trunk, particularly those supplied by the median and ulnar nerves. Unlike the rare and well-defined true TOS, neurogenic TOS is a condition commonly misdiagnosed as TOS, which has various UE sensorimotor symptoms but no consistent clinical history. Patients said to have this form of TOS have no objective neurologic abnormalities and no abnormalities on EDS. This form of TOS has been aptly referred to as "disputed" neurogenic TOS, and

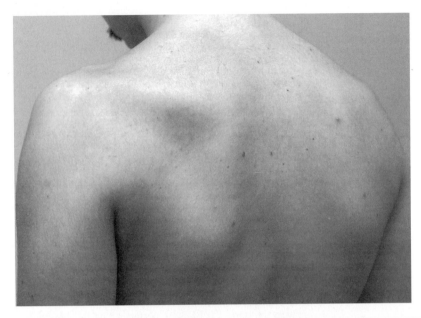

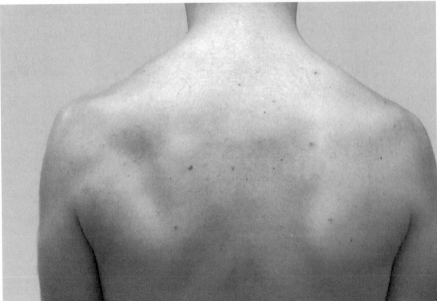

FIG. 24.1 A 25-year-old man developed abrupt onset of severe left shoulder pain followed by persistent weakness of arm external rotation. Examination 2 years after onset showed atrophy of the left deltoid, supraspinatus, and infraspinatus muscles. The latissimus dorsi, serratus anterior, and rhomboid muscles were normal. The supraspinatus and infraspinatus muscles showed fibrillation potentials and abnormal motor unit potentials suggesting partial reinnervation. The findings were consistent with nonfamilial Parsonage–Turner (neuralgic amyotrophy) syndrome. **Top:** Oblique view of left shoulder, showing atrophy of supraspinatus and infraspinatus muscles. **Bottom:** Direct view of back, showing asymmetric atrophy of the left supraspinatus and infraspinatus muscles. (Courtesy of José Biller, M.D.)

its existence as an entity remains controversial. Patients erroneously given the diagnosis of this type of TOS often undergo first-rib resection, and severe brachial plexopathy can be a complication.

   c. **Brachial plexopathy in patients with malignant disease**

      (1) **Anatomy and etiology.** Metastasis to the brachial plexus must be considered whenever a patient with a history of malignant disease, especially breast or lung cancer, has UE pain or sensorimotor symptoms. Brachial plexopathy usually is not the presenting feature of malignant disease, except in Pancoast's syndrome, in which apical lung carcinoma invades the lower trunk of the brachial plexus. Brachial plexopathy from radiation injury can occur months to many years after radiation therapy to the chest wall.

      (2) The **clinical features** of brachial plexopathy resulting from tumor invasion are pain, weakness, and sensory changes that can involve the upper or lower plexus. Unlike idiopathic brachial plexopathy, malignant brachial plexopathy has a gradual onset of symptoms, and lymphedema of the arm is common. In Pancoast's syndrome, patients usually first have pain in the medial aspect of the arm and may have sensorimotor abnormalities in the lower-trunk distribution. Horner's syndrome (ipsilateral ptosis, miosis, and facial anhidrosis) often results from tumor invasion of the inferior cervical sympathetic ganglion. Malignant plexopathy may be more likely than radiation plexopathy to be painful and involve the lower trunk, but this generalization is not reliable.

      (3) **Diagnosis.** A patient with a history of malignant disease and new-onset UE sensorimotor symptoms or pain needs EDS to exclude common conditions such as mononeuropathy or radiculopathy, which can cause symptoms identical to those of brachial plexopathy. The EDS can help determine whether there is evidence of brachial plexopathy and clarify the locations of abnormalities within the plexus. This information can help in planning and interpreting MRI studies of the plexus, which should be performed to look for evidence of tumor. Patients with lower-trunk plexopathy need apical view chest radiographs obtained to look for an apical lung tumor. Myokymic discharges detected at EDS in patients who have undergone radiation therapy to the chest wall support a diagnosis of radiation plexopathy but do not conclusively exclude tumor metastasis.

  3. Cervical radiculopathy. The clinical and EDS features of cervical radiculopathy are described in (3) and reviewed in Chapter 22, section **III.**

B. Musculoskeletal disorders share the predominant symptom of pain and an absence of other neurologic manifestations. In general, results of EDS are normal when MSK disorders are the cause of UE pain symptoms. However, it is common for an underlying neurologic disorder that affects the PNS to result in a secondary MSK disorder, in which case results of EDS can be abnormal because of the underlying neurologic disorder.

  1. Rotator cuff injury. The rotator cuff comprises the tendons of the supraspinatus, infraspinatus, teres minor, and subscapularis muscles, which fix the humeral head in the glenoid fossa during shoulder abduction and provide internal and external arm rotation. Rotator cuff inflammation (tendinitis) and tear are common causes of shoulder pain. Tendinitis results from repetitive minor trauma to the cuff, and tear can occur as a chronic stage of this degenerative process or acutely from abrupt trauma. With tendinitis or tear, there is shoulder pain on arm abduction or on internal or external arm rotation. With tear, there can be weakness of rotator cuff function, but EMG findings are normal. Plain radiographs may reveal tendon or subacromial bursa calcifications. Ultrasonography or arthrography of the shoulder can confirm a rotator cuff tear.

  2. Bicipital tendinitis. Inflammation of the biceps tendon (tendinitis) causes pain and tenderness in the anterior shoulder region. The pain may be reproduced by supination of the forearm against resistance or by flexion and extension of the shoulder. There are no neurologic abnormalities, and the diagnosis is established clinically.

3. **Adhesive capsulitis (frozen shoulder).** Loss of motion at the shoulder joint can result in adhesion of the joint capsule to the humerus. Usually, shoulder pain from any cause leads to immobility and subsequent adhesive capsulitis. Sometimes, however, weakness of shoulder girdle muscles from either PNS or CNS disorders can cause this problem. Whatever the cause, the joint becomes stiff, and attempted motion causes severe shoulder pain. Muscle atrophy can result from PNS disease or secondarily from disuse. The diagnosis usually is made with the clinical features.

4. **Lateral epicondylitis (tennis elbow).** Overuse of the extensor carpi radialis muscles (wrist extensors) or direct trauma to their tendinous insertion on the lateral epicondyle can lead to inflammation, degeneration, or tear of the tendons. This produces pain localized over the lateral epicondyle, which can be exacerbated by use of the forearm and wrist extensor muscles.

V. Referral. Patients should be referred to a reliable EMG laboratory for EDS, because these studies facilitate accurate diagnosis. Establishing the diagnosis guides subsequent diagnostic testing and treatment decisions. In addition, EDS can help estimate the severity of the abnormality, which can help in prognosis. Neurologic consultation for UE pain or sensorimotor symptoms is appropriate at any stage of the evaluation if there are questions concerning diagnosis or management.

Recommended Readings

Cailliet R, ed. *Neck and arm pain,* 2nd ed. Philadelphia: FA Davis Co, 1981.

Dawson DM. Entrapment neuropathies of the upper extremities. *N Engl J Med* 1993;329: 2013–2018.

Nakano KK. The entrapment neuropathies. *Muscle Nerve* 1978;1:264–279.

Pécina MM, Krmpotíc-Nemaníc J, Markiewitz AD. Tunnel syndromes, 2nd ed. Boca Raton, FL: CRC, 1997.

Stewart JD. *Focal peripheral neuropathies,* 2nd ed. New York: Raven Press, 1993.

25. APPROACH TO THE PATIENT WITH LOWER EXTREMITY PAIN AND PARESTHESIAS AND ENTRAPMENT NEUROPATHIES

Gregory Gruener

Lower extremity pain and paresthesia are common symptoms and in general reflect peripheral nervous system disorders that result from involvement of specific peripheral nerves, lumbosacral plexus or roots, or polyneuropathy. Diagnosis of a mononeuropathy requires that the motor, reflex, and sensory changes be confined to a single nerve and often is supported by the results of electrodiagnostic studies.

The diagnosis and management of peripheral nervous system disorders once rested on the skill of specialists. However, reemergence of generalists in health care has resulted in at least two major effects. The first, as expected, is that persons with these disorders are no longer under the sole care of a specialist. The second, somewhat unexpected, effect is that although specialists may not be replaced, their role has become more demanding. Specialists will have to develop greater proficiency in differentiating neuropathy from radiculopathy, plexopathy, and other nonneurologic syndromes of pain, disturbed sensation, or weakness. Such increasing competency will have to occur in the setting of fewer and more carefully selected laboratory evaluations.

Fortunately, recognition of neuropathy has always necessitated that adequate attention be paid to both the history and examination, skills that can be developed by both specialists and generalists. Once performed, the history and examination allow preliminary anatomic localization, ranking of potential causes, and finally, planning of further diagnostic evaluation.

This chapter is a descriptive outline of common as well as some infrequent forms of lower extremity neuropathy. Symptoms and findings are emphasized, and the most frequent etiologic considerations reviewed. The importance of bedside examination is assumed throughout, but the application of diagnostic tests also is reviewed.

I. **Evaluation**
    A. **History.** Various aspects of the history need to be taken into account in determining the cause of a specific case of mononeuropathy. The nature of onset (abrupt or insidious), preceding events (injury, surgery, or illness), associated symptoms (fever, weight loss, or joint swelling), and aggravating or alleviating features (joint position or specific activities) all are important in diagnosis. Because the observed deficit can be similar regardless of the cause, historical information is instrumental in defining or limiting the possible etiologic factors.
    B. **Physical examination.** Although motor and sensory symptoms and signs must correspond to the distribution of a single peripheral nerve or its branch, the degree of the deficit and constellation of findings can vary. Motor signs may be clinically absent, or varying degrees of weakness, atrophy, or fasciculation found. Likewise, sensory symptoms can be positive (e.g., tingling, pricking, burning) or negative (hypesthesia), and while corresponding to the sensory distribution of a nerve, they are frequently most pronounced in the distal distribution. Therefore the sensory examination should begin with the **patient's description** of the area of involvement and can be more helpful than routine testing in identifying the pattern of sensory deficit. The **course of the nerve** should be evaluated and local areas of discomfort or the presence of a Tinel's sign (pain or paresthesia in the cutaneous distribution of a nerve elicited by light percussion over the nerve) sought. The relationships of these sites of discomfort to adjacent anatomic structures can later help in determining the cause of mononeuropathy.
    C. **Diagnostic studies.** Further evaluation often is necessary, not only to confirm the presence and severity of a mononeuropathy but also to help exclude more proximal sites of involvement (plexus or root) that can masquerade clinically as mononeuropathy.
        1. **Electrodiagnostic studies.** Electromyography (EMG) and nerve stimulation studies (NSS) are quite useful in the evaluation of mononeuropathy. They can aid in localization, defining severity, and detecting bilateral but asymmetric processes and provide prognostic information.

2. **Laboratory testing** usually is directed at identification of a systemic or generalized disease that may be a predisposing factor or indirectly be responsible for mononeuropathy. (Owing to the practical nature of this section, full discourse on the multiple medical or systemic diseases that can manifest as mononeuropathy is not provided. The Recommended Readings can be consulted once initial localization has been made. They provide a thorough list of frequent as well as unusual causes of specific types of mononeuropathy.)

3. **Imaging studies.** Radiographic testing usually is conducted in an attempt to identify intrathoracic, abdominal, retroperitoneal, or pelvic masses that may lead to nerve-root or plexus injury. The role of imaging studies is less clear in delineating causes of neuropathy localized to a limb, unless a focal site of involvement is suspected (entrapment or mass lesion). In such cases, testing usually is conducted with computed tomography (CT) or, increasingly, magnetic resonance imaging (MRI). Routine x-ray studies now play a less significant role.

II. Specific forms of mononeuropathy

A. Femoral and saphenous neuropathy. Formed within the psoas muscle by fusion of the posterior divisions of the ventral rami of the L2-4 spinal nerves, the femoral nerve exits from its lateral border and descends between the psoas and iliacus muscles (which it may also innervate) and under the fascia of the iliacus. Emerging under the inguinal ligament, lateral to the femoral artery, the nerve divides into motor branches, which supply the quadriceps muscles, and sensory branches to the anterior portion of the thigh. One major division, the saphenous nerve, descends medially into Hunter's (adductor) canal, accompanying the femoral artery. At the medial and superior aspects of the knee, the saphenous nerve emerges from the canal and then, accompanying the saphenous vein, descends medially down the leg, ending at the medial aspect of the foot. The saphenous nerve supplies the sensory innervation to the medial aspect of both the leg and the foot.

1. **Etiology. Femoral neuropathy** usually is caused by trauma from surgery (intrapelvic, inguinal, or hip operations), stretch or traction injuries (prolonged lithotomy position in childbirth), or direct compression (hematoma within the iliacus compartment). Although diabetes mellitus is described as a frequent etiologic factor, such cases are usually misnomers and often represent restricted plexopathy or more widespread lesions with predominantly femoral nerve dysfunction. **Saphenous neuropathy** most often is attributable to injury following surgery (arterial surgery, saphenous vein removal, or knee operations).

2. **Clinical manifestations**
   a. **History.** The patient initially reports leg weakness (as if the leg will "fold under") on attempting to stand or walk. Pain in the anterior part of the thigh is a frequent accompaniment in cases resulting from iliacus hematoma and, when accompanied by the abrupt onset of leg weakness, should lead to suspicion of this condition. A similar pattern of pain, but usually subacute in onset, can be observed in cases of "femoral neuropathy" occurring in diabetes mellitus. With the exception of pain, sensory involvement tends to be an infrequent and minimal symptom of femoral neuropathy.

   Because of its association with surgical injury, sensory loss in saphenous neuropathy may initially go unnoticed and often is of little concern to the patient. However, pain may be prominent, and in such cases, it usually appears some time after the assumed injury to the nerve.

   b. **Physical examination**
      (1) **Neurologic.** A neurologic examination reveals weakness of the quadriceps muscles, absent or diminished patellar reflex, and sensory loss over the anterior thigh and, with saphenous nerve involvement, the medial aspect of the leg and foot.
      (2) **General.** Examination or palpation within the inguinal region and, in cases of saphenous nerve involvement, the medial aspect of

the knee may be fruitful in identifying focal areas of pain and perhaps the site of involvement. The proximity of a surgical scar or point of injury can provide additional etiologic information. In cases in which retroperitoneal hemorrhage is suspected, peripheral pulses may be normal, but there is characteristic posturing of the leg (held flexed at the hip), and attempts to extend or perform a reverse straight-leg test exacerbate the pain.

3. **Differential diagnosis.** The most productive test for localization is evaluation of hip adduction strength. Impairment suggests a more proximal process, either plexus or root as the site of involvement, although a superimposed obturator neuropathy cannot be excluded.

4. **Evaluation**
   a. **Electrodiagnostic.** Nerve conduction studies (NCS) are not as helpful as EMG in evaluation for suspected femoral neuropathy. EMG in such cases involves a careful search of both L2-4 innervated muscles and paraspinal muscles, because neither should be involved in isolated femoral neuropathy.
   b. **Imaging.** CT or MRI of the retroperitoneum best identifies cases resulting from retroperitoneal hemorrhage or suspected mass lesion.

B. **Obturator neuropathy.** Arising within the psoas muscle, from ventral divisions of the L2-4 spinal nerves, the obturator nerve exits from the psoas muscle at its lateral margin, descends into the pelvis, and exits through the obturator foramen. It innervates the adductor magnus, longus, and brevis muscles and supplies sensation to the upper medial aspect of the thigh.

1. **Etiology.** Isolated neuropathy of the obturator nerve is unusual. In cases resulting from pelvic or hip fracture, involvement of other nerves to the lower extremity or lumbosacral plexus also occurs. Both benign and malignant pelvic masses can result in obturator neuropathy, as can surgical procedures performed on these masses or within the pelvis.

2. **Clinical manifestations**
   a. **History.** Leg weakness and difficulty walking are the most common first symptoms and usually overshadow sensory loss, if present.
   b. **Physical examination**
      (1) **Neurologic.** Motor evaluation shows weakness of hip adduction, and sensory loss may be found along the upper medial thigh. The patellar reflex should be intact.
      (2) **General.** Careful pelvic and rectal examinations to identify an intrapelvic tumor are needed when obturator paralysis occurs without trauma.

3. **Differential diagnosis.** The clinical examination must be carefully directed at detecting, because of its infrequency, sensory or motor involvement other than that which could be attributed to the obturator nerve. The presence of hip flexor or knee extensor weakness or an impaired patellar reflex suggests lumbosacral plexopathy or L3-4 radiculopathy. In addition, sensory loss, which extends below the knee, is inconsistent with the sensory deficit of obturator neuropathy.

4. **Evaluation**
   a. **Electrodiagnostic.** NCS are not as helpful as EMG in the evaluation of suspected obturator neuropathy. Evidence of involvement of other L2-4 muscles or paraspinal muscles suggests a more proximal lesion.
   b. **Imaging.** When obvious trauma is not a consideration, further evaluation may be needed. Imaging of the pelvic cavity with CT or MRI is helpful in identifying a mass or infiltrative lesion.

C. **Lateral femoral cutaneous neuropathy.** Dorsal divisions of the ventral primary rami of the L2-3 spinal nerves contribute to the lateral femoral cutaneous nerve, which emerges from the lateral border of the psoas major muscle. It then crosses laterally, within the fascia of the iliacus muscle, and crosses over the sartorius muscle before passing under the lateral border of the inguinal ligament. Piercing the fascia lata, it divides into anterior and posterior branches that provide sensory innervation to the anterolateral aspects of the thigh. Anatomic variations are frequent in regard to the origin of this nerve (it can arise as a branch of the femoral or genitofemoral nerve), its course after arriving at the inguinal ligament, and the extent of its sensory innervation.

1. **Etiology.** In most cases, entrapment or compression at or near the inguinal ligament is the assumed etiologic factor. However, entrapment or compression at other sites, such as a retroperitoneal mass, surgical procedures (especially those involving retroperitoneal structures, pelvis, or inguinal sites), and trauma to the thigh, also can injure the lateral femoral cutaneous nerve.

2. **Clinical manifestations**

   a. **History.** Pain, burning, or a "crawling" sensation with variable loss of sensation on the anterolateral aspects of the thigh exacerbated by walking or getting up and out of a chair is a frequent presentation (meralgia paresthetica). Frequently, the patient rubs the thigh for relief, and this can serve as a diagnostic clue.

   b. **Physical examination**

      (1) **Neurologic.** The area of sensory change usually is small and over the lateral aspect of the thigh.

      (2) **General.** Careful palpation along the inguinal ligament and anterior pelvic brim may help detect a localized area of tenderness and precipitate symptoms, helping to confirm the diagnosis.

3. **Differential diagnosis.** The primary differential diagnosis is femoral neuropathy. Lumbar plexopathy and L2 radiculopathy also are considerations but are unlikely to be points of confusion. Limited sensory impairment, lack of motor involvement, and intact reflexes help in excluding these other possibilities.

4. **Evaluation.** Although clinical features usually provide enough support for a diagnosis, when uncertainty or a preexisting illness complicates the issue (retroperitoneal mass), further testing may be needed.

   Unlike the situation with other entrapment syndromes, responsiveness to treatment may help to "confirm" the diagnosis of lateral femoral cutaneous neuropathy. With this in mind, one can consider subcutaneous injection of an anesthetic agent at the assumed exit point of the lateral femoral cutaneous nerve (medial to the anterior superior iliac spine and under the inguinal ligament) or at a site of local tenderness. A response to such treatment not only supports the diagnosis but also can result in alleviation of symptoms.

   a. **Electrodiagnostic.** Difficulty in eliciting a response from healthy or control subjects during NSS has appropriately limited use of this modality in the evaluation of patients believed to have lateral femoral cutaneous neuropathy. However, EMG studies play a role in evaluating patients with unusual or unclear symptoms, because detection of clinically silent motor involvement implies involvement of more than the lateral femoral cutaneous nerve.

   b. **Imaging.** Unless there is a strong clinical suspicion of a retroperitoneal or pelvic mass resulting in lateral femoral cutaneous nerve entrapment, radiographic evaluation is not necessary. However, unexplained or concomitant gastrointestinal or urogenital symptoms should raise suspicion of such a process. In such cases, further evaluation is appropriate.

D. **Sciatic neuropathy.** The sciatic nerve arises from the ventral rami of the L4-5 spinal nerves, which, by way of the lumbosacral trunk, fuse with those from S1-3. Passing along the inner wall of the pelvis, the nerve exits through the sciatic notch and passes under the piriformis muscle, where it lies between the ischial tuberosity and greater trochanter. Remaining in this deep location, the sciatic nerve descends into the thigh and, proximal to the knee, divides into the peroneal and tibial nerves. The sciatic nerve itself is clearly divisible into two trunks—the medial, which receives contributions from the L4-S3 rami and gives rise to the tibial nerve, and the lateral, the contributions of which are from L4-S2 and from which the common peroneal nerve is derived. The sciatic nerve itself has no sensory branches. The lateral trunk provides innervation to the short head of the biceps femoris muscle and, by way of the medial trunk, the semitendinosus, semimembranosus, and long head of the biceps femoris muscles. With the obturator nerve, the adductor magnus muscle also is innervated.

1. **Etiology.** Most cases of sciatic neuropathy, whether involved at the gluteus muscles or the thigh, are secondary to trauma. The sciatic nerve is possibly second only to the peroneal nerve in regard to frequency of involvement. This includes involvement secondary to injury to adjoining or neighboring structures from fracture of the pelvis, hip, or femur or from gunshot wounds. Injection injuries are no longer as frequent a cause as in the past, but compression injuries are increasing and often occur in the setting of prolonged immobility, such as in various operative procedures, such as cardiac bypass graft surgery. Miscellaneous causes include entrapment by fibrous constricting bands, local hematoma, or tumor.

   Mention must be made of the so-called piriformis syndrome. At this time, few cases rigorously support the assumed pathogenesis of this syndrome—compression of the sciatic nerve by the overlying piriformis muscle—although it remains a frequent clinical diagnosis. Point tenderness of the sciatic nerve at the level of the piriformis muscle also is found among patients with plexopathy or lumbosacral radiculopathy and does not necessarily confirm pathologic compression of the sciatic nerve by the piriformis muscle.

2. **Clinical manifestations**
   a. **History.** Complete lesions, which fortunately are infrequent, are associated with paralysis of the hamstring muscles and all muscles below the knee. Sensory loss occurs in the tibial and peroneal distributions. Partial lesions, especially those of the lateral trunk, make up most cases of sciatic neuropathy and often manifest as foot drop.
   b. **Physical examination**
      (1) **Neurologic.** Although paralysis of varying degrees in muscles innervated by both the medial and lateral trunks can be present, involvement of muscles innervated by the lateral trunk tends to be the most frequent presentation. Sensory loss is variable but restricted to the distribution of the sensory branches of the peroneal and tibial nerves. The muscle stretch reflexes of the hamstring and Achilles tendons can be depressed.
      (2) **General.** Palpation along the course of the nerve can help identify masses or locate points of pain and tenderness but does not entirely exclude more proximal nerve lesions.

3. **Differential diagnosis.** Care must be taken to ensure that radiculopathy (especially L5-S1) is not masquerading as sciatic neuropathy. The straight-leg-raise test, frequently positive in radiculopathy, also can be elicited in cases of lumbosacral plexopathy and sciatic neuropathy. A careful rectal and pelvic examination is indicated when sciatic neuropathy is suspected, because involvement of the sacral plexus by pelvic masses may not otherwise be identified. Finally, isolated common peroneal or tibial neuropathy must be considered as causes of the symptoms.

4. **Evaluation**
   a. **Electrodiagnostic.** Both NSS and EMG studies are useful in differentiating sciatic mononeuropathy from L5-S2 radiculopathy or plexopathy, but they necessitate careful screening of the paraspinal and gluteal muscles. However, just as the lateral division of the sciatic nerve can be the most involved clinically, EMG findings may show a similar pattern. In these cases of sciatic mononeuropathy, a pattern of abnormal results of motor and sensory studies of the peroneal nerve with normal results of tibial nerve studies is not an infrequent finding.
   b. **Imaging.** In cases in which radiculopathy and plexopathy cannot be excluded, further neuroradiographic studies can provide useful information. In addition, in cases in which only sciatic nerve involvement is found, MRI with gadolinium may effectively depict the course of the nerve and help in identifying focal abnormalities.

E. Peroneal neuropathy. Arising from posterior divisions of the L4-S2 ventral rami of spinal nerves, the common peroneal nerve descends into the leg as the lateral division of the sciatic nerve. At the level of the popliteal fossa, it branches from the sciatic nerve and moves toward the lower lateral portion of the popliteal fossa. Two cutaneous sensory branches arise at this point, one to the sural nerve and the other, the lateral cutaneous (sural) nerve of the calf, providing sensation to the upper lateral calf. Exiting laterally from the popliteal space, the peroneal nerve is in close juxtaposition to the fibula, winds below its head, and passes through a tendinous arch formed by the peroneus longus muscle. At its exit from the arch, the peroneal nerve divides into the superficial and deep peroneal nerves. The superficial peroneal nerve descends adjacent to the peroneus longus and brevis muscles, which it innervates, and in the distal third of the leg it pierces the fascia. The terminal branches (medial and lateral) of the superficial peroneal nerve provide sensation to the lateral dorsal surface of the foot. The deep peroneal nerve enters the extensor compartment of the leg and with the tibial artery descends on the interosseous membrane, innervating the tibialis anterior, extensor hallucis longus, and extensor digitorum longus muscles. The terminal portion of this nerve then passes under the extensor retinaculum at the ankle, where a lateral branch innervates the extensor digitorum brevis muscle and a medial branch provides sensory innervation to the first and second toes.

1. **Etiology.** Most cases of peroneal neuropathy are caused by external compression (anesthesia and casts) and trauma (blunt injury, arthroscopic knee surgery, and fractures) despite numerous but less frequent causes (e.g., tumor, constriction by adjacent structures, involvement in systemic disease, and traction injuries from severe ankle strain).

2. **Clinical manifestations**
   a. **History.** Most patients have foot drop, and sensory disorders are usually minimal or of no concern. Less prominent degrees of weakness or weakness affecting only intrinsic foot muscles may not elicit alarm in the patient. On review of the history, careful attention needs to be paid to possible episodes of trauma, compression, or unusual sustained postures that may have preceded the problem (e.g., squatting, kneeling).
   b. **Physical examination**
      (1) **Neurologic.** The characteristic presentation is foot drop, and in a complete lesion of the common peroneal nerve, there is paralysis of ankle dorsiflexion, ankle eversion, and toe extension (dorsiflexion). Sensory loss occurs in the anterolateral lower leg and the dorsum of the foot and toes.
      (2) **General.** Palpation in the popliteal fossa and along the fibular head may elicit signs of tenderness or discovery of a mass, further define the site of involvement, and suggest possible etiologic factors. Examination of the dorsum of the ankle and distal lateral leg, where the terminal branch of the deep peroneal nerve emerges, may reveal similar signs and suggest a distal injury. The most common sites at which focal pathologic processes can affect the nerve or its branches include the fibular head and its proximal neck, the outer compartment of the leg, and the superior and inferior extensor retinaculum at the ankle, beneath which branches of the peroneal nerve pass. However, the peroneal nerve also serves as a reminder that in cases of focal compression, there can be variable fascicular involvement. Motor impairment of only the deep or superficial component, sensory dysfunction only, or various combinations may be the result of nerve compression at the fibular head.

3. **Differential diagnosis.** The primary differential diagnoses in these cases are other causes of foot drop. Involvement of the L5 root, the lumbosacral trunk, and the lateral division of the sciatic nerve all can produce foot drop.

4. **Evaluation.** The extent of evaluation depends on the history. In cases in which an identifiable episode of compression is present, observation, after elimination of the compression, is often all that is needed. When disruption

of the nerve (laceration) is suggested, the onset of the problem is insidious, or physical findings at EMG are inconclusive (incomplete common peroneal neuropathy), further evaluation is indicated.

   a. Electrodiagnostic. NCS can allow identification of both the site of involvement and the extent of axonal injury. Such studies may have to be performed on the asymptomatic leg, because the discovery of bilateral but asymmetric nerve involvement suggests a systemic illness (diabetes) as the etiologic factor. EMG helps to further define the extent of axonal injury or evidence of another cause of the patient's symptoms, if abnormalities are found in other L4-5 innervated muscles or paraspinal muscles.

   b. Imaging. X-ray studies can be useful when joint trauma or a mass is detectable at examination. However, CT and MRI are more useful in defining lesions of the nerve and delineating the relation of adjacent structures to the nerve.

F. Tibial neuropathy. Ventral rami from the L5-S2 spinal nerves contribute to the tibial nerve, which descends into the thigh as part of the medial trunk of the sciatic nerve. At the distal portion of the thigh, the sciatic nerve bifurcates into both the tibial and peroneal nerves. Entering the calf, it descends to the depth of the gastrocnemius, which it innervates, and provides innervation to the soleus, tibialis posterior, flexor digitorum, and hallucis longus muscles as it continues its descent. Finally, at the level of the ankle, it divides into its terminal branches (plantar nerves), which provide innervation to all intrinsic foot flexor muscles as well as sensation to the sole.

   1. Etiology. Tibial neuropathy is infrequent, in part because of the deep anatomic location of the nerve. Although tibial neuropathy occurs less frequently than does peroneal neuropathy, severe ankle injuries can cause more proximal tibial nerve injuries. Major knee trauma is a surprisingly infrequent cause of severe tibial nerve injury.

   2. Clinical manifestations

   a. History. Sensory loss usually is evident along the side of the foot and extending proximally if the contribution of the tibial nerve to the sural nerve is involved. Weakness may not be noticed unless ankle plantar flexion is involved.

   b. Physical examination

   (1) **Neurologic.** Sensory loss usually is present along the sole of the foot. Weakness may be limited to intrinsic toe flexor muscles, or, with more proximal muscle involvement, ankle dorsiflexion and inversion weakness may be found.

   (2) **General.** Careful palpation of the course of the nerve, especially within the popliteal space, should be performed. The finding of a mass or precipitation of paresthesia or pain, in addition to helping localize the involvement, suggests the cause, because tumors involving the tibial nerve may increase its sensitivity to such maneuvers.

   3. Differential diagnosis. Because of its infrequent occurrence, any suspicion of tibial neuropathy should prompt a search for another cause or more proximal lesion. Radiculopathy, plexopathy, or sciatic neuropathy can manifest clinically as isolated tibial neuropathy. Careful examination of more proximal muscles and reflexes, as well as the sensory examination, can help identify or suggest these conditions as more appropriate diagnoses.

   4. Evaluation

   a. Electrodiagnostic studies play a crucial role in identifying as well as excluding tibial neuropathy. Involvement of other nerves on NSS, EMG identification of muscles other than those innervated by the tibial nerve, or paraspinal muscle involvement suggests another cause. At times, plantar nerve involvement rather than more proximal tibial lesions can be identified as the cause of the sensory or motor deficits.

   b. Imaging. Identification of a mass or point of tenderness in cases of unclear causation may necessitate MRI to identify the anatomic structure of the nerve and its relations to adjacent structures.

G. Medial and lateral plantar neuropathy. At the level of the ankle, the terminal portion of the tibial nerve is medial to the Achilles tendon. As it descends, the nerve passes under the flexor retinaculum, which composes the roof of the tarsal tunnel. Within the tunnel, the tibial nerve divides into medial and lateral plantar nerves, which descend toward the foot, and a calcaneal or sensory branch, which provides sensation to the heel. Both plantar nerves then cross under the abductor hallucis muscle (which the medial plantar nerve innervates) and go on to innervate all the muscles of the sole as well as providing sensation to the sole and the toes (the medial nerve supplies the medial portion and the lateral nerve supplies the lateral portion) through their distal divisions, which give rise to the digital nerves. Muscles innervated by the medial plantar nerve include the flexor hallucis brevis and digitorum brevis. The lateral plantar nerve innervates the interossei, the flexor and abductor digiti minimi, and the adductor hallucis.

1. **Etiology.** The proximity of the plantar nerves to osseous and fibrous structures results in injury or compression as a direct result of disorders of those structures. At the level of the tarsal tunnel, external compression and ankle injury are the most frequent etiologic factors. A multitude of other less frequent structural abnormalities (synovial or joint changes and mass lesions) also can lead to nerve injury. Within the foot itself, the medial and lateral plantar nerves are susceptible to the effects of trauma to or fracture of the foot bones.

2. **Clinical manifestations**
   a. **History.** The first recognition of disorders of these nerves occurs when sensory impairment develops, because foot pain or discomfort more frequently has an orthopedic origin. Sensory loss can be present in the sole or heel and at times can be precipitated by specific foot positions. Weakness of foot muscles usually produces no significant symptoms.
   b. **Physical examination**
      (1) **Neurologic.** Sensory loss in the distribution of the plantar nerves or their distal divisions (digital nerves) should be sought. If foot involvement is asymmetric, changes in foot muscle bulk can be appreciated, as can weakness, although usually only toe flexion can be reliably evaluated clinically.
      (2) **General.** Careful examination of the course of the nerve at the ankle and attempts to elicit a Tinel's sign by means of light percussion over its course help confirm the presence of a plantar neuropathy. Joint changes, deformity, or swelling also can help determine a site of nerve involvement.

3. **Differential diagnosis.** One needs to consider more proximal nerve (tibial) or root (S1) lesions that also can cause foot pain or paresthesia. Motor and reflex changes should aid in this distinction. Although polyneuropathy can enter into it, bilaterality, distal reflex depression, and sensory involvement of more than the plantar sensory nerve distribution should aid in the differential diagnosis.

4. **Evaluation**
   a. **Electrodiagnostic** studies are helpful in demonstrating findings consistent with nerve entrapment (tarsal tunnel) and the sensory or motor changes that can be expected with involvement of medial or lateral plantar as well as calcaneal nerves. Because of the nature of such recordings, further study of asymptomatic or contralateral nerves sometimes is necessary for clear interpretation of electrodiagnostic findings. Once again, EMG may be needed to exclude more proximal difficulties (tibial neuropathy, sciatic neuropathy, or radiculopathy).
   b. **Imaging.** Studies of possible sites of involvement (ankle) are not usually indicated. However, in cases of marked discomfort or disability, such studies can identify orthopedic or joint abnormalities and guide treatment.

H. Iliohypogastric, ilioinguinal, and genitofemoral neuropathy. The iliohypogastric, ilioinguinal, and genitofemoral nerves can be described as a group because of the similarity of their origins, sites of innervation, and causes of dysfunction. These nerves arise from the L1 spinal roots (the genitofemoral nerve also has an L2 root contribution) and first pass through and then close to the psoas muscle in their intraabdominal course. The iliohypogastric nerve emerges above the iliac crest and supplies sensation to an area of skin of the upper buttock and another near the pubis. The ilioinguinal nerve enters the inguinal canal at its lateral border and supplies the area above the inguinal ligament and the base of the genitalia. Both the iliohypogastric and ilioinguinal nerves also supply the muscles of the lower abdominal area. After it emerges from the psoas muscle, the genitofemoral nerve is retroperitoneal and descends to the inguinal ligament while resting on the surface of the psoas muscle. It supplies sensation to a small area over the proximal genitalia and anterior proximal thigh.

1. **Etiology.** Because of the location and course of these nerves, neuropathy usually results from surgical procedures, especially inguinal herniorrhaphy. The development of neuralgia is not infrequent after injuries to these nerves.
2. **Clinical manifestations**
   a. **History.** Patients have varying sensory problems, including numbness, paresthesia, or pain within the ipsilateral inguinal and perineal areas. If the cause is related to surgery, these difficulties may be evident immediately after the operation or may not become evident for several weeks.
   b. **Physical examination**
      (1) **Neurologic.** Iliohypogastric neuropathies are infrequent. They cause sensory loss over the suprapubic and upper buttock areas. Ilioinguinal impairment results in sensory loss over the inguinal area and the base of the genitalia but typically resolve or result in minimal disability. In other cases, pain may appear both here and in the inferior abdomen and upper thigh and be worsened or precipitated by changes in leg position. Genitofemoral neuropathy usually accompanies inguinal nerve involvement because of the anatomic proximity of the genitofemoral and inguinal nerves. Symptoms and precipitating factors are similar as well, but sensory problems can extend into the medial and proximal areas of the genitalia.
      (2) **General.** In ilioinguinal and genitofemoral neuropathy, areas of tenderness that often conform to the site of injury may be found in the inguinal region.
3. **Differential diagnosis.** In these cases, nerve involvement predominantly causes sensory impairment, and the differential diagnosis is directed at detecting other causes of sensory impairment outside the typical boundaries of these nerves, including abnormalities in the medial thigh (obturator nerve), anterior thigh (femoral nerve), and lateral thigh (lateral femoral cutaneous nerve), as well as dermatomal involvement caused by T12 or L1 radiculopathy. Because of these overlapping sensory innervations, the presence of motor deficits or reflex changes provides the strongest clue to the presence of one of these other disorders. Back pain, which can suggest a radiculopathy, or the absence of a previous operative procedure, which is the usual cause of such neuropathy, suggests another etiologic factor.
4. **Evaluation**
   a. **Electrodiagnostic** studies play little role in the identification of these types of neuropathy. However, they become indispensable in helping to identify either more proximal lesions (plexus or root) or other forms of neuropathy (femoral) that may clinically resemble iliohypogastric, ilioinguinal, or genitofemoral neuropathy in regard to sensory innervation.
   b. **Imaging** is performed only if there is suspicion of radiculopathy or if a retroperitoneal, intraabdominal, or pelvic lesion is suspected as a cause of the sensory symptoms.
I. **Miscellaneous neuropathy.** For the sake of completeness, the following nerves are discussed briefly. This grouping is based on both infrequent occurrence and the infrequency of isolated involvement of these nerves.

1. **Superior gluteal neuropathy.** Arising from, and receiving its contributions from the L4-S1 components of the sacral plexus, the superior gluteal nerve passes through the sciatic notch above the piriformis muscle and innervates the gluteus medius and minimus muscles. Its isolated involvement is unusual and is most often the result of injury by misplaced injection.
2. **Inferior gluteal neuropathy.** The inferior gluteal nerve arises from the L5-S2 divisions of the sacral plexus and exits through the sciatic notch. Its proximity to the sciatic, pudendal, and posterior cutaneous nerves of the thigh results in concomitant injury to these nerves.
3. **Neuropathy of the posterior cutaneous nerve of the thigh.** Arising from the S1-3 components of the sacral plexus, the posterior cutaneous nerve of the thigh descends through the sciatic notch close to the sciatic nerve and supplies sensation to the posterior portion of the buttock and thigh. At times it is susceptible to local compression, but its isolated involvement is unusual.
4. **Pudendal neuropathy.** Derived from the S2-4 components of the sacral plexus, the pudendal nerve passes through the sciatic notch and descends toward the perineum. Supplying muscles of the perineum, including the anal sphincter and erectile tissue, it also provides sensory innervation to the perineum. Its deep location protects it, but prolonged compression can cause dysfunction. Dysfunction attributable to stretch injuries and related to prolonged labor can occur and manifest as fecal and urinary incontinence.

III. **Referrals**
  A. **Indications for and purposes of neurologic consultation**
    1. Site of involvement unclear from examination or history
    2. Identification of a diffuse disorder without a clear cause or with a discrepancy between the severity of the underlying disease and the neuropathy
    3. Progressive deterioration despite appropriate treatment
    4. Problem precipitated by trauma or injury
    5. Preparation for more expensive or invasive evaluation (MRI or nerve biopsy) or recommending more aggressive intervention (surgery)
    6. Confirmation of diagnosis, etiologic factor, or treatment plan
  B. **EMG and NCS evaluation**
    1. Basic tenets of such testing
      a. Testing is an extension of the clinical examination and not a replacement for a careful history and examination.
      b. Testing is intended to clarify the clinical question to be answered or addressed (e.g., carpal tunnel syndrome or C6 radiculopathy).
      c. Sensitivity and specificity vary according to the etiologic factor and process in question.
    2. **Role in the evaluation of neuropathy**
      a. Confirmation of diagnosis or characterization, localization, and quantification of a disease process
      b. Prognosis
      c. Detection of subclinical disease
      d. Planning of treatment or determination of the need for further evaluation or consultation

Recommended Readings

Dawson DM, Hallet M, Millender LH. *Entrapment neuropathies,* 3rd ed. Boston: Little, Brown, 1999.

Medical Research Council of the U.K. *Aids to the examination of the peripheral nervous system.* London: Bailliere Tindall, 1986.

Mumenthaler M, Schliak H, eds. *Peripheral nerve lesions: diagnosis and therapy.* Stuttgart: Thieme, 1990.

Pécina MM, Krmpotíc-Nemaníc J, Markiewitz AD. *Tunnel syndromes,* 2nd ed. Boca Raton, FL: CRC, 1997.

Stewart JD. *Focal peripheral neuropathies,* 3rd ed. New York: Raven Press, 2000.

26. APPROACH TO THE PATIENT WITH FAILED BACK SYNDROME

Michael W. Groff

The **failed back syndrome** (FBS) is a clinical condition experienced by patients who undergo a surgical procedure, typically in the lumbosacral region, with unsatisfactory results. Back pain is the second most common reason, behind asthma, for patients to seek medical help. It has been estimated that 300,000 laminectomies were performed last year. With the advent of modern instrumentation systems, an increasing number of lumbar fusions are being performed each year. Unfortunately, not every operation is successful, the success rate ranging from 50% to nearly 100% depending on the indication. Consequently the prevalence of FBS is quite high.

I. By definition, FBS implies previous surgery and the first priority in the evaluation of these patients is to understand the indication for the original operation. If the original indication for surgery is suspect, it is extremely unlikely that further surgical intervention will be helpful.
  A. **Radiculopathy** is pain that shoots like a jolt of electricity and follows a particular dermatomal distribution. This is most often caused by a herniated disk, but not exclusively so. Many times there is associated sensory loss in the same dermatome. The associated myotome can manifest weakness in some cases. Abnormal reflexes also can help to localize the level of involvement in the spinal canal.
    1. Imaging is helpful in this context to confirm the level implicated by the history and physical examination findings. However, it has been well shown that healthy persons without back pain can harbor disks that would be concerning from a purely radiographic perspective. Therefore imaging findings without a clinical correlate can typically be ignored.
    2. The most common cause of the pathogenesis of radiculopathy is herniation of a disk followed closely by degenerative foraminal stenosis. Other entities, such as synovial cyst, are distinctly less common.
    3. Whatever the cause, surgery for radiculopathy is focused on decompressing the affected nerve root. The prognosis is quite good; early good results are achieved in more than 95% of cases.
    4. When this type of surgery is unsuccessful, strong consideration should be given to the possibility that the diagnosis was incorrect, the wrong level was operated on, or the patient has secondary issues that are preventing improvement.
    5. Radiculopathy can be confused with hip disease in some cases. A positive **Patrick's test** should be followed with an evaluation to rule out hip arthrosis.
  B. **Claudication** is cramping pain caused by exertion. Most patients report the onset of symptoms after walking a particular distance. The pain typically abates after several minutes of rest, such that the person can continue.
    1. It is important not to confuse **neurogenic** and **vascular** claudication. Putting patients on an exercise bicycle is a good test for establishing the cause of claudication. The flexed posture of the spine on the bicycle opens up the spinal canal, and therefore patients with neurogenic claudication do much better on the bicycle than they would walking. Patients with vascular claudication show no such improvement.
    2. **Neurogenic claudication** is most commonly managed with lumbar laminectomy over the stenotic levels. This has led to the incorrect impression that the compression is due to a change in the diameter of the bony canal. In fact, this is a degenerative disease whereby the canal is progressively occupied by more and more hypertrophied ligamentum flavum, facet capsule, and synovium. For this reason bilateral laminotomy has been advocated and may be preferable to conventional laminectomy because it has less chance of introducing iatrogenic instability.
    3. Imaging with either **magnetic resonance imaging** (MRI) or **computed tomographic (CT) myelography** shows a markedly compressed thecal sac with a characteristic trefoil configuration.

C. **Instability** is another common indication for lumbar surgery. From both a theoretical and a practical standpoint, instability is distinct from stenosis and radiculopathy. Management of radiculopathy and stenosis is decompression; management of instability is fusion. The success of fusion operations is distinctly less than that of decompression. For this reason, many patients with FBS have experienced failed fusion.

   1. **Instability** is defined as the ability of the bony components of the spine to withstand physiologic loads without compromising the function of the neural elements.

   2. Although instability often is thought of in a binomial way as either present or absent, in clinical practice there is a spectrum of instability ranging from **gross instability,** most often the result of trauma, to **microinstability,** which is found in the context of degenerative disease.

   3. The underlying hypothesis in offering fusion to patients with degenerative spondylosis is that instability represents abnormal movement of the joint, which in turn causes mechanical back pain. It is not responsible for radiculopathy. The pain is characteristically exacerbated by prolonged sitting or standing and often is relieved by recumbency. Because the pain does not radiate, it is not possible to localize the responsible spinal level by means of history or physical examination.

   4. The pathogenesis of mechanical back pain is controversial and likely is multifactorial. There is evidence implicating the disk space as well as the facet joints. Unfortunately, the pain generator remains unknown.

   5. If **flexion–extension radiographs (dynamic radiographs)** show movement of more than 4 mm, the diagnosis is more certain. However, a large number of patients with movement in excess of 4 mm do not have mechanical pain. Plain radiographs can provide indirect evidence of instability in the form of traction spurs that result from the tension placed on the bone from the **Sharpy's fibers** of the annulus or loss of disk height indicative of disk degeneration. MRI often shows **Modic changes** at the interspace thought to represent inflammatory reaction in the adjacent vertebral bodies secondary to disk disruption. Many of these findings are present in patients who are pain free, and therefore the utility is suspect.

   6. In an attempt to better determine whether instability is present in a particular patient and whether it is responsible for the back pain being reported, several strategies have emerged.

      a. Use of an **external orthosis (TLSO)** has intuitive appeal because it arrests, albeit incompletely, the movement thought to be responsible for the back pain.

      b. **Provocative diskography** has been championed because it shows the disk disruption anatomically and functionally with the presence of concordant pain.

      c. Percutaneous placement of **pedicle screws** and immobilization with an external connector has been studied.

      d. TLSO trials and provocative diskography have been shown to be unsuccessful in prognosticating the outcome of lumbar fusion. The morbidity and invasiveness of percutaneous pedicle screw placement probably exceeds that of the instrumented fusion being considered.

   7. At present, it is not possible to predict who will benefit from lumbar fusion and who will not. This explains, in part, the relative lack of success with fusion operations compared with decompression operations for radiculopathy or stenosis. Most series have favorable outcome in 50% to 70% of cases when lumbar fusion is performed for degenerative disease.

   8. If the indication for fusion was not present at the time of the first operation, revision surgery will be futile. Moreover, even when the original procedure is well conceived, revision surgery is effective only if a problem amenable to surgical correction is identified preoperatively. Examples consistent with a successful operation include pseudoarthrosis and degeneration at the level adjacent to the fusion. The plan should be well defined preoperatively. In the era of modern imaging, it is unwise to perform **exploratory** lumbar surgery.

II. Many somatic problems not related to the spine can manifest as back pain. These must be excluded in a thorough review of systems.

  A. Abdominal causes include aortic aneurysm, cholelithiasis, and pancreatitis. Pyelonephritis most often manifests as flank pain but can also lead to referred back pain.

  B. In female patients, **endometriosis** can manifest as back pain.

  C. Osteoarthritis of the hip can be easily confused with back pain radiating into the buttock. A Patrick's test is useful to differentiate the two. **Sacroiliac joint pain** also has been implicated.

  D. Major depression has been shown to exacerbate the severity of back pain. It is also a poor prognostic sign for outcome after surgical intervention. Ongoing worker's compensation litigation also has been shown to be an independent predictor of poor outcome.

III. After the rationale for the primary operation or previous operations is understood, emphasis should be given to nonsurgical modalities. In any cohort of patients with FBS, only a small number should ever come to revision surgery. This emphasis is correct before the first operation and becomes increasingly important with each subsequent operation.

  A. It should be well understood that **lumbar spondylosis** is a degenerative disease. As such, surgery can ameliorate the most severe manifestations of the problem but it can never address the underlying cause. For this reason, treatment such as weight loss, smoking cessation, and physical therapy offers the patient a better outcome, if successful, and can often make surgery unnecessary. Moreover, even when surgery is entertained, it should only be in the context of a complete treatment plan that embraces these other aspects of care.

  B. At the same time, the efficacy of surgery decreases with each operation. Some authors have suggested that **revision lumbar fusion,** which is only indicated when a technical error has been identified, is only one-half as successful as primary surgery.

  C. In most cases of FBS, the patient comes to medical attention with the chief symptom of pain. Pain is a subjective symptom. Considerable progress has been made in the development of **outcome instruments** used in an attempt to quantify pain and functional level in an objective way. This has given spine specialists a better understanding of the effect of various interventions.

  D. The pain that patients report and the disability they experience has a great deal to do with their expectations. Pain is ordinarily an important protective phenomenon. When pain becomes chronic, as in FBS, the noxious percept that reaches consciousness serves no productive purpose. The assumption of many patients that the pain they are experiencing is evidence of ongoing damage is incorrect. When patients understand this, their perception of pain can become less noxious, and their functional abilities improve. In one study, use of an informational booklet that emphasized the concept that back pain should not be equated with damage to tissue was shown to have a statistically significant correlation with improvement in pain perception compared with a more traditional explanation.

  E. As a clearer understanding emerges of the nature of pain in FBS, more effective, interdisciplinary treatments are being developed. It is increasingly recognized that depression not only exacerbates the symptoms of FBS but also is a consistent consequence of FBS. Preoperative evaluation should include psychiatric assessment. If they are found, substantive problems should be addressed before surgical intervention is planned.

IV. The nonsurgical therapies discussed in **III.** address the causes of FBS in just as direct a manner as surgery does. In some cases, indirect measures can be considered purely with the intent of ameliorating a patient's pain. Although these modalities are not directed at the underlying cause, they do enhance functional ability and improve quality of life.

  A. There is increasing experience with **narcotics** in the management of chronic pain of a nonmalignant causation, such as FBS. This is an expansion of experience with **cancer pain.** The original motivation for use of long-term administration of narcotics in the context of cancer pain was that patients would die of disease before or soon after addiction developed. As survival times improved and indications were liberalized, a large number of these patients were using narcotic analgesics for increasing durations. It was found that addiction was rare in this population. It has been suggested that chronic pain, for reasons that remain unclear, prevents the development of addiction. Subsequently, some authors have expanded the indications to include patients with **chronic pain of benign causation.** The initial experience has been similar, and addiction is similarly rare. Because the life expectancy of patients with FBS is much longer than that of patients with cancer, the duration of treatment is considerably longer. These patients must be followed for the development of toleration and habituation. Serum chemistries with liver function tests should be checked on a regular schedule. This strategy requires a stringent monitoring program. Moreover, it has been estimated that as many as 45% of patients with FBS are being medicated excessively, and this treatment remains controversial.

B. **Intrathecal pumps** for the administration of opioids have been used to minimize the side effects of systemic opiate therapy, such as sedation, lethargy, and decreased libido. Because the drug is delivered directly to the opiate receptors within the dorsal horn of the spinal cord, effective analgesia can be obtained at much lower doses. This leads to a much lower incidence of side effects. A full range of analgesics is available. **Morphine** typically is chosen as a first-line drug. Its hydrophilic properties make it more difficult for it to diffuse out of the subarachnoid space and thereby dilute its effect. **Hydromorphine** and **fentanyl** also have been used effectively. Once successfully implanted, drug pumps have to be refilled every 2 to 12 weeks. Although the incidence of side effects is decreased, constipation, myoclonus, amenorrhea, decreased libido, and dependent edema have been reported.

C. The **gate-control theory** of pain proposed by Melzack and Wall was the inspiration for **spinal cord stimulation.** Early attempts were frustrated by the technology of the day. Current systems are much more effective and easier to insert. At present, most stimulators are inserted percutaneously in a pain clinic in the anesthesia department. The success rate is as high as 75% over the short term and decreases to 50% in long-term follow-up studies. The complication rate is low, neurologic injury occurring in less than 1% of patients. The most common complication is wound infection, which has an incidence of 5%.

V. When conservative therapy is unsuccessful, operative intervention should be considered. Zeidman and Long have suggested considering the length of time from the original operation to the reappearance of symptoms. Patients are thereby divided into three groups.

A. In cases of **immediate failure,** the patients never improve after surgery. This universally implies an **error in diagnosis** or a **technical deficiency** with the surgery. After the protocol outlined in **III.** and **IV.** has been implemented, these patients should need MRI with and without contrast material. The prognosis for these patients is very good when the error is identified. If no deficiency is found, the outcome is considerably more discouraging. Surgery has no role in those cases.

B. The next group of failures manifests **days to weeks** after surgery. It is quite common, however, for patients who have initial improvement postoperatively in the hospital to experience a setback as they become more active on arriving home. This is a normal, although not universal, finding and is best managed expectantly. Patients who experience initial improvement and then experience clear deterioration need a more deliberate evaluation. These cases can represent **recurrent disk herniation** or **iatrogenic instability.** The physical examination and pain signature favor one diagnosis over the other. The former is best evaluated with MRI with and without contrast material. The later should be evaluated with CT to assess the bony removal and flexion–extension plain radiographs to show gross instability if present. In this time frame, some patients have progressive **causalgia-type pain.** This is often the result of a battering of nerve root during surgery. This condition is very refractory. Gabapentin has been tried with limited success.

C. Another group of failures manifests **weeks to months** after surgery. The description of clear radiculopathy suggests recurrent herniation. **Arachnoiditis** manifests most often at this time. Patients often describe back and leg pain, which can be similar to the presenting problem. Classic cases manifest as symptoms of claudication or lower extremity causalgia. CT myelography is the study of choice and typically shows clumping of nerve roots and restricted flow of intrathecal contrast material. Surgery directed at the arachnoiditis is largely unsuccessful and should be reserved for cases of progressive neurologic deterioration. There has been some success with spinal cord stimulators in these cases. This is a difficult problem to treat. The incidence has decreased dramatically with the advent of water-soluble contrast agents and the relatively infrequent use of myelography in the MRI era.

A problem that has not abated is **epidural fibrosis.** This continues to be a problem although many different strategies have been directed against it over the years. Fat grafts once were used, and the recent enthusiasm for nonadhesive barriers such as carbohydrate polymer gel (Adcon-L; Gliatech, Cleveland, OH, U.S.A.) has waned somewhat. Epidural fibrosis can cause nondermatomal causalgia. The diagnosis often is made by means of MRI with contrast material. At present, there is no effective procedure to free nerves trapped in epidural fibrosis, and symptomatic treatment is offered.

D. The last group of failures manifests after a pain-free interval of **months to years.**

1. Many of these cases have developed either iatrogenic lumbar instability because decompression was too wide or lumbar instability caused by the intrinsic disease. The incidence of **postlaminectomy spondylolisthesis** is somewhere between 2% and 10%. Even simple diskectomy has been associated with a 3% incidence of postoperative instability that necessitates subsequent fusion. It has been widely circulated that the medial half of the facet joint can be removed bilaterally without inducing instability. However, this admonishment is not consistent with the fact that the medial half of the joint comprises the descending facet almost exclusively and that removal of the medial half can leave the facet completely incompetent. There is consensus that complete laminectomy and bilateral facetectomy consistently produce instability. In cases in which this extent of resection is needed to accomplish decompression, fusion should be incorporated into the surgical plan.

2. **Pseudoarthrosis** after lumbar fusion manifests in a time frame similar to that of postlaminectomy spondylolisthesis. In part, the timing of presentation may represent the fact that most spine surgeons are not prepared to give up on a fusion for 9 to 12 months after surgery. There also are no commonly accepted criteria for diagnosis of pseudoarthrosis. Flexion–extension radiographs often appear normal, and bone scans are equivocal. The incidence of symptomatic pseudoarthrosis after a posterolateral lumbosacral fusion is between 5% and 15%. The cause can be either technical deficiency of the surgery or biologic deficiency of the patient. There is good evidence that smoking negatively affects the rate of fusion, but this effect may not be as large as was previously thought. The rate of pseudoarthrosis increases with the number of levels of arthrodesis. Bone stimulators can be implanted at the time of surgery when significant risk factors are present or applied transdermally when the fusion mass on postoperative radiographs is unsatisfactory.

VI. **Radiography plays an important role in the evaluation of FBS.**

A. In the evaluation of recurrent disk herniation, **contrast-enhanced CT** or **MRI** is vital. Postoperative scar becomes homogeneously enhanced. A herniated disk may have some peripheral enhancement, but because it is avascular, the disk does not become centrally enhanced. Although scar and disk can both cause compressive symptoms, surgery to remove scar tissue often results in increased scar tissue postoperatively.

B. Radiographic evaluation of a fusion is more difficult. In short, there is no universally accepted way to assess successful fusion after arthrodesis.

1. **Flexion and extension radiographs** are specific for instability if motion is detected. However, these studies are very insensitive. Fibrous nonunion or the instrumentation itself can prevent the flexion–extension radiographs from appearing abnormal even though instability exists.

2. **Plain radiographs** can show a robust fusion mass, but it is often impossible to know whether the bony mass is in continuity. Lucency or halos around pedicle screws suggest instability. CT with sagittal and coronal reconstruction can be helpful. Special techniques must be used to minimize artifact of the instrumentation.

3. **Bone spectroscopy** has been advocated, but this modality is unreliable for at least several years after surgery.

4. **Three-dimensional CT** has been advocated by some authors in the evaluation of FBS. It has the advantage of clearly imaging the bony resection and can clearly delineate the extent of bony fusion.

VII. Referrals

A. Referral to a neurologist or spine surgeon is indicated for any patient with a new neurologic deficit. In the context of FBS and chronic pain, it is important not to miss this dramatic change in the patient's course.

B. Imaging should be performed only in response to a significant change in the symptoms. When dramatic changes are found at imaging studies, patients with FBS should be reevaluated.

C. Often the job of weaning narcotics is left to an internist or general neurosurgeon. This can be appropriate; however, when reduction goals are not being met and the program becomes stalled, these patients should be referred to specialized centers. Long-term use of narcotic analgesics can be acceptable treatment in some cases, but it should be chosen explicitly, not as an ad hoc default.

D. FBS is a difficult management problem, and all these patients should be seen by a spine surgeon or pain center. In general, patients with FBS should be cared for by a multidisciplinary team.

Recommended Readings

Burchiel KJ, Anderson VC, Brown FD, et al. Prospective, multicenter study of spinal cord stimulation for relief of chronic back and extremity pain. *Spine* 1996;21:2786–2794.

Burton AK, Waddell G, Tillotson KM, et al. Information and advice to patients with back pain can have a positive effect. *Spine* 1999;24:2484–2491.

Hassenbusch SJ, Stanton-Hicks M, Covington EC. Spinal cord stimulation versus spinal infusion for low back and leg pain. *Acta Neurochir* 1995; 64:109–115.

Melzack R, Wall PD. *The challenge of pain.* New York: Basic Books, 1983.

North RB, Campbell JN, James CS, et al. Failed back surgery syndrome: 5 year follow-up in 102 patients undergoing repeated operation. *Neurosurgery* 1991;28:685–690.

Weber H. Lumbar disc herniation: a controlled, prospective study with ten years of observation. *Spine* 1983;8:131–140.

Zeidman SM, Long DM. Failed back surgery syndrome. In: Menezes AH, Volker KH, eds. *Principles of spinal surgery.* New York: McGraw–Hill, 1996:657–678.

Zinreich SJ, Long DM, Davis R, et al. Three-dimensional CT imaging in postsurgical "failed back" syndrome. *J Comput Assist Tomogr* 1990;14:574–580.

27. APPROACH TO THE PATIENT WITH ACUTE SENSORY LOSS

David H. Mattson
Oldrich J. Kolar

Acute sensory loss can result from pathologic processes involving sensory fibers in individual peripheral nerves (**mononeuropathy**), multiple individual peripheral nerves (**mononeuropathy multiplex**), multiple generally symmetrically affected peripheral nerves (**polyneuropathy**), individual nerve roots (**monoradiculopathy**) or multiple nerve roots (**polyradiculopathy**), cervicobrachial or lumbosacral plexus (**plexopathy**), the spinal cord, the brainstem, the thalamus, or the cerebral hemispheres.

Acute sensory loss can be **transient, recurrent, or progressive.** Changes in the quality of sensory disturbances noticed over hours or days suggest progressive neurologic problems. In advancing processes involving the peripheral nervous system (PNS), increased sensation with or without discomfort to touch or to simple contact with bed sheets or clothing may in several hours or days be followed by progressive decreases in sensation modalities. The reverse also can be true, acute numbness being followed by abnormally increased and uncomfortable sensation.

I. **Etiology.** Localization of the pathologic processes resulting in acute sensory loss can be helpful in differential diagnostic considerations and in the selection of proper paraclinical investigations.

A. **Sensory receptors.**

1. **Exteroceptors,** which are localized in the skin, represent superficial sensation modalities to pain, touch, cold, and warmth. The cutaneous sensory fibers run in sensory or mixed sensory and motor nerves. All the sensory neurons have their cell bodies in the dorsal ganglia with their central projections to the posterior roots.

2. **Proprioceptors,** which are localized in deeper somatic structures, including tendons, muscles, and joints, transduce columns of the spinal cord and terminate in the gracile and cuneate nuclei of the medulla. The secondary afferent fibers from these nuclei cross the midline in the medulla and ascend in the brainstem as the medial lemniscus to the posterior thalamic complex. Unconscious proprioceptive information is carried through the spinocerebellar tracts in the lateral columns and in the cuneocerebellar and rostrocerebellar tracts in the dorsal columns of the cord.

B. **Peripheral nerve.** Decreased pain sensation resulting from compression of a single root can be detected in segments oriented longitudinally in the extremities and horizontally over the trunk. Overlapping in sensory zones from one nerve root to another is expressed more for touch than for pain. There also is a 2 to 3 cm crossover in perception of sensory modalities at the midline over the chest and abdomen.

C. **Spinal cord.** Most fibers conducting pain and temperature sensation decussate over several segments by way of the ventral white commissure and ascend in the lateral columns of the cord as the lateral spinothalamic tract. Fibers conducting light touch and two-point discrimination ascend in the ipsilateral posterior column of the spinal cord and decussate in the medial lemniscus of the medulla.

D. **Cranial nerve and brainstem.** Cutaneous sensation from the face is carried to the brainstem by the trigeminal nerve. After entering the pons, part of the sensory fibers descend as a bundle to form the spinal tract of the trigeminal nerve, which reaches the upper cervical segment of the spinal cord. The spinal tract of the trigeminal nerve gives off fibers to the medially located nucleus of the spinal tract of the trigeminal nerve, which also descends into the upper cervical cord. The nucleus of the spinal tract of the trigeminal nerve receives fibers conducting sensations of pain, temperature, and light touch from the face and mucous membranes. Ascending fibers from the spinal nucleus travel mainly ipsilaterally in the trigeminothalamic tract and terminate in the ventral thalamus. The spinothalamic tract has connections with the brainstem reticular formation. It joins the medial lemniscus at the midbrain level and terminates in the posterior ventral complex of the thalamic nuclei.

E. Cortex. The cortical projections of the posterior ventral thalamic complex ascend through the medial portion of the internal capsule to reach the postcentral cortex in a somatotopic arrangement similar to the precentral motor cortex with the face in the lowest area and the leg in the parasagittal region. In addition to the postcentral cortex, the cortical thalamic projections include the superior parietal lobule, which is considered to represent sensations of numbness and tingling over the contralateral or bilateral aspects of the body. The fine sensory discrimination and fine location of pain, temperature, touch, and pressure (so-called primary modalities) require normal functioning of the sensory cortex. The cerebral cortex of the postcentral gyrus also subserves cortical sensory processes, including perception of sizes and shapes of objects (stereognosis), ability to recognize numbers or letters drawn on the patient's skin (graphesthesia), and two-point discrimination.

II. Clinical manifestations

A. Examination of sensory modalities in acute sensory loss. In examination of patients reporting acute sensory loss, the **location, extent,** and **quality** of the sensory deficit can help localize the lesion and narrow the differential diagnosis. In rare instances, patients reporting numbness in the extremities actually refer to muscle weakness. Particularly at the early stage of an acute neurologic disorder resulting in sensory deficits, the patient may experience ill-defined sensations of tightness, pressure, or a "bandlike" feeling at the level of the upper chest, lower chest, waist, or extremities. If the patient reports acute onset of a burning sensation usually associated with discomfort or pain, early involvement of the autonomic (sympathetic) nervous system should be considered.

In many instances, no sensory impairment can be found in persons reporting acute sensory disturbances. Conversely, the neurologic examination may show sensory deficits of which the patient is unaware. The patient's alertness, willingness to cooperate, intelligence, and suggestibility can influence the result of the examination. If the patient is tired after a lengthy examination, evaluation of sensory modalities may show suboptimal reproducibility.

1. **Touch sensation** is tested with a wisp of cotton or the light touch of a finger. The stimulus applied to the area being tested should be compared with that applied to the contralateral area with expected normal sensation. A heavier stimulus usually has to be applied over cornified areas, particularly over soles and palms. Perception of moving contact with cotton or the examiner's fingertips is more sensitive than perception of a stationary stimulus.

2. In testing of **pain sensation,** the patient is expected to indicate the intensity of the pinprick sensation in comparison with that in a corresponding area with normal pain sensation. The individual pinprick stimuli should be applied in intervals longer than 1 second to avoid excessive pain secondary to summation of the successive stimuli. If reproducible demarcation of the decreased sensation can be obtained, one has to determine whether the distribution suggests nerve root or peripheral nerve involvement. Dermatomal charts showing typical peripheral nerve or nerve root distributions vary somewhat from one book or study to another, and there can be variability among patients. Should the pinprick sensation indicate a decrease or loss of pain sensation at a certain level of the chest or abdomen, the demarcation is determined more reliably by means of proceeding from the area of decreased or absent sensation to the level of normal sensation.

3. In testing **thermal modalities,** one should realize that perception is relatively delayed. The test tubes with cold and warm water should remain in contact with the tested skin area for several seconds. In the warm range, a healthy person recognizes differences between 35°C and 40°C and in the cold range between 10°C and 20°C. Exposure to temperatures below 10°C and above 50°C can be confused with pain. To determine the demarcation of the thermal sensation deficit, one should move the test tube from the areas of decreased sensation to the normal areas.

4. **Position sense** in fingers or toes is examined by holding the digit at the side opposite the direction of movement, which is flexion or extension. The patient

is asked to identify the directions of passive movements. In testing of lateralized postural sense in the extremities, the patient is asked to place the extremity being tested in the position corresponding to that of the opposite limb as the opposite limb is passively manipulated by the examiner.

5. **Vibration sense** is a composite sensation requiring preserved touch and deep pressure sensation with fibers ascending in the dorsal columns of the spinal cord. Vibration and position senses usually decrease together. A tuning fork with a low rate and long duration of vibration (128 dv) should be used for a routine examination. The tuning fork is placed over a bony prominence, and the fork is moved quickly to the corresponding point on the opposite limb when the vibration is no longer perceived in the tested area.

B. **Positive and negative sensory symptoms**
   1. **Positive symptoms**
      a. **Paresthesia** means spontaneous abnormal sensation frequently described by the patient as tingling, prickling, or "pins and needles."
      b. **Dysesthesia** is discomfort or pain triggered by painless stimuli such as soft touch or mild pressure.
      c. **Hyperesthesia** indicates abnormally increased sensitivity on examination of light touch, pinprick, or thermal sensation that is not infrequently followed in the same area by hypesthesia, or decreased sensation.
   2. **Negative symptoms. Numbness. Anesthesia** designates complete loss of sensation. **Thermohypesthesia,** which is decreased sensation for cold and warmth, can progress to thermoanesthesia, which indicates complete loss of thermal sensation. **Pallesthesia** indicates loss of vibratory sense.
   3. **Neuropathic pain.** Pain from nerve contusion, crush, demyelination with ephaptic nerve transmission to adjacent demyelinated axons, or partial remyelination can cause a deep, nonlocalizing pain. This pain can be burning, searing, aching, or lancinating. It is less typically part of acute nerve injury.

C. **Functional sensory loss.** In practice, one may encounter persons with functional sensory loss. However, it often is difficult to establish with certainty that the sensory impairment is functional. Functional sensory loss frequently occurs in a nonanatomic distribution, but then so can central nervous system (CNS) inflammatory demyelinating sensory loss. Demarcation of the losses of touch, pinprick, and vibration sensation is indicated exactly at the midline over the chest or abdomen or in the entire limb with sharp delineation of the sensory loss. Repeated examination usually reveals significant differences in the demarcation of the sensory deficits. Because examination of such patients can be time-consuming, it is helpful to provide them with a dermograph and ask them to draw a line demarcating the area of the sensory deficit themselves.

III. **Pathologic processes manifested by acute sensory loss.** Most patients with acute sensory impairment fall into four general diagnostic categories represented by (1) infectious–parainfectious, (2) inflammatory–demyelinating, (3) ischemic–hemorrhagic, and (4) traumatic–compressive. Neurologic disorders secondary to metabolic or toxic derangements rarely manifest as acute sensory loss.

A. **Infectious–parainfectious neurologic diseases** are preceded by or associated with symptoms of acute, often febrile disease involving the upper respiratory or gastrointestinal system or the lower urinary tract. Parainfectious involvement of the CNS or PNS typically follows the onset of clinical symptoms of the infectious process by 1 to 3 weeks.

B. **Inflammatory–demyelinating disease** can be parainfectious or postinfectious but also can be idiopathic or autoimmune, including multiple sclerosis or transverse myelitis that is not part of multiple sclerosis.

C. **Ischemic–hemorrhagic neurologic disorders** manifesting as acute CNS or PNS involvement usually occur among older persons with vascular risk factors.

D. **Traumatic–compressive lesions** of the CNS and PNS can manifest as acute sensory loss. Complications of surgical procedures, venipuncture, or intravascular injection should be considered as causes of acute sensory loss, usually secondary to peripheral nerve damage.

IV. Clinical aspects of acute sensory loss by somatotopic localization. Pure sensory loss, acute or chronic, is unusual. Accompanying signs referable to other cranial nerves, motor loss, cortical modalities including visual field loss, and reflexes can help localize a lesion and narrow the diagnostic considerations and evaluation.

    A. Acute sensory loss in the face. Sensory disturbance solely in the face usually indicates a lesion in a branch or branches of the trigeminal nerve, the trigeminal nucleus in the brainstem, or in the lemniscal pathways of the brainstem. It would be less typical to have pure facial sensory disturbance from a lesion in the thalamus, cortical projections, or somatosensory cortex, all of which would typically involve more than the face (see **IV.B.**).

        1. **Acute onset of facial paresthesia** manifesting as numbness, tingling, or ill-defined discomfort is frequently encountered in clinical practice. If the paresthesia lasts only several seconds or minutes, or if the person is young, tense, nervous, or exposed to stressful circumstances, often no specific pathologic condition is identified. Paresthesia, especially in the perioral area, can be reproduced by hyperventilation. The paresthesia usually regresses completely.

        2. Some patients with acute onset of **idiopathic peripheral facial nerve (Bell's) palsy** may describe numbness or abnormal sensation over the paretic facial muscles. In case of isolated facial nerve involvement, the abnormal facial sensation ceases with regression of the muscle weakness. Pathologic processes involving the first division of the trigeminal nerve result in sensory impairment in the corresponding forehead area. Corneal, conjunctival, and sneeze reflexes are decreased or absent.

        3. Decreased or absent corneal reflex with alteration in sensory modalities in the ophthalmic division of the trigeminal nerve accompanying abrupt onset of fever, proptosis, chemosis, diplopia, and papilledema suggests **cavernous sinus thrombosis.** Suppurative processes involving the upper half of the face, orbits, or nasal sinuses usually are present. Septic cavernous sinus thrombosis represents a life-threatening process necessitating immediate hospitalization. Sensory deficit in the area of the first division of the trigeminal nerve also can accompany acute onset of meningitis.

        4. A relatively sudden onset of numbness over the first two divisions of the trigeminal nerve associated with dysesthesia or hypesthesia to pinprick can represent a low-grade inflammatory process involving the cavernous sinus (**Tolosa–Hunt syndrome**). There is lateralized retroocular or periorbital pain and diplopia. The corneal reflex may be absent or decreased. Diplopia is most frequently secondary to involvement of the abducens nerve in the lateral wall of the cavernous sinus.

        5. Patients with recurrent or chronic frontal or maxillary sinusitis may occasionally describe numbness or a dull sensation in the area of the forehead or infraorbital region. Sensory disturbances frequently are associated with pain and decrease in pinprick or light touch sensation suggestive of symptomatic neuralgia of the ophthalmic or maxillary nerve. An ear, nose, and throat consultation and aggressive management of the sinusitis usually result in complete regression of the neurologic symptoms.

        6. Decreased sensation in the first, second, or third division of the trigeminal nerve associated with a clinical history of acute injury involving the head can result from involvement of the trigeminal nerve secondary to skull fracture, contusion, or hematoma.

        7. Acute onset of persistent sensory impairment usually manifesting as numbness or ill-defined dysesthesia in the infraorbital area corresponding to the maxillary division can be an early sign of multiple sclerosis. If the sensory disturbances are persistent, extend over the entire half of the face or to the contralateral aspect, and become associated with discomfort or pain and if the patient is young or middle-aged, a demyelinating process should be considered.

        8. Acute decrease or absence of pinprick, light touch, or thermal sensation in the area of the mandibular division of the trigeminal nerve can reflect inflammatory or traumatic events involving the mandible or fracture of the base of the skull in the area of the foramen ovale.

9. Osteomyelitis of the mandible, usually complicating progressive dental pathologic processes, can manifest as a relatively abrupt onset of numbness with or without hypalgesia in the area of the chin suggestive of neuritis affecting the mental nerve. Acute presentation of the **numb chin syndrome** may be a paraneoplastic manifestation among persons with lymphoma, breast or prostate cancer, or melanoma. Orthodontic consultation should exclude malfitting dentures.

B. **Facial sensory disturbance in association with hemibody sensory disturbance, either ipsilateral or contralateral**

1. Abrupt onset of hypalgesia and thermoanesthesia over the entire half of the face accompanied by hypalgesia and thermoanesthesia over the contralateral half of the trunk and extremities indicates involvement of the lateral medulla. The acute sensory loss often is associated with dysphagia, dysarthria, vertigo, vomiting, ipsilateral cerebellar signs, and ipsilateral Horner's syndrome. The most frequent cause of the lateral medullary (Wallenberg's) syndrome is occlusion of the intracranial vertebral artery. Less common causes include vertebral artery dissection, hematoma, demyelination, metastatic disease, and abscess.

2. Acute onset of bilateral or unilateral facial numbness rapidly extending into the contralateral half of the face and associated with or followed by progressive weakness of facial muscles, can be the earliest manifestation of acute demyelinating polyneuropathy. Cases that begin in the face and descend are called the **Fisher variant of the Guillain–Barré syndrome (GBS).** Typical GBS starts with numbness, paresthesia, and weakness in the distal portion of the legs and ascends to eventually involve the face. Fisher variant GBS tends to involve the respiratory centers of the brainstem more quickly than typical GBS, making surveillance of respiratory status particularly important in Miller Fisher variant GBS. The diagnosis of GBS should be particularly considered in evaluation of persons with histories of respiratory or gastrointestinal viral infection, immunization, or surgical procedures preceding the onset of neurologic symptoms.

3. Recurrent sensory disturbances in hemifacial distribution, particularly among older patients with a clinical history of arterial hypertension, cardiovascular disease, diabetes, and cigarette smoking, may represent a carotid artery territory transient ischemic attack (TIA). Patients may report numbness or a feeling of dullness or tingling involving the entire half of the face. The TIA episodes are of variable duration, usually lasting less than 20 to 30 minutes.

4. Loss of pain sensation and thermodysesthesia with preserved light touch sensation suggest **syringobulbia.** In these patients, an expanding syrinx involving the spinal nucleus of the trigeminal nerve may be found at magnetic resonance imaging (MRI).

5. The rostral part of the nucleus of the spinal tract of the trigeminal nerve represents the midline facial areas, whereas the sensation fibers from the lateral facial areas terminate in the more caudal part of the nucleus at the level of the medulla and spinal cord. In acute intraparenchymal processes involving the brainstem, facial sensory loss can occur in an "onionskin" distribution with decreased sensation in the central facial areas, indicating a pontine or pontomedullary lesion. Acute presentation of **"onionskin-like" sensation deficits** in the face can accompany acute brainstem encephalitis. These patients usually have flulike symptoms, headaches, nausea, dizziness, and facial numbness. In some instances, peripheral facial palsy is observed. Involvement of the trigeminal nerve by tumor, vascular malformation, or connective tissue disease rarely manifests as acute sensory loss in the face.

C. **Acute sensory loss over the scalp and neck.** Not infrequently, a tense and anxious patient reports acute onset of numbness in the "top of the head." Such patients also commonly describe discomfort or pain on combing the hair. Associated problems may include sleeping difficulties, generalized fatigue, light-headedness, and recurrent bioccipital or diffuse pressurelike headaches.

1. Some patients, after exposure to cold or with no obvious reasons, may experience the sudden onset of lateralized discomfort or pain associated with decreased sensation in the occipital area. The pain has a tendency to radiate proximally into the ipsilateral parietal region. There may be discomfort on compression and decreased pinprick sensation in the distribution of the greater or lesser occipital nerves.

2. Acute sensory impairment in the area over the angle of the mandible, the lower part of the external ear, and the upper neck below the ear suggests neuropathy involving the great auricular nerve.

D. **Acute sensory loss over half of the face, trunk, and corresponding extremities.** Acute primary modality sensory loss over the entire half of the body often is a manifestation of a stroke. A traumatic CNS lesion also should be considered when the clinical history indicates injury.

1. Sensory loss in half of the body can be transient or permanent when indicative of irreversible tissue damage rostral to the upper brainstem up to the postcentral gyrus and parietal area of the cerebral hemisphere contralateral to the side of the sensory deficit.

2. Acute onset of numbness, tingling, prickling, or a crawling sensation starting in the lips, fingers, or toes and spreading in seconds over half of the body may represent a partial seizure with somatosensory manifestations. The abnormal sensation may follow a rather stereotypical pattern, usually lasting less than 1 minute. The onset of focal seizures among adults frequently reflects a focal pathologic condition such as a tumors or vascular malformation involving the contralateral hemisphere.

3. With normal findings at evaluation of patients with recurrent hemisensory impairment for focal sensory seizures, early symptoms of TIAs should be considered. The transient sensory impairment in TIAs usually lasts longer than do sensory disturbances representing partial somatosensory epilepsy. The diagnosis of TIA is more probable if the episodic subjective hemisensory impairment is accompanied by motor deficits in the extremities.

4. A patient with an acute vascular event in the area of the nondominant, right parietal lobe may be unable to give a reliable history because of decreased ability to appreciate motor or sensory deficits in the contralateral extremities **(anosognosia).** Besides diminished light touch and pain sensations, ischemic lesions involving the contralateral postcentral gyrus can cause decreased or absent perception of sizes and shapes of objects **(astereognosis),** inability to recognize numbers or letters drawn on the patient's skin **(agraphesthesia),** or altered **two-point discrimination.**

5. Acute onset of hemisensory impairment that manifests as a tingling sensation, numbness, or ill-defined pain can accompany an acute vascular lesion involving the contralateral thalamus. Patients often have midline demarcation of the sensory disturbances in the absence of reproducible abnormalities at examination. Patients may be unaware of the profound sensory loss in the involved areas. There may be a feeling of deformation or enlargement of the involved extremities. Thalamic paresthesia and pain often are disabling and difficult to manage. Vascular lesions of the thalamus typically are lacunar infarcts of small thalamoperforate vessels coming off the vasculature of the circle of Willis.

E. **Clinical aspects of acute sensory loss in the area of the trunk.** Acute unilateral or bilateral sensory loss with a horizontal sensory level over the chest or abdomen localizes a lesion to the spinal cord and necessitates emergency evaluation to minimize residual neurologic impairment secondary to a possible spinal cord lesion. Particularly with a clinical history of a potential spinal cord injury, expedient decisions may be crucial in optimizing outcome.

1. **Complete transection of the spinal cord** is relatively easy to diagnose. Muscle weakness is present in both lower or the upper and lower extremi-

ties. All forms of sensation are lost one to two segments below the level of the lesion. Absence of vibration sense at the spinous process below the lesion can be helpful in localizing the spinal cord damage. A zone of increased pinprick or light touch sensation at the upper border of the anesthetic zone may be established. Urinary and fecal incontinence is present.

2. In the case of an acute spinal cord lesion extending over the entire lateral half of the cord, a **syndrome of cord hemisection (Brown-Séquard's syndrome)** may be identified. There is contralateral loss of pain and thermal sensation one or two segments below the lesion with muscle weakness in the lower extremity on the side of the spinal cord lesion.

3. Acute loss of pain and temperature sensation can accompany **occlusion of the anterior spinal artery.** Light touch, position, and vibration senses remain intact. Anterior spinal artery syndrome can occur during aortic surgery or in advanced atherosclerotic disease of the aorta. It also can develop in the course of meningovascular syphilis or as a manifestation of collagenvascular disease. Dissociated sensory deficits also can occur in association with acute spinal cord infarction in the "watershed" areas (T1-4 and T12-L1 levels).

4. Occasionally after falls that involve landing on the buttocks, patients may have loss of pain and temperature sensation with preserved tactile sensation one to two segments below the level of the expected spinal cord involvement. Expanding hematomas in the spinal cord gray matter compromise the ventral white commissure conducting fibers for pain and temperature sensation. Light touch and vibration senses remain intact. The dissociated sensory deficit can extend over several segments.

5. Acute ascending sensory loss for pain, soft touch, and temperature can be a manifestation of an acute spinal cord inflammatory process. In **acute transverse myelitis,** the sensory level is most frequently found at the T4-6 and T10-12 levels. Decreased or absent vibration and position senses below the level of the spinal cord involvement and functional alteration in sphincters with urinary and fecal incontinence can be present. Symmetric, severe muscle weakness in the lower extremities can develop over hours. Viral diseases or vaccinations may precede the onset of neurologic symptoms by 1 to 3 weeks. Postinfectious isolated transverse myelitis typically causes fairly dense sensory and motor deficits, compared with the partial patchy sensory and motor deficits of the transverse myelitis that is part of multiple sclerosis. In postinfectious transverse myelitis, there typically is much more cerebrospinal fluid (CSF) inflammation (50 to 100 lymphocytes per cubic millimeter), and demyelination extends over several spinal cord segments. In the transverse myelitis of multiple sclerosis, there are typically no or mild CSF inflammation (fewer than 20 lymphocytes per milliliter) and much smaller segments of spinal cord demyelination. Approximately 10% to 50% of patients with transverse myelitis eventually have additional attacks of demyelination in other locations in the brain or spinal cord. The condition then is diagnosed as multiple sclerosis. The Presence of subclinical white matter lesions in the brain at MRI performed during a clinically isolated bout of transverse myelitis indicates increased risk of development of multiple sclerosis.

6. **Acute "saddle" sensory loss** localizes a lesion to the tip of the spinal cord, at the conus medullaris. Sphincteric disturbance of bowel and bladder function often is associated.

F. Acute sensory loss in individual extremities can be established in longitudinal zones corresponding to individual nerve roots, in various areas supplied by individual nerve roots, in various areas corresponding to trunks or branches of the brachial or lumbosacral plexus, or in various areas supplied by individual nerves. Individual nerve roots typically are affected by trauma from spondylotic vertebral bone spurs or herniated disk protrusions. The brachial plexus can be affected by local trauma, either during operations in the area or in accidents involving the shoulder, including birth injuries, and can become inflamed. The lumbosacral plexus can be affected by operations in the area, including those that cause retroperitoneal hematoma. Peripheral nerves are susceptible to trauma or compression in certain classic areas, including the radial nerve in the upper arm, the ulnar nerve at the elbow, the median nerve at the wrist, the peroneal nerve at the knee, and the tibial nerve at the medial malleolus.

1. **Nerve roots**

   a. In the upper extremities, diminished or lost pinprick or light touch sensation over the thumb and the radial aspect of the arm suggests involvement of the C6 nerve root. Decreased pinprick sensation over the ring and little fingers and the ulnar aspects of the forearm and arm indicates involvement of the C8 nerve root. If there is decreased pinprick sensation over the index and middle fingers, and sometimes over the radial aspect of the ring finger, damage to the C7 nerve root should be considered.

   b. In the lower extremities, acute loss of pinprick and light touch sensations involving the L1 nerve root can be established as a longitudinal zone at the level of the groin followed distally by the L2 and L3 nerve roots involving the anterior aspect of the thigh, extending proximally at the left above the buttocks. Sensory deficits along the medial and lateral aspects of the shin correspond, respectively, to the L4 and L5 nerve roots. Involvement of the S1 and S2 nerve roots manifests as decreased sensation in the posterior aspects of the thigh and calf.

2. **Peripheral nerves**

   a. **Axillary nerve.** Besides instances of acute sensory loss accompanying nerve-root involvement, localized sensory deficits suggestive of a peripheral nerve lesion may be encountered. Dislocation of the shoulder joint, injury to the humerus, or prolonged pressure, stretching, or traction involving the arm during anesthesia or sleep can result in lesions of the axillary nerve. Localized pinprick and light touch deficits over the lower portion of the deltoid muscle allow the examiner to identify the nerve involved.

   b. **Median nerve.** Diminished or absent sensation over the palmar aspects of the first three and one-half fingers and the dorsal aspects of the terminal phalanges of the second and third fingers and half of the fourth finger indicates damage to the median nerve. Acute sensory loss in the area of the median nerve is caused predominantly by injuries involving the arm, forearm, wrist, and hand, including stab and bullet wounds. Procedures involving needle insertion, particularly in the cubital fossa, also can result in median nerve damage manifested by sensory deficits and pain, frequently with a burning, causalgic component. In rare instances, prolonged compression during anesthesia or sleep can cause acute median nerve involvement that manifests as sensory and motor deficits. Numbness and tingling in the distribution of the median nerve that wakes a person from sleep and are relieved by shaking the hand and arm are a classic sign of carpal tunnel syndrome, which typically results from repetitive motion injury around the wrist. Persons with diabetes, hypothyroidism, arthritis, or acromegaly or those who are pregnant are particularly predisposed to development of carpal tunnel syndrome.

   c. **Ulnar nerve.** Acute sensory impairment indicating ulnar nerve damage manifests as paresthesia followed by decreased light touch and pinprick sensation over the fifth and ulnar half of the fourth finger and the ulnar portion of the hand to the wrist. Fractures and dislocations of the humerus involving the elbow, lacerating wounds, and pressure on the nerve during anesthesia, or drunkenness ("Saturday night palsy") are the most frequent causes of acute ulnar nerve damage.

   d. **Radial nerve.** Among patients with acute radial nerve lesions, the sensory deficit may be established over the posterior aspect of the arm if the nerve damage occurs in the axilla. Radial nerve lesions proximal to the spiral groove of the humerus lead to decreased sensation over the distal extensor aspect of the forearm. The superficial branch of the radial nerve gives origin to the dorsal digital nerve in the distal forearm and supplies the skin on the dorsal and radial aspects of the hand and the dorsa of the first four digits. The radial nerve is probably the most commonly injured peripheral nerve. Injuries including dislocation and fracture of the shoulder, extended pressure on the nerve (particularly at the groove of the nerve), and fractures of the neck of the radius are the most frequent causes of radial nerve damage.

  e. **Femoral nerve.** An acute lesion of the femoral nerve manifests as decreased sensation over the anterior and medial aspects of the thigh and in the area of the saphenous nerve in the medial aspect of the lower leg. Acute femoral nerve injury may follow fractures of the pelvis and femur, dislocation of the hip, pressure or traction during hysterectomy, forceps delivery, or pressure in hematoma in the area of the iliopsoas muscle or groin. Paresthesia and sensory loss in the area of the saphenous nerve can occur as a result of injury in the area above the medial aspect of the knee in medial arthrotomy or as a complication of coronary artery bypass graft surgery.

  f. **Obturator nerve.** Sensory loss in obturator nerve injury is found over a small area of skin over the medial aspect of the thigh. The nerve can be damaged during surgical procedures involving the hip or pelvis, in cases of obturator hernia, or secondary to iliopsoas hematoma.

  g. **Lateral femoral cutaneous nerve.** Abrupt onset of tingling, numbness, and discomfort in the lateral and anterolateral aspects of the thigh is typical of involvement of the lateral femoral cutaneous nerve (meralgia paresthetica). Pinprick hyperesthesia is followed by hypesthesia for pain and soft touch. The discomfort or pain can be bilateral. The nerve can be damaged by compression by the inguinal ligament, in iliopsoas hemorrhage, or by tightly fitting garments on obese individuals.

  h. **Sciatic nerve.** Acute sensory impairment involving the outer aspect of the shin and over the dorsal, plantar, and inner aspects of the foot occurs in acute sciatic nerve lesions. The distribution of the sensory deficits reflects the areas of skin sensation supplied by the two branches of the sciatic nerve—the peroneal nerve and the tibial nerve. Acute sciatic nerve damage can occur in association with fractures or dislocations of the hip, hip joint surgery, other pathologic conditions of the pelvis including gunshot wounds, or injections in the vicinity of the sciatic nerve.

  i. **Peroneal nerve.** With injury to the common peroneal nerve at the level of the fibular head, impaired sensation in the lateral aspect of the shin and over the dorsum of the foot is established. Sometimes only the superficial branch of the peroneal nerve is damaged, manifesting as decreased pinprick or light touch sensation in the more distal portion of the lateral aspect of the shin. A small patch of skin hypesthesia for pinprick or soft touch may be established between the first and second toes in instances of deep peroneal nerve lesion. Most peroneal nerve lesions are traumatic, including those caused by compression exerted at the upper and outer aspects of the leg, stretching of the hip and knee, or surgical procedures involving the knee joint.

  j. **Tibial nerve.** Acute damage to the tibial nerve results in sensory disturbances in the lateral aspect of the calf supplied by its branch, the medial sural cutaneous nerve. Additional branches of the tibial nerve supply sensation to the skin of the lateral aspect of the heel, the lateral aspect of the foot (sural nerve), and the sole, the medial two thirds of the sole being innervated by the median plantar nerve and the lateral third by the lateral plantar nerve. The tibial nerve is injured mostly in the popliteal fossa at the level of the ankle or foot. Injury at the tarsal tunnel where the nerve crosses the medial malleolus causes sensory loss in the toes and dorsum of the foot.

3. **Plexopathy.** Acute sensorimotor deficits indicating multiple nerve involvement in the individual upper or lower extremities suggest plexopathy.

  a. **Brachial plexus.** Acute onset of tingling, numbness, and pain, usually followed in several hours or days by muscle weakness and patchy hypesthesia in the area of the shoulder girdle and proximal arm muscles, is typical of brachial plexus neuritis (neuralgic amyotrophy). Acute brachial plexopathy can be caused by trauma in which the arm is hyperabducted or can be secondary to traction involving the arm, including birth injuries. Brachial plexus neuritis can occur in epidemic form. Brachial plexus neuritis can follow infection, vaccination, or parenteral administration of serum. Brachial plexopathy can occur as a complication of coronary artery bypass surgery. In some patients, no apparent cause of plexopathy is established.

   b. **Lumbosacral plexopathy** is recognized when there are sensorimotor deficits and pain in the lower extremities. In acute lumbar plexopathy, a common etiologic factor other than trauma is retroperitoneal hemorrhage.

G. **Clinical aspects of acute sensory loss in both feet or both hands.** Some patients describe tingling, prickling, numbness, or "stiffness" in the hands and feet. The acroparesthesia may be of variable duration, frequently is more pronounced at night, and may be associated with decreased sensation in the fingertips. The underlying pathologic condition usually is of no imminent severity. Should the paresthesia increase in intensity and be accompanied by decreased ability to move the toes or fingers, close patient observation is indicated to exclude GBS. Less frequently, the sensorimotor disturbances start in both hands or manifested as facial numbness. For some patients, the sensory disturbances are minimal in comparison with the severity of muscle weakness, or the ascending sensory deficits remain localized only in the lower extremities. In patients with GBS, deep sensory modalities, including position and vibration senses, are more impaired than is superficial sensation.

V. **Diagnostic approaches to acute sensory loss.** Evaluation for acute sensory loss is driven by both the localization of the lesion to the PNS, nerve root, spinal cord, or brain, as determined by the findings at neurologic examination, and by the suspected etiologic factor, including infectious–parainfectious, inflammatory–demyelinating, vascular–hemorrhagic, or traumatic–compressive.

   A. **PNS evaluation.** If a lesion localizes to a particular peripheral nerve, the extremity and nerve can be specifically evaluated radiographically and electrophysiologically.

      1. Radiographs of the involved limb can help identify fractures or bony deformities that can cause focal compression of damage to the nerve. CT or MRI of the brachial or lumbosacral plexus can be useful in identifying damage or structures that cause damage.

      2. **Electromyography (EMG)** with nerve conduction studies can be helpful in both documenting damage to a peripheral nerve, a plexus, or a nerve root, in localizing where the damage has occurred, and in providing prognostic information about recovery from the documented damage. In a traumatized nerve or root, abnormalities may not appear immediately on nerve conduction studies. It also takes approximately 2 weeks for denervative change to occur in muscles innervated by damaged nerves, so an initially unremarkable or borderline EMG must be repeated if there is continued suspicion of damage. In the acute period, a demyelinated nerve can show slowing of nerve conduction, conduction block across demyelinated nerve segments, and slowing of F waves that reflect proximal nerve root damage. The degree of denervation and axonal dropout found at subacute EMG studies is prognostically useful.

   B. **Spinal cord evaluation.** Localization of a lesion to the spinal cord necessitates neuroimaging of the cord. Traumatic lesions necessitate immediate imaging of an immediately stabilized spine by means of traditional radiographs and subsequent imaging of the spinal cord parenchyma by means of CT myelography, MRI, or both.

      1. **MRI** is the preferred technique for imaging the spinal cord parenchyma, and use of gadolinium can be helpful in identifying acute inflammatory lesions or syringomyelic cavities. In general, MRI provides the best images if only a segment of the cord is targeted—cervical, thoracic, or lumbosacral. If the first imaged segment does not provide a diagnosis, other segments should be

examined. Some total spine MRI imaging techniques can effectively "clear" the cord or help target a segment of the cord for more precise imaging.

2. Traditional myelography is essentially obsolete, but **CT myelography** can be used to examine segments of the cord for suspected pathologic conditions. CT myelography is especially good at depicting bone, disk, and ligamentous structures that may be impinging on the spinal cord.

3. Another useful test for evaluating spinal cord function, is **somatosensory evoked responses,** which can help determine whether there is slowed conduction of somatosensory stimuli from arms or legs in the somatosensory pathways from spinal cord to cortex and can crudely localize the lesion. Testing of somatosensory evoked responses occasionally can help identify a peripheral nerve lesion, which is then better localized by means of nerve conduction studies.

4. For suspected vascular lesions in the spinal cord, **MR angiography** can occasionally noninvasively help identify a lesion. Traditional angiography of spinal vessels is occasionally performed to try to identify lesions.

C. **Brain evaluation.** Acute sensory loss that localizes to the brain, including cerebral cortex or brainstem, is best evaluated by means of neuroimaging with occasionally focused views of the base of the skull, the brainstem, or the orbits.

1. Traditional **radiographs,** including sinus radiographs, can be helpful.

2. For acute suspected vascular lesions, including hemorrhage or stroke, the best technique is **CT.**

3. Follow-up imaging by means of **MRI** can more precisely localize the lesion, help assure there is no hemorrhage into a tumor, and can include MR angiography to examine blood vessels. For suspected inflammatory–demyelinating or postinfectious processes, MRI is the procedure of choice. Gadolinium contrast material can be administered to assess whether there is acute enhancement, which suggests active inflammation and breakdown of the blood–brain barrier.

4. **MR angiography** can depict the larger vessels of the anterior and posterior cerebral circulation and the carotid arteries. **MR venography** can depict and aid in the diagnosis of cortical sinus thrombosis.

5. **Cerebral angiography** may be necessary to diagnose vascular abnormalities such as ruptured aneurysm, atherosclerotic narrowing, vasculitis, and sinus thrombosis.

6. **Electroencephalography** can aid in the diagnosis of seizures.

D. **Vascular–hemorrhagic and traumatic–compressive processes** are largely addressed with the previously discussed neuroimaging and electrophysiologic techniques. Vascular–hemorrhagic processes also can necessitate further blood work, including assessment for hypercholesterolemia or hypercoagulable or prothrombotic states.

E. **Inflammatory–demyelinating and parainfectious–postinfectious processes** necessitate evaluation with neuroimaging techniques as discussed earlier but also necessitate extensive blood work and sampling of CSF. Fever and meningismus raise suspicion of infection.

1. Blood work is performed in an attempt to identify infectious or inflammatory conditions that can cause acute sensory loss, including complete blood cell count, blood cultures when indicated, erythrocyte sedimentation rate, antinuclear antibodies, rheumatoid factor, angiotensin-converting enzyme level, rapid plasma reagent test, Lyme titer, antineutrophil cytoplasm autoantibodies, glucose level, and hemoglobin A_{Ic}.

2. Examination of spinal fluid can show whether there is acute protein elevation, glucose depression, or white blood cell elevation suggestive of infectious or inflammatory causes of for acute sensory loss. Hypoglycorrhachia can indicate the need for further attempts to isolate certain infectious agents such as fungi or acid-fast bacilli. The nature of CSF pleocytosis can dictate further evaluation; the most typical inflammatory causes of postinfectious sensory loss cause lymphocytic pleocytosis. To further pursue postinfectious and demyelinating etiologic factors, spinal fluid should be examined for IgG

level and IgG index, both of which are elevated in multiple sclerosis and often in transverse myelitis, and for the presence of oligoclonal IgG bands in CSF but not serum. These bands are present in most cases of multiple sclerosis and in many forms of parainfectious or postinfectious encephalomyelitis. Myelin basic protein levels in CSF can indicate ongoing demyelination. For suspected infectious causes, cultures and smears for bacteria, acid-fast bacilli, and fungus are important. Serologic and polymerase chain reaction tests also can be done for many viruses, including herpes simplex types 1 and 2, Epstein–Barr virus, cytomegalovirus, human herpesvirus type 6. A CSF Venereal Disease Research Laboratory test and angiotensin-converting enzyme level are useful.

VI. Referrals. Cases of acute sensory loss should be referred to a neurologist if
  A. Sudden onset or resolution suggests TIAs.
  B. Radiculopathy is suspected and focal neurologic deficits are present (weakness, reflex loss).
  C. Fever is present and there is a suspicion of encephalitis or cortical sinus thrombosis.
  D. Deficits worsen or evolve to include motor signs and symptoms.
  E. Acute deficit is present with spinal cord localization. A neurosurgeon also should be informed.

Recommended Readings

Brazis PW, Masdeu JC, Biller J. *Localization in clinical neurology,* 3rd ed. Boston: Little, Brown, 1996.

Carpenter, MB. *Core text of neuroanatomy.* Baltimore: Williams & Wilkins, 1975.

Fisher CM. Pure sensory stroke and allied conditions. *Stroke* 1982;13:434–447.

Haerer AF, ed. *DeJong's The neurologic examination,* 5th ed. Philadelphia: JB Lippincott Co., 1992.

Kimnra J. *Electrodiagnosis in diseases of nerve and muscle.* Philadelphia: FA Davis Co, 1984.

Koski CL. Guillian Barre syndrome and chronic inflammatory demyelinating polyneuropathy: pathogenesis and treatment. *Semin Neurol* 1994;14:123–130.

Mayo Clinic and Mayo Foundation. *Clinical examinations in neurology,* 6th ed. St. Louis: Mosby, 1991.

Noseworthy JH, Lucchinetti C, Rodriguez M, et al. Multiple sclerosis. *N Engl J Med* 2000; 343:938–952.

Patten J. *Neurological differential diagnosis.* New York: Springer-Verlag, 1980.

Scott TF, Bhagavatula K, Snyder PJ, et al. Transverse myelitis: comparison with spinal cord presentations of multiple sclerosis. *Neurology* 1998;50:429–433.

28. APPROACH TO THE HYPERKINETIC PATIENT

Allison Brashear

The patient who presents with a **hyperkinetic movement disorder** experiences excessive movement. The patient may state that it interferes with the activities of daily living, or the patient may be unaware of the problem and the family may prompt the evaluation. The correct diagnosis depends on the character of the movement, that is, when it occurs, its speed, its location, and contributing factors. The more common disorders include dystonia, tremor, chorea, tics, myoclonus, and tardive dyskinesia (Table 28.1).

I. **Dystonia**
   A. Definition. Dystonia is a disorder consisting of intermittent or sustained, often painful, twisting, repetitive muscle spasms that may occur in one part of the body (focal dystonia) or throughout the entire body (generalized dystonia).
      1. Initially, the movements may be triggered by a specific act, such as writing, and are made worse by movement of other parts of the body.
      2. There may be superimposed tremor or myoclonic jerks.
      3. The patient may use a "sensory trick"—a tactile stimulus—that can decrease the muscle contractions.
      4. The movements may be painful.
   B. Classification
      1. Dystonia is classified by the part of the body affected (focal versus generalized dystonia), by the age of onset (adult-onset versus childhood-onset dystonia), and by contributing factors (idiopathic versus secondary dystonia).
      2. Psychogenic dystonia. Dystonia was once diagnosed as hysteria or malingering, and patients were often referred to a psychiatrist for evaluation. Psychogenic dystonia can be differentiated from idiopathic or secondary dystonia only with a detailed history and physical examination. Sensory tricks and variations in weakness are common in idiopathic dystonia, and referral to a specialist may be needed to discern idiopathic dystonia from the psychogenic form. Clues to psychogenic dystonia include inconsistent movements and postures, false weakness and sensory symptoms, and overt psychiatric disease.
   C. Pathophysiology
      1. Idiopathic dystonia is not associated with any particular brain lesion. Secondary dystonia is most often observed in patients with lesions in the basal ganglia, such as the putamen, and their connections with the thalamus and cortex.
      2. Genetics. The prevalence of familial generalized dystonia is 1 in 160,000 in the general population, and in the Ashkenazi Jewish population it is 1 in 15,000 to 1 in 23,000. The gene for primary torsion dystonia has been found on chromosome 9. Persons with the DYT1 gene usually have onset before 26 years of age and generally have lower limb symptoms. The testing guidelines for DYT1 gene testing suggest that using a cutoff of symptoms by the age of 26 years gives a sensitivity of 100% but a specificity of 54%. Onset up to 44 years of age has occurred in individuals with the gene, although most of these are of limb onset. The DYT1 gene is more common among persons of Ashkenazi Jewish descent, although it has been found in non-Jewish persons.
      3. Testing. The genetic test for DYT1 is commercially available. There is no clinical confirmatory test. A detailed neurologic history and examination are the best method of diagnosis.
   D. Generalized dystonia. The spasms of generalized dystonia affect most of the body. They can manifest in one part of the body, particularly the foot, but rapidly spread to contiguous parts and usually involve the limbs, trunk, and neck. Generalized dystonia more commonly manifests among children and young adults. Onset is typically in the legs and spreads to contiguous body parts.
   E. Focal dystonia is isolated to one part of the body. Table 28.2 lists the types and areas affected.

Table 28.1 Hyperkinetic movement disorders

Term	Clinical manifestations
Dystonia	Sustained muscular spasms that can be focal or generalized
Tremor	Rhythmic oscillation of agonist and antagonist muscles
Chorea	Quick, irregular, often semipurposeful movements
Hemiballismus	Violent type of flinging movements occurring on one side of the body
Tics	Sudden, fast, irregular movements, usually in the same muscle group
Myoclonus	Sudden, fast movements, usually repeated in the same body part
Tardive dyskinesia	Combined chorea and dystonic movements, usually in the face and lower jaw, but may be generalized; history of use of neuroleptic agents

F. Etiology. Dystonia can be idiopathic (primary) or have a known cause (secondary).
   1. Idiopathic (primary) dystonia
      a. Idiopathic dystonia has no known cause.
      b. Birth history is normal, and the examination findings are normal except for dystonia. Ceruloplasmin and brain imaging are normal.
      c. Types of idiopathic dystonia include focal and generalized forms. Regardless of a focal or generalized presentation, dystonia can be genetic, such as autosomal dominant (DYT1), X-linked (Lubag syndrome), or sporadic.
   2. Secondary dystonia. The most common known metabolic defect causing secondary dystonia is Wilson's disease.
      a. Known metabolic defect. Wilson's disease is an inherited deficit in copper metabolism.
         (1) Neurologic symptoms affecting the basal ganglia, including bradykinesia, dysarthria, dystonia, tremor, ataxia, and abnormal gait, occur in 40% to 60% of patients. Spasmodic dysphonia (involving the vocal chords) is a common form.
         (2) Rare autosomal recessive disease located on the long arm of chromosome 13.
         (3) Exclude with slit-lamp eye examination for Kayser–Fleischer rings and determination of serum ceruloplasmin level in patients younger than 50 years. Treatment can reverse the liver involvement in Wilson's disease and prevent severe neurologic sequelae.

Table 28.2 Types of focal dystonia

Term	Clinical manifestations
Blepharospasm	Involuntary spasms of the orbicularis oculi (around the eyes), resulting in eye closure
Limb dystonia	Writer's cramp or intermittent spasms of the foot or hand
Oromandibular dystonia	Facial grimacing, sometimes isolated to jaw opening or closing; Meige's syndrome when eyes and lower jaw are both involved
Spasmodic dysphonia	Intermittent spasms of the vocal chords, resulting in a strain and strangle quality to the voice (adductor type); rarely presents a breathy voice (abductor type)
Torticollis (cervical dystonia)	Involuntary twisting, turning, and tilting of the neck, often associated with pain and tremor

(4) Wing-beating tremor is classically described in patients with Wilson's disease. This tremor is absent at rest and develops after the arms are extended.

b. Other neurologic syndromes manifesting as secondary dystonia are those with **unknown metabolic defects,** including degenerative disease, a juvenile variant of Huntington's disease, dystonia with parkinsonian symptoms, early-onset Parkinson's disease, rapid-onset dystonia–parkinsonism, and dopamine-responsive dystonia (hereditary).

3. Acquired dystonia occurs as a result of an injury, treatment, or other disease process. These can include

a. Prenatal injury resulting in an ischemic event manifesting as dystonia.

b. Exposure to toxins (carbon monoxide, manganese) resulting in structural changes to the basal ganglia.

c. Anoxic injury to the cerebral cortex or basal ganglia resulting in dystonic posturing.

d. Tardive syndrome from dopamine blockers (phenothiazine, metoclopramide). Tardive dystonia generally occurs during treatment or within 3 months of discontinuation of therapy.

e. Focal brain lesions (stroke, tumor, demyelinating, postinfectious, posttraumatic), regardless of the cause, can manifest as dystonia.

f. Peripheral nerve injury to the neck or limbs can result in dystonic posturing of that body part. Why this causes dystonia has not been determined.

g. Psychogenic dystonia remains a diagnosis of exclusion. Irregular spasms, unusual triggers, and bizarre postures may be clues.

G. Clinical manifestations of dystonia

1. Focal dystonia

a. Blepharospasm is a disorder that consists of uncontrollable involuntary spasms of the eyelids causing spontaneous closure. It often interferes with vision, resulting in functional blindness. It may be worsened by bright light or stress.

b. Oromandibular dystonia consists of grimacing of the lower part of the face, usually involving the mouth, jaw, and platysma muscle. If associated with blepharospasm, it is called *Meige's syndrome.*

c. Spasmodic torticollis or cervical dystonia consists of intermittent, uncontrollable spasms of the neck muscles, often associated with severe pain. The neck may involuntarily turn, tilt, or rotate forward, sideways, or backward.

d. Spasmodic dysphonia involves only the vocal cords. There are two types of spasmodic dysphonia. With **adductor-type** spasmodic dysphonia, hyperadduction of the cords produces an intermittent strain and strangle quality to the voice. Often patients also report tightness in the throat during the spasms. With the more rare **abductor type** of spasmodic dysphonia, there is a whispering quality to the voice, similar to the movie star Marilyn Monroe's voice.

e. Occupational dystonia. Writer's cramp is the most common and most underdiagnosed form of limb dystonia. Dystonic posturing may be noticed in the hand or foot. Early in the course of the disease, the movement may be brought out by performing a specific task such as writing, typing, or playing a musical instrument. Examples of this include an auctioneer who has jaw dystonia only during an auction, a secretary who has dystonic hand cramps while typing, and a violinist who has finger spasms only while playing.

2. Hemidystonia involves one side of the body and almost always results from a focal lesion (vascular, neoplastic, or traumatic).

3. Generalized dystonia. Spasms occur in two or more limbs, and usually also in the trunk and neck. Symptoms usually begin in the legs and progressively involve other parts of the body.

H. Evaluation of dystonia
1. Focal dystonia
a. Onset after 50 years of age
(1) Magnetic resonance imaging (MRI) of the brain
(2) Family history
(3) Search for medication as a cause (e.g., dopamine receptor blocking drugs such as phenothiazines or metoclopramide).
b. Onset before 50 years of age
(1) MRI of the brain
(2) Ceruloplasmin and slit-lamp examination for Kayser–Fleischer rings
(3) Screen for medication as a cause
(4) Persons with onset before 26 years of age should be considered for genetic testing for the DYT1 gene. A detailed family history should be obtained.
2. Hemidystonia
a. MRI of the brain to rule out structural causes (neoplastic, vascular, infectious, or traumatic)
b. Ceruloplasmin and ophthalmologic examination with a slit lamp for Kayser–Fleischer rings
3. Generalized dystonia
a. Family and medication history
b. MRI of the brain
c. Ceruloplasmin and ophthalmologic examination with a slit lamp for Kayser–Fleischer rings
d. DTY1 gene testing

II. Tremor
A. Definition.
Tremor consists of rhythmic, oscillating movements of agonist and antagonist muscles. The movements are equal in amplitude and frequency. Symptoms are made worse by anxiety and disappear with sleep.
B. Classification
1. **Physiologic tremor** is a low-amplitude (8 to 12 Hz) tremor that is most prominent in outstretched hands and that under certain circumstances is present in all persons.
2. **Essential tremor** is a postural or action-involved tremor that rarely is present at rest. The frequency usually is 4 to 12 Hz but may decrease with age. Data suggest that different anatomic locations (arm tremor only versus head and arm tremor versus isolated head tremor) may have clinically different presentations. Most subjects progressed slowly, but a small subgroup had a more rapid progression. The more rapid progression appeared to be associated with a higher age at onset and the presence of concomitant head and arm tremor.
3. **Cerebellar tremor** is most prominent in voluntary movements and has a frequency of 3 to 4 Hz. Patients perform poorly on finger-to-nose and heel-to-shin testing. The tremor may involve only the trunk in some patients.
4. **Rest tremor (parkinsonian tremor)** occurs at 3 to 7 Hz and is most obvious when the limb is fully supported and at rest. Rest tremor is reduced by action and intention.
C. Etiology
1. **Physiologic tremor** is exacerbated by excited mental states, metabolic or endocrine derangements, fever, drugs (thyroid, lithium, β-agonists, theophylline, and sodium valproate), alcohol withdrawal, and caffeine use.
2. **Essential tremor**
   a. The cause of essential tremor is unclear.
   b. Most patients have strong family histories.
   c. An association with Parkinson's disease and dystonia has been suggested.
   d. The diagnosis can be confirmed by means of suppression of the tremor through ingestion of a small amount of alcohol. Lack of response does not exclude the diagnosis.
3. **Cerebellar tremor** is typically observed with a lack of feedback of the cerebellum to the motor cortex. The cause of a cerebellar tremor include demyeli-

nating disease (such as multiple sclerosis), a space-occupying lesion, or an ischemic, toxic, or infectious disorder.

4. **Rest tremor** is part of the clinical features of Parkinson's disease. However, some patients come to medical attention with this type of tremor and may not have other symptoms of Parkinson's disease, such as bradykinesia, postural instability, and cogwheel rigidity. The cause of a resting tremor is generally considered to be in the central nervous system (CNS), but the exact anatomic lesion is unknown.

   D. Evaluation
   1. **Physiologic tremor**
      a. Medication (most common cause)
      b. Drug or alcohol withdrawal
      c. Assess for anxiety
      d. Perform thyroid function tests to rule out hyperthyroidism
   2. **Essential tremor**
      a. Hyperthyroidism can worsen an existing essential tremor.
      b. Use of drugs such as lithium or sodium valproate or alcohol withdrawal can exacerbate an essential tremor.
   3. **Cerebellar tremor.** Patients with a cerebellar tremor should be evaluated with MRI of the brain, including the posterior fossa, to rule out a mass, ischemic, or demyelinating lesions as the cause.
   4. **Resting tremor.** A patient with a rest tremor should be given a trial of medication for Parkinson's disease. Rest tremor may be the manifesting symptom of Parkinson's disease.

III. Chorea
   A. Definition. Chorea is hyperactive, fast, arrhythmic, often semipurposeful movement. It can affect the limbs, face, or trunk.
   B. Classification
   1. Adult-onset chorea
      a. Positive family history
         (1) Huntington's disease
            (a) Huntington's disease is a progressive neurodegenerative disease with autosomal dominant inheritance localized to chromosome 4.
            (b) Patients with positive family histories often come to medical attention with chorea. The mean age at onset is 40 years, but the onset can be any time from childhood to old age. Some patients may notice problems with control of fine movement, dropping of objects, or incoordination before the onset of chorea.
            (c) Cognitive deficits manifest as problems of concentration, attention, and coordination of spatial motor acts rather than problems of memory. Subtle findings, such as changes in job performance or interests, may be revealed when the patient visits the physician. Memory problems often are short-term problems, and unlike patients with Alzheimer's disease, patients with end-stage Huntington's disease may retain recognition of family and familiar surroundings.
         (2) **Wilson's disease.** See I.F.2.a.
      b. **No family history.** A focal brain lesion, such as a mass, infection, or vascular lesion can cause chorea in someone without a family history of chorea.
      c. **Other causes of chorea**
         (1) Pregnancy. Chorea gravidarum or chorea caused by hormone replacement in a pregnant patient should be investigated.
         (2) Encephalitis
         (3) Drugs. Levodopa, oral contraceptives, anticonvulsants, lithium
         (4) Metabolic and autoimmune disorders. Consider systemic lupus erythematosus, antiphospholipid antibody syndrome, or lupus anti-

coagulant, thyrotoxicosis Sydenham's chorea, polycythemia rubra vera, and hypoparathyroidism.

(5) Infection. Lesions due to toxoplasmosis have been reported.

2. Childhood-onset chorea

  a. Positive family history

(1) **Wilson's disease.** See I.F.2.a.

(2) **Huntington's disease** can occur among children whose fathers have Huntington's disease.

(3) A history of rheumatic fever suggests a diagnosis of Sydenham's chorea.

(4) A history of progressive cerebellar ataxia, choreoathetosis, ocular motor apraxia, and telangiectasias of the conjunctiva and skin in a child or adolescent suggests a diagnosis of ataxia telangiectasia (Louis–Barr syndrome).

  b. History of birth trauma or CNS infection. Childhood-onset chorea can develop in children with a history of birth injury or as a result of encephalitis.

C. Evaluation

  1. Positive family history

  a. Abnormal findings at slit-lamp examination for Kayser–Fleischer rings suggests the presence of Wilson's disease.

(1) Seek neurologic consultation for treatment.

(2) Seek genetic counseling.

  b. Computed tomography (CT) or MRI of the brain that shows atrophy of the caudate nucleus suggests the presence of Huntington's disease. Genetic counseling should be sought. The asymptomatic gene carrier state and symptomatic cases can be confirmed with testing. The test is commercially available. Because the penetrance of Huntington's disease is 100%, testing of persons without symptoms who have a family history is not routinely recommended. If such testing is pursued, it should be performed in conjunction with psychological counseling and support.

  2. Negative family history

  a. CT of the head

  b. Birth history

  c. History of drug use

  d. Thyroid, calcium tests

  e. Pregnancy test

  f. Cerebrospinal fluid examination

IV. Hemiballismus

  A. Definition. Hemiballismus is a rare disorder involving violent flinging of the arm or leg on one side of the body.

  B. Etiology. Caused by destruction of part of the contralateral subthalamic nucleus that results in disinhibition of the output of the globus pallidus. The cause usually is hemorrhagic or ischemic infarction but also can be previous surgery or an undiagnosed tumor.

V. Tics

  A. Definition. Tics are sudden, brief movements or vocalizations that appear irregularly in a group of muscles. A tic can be a simple movement, such as a head jerk or shoulder shrug, or a complicated task that appears to mimic a voluntary act, such as an obscene gesture.

  B. Types of tic disorders

  1. Motor tics are abrupt, simple motor tasks, such as rapid head jerks.

  2. Vocal tics are repetitive vocalizations, such as grunting and throat clearing.

  3. Complicated motor and vocal tics

  a. Complicated motor tics are semipurposeful movements.

  b. Complicated vocal tics are repeated words or sentences. They can be made-up or obscene words.

  4. Tourette's syndrome (TS)

  a. Patients with TS have multiple motor tics with one or more vocal tics.

      b. Onset of symptoms occurs before 21 years of age.

      c. The estimated prevalence of TS is 1 to 10 cases per 10,000 persons. However, because the diagnosis of TS can be missed in the mildest form, this may be a gross underestimation.

      d. Symptoms persist for at least 12 months.

      e. Behavioral disturbances

          (1) Obsessive–compulsive disorder is characterized by repetitive, stereotyped behaviors or thoughts.

          (2) Attention-deficit hyperactivity disorder (with or without hyperactivity) manifests as poor attention span, restlessness, poor concentration, and low impulse control.

      f. Learning disabilities. In addition to obsessive–compulsive disorder and attention-deficit hyperactivity disorder, some patients with TS have problems with classroom learning and academics.

      g. Sleep disturbances include somnambulism, nightmares, insomnia, and restlessness. These disturbances may be related to treatment, environment, or superimposed psychiatric disease.

C. Etiology

   1. Tics involve **inherited changes in synaptic transmission.**

   2. The **dopamine hypothesis** involves both presynaptic and postsynaptic function. It has been proposed that TS is caused by supersensitivity of the postsynaptic dopamine receptors, dopamine hyperinnervation, abnormal presynaptic function, or excessive phasic release of dopamine.

   3. TS is generally hereditary. The gene and the biochemical defect are unknown. There is strong evidence that monozygotic twins have a 86% concordance rate of TS compared with a 20% rate among dizygotic twins. A gene has not been identified.

   4. Other causes

      a. Tics may be observed after head trauma, toxin exposure, and encephalitis.

      b. Tics can occur in association with other primary neurologic disorders, such as Huntington's disease, Parkinson's disease, dystonia, and side effects of medications such as methylphenidate.

VI. Myoclonus

A. Definition. Myoclonus is defined as sudden, brief, involuntary jerks or contractions, either rhythmic or irregular, of single muscles or groups of muscles. It can occur at rest or in response to touch, auditory, or visual stimulation.

B. Types of myoclonic disorders. Myoclonus can be divided into epileptic, non-epileptic, and inherited types.

   1. Epileptic myoclonus comprises generally progressive degenerative disorders affecting the nervous system. Myoclonus can occur in association with ataxia, dementia, or other seizure types.

      a. Progressive myoclonic epilepsy. Myoclonic and tonic–clonic seizures occur among patients with progressive neurologic decline.

          (1) Progressive myoclonic epilepsy is associated with ataxia and dementia.

          (2) Neuropathologic studies can help differentiate the subgroups of neurologic syndromes associated with myoclonus.

             (a) Myoclonic epilepsy with ragged red fibers (MERRF) manifests in the second decade with myoclonic seizures and possibly hearing loss, optic atrophy, neuropathy, or hypoventilation. The diagnosis is triggered by detection of ragged red fibers during muscle biopsy.

             (b) Lafora's myoclonic epilepsy (Lafora's bodies) is an autosomal recessive storage disease diagnosed by means of skin biopsy. Dementia always is present and is accompanied by myoclonus and seizures. The mean age at presentation is 14 years, and the disorder can manifest as a behavioral change or school problem.

      (c) Baltic myoclonus (Unverricht–Lundborg disease) has autosomal recessive inheritance, and the mean age at presentation is 10 years. Myoclonus always is present, can be provoked by sound or touch, and can provoke a generalized seizure. There is no test for this disorder. Gait ataxia, dysarthria, tremor, and mild dementia eventually develop.

  b. Infection of the CNS

    (1) Creutzfeldt–Jakob disease manifests a rapid onset of dementia and associated neurologic findings of myoclonic jerks, ataxia, pyramidal and extrapyramidal signs, and akinetic mutism. Cases of slowly progressive dementia have been reported without all of these clinical features. The characteristic electroencephalogram (EEG) shows periodic lateralized epileptiform discharges (PLEDs). The recent finding of protein 14-3-3 in cerebrospinal fluid may improve the ability to diagnose this disease. However, absence of this protein does not exclude this disease as a diagnosis.

    (2) Subacute sclerosing panencephalitis is a rare sequela of measles. The onset usually occurs before 2 years of age and is followed by a silent period as long as 8 years. Myoclonus is preceded by intellectual decline, personality changes, ataxia, and hyperactive reflexes. The EEG shows PLEDs, and cerebrospinal fluid may contain oligoclonal bands and antibodies to the measles virus.

  c. Drug-related conditions. Myoclonus has been found among patients treated with levodopa, bromocriptine, tricyclic antidepressants, and narcotics.

  d. Toxic and metabolic conditions. Myoclonus can occur in a confused patient as either large rhythmic movements or small irregular jerks and may be stimulus induced. Myoclonic movements can be confused with seizures, particularly if the patient is acutely ill, and ruling out seizures may necessitate an EEG. The most common cause is severe renal or hepatic disease. Systemic infection or drug intoxication also can cause myoclonic jerks. In rare instances, heavy metal intoxication can cause myoclonus.

2. Nonepileptic myoclonus. Nonepileptic myoclonic disorders are nonprogressive. EEG correlation is found in some cases of epilepsia partialis continua and juvenile myoclonic epilepsy.

  a. Action myoclonus is induced by a voluntary movement or stimulus, such as a loud noise, and is common after hypoxic injury.

  b. Palatal myoclonus consists of regular, rhythmic movement of the palate that can spread to the throat, face, and diaphragm. Movement persists during sleep. The neuropathologic lesion involves the red nucleus, the inferior olive, and the dentate nucleus (triangle of Guillain–Mollaret). This lesion often is ischemic, but it can be neoplastic, inflammatory, or degenerative.

  c. Segmental myoclonus may arise in an arm or leg secondary to peripheral nervous system or CNS trauma, infection, or inflammation. It also can accompany renal failure, neuropathy, or acquired immunodeficiency syndrome.

  d. Sleep myoclonus occurs soon after going to or arousing from sleep. It can be confused with seizure, particularly among infants. This benign form of myoclonus can be difficult to differentiate from infantile spasms. EEG findings are normal.

  e. Epilepsia partialis continua manifests as regular myoclonic jerking associated with a cortical discharge and no change in level of consciousness.

  f. Juvenile myoclonic epilepsy. Among children, jerks can precede a seizure. A family history and abnormal EEG findings establish the diagnosis.

g. Opsoclonus–myoclonus among children

(1) Neural crest tumors may be seen on chest radiograph, or chest CT may be needed. Elevated levels catecholamine metabolites are present in the urine.

(2) Opsoclonus–myoclonus also can occur in postinfectious syndromes.

3. **Inherited myoclonus–dystonia** is a new term used to describe cases of myoclonus that begin in the first two decades of life, are autosomal dominant with variable penetrance and little or no progression, are responsive to alcohol ingestion, and are associated with dystonia. This disorder has been linked to the site of the dopamine D2 receptor gene on chromosome 11 in some families, but the gene has not been located. In addition, other families with this syndrome do not link to this region of chromosome 11. Eight families have been linked to a region on chromosome 7q. The likelihood is that inherited myoclonus–dystonia is a phenotype with several genotypes depending on the family studied.

VII. Tardive dyskinesia

A. Definition. Tardive dyskinesia is a disorder that manifests as involuntary movements among some patients after they receive prolonged neuroleptic drug therapy.

B. Classification

1. **Classic** tardive dyskinesia manifests as choreoathetoid movements of the face, limbs, and trunk.

2. **Variable forms**

   a. **Tardive dystonia** manifests as spasms similar to those observed in torticollis, blepharospasm, or Meige's syndrome.

   b. **Tardive akathisia** manifests as persistent motor restlessness.

C. Etiology

1. Tardive dyskinesia must be differentiated from other drug-induced syndromes.

   a. **Acute extrapyramidal syndrome.** Anticholinergic drugs relieve acute extrapyramidal syndrome but leave a tardive syndrome unchanged or worse.

   b. Dopamine agonists and levodopa can cause hyperkinetic dyskinesia.

2. **Risk factors for tardive dyskinesia**

   a. Age older than 65 years

   b. Severity may be greater in affective disorders than in schizophrenia.

   c. Long-term use of antiemetic drugs, such as prochlorperazine and metoclopramide

   d. The relation between total dosage and duration is unclear.

VIII. Referrals

A. Dystonia. For diagnosis and planning of treatment, patients with focal or generalized dystonia should be referred to a neurologist with expertise in movement disorders.

B. Tremor

1. **Physiologic tremor** does not necessitate neurologic evaluation.

2. **Essential tremor** can be diagnosed at clinical examination. Referral is recommended for patients who do not respond to β-blockers.

3. **Cerebellar tremor** necessitates no referral if symptoms follow the description in **II.B.3.**

4. **Rest tremor.** Treatment can be initiated by the primary care physician. Patients with refractory cases should be referred to a neurologist.

C. Chorea

1. **Huntington's disease.** Patients with suspected Huntington's disease should see a neurologist for a second opinion. Issues of genetic counseling and experimental clinical trials are best answered by a neurologist experienced in treating patients with this disease. Genetic testing without counseling is not recommended.

2. **Other forms of chorea.** Drug-induced, metabolic, or pregnancy-associated chorea can be managed by a primary care physician. Patients with refractory or unclear cases should be referred to a neurologist.

D. Hemiballismus. The diagnosis of hemiballismus should be made by an experienced neurologist.

   E. Tics. Most tics can be diagnosed and managed by a primary care physician. Referrals should be made for unclear or refractory cases.
   F. Myoclonus. Most cases of myoclonus should be evaluated by a neurologist. An experienced neurologist can differentiate the epileptic and nonepileptic forms.
   G. Tardive dyskinesia. Patients with tardive dystonia should be under the care of a psychiatrist. Antipsychotic medications should be adjusted to decrease the risk of further dystonia.

Recommended Readings

Bressman SB, Greene PE. Dystonia. *Current Treatment Options in Neurology* 2000;2:275–285.
Bressman SB, Sabatti C, Raymond D, et al. The DYT1 phenotype and guidelines for diagnostic testing. *Neurology* 2000; 54;1746–1752.
Brewer G. Wilson's disease. *Current Treatment Options in Neurology* 2000;2:193–204.
Butler I. Movement disorders of children. *Pediatr Neurol* 1992;39:727–742.
Jankovic J. Essential tremor: clinical characteristics. *Neurology* 2000;54[Suppl 4]:S21–S25.
Quinn N, Schrag A. Huntington's disease and the other choreas. *J Neurol* 1998;245:709–716.
Singer HS. Current issues in Tourette syndrome. *Mov Disord* 2000;15:1051–1063.

29. APPROACH TO THE HYPOKINETIC PATIENT

Robert L. Rodnitzky
Ergun Y. Uc

Hypokinesia is defined as a decrease in the normal amount, amplitude, or speed of automatic or volitional movements. The term **bradykinesia** often is used when the predominant movement abnormality is slowness. The term **akinesia** sometimes is used to imply a severe reduction in the amount or amplitude of movement. In truth, it is rare for any of these three parameters of movement to be affected in isolation. Thus, a patient with bradykinesia typically manifests a decreased amount and amplitude of movement in addition to a striking slowness of movement. The movement of patients with hypokinesia often is referred to as parkinsonian because bradykinesia is so common in Parkinson's disease. However, bradykinesia is only one of four cardinal features of Parkinson's disease, the others being rigidity, rest tremor, and postural imbalance. Bradykinesia in the absence of the other features is not sufficient to make a diagnosis of Parkinson's disease. The term **parkinsonism** is used to infer a condition characterized by one or more of these cardinal signs that clinically resembles idiopathic Parkinson's disease (IPD) but is histologically different and often accompanied by additional neurologic signs and symptoms.

Hypokinesia can be used to describe both slowed volitional movements, such as reaching for an object, and automatic movements, such as eye blinking or arm swing while walking. Surprisingly, when hypokinesia develops over a period of several months or longer, the patient and family members may be relatively unaware of the problem. A striking and remarkable decrease in blink frequency often goes unnoticed until brought to the attention of the patient or family members. When hypokinesia begins to result in functional disability, patients become aware of a problem in motor function, but rather than attribute it to the speed or amplitude of their movement, they more commonly describe the difficulty as "weakness." Through careful questioning, the clinician can discern a history of weakness from that of hypokinesia. Once the distinction is made, it is important to determine whether slowness or lack of movement is due to an extrapyramidal system disorder (e.g., Parkinson's disease) or to certain psychiatric disorders (catatonia or severe depression). One final differentiation must be made from neuromuscular disorders producing severe stiffness with associated slowness of movement.

Hypokinesia related to abnormalities of the motor system is seldom life threatening except in extreme form, in which severe immobilization can result in serious complications such as pneumonia or pulmonary embolism. Yet hypokinesia always merits serious attention because it often results in considerable functional and social disability.

I. Etiology
   A. **Basal ganglia abnormalities.** Dysfunction of the basal ganglia is the most common cause of hypokinesia. Among basal ganglia disorders, those in which there is dysfunction of the striatum are most likely to produce a parkinsonian syndrome. IPD, in which the nigrostriatal pathway is involved, is a classic example of striatal dysfunction that leads to hypokinesia. It is believed that the decrease in motor activity in this instance results from diminished excitatory drive of the motor cortex due to dysfunction in the striatopalidothalamic pathways. Sometimes hypokinesia can be corrected by means of pharmacologic alteration of critical neurotransmitters in these pathways or less commonly by means of stereotactic lesioning of component structures in the hope of restoring the critical balance of inhibitory and excitatory influences in motor systems. The following are possible mechanisms whereby the basal ganglia or their neurotransmitter systems become affected.
      1. **Degenerative disorders** of the basal ganglia typically result in a loss of specific groups of cells often linked by their neurotransmitter content or physiologic role.
      2. **Pharmacologic agents** can produce hypokinesia by altering the release or reuptake of basal ganglia neurotransmitters or by blocking their receptors. This is especially true of agents that affect the neurotransmitter dopamine.
      3. **Vascular disorders** can result in isolated infarction that affects one or more basal ganglia structures. More commonly, hypokinesia results from a

multiinfarct state consisting of multiple smaller ischemic lesions scattered throughout both hemispheres and diffusely affecting basal ganglia structures and their connections.

4. **Trauma** can cause basal ganglia dysfunction in several ways. Direct trauma such as a gunshot wound to the basal ganglia is one potential mechanism. Repetitive head trauma over a period of months or years often results in a parkinsonian state, presumably caused by the cumulative effect of shearing forces on midbrain structures and blood vessels produced by rapid and severe blows to the head. This damage impairs the substantia nigra and its striatal projection fibers. This condition, often occurring among boxers, is referred to as *pugilistic encephalopathy.*

5. **Toxins** can cause basal ganglia dysfunction as part of a generalized toxic encephalopathy but do so even more commonly by targeting specific neurons in the basal ganglia or a connecting structure such as the substantia nigra.

6. **Central nervous system (CNS) infection** can impair basal ganglia function as a result of localized lesions such as an abscess involving these structures. Delayed onset of dysfunction can occur months to decades after a viral infection, as illustrated by the late appearance of parkinsonism after an epidemic form of encephalitis (encephalitis lethargica) that occurred in the early part of the twentieth century.

B. **Psychiatric syndromes** can result in marked slowness or reduction in motor activity.

1. **Depression** is classically associated with psychomotor retardation in which spontaneous movement may be both reduced and slowed.

2. **Catatonia** is characterized by severe reduction in spontaneous movement and a tendency to remain unmoving in a single position for a protracted period even when passively placed in that position by the examiner. This phenomenon is known as **waxy flexibility.**

C. **Metabolic disorders,** notably hypothyroidism, can result in global slowing of motor function.

D. **Neuromuscular disorders** that result in extreme muscle rigidity or stiffness retard the speed of movement, especially of axial and appendicular muscles but seldom of facial muscles.

II. The **clinical manifestations** of hypokinesia result from different combinations of reduction in the speed, frequency, and amplitude of spontaneous or automatic movement.

A. **Hypomimia** is a decrease in facial expression. The diminished range of facial response to emotional stimuli gives rise to the term **expressionless facies.** The reduced eye blink rate results in an appearance resembling a constant stare.

B. **Diminished automatic movement** is noticeable as a decrease in gesticulation and head movement during conversation, a reduction in the automatic repositioning of limbs while sitting in a chair or reclining in bed, and as a decrease in the amplitude of arm swing while walking. In severe hypokinesia, affected arms may not swing at all but be held in a semiflexed posture across the front of the trunk. Among patients with asymmetric hypokinesia, as is often the case in Parkinson's disease, reduction in arm swing is greatest on the more involved side.

C. **Impairment of repetitive movements** is particularly prominent among patients with hypokinesia. The patient may state that activities such as handwriting or buttoning a shirt are particularly difficult. Not only are repetitive movements performed slowly, but also the amplitude of each successive movement typically becomes progressively smaller. This may account for the progressively smaller letters (micrographia) seen when a hypokinetic patient is asked to write a long sentence or for increasing difficulty with the successive fine movements required to successfully place a button through a button hole.

D. **Impaired initiation of movement** manifests as difficulty in arising from a chair or hesitancy in taking the first step while attempting to walk. Many patients with Parkinson's disease have difficulty initiating two motor acts simultaneously, such as standing up and shaking hands.

E. **Freezing** is a sudden involuntary cessation of a motor act, usually walking, while other functions remain intact. This phenomenon is confined to basal ganglia disorders. Freezing can occur spontaneously or be provoked by external circumstances, such as attempting to turn in mid gait or pass through a narrow space such as a doorway. Emotional stimuli, including anger or fear, can provoke freezing, as can the prospect of entering a room filled with people. A variety of sensory or motor tricks such as marching to a cadence are effective in overcoming freezing.

F. Hypophonia is characterized by diminished amplitude and inflection of speech. In its most severe form, it results in a muffled pattern of articulation. **Tachyphemia** is an excessively rapid speech pattern that is a common accompaniment of hypophonia, making such speech even more unintelligible.

III. Evaluation

A. History

1. **Direct motor symptoms of hypokinesia.** It is important to carefully analyze all motor symptoms in the history because what the patient represents as weakness or poor balance may actually be a manifestation of hypokinesia. Conversely, a report of slowness in performing motor functions, such as dressing, walking, feeding or writing, must be clarified to determine whether the slowing is actually a secondary phenomenon related to incoordination, weakness, or dementia. Specific symptoms that are particularly common among patients with hypokinesia should be recorded. These include difficulty in rising from a chair, hesitancy in initiating gait, and a change in the legibility and size of handwriting. If there have been frequent falls, it should be determined whether they are related to freezing. Because a change in facial expression may not be apparent to the patient, friends and family should be asked to comment on this symptom.

2. **Associated neurologic symptoms.** The identity of the underlying neurologic condition that has resulted in the hypokinetic state often is suggested by the constellation of other associated neurologic symptoms that the patient relates. Thus IPD is suggested when hypokinesia is associated with the symptoms of rest tremor, stiffness (rigidity), and postural imbalance in the absence of other neurologic symptoms. On the other hand, the association of hypokinesia with neurologic symptoms outside the motor realm usually suggests a condition other than IPD. Such symptoms include seizures, sensory loss, paresthesia, headache, early dementia, visual loss, apraxia, and early or severe autonomic symptoms, such as impotence, orthostatic hypotension, or urinary incontinence. Another useful historical fact in differentiating IPD from other forms of parkinsonism is the sequence in which otherwise typical parkinsonian symptoms appear. Whereas postural imbalance and severe gait disturbance often appear late in the course of IPD, their appearance as initial symptoms in a patient with hypokinesia suggest a different cause of parkinsonism.

3. **Toxic exposure.** Exposure to toxins such as manganese (as occurs among welders) or carbon monoxide must be ascertained because both can result in parkinsonism. Less common causes include mercury, carbon disulfide, methanol, and cyanide.

4. **Medication usage.** Patients must be asked whether they are currently taking or have recently been treated with antidopaminergic drugs such as neuroleptics, reserpine, or metoclopramide. Any history of illicit drug use should be ascertained.

5. **Family history.** Because IPD is a common disorder, it is not uncommon for patients to have a family member who carries the same diagnosis. Although there appear to be genetic factors that contribute to the development of this disorder, a mendelian pattern of inheritance has been observed in only a few families worldwide and in patients with onset of the condition at a very young age. Therefore, a family history of a hypokinetic disorder in more than one first-degree relative or a clear mendelian pattern of inheritance should raise the question of a neurologic disorder other than Parkinson's disease (although rare instances of autosomal dominant IPD have been reported). Heritable disorders that can mimic Parkinson's disease include Wilson's disease (autosomal recessive), juvenile Huntington's disease (autosomal dominant), and essential tremor (autosomal dominant with variable penetrance).

6. **Psychiatric symptoms.** Determine whether there have been symptoms suggestive of depression, such as suicidal thoughts, feelings of guilt or self deprecation, or vegetative symptoms such as anorexia and disturbed sleep. If hallucinosis is present, it must be determined whether it began early or late in the illness and whether it appeared in response to the institution or escalation of an antiparkinson drug. Although depression can occur at any stage of Parkinson's disease, hallucinations are not present in the early stages of the illness and should not appear any time in the absence of concurrent treatment with antiparkinson medications. Very early appearance of hallucinations in parkinsonism or their presence in an untreated patient with parkinsonism, raises the probability of dementia with Lewy bodies.

7. **Cognitive symptoms.** Document whether there have been any changes in memory, orientation, judgment, and intellectual function. Severe, early abnormalities of this type can indicate a primary dementing disorder such as Alzheimer's disease or the presence of a multiinfarct state. Mild to moderate cognitive symptoms are present in most of the Parkinson's-plus syndromes, but are seldom the initial symptom. Dementia appears in approximately 30% of patients with IPD but usually when the illness is moderately advanced.

8. **Response to medications.** Determine whether there has been a previous trial of therapy with dopaminergic agents and if so whether they produced objective improvement. In a patient with parkinsonism, absence of benefit from adequate dosages of dopaminergic drugs, especially levodopa, casts doubt on the diagnosis of IPD and suggests a diagnosis of secondary parkinsonism or one of the Parkinson's-plus syndromes. Equally important is determining whether, early in the illness, these medications produced psychiatric side effects, such as hallucinations, or autonomic symptoms such as severe orthostatic hypotension, the former suggesting the possibility of dementia with Lewy bodies and the latter indicating possible multiple system atrophy. In IPD, psychiatric and autonomic side effects from dopaminergic drugs are not uncommon but usually appear when the illness is at least moderately advanced.

IV. **Physical examination**
  A. **Clinical findings of parkinsonism**
   1. **Gait and posture** should be evaluated by having the patient walk a distance of at least 20 feet (6 m) in an area free of obstacles. Patients with parkinsonism have a reduced length of stride. The arms do not swing and may be held flexed across the front of the trunk. The upright posture is commonly flexed in IPD. There may be difficulty in initiating gait, and turns may be accomplished with several small steps or with the body moving as a single unit (en bloc turning). The gait in IPD occasionally is characterized by progressively more rapid, small steps as the body leans forward (festination). On the other hand, the patient's feet may "freeze" in mid gait.
   2. **Rising from a chair** is tested by asking the patient to rise with arms crossed in front of the body to prevent pushing off. A patient with hypokinesia may need several attempts to succeed or may be totally unable to rise without using the arms. If the patient is unable to rise without assistance, a judgment must be made whether the cause is weakness (which can be tested independently) or bradykinesia.
   3. **Postural reflexes** are evaluated by asking the patient to establish a comfortable base, with feet slightly apart. While standing behind the patient, the examiner applies a brisk backward sternal perturbation. A normal response is to take a corrective step backward to prevent falling. When postural reflexes are impaired, more than one step is needed before balance is reestablished. When postural reflexes are absent, the patient continues to reel backward and falls if not stopped by the examiner.
   4. **Rigidity.** If rigidity is present, it must be determined whether it is predominant in axial muscles (neck or trunk), in the limbs, or equally severe in both. Increased resistance to passive movement of the involved body part is easily appreciated when rigidity is severe. When subtle, rigidity can be rein-

forced by asking the patient to alternately open and close the fist of the hand on the side opposite of the arm or leg being tested. The presence of tremor in the limb demonstrating rigidity gives rise to a ratchet-like sensation referred to as **cogwheel rigidity.**

5. **Tremor** may appear in one or more forms among patients with parkinsonism.

   a. **Resting tremor,** the hallmark of IPD and also present in some other forms of parkinsonism, is most common in the hands and occurs to a slightly lesser extent in the lower extremities and mandible. Rest tremor rarely involves the head and never affects the voice. It appears at a frequency of 4 to 5 Hz and often is at least temporarily extinguished by volitional movement. Because it is well known that rest tremor is enhanced by stress or anxiety, a subtle tremor can be uncovered by asking the patient to perform difficult mental arithmetic, a mildly stressful task. Rest tremor is the hallmark of IPD, and its absence casts doubt on the diagnosis but certainly does not rule it out.

   b. **Action tremor** can be present in Parkinson's disease as well as in other parkinsonian syndromes, especially those associated with cerebellar dysfunction. It can be present as a **postural tremor** while the arms are outstretched in front of the patient or as a **kinetic tremor** while the patient is performing a task such as the finger-to-nose test. Postural tremor alone, in the absence of parkinsonian signs, suggests a diagnosis of essential tremor.

   c. **Positional tremor.** Some tremors are particularly prominent when the involved body part is placed in a specific position. The **wing-beating tremor** of Wilson's disease is an example of this phenomenon. This tremor is noticed when the arms are abducted at the shoulders while flexed at the elbow.

6. **Bradykinesia** can be documented by simply observing the speed, amplitude, and amount of ordinary movements made by the patient, such as gestures or shifting of body position. Specific tasks such as the finger-to-nose test also provide an opportunity to observe the speed of movement. Repetitive motion tasks such as tapping the index finger against the thumb demonstrate slowness of movement and a progressive loss of amplitude as the movement is repeated.

7. **Facial expression.** The **diminished facial expression** typical of IPD is characterized by a constant neutral countenance with infrequent eye blinking. A **fixed facial expression,** often present in progressive supranuclear palsy, consists of an unchanging expression, such as surprise in which the forehead may be furrowed, the eyelids retracted, and the nasolabial folds deepened. **Myerson's sign** is present in Parkinson's disease and a variety of other basal ganglia disorders. It consists of persistent reflex blinking to repetitive finger taps applied to the glabella just superior to the bridge of the nose. Among healthy persons, there is rapid habituation to this stimulus, so that no blinking occurs after the fourth or fifth tap.

B. **Nonparkinsonian neurologic signs.** Several neurologic findings are associated with one or more forms of parkinsonism, but most of these signs are uncommon in IPD.

   1. **Apraxia** should be tested independently in both upper extremities. The patient should be asked to perform tasks such as saluting, throwing a kiss, or demonstrating how to use an imaginary toothbrush. Inability to perform these tasks in the face of normal strength and coordination or the use of a body part such as a finger in place of an imagined implement suggests apraxia. The most common syndromes that can combine a parkinsonian appearance with apraxia are corticobasal degeneration and Alzheimer's disease.

   2. **Cortical sensory functions** such as graphesthesia, stereognosis, and tactile localization should be assessed. These sometimes are abnormal in corticobasal degeneration.

   3. **The alien limb phenomenon** is present when a patient manifests uncontrollable grasping and manipulating of objects or when a hand exhibits interfering involuntary movement with one of the other limbs (intermanual

conflict). This phenomenon can be present in corticobasal degeneration, ischemic stroke, or Creutzfeldt–Jakob disease, all of which can be associated with a parkinsonian appearance.

4. **Ocular motility abnormalities** occur in some forms of parkinsonism. Inability to generate normal eye movements, especially downward, with preservation of the same movements when eliciting the oculocephalic reflex indicates a **supranuclear gaze palsy.** This finding is most characteristic of progressive supranuclear palsy, but it can be found in other forms of parkinsonism as well. It is important to remember that limited upgaze is not an uncommon finding among healthy elderly patients, but impaired downgaze always is abnormal. Subtle abnormalities of saccadic eye movement can be uncovered by evoking saccades in the form of optokinetic nystagmus. In some basal ganglia disorders, such as Huntington's disease, the saccadic excursion may be complete, but the speed of eye movement is slowed. It is important to observe the patient for the presence of **macro square wave jerks.** This ocular movement abnormality consists of spontaneous, repetitive, alternate right then left, 5 to 10 degree horizontal deviations of the eyes from the midline. This finding also is associated with progressive supranuclear palsy.

5. **Reflex myoclonus** is elicited by tapping the arm, leg, or fingertip with the examiner's own fingertip or with a percussion hammer.

6. **Blood pressure measurements** must be measured in the recumbent and standing positions while the concurrent heart rate is recorded. Orthostatic hypotension is an early and common manifestation of multiple system atrophy. It occurs later in the course of IPD, especially when dopaminergic or anticholinergic drugs are being taken.

7. **Mental status evaluation** should include functions such as immediate and short-term recall, orientation, constructional praxis, calculation, and comprehension of three-step commands. The standardized mini–mental state examination suffices for this purpose.

8. **Other neurologic signs.** To determine the extent of involvement of the CNS, a complete neurologic examination should be performed to establish the presence of hyperactive or hypoactive stretch reflexes, sensory loss, cranial nerve dysfunction, cerebellar signs, pathologic reflexes (especially the Babinski sign), weakness, or muscle atrophy.

V. **Laboratory studies**
   A. **Neuroimaging**
      1. **Typical Parkinson's disease.** In classic IPD, the diagnosis of which is strongly suggested by the history and physical examination, neuroimaging is not necessary. Parkinson's disease is commonly somewhat asymmetric, but if symptoms or signs of parkinsonism are remarkably asymmetric resulting in severe involvement on one side and almost no involvement on the other, a CNS imaging study, preferably magnetic resonance imaging (MRI), is indicated to evaluate for the possibility of a unilateral structural basal ganglia lesion such as a neoplasm, arteriovenous malformation, or infarct or the presence of brain hemiatrophy.
      2. **Other forms of parkinsonism.** In patients with insufficient findings to make a diagnosis of IPD (e.g., a patient with hypokinesia only) or with additional neurologic findings not usually seen in Parkinson's disease, a brain imaging procedure is indicated, preferably MRI. Not all degenerative forms of parkinsonism are associated with demonstrable MRI abnormalities and those that are may have the characteristic abnormality infrequently or only in the advanced stages of the illness (see **VIII.C.**). Therefore, normal findings on MRI or computed tomography (CT) of the brain do not rule out syndromes such as progressive supranuclear palsy or multiple system atrophy but do usually eliminate from consideration conditions such as normal pressure hydrocephalus, brain tumor, or stroke.
   B. **Laboratory and genetic tests** are not useful in establishing a diagnosis of IPD but can be of benefit in diagnosing several other causes of parkinsonism (see **VIII.**).

VI. Differential diagnosis (Fig. 29.1)

    A. IPD is the most common cause of parkinsonism. It is a degenerative disorder of unknown but probable multifactorial causation (environmental and hereditary). There is increasing evidence that genetic factors play an important role in Parkinson's disease. There is a high rate of concordance among monozygotic twins when one twin has young-onset disease. Mutations in a gene on chromosome 4, coding for the synaptic protein α-synuclein have been identified in families with a rare autosomal dominant inheritance pattern of the disease. A gene on chromosome 6 for an autosomal recessive variant of parkinsonism encodes parkin, a protein of unknown function. However, further studies in other kindreds and with patients who have sporadic IPD suggested that IPD is only rarely caused by such mutations. Metabolic dysfunction of mitochondrial complex I has been found in Parkinson's disease, whether acquired or hereditary. The predominant abnormality is in the substantia nigra pars compacta and nigrostriatal pathway leading to dopamine deficiency in the striatum. The wide spectrum of symptoms and the resistance of some symptoms, such as depression, to levodopa support pathologic observations that the degenerative process also involves other brainstem nuclei and subcortical structures.

        1. Clinical features. The cardinal symptoms are resting tremor, bradykinesia, rigidity, and impairment of balance. The onset usually is asymmetric, and tremor is the most common initial sign. Postural instability, gait difficulty, and dysautonomia appear with progression of the disease. Approximately 30% of patients have dementia, but it is seldom severe and never is the initial symptom. The incidence of IPD increases sharply with age, although the disease can occur at any age. Patients with onset of IPD between 21 and 39 years of age are arbitrarily classified as having young-onset IPD. They have gradual progression of symptoms and are more likely to experience dystonia as an early sign. Levodopa-induced dyskinesia and motor fluctuations that can occur in IPD at any age are more frequent in this age group. The differential diagnosis of juvenile parkinsonism (before 21 years if age) is broad and includes hereditary and metabolic conditions.

        2. Neuroimaging. Findings at MRI and CT of the brain usually are unremarkable in IPD. Positron emission tomography (PET) shows decreased fluorodopa uptake in the striatum but no striatal abnormality on deoxyglucose scans.

        3. Neuropathologic examination. Lewy bodies (eosinophilic intracytoplasmic inclusions), mainly in the substantia nigra, are the pathologic hallmark of Parkinson's disease. In IPD, these inclusions stain for α-synuclein, the protein produced by the mutant gene in the rare autosomal dominant form of Parkinson's disease.

        4. Other tests. There is no specific test for the diagnosis of IPD.

    B. Secondary parkinsonism. Parkinsonism can be induced by a wide spectrum of disease processes that affect the brain, especially the basal ganglia. These include infection, cerebrovascular disorders, exposure to toxins, metabolic disorders, trauma, neoplasm, drug effects, hypoxemia, and hydrocephalus. Selected causes are as follows.

        1. Drug-induced parkinsonism. Neuroleptics and metoclopramide block striatal D2 dopamine receptors, and reserpine depletes dopamine from presynaptic vesicles. Each of these drugs can produce motor symptoms indistinguishable from those of IPD. The "atypical" neuroleptic clozapine mainly blocks extrastriatal (D4) receptors and does not cause parkinsonism. Another atypical agent, quetiapine, also seems to have low potential to cause this adverse effect. Other atypical neuroleptics, such as risperidone and olanzapine, can cause parkinsonism, especially when high dosages are used. An underlying predisposition to Parkinson's disease may be responsible in part for the emergence of this syndrome. The resolution of drug-induced parkinsonism can take several months after discontinuation of the offending medication.

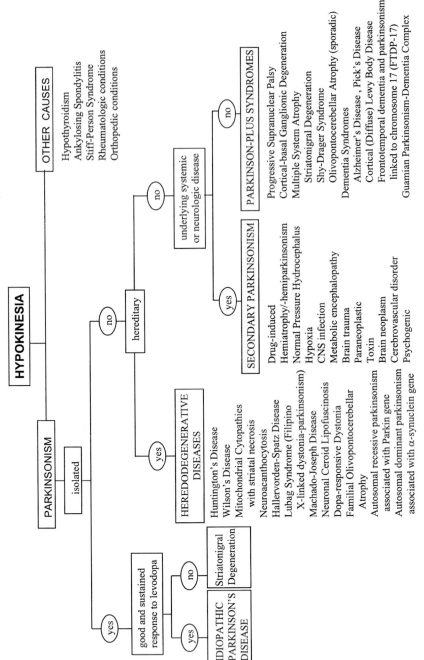

FIG. 29.1 Algorithm for differential diagnosis of hypokinesia.

2. **Normal pressure hydrocephalus (NPH)**
    a. **Clinical features.** NPH is a form of communicating hydrocephalus. Approximately one third of patients with this disorder have a history of spontaneous or traumatic subarachnoid hemorrhage or meningitis that might have led to impairment of cerebrospinal fluid (CSF) absorptive mechanisms over the surface of the brain. Although, as measured by means of lumbar puncture, CSF pressure is normal, excessive force on the walls of the dilated lateral ventricles, especially the frontal horn, leads to compression of surrounding structures. The clinical triad of NPH consists of gait apraxia ("magnetic gait"), subcortical dementia (which may later include cortical features), and urinary incontinence, often appearing late in the illness. The hesitant gait may resemble that of IPD, but the absence of rest tremor, the appearance of incontinence, and the absence of significant benefit from levodopa allow the two conditions to be differentiated. Early recognition of this syndrome is important because in some cases shunting the ventricles can reverse it.
    b. **Neuroimaging.** Enlarged lateral ventricles, especially the frontal and lateral horns, which are disproportionate to cortical atrophy, are seen. Proton-density MR images reveal periventricular hyperintensity suggesting transependymal flow. In the care of elderly patients, separating this finding from nonspecific periventricular white matter changes on T2-weighted images can be difficult. The results of isotope cisternography, although demonstrating impaired CSF absorption in some patients, are not considered a reliable predictor of response to shunting.
    c. **Other tests.** The Fisher test consists of removing 30 to 50 mL of CSF and observing for improvement in symptoms over the next 24 hours. It is a useful test and does not require sophisticated laboratory techniques. Intracranial pressure monitoring allows demonstration of periods of high CSF pressure (b waves) and is used widely as a predictor of response to shunting.
3. **Hemiatrophy–hemiparkinsonism.** Patients with this disorder come to medical attention at a relatively early age with markedly asymmetric parkinsonism affecting the side of the body that manifests hemiatrophy. The patients may have a history of abnormal birth and contralateral hemisphere hemiatrophy, both of which raise the possibility of an early childhood brain insult that later in life manifests as delayed-onset parkinsonism. The slow progression of this disorder, its occasional association with dystonia, and the striking asymmetry form the basis of its distinction from IPD.
4. **Toxins**
    a. **MPTP** (1-methyl-4-phenyl-1,2,3,6-tetrahydropyridine) is a toxin inadvertently self-administered by several substance abusers resulting in an acute and severe parkinsonian state. The use of MPTP in the laboratory led to the most widely used animal model of IPD. New cases of human MPTP parkinsonism are rare.
    b. **Carbon monoxide (CO).** Parkinsonism can result from acute or chronic CO poisoning. This toxin causes globus pallidus or striatal necrosis. The onset can be immediate after the incident, but more commonly the disorder develops days to weeks after initial recovery from coma. The history of CO-induced coma and poor or absent response to levodopa suggest the diagnosis.
    c. **Manganese** intoxication can result in a parkinsonian state. It also often is associated with unusual behavioral symptoms such as hallucinations and emotional lability or other movement disorders such as dystonia.
    d. **Cyanide** and **methanol** intoxication can cause bilateral basal ganglia necrosis and parkinsonism.
5. **Cerebrovascular disease.** Either a lacunar state with multiple small infarcts of the basal ganglia or subacute arteriosclerotic encephalopathy affecting basal ganglia connections can lead to parkinsonism. In either condition, dementia is common. Resting tremor usually is absent in these patients.

Gait disorder can be prominent and occasionally constitutes the only neurologic symptom, giving rise to the term *lower body parkinsonism*. The response to levodopa is limited.

6. **Trauma.** Pugilistic encephalopathy is a progressive neurologic syndrome characterized by parkinsonism, dementia, and ataxia. It occurs among boxers with a history of repeated head trauma. Treatment usually is unsatisfactory. Focal acute injury to the midbrain and substantia nigra and subdural hematoma are two other possible causes of posttraumatic parkinsonism.

7. **Aftermath of encephalitis.** Fifty percent of the survivors of the encephalitis lethargica epidemic of 1917 to 1925 eventually had parkinsonism, often as long as decades after the acute infection. This form of encephalitis has not reappeared in epidemic form. Accordingly, new cases of postencephalitic parkinsonism are rare in the modern era.

C. **Parkinson's-plus syndromes.** This is a group of parkinsonian syndromes differentiated from IPD by the presence of additional prominent neurologic abnormalities. In these conditions, there can be cerebellar, autonomic, pyramidal, oculomotor, cortical sensory, bulbar, cognitive, and psychiatric dysfunction as well as apraxia and movement disorders not typical in unmanaged IPD, such as myoclonus, dystonia, or chorea. Any of these neurologic or psychiatric abnormalities can appear early in the course of the illness. Early falls with gait disturbance or postural instability, absence of resting tremor, early dementia and supranuclear gaze palsy are signs that always should prompt consideration of a Parkinson's-plus syndrome. The parkinsonian components of these disorders, such as akinesia and rigidity, are usually not responsive to levodopa, although early transient responsiveness can be observed. The onset of these diseases is generally in the fifth or sixth decade of life with an average survival period of 5 to 15 years. The cause of death usually is pneumonia, other intercurrent infections, or sepsis. The etiopathogenesis of this entire group of disorders is largely unknown.

Despite the apparent clinical differences between IPD and the Parkinson's-plus syndromes, differentiation between the two can be difficult. In a clinicopathologic study, 24% of patients given the clinical diagnosis of IPD were found to have a different type of parkinsonism at autopsy. In Parkinson's-plus syndromes, the findings at head CT or brain MRI can be unremarkable, can show generalized cerebral or cerebellar atrophy, or occasionally reveal focal changes in structures such as the caudate, putamen, cerebellum, or midbrain. Blood cell count, blood chemistry, serology, electromyography (EMG), and evoked potentials usually are not helpful. Electroencephalography may show nonspecific abnormality, such as slowing of the background activity. The specific features of individual Parkinson's-plus syndromes are as follows. Although each of these conditions has characteristic clinical findings, it is important to remember that there is considerable overlap in signs and symptoms.

1. **Progressive supranuclear palsy (PSP)**
   a. **Clinical features.** Early onset of gait difficulty, loss of postural reflexes resulting in backward falls, and freezing of gait, coupled with supranuclear gaze palsy (initially downgaze) are suggestive of PSP. Axial rigidity and nuchal dystonia with extensor posture of the neck, generalized bradykinesia, "apraxia" of eyelid opening and closing, blepharospasm, a furrowed forehead leading to a fixed facial expression, and a monotonous but not hypophonic voice are additional features suggesting the diagnosis. There is variable, but often mild, cognitive decline, especially in executive functions. The presence of prominent bradykinesia in association with the typical fixed facial expression raises the possible diagnosis of Parkinson's disease for these patients, but the ocular motility abnormalities, the frequent absence of tremor, and the absence or loss of levodopa response suggest the correct diagnosis.
   b. **Neuroimaging.** Midbrain and, later, pontine atrophy are sometimes apparent at MRI or CT.
   c. **Neuropathologic examination.** Globose neurofibrillary tangles are present and affect mainly the cholinergic neurons of the basal ganglia

and brainstem nuclei with apparent sparing of the cortex. Cytoplasmic neuronal inclusions consisting of aggregated hyperphosphorylated tau protein are present.

2. Cortical–basal ganglionic degeneration

    a. Clinical features. This syndrome can manifest as a strikingly asymmetric or unilateral akinetic–rigid syndrome associated with limb apraxia, alien limb phenomenon, cortical sensory signs, stimulus sensitive myoclonus, dystonia, and postural or action tremor. Supranuclear gaze palsy, cognitive impairment, and pyramidal tract signs also can be present.

    b. Neuroimaging. Findings at MRI or CT of the brain are abnormal in some cases and reveal asymmetric frontoparietal atrophy.

    c. Neuropathologic examination. Neuronal loss and gliosis are found in the frontoparietal regions and substantia nigra pars compacta. Swollen achromatic neurons and basophilic nigral inclusions, which represent an overlap with Pick's disease, are characteristic. Abundant cytoplasmic inclusions consisting of aggregated hyperphosphorylated tau protein are found.

3. Multiple system atrophy (MSA)

    a. Clinical features. This degenerative disorder consists of three component syndromes that can occur individually or in various combinations.

        (1) Striatonigral degeneration. In this syndrome, akinetic–rigid parkinsonism is predominant, but tremor is seldom present. It usually is not responsive to levodopa because the degenerative process involves the postsynaptic dopamine receptors.

        (2) Sporadic olivopontocerebellar atrophy. Cerebellar signs, especially ataxia and dysarthria, are the prominent findings in this syndrome, although they seldom exist in isolation. Other associated signs include gaze palsy, hyperreflexia, an extensor plantar response, and most important, features of parkinsonism.

        (3) Shy–Drager syndrome. In this syndrome, dysfunction of the autonomic nervous system results in symptoms such as disabling orthostatic hypotension, bowel and bladder dysfunction, and impotence.

        It is not clear whether these three disorders are distinct entities or represent different clinical presentations of the same basic condition, but they commonly occur together and share the pathologic features described in **c.** From a diagnostic point of view, the syndrome of MSA always should be suspected when a patient with hypokinesia has little response to levodopa and has prominent autonomic or cerebellar dysfunction.

    b. Neuroimaging. MRI of the brain shows putaminal hypointensity in striatonigral degeneration, probably caused by excessive iron deposition in this structure. Cerebellar atrophy can be seen in sporadic olivopontocerebellar atrophy.

    c. Neuropathologic examination. Common to all the MSA syndromes is the presence of characteristic glial cytoplasmic inclusions. Like Lewy bodies in IPD, these inclusions stain for the protein α-synuclein. Especially in Shy–Drager syndrome, additional neuronal loss and gliosis are seen in the structures responsible for autonomic functions, such as the intermediolateral cell column of the spinal cord and the dorsal motor nucleus of the vagus.

4. Dementia syndromes. Alzheimer's disease, Pick's disease, and dementia with Lewy bodies are degenerative CNS diseases the predominant manifestation of which is dementia. Familial frontotemporal dementia and parkinsonism linked to chromosome 17 are associated with mutations in the tau gene. Although the degenerative process in these disorders has a predilection for certain cortical regions, subcortical structures also may be involved. This involvement leads to extrapyramidal manifestations, including parkinsonism. The key to identifying a primary dementia disorder as a cause of parkinsonism is the early appearance of dementia, which often antedates the onset of hypokinesia or rigidity.

D. Heredodegenerative diseases

1. **Wilson's disease,** an autosomal recessive condition associated with impairment of copper excretion, results in copper accumulation in different organ systems, including the CNS, liver (cirrhosis), cornea **(Kayser–Fleischer ring),** heart, and kidney.

   a. **Clinical features.** The age at onset ranges from 5 to 50 years, peaking between 8 and 16 years. Neurologic symptoms are present at the onset of the disease in about 40% of patients. Extrapyramidal symptoms such as dystonia, rigidity, and bradykinesia are more common among children whereas tremor and dysarthria are more likely to appear among adults. A variety of psychiatric symptoms can be seen in Wilson's disease. An especially important clue to the diagnosis is the presence of liver dysfunction such as cirrhosis or chronic active hepatitis, especially in a young patient. The combination of bradykinesia and tremor in these patients can suggest Parkinson's disease, but the very young age at onset and the presence of psychiatric symptoms, liver dysfunction, or dystonia should prompt a search for laboratory signs of Wilson's disease. Because the consequences of Wilson's disease are preventable, and the neurologic symptoms are reversible with early treatment with copper chelating drugs, this condition should always be kept in the differential diagnosis of atypical parkinsonism, especially that appearing before the age of 50 years.

   b. **Neuroimaging.** MRI of the brain shows ventricular dilatation as well as cortical and brainstem atrophy. The basal ganglia, especially the putamen, can appear either hypointense or hyperintense on T2-weighted studies and hypodense on CT scans. Occasionally there is the characteristic "face of the giant panda" appearance of the midbrain on MR images.

   c. **Neuropathologic examination.** There is generalized brain atrophy. The putamen, globus pallidus, and caudate are cavitated and display a brown pigmentation that reflects copper deposition.

   d. **Other tests.** Measurement of ceruloplasmin in the plasma is the most useful screening test. The results usually is less than 20 mg/dL (normal, 25 to 45 mg/dL). Plasma copper level is decreased, and 24-hour urinary copper excretion is increased. Slit-lamp examination of the cornea reveals a Kayser–Fleischer ring in almost all patients with neurologic symptoms and represents a highly specific but not pathognomonic finding. If one or more of these test results are normal and the diagnosis is in doubt, the diagnosis is confirmed with liver biopsy results that show increased copper content.

2. **Huntington's disease** is a relentlessly progressive autosomal dominant disorder characterized by dementia, psychiatric disturbance, and a variety of movement disorders.

   a. **Clinical features.** The major clinical components of Huntington's disease are cognitive decline, various psychiatric abnormalities (personality changes, depression, mania, psychosis), and movement disorder. Although chorea is the most common motor symptom, bradykinesia usually coexists with chorea and may explain the occasional exacerbation of motor impairment when control of chorea is attempted with antidopaminergic medications. An abnormality of saccadic eye movement, particularly slow saccades, is often one of the earliest neurologic signs of this disorder. The typical age at onset is in the fourth or fifth decade, but 10% of patients have symptoms before 20 years of age (juvenile Huntington's). Successive generations may have symptoms at a progressively earlier age, especially if they have inherited the disease from their father, reflecting the genetic phenomenon of anticipation. The juvenile form manifests as a combination of a progressive akinetic–rigid syndrome (the Westphal variant), dementia, ataxia, and seizures. These akinetic–rigid patients are most likely to be confused with those with IPD, but the autosomal dominant inheritance pattern, the early age at onset, and the presence of seizures should suggest the correct diagnosis. There is a general inverse correlation between the age at onset and the rapidity of progression. The duration of illness from onset to death is approximately 15 years for adult-onset Huntington's disease and 8 to 10 years for those with onset in childhood.

b. Neuroimaging. Atrophy of the head of the caudate is the principal finding at neuroimaging. It can be appreciated on either MRI or CT.

c. Neuropathologic examination. There is loss of medium spiny striatal neurons as well as gliosis in cortex and striatum, particularly the caudate. This striatal neuronal loss accounts for the drastic decrease in the two neurotransmitters associated with these cells, γ-aminobutyric acid, and enkephalin.

d. Other tests. Huntington's disease can be diagnosed, and presymptomatic cases can be identified with great certainty by means of DNA testing. The genetic abnormality has been localized to chromosome 4 and consists of an expansion of the usual number of repeats of the trinucleotide sequence CAG. The presence of 40 or more CAG repeats confirms the diagnosis of Huntington's disease. The age at onset usually is inversely proportional to the number of CAG repeats. Because of the ethical, legal, and psychologic implications of presymptomatic predictive testing, it should be performed only by a team of clinicians and geneticists fully sensitive to these issues and aware of published guidelines.

3. **Other neurologic conditions** occasionally associated with parkinsonism include neuroacanthocytosis, Hallervorden–Spatz disease, Machado–Joseph disease, and familial calcification of the basal ganglia.

VII. Diagnostic approach

A. Clinical features. Careful history taking and physical examination are essential. A meticulous survey of the medical and psychiatric history, family history, and occupational or environmental exposure to toxins reveals most causes of secondary parkinsonism. Disease onset at a young age, a strong family history of the same disorder, lack of resting tremor, absent response to levodopa and early appearance of postural instability, gait disorder, dysautonomia, or dementia should be considered red flags in the history that suggest a diagnosis other than IPD. The general physical examination is important because it may reveal signs of a systemic disease contributing to secondary parkinsonism. Neurologic examination establishes whether parkinsonism (resting tremor, bradykinesia, rigidity) is isolated or associated with involvement of other neuronal systems in the CNS. The presence of aphasia, apraxia, supranuclear gaze palsy, cortical sensory loss, alien limb phenomenon, pyramidal signs, lower motor neuron findings, myoclonus, chorea, or dystonia indicate more widespread involvement of the CNS than is the case in IPD.

B. General laboratory tests

1. **Complete blood cell count and peripheral blood smear.** Acanthocytes are found on a fresh peripheral blood smear in neuroacanthocytosis. A low hemoglobin and elevated reticulocyte count consistent with hemolytic anemia may be present in Wilson's disease.

2. **Blood chemistry.** Abnormal results of liver function tests are found in Wilson's disease. Hypocalcemia, hypomagnesemia, and a low parathormone level are present in hypoparathyroidism. An elevated creatine kinase level is associated with neuroacanthocytosis, and an elevated serum lactate level, suggesting lactic acidosis, is found in mitochondrial cytopathy. Low levels of thyroxine and high levels of thyroid-stimulating hormone levels point to hypothyroidism.

3. **Serologic testing.** Elevated erythrocyte sedimentation rate, C-reactive protein level, or rheumatoid factor level may be found in inflammatory or rheumatologic conditions that can induce hypokinesia by affecting the musculoskeletal system. Antibodies against glutamic acid decarboxylase are present in stiff person syndrome.

C. Radiology

1. **Plain radiographs.** Spinal radiographs may reveal ankylosing spondylitis or osteoarthritis as the cause of mechanical limitation of movement.
2. **CT or MRI of the brain.** CT may depict a neoplasm, cerebrovascular disease, hydrocephalus, basal ganglia calcification, atrophy, or sequelae of trauma. Contrast enhancement is recommended to evaluate mass lesions. CT has limitations in that resolution is not always adequate to evaluate density changes or storage materials in the basal ganglia, and brainstem or cerebellar sections may suffer from bone artifact. In these circumstances, MRI of the brain, although more expensive than CT, is more desirable. The following characteristic MRI patterns suggest specific hypokinetic disorders:

   Many lacunes: vascular parkinsonism
   Large ventricles out of proportion to cerebral atrophy, transependymal flow: NPH.
   Caudate atrophy : Huntington's disease
   Decreased T2 signal in striatum: MSA
   Homogeneous decreased T2 signal or decreased T2 signal with a central hyperintensity ("Tiger's eye") in the globus pallidus: Hallervorden–Spatz syndrome
   Striatal necrosis: Wilson's disease, Leigh's disease, CO intoxication
   Midbrain atrophy: PSP
   Asymmetric frontoparietal atrophy: cortical–basal ganglionic degeneration

3. **PET or single photon emission computed tomography (SPECT).** These modalities can be useful in differentiating IPD from Parkinson's-plus syndromes by characterizing the regional cerebral metabolism pattern and in determining whether the nigrostriatal abnormality is presynaptic or postsynaptic (Parkinson's plus). The status of nigral dopaminergic neurons can be determined with fluorodopa (PET) or [^{123}I]β carbomethoxy-3 β-(4-iodophenyl)tropane [^{123}I]β-CIT (SPECT). In IPD either of these two modalities shows a loss of dopaminergic nigral cells. Striatal dopamine D2 receptors can be imaged with [^{11}C]raclopride (PET) or [^{123}I]iodobenzamide (SPECT). Findings with these two modalities are most likely to be abnormal in conditions such as MSA that feature primary striatal pathologic changes. Regional cerebral metabolism patterns can be identified with [^{18}F]fluorodeoxyglucose (PET). In IPD, the findings with this study tend to be normal, whereas in many other parkinsonian conditions, abnormally low striatal metabolism is found.

D. Electrophysiology

1. **Electrocardiogram.** Heart block may be present in mitochondrial cytopathy.
2. **Electroencephalography.** Epileptic activity or focal slowing may appear with focal lesions (stroke, tumor). Slow background activity is seen in some forms of primary dementia. Periodic triphasic complexes are present in Creutzfeldt–Jakob disease.
3. **EMG and nerve conduction testing.** Mild nerve conduction slowing suggestive of axonal polyneuropathy occurs in neuroacanthocytosis. EMG findings consistent with myopathy may be present in mitochondrial cytopathy.

E. Neuropsychologic testing.
If there is clinical suspicion of dementia, formal testing should be used to plot the profile of cognitive decline.

F. CSF analysis.
An elevated protein level and pleocytosis can be detected if there is CNS infection. The presence of high levels of 14-3-3 protein in the CSF is highly suggestive of Creutzfeldt–Jakob disease. A large volume of CSF can be removed (Fisher test) with observation for improvement in neurologic signs as one means of corroborating the diagnosis of NPH.

G. Special diagnostic tests

1. **Huntington's disease.** DNA testing is performed to measure CAG triplet expansion. Genetic and psychologic counseling is advised before testing persons at risk who do not have symptoms.
2. **Wilson's disease.** Low ceruloplasmin level, low serum copper level, increased 24-hour urinary copper excretion, and a Kayser–Fleischer ring at slit-lamp

examination of the cornea all suggest Wilson's disease. Liver biopsy for copper content is performed only if the diagnosis is in question.
3. **NPH.** Intracranial pressure monitoring shows episodic appearance of high pressure waves.

VIII. Referrals. Patients with new-onset hypokinesia who have the following characteristics are less likely to have IPD and would benefit from referral to a movement disorders specialist:

Early onset, such as before 50 years of age
Early gait difficulty and postural instability
Prominent dementia
Family history of parkinsonism
Supranuclear gaze palsy
Apraxia, alien limb phenomenon, cortical sensory loss, myoclonus, marked asymmetry of neurologic involvement
Bulbar, cerebellar, or pyramidal dysfunction
Marked dysautonomia
Absent, limited, or unsustained response to levodopa

Recommended Readings

Gilman S, Low PA, Quinn N, et al. Consensus statement on the diagnosis of multiple system atrophy. *J Neurol Sci* 1999;163:94–98.

Jankovic J, Tolosa E, eds. *Parkinson's disease and movement disorders,* 3rd ed. Baltimore: Williams & Wilkins, 1998.

Lang AE, Lozano AM. Parkinson's disease. *N Engl J Med* 1998;339:1044–1053.

Litvan I, Agid Y, Goetz C, et al. Accuracy of the clinical diagnosis of corticobasal degeneration: a clinicopathologic study. *Neurology* 1997;48:119–125.

Litvan I, Grimes DA, Lang AE, et al. Clinical features differentiating patients with postmortem confirmed progressive supranuclear palsy and corticobasal degeneration. *J Neurol* 1999;46[Suppl 2]:II1–II5.

Litvan I, MacIntyre A, Goetz CG, et al. Accuracy of the clinical diagnoses of Lewy body disease, Parkinson disease, and dementia with Lewy bodies: a clinicopathologic study. *Arch Neurol* 1998;55:969–978.

Lucking CB, Durr A, Bonifati V, et al. Association between early-onset Parkinson's disease and mutations in the parkin gene. French Parkinson's Disease Genetics Study Group. *N Engl J Med* 2000;342:1560–1567.

Martin JB. Molecular basis of the neurodegenerative disorders. *N Engl J Med* 1999;340: 1970–1980.

Purdon SE, Mohr E, Ilivitsky V, et al. Huntington's disease: pathogenesis, diagnosis and treatment. *J Psychiatry Neurosci* 1994;19:359–367.

Schrag A Ben-Shlomo Y, Brown R, et al. Young-onset Parkinson's disease revisited: clinical features, natural history, and mortality. *Mov Disord* 1998;13:885–894.

Spillantini MG, Goedert M. Tau protein pathology in neurodegenerative diseases. *Trends Neurosci* 1998;21:428–433.

Yarze JC Martin P, Munoz SJ, et al. Wilson's disease: current status. *Am J Med* 1992;92: 643–654.

30. APPROACH TO THE PATIENT WITH ACUTE MUSCLE WEAKNESS

Rahman Pourmand
Holli A. Horak

Muscular weakness implies lack or diminution of muscle strength, which leads to an inability to perform the usual function of a given muscle or group of muscles. Muscle weakness should be differentiated from fatigue, which is the subjective perception of weakness. In other words, weakness is the objective evidence of lack of strength, and fatigue is a subjective symptom. After the existence of "true" weakness is established, an etiologic search should be conducted. Muscular weakness has diverse causes. This chapter emphasizes the diagnostic evaluation and differential diagnosis of the leading neurologic causes of weakness, particularly as they relate to peripheral nervous system (PNS) involvement.

I. **Evaluation**
   A. **History.** Determination of the onset, course, and distribution of weakness and associated neurologic findings (such as cranial nerve involvement) is important. A history of recent febrile illness, changing of medications, or exposure to toxic agents should be elicited.
   B. **General physical examination.** Examination of the skin is helpful in dermatomyositis or collagen vascular disease, which can manifest as myopathic weakness. Signs of hyperthyroidism can be helpful in examinations of patients with suspected myopathy or myasthenia gravis. Respiratory muscle dysfunction is paramount in the evaluation of any patient with acute muscle weakness.
   C. **Neurologic examination.** Only the neurologic examination dealing primarily with the evaluation of acute muscle weakness resulting from PNS involvement is highlighted.
      1. **Distribution of weakness**
         a. **Proximal symmetric muscle weakness** usually is found among patients with primary muscle disease such as polymyositis or dermatomyositis (PM/DM) or in patients with acute polyradiculoneuropathy, such as the Guillain–Barré syndrome (GBS).
         b. **Proximal asymmetric muscle weakness** occurs among patients with acute brachial plexopathy or acute lumbosacral plexopathy. Acute focal myositis and myasthenia gravis also can manifest as asymmetric limb weakness.
         c. Predominantly **distal asymmetric muscle weakness** occurs in patients with acute mononeuropathy such as foot drop secondary to peroneal nerve palsy or wrist drop resulting from radial nerve palsy. Mononeuritis multiplex (vasculitis of the PNS) manifests as a multifocal asymmetric peripheral weakness. Focal weakness also occurs with anterior horn cell involvement such as acute anterior poliomyelitis.
         d. **Acute diffuse muscle weakness** is found among patients with GBS, myasthenia gravis, periodic paralysis, or tick paralysis.
      2. **Muscle bulk.** Muscle bulk is preserved in many adult neuromuscular diseases. Decreased muscle bulk is commonly present in patients with muscular dystrophy, motor neuron disease (MND), or chronic neuropathy. Muscle bulk usually is normal during the acute stage of polymyositis, myasthenia gravis, MND, or acute polyneuropathy.
      3. **Muscle tone** often is normal in patients with polymyositis or myasthenia gravis. Tone is decreased (flaccid) in MND and GBS.
      4. **Key muscles.** Examination of selected muscles is key for differentiating upper and lower motor neuron weakness. For example, neck flexor and hip flexor muscles are compromised early in myasthenia gravis and polymyositis.
      5. **Sensory features.** Sensory symptoms are common among patients with polyneuropathy or plexopathy. The best examples are GBS and plexopathy, which have sensory manifestations. Findings at sensory examination usually are normal among patients with primary muscle disease or neuromuscular junction disease.

6. Muscle stretch reflexes are normal in patients with neuromuscular junction disease or primary muscle disease and are diminished or absent in patients with GBS, acute polyneuropathy, or acute MND.

II. **Laboratory studies** (Table 30.1)

A. **Blood tests.** If myositis is suspected, measurement of serum creatine kinase, aldolase, erythrocyte sedimentation rate (ESR), lactic acid dehydrogenase, and aspartate aminotransferase are useful. Anti-Jo antibody test results are positive in approximately 30% of cases of polymyositis. The presence of this antibody is a marker of risk for pulmonary involvement. Other autoantibodies associated with inflammatory myopathy are insensitive and not diagnostically useful.

If vasculitis is suspected, measure ESR, serum complement, antinuclear antibodies, antineutrophil cytoplasmic antibodies, and cryoglobulins and evaluate for hepatitis C infection. If myasthenia gravis is suspected, check acetylcholine receptor antibody titers and thyroid function tests.

In conditions such as periodic paralysis, serum potassium and thyroid function tests are critical. Genetic testing for the underlying channelopathy of periodic paralysis is commercially available only for hypokalemic periodic paralysis. This genetic defect involves an L-type Ca^{2+} channel.

Autoantibodies are associated with a variety of peripheral neuropathy syndromes, few of which are associated with acute neuropathy. The importance of most of these antibodies is yet to be defined. One possible exception is anti-GM1 ganglioside antibody seen with GBS. This antibody is associated with considerable axonal involvement and a worse prognosis with long-term disability.

Table 30.1 Diagnostic differentiation among acute polyneuropathy, polymyositis, and myasthenia gravis

Features	Polyradiculo-neuropathy	Polymyositis	Myasthenia gravis
Clinical			
Weakness	Greater distal	Greater proximal	Greater oculobulbar
Fatigability	–	–	+
Wasting	–	–	–
Sensory loss	+	–	–
Muscle stretch reflexes	Decreased or absent	N	N
Fasciculations	–	–	–
Laboratory			
Cerebrospinal fluid protein	Increased	N	N
Needle electromyography			
Fibrillations	+	+	–
Fasciculations	±	–	–
Recruitment	Decreased	Increased or N	N
Slow nerve conduction velocity	+	–	–
Muscle enzymes	N	Increased	N
AChR Ab	N	N	+
Muscle biopsy	N[a]	Necrosis, regeneration, inflammation	N[a]

–, absent; +, present; ±, may or may not be seen; N, normal; AChR Ab, acetylcholine receptor antibody
[a], not necessary for diagnosis.

The anti-GQ1b ganglioside antibody is both sensitive and specific for the Miller Fisher variant of GBS. This variant manifests as ophthalmoparesis, ataxia, and areflexia. Patients with typical GBS with recent gastrointestinal illness may have detectable *Campylobacter jejuni* infection.

   B. Lumbar puncture is indicated in the evaluation patients with suspected GBS, in which cerebrospinal fluid (CSF) may show protein elevation with minimal or absent pleocytosis (albuminocytologic dissociation). In the evaluation of patients with acute poliomyelitis, lumbar puncture may show lymphocytic pleocytosis and protein elevation.

   C. Electrodiagnostic studies. Electromyography (EMG) and nerve conduction studies (NCS) are extremely useful in the evaluation of disorders of motor neurons, peripheral nerves, neuromuscular junctions, and muscles. The yield increases when an history has been obtained and a careful clinical examination has been performed. The value of electrodiagnostic tests is discussed in Chapter 33.

   D. Muscle biopsy. Muscle tissue can be obtained by means of open incision. The site of muscle biopsy should involve a weak but not atrophic muscle. Two-site muscle biopsy occasionally is necessary to increase diagnostic yield. Specimen handling and interpretation of muscle biopsy findings by an experienced pathologist are crucial. Muscle biopsy aids in diagnosis of acute PM/DM and acute vasculitis.

   E. Nerve biopsy is commonly performed on the sural nerve. This procedure should be performed only when the biopsy results will influence management. One of the leading indications for nerve biopsy is the suspicion of vasculitic polyneuropathy, particularly when the manifestation are similar to those of mononeuritis multiplex or overlapping polyneuropathy.

III. Differential diagnosis. A useful approach to evaluation of acute muscle weakness associated with PNS involvement is to localize the site of lesion along the "motor unit," which consists of all the muscle fibers innervated by a single anterior horn cell. This discussion is limited to the most frequent conditions causing acute muscle weakness, particularly those leading to generalized muscle weakness.

   A. Acute anterior horn cell disease. Acute anterior poliomyelitis commonly affects children and often is caused by a group of polioviruses. Most persistent paralytic cases have been caused by type 1 poliovirus. In the United States, oral polio vaccine strains represent a major source of acute paralytic poliomyelitis. It typically follows a prodrome of systemic symptoms such as fever, nausea, vomiting, constipation, muscle pain, and headaches. Muscle weakness develops a few days after the prodromal stage with asymmetric weakness of the lower extremities. Bulbar palsy and respiratory failure may occur. Muscle stretch reflexes are decreased or absent. Some patients describe muscle pain in the acute stage. For confirmation of diagnosis, CSF examination is helpful. EMG findings usually are normal in the acute period.

   B. Acute polyradiculoneuropathy. GBS is acute inflammatory demyelinating polyradiculoneuropathy. It begins with lower-extremity paresthesia followed by ascending symmetric muscle weakness. Proximal muscles are initially involved more often than are their distal counterparts.

   Muscle stretch reflexes are universally absent or diminished. Bifacial peripheral-type weakness is frequent. Labile blood pressure, tachycardia, and other autonomic disturbances may occur as a result of involvement of the autonomic nervous system. Early in the course of the disease, the only EMG abnormality is absence of F waves as a result of proximal root involvement; later, the EMG shows changes consistent with segmental demyelination. CSF examination shows elevation of protein with minimal or no pleocytosis.

   C. Acute plexopathy
      1. Acute idiopathic brachial plexopathy is an uncommon disorder characterized by shoulder pain followed by weakness of shoulder girdle muscles. Pain is a very important part of this syndrome. There are familial and sporadic cases. A history of a preceding febrile illness resulting from viral infection or vaccination is common. Patients usually have good prognoses. The diagnosis is confirmed by clinical presentation and EMG.

2. **Acute lumbosacral plexopathy,** or diabetic amyotrophy or acute femoral neuropathy, is an acute inflammatory lesion of the lumbosacral plexus. Patients have weakness, sensory changes, and severe neuropathic pain, which can be asymmetric, due to unequal involvement of the various roots within the plexus. It occurs most often in the setting of poorly controlled diabetes, but it can be a sign of carcinomatous infiltration or vasculitis and rarely may be idiopathic. Diagnosis is made with clinical examination, EMG, and lumbar puncture. Treatment with a 5-day course of high-dose steroids can reduce the inflammation and decrease the acute pain. Recovery from weakness is prolonged, requiring regeneration and remyelination of axons.

3. **Other acute forms of plexopathy.** Acute plexus lesions can occur in patients who have sustained closed or open trauma to the brachial plexus, as in traction injuries. Neoplasia radiation and orthopedic procedures also can cause plexus damage. Traumatic plexus injuries may follow gunshot wounds, needle punctures, and insertion of intravenous lines.

D. **Acute neuropathy**

1. **GBS.** See III.B.

2. **Lyme disease.** Acute demyelinating polyneuropathy can occur among patients with Lyme disease. Lyme disease often manifests as cranial neuropathy such as peripheral facial palsy and an ascending-type paralysis from the lower extremities, such as in patients with GBS. CSF is abnormal, showing elevation of protein, but unlike the findings in GBS, there is a moderate degree of lymphocytic pleocytosis. NCSs show evidence of demyelination.

3. **Human immunodeficiency virus (HIV) infection.** Acute inflammatory demyelinating polyneuropathy similar to GBS occurs among in patients with HIV infection. CSF pleocytosis is common.

4. **Cytomegalovirus (CMV) radiculitis.** Active CMV infection within the spinal canal, at the level of the nerve roots results in multiple radiculopathy, with sensory loss and weakness in the involved nerve roots. This can manifest as a cauda equina syndrome, with sacral involvement and bowel and bladder dysfunction. CMV radiculitis often occurs in the setting of HIV infection. Active CMV infection should be considered in the evaluation of any immunocompromised patient who has asymmetric, painful, acute lower extremity weakness.

5. **Mononeuritis multiplex.** An asymmetric form of acute generalized sensorimotor polyneuropathy is common among patients with vasculitis. EMG shows evidence of multiple mononeuropathy. The diagnosis is established by clinical presentation, EMG, nerve biopsy, and appropriate laboratory evaluation for vasculitis, including HIV infection and hepatitis C.

6. **Acute motor axonal neuropathy** was first recognized in northern China and was referred to as the *Chinese paralytic syndrome*. This condition has many similarities to GBS. Pathologically, it is an axonopathy without inflammation and demyelination. CSF examination shows few cells but an increasing protein level. Patients have flaccid, symmetric paralysis and areflexia. The clinical course usually is progressive and often causes respiratory failure. EMG shows evidence of normal motor conduction velocity and latency, but the amplitudes of compound muscle action potentials are decreased. Sensory nerve action potentials and F waves are within normal ranges. Rare variants include acute motor and sensory neuropathy, which includes sensory involvement.

7. **Acute intermittent porphyria (AIP).** Weakness usually starts in the proximal upper extremities, but eventually all muscles become involved. Patients may become quadriparetic. Muscle tone is reduced. There is areflexia or hyporeflexia, except for ankle jerks, which may be preserved. Weakness of bulbar muscles is uncommon. Paresthesia and autonomic dysfunction are frequently present. Attacks of AIP usually are associated with abdominal pain and cramping. Confusion or seizures may occur. Attacks of AIP may be precipitated by fasting or by various drugs or infections. During attacks

there are increases in urinary excretion of both δ-aminolevulinic acid and porphobilinogen (PBG), measurement of which should be supplemented with quantitative examination of urinary PBG excretion. The increase in PBG excretion (in milligrams per gram of creatinine) is greater than the increase in aminolevulinic acid excretion. The reverse is true in other forms of porphyria. Between attacks or in the recovery phase, erythrocytes may show a low level of uroporphyrinogen I synthase. NCSs show amplitude reduction of motor and sensory nerve action potentials, with preservation of conduction velocities and F waves. Needle examination shows evidence of denervation consistent with axonal neuropathy. The CSF is usually normal, but protein content may be elevated.

8. **Barium salt toxicity** can produce generalized weakness and areflexia. Muscle stretch reflexes usually are absent. Muscle fasciculations, perioral paresthesia, and dry mouth are common. Testicular pain is characteristic of barium intoxication. Onset of weakness usually is associated with a low serum potassium level.

9. **Acute critical illness neuropathy** often manifests in the intensive care unit as failure to wean from the ventilator. The patient has weakness and atrophy with amplitude loss on EMG and NCSs. Overlap with acute quadriplegic myopathy may be present (see **III.F.5.**).

E. **Acute neuromuscular junction disorders**
1. **Presynaptic disorders.** Only selective disorders are considered. Eaton–Lambert myasthenic syndrome, which has a more insidious presentation, is not discussed.
   a. **Botulism** is caused by ingestion of toxins produced by *Clostridium botulinum*. This disease often manifests as weakness of extraocular muscles followed by dysarthria and limb and respiratory muscle weakness. This diagnosis is suggested by a history of ingestion of contaminated food. Incremental responses are observed with repetitive nerve stimulation at high frequency rates. Results of NCSs are usually normal. Botulism intoxication occurs most often among infants, whose gastrointestinal tract can be colonized by *C. botulinum*.
   b. **Tick paralysis** is a rare disease caused by the female tick *Dermacentor andersoni*. Neurologic symptoms begin with walking difficulty and imbalance followed by ascending flaccid paralysis and areflexia. Ocular and bulbar muscles may be involved. EMG shows reduced amplitude of muscle action potentials and an incremental response to a higher rate of stimulation, particularly during the acute stage. Some degree of slowing of conduction of motor and sensory nerves may be observed. A careful search for a tick in the scalp hair or pubic area is recommended.
   c. **Organophosphate poisoning** causes predominantly proximal lower-extremity muscle weakness. Extraocular and bulbar muscles may show signs of fatigue and weakness. Muscarinic symptoms such as miosis, increased salivation, and generalized fasciculations are often present. EMG findings usually are normal. Repetitive nerve stimulation may elicit incremental responses at higher rates of stimulation.
   d. **Drug-induced myasthenia gravis.** Certain medications adversely affect neuromuscular transmission. Weakness usually involves proximal limb muscles rather than ocular or bulbar muscles. Drug-induced myasthenia gravis may be associated with the use of kanamycin, gentamicin, procainamide, primidone, or hydantoins.
2. **Postsynaptic disorders: myasthenia gravis.** Adult onset of autoimmune acquired myasthenia gravis commonly begins with fluctuating and asymmetric weakness of extraocular and eyelid muscles followed by bulbar and limb weakness. The usual initial features are unilateral or bilateral and include eyelid ptosis followed by dysarthria, dysphagia, proximal limb weakness, and respiratory muscle dysfunction. There is also fatigability induced by repetitive exercise. Muscle tone, bulk, reflexes, and sensory examination are normal. Diagnosis is based on clinical examination, edrophonium (Ten-

silon; ICN Pharmaceuticals, Costa Mesa, CA, U.S.A.) testing, single-fiber EMG, repetitive nerve stimulation, and determination of the presence of serum acetylcholine receptor antibodies.

F. Primary myopathy

1. **PM/DM.** Acute inflammatory myopathy usually begins with proximal symmetric weakness involving the muscles of the shoulder and hip girdle. Muscle tone, bulk, and muscle stretch reflexes are normal. There are no sensory deficits. Polymyositis usually is painless. If a typical skin lesion (erythematous rash in the periorbital, malar, forehead, or chest region, and particularly a scaly erythematous rash over the knuckles and extensor surfaces) exists with weakness, dermatomyositis should be considered. Serum creatine kinase, aldolase, lactic acid dehydrogenase, and aspartate aminotransferase levels often are elevated. ESR usually is high. NCS and amplitude are normal. Needle examination of the muscles shows increased numbers of spontaneous potentials, such as fibrillations, positive sharp waves, bizarre high-frequency discharges, and small, polyphasic, short-duration, low-amplitude voluntary motor unit potentials. Muscle biopsy shows an inflammatory response involving the perimysium and endomysium associated with muscle fiber necrosis and a variable degree of muscle fiber regeneration.

2. **Acute infectious myositis.** Postviral myositis often is associated with myalgia and weakness. In severe cases, there also is generalized weakness. Parasitic infections such as trichinosis and HIV infection can manifest as evidence of proximal muscle weakness.

3. **Acute toxic myopathy.** Acute alcoholic myopathy manifests as generalized symmetric weakness. Hypermagnesemia also produces acute generalized weakness, particularly in alcoholic patients and in patients receiving hyperalimentation with magnesium. Amiodarone and L-tryptophan can cause acute myopathy, and L-tryptophan causes generalized myalgia, weakness, and eosinophilia.

4. **Acute periodic paralysis** is a group of primary muscle diseases associated with a normal potassium (normokalemic), elevated potassium (hyperkalemic), or low potassium (hypokalemic) level. Hyperkalemic periodic paralysis often follows ingestion of a low- or high-carbohydrate diet after vigorous exercise. Hyperkalemic periodic paralysis manifests as generalized weakness with sparing of cranial nerves and respiratory muscles. During attacks, muscle stretch reflexes are absent. The diagnosis is suspected if the patient has a history of intermittent weakness induced by exertion or a high-carbohydrate diet, a family history, and abnormal serum potassium levels during attacks. EMG during an attack may show no abnormalities, but a decrement in motor nerve amplitude may be seen after exercise. Muscle biopsy may show a vacuolar myopathy, particularly if the specimen is obtained during the attack.

5. **Acute steroid quadriplegic myopathy** often occurs among patients treated for status asthmaticus with high-dose steroids and neuromuscular blockade agents. After the status asthmaticus has been brought under control, the patient remains weak and may even become ventilator dependent. EMG shows evidence of neurogenic and myopathic features. Muscle biopsy typically shows loss of myosin filaments at electron microscopic examination.

IV. Diagnostic approach. Diagnosis begins with establishing the presence of weakness and then determining whether the weakness reflects upper or lower motor neuron involvement. After exclusion of upper motor neuron weakness, further localization to the lower motor neuron is needed, as suggested by the algorithm presented in Fig. 30.1. Diagnosis often requires support by laboratory studies. Of these, the most confirmatory and cost-effective test is EMG. Muscle biopsy is recommended for evaluation of PM/DM. Nerve biopsy is indicated mainly in cases of vasculitic neuropathy.

V. Referrals. Patients with acute onset of generalized neuromuscular-type weakness need to be hospitalized, particularly those with acute paralysis or paresis. If respiratory or bulbar muscles are compromised, patients need admission to an intensive care unit. Bedside pulmonary function tests, including forced vital capacity and negative inspiratory force, are

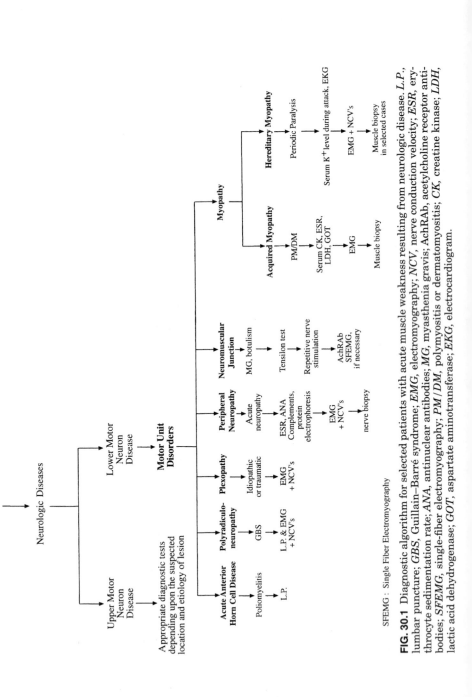

SFEMG : Single Fiber Electromyography

FIG. 30.1 Diagnostic algorithm for selected patients with acute muscle weakness resulting from neurologic disease. *L.P.*, lumbar puncture; *GBS*, Guillain–Barré syndrome; *EMG*, electromyography; *NCV*, nerve conduction velocity; *ESR*, erythrocyte sedimentation rate; *ANA*, antinuclear antibodies; *MG*, myasthenia gravis; *AchRAb*, acetylcholine receptor antibodies; *SFEMG*, single-fiber electromyography; *PM/DM*, polymyositis or dermatomyositis; *CK*, creatine kinase; *LDH*, lactic acid dehydrogenase; *GOT*, aspartate aminotransferase; *EKG*, electrocardiogram.

used to monitor respiratory function. Worsening function over time, especially a forced vital capacity less than 1 L, indicates impending respiratory failure, and intubation should be considered. Neuromuscular diseases with a subacute onset can be diagnosed and managed in the outpatient setting. Many of the therapies for neuromuscular weakness require careful monitoring and follow-up assessment, especially if steroids and immunosuppressive agents are used.

Recommended Readings

Al-Lozi MT, Pestronk A, Yee WC, et al. Rapidly evolving myopathy with myosin-deficient fibers. *Ann Neurol* 1994;35:273–279.

Asbury AK, Cornblath DR. Assessment of current diagnostic criteria for Guillain–Barré syndrome. *Ann Neurol* 1990;27[Suppl]:S21–S24.

Buruma OJS, et al. Periodic paralysis. In: PA Vinken, GW Bruyn, eds. *Handbook of clinical neurology*. Amsterdam: North Holland, 1979:147–174.

Dalakas MC, et al. The postpolio syndrome. In: Plum F, ed. *Advances in contemporary neurology*. Philadelphia: FA Davis Co, 1988:51–94.

DeVere R, Bradley WG. Polymyositis: its presentations, morbidity and mortality. *Brain* 1975; 98:637–666.

Flanagan KM. Genetic testing in the neuromuscular clinic. *J Neuromusc Dis* 2000;1:205–213.

Gould DB, Sorrell MR, Lupariello AD, et al. Barium sulfide poisoning. *Arch Intern Med* 1973; 132:891–894.

Hirano M, Ott BR, Raps EC, et al. Acute quadriplegic myopathy: a complication of treatment with steroids, nondepolarizing blocking agents or both. *Neurology* 1992;42:2082–2087.

Hudgson P. Polymyositis and dermatomyositis in adults. *Clin Rheum Dis* 1984;10:85–93.

Hughes JM, Blumenthal JR, Merson MH, et al. Clinical features of type A and B food-borne botulism. *Ann Intern Med* 1981;95:442–445.

Kaminski HJ, et al. Autoantibody testing in neuromuscular disorders, II: neuromuscular junction, hyperexcitability, and muscle disorders. *J Clin Neuromuscul Disord* 2000;2:96–105.

Kissel JT. The use and misuse of autoantibodies in peripheral neuropathy evaluations. *Semin Neurol* 1998;18: 83–94.

Kissel JT, et al. The spectrum of peripheral neuropathies with necrotizing angiopathy. *Ann Neurol* 1983;14:122–123.

Leger JM, Bouche P, Bolgert F, et al. The spectrum of polyneuropathies in patients infected with HIV. *J Neurol Neurosurg Psychiatry* 1989;52:1369–1374.

Oh SJ, Kim DE, Kuruoglu R, et al. Diagnostic sensitivity of the laboratory tests in myasthenia gravis. *Muscle Nerve* 1992;15:720–724.

Oosterhuis HJGH. Diagnosis and differential diagnosis. In: DeBaets H, Oosterhuis NJGH, eds. *Myasthenia gravis*. Boca Raton, FL: CRC, 1993:203–234.

Parry GJ. Peripheral neuropathies associated with human immunodeficiency virus infection. *Ann Neurol* 1988;23[Suppl]:S49–S53.

Pearn J. Neuromuscular paralysis caused by tick envenomation. *J Neurol Sci* 1977;34:37–42.

Reik RJ. Peripheral neuropathy in Lyme disease. In: Dyck PJ, Thomas PK, eds. *Peripheral neuropathy*. Philadelphia: WB Saunders, 1993:1481–1511.

Ridley A. The neuropathy of acute intermittent porphyria. *Q J Med* 1969;38:307–333.

Ropper AH, et al. Clinical features of the typical syndrome. In Ropper AH, Wijdicks EFM, Truax B, eds. *Guillain–Barré syndrome*. Philadelphia: FA Davis Co, 1991:73–105.

Senanayake N, Karalliedde L. Neurotoxic effects of organophosphorous insecticides: an intermediate syndrome. *N Engl J Med* 1987;316:761–763.

Shankle R, Keane JR. Acute paralysis from inhaled barium carbonate. *Arch Neurol* 1988;145: 579–588.

Swift TR, Ignacio OJ. Tick paralysis: electrophysiological studies. *Neurology* 1975;25: 1130–1133.

Wadia RS, Sadagopan C, Amin RB, et al. Neurological manifestations of organophosphorous insecticide poisoning. *J Neurol Neurosurg Psychiatry* 1974;37:841–847.

Windebank AJ. Mental neuropathy. In: Dyck PJ, Thomas PK, eds. *Peripheral neuropathy*. Philadelphia: WB Saunders, 1993:1549–1570.

Wolfe GI, Kaminski HJ. Autoantibody testing in neuromuscular disorders, 1: peripheral neuropathies. *J Clin Neuromuscul Disord* 2000;2:85–95.

31. APPROACH TO THE PATIENT WITH BLADDER, BOWEL, OR SEXUAL DYSFUNCTION AND OTHER AUTONOMIC DISORDERS

Bhuwan P. Garg

I. **Urinary incontinence**
   A. **Introduction.** A wide range of neurologic diseases are associated with urinary bladder dysfunction. Common conditions are stroke, dementia, Parkinson's disease, multiple sclerosis, diabetes mellitus, and other forms of neuropathy with autonomic involvement. Knowledge of normal bladder function is essential in understanding the pathology of the urinary bladder in neurologic disorders.
   B. **Anatomy and nerve supply**
      1. The urinary bladder is a hollow viscus with the primary function of urine storage with periodic evacuation. Micturition, an intricate and well-coordinated activity, is primarily a parasympathetic function. The sympathetic nervous system is involved in urine storage and bladder capacity. Volitional control over micturition is exerted through the corticospinal pathways and spinal nerves innervating the external sphincter, periurethral muscles, and other abdominal and pelvic muscles. Cerebral cortex, basal ganglia, cerebellum, and brainstem pontine detrusor nuclei exert suprasegmental influence over the sacral spinal nuclei involved in urinary bladder innervation by means of the peripheral nerves.
      2. The various neuroanatomic connections that are important in urinary bladder control have been termed *circuits* (or *loops*) by Bradley.
         a. The **first circuit** connects the dorsomedial frontal lobe to the pontine detrusor nucleus with additional connections to the basal ganglia and provides the volitional control over micturition.
         b. The **second circuit** (the spinobulbospinal pathway) is a reflex arc that starts in the sensory nerves of the urinary bladder and projects to the pontine detrusor nucleus and its outflow connections to the spinal sacral motor nuclei that make up the detrusor motor axons. This circuit constitutes the **parasympathetic innervation.**
         c. The **third circuit** is a spinal segmental reflex arc consisting of afferent nerve fibers from the detrusor muscle that synapse with the cells in the pudendal nucleus and its efferent nerve fibers to the striated sphincter muscles.
         d. The **fourth circuit** has a supraspinal component consisting of afferent fibers running in the dorsal nerve of the penis and the posterior columns to the cerebral cortex and efferent fibers by means of the corticospinal tracts to the sacral motoneurons. The spinal segment of this circuit is the sensory input from the external urethral sphincter and perhaps from muscle spindles in the other striated muscles of the periurethral area. The efferent arc of this circuit is formed by the axons of the α and γ motoneurons in the sacral spinal cord that travel in the pudendal nerve and innervate the external urinary sphincter.
      3. Circuit 2 exerts brainstem control over micturition, whereas circuits 1 and 4 provide the voluntary control. The sympathetic motor nerve supply to the bladder is carried by the hypogastric nerves; the cell bodies are situated in the intermediolateral column of the spinal cord extending from T11 to L2.
   C. **Clinical evaluation**
      1. **History.** A careful and detailed history is essential (Table 31.1). The patient should be questioned regarding urinary incontinence, pattern of incontinence if present, changes in urinary habits, and frequency and urgency of urination. Desire to void, ability to initiate and terminate urination, force of urinary stream and urine volume, and sensations associated with urination are important aspects of the history. In spinal cord lesions, the level of lesion determines the symptoms and signs. Particular attention must also be paid to the drugs that the patient may be taking.

Table 31.1 Factors in history-taking for bladder, bowel, and sexual dysfunction

Bladder Dysfunction
Onset
  Acute, remittent, or progressive
Voiding
  Frequency: day and night
  Stream: slow, interrupted, or normal
  Initiation: voluntary or involuntary
  Termination: dribbling, abrupt, or normal
  Ability to stop on command
  Volume of urine passed
  Associated symptoms, e.g., headache, sweating
Sensation
  Sensation of bladder fullness
  Urge to void
  Passage of urine in urethra
  Effect of posture, cough, strain, etc.

Bowel Dysfunction
Continence or incontinence
Stool consistency
Constipation
Sensation of urge to void
Ability to discriminate between stool and flatus
Urgency, ability to hold
Drug use, e.g., laxatives, antacids

Sexual Dysfunction
Libido: normal or reduced
Erection: present or absent, duration, spontaneous, nocturnal, psychogenic
Ejaculation: normal, absent, or premature

Drug histories should be obtained for all patients.

    2. Examination. Neurologic examination indicates the nature, site, and extent of the neuroanatomic lesion. The examination also may make it evident how much the patient can participate in his or her own care, such as in cases of dementia and Parkinson's disease. In frontal lobe lesions and suprasegmental spinal cord lesions, there are increased frequency and urgency of urination with reduced bladder capacity. Bladder sensation may be preserved in incomplete spinal cord lesions. This condition is called *neurogenic bladder*. Table 31.2 presents clinical features of lower spinal cord lesions. In cauda equina lesions, if the motor nerves are preferentially involved, volitional voiding may be severely compromised even though bladder sensation may be largely preserved. This condition is called *motor paralytic bladder.*
  D. Laboratory evaluation. Laboratory studies are selected to clarify the nature of the bladder dysfunction and to detect any other associated abnormalities, such as renal dysfunction. Magnetic resonance imaging (MRI) of the spine, and sometimes of the brain if indicated, is essential in the evaluation for neurogenic urinary incontinence. Bladder neck obstruction must be excluded, especially in the motor paralytic type of bladder dysfunction. Consultation with a urologist is desirable in the evaluation and management of bladder dysfunction.
    1. Urine studies. Urinalysis and urine culture with appropriate sensitivity studies should be done. Many patients with neurourologic dysfunction have associated urinary tract infection, which should be managed adequately and promptly with appropriate antibiotics.

Table 31.2 Features of lower spinal cord lesions

Feature	Conus medullaris	Cauda equina
Location	S3–Cocc 1	L3–Cocc 1 roots
Onset	Often sudden and bilateral	Usually gradual and unilateral
Motor	Mild dysfunction; fasciculations may be present	Marked dysfunction; fasciculations are rare
Sensory	Symmetric, bilateral saddle-type distribution; mild pain if present	Asymmetric, unilateral saddle-type distribution; radicular pain may be present
Reflexes	Variable loss of Achilles tendon reflexes	Variable loss of patellar and Achilles tendon reflexes
Bladder	Paralytic, atonic bladder with increased capacity, incontinence	Paralytic, atonic bladder with increased capacity, incontinence, variable severity
Rectum	Patulous anus; decreased sphincter tone	Patulous anus; decreased sphincter tone; variable severity

2. **Renal function studies**
   a. Blood urea nitrogen, creatinine, creatinine clearance, glomerular filtration rate, and other renal function studies should be performed as indicated to detect initial and subsequent impairment.
   b. **Intravenous pyelography** is a useful study in the initial and follow-up evaluation of patients with neurogenic bladder dysfunction.
3. **Urodynamic investigations**
   a. **Cystometry** is an investigation of prime importance in the evaluation of patients who have incontinence and voiding difficulties resulting from neurologic causes. Cystometry provides information about the pressure–volume relation on filling (bladder compliance), bladder capacity, volume at first sensation and at urge to void, voiding pressure, and the presence of uninhibited detrusor contractions. A normal adult bladder can usually be filled with 500 mL of fluid without the pressure increasing to more than 10 cm of water. Urodynamic findings in various types of neurogenic bladder dysfunctions are listed in Table 31.3.
   b. **Micturating cystourethrography** often if combined with cystometry. Sphincter dyssynergia, position and opening of the bladder neck, and urethral anomaly and stricture as well as ureteric reflux can be visualized.
   c. **Cystourethroscopy** is used to assess the structural integrity of the lower urinary system, which consists of the urethra, bladder, and ureteral orifices. It is not used to examine the bladder during the voiding state and is not useful for diagnosis of functional disorders.
   d. **Retrograde urethrography** is used as a supplement to cystourethrography for delineation of urethral strictures, valves, diverticula, and false passages.

Table 31.3 Urodynamic findings in various types of neurogenic bladder dysfunction

Spastic bladder	Atonic bladder	Sphincter dyssynergia
Decreased capacity	Increased capacity	Fluctuating voiding pressure
Reduced compliance	Increased compliance	Intermittent flow rate
Uninhibited detrusor contractions	Low voiding pressure and flow rate	

4. Neurophysiologic studies. Sphincter and pelvic floor electromyography (EMG) is a specialized technique useful when performed by experienced examiners in detecting denervation potentials in selected muscles in lesions of the anterior horn cells in the spinal cord. Increased terminal latency on pudendal nerve stimulation can be observed in neuropathic causes of incontinence. Results of pudendal nerve conduction velocity studies may be abnormal in neuropathic causes. It is technically difficult to record from the urethral sphincter (mainly S3 innervation), and hence the anal sphincter (mainly S4 innervation) often is used instead.

E. Management of urinary incontinence

1. Incontinence with urgency

a. Patients with urinary incontinence with urgency usually have upper motor neuron signs at neurologic examination. Table 31.4 lists some causes of this type of incontinence. Frequency of micturition often is present in these patients, and bladder capacity usually is reduced. The nonneurologic cause of urgency usually is cystitis secondary to infection or inflammation with another cause. Cystitis may be present in patients with neurogenic incontinence, and urinalysis and urine culture should be performed when appropriate.

b. Methods used in management

(1) Bladder training. Timed bladder emptying, intermittent catheterization, and biofeedback techniques are used.

(2) Pharmacotherapy. Many classes of drugs are useful. Such drugs include anticholinergics, musculotropics, calcium antagonists, β-adrenergic agonists, and tricyclic antidepressants. Table 31.5 provides the dosages.

(3) Surgical methods. Dorsal root rhizotomy, selective sacral root rhizotomy, peripheral bladder denervation, and cystoplasty to increase bladder capacity all have been used. Residual urine volumes should be checked for all patients, because large residuals predispose to further complications.

2. Atonic bladder with overflow incontinence occurs in cases of spinal shock, conus medullaris and cauda equina lesions, and neuropathy of various types (Table 31.6). It also occurs in the course of some progressive neurologic diseases, such as multiple system atrophy (MSA). Bladder capacity increases. The goal of therapy is to improve bladder tonus and to reduce bladder capacity. The following methods are used.

a. Credé's maneuver or a Valsalva maneuver can be used to empty the bladder.

b. Intermittent self-catheterization is perhaps the mainstay of long-term treatment. Aseptic technique is taught to the patient to prevent infection.

c. Pharmacotherapy usually is not an effective treatment modality. Drugs such as bethanecol in a dosage range of 25 to 100 mg four times a day can be used, but often there are unacceptable side effects.

3. Detrusor sphincter dyssynergia is a condition in which the external urethral sphincter fails to relax when there is constriction of the detrusor

Table 31.4 Selected neurologic causes of urinary incontinence with urgency

Alzheimer's disease	Cervical spondylosis
Parkinson's disease	Spinal cord tumor
Other diseases with dementia	Spinal cord injury
Myxedema	Spinal cord compression
Hydrocephalus	Syphilis
Bilateral frontal lobe lesions	Sacral agenesis
Parasagittal tumors	Tethered cord syndromes
Multiple sclerosis	Myelomeningocele
Transverse myelitis	

Table 31.5 Drugs used to manage neurogenic bladder dysfunction

Class of drug	Drug name	Dosage
Anticholinergics	Propantheline bromide	15–30 mg every 4–6 h
	Glycopyrrolate	1.0 mg two or three times a day
Musculotropics	Oxybutynin	5 mg three or four times a day
	Flavoxate	100–200 mg three or four times a day
	Dicyclomine	20 mg three times a day
Calcium antagonists	Terodiline	12.5 mg two or three times a day
β-Adrenergic agonists	Terbutaline	5.0 mg three times a day
Tricyclic antidepressants	Imipramine	25 mg three or four times a day

muscles during voiding. This failure can be intermittent and incomplete or occur after a delay. There is often increased residual urine volume with low flow and an intermittent pattern of voiding (Table 31.3). Urodynamic studies such as cystometry are useful in the diagnosis.

   II. Fecal incontinence. The anatomy of the rectum, the anus, and the anal sphincters and the associated neuromuscular reflex mechanisms are important in maintaining fecal continence.

   A. Nerve supply. The innervation of the rectum parallels that of the urinary bladder. The external anal sphincter is innervated from sacral segments S2 to S4 by the pudendal nerves. The internal anal sphincter receives its innervation from the sympathetic system by means of the hypogastric plexus, the nerve cell bodies being situated at the L1–2 level. Somatic sensations of light touch, pain, and temperature reach the sacral cord through the pudendal nerves. In general, the parasympathetic system controls bowel emptying whereas the sympathetic system modulates rectal filling.

   B. Clinical evaluation

   1. History. A careful history is essential and should include an inquiry into the circumstances at the onset, alterations in bowel habits, and stool frequency, consistency, and mass (Table 31.1). The patient should be questioned to establish whether there is preservation of rectal sensation as manifested by the ability to feel the pressure of fecal volume and the need to defecate, whether there is ability to differentiate the passage of flatus and the passage of feces, whether the patient can voluntarily inhibit defecation, and whether there is urgency.

   2. Examination. The neurologic examination indicates the site and extent of the lesion responsible for bowel incontinence, as in the case of urinary incontinence. In upper motor neuron lesions rostral to the sacral cord, there is fecal retention, loss of voluntary control, increased anal sphincter tone, and inability to relax or contract the sphincter on command. Lesions of the sacral cord, conus medullaris, or cauda equina result in a weak and areflexic anal

Table 31.6 Selected causes of atonic bladder

Acute spinal shock	Guillain–Barré syndrome
Acute transverse myelitis	Amyloid neuropathy
Conus medullaris lesions	Tabes dorsalis
Cauda equina lesions	Multiple system atrophy
Peripheral neuropathy	Friedreich's ataxia
Diabetes mellitus	Pelvic radiation
Alcoholic neuropathy	Acute intoxication (e.g., alcohol)
Heavy metal toxicity	Plexopathy

sphincter with a patulous anus. There may also be associated sensory loss. The extent of the sensory deficit and its recovery is important in determining bowel control.

C. Laboratory evaluation. The laboratory studies used in the investigation of fecal incontinence are limited.

   1. Endoscopic studies. Proctoscopy and other endoscopic studies, as indicated, demonstrate structural abnormalities.

   2. Radiologic studies

      a. MRI of the spine is essential in spinal cord lesions.

      b. Pelvic computed tomography may be indicated for some patients with malformations and other structural abnormalities.

      c. Barium enema radiographic examination is helpful in demonstrating obstruction and some structural abnormalities.

   3. Neurophysiologic studies. Anal sphincter and puborectalis muscle EMG and pudendal nerve conduction studies, as discussed in **I.D.4.**, may provide discriminative evidence of the type of neurologic disorder (Table 31.2).

D. Management of fecal incontinence. First, overflow incontinence as a result of fecal impaction must be excluded. The history should have excluded overuse of laxatives or other medications such as magnesium-containing antacids as a cause of incontinence that responds to cessation of the offending medication. Rectal prolapse, if present, should be managed. Table 31.7 lists some diagnostic considerations.

   1. Dietary management. The goal is to increase the volume of the colonic contents and maintain them at near-normal consistency.

      a. Diet high in fiber content

      b. Docusate sodium to prevent stool hardening

      c. Psyllium types of dietary fiber to decrease stool viscosity and increase volume

   2. Techniques for achieving orderly defecation

      a. A Valsalva maneuver and abdominal pressure work for some patients who have preservation of some rectal sensation and feel the urge to defecate.

      b. Glycerine suppositories and digital stimulation of the rectum with a gloved finger work for some patients. These methods are most effective with the patient in the sitting position.

      c. Neural stimulators. Anterior sacral root stimulators are under investigation.

Table 31.7 Selected causes of fecal incontinence

Structural	Frontal lobe lesions including tumors
Rectal prolapse	Alzheimer's disease
Carcinoma of the anal canal	Lower motor lesions
Carcinoma of the lower rectum	Myelodysplasia
Pelvic fracture	Meningomyelocele
Trauma to the anal sphincter	Cauda equina tumors
Obstetric injury to the anal sphincter	Conus medullaris tumors and compression
Aftermath of anorectal surgery	Sacrococcygeal teratoma, lipoma, and other
Imperforate anus	tumors
Caudal regression syndrome	Neuropathy and reduced rectal sensation
Sacral agenesis	
	Fecal Impaction
Neurogenic	Chronic constipation
Upper motor neuron lesions	Delayed colonic mobility
Multiple sclerosis	Severe decreased muscle tone
Transverse myelitis	Prolonged immobility
Spinal cord injury	Dementia
Spinal cord tumor, compression	

   d. Surgical intervention. Formation of a replacement sphincter and pelvic floor reconstruction may be considered in suitable cases.

   3. Biofeedback. EMG feedback training has been effective for some patients with fecal incontinence.

III. Sexual dysfunction

   A. The sexual response cycle of excitement, plateau, orgasm, and resolution is mediated through the integrated and coordinated activity of the somatic and autonomic nervous systems innervating the reproductive system. Sexual dysfunction of men is better understood than that of women.

   Male sexual dysfunction can manifest as diminished libido, impaired penile erection, or failure to ejaculate. Psychogenic causes of sexual dysfunction are common and may be the primary cause. Patients with organic sexual dysfunction often have secondary psychogenic factors. Depression and anxiety are the most common psychological causes of sexual dysfunction, whereas chronic ill health is probably the most common cause of organic sexual dysfunction. Organic causes of sexual dysfunction include vascular, endocrine, and neurologic abnormalities. Neurologic causes involve impairment of the somatic, sympathetic, and parasympathetic nervous systems.

   B. Anatomy of and nerve supply to the sexual organs

   1. Somatic motor and sensory nerve supply. The pudendal nerve carries both the motor and sensory fibers that innervate the penis and clitoris. Motor nerve fibers that reach the pudendal nerve by way of the sacral plexus arise from cells in the medial part of the nucleus of Onufrowicz (Onuf's nucleus) situated at the sacral S2–4 level. The sensory fibers also reach the same sacral levels. There are three branches of the pudendal nerve. The first branch, the inferior rectal nerve, innervates the external anal sphincter. The second branch, the perineal nerve, supplies the external urethral sphincter, the bulbocavernosus and ischiocavernosus muscles and other muscles of the perineum, as well as the skin of the perineum and scrotum in men and the labia in women. The third branch is the dorsal (sensory) nerve of the penis or clitoris.

   2. Parasympathetic nerve supply. The parasympathetic nerves have their cell bodies in the sacral cord. The preganglionic fibers exit and travel with sacral ventral roots S2–4 in the cauda equina and form the pelvic nerves that join the inferior hypogastric or pelvic plexus. The postganglionic fibers from this plexus innervate the erectile penile and clitoral tissues, the smooth muscles in the urethra, and the seminal vesicles and prostate in men and vagina and uterus in women. They also innervate the blood vessels in the pelvic structures involved in sexual function.

   3. Sympathetic nerve supply. The sympathetic nerves arise from cells in the intermediolateral cell column in the lower thoracic and upper lumbar spinal cord. The preganglionic fibers leave the cord at the T11–12 level with the ventral nerve roots and enter the sympathetic chain and the inferior mesenteric and superior hypogastric plexus. The postganglionic fibers travel in the hypogastric nerves and innervate the same structures as do the parasympathetic nerves.

   C. Clinical evaluation

   1. History. Tables 31.8 and 31.9 list various causes of diminished libido and erectile impotence. The history should be directed at eliciting the appropriate information. Particular attention should be paid to the history of medication use, alcohol intake, symptoms of leg claudication, and psychological symptoms.

   2. Examination can disclose evidence of liver dysfunction, testicular atrophy and hypogonadism, or vascular insufficiency. Neurologic examination can provide evidence of cerebral, spinal cord, or peripheral nerve dysfunction.

   D. Laboratory evaluation of sexual dysfunction is an adjunct to clinical evaluation and is used to confirm a precise cause and formulate a course of treatment.

   1. Endocrine evaluation. Fasting blood sugar and a glucose tolerance test if necessary, liver function tests, and appropriate endocrine tests such as thyroid function and prolactin level tests may help establish the diagnosis. Consultation with an endocrinologist should be sought if necessary.

Table 31.8 Causes of diminished libido

Chronic ill health	Drugs (continued)
Addison's disease	Cimetidine
Hypothyroidism	Tricyclic antidepressants
Hypogonadism	Monoamine oxidase inhibitors
Excessive estrogen in men	Sedatives and narcotics
Chronic hepatic disease	Alcohol
Drugs	Depression
Reserpine	Anxiety
Propranolol	

Drug history is important, and any medicine the patient is taking should be excluded as a cause.

2. **Neurophysiologic tests.** Specialized sleep studies, EMG (especially in suspected cases of MSA), and somatosensory evoked potentials in some cases of myelopathy can be useful to selected patients.
3. **Vascular studies**
   a. Low-dosage injection of vasoactive agents such as papaverine into the corpora cavernosa of the penis can help differentiate vascular from other causes. The response to injection of a vasoactive agent is poor in erectile impotence resulting from vascular causes.
   b. Arteriography of the major leg and pelvic vessels sometimes is indicated.
4. **Psychiatric evaluation.** Psychiatric consultation should be obtained in appropriate cases.
E. **Management of sexual dysfunction.** Endocrine, metabolic, vascular, and psychogenic causes can must be managed when present. When drugs are the etiologic factor, changes in medication may be beneficial. Other specialized treatment modalities consist of cavernosal unstriated muscle relaxant injection, penile implants, sacral root stimulation, pharmacologic treatment, and use of a vibrator. Sildenafil can be effective in the care of appropriately selected patients with erectile dysfunction. Consultation should be obtained from physicians familiar with these techniques.
IV. **Generalized autonomic failure**
A. Primary autonomic failure occurs in two neurodegenerative conditions of unknown causation. These are pure autonomic failure and MSA. Autonomic failure also develops in some patients with Parkinson's disease. Patients with Parkinson's disease usually have motor dysfunction. Either autonomic or motor dysfunction can be the initial symptom among patients with MSA. α-Synuclein accumulates in all three conditions in the neuronal cytoplasmic inclusions. The relation of these three conditions to one another, if any, is yet to be elucidated.

Table 31.9 Causes of erectile impotence

Conus medullaris lesion	Hyperprolactinemia
Cauda equina lesion	Antihypertensive medications
Spinal cord injury	Anticholinergic medications
Myelopathy	Antipsychotic medications
Multiple sclerosis	Antihistamines
Peripheral neuropathy	Alcohol
Diabetes mellitus	Syphilis
Amyloid neuropathy	Arteriosclerosis
Vitamin B_{12} deficiency	Excessive venous leakage (venous leakers)
Sacral plexus lesion	Depression
Multiple system atrophy	Anxiety
Pure autonomic failure	

Drug history is important, and any medicine the patient is taking should be excluded as a cause.

1. **MSA,** initially described by Shy and Drager, is characterized by autonomic failure and motor abnormalities. It is often confused with Parkinson's disease, from which it must be differentiated. The onset of symptoms occurs in the fifth to seventh decades of life. The condition may be more common than is usually recognized, with an estimated prevalence of 5 to 15 cases per 100,000 persons.

2. **Pure autonomic failure** is a clinical condition in which there is autonomic failure without other associated neurologic or motor abnormalities except for bladder and sexual dysfunction in some patients.

B. **Clinical evaluation**

1. **Autonomic failure.** Patients have orthostatic hypotension, urinary and rectal incontinence, loss of sweating, iris atrophy, and impotence. There is usually an atonic bladder and decreased rectal sphincter tone. Pupils may show alternating anisocoria. In men, sexual dysfunction is an early sign, first with failure of erection followed later by failure of ejaculation. MSA should be considered in the evaluation of patients with impotence who also have signs and symptoms of bladder and bowel dysfunction. Sympathetic cardiac innervation is selectively affected in pure autonomic failure and Parkinson's disease and not in MSA.

C. **Motor abnormalities** can be categorized into the following three types.

1. **Striatonigral degeneration.** Clinical features may superficially resemble those of Parkinson's disease. However, patients with MSA have a predominance of rigidity without much tremor. There is limb akinesia and rigidity without the classic cogwheel or lead pipe type of phenomenon that is common in Parkinson's disease. Patients have difficulty standing, walking, and turning. Gait is slow and clumsy. There is progressive loss of facial expression with associated slurred speech, which is faint. Salivation is reduced. Patients have stooping posture with excessive cervical flexion, which makes forward gaze difficult.

2. **Pyramidal and peripheral motor abnormalities.** Spastic muscle tone can be difficult to detect in the presence of other extrapyramidal signs. Muscle stretch reflexes are increased, and primitive reflexes such as palmomental reflexes may be present. Conjugate extraocular movements may be restricted. Muscle atrophy of a mild nature, especially in the distal muscles, can be associated with fasciculations. Results of EMG suggest involvement of the anterior horn cells.

3. **Cerebellar dysfunction** is characterized by prominent truncal ataxia and gait disturbance that make it difficult for the patient to stand. Action tremor of mild to moderate intensity is present. Speech is markedly slurred and has a cerebellar quality. The cerebellar deficit resembles that seen in olivopontocerebellar atrophy, although associated optic atrophy, retinitis pigmentosa, chorea, or cataracts are not present.

D. **Laboratory evaluation**

1. **Orthostatic hypotension.** Demonstration of orthostatic hypotension is crucial to the diagnosis of MSA. Blood pressure is measured in the supine and upright positions. A decrease in systolic blood pressure of 20 mm Hg or more or a decrease in diastolic pressure of 10 mm Hg or more in response to upright posture is abnormal. This decrease in blood pressure occurs within 3 minutes of standing; rarely it may not occur until after 10 minutes of standing. The patient may report weakness, dizziness, or faintness or may have a syncopal episode.

2. **Pharmacologic tests.** There is failure of the increase in plasma norepinephrine levels as a result of head-up tilt. Plasma norepinephrine concentration in the supine position is normal in patients with MSA (because postganglionic neurons are normal) and low in patients with pure autonomic failure. Clonidine-induced growth hormone response is blunted in patients with MSA but not in pure autonomic failure and Parkinson's disease.

3. **EMG** may show signs of denervation in limb muscles, suggesting involvement of the anterior horn cells in MSA.

4. MRI. Decreased signal intensity may be observed in the posterolateral aspect of the putamen on T2-weighted images only in patients with MSA and not in pure autonomic failure or Parkinson's disease. Cerebellar atrophy may be present in some patients even without clinical cerebellar signs.

5. Bladder, bowel, and sexual dysfunction. Evaluation and management of these abnormalities are as described in **I.** through **III.**

E. Management. Only symptomatic treatment is available. Rigidity, bradykinesia, and motor symptoms usually do not respond to levodopa, although it may be worth a try. Side effects, especially accentuation of hypotension, must be kept in mind.

1. Orthostatic hypotension

  a. Nighttime measures

    (1) Posture. Elevation of the head of the bed 6 to 12 inches (15 to 30 cm) at night often is helpful. Patients tolerate this rather uncomfortable position once they experience the benefits. Sitting on the edge of the bed for a short time after awakening in the morning also can minimize symptoms.

    (2) Desmopressin is given at night as either a nasal spray or an intramuscular injection. A single dose of 5 to 40 mg often is sufficient to prevent nocturia and morning postural hypotension. It is best to start treatment in the hospital under close supervision to establish an appropriate dosage that does not cause side effects. Plasma sodium concentration and osmolality should be monitored on a regular, outpatient basis.

  b. Daytime measures

    (1) Fludrocortisone in oral doses of 0.1 to 0.4 mg/d with adequate hydration and dietary intake of at least 150 mEq of sodium often is helpful. Small, frequent meals prevent postprandial aggravation of orthostatic hypotension.

    (2) Midodrine in a dose of 5 to 10 mg up to four times a day may benefit some patients who have responded poorly to fludrocortisone.

    (3) Ephedrine or **phenylpropanolamine** in a dosage of 12.5 to 75 mg three times a day as tolerated may be effective for some patients and is worth trying. Some patients may tolerate 5 to 10 mg three times a day of methylphenidate, although it may disturb sleep if the last dose of the day is given late in the evening.

    (4) Elastic support garments have long been used to manage orthostatic hypotension, and some patients find them beneficial. They rarely are of much long-term benefit.

    (5) Mild exercise can help by maintaining and improving muscle tone and thereby facilitating venous return.

    (6) Bladder, bowel, and sexual dysfunction is managed as outlined in secs. **I** through **III.**

V. Acute autonomic dysfunction

A. Autonomic crises. Acute autonomic dysfunction occurs in many conditions and a hypersympathetic state is most often encountered. Examples of such neurologic conditions are as follows.

1. Cerebral lesions: ischemic stroke, cerebral hemorrhage, subarachnoid hemorrhage, Cushing response, intracranial mass lesion

2. Spinal cord lesions

3. Peripheral nerve disease: Guillain–Barré syndrome

4. Systemic diseases: tetanus, acute episode of porphyria

5. Drug-related conditions: neuroleptic malignant syndrome, sympathomimetic drug overdose, tricyclic antidepressant overdose

B. Autonomic dysreflexia is a sympathetic storm that occurs in cases of spinal cord transection. The spinal cord lesion usually is above the midthoracic level. The episodes are paroxysmal and start several months after the acute spinal cord injury as recovery occurs. The episodes are characterized by sudden onset of severe hypertension, headache, sweating and flushing, piloerection, and sometimes chills. A precipitating cause can most often be identified and is a noxious stimulus. Urinary bladder distention and fecal impaction are common causes. Elimination of the precipitating cause often results in resolution of the episode. Prevention is the best therapy. Drugs such as propantheline or oxybutynin, both of which have anticholinergic effects, sometimes can be used.

VI. Indications for referral
    A. Referral to a specialist should be considered when bladder or bowel dysfunction is associated with numbness, tingling, pain, or weakness or when the findings at neurologic examination are abnormal. For example, a 5-year-old boy with enuresis and normal neurologic findings may not need neurologic consultation, but if this patient also reports back pain and has abnormal neurologic findings, referral is appropriate.
    B. Patients with autonomic dysfunction associated with abnormal findings at neurologic examination need evaluation by a neurologist.
    C. Patients with bladder, bowel, or sexual dysfunction who have progressive neurologic dysfunction or do not respond to treatment need referral to a specialist.
    D. Patients with preexisting neurologic disease who have new bladder, bowel, or autonomic dysfunction need evaluation or reevaluation by a neurologist.
    E. Patients with bladder, bowel, or sexual dysfunction after trauma need evaluation by a specialist.

Recommended Readings

Banwell JG, Creasey GH, Aggarwal AM, et al. Management of the neurogenic bowel in patients with spinal cord injury. *Urol Clin North Am* 1993;20:517–526.

Benarroch EE. Neurogenic orthostatic hypotension. In: Johnson RT, Griffin JW, eds. *Current therapy in neurologic disease,* 5th ed. St. Louis: Mosby, 1997.

Betts CD, Jones SJ, Fowler CG, et al. Erectile dysfunction in multiple sclerosis: associated neurological and neurophysiologic deficits, and treatment of the condition. *Brain* 1994;117:1303–1310.

Campbell MF, Retik AB, Darraco Vaughn E, et al, eds. *Campbell's urology,* 7th ed. Philadelphia: WB Saunders, 1997.

Fowler CJ. Neuro-urology. In: WG Bradley, Daroff RB, Fenichel GM, et al, eds. *Neurology in clinical practice: principles of diagnosis and management,* 2nd ed. Boston: Butterworth–Heinemann, 1996:659–672.

Fowler CJ. Electrophysiologic evaluation of sexual dysfunction. In: PA Low, ed. *Clinical autonomic disorders, evaluation and management,* 2nd ed. Philadelphia: Lippincott–Raven, 1997.

Garg BP. Disorders of micturition and defecation. In: Swaiman KF, Ashwal S, eds. *Pediatric neurology: principles and practice,* 3rd ed. St. Louis: Mosby, 1999.

Low PA, Bannister RG. Multiple system atrophy and pure autonomic failure. In: PA Low, ed. *Clinical autonomic disorders, evaluation and management,* 2nd ed. Philadelphia: Lippincott–Raven, 1997.

Resnick WM, Yalla SV. Management of urinary incontinence in the elderly. *N Engl J Med* 1985;313:800–805.

Rushton DN. Sexual and sphincter dysfunction. In: WG Bradley, Daroff RB, Fenichel GM, et al, eds. *Neurology in clinical practice: principles of diagnosis and management,* 2nd ed. Boston: Butterworth–Heinemann, 1996:407–420.

Shy GM, Drager GA. A neurological syndrome associated with orthostatic hypotension: A clinical-pathologic study. *Arch Neurol* 1960;2:511–527.

Stewart JD. Management of male sexual dysfunction. In: PA Low, ed. *Clinical autonomic disorders, evaluation and management,* 2nd ed. Philadelphia: Lippincott–Raven, 1997.

Wein AJ. Practical uropharmacology. *Urol Clin North Am* 1991;18:269–281.

Young CC, Bradley WE. The diagnosis and treatment of urinary bladder dysfunction. In: PA Low, ed. *Clinical autonomic disorders, evaluation and management,* 2nd ed. Philadelphia: Lippincott–Raven, 1997.

32. NEUROIMAGING OF COMMON NEUROLOGIC CONDITIONS

Steven J. Willing
Shane J. Rose

I. **Headaches.** Headaches are one of the most common afflictions of humankind; those among us who have never experienced a single event are few and far between. Only a tiny fraction seeks medical attention.

A. **Chronic headaches and migraine.** A number of prospective and retrospective studies have been performed examining the incidence of relevant new and treatable intracranial pathologic conditions uncovered by computed tomography (CT) for sporadic, nontraumatic headache. Overall, the true-positive rate in an otherwise healthy population is approximately 0.4%, leading most to conclude that routine imaging is not warranted. With such a low incidence of true-positive results, there is an increase in the relative likelihood that false-positive findings will generate additional procedures.

Sinusitis (including mastoiditis) is another common human affliction and is often a cause of headaches. Primarily this is a clinical diagnosis based on symptoms and direct visualization of the nasal cavity. Sinus CT has superseded the largely unreliable sinus radiographs in cases in which imaging is deemed necessary. Sinusitis also is a common finding in head CT performed for headache, although proper head CT technique should spare the ocular lens and therefore should not span the maxillary sinuses.

Among selected populations with a higher prevalence of true-positive findings, notably the immunocompromised and patients with known primary malignant tumors, the likelihood of positive findings is considered sufficient to justify imaging for new-onset headache with either CT or magnetic resonance imaging (MRI).

B. **Acute headache.** The acute onset of severe headache in a patient without migraines, possibly accompanied by photophobia and meningismus, often signals the onset of subarachnoid hemorrhage (SAH). Among this subgroup of patients, the frequency of positive findings approaches 50% and CT is clearly appropriate. MRI is significantly less effective in the detection of acute SAH. Although CT is highly sensitive in the acute phase (>90%), the sensitivity declines rapidly over the ensuing 2 to 3 days. Normal findings at CT do not exclude SAH, and lumbar puncture should be performed if the CT findings are normal.

Acute onset of a severe unilateral headache radiating down the side of the neck, possibly with acute Horner's syndrome, may herald acute carotid or vertebral dissection. In this situation, MRI, particularly MR angiography (MRA), is most useful. Diagnostic angiography should be reserved for ambiguous cases or cases refractory to medical therapy for which endovascular repair is contemplated.

1. **SAH and aneurysms.** If nontraumatic SAH is detected at CT, it is necessary to identify the source of the hemorrhage. Approximately 85% of cases of acute SAH are caused by a ruptured berry aneurysm. Less common causes include arteriovenous malformation (AVM), idiopathic perimesencephalic SAH, dural fistula, moyamoya disease, vertebral dissection, spinal AVM, or tumor.

Although it is likely that at some point in the future noninvasive modalities such as MRA or CT angiography (CTA) will become acceptable for diagnosis, at present **catheter-based cerebral angiography** remains the standard for evaluation of SAH (Fig. 32.1). Properly performed angiography is highly sensitive for aneurysms as well as AVM and dural fistula, which are frequently undetectable at MRI. The risk of permanent neurologic deficit from angiography should be well below 1.0%, particularly in this group of patients who are younger on average and less likely to have serious atheromatous disease.

2. **Intracerebral hemorrhage.** There are many causes of acute nontraumatic cerebral hemorrhage, the most common including hypertension cerebral, amyloid angiopathy, hemorrhagic infarction, tumor, and AVM. **CT** is both quick and sensitive for the diagnosis of cerebral hemorrhage, thus its National Institutes of Health–approved role in excluding hemorrhage before adminis-

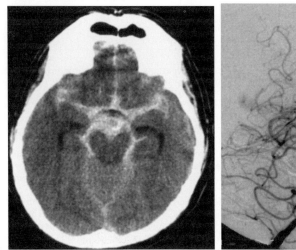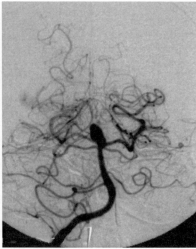

A   B

FIG. 32.1 Ruptured aneurysm. **A:** Axial computed tomographic scan shows high attenuation (*bright*) in the basal cisterns representing acute subarachnoid hemorrhage. **B:** Vertebral angiogram filling the basilar artery (anteroposterior projection) shows a large aneurysm protruding upward from the basilar bifurcation.

tration of intravenous tissue plasminogen activator for stroke. In the care of patients with uncontrolled hypertension who have acute cerebral hematoma in the customary deep location, no further imaging may be necessary. In other cases, the diagnostic evaluation is not complete until the cause of the hemorrhage is established. **MRI** is more effective than CT in the diagnosis of underlying tumor or AVM. **Cerebral angiography** remains the standard for diagnosis of AVM, fistula, and aneurysm. (It is not rare for ruptured aneurysms to bleed into cerebral parenchyma or ventricles, and subarachnoid blood may be undetectable at first).

   II. Seizures. Seizures result from a focal or generalized abnormal discharge of neurons that have been released from normal physiologic control. The goal of imaging in epilepsy is to determine whether the loss of normal control is caused by a structural abnormality and to delineate the location of the abnormality and surrounding structures in an effort to plan surgical intervention. **High-field MRI** is the modality of choice in almost all forms of epilepsy. The superior resolution, soft tissue contrast, absence of beam hardening, and multiplanar capabilities of MRI make it far more sensitive in all but the most acute instances. In instances in which infection, trauma, or malignant disease requires fast and accurate diagnosis for adequate management of acute seizures, CT may be sufficient. Positron emission tomography (PET) and single photon emission computed tomography (SPECT) imaging have proved helpful in evaluating the primary focus of seizure activity when a radiopharmaceutical is injected in the intraictal or periictal phase.

   A. New onset
      1. Infant. Neonatal seizures are most commonly associated with intracranial hemorrhage, infection, migrational anomalies, and perinatal ischemia. Although congenital malformations have been diagnosed with increasing frequency with fetal ultrasonography and MRI, most disorders are diagnosed postnatally. Although CT may be adequate to diagnose large structural defects and some migrational disorders, MRI is generally more sensitive and should be the primary means of evaluation. The purpose of neuroimaging at this age is to exclude disorders that require quick and accurate diagnosis and treatment such as hemorrhage, hypoxic–ischemic injury, and infection.

2. **Child.** Childhood onset of seizures is less likely to result from a detectable structural abnormality. Imaging in this age group should generally be limited to children with abnormal physical findings, delayed development, or specific seizure types commonly linked to structural abnormalities. Imaging is generally not indicated for absence (petit mal) seizures or febrile seizures. Benign focal epilepsy usually is identified by means of history and electroencephalographic findings and is unlikely to result from a lesion identifiable on images. In some cases, a diagnosis of infantile spasms and seizure onset (usually before 4 years of age) is made during early childhood (Lennox–Gastaut syndrome). In cases in which neuroimaging has not already been performed, MRI may be useful in evaluating these patients given the high likelihood of intracranial abnormality. Juvenile myoclonic epilepsy, which typically develops between the ages of 8 and 20 years, usually requires imaging only in cases with a focal deficit or seizure focus.

3. **Adult.** New-onset seizures in an adult may result from a plethora of conditions, including both primary and secondary tumor, vascular malformation, inflammatory conditions, stroke, hypertension, vasculitis, or gliosis from previous insult (e.g., trauma, infarction). In general, all patients older than 18 years with new-onset seizures need neuroimaging. Imaging can help detect abnormalities in patients with head injury several years after the event. Penetrating injuries substantially increase the risk of subsequent seizures; some series have had an increase in occurrence as high as 34%. Mild head injury (without skull fracture, hemorrhage, contusion, or extended loss of consciousness) does not increase the risk of seizures, and therefore imaging is rarely indicated. Patients with signs of temporal lobe epilepsy may benefit from MRI with special attention to the hippocampus, including labor-intensive and seldom used volumetric analysis. Adults have a higher incidence of neoplasm with increasing age, and patients with relatively late-onset seizures should be carefully evaluated for both primary and secondary neoplasms.

4. **Evaluation for surgical correction.** The surgical options for control of medically intractable seizures include anterior temporal lobectomy for mesial temporal sclerosis and, rarely, resection of cortical dysplasia. Evaluation for surgical resection requires strong evidence that the seizures originate from a single focus and that the area can be resected safely. The most relevant MRI abnormality is the presence of hyperintensity on T2-weighted images and volume loss in the hippocampus indicating mesial temporal sclerosis. For this condition, MRI with a variety of field strengths and techniques has a sensitivity of 55% and a specificity of 78%.

The decision to operate should be based on the concordance of electroencephalographic and MRI findings. In cases in which MRI findings are negative or equivocal, researchers have found benefit from functional imaging such as PET, SPECT, or magnetic source imaging. A seizure focus is generally characterized by diminished perfusion and metabolism in the interictal period and increased perfusion and metabolism during the ictus. The addition of intraictal or postictal injection of a radiopharmaceutical may help in localizing the focus during PET and SPECT. Ictal SPECT and interictal PET both are highly sensitive for localization of temporal lobe foci and are superior to MRI.

Although not primarily an imaging tool, diagnostic angiography followed by intracarotid injection of amobarbital or methohexital can be used to evaluate language and memory hemispheric dominance before temporal lobectomy (Wada test). The purpose of diagnostic angiography is to exclude vascular anomalies such as a persistent trigeminal artery that would preclude amobarbital injection.

III. Dementia. Dementia can be caused by a primary dementing disorder (Alzheimer's disease, Pick's disease, vascular dementia) or can be secondary to tumor, chronic subdural hematoma, or stroke. The primary objective of imaging in evaluation of these patients is to exclude correctable disorders causing mass effect or hydrocephalus, which occur among approximately 5% of patients with dementia without clinical evidence predictive of a mass lesion. A secondary objective is to diagnose the specific dementing disorder. It remains to be proved that the use of imaging to obtain a specific diagnosis results in meaningful therapeutic benefit, although this can be helpful in clinical trials or in specific situations. In all cases, MRI without contrast enhancement is recommended for initial imaging evaluation.

MRI may show findings specific for vascular dementia or normal pressure hydrocephalus. In evaluation for the most common cause of dementia, Alzheimer's disease, routine MRI lacks sensitivity and is performed primarily to exclude other conditions. However, with MRI one can obtain a volumetric analysis of the hippocampal formation that can be quite specific, showing reduced volume in Alzheimer's disease relative to simple atrophy. The highest sensitivity and specificity for Alzheimer's disease have been reported with PET with fluorine-18-fluorodeoxyglucose. Patients with Alzheimer's disease have reduced glucose metabolism in the parietal, temporal, and posterior cingulate regions.

IV. Altered consciousness. Emergent evaluation of altered levels of consciousness is one of the most common indications for neuroimaging in the acute setting. Quickly determining the cause of impaired consciousness has far-reaching implications in the evaluation and management of myriad disorders. The difficulty in evaluation of acutely altered consciousness cannot be overstated. Although histories often are inadequate or nonexistent, the clinician is asked to diagnose and manage a generally vague symptom, such as confusion or coma, that can be caused by any number of medical problems. Common causes of impaired consciousness include chemical ingestion, metabolic disorders, structural abnormalities, primary and metastatic malignant tumors, trauma, hemorrhage, or cerebral infarction.

  A. The speed and widespread availability of **CT** has made it the most common imaging method in the acute setting. The sensitivity of CT in evaluating for acute intracranial hemorrhage far surpasses that of MRI. Although "normal" CT findings may be seen up to 24 hours after ischemia, careful examination with appropriate history often can help in evaluation. Again, the basic role of imaging is to exclude the causes that are easily recognizable and can be managed immediately, such as subdural or epidural hematoma. Although "normal" findings do not rule out a serious pathologic condition, it does in most cases obviate immediate surgical intervention. This allows the clinician to continue an evaluation that includes lumbar puncture, which is necessary to evaluate for other correctable causes such as infection.

  B. MRI is indicated when CT does not provide enough information for a diagnosis and another cause cannot be determined. Changes not seen with CT often can be evaluated in a more specific way with MRI. For example, specific patterns of subcortical white matter changes in hypertensive encephalopathy can be diagnosed and followed with MRI, whereas CT often does not depict these changes. These findings may encourage more aggressive control of hypertension and allow the physicians to relay a better prognosis to the family. With a combination of MRI and MRA, basilar artery stenosis and occlusion can be quickly identified, with the possibility of benefit from thrombolysis or angioplasty.

V. Acute and chronic cerebral ischemia. Acute onset of neurologic deficit is most often related to ischemia or stroke. Although ischemia may be related to the transient decrease in blood flow to the brain in whole or in part, stroke is generally thought of in terms of a complete or nearly complete occlusion of an arterial bed either by embolus or thrombosis. The deficit is focal and attributable to the specific region of brain supplied by the corresponding vascular territory. The spectrum of neurologic findings correlates with the amount and location of cerebral tissue involved, and this corresponds to the arterial territory and extent of embolization. Larger or more involved deficits correspond to more proximal arterial occlusion. Very large infarcts may be secondary to thrombosis rather than embolization. One caveat concerns involvement of deep gray or white matter structures. In this instance, a very small occlusion of a tiny branch can cause severe deficits and mimic the infarction of a larger arterial territory. Strokes involving the internal capsule, thalamus, and brainstem can cause minimal cell death but severe deficit owing to the crucial structures involved.

  A. Acute onset neurologic deficit. Before the advent of thrombolysis, there was little that a clinician could do in the management of embolic or thrombotic stroke. With the increasing use of thrombolysis in acute stroke, imaging becomes critical in excluding hemorrhage (an absolute contraindication to use of thrombolytic agents) and can be useful in discriminating dead from salvageable tissue. CT remains the mainstay for evaluation of stroke in the acute phase. Its role is exclusion to diagnose hemorrhage, previous stroke, and masses that preclude administration of thrombolytic agents.

In most centers that do not offer intraarterial thrombolysis, intravenous thrombolysis is the only therapeutic option in the acute stage of a stroke. In this case, the main objective of imaging is to exclude hemorrhage. and CT is both fast and sensitive. Where intraarterial thrombolysis is available, the picture is much more complicated. It is desirable to identify noninvasively patients who do not have major vascular occlusions to avoid calling in personnel unnecessarily. Plain CT cannot do this, but other forms of imaging such as CTA, MRA, or perfusion MRI can help identify patients without vascular occlusion. On the other hand, some investigators believe that some patients still have salvageable brain beyond the usual therapeutic window of 6 hours for intraarterial thrombolysis. Functional imaging methods such as diffusion–perfusion MRI or SPECT may be able to help differentiate brain that is merely ischemic and brain that is infarcted and dead (Fig. 32.2).

B. **Intermittent and chronic deficits**
  1. **Brain imaging.** With both transient ischemic attacks and chronic deficits, MRI is generally preferred. Although CT is sensitive for chronic infarcts, MRI is more sensitive both for the smaller lesions and for posterior fossa lesions. With true transient ischemic attacks, the findings at imaging studies should be normal. Various disorders that mimic ischemia must be ruled out, such as tumors or multiple sclerosis. MRI has the added advantage that vascular imaging can be performed concurrently.
  2. **Vascular imaging.** Evaluation of the possible sources of emboli begins with evaluation of the carotid arteries. Doppler sonography is the screening test of choice because it is quick, sensitive, and inexpensive, but evaluation of the arteries with other methods has increased as well. Until recently, one advantage of MRI was that it could be used to evaluate vasculature by means of MRA. However, with the introduction of high-speed, thin-section helical CTA, this may become less of an issue. In fact, owing to the speed with which CTA can be completed, it has been suggested that CTA may supplant MRA altogether.

     Vascular stenosis on any of these screening examinations may prompt catheter-based angiography for more precise evaluation. MRA tends to exaggerate stenosis, making accurate evaluation critical because carotid endarterectomy may be recommended for selected patients with asymptomatic stenosis of 60% or greater. However, if the stenosis is not 60% but merely 50%, data suggest that patients are more likely to have a stroke from the surgery than from the stenosis.

VI. **Hearing loss and tinnitus**
  A. **Conductive hearing loss.** Any disturbance of sound transmission along the pathway from outside environment to the cochlear apparatus results in conductive hearing loss. The most common cause is fluid in the middle ear from effusion or otomastoiditis. These conditions are diagnosed by means of otoscopy, are easily managed, and usually are self-limited. Otosclerosis is a common disorder and usually is diagnosed on the basis of the appropriate history in conjunction with auditory testing. Imaging is generally indicated when the findings of the history and auditory testing are atypical or inconclusive. Of other possible etiologic factors, the more common ones include ossicular dislocation (trauma), cholesteatoma, and tympanic paraganglioma (glomus tympanicum). High-resolution CT with 1 to 2 mm sections is fast, highly sensitive, and relatively specific for most disorders in this area. MRI is severely limited because air and bone, the two principle substances in this region, produce no detectable signal.
  B. **Sensorineural hearing loss.** Sensorineural hearing loss (SNHL) results from any disruption of transmission from the auditory vestibule, through cochlea and cochlear nerve, to the auditory cortex. Among infants and children, most cases result from congenital anomalies of the inner ear, and CT is the procedure of choice because it provides superior bone detail. Among adults, most cases of SNHL

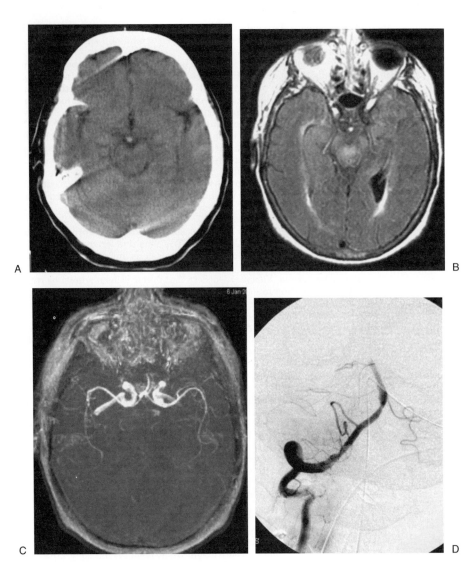

FIG. 32.2 Stroke. **A:** Axial computed tomographic scan shows high attenuation in the basilar artery representing acute thromboembolus. **B:** Axial magnetic resonance image [fluid-attenuated inversion recovery (FLAIR) sequence] shows hyperintensity within the central pons representing early infarction. **C:** Magnetic resonance angiogram in the axial projection shows both carotid arteries but no flow from the vertebrobasilar system. **D:** Right vertebral angiogram shows abrupt termination of the basilar artery in its midsegment.

develop with advancing age and often are related to a lifetime of overexposure to loud noise. Among structural disorders that can be diagnosed with imaging, the most common is acoustic neuroma (vestibular schwannoma). Contrast-enhanced MRI is highly sensitive for this rather uncommon condition and is the procedure of choice. As an added benefit, MRI is also highly sensitive for ischemic or demyelinating lesions along the auditory pathways or for other mass lesions in the cerebellopontine angle or brainstem that also can cause SNHL.

C. **Tinnitus.** The algorithm for the differential diagnosis of tinnitus begins with whether the tinnitus is pulsatile or nonpulsatile.

   1. **Pulsatile tinnitus** can be caused by carotid stenosis, tympanic paraganglioma, aberrant carotid artery or dehiscent jugular vein, or dural arteriovenous fistula. CT is an effective modality for initial evaluation and to exclude the most common causes. Only catheter-based cerebral angiography is sufficiently sensitive to exclude dural arteriovenous fistula when all other causes have been eliminated.

   2. The most common causes of **nonpulsatile tinnitus** are Ménière's disease, middle-ear effusion, and otosclerosis. Imaging usually is not necessary, although CT can be helpful in ambiguous cases.

VII. **Vertigo and ataxia.** Some of the most common causes of vertigo are medical inner ear disorders such as Ménière's disease and viral labyrinthitis. Although imaging abnormalities frequently are demonstrable, that does not mean imaging is particularly necessary. When vertigo or ataxia is progressive or the cause is unknown, MRI is far superior to CT in diagnosis of the usual causes. Contrast-enhanced MRI or very thin T2-weighted sections are both extremely sensitive for acoustic neuroma. T2-weighted or fluid-attenuated inversion recovery (FLAIR) sequences are highly sensitive for demyelinating or ischemic lesions of the brainstem and cerebellum. Olivopontocerebellar atrophy and related degenerative conditions result in atrophic changes of the involved structures. The MRI findings are rarely specific, but MRI remains far superior to CT in sensitivity for such changes.

VIII. **Disturbances of vision**

A. **Visual deficit.** Most cases of visual impairment result from common primary ocular disorders, including refractive impairment and cataracts. Conditions that may point to extraocular pathologic conditions include visual field deficits, acute onset of deficit, or visual deficits with normal ocular examination.

   In nearly all cases in which imaging is indicated, contrast-enhanced MRI is preferred over CT. The superior soft-tissue characterization of MRI allows improved detection of ischemic or demyelinating lesions along the optic pathway. The multiplanar capability of MRI allows improved visualization of the optic chiasm, nerves, and tracts. Intravenous administration of contrast medium may be needed to demonstrate enhancement of the optic nerve pathways in optic neuritis.

   Intermittent episodes of monocular blindness or impairment are known as **amaurosis fugax** and often herald the presence of significant carotid artery disease, most commonly in the neck at the origin of the internal carotid artery. Evaluation of these patients should be directed at the carotid arterial system. Duplex ultrasonography is very sensitive for internal carotid origin or common carotid stenosis but is ineffective for high cervical or intracranial stenosis, is highly operator dependent, may be totally unreliable in some sites, and in the best of hands gives only a fair approximation of the severity of stenosis. Abnormal findings at carotid Doppler examination should be corroborated with another noninvasive study, either MRA or CTA, or by means of catheter angiography.

B. **Motility impairment.** Ocular motility impairment can be caused by disorders occurring anywhere from the brainstem nuclei of cranial nerves III, IV, and VI to the anatomic structure of the orbit itself. In many cases, such as diabetic neuropathy, no imaging abnormality is present or at least discernible. Common causes of motility impairment that can be seen at imaging include orbital blowout fractures, masses of the orbital apex, superior orbital fissure, cavernous sinus, or cranial nerves, and ischemia, demyelination, or tumor of the brainstem. If there is a history of trauma, CT is best suited for evaluation because of its superior depiction of bony anatomy. In most other cases, contrast-enhanced MRI is preferred. Such an examination should be tailored to this problem with thin coronal sections from the back of the globe to the brainstem. MRA should be considered in cases of oculomotor nerve impairment because of its association with posterior communicating artery aneurysm.

IX. Trauma

A. Closed head injury is one of the most common indications for head CT in any hospital with a busy trauma service. With moderate to severe head injury or low Glasgow Coma Scale scores, head CT is the imaging procedure of choice both for emergency evaluation and in case of subsequent clinical deterioration. With minor or mild head injury, CT may still be indicated despite a low yield. The cost of a CT nearly always is less than the cost of admission and a period of observation. Attempts to identify factors predictive of abnormal CT findings in this group have been largely unsuccessful. The realm of common CT findings includes epidural and subdural hematoma, SAH, hemorrhagic contusion, subdural hygroma, fractures, and herniation. The CT scans must be reviewed with both soft tissue and bone window settings to detect all important findings. CT may provide useful prognostic information as well, because poorer outcomes have been associated with midline shift over 10 mm.

Posttraumatic cerebral edema is somewhat of a misnomer, because the cerebral swelling in this condition has been traced to increased blood volume rather than interstitial or intracellular water. In this condition, cerebral swelling results in small ventricles and cisterns but a normal gray–white junction. Generalized loss of the gray–white junction is an ominous finding, usually indicating generalized anoxia from shock and hypoperfusion.

MRI may be helpful in the subacute and chronic phase, although more as a prognostic tool. MRI is much more sensitive for nonhemorrhagic contusion and white matter shearing injuries. The severity of white matter injury may be predictive of recovery or a chronic vegetative state.

Some patients may come to medical attention with headaches or seizures days or weeks after blunt head injury. In this case, MRI is preferred, because by this time blood has become isodense on CT but is easily visible at MRI. It is not altogether rare to image a patient weeks after a mild head injury only to discover previously undiagnosed hemorrhagic contusions. When chronic hematoma is found in the characteristic subfrontal or anterior temporal cortical regions, posttraumatic contusion can be diagnosed with reasonable confidence.

B. Penetrating head injury. CT is the preferred modality for imaging of penetrating injury to the head. It is highly effective in demonstration of fractures, displaced bone fragments, hemorrhage, edema, mass effect and herniation, secondary infarcts, and presence and location of foreign bodies and shrapnel. This information is useful to both guide therapy and assess the prognosis for survival or recovery.

C. Cervical spinal injury. Plain radiography of the cervical spine remains the mainstay for diagnosis of cervical spinal injuries. As a screening tool, it is accurate and effective. A standard cervical spinal series should include anteroposterior, lateral, odontoid, and both oblique views. CT is used for further evaluation of known fractures and for diagnosis in ambiguous cases such as severe neck pain despite normal radiographs.

MRI is preferred for evaluation of injury to the spinal cord proper. Hyperintensity on T2-weighted images may denote cord contusion, whereas hypointensity on T2-weighted and gradient echo images usually indicates hemorrhage. Cord contusion can exist with or without posterior bony displacement or canal compromise. Data suggest that the presence of hemorrhage is predictive of a worse prognosis (Fig. 32.3).

D. Vascular injury

   1. For **blunt injury** to the neck, if the patient's condition is stable, MRA or CTA may be sufficient to diagnose dissection. In the presence of expanding hematoma, uncontrolled bleeding, or neurologic deficit, emergency angiography is indicated (unless the patient goes straight to surgery) and may lead to therapeutic endovascular intervention in the same session.

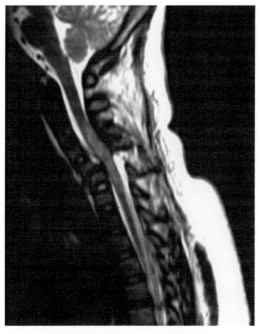

FIG. 32.3 Cervical fracture with cord contusion. Sagittal T2-weighted magnetic resonance image shows a fracture–dislocation of the cervical spine at C5–6. The spinal cord is enlarged and hyperintense with severe edema. Tiny darker spots in the involved cord may be hemorrhage.

   2. For **penetrating injury,** CT of the neck is first indicated to assess the depth of injury and the presence of fractures or foreign bodies. CTA or MRA may be performed to exclude dissection or pseudoaneurysm. Emergency angiography may be reserved for the same exceptions as for blunt injury.
   X. Neck pain and cervical radiculopathy. Degenerative disorders of the cervical spine are extremely common in the middle-aged and older populations. The condition of cervical spondylosis manifests as cervical disk degeneration, osteophyte formation at the disk margins, and hypertrophic degenerative changes of the cervical facet joints. These changes conspire to cause stenosis of the cervical spinal canal with resulting cord compression or stenosis of cervical foramina with nerve root compression. Acute disk herniation may be seen in patients at any age after childhood. Less common causes of cervical cord abnormalities include Chiari I malformation, syrinx, meningioma, or schwannoma.
   The imaging evaluation for these conditions generally begins with MRI of the cervical spine. MRI has the advantage of being able to accurately depict tonsillar herniation and a multitude of cord disorders such as syrinx, myelomalacia, demyelination, or the rare tumor. For degenerative disorders, MRI is less useful here than in the lumbar spine because the structures are much smaller and this area is more prone to artifact. Many reports show that CT myelography is superior to MRI for evaluation of osteophytes and foraminal stenosis, but it has declined in popularity because it is an invasive procedure requiring lumber or cervical spinal puncture with injection of iodinated contrast material. Some of the deficiencies of MRI can be overcome by performing complete radiography of the cervical spine, including both oblique views to show the bony anatomy of the foramina.
   XI. Back pain and sciatic radiculopathy
      A. New onset or presentation. It is estimated that at least 85% of the adult population has experienced clinically significant back pain at some point. Many if not most cases are due to muscle strain, mild trauma, obesity, poor posture,

or osteoarthritis. Imaging shows either mild alignment abnormalities or no abnormalities at all. The imaging evaluation for back pain is a subject that has generated a great deal of debate because of the prevalence of the disorder, a widely perceived overuse of imaging, and the confusing array of imaging options. Whether to pursue imaging at all is a matter of judgment for the individual clinician, but there is medical consensus for not performing imaging in straightforward, uncomplicated cases. Clinical findings that should prompt early imaging include neurologic deficit, sudden onset, age older than 70 years, steroid use, osteoporosis, unrelenting progression, radiation of pain, fever, or a history of surgery, sepsis, malignant disease, or trauma.

When imaging is thought indicated, the clinician is faced with the options of plain radiography, CT, myelography, CT plus myelography, radionuclide bone scan, or MRI. **Plain radiography** of the spine is widely available and can specifically depict an assortment of conditions, including spondylolysis and spondylolisthesis, stenosis, arthritic and disk degeneration, tumors, compression or other fractures, advanced osteomyelitis, or paraspinal abnormalities such as renal calculi. The main limitation is a lack of sensitivity for purely soft tissue abnormalities, including but not limited to disk herniation, spinal stenosis, early osteomyelitis, and spinal metastatic lesions.

Because of its superior soft tissue discrimination and ability to characterize bone marrow, **MRI** is superior to CT for evaluation of osteomyelitis and metastasis. MRI has the added bonus of showing the presence or absence of cord or cauda equina compression without the need for contrast injection into the subarachnoid space. In the evaluation of disk disease, the advantage of MRI is not so clear-cut. MRI is comparable with CT myelography and only slightly better than plain CT in evaluation for disk disease. From a patient's standpoint, however, only the most severely claustrophobic would prefer myelography and CT to MRI.

MRI is relatively insensitive for spondylolysis without spondylolisthesis, for stress fractures, or nondisplaced fractures of the spinal column. In these cases, **plain CT** or **bone scans** are useful for diagnosis.

B. **Failed back syndrome.** In patients who have undergone surgery for disk disease and later have recurrent or unremitting pain, the imaging findings can be confusing owing to postoperative scar and granulation tissue masquerading as disk. Contrast-enhanced CT was the first imaging test able to differentiate the two conditions, but this has since been supplanted by MRI. For the typical patient with back pain and sciatica, MRI without contrast administration is sufficient. However, most neuroradiologists consider intravenous contrast imaging a necessity when there has been previous surgery. As a rule, granulation tissue enhances whereas herniated disk does not. Correlation with surgical findings has shown MRI generally accurate in differentiation of disk from "scar." However, certain caveats apply, the most important being that in the first 3 to 6 months after surgery, this distinction is significantly less reliable.

XII. **Myelopathy.** In the realm of spinal cord imaging, MRI was a true breakthrough. Although we could define the outlines of the cord with myelography and later CT, and occasionally see filling of a syrinx on postmyelography CT, direct visualization of cord lesions was not possible until the advent of MRI. With MRI, we can evaluate the presence of cord compression from trauma or tumor, congenital anomalies such as tethered cord or diastematomyelia, cord contusion and hemorrhage from trauma, spinal cord tumors, and inflammatory and demyelinating conditions. MRI with contrast enhancement is sensitive as a screening tool for vascular disorders such as AVM and fistula, so that only abnormal findings on images necessitate spinal angiography for definitive evaluation and treatment planning.

Inflammatory conditions, including transverse myelitis and multiple sclerosis, exhibit hyperintensity in the cord on T2-weighted images with enhancement often present in acute stages. Spinal cord tumors show cord enlargement and hyperintensity on T2-weighted images and nearly always become enhanced.

One of the most common causes of myelopathy among the elderly is extrinsic compression of the cord from vertebral body metastasis. In a significant percentage of such patients, myelopathy is the initial symptom and there is no history of known malignant disease. MRI of the entire spine (cervical, thoracic, and lumbar) is the procedure of choice for evaluation for cord compression and has supplanted myelography, which often was a cumbersome and painful ordeal for both physician and patient. Intravenous contrast imaging is of little value in evaluating extrinsic cord compression but usually is performed to detect the occasional case of meningeal carcinomatosis.

The most important pitfall in evaluation of the spinal cord is the preponderance of artifactual hyperintensity through this region on T2-weighted images. These artifacts result from patient activity, respiration, cardiac pulsations, aortic flow, and cerebrospinal fluid flow. We will have to rely on future advances in technology to reduce the effects of these factors on spinal cord imaging.

Recommended Readings

American College of Radiology. ACR appropriateness criteria 2000. *Radiology* 2000;215: 415–606.

Biller J, Feinberg WM, Castaldo JE, et al. Guidelines for carotid endarterectomy. *Circulation* 1998;97:501–509.

Frishberg BM. Neuroimaging in presumed primary headache disorders. *Semin Neurol* 1997; 17:373–382.

Knopman DS, DeKosky ST, Cummings JL, et al. Practice parameter: diagnosis of dementia (an evidence-based review). *Neurology* 2001;56:1143–1153.

Silberstein SD. Practice parameter: e-based guidelines for migraine headache (an evidence-based review). *Neurology* 2000;55:754–762.

33. APPROACH TO THE SELECTION OF ELECTRODIAGNOSTIC, SPINAL FLUID, AND OTHER ANCILLARY TESTING

Paul W. Brazis

Neurophysiologic electrodiagnostic studies define alterations in the functions of the nervous system that may not be visualized with imaging procedures. The major areas of study include electroencephalography (EEG), nerve conduction studies (NCS) and electromyography (EMG), and evoked potentials. A discussion of the clinical usefulness of these examinations is followed by brief descriptions of other ancillary neurologic tests, such as polysomnography and the multiple sleep latency test, and of the indications, contraindications, and clinical worth of lumbar puncture (LP) for cerebrospinal fluid (CSF) analysis.

Electroencephalography

   I. EEG involves recording of the spontaneous electrical activity of the brain from the scalp and activity elicited by activation procedures, including sleep, hyperventilation, and photic stimulation. Small metal disks containing conductive gel are attached to the scalp and ear lobes according to a system of measurements and are connected by flexible wires to a recording instrument that amplifies brain activity approximately 1 million times. The EEG is sampled on moving paper or on a computer simultaneously from 16 or 21 pairs of electrodes (derivations) in selected combinations (montages).
   II. **Normal EEG activity**
   A. **EEG rhythms.** The EEG is a composite of several different types of activity, each with characteristic factors of frequency, amplitude, morphology, reactivity, topography, and quantity. The frequency bands of activity are as follows.
   1. **Delta activity** (<4 Hz)
   2. **Theta activity** (4 to <8 Hz)
   3. **Alpha activity** (8 to 13 Hz)
   4. **Beta activity** (>13 Hz)
   B. The most characteristic feature of a normal EEG in an adult during relaxed wakefulness is the **alpha rhythm,** which occurs over the posterior regions of the head while the eyes are closed (Fig. 33.1). Judgments of normality for various EEG activities depend on the age and state of alertness of the subject. Complex changes in EEG patterns occur throughout life, and patterns evolve when going from wakefulness through different stages of sleep.
   C. **Activation procedures** are used to elicit abnormal activities that may not occur spontaneously.
   1. **Hyperventilation** for 3 minutes is most effective for activating generalized seizure activity, such as the spike–wave paroxysms of absence (petit mal) seizures. Hyperventilation may less frequently activate focal abnormalities (e.g., slowing) and focal epileptiform activity. Hyperventilation is contraindicated if the patient has cardiac infarction, recent subarachnoid hemorrhage, or significant pulmonary disease.
   2. **Photic stimulation** consists of repetitive brief flashes of light generated by an electronic apparatus and delivered at frequencies of 1 to 30 Hz. This procedure evokes responses over the occipitoparietal regions (photic driving). The most frequent abnormal response is diffuse paroxysms of spike–wave complexes (photoparoxysmal or photoconvulsive response) that often indicate a seizure propensity.
   3. **Sleep recordings** are most useful for recording paroxysmal abnormalities in patients with epilepsy. Sleep may activate focal or generalized epileptiform activity. Sleep deprivation the night before the study may facilitate sleep, and the deprivation itself may activate epileptiform activity.
   III. **Abnormal EEG activity.** Many EEG changes are nonspecific, but some are highly suggestive of specific entities, such as epilepsy, herpes encephalitis, and metabolic encephalopathy. In general, neuronal damage or dysfunction is suggested by the presence of **slow waves** (activity in the theta or delta range) in a focal or diffuse location. The presence of **sharp waves** or **spikes** (epileptiform activity) in a focal or diffuse pattern suggests a seizure tendency. Localized slowing is highly sensitive and significant for local neuronal dysfunction

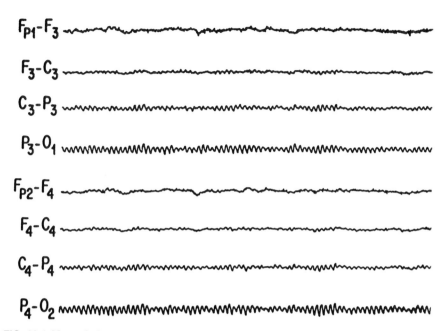

FIG. 33.1 Normal electroencephalogram (EEG) of a man at rest with eyes closed. *Top four rows:* EEG activity from frontal to occipital regions on left. *Bottom four rows:* EEG activity from frontal to occipital regions on right. Normal alpha activity is evident over posterior head regions.

or focal brain damage but is quite nonspecific because it cannot help differentiate the pathologic type of lesion. Thus cerebral infarction, tumor, abscess, and trauma all can cause similar focal EEG changes. Diffuse slowing also indicates organic rather than psychiatric disease but again is nonspecific because such slowing can occur with significant toxic, metabolic, degenerative, or even multifocal disease process. EEG is useful in following the courses of patients with altered states of consciousness and can, in certain circumstances, provide prognostic information. Finally, EEG is important in the determination of brain death.

    A. Epilepsy

        1. Some types of interictal EEG patterns are called *epileptiform* because they have a distinct morphology and occur in a high proportion of EEGs from patients with seizures but rarely in records from patients without symptoms. Such patterns include **sporadic spikes, sharp waves,** and **spike- and slow-wave complexes.** Not all spike patterns indicate epilepsy: 14-Hz and 6-Hz positive spikes, sporadic sleep spikes, wicket spikes, 6-Hz spike–wave complexes, and the psychomotor variant pattern are all spike patterns that are of no proven clinical significance. Interictal findings must always be interpreted with caution. Although certain patterns of abnormality can be useful in supporting a diagnosis of epilepsy, even epileptiform discharges, with few exceptions, correlate poorly with the frequency and likelihood of recurrence of epileptic seizures. One must always treat the patient and never "treat" the EEG.

        2. A substantial portion of patients with unquestioned epilepsy have normal EEG findings. However, epileptiform activity has a high correlation with clinical epilepsy. Only approximately 2% of patients without epilepsy have epileptiform EEG activity, in contrast to 50% to 90% of patients with epilepsy, depending on the circumstances of recording and on whether more than one EEG has been obtained. The most conclusive proof of an epileptic basis of episodic symptoms is obtained by recording an EEG seizure during a typical behavioral episode.

3. The EEG helps establish whether the seizure originates from a limited or focal area of the brain (**focal or partial seizures**) (Fig. 33.2) or involves the brain as a whole from the onset (**generalized seizures**). This distinction is important because of the different possible causes of these two basic types of epilepsy and because the clinical manifestations of both types can be similar.

4. In general, epileptiform activity on an EEG may be helpful in classifying seizure type.

   a. Generalized seizures of nonfocal origin usually are associated with bilaterally synchronous bursts of spikes and spike–wave discharges.

   b. Consistently focal epileptiform activity correlates with partial or focal epilepsy.

       (1) Anterior temporal spikes correlate with complex partial seizures.

       (2) Rolandic spikes correlate with simple motor or sensory seizures.

       (3) Occipital spikes correlate with primitive visual hallucinations or diminished visual function.

5. EEG analysis can allow further discrimination of several relatively **specific electroclinical syndromes.**

   a. Hypsarrhythmia refers to a high-voltage, arrhythmic EEG pattern with a chaotic admixture of continuous, multifocal spike–wave and sharp-wave discharges and widespread, high-voltage, arrhythmic slow waves. This infantile EEG pattern usually occurs in association with infantile spasms, myoclonic jerks, and mental retardation (West's syndrome). It usually indicates severe diffuse cerebral dysfunction. **Infantile spasms** consist of tonic flexion or extension of the neck, body, or extremities with the arms flung outward and typically last 3 to 10 seconds. The EEG and clinical findings do not correlate with a specific disease entity but reflect a severe cerebral insult occurring before 1 year of age.

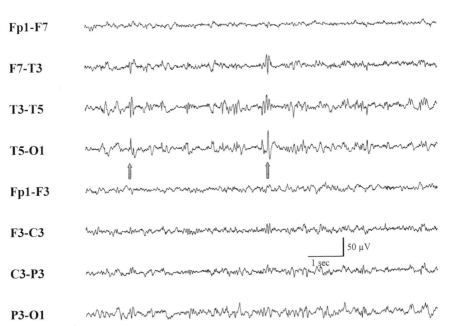

FIG. 33.2 Focal epileptiform activity (spike) (*arrows*) in left posterior temporal region of an adult with partial seizures.

    b. 3-Hz spike–wave activity is associated with typical absence attacks
(petit mal epilepsy) (Fig. 33.3). This pattern most often occurs among
children between the ages of 3 and 15 years and is enhanced by hyperventilation and hypoglycemia. These bursts are typically accompanied
by clinical signs such as staring, brief clonic movements, unresponsiveness, and motor arrest.

    c. Generalized multiple spikes and waves (polyspike–wave pattern)
are typically associated with myoclonic epilepsy or other generalized
epilepsy syndromes (Fig. 33.4).

    d. Generalized slow spike–wave patterns at a frequency of 1 to 2.5 Hz
occur in children between the ages of 1 and 6 years who have underlying diffuse cerebral dysfunction. Most of these children have mental
retardation and poorly controlled seizures. The clinical triad of mental
retardation, severe seizures, and slow spike–wave pattern is called
Lennox–Gastaut syndrome.

    e. Central–midtemporal spikes occur in childhood and are associated
with benign rolandic epilepsy. These seizures often are nocturnal and
consist of focal clonic movements of the face or hand, tingling in the side
of the mouth, tongue, cheek, or hand, motor speech arrest, and excessive
salivation. The spells are easily controlled with anticonvulsants and disappear by 12 to 14 years of age.

    f. Periodic lateralized epileptiform discharges are high-voltage,
sharply contoured complexes that occur over one cerebral hemisphere
with a periodicity of one complex every 1 to 4 seconds. These complexes
are not necessarily epileptiform and correlate with acute destructive
cerebral lesions, including infarction, rapidly growing tumors, and herpes simplex encephalitis.

6. Focal slowing (delta activity) in the interictal period usually indicates
an underlying structural lesion of the brain as the cause of the seizures.
However, such focal slowing may be the transient aftermath of a partial
seizure and may not indicate a gross structural lesion. Such slowing may
correlate with a clinical transient postictal neurologic deficit (Todd's phenomenon) and subsides within 3 days after the ictus.

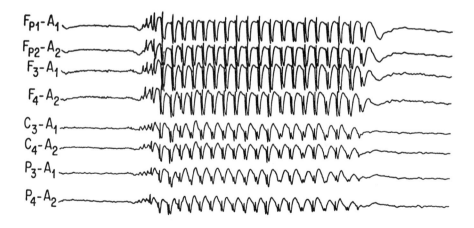

FIG. 33.3 Burst of generalized 3 per second spike–wave discharges in a child with absence
(petit mal) seizures.

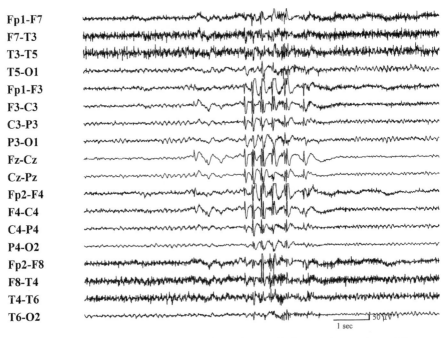

Fp1-F7
F7-T3
T3-T5
T5-O1
Fp1-F3
F3-C3
C3-P3
P3-O1
Fz-Cz
Cz-Pz
Fp2-F4
F4-C4
C4-P4
P4-O2
Fp2-F8
F8-T4
T4-T6
T6-O2

1 sec

FIG. 33.4 Burst of generalized multiple spike and wave discharges in a patient with generalized tonic–clonic seizures.

7. The EEG can make a critical contribution to the diagnosis when a patient is obtunded and prolonged epileptiform discharges with only brief interruptions are recorded. These signify **nonconvulsive status epilepticus.**
8. **Ambulatory EEG monitoring** is the recording of an EEG for a freely mobile patient outside the EEG laboratory. It is similar to Holter monitoring for electrocardiographic (ECG) recording. The main indication is to determine whether a spell is a seizure or another phenomenon, especially when spells occur at unusual times or in association with specific events or activities. The yield depends on the type of patient selected, but the absence of EEG seizure activity during a spell does not fully exclude a seizure disorder, because surface electrodes may not record some mesial temporal, basal frontal, or deep midsagittal seizure discharges.
9. Patients with intractable focal seizures are sometimes candidates for surgical removal of the area of abnormality. Precise identification of the epileptogenic brain area requires special inpatient monitoring facilities for **simultaneous closed-circuit television (CCTV) and EEG recording.** Prolonged CCTV–EEG monitoring is often used to document whether a patient's clinical spells are epileptic or functional (psychogenic).

B. **Altered states of consciousness**
1. For most causes of acute encephalopathy (e.g., toxic–metabolic disease), the EEG changes are nonspecific, consisting of diffuse slowing. There is, however, generally good correlation between the degree of EEG abnormality and the clinical state.
2. Abnormal EEG findings confirm an organic rather than a psychogenic cause of an altered state of consciousness. It is also required to document unrecognized epileptic activity as a cause of depressed consciousness (nonconvulsive status epilepticus).

3. Certain EEG patterns increase the likelihood of specific metabolic disorders.
   a. Prominent **generalized fast (beta) activity** on the EEG recording of a comatose or obtunded patient should raise the suspicion of drug intoxication.
   b. Broad **triphasic waves** that are bilaterally symmetric and synchronous and have a frontal predominance may occur during an intermediate stage of hepatic encephalopathy. However, such a pattern also can occur with other metabolic disorders.
   c. Severe generalized voltage depression may suggest hypothyroidism if anoxia and hypothermia can be excluded.
   d. Patients with uremia, uremic patients undergoing hemodialysis, and patients with hyponatremia may have paroxysmal spike–wave discharges and a photoparoxysmal response to photic stimulation in addition to the diffuse slow-wave abnormality.
   e. Focal epileptiform activity is common in hyperosmolar coma.
4. **Cerebral hypoxia** produces diffuse nonspecific slow-wave abnormalities that may be reversible. More severe hypoxia can cause EEG abnormalities that can be paroxysmal and associated with clinical myoclonus. An EEG obtained 6 hours or more after a hypoxic insult may show patterns of prognostic value in determining the likelihood of neurologic recovery. A poor neurologic outcome is suggested by the presence of the following abnormalities.
   a. **Alpha coma** refers to the apparent paradoxic appearance of monorhythmic alpha frequency activity in the EEG of a comatose patient. However, unlike normal alpha activity, the activity of alpha coma is generalized, often most prominent frontally, and completely unreactive to external stimuli.
   b. The **burst–suppression pattern** consists of occasional generalized bursts of medium- to high-voltage, mixed-frequency slow-wave activity, sometimes with intermixed spikes, and intervening periods of severe voltage depression or cerebral inactivity. The bursts may be accompanied by generalized myoclonic jerks.
   c. The **periodic pattern** consists of generalized spikes or sharp waves that reoccur at a relatively fixed periodicity of one or two per second. The periodic pattern usually is accompanied by myoclonic jerks.
   d. **Electrocerebral silence.** See **III.C.1.**
5. **Infectious diseases** of the central nervous system (CNS) produce predominantly diffuse and nonspecific slow-wave activity. However, certain EEG patterns assist in the diagnosis of specific infectious causes.
   a. The EEG is extremely important in the initial assessment of **herpes simplex encephalitis,** often showing abnormalities before lesions detected with computed tomography (CT) or magnetic resonance imaging (MRI) are recognized. Most patients have temporal or frontotemporal slowing that can be unilateral or, if bilateral, asymmetric. **Periodic sharp complexes** over one or both frontotemporal regions add relative specificity to the EEG findings. These diagnostic features usually appear between the second and fifteenth days of illness and are sometimes detected only on serial tracings.
   b. **Subacute sclerosing panencephalitis** has a distinctive EEG pattern of periodic bursts of stereotyped slow-wave and sharp-wave complexes occurring at intervals of 3 to 15 seconds.
   c. **Creutzfeldt–Jakob disease** is associated with a relatively specific EEG pattern of diffuse high-voltage diphasic and triphasic sharp-wave complexes occurring at a periodicity of approximately one per second (Fig. 33.5).

C. **Brain death**
   1. Because the EEG is a measure of cerebral, especially cortical, function, it has been widely used to provide objective evidence of loss of that function. With cortical death, the EEG shows complete loss of brain-generated activity— **electrocerebral silence.** The determination of electrocerebral silence is

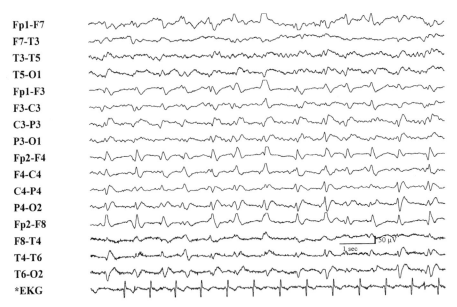

Fp1-F7
F7-T3
T3-T5
T5-O1
Fp1-F3
F3-C3
C3-P3
P3-O1
Fp2-F4
F4-C4
C4-P4
P4-O2
Fp2-F8
F8-T4
T4-T6
T6-O2
*EKG

FIG. 33.5 Generalized periodic (approximately one per second) diphasic and triphasic sharp waves seen in a patient with biopsy-proven Creutzfeldt–Jakob disease.

technically demanding and requires strict adherence to a standard special recording protocol.

2. In rare instances, temporary and reversible loss of cerebral electrical activity may be observed immediately after cardiorespiratory arrest, overdose of CNS depressants, and severe hypothermia. Therefore, electrocerebral silence in these circumstances does not indicate irreversible cortical dysfunction.

3. Patients in a chronic vegetative state with preserved brainstem function may have isoelectric EEG findings, which probably reflect total neocortical death.

4. Establishment of **brain death** (cerebral plus brainstem death) requires the following criteria:
   a. Irreversible structural brain damage
   b. Apneic coma
   c. Loss of brainstem reflexes and signs of brainstem function
   d. Electrocerebral silence on EEG (best viewed as a confirmatory test)

Nerve Conduction Studies and Electromyography
I. Introduction
A. **NCS** are a simple and reliable method of testing peripheral nerve function. An impulse initiated by means of electrical stimulation of the nerve travels along motor, sensory, or mixed nerves. The conduction characteristics of the impulse are assessed by means of recording potentials either from the muscle innervated by the motor nerve or from the nerve itself.

B. The **motor unit** consists of a single lower motor neuron and all of the muscle fibers it innervates. **Motor nerve conduction studies** are techniques used to assess the integrity of the motor unit. Information about the function and structural status of the motor neuron, nerve, neuromuscular junction, and muscle is acquired. Quantitative information can be obtained regarding the location, distribution, time course, and pathophysiologic characteristics of lesions affecting the peripheral nervous system (PNS). Prognosis, response to treatment, and the status of repair of the motor unit also can be assessed. In motor conduction studies, recording electrodes are placed on the skin over the motor point of a muscle and over the tendon of the muscle, and stimulating electrodes are placed over the skin along the course of the nerve to be tested. The response of the muscle to electrical stimulation can be measured by recording compound muscle action potential (CMAP), which is the summation of the electrical potentials of all muscle fibers that respond to stimulation of the nerve (Fig. 33.6). The time it takes for the electrical impulse to travel to the muscle (latency) can be measured. By means of stimulating the nerve at various locations and measuring the distance the stimulus travels, motor nerve conduction velocities are obtained. Motor nerve conduction studies can be used for the following purposes:

1. To obtain objective evidence of disease of motor units
2. To identify and localize sites of compression, ischemia, and other focal lesions of nerves that can manifest as conduction block, slow conduction at the site of the lesion, or abnormal conduction proximal or distal to the lesion
3. To detect widespread involvement of nerves in patients with involvement of a single nerve (mononeuropathy)
4. To differentiate peripheral neuropathy from myopathy and lower motor neuron disease (e.g., amyotrophic lateral sclerosis) in patients with weakness
5. To detect disease before development of significant clinical signs (e.g., familial neuropathy)

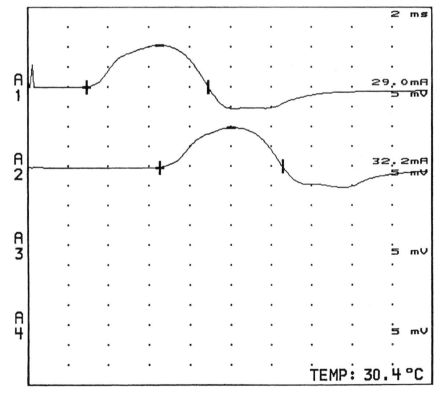

FIG. 33.6 Compound muscle action potentials (CMAPs) recorded from the thenar muscles with stimulation of the left median nerve at the wrist (*upper potential at A1*) and forearm (*lower potential at A2*).

C. **Diseases of the neuromuscular junction** (e.g., myasthenia gravis) can be assessed by means of **repetitive stimulation of motor nerves.** With fatigability of the neuromuscular junction, if a CMAP is recorded and compared with subsequent CMAPs, a decline in amplitude of the potential may be observed as progressively fewer muscle fibers respond to the stimuli, even though the nerve is stimulated at rates that a normal muscle could endure for long periods.

D. In **sensory nerve conduction studies** electrical stimulation is used to record the action potential evoked in a cutaneous nerve (Fig. 33.7). Selective sensory nerve conduction studies can be performed by means of stimulating nerves that have only sensory components (e.g., the sural nerve). An alternative is selective stimulation of only the sensory components of a mixed nerve. The latter can be done by means of isolating the sensory components anatomically (stimulating the digits of the hand and recording over the mixed nerve at the wrist or elbow) or stimulating the mixed nerve and recording over the digits where only sensory axons are present for the most part. Sensory nerve conduction studies may be valuable for the following purposes.

   1. In diffuse disorders affecting the sensory system, for determining which population of sensory nerves is involved (e.g., small fibers carrying pain and temperature sensation or large fibers conveying proprioception), determining whether the disorder is predominantly affecting the axon or the myelin

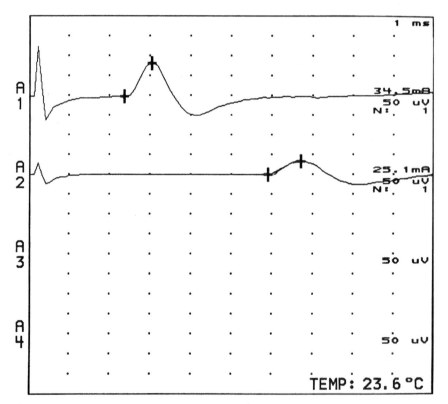

FIG. 33.7 Sensory nerve action potentials obtained by means of recording over the index finger with stimulation of the left median nerve at the wrist (*upper response at A1*) and forearm (*lower response at A2*).

of the peripheral nerve, or determining whether the peripheral sensory nerves are involved at all

    2. In focal neuropathy, for demonstrating a site of injury or block, particularly when only sensory nerves are affected

    3. For confirmation or quantification when sensory abnormalities appear earlier than motor changes in peripheral neuropathy or before objective clinical signs are present.

    4. For predicting whether a lesion is proximal or distal to the dorsal root ganglion (e.g., for differentiating brachial plexus from nerve-root injury)

E. **EMG** usually is performed along with nerve conduction studies and yields complementary information. A needle electrode is inserted into the muscles of interest, and the action potentials generated by groups of muscle fibers [**motor unit potentials (MUPs)**] are observed and recorded (Fig. 33.8). The muscle is tested at rest, with slight contraction, and with stronger contraction. Normally the muscle is silent at rest. In **active neuropathic processes** or in severe or inflammatory myopathy, spontaneous action potentials from single muscle fibers (fibrillation potentials) can occur. In certain neurogenic processes, especially motor neuron disease, spontaneous contractions of groups of muscle fibers (fasciculation potentials) may be observed. Characteristic changes in MUP parameters and recruitment can occur in neurogenic or myopathic processes. In **neuropathic conditions,** the MUPs often are of increased amplitude, duration, and degree of polyphasia with poor recruitment of fibers with increased effort. In **myopathic processes,** the MUPs may be of decreased amplitude and duration with increased polyphasia and rapid recruitment. Single-muscle-fiber action potentials can be studied with a technically more difficult method, **single-fiber EMG.**

F. In general, EMG and NCS are used to study and diagnose motor neuron disease (e.g., amyotrophic lateral sclerosis), processes affecting the plexus or nerve roots, entrapment neuropathy, peripheral polyneuropathy, disease of the neuromuscular junction (e.g., myasthenia gravis), and disease of the muscle. Because it involves electrical shocks and the insertion of needles into several muscles, an EMG/NCS study is uncomfortable. The study is safe as long as electrical safety techniques are used. A tendency toward bleeding may limit EMG studies.

II. EMG/NCS abnormalities

    A. An EMG/NCS study is essential for evaluation and electrophysiologic diagnosis of **motor neuron disease** (e.g., amyotrophic lateral sclerosis). In general, findings at NCS are normal except perhaps for a decrease in CMAP amplitudes (because the disease is purely motor, results of sensory conduction studies are normal). Needle EMG shows diffuse evidence of neurogenic damage from anterior horn cell injury, including abnormal spontaneous activity (fibrillations and

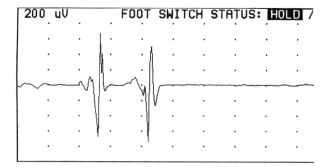

FIG. 33.8 Motor unit potentials recorded with needle insertion into the right biceps muscle during minimal muscle contraction.

fasciculations), abnormal MUP parameters (large, wide, polyphasic MUPs), and poor recruitment of MUPs with effort. Often the EMG study suggests active neurogenic damage, even in muscles or limbs that appear to have little or no clinical involvement. The needle examination can provide information about prognosis, and the EMG may assist in the diagnosis of other diseases of the anterior horn cells, such as postpolio syndrome and spinal muscular atrophy.

B. **Radiculopathy** comprises a constellation of symptoms and signs resulting from transient or permanent damage to the nerve at the anatomic level where the nerve exits the spinal canal in the spinal foramina. Findings at NCS generally are normal. The EMG shows evidence of neurogenic changes (e.g., fibrillation and MUP changes) in muscles innervated by a specific root, other muscles innervated by uninvolved roots being spared. The pattern of neurogenic changes depends on the severity of the process, the duration of the disease, and the degree of neurogenic repair (reinnervation). EMG can be helpful in the following ways.

   1. EMG study is useful for identifying the location of disease and confirming that it is at the level of the root. In studies of patients with surgically detected cervical or lumbosacral radiculopathy, EMG findings are abnormal only approximately 90% of the time. Normal results do not preclude the presence of radiculopathy.
   2. EMG provides further localization by determining which root or roots are affected.
   3. EMG study is useful in determining whether there is active denervation (indicated by the presence of fibrillation potentials).
   4. EMG can help determine the time elapsed since the onset of the radiculopathy (acute, subacute, chronic, or old).
   5. EMG may provide information about the severity of the radiculopathy.
   6. EMG may reveal other abnormalities that explain the symptoms.
   7. EMG may help to determine whether an abnormality on an MR image or myelogram has any physiologic significance.

C. Brachial and lumbosacral **plexopathy** and **entrapment neuropathy** (e.g., carpal tunnel syndrome, ulnar neuropathy at the elbow, and peroneal neuropathy at the fibular head) are localized and diagnosed with EMG/NCS.

D. **Peripheral polyneuropathy** often is investigated with EMG/NCS. The electrophysiologic characteristics of the neuropathic disorder serve as additional sources of information to help characterize the disease and allow narrowing of the differential diagnostic possibilities. EMG/NCS allows evaluation of the amount of motor and sensory involvement, helps determine whether the lesion is primarily the result of damage to the myelin sheath or to the axon, indicates whether the lesion is focal or diffuse, helps determine whether the process is distal or proximal, and gives information concerning the severity and temporal profile of the process. Prolonged distal sensory and motor latencies, slowed conduction velocities, abnormalities of sensory responses and MUPs, and "neurogenic" EMG changes occur. Abnormal findings confirm the presence of a neuropathy; however, small-fiber sensory neuropathy (that affecting only sensory nerve fibers conveying pain and temperature sensation) often is associated with normal results. EMG/NCS can help separate generalized sensorimotor peripheral polyneuropathy from multiple mononeuropathy at sites of common compression (e.g., median and ulnar neuropathy at the wrist). Peripheral polyneuropathy may be divided by electrophysiologic patterns into the following categories:

   1. Uniform demyelinating mixed sensorimotor neuropathy, including certain hereditary forms of neuropathy, metachromatic leukodystrophy, Krabbe's disease, and Tangier disease
   2. Segmental demyelinating motor sensory polyneuropathy, including inflammatory neuropathy (e.g., Guillain–Barré syndrome) and neuropathy associated with gammopathy, hypothyroidism, carcinoma or lymphoma, acquired immunodeficiency syndrome (AIDS), Lyme disease, and certain toxins
   3. Axonal motor sensory polyneuropathy, including porphyria, certain hereditary forms of neuropathy, lymphomatous neuropathy, and certain toxic forms of neuropathy

    4. Axonal sensory neuronopathy, including certain hereditary forms of neuropathy, primary amyloidosis, Sjögren's syndrome, paraneoplastic neuropathy, and neuropathy caused by drugs or vitamin B_{12} deficiency

    5. Mixed axonal demyelinating sensorimotor polyneuropathy resulting from uremia or diabetes mellitus

    6. Axonal sensorimotor polyneuropathy, including neuropathy caused by nutritional deficiencies, alcohol, sarcoidosis, connective tissue diseases, toxins, heavy metals, and drugs

  E. Disease of the neuromuscular junction can be diagnosed with repetitive stimulation studies. Repetitive stimulation of motor nerves is used chiefly in the diagnosis of **myasthenia gravis.** In this disease, a characteristic progressive decline in amplitude of the first few responses to stimulation is revealed at a stimulation rate of two per second. The defect can be further characterized by the way it is altered after a brief contraction of the muscle. For some patients with myasthenia gravis who have normal results of repetitive stimulation studies, the diagnosis can be assisted with single-fiber EMG. Repetitive stimulation studies are invaluable in the diagnosis of the Lambert–Eaton myasthenic syndrome. In the myasthenic syndrome, the initial action potential evoked in the rested muscle by one maximal nerve stimulation is greatly reduced in amplitude. A further reduction in amplitude can occur with repetitive stimulation at low rates, but striking facilitation (enlargement of the MUPs) occurs during stimulation at higher rates. Unusual fatigability of the peripheral neuromuscular system occasionally is found in other diseases, such as amyotrophic lateral sclerosis, but this abnormality is of little diagnostic value.

  F. Electrodiagnostic studies show a wide variety of abnormalities in patients with **myopathy.** The NCS findings are essentially normal, except for occasional reductions in CMAP amplitudes. The EMG may reveal fibrillation potentials in severe myopathy or in inflammatory myopathy (e.g., polymyositis). "Myopathic" MUPs are of decreased amplitude and duration with increased polyphasia and rapid recruitment out of proportion to the degree of contraction effort. EMG studies usually are not sufficient to identify a specific disease, but the pattern of findings can be associated with groups of muscle disorders. Toxic and endocrine myopathy may produce little or no EMG abnormalities. An EMG/NCS examination does or helps with the following:

    1. Differentiate neurogenic from myopathic disorders as causes of weaknes.

    2. Provide clues to the cause of myopathy

    3. Estimate the severity and acuteness of the process

    4. Assess the activity and course of the disease

    5. Provide important information on the distribution of involvement to guide selection of a biopsy site (muscle biopsy must not be performed on a muscle that has been needled but in a corresponding muscle in the opposite extremity)

    6. Detect abnormalities even if not clinically apparent

Evoked Potentials

  I. Evoked potentials are electrical signals generated by the nervous system in response to sensory stimuli. The timing and location of these signals are determined by the sensory system involved and the sequence in which different neural structures are activated. Identical sensory stimuli are presented repeatedly while a computer averages the time-locked low-voltage responses from the brain or spinal cord and unrelated electrical noise and background EEG activity are averaged out.

  II. Visual evoked potentials (VEPs)

    A. Disorders of central visual pathways are tested with VEPs, which are the cortical responses to visual stimuli. Stroboscopic flashes of light or, more commonly, black-and-white checkerboard patterns evoke potentials over the occipital lobes that are detected with scalp electrodes. The major positive deflection at a latency of approximately 100 milliseconds (**P100 response**) (Fig. 33.9) is most useful for clinical application. Delays in this latency suggest damage to visual conducting pathways.

    B. Unilateral prolongation of the P100 response implies an abnormality anterior to the optic chiasm (usually in the optic nerve) on that side. Bilateral P100 delay

Normal
F Age: 47

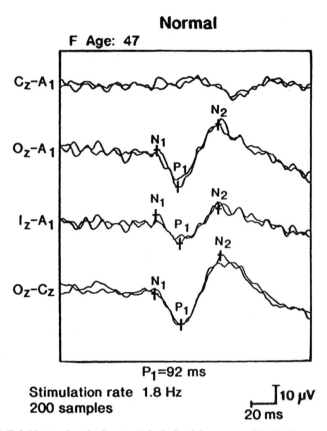

P_1=92 ms

Stimulation rate 1.8 Hz
200 samples

10 μV
20 ms

FIG. 33.9 Full-field visual evoked potential of a healthy person. *P1,* P100 response.

can be caused by bilateral lesions either anterior or posterior to the chiasm or by a lesion within the chiasm itself.

C. **Uses of VEPs**
    1. VEPs can aid in the detection of a clinically "silent" lesion in a patient believed to have multiple sclerosis (MS). The VEP is a sufficiently sensitive indicator of optic nerve demyelination that it can reveal asymptomatic and clinically undetectable lesions. VEPs reveal abnormalities in 70% to 80% of patients with definite MS who do not have histories of optic neuritis or visual symptoms. Abnormalities are not specific for MS and can be abnormal in a variety of other diseases, including certain ocular diseases, compressive lesions of the optic nerve, nutritional and toxic optic neuropathy, including pernicious anemia, and diffuse CNS diseases such as adrenoleukodystrophy and some forms of spinocerebellar degeneration.
    2. The VEP is helpful in differentiating functional (e.g., psychogenic) visual impairment from true blindness or bilateral optic nerve disease. A normal VEP strongly favors functional illness. It should be mentioned, however, that rare patients have been described with blindness from severe bilateral destruction of the occipital lobes who had essentially normal VEP studies. In addition, some patients with functional problems can voluntarily suppress the VEP response by means of strategies such as transcendental meditation, concentration beyond the plane of the checks, or ocular convergence.

3. VEPs can be of some assistance in evaluating the vision of pediatric patients, for example, in evaluating infants at high risk and in the detection of amblyopia.

III. Brainstem auditory evoked potentials (BAEPs)

A. BAEPs are a series of evoked potentials elicited by auditory clicks and generated by sequential activation of the brainstem auditory pathways. Although five waveforms (I through V) are usually resolved (Fig. 33.10), the most stable and important waveforms are I, III, and V. The I–III interpeak latency is a measure of auditory conduction of the more caudal segment of the brainstem (acoustic nerve to lower pons), whereas the III–V interpeak latency is a measure of conduction in the more rostral pontine and lower midbrain pathways. The I–V interpeak latency is a measure of the total conduction time within the brainstem auditory pathways.

B. Abnormality is based on prolongation of interpeak latencies, especially asymmetric prolongations, as well as reduction in amplitude or absence of certain waveforms. Prolonged I–III interpeak latency indicates a lower pontine lesion, whereas prolonged III–V interpeak latency indicates a lesion of the upper pons–lower midbrain level.

C. BAEPs can be clinically helpful in the following circumstances.

1. BAEPs, like VEPs, can be very sensitive to white matter disease and can help confirm or document a lesion within the brainstem, even if there are no brainstem signs or symptoms, when MS is suspected clinically and the patient has a lesion outside the brainstem. Approximately 50% of patients with definite MS have abnormal BAEPs. However, VEPs and somatosensory evoked potentials (SEPs) (see **IV.**) are more sensitive than are BAEPs in detecting abnormalities in patients with MS. Other demyelinating processes affecting the brainstem, such as central pontine myelinolysis, metachromatic leukodystrophy, and adrenoleukodystrophy, also can cause BAEP abnormalities.

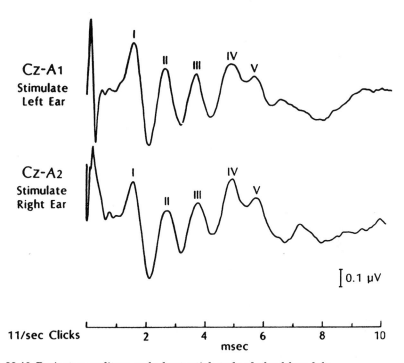

FIG. 33.10 Brainstem auditory evoked potential study of a healthy adult.

2. A **posterior fossa tumor** or other mass within or outside of the brainstem can produce abnormal BAEPs through direct involvement of the brainstem auditory pathways or secondary brainstem compression. BAEPs are highly sensitive screening procedures for acoustic neuroma and other cerebellopontine angle tumors.

3. BAEPs can assist in determination of **brain death.** Preservation of wave I with loss of all subsequent response supports brainstem death of a comatose patient. The BAEP does not, however, provide information about the cortical function of a patient in a coma.

4. BAEPs can be used to assess the **hearing of young children** and of patients otherwise unable to cooperate during standard audiometry. BAEP testing can be used to estimate hearing threshold and may help differentiate conductive hearing loss from sensorineural hearing loss.

IV. **Somatosensory evoked potentials (SEPs)**

A. After electrical stimulation of a peripheral nerve (usually the median or ulnar nerve at the wrist or the tibial nerve at the ankle), recording electrodes placed over the spine and scalp reveal a series of electrical potentials that correspond to sequential activation of neural structures along the dorsal column–lemniscal pathway. These SEPs are named according to their polarities and their times of occurrence in healthy persons. Because SEP latencies vary considerably with body height and limb length, absolute latency values are of limited use. Interpeak latencies, which are measures of the time intervals between successive peaks in the sensory pathways, are incorporated in clinical studies.

B. SEPs yield information concerning PNS abnormalities but are not as effective as conventional NCS in identifying and localizing peripheral disorders. Therefore, although SEPs have been used to study plexopathy and radiculopathy, their use is limited for these conditions.

C. **Uses of SEPs**

1. SEPs can be used to confirm the presence of a clinically "silent" spinal cord lesion in a patient believed to have MS. Median SEPs are abnormal in approximately two thirds of patients with definite MS. Lower-limb SEPs have somewhat greater abnormality rates, probably because of the greater length of white matter traversed. Prolonged central conduction times do not necessarily indicate demyelination, because abnormal interpeak latencies can occur with hereditary spastic paraplegia, olivopontocerebellar atrophy, and subacute combined degeneration resulting from vitamin B_{12} deficiency.

2. Abnormally large ("giant") cortical SEPs are characteristic of some relatively rare neurologic conditions, such as progressive myoclonic epilepsy, late infantile ceroid lipofuscinosis, and some other disorders associated with myoclonus.

3. SEPs may be helpful in demonstrating intact central sensory pathways in patients with functional (e.g., hysterical) sensory loss.

4. SEPs have been especially helpful in monitoring spinal cord function during surgery (e.g., surgery for correction of spinal scoliosis).

Other Ancillary Neurologic Studies

I. **Polysomnography**

A. Polysomnography consists of continuous monitoring of several biologic variables during nocturnal sleep. Eye movements (electrooculography), EEG activity, submental EMG, the ECG, and limb movements are routinely monitored. Respiration is monitored with intraesophageal pressure gauges, intercostal surface EMG, rib cage and abdominal strain gauges, oronasal thermistors or carbon dioxide detectors, ear or finger oximetry, and other means of determining the presence of central, peripheral, or mixed apnea syndromes. A microphone attached to the throat helps detect snoring. Each 30-second epoch of the polysomnogram is scored as awake, stage I–IV non–rapid eye movement (non-REM) sleep, or REM sleep.

B. Polysomnography is used to investigate two types of problems: sleep disorders, such as too much or too little sleep, and risk factors or specific syndromes induced by or linked to sleep or specific sleep states. These disorders include the following:

1. Sleep apnea syndromes, which can be obstructive, central, or mixed
2. Narcolepsy
3. Idiopathic CNS hypersomnia
4. Periodic movements of sleep and sleep-related myoclonus
5. REM behavioral disorder
6. Disorders of the sleep–wake cycle
7. Parasomnia, such as sleepwalking, nightmares, night terrors, and head banging

II. **Multiple sleep latency test**

A. The multiple sleep latency test consists of five 20-minute attempts, one every 2 hours, to fall asleep throughout the day. The aim is to determine the sleep latency and whether REM sleep episodes are recorded during the nap. Patients should not take sleep-related medications for 10 to 15 days. The study usually follows polysomnography because knowledge of the patient's previous night's sleep is required for appropriate interpretation. During the study, the EEG, submental EMG, ECG, and eye movements are monitored. Healthy persons have mean sleep latencies greater than 10 minutes and fewer than two sleep-onset REM periods during the study.

B. The multiple sleep latency test is designed to evaluate the following:

1. **Excessive daytime somnolence** by quantifying the time needed to fall asleep. Pathologic sleepiness is manifested by a mean sleep latency of less than 5 minutes.

2. The possibility of **narcolepsy** by checking for abnormally short latencies to REM sleep. The occurrence of two or more sleep-onset REM periods during the study is strong evidence of narcolepsy, as long as sleep apnea and withdrawal from stimulants and alcohol have been ruled out.

Lumbar Puncture

I. LP should be considered only after a thorough evaluation of the patient and serious consideration of the potential value and hazards of the procedure.

II. **Indications for CSF examination and LP**

A. CSF examination is key to the diagnosis and management of various CNS infections, including acute and chronic meningitis and encephalitis. In many patients with fever of unknown origin, even in the absence of meningeal signs, early LP is commonly of value, especially because meningeal signs may be minimal or absent in very young or elderly patients. Meningeal infection especially should be sought in patients with fever and impaired sensorium or an immunocompromised state (e.g., patients with AIDS). If a patient has unexplained acute confusion, stupor, or coma, even if afebrile, CSF examination is necessary for evaluation for meningoencephalitis. In most clinical settings, CT of the brain or other neuroimaging should be performed before LP to rule out a possible intracranial mass (e.g., hemorrhage or abscess), which would make LP a potentially lethal procedure. However, if the patient is extremely ill and acute meningitis, such as meningococcal meningitis, is suspected, LP should be performed without delay to avoid losing valuable time in beginning appropriate therapy.

B. In patients with suspected subarachnoid hemorrhage, urgent CT is indicated to evaluate for the presence of blood. However, in approximately 10% of patients with **subarachnoid hemorrhage,** CT does not show blood, and a spinal tap is indicated. If the diagnostic LP shows subarachnoid blood or xanthochromia, cerebral angiography is needed to determine the source of the hemorrhage.

C. In patients with **unexplained dementia,** CSF examination may be necessary to evaluate for CNS vasculitis, infection, or granulomatous disease. The CSF should always be examined if the patient has dementia and a positive result of a fluorescent treponemal antibody absorption test. Patients with radiographic hydrocephalus also may need a CSF study to exclude chronic meningitis as a cause of symptomatic hydrocephalus. In patients with suspected Creutzfeldt–Jakob disease, a positive result of radioimmunoassay of the CSF for "prion protein" (14-3-3 protein) is a sensitive and relatively specific marker for prion disease, although false-positive results have been described with encephalitis and with recent stroke.

D. CSF examination usually is not warranted for and can be dangerous for most patients with stroke. However, CSF analysis can assist in the etiologic diagnosis of **unexplained stroke in young or middle-aged patients** who lack atherosclerotic risk factors. Causes such as CNS vasculitis, meningovascular syphilis, and AIDS may be diagnosed.

E. CSF studies can aid in the diagnosis of **MS,** although there is no specific CSF marker for this disease. Elevated CSF immunoglobulin G (IgG) levels with normal serum IgG levels and the presence of oligoclonal bands in the CSF are characteristic but not specific for MS. An elevated CSF gamma globulin level can occur in neurosyphilis, viral meningoencephalitis, and subacute sclerosing panencephalitis.

F. CSF analysis often is necessary, after appropriate neuroimaging, in the evaluation of patients admitted with an **initial tonic–clonic seizure or status epilepticus** to exclude active CNS infection or hemorrhage.

G. LP is necessary to confirm the clinical suspicion of **carcinomatous or leukemic meningitis.** Numerous LPs sometimes are needed. The typical CSF pattern is pleocytosis with elevated protein, low glucose, and a positive cytologic results for a malignant tumor.

H. CSF studies can aid in the diagnosis of certain **inflammatory or demyelinating forms of neuropathy,** such as Guillain–Barré syndrome or chronic idiopathic demyelinating polyradiculoneuropathy. The CSF protein level often is elevated without an abnormal cellular response.

I. Although LP is generally contraindicated in the evaluation of patients with papilledema, LP is indicated to document increased intracranial pressure in a patient with suspected **idiopathic intracranial hypertension (pseudotumor cerebri)** after results of neuroimaging studies have proved normal. The spinal fluid is under increased pressure but is otherwise normal in this entity, except for occasional decreases in CSF protein level. LP is needed to document low CSF pressure in rare low-pressure syndromes in a patient with headaches that occur on standing and are relieved by lying down.

J. LP can be used to deliver **intrathecal antibiotics and chemotherapy** in the management of certain CNS infections and meningeal malignant tumors. LP also is needed in certain diagnostic procedures, such as myelography and cisternography.

III. Contraindications to LP

A. LP is contraindicated in evaluation of any patient with **increased intracranial pressure,** except idiopathic intracranial hypertension, because of the real danger of cerebral herniation and death.

B. LP is contraindicated if there is **suppuration in the skin or deeper tissues overlying the spinal canal** because of the danger of inducing purulent meningitis.

C. LP is dangerous in the presence of **anticoagulation therapy or a bleeding diathesis.** Heparin administration should not be reinstituted for a minimum of 2 hours after LP is performed. In general, LP is hazardous if the platelet count is less than 50,000/mL, or especially if it is less than 20,000/mL. In such cases, platelet transfusions should be initiated if possible before LP.

D. LP should not be performed when a **spinal mass** is suspected unless the procedure is part of a myelogram with neurosurgical assistance readily available. A dramatic deterioration in spinal cord or cauda equina function can occur after LP.

IV. Complications of LP

A. Brain herniation and death can occur if an LP is performed on a patient with increased intracranial pressure from a cerebral mass lesion. LP is contraindicated in the evaluation of any patient believed to have an intracranial mass.

B. Headache of low-pressure type occurs in as many as 10% of patients after LP (spinal headache). This type of headache occurs only on standing and is relieved by lying down. It usually is self-limiting, but it can require an epidural autologous blood patch for relief. Post-LP headache is most common among young women with lower body mass. Use of a higher-gauge (smaller diameter) needle, needle insertion parallel to dural fibers (bevel up with patient on side), and replacing the stylet before needle removal may help prevent post-LP headache. The occurrence of post-LP headache is unrelated to CSF opening pressure, cells, and protein; patient position during LP; duration of recumbency after LP; amount of CSF removed; or hydration after LP.

C. **Diplopia,** which usually results from unilateral or bilateral cranial nerve VI palsy, occurs rarely and usually is self-limiting.

D. **Aseptic meningitis** occurs rarely and is characterized by posterior neck pain, headache, and neck stiffness. This process usually is self-limiting.

E. **Spinal epidural, subdural, and subarachnoid hematoma** can occur, especially in patients taking anticoagulants or with bleeding diatheses. Such hematomas usually are self-limiting and can cause local pain and meningeal irritation. However, in rare instances, epidural hematoma causes flaccid and potentially irreversible paraplegia that necessitates emergency surgical evacuation.

V. **General comments on evaluation of LP results**

A. Normal **CSF pressure** is 70 to 180 mm of water in the lateral recumbent position. Pressure should be greater than 200 mm of water to be considered elevated. In an obese patient with possible idiopathic intracranial hypertension, the pressure should be greater than 250 mm of water to establish this diagnosis.

B. Normal **CSF glucose** level is approximately two-thirds the serum glucose level, which must be measured at the time of the LP. Hypoglycorrhachia (low CSF glucose) with few white blood cells suggests fungal infection. Many white cells suggest bacterial infection. Abnormal (malignant) cells suggest a malignant meningeal tumor.

C. The **CSF protein** level may be increased (>100 mg/dL) in many CNS infectious and malignant processes. Causes of elevation of CSF protein level with normal findings at neuroimaging include myxedema, inflammatory demyelinating polyneuropathy, diabetic polyneuropathy, neurofibroma within the CSF pathways, resolving subarachnoid hemorrhage, gliomatosis cerebri, CNS vasculitis, and any process that causes spinal compression or obstruction of CSF flow.

D. Normally, the CSF can contain up to five lymphocytes or mononuclear cells per milliliter. **Pleocytosis** causes CSF clouding when there are at least 200 cells/mL. White blood cell count increases with subarachnoid infection, hemorrhage, chemical meningitis, or meningeal neoplasms. Pleocytosis also can occur for approximately 24 hours after a generalized seizure.

E. If initial spinal fluid appears bloody, one must attempt to determine whether the source of the blood is a traumatic tap or subarachnoid hemorrhage. If the initial tube of fluid is bloody and subsequent tubes are progressively clear, it is most likely that the tap was traumatic. One should then immediately centrifuge the fluid to see whether the supernatant is clear, which suggests a traumatic tap. If the supernatant fluid is xanthochromic (yellow-tinged), it is likely that the blood has been present in the CSF for a few hours. Xanthochromia occurs several hours after subarachnoid hemorrhage, reaches its greatest intensity at the end of 1 week, and clears in approximately 2 to 4 weeks. Xanthochromia also can be observed in jaundice and hypercarotenemia.

F. Polymerase chain reaction testing of the CSF has been found to have great utility in the diagnosis of several CNS infections. These include

1. Herpes simplex virus I (herpes simplex encephalitis)
2. Herpes simplex II (herpes simplex encephalitis in neonates, recurrent meningitis)
3. JC virus (progressive multifocal leukoencephalopathy)
4. Cytomegalovirus (CMV ependymitis and polyradiculopathy associated with AIDS)
5. *Borrelia burgdorferi* (Lyme disease)
6. *Tropheryma whippleii* (Whipple's disease of the CNS)
7. Toxoplasmosis (CNS toxoplasmosis in AIDS)
8. *Mycobacterium tuberculosis* (tubercular meningitis)
9. Other viruses causing encephalitis, including enteroviruses, varicella-zoster virus, Epstein–Barr virus, and herpesvirus type 6

Referrals

All clinical neurophysiologic tests should be performed and interpreted by clinicians with expertise and special training in clinical neurophysiology. Laboratories performing these studies must follow the clinical and technical guidelines published by neurophysiologic societies, the American Academy of Neurology, and other organizations. Strict adherence to these guidelines is mandatory to ensure patient safety and meaningful clinical interpretation. Neurologic consultation is suggested whenever LP reveals abnormalities suggesting CNS infection, increased or decreased intracranial pressure, or subarachnoid hemorrhage.

Recommended Readings

Aminoff MJ. *Electrodiagnosis in clinical neurology,* 2nd ed. New York: Churchill–Livingstone, 1986.

Brown WF, Bolton CF. *Clinical electromyography,* 2nd ed. Boston: Butterworth–Heinemann, 1993.

Daly DD, Pedley TA. *Current practice of clinical electroencephalography,* 2nd ed. New York: Raven Press, 1990.

Daube JR. *Clinical neurophysiology.* Philadelphia: FA Davis Co, 1996.

Donofrio PD, Albers JW. Polyneuropathy: classification by nerve conduction studies and EMG. *Muscle Nerve* 1990;13:889–903.

Fishman RA. *Cerebrospinal fluid in diseases of the nervous system,* 2nd ed. Philadelphia: WB Saunders, 1992.

Kimura J, Dickins QS. Electrodiagnosis of neuromuscular disorders. In: WG Bradley, ed. *Neurology in clinical practice.* Boston: Butterworth–Heinemann, 1991:452–467.

Kuntz KM, Kokmen E, Stevens JC, et al. Post-lumbar puncture headaches: experience in 501 consecutive procedures. *Neurology* 1992;42:1884–1887.

Members of the Department of Neurology, Mayo Clinic and Mayo Foundation for Medical Education and Research. *Clinical examinations in neurology,* 6th ed. St. Louis: Mosby, 1991.

Parkes JD. Disorders of sleep. In: Bradley WG, ed. *Neurology in clinical practice.* Boston: Butterworth–Heinemann, 1991:1479–1506.

Pedley TA, Emerson RG. Electroencephalography and evoked potentials. In: Bradley WG, ed. *Neurology in clinical practice.* Boston: Butterworth–Heinemann, 1991:429–451.

Roos KL, ed. *Central nervous system infectious diseases and therapy.* New York: Marcel Dekker, 1997.

34. APPROACH TO COMMON OFFICE PROBLEMS OF PEDIATRIC NEUROLOGY

David W. Dunn
Hema Patel

Delayed Development

I. Definition. A child with developmental delay has not met expected milestones in one or more areas. This can be determined with a screening test such as the Denver Developmental Test, with more specific intelligence tests such as the Wechsler Intelligence Scale for Children (WISC-III), or with achievement tests such as the Wide Range Achievement Tests–Revised (WRAT-R) or the Peabody Individual Achievement Tests. Both tests of intelligence and tests of achievement require referral to a psychologist or other professional trained to administer these assessments. The causes of delay fall into two main categories—nonprogressive and progressive retardation.

II. Static encephalopathy. Nonprogressive causes of retardation or delay are also called *static encephalopathy*. The child may have delays obvious at birth or may not reach milestones at the expected rate. The child continues to progress, although at a reduced rate, and does not lose previously acquired skills. Such children do not reach a level of normal functioning. However, their developmental curves seem to parallel those of children without difficulties in acquiring milestones.

III. Causes of static encephalopathy
   - **A. Nonprogressive delays involving multiple functional areas.** Chromosomal disorders, brain malformations, intrauterine infections, and perinatal insults to the brain are potential causes of static encephalopathy. This disorder also can follow acquired damage to the brain from meningitis, encephalitis, hypoxia, and head trauma.
   - **B. Nonprogressive delay in a single functional area.** Nonprogressive motor delay can be observed in some children with cerebral palsy and in some children with congenital myopathy. Nonprogressive isolated speech delay can accompany deafness, autism, and developmental speech disorders.

IV. Progressive retardation. A child with progressive retardation first slows in the acquisition of new skills, then stops developing, and finally loses developmental milestones. The differential diagnosis is extensive, including degenerative, metabolic, infectious, and mass lesions. The constellation of symptoms and signs with which the child presents determines the evaluation. Some children may have disorders that diffusely involve the central nervous system (CNS). They have dysfunctions in both cognitive and motor areas. In the beginning of the illness, there may be predominantly motor or cognitive symptoms and signs, but with time, the patient progressively loses function in other areas. In some children, the regression may be limited to a single area of the neuromuscular system. For example, children with cerebellar degenerative disorders may have progressive loss of coordination with preservation of cognitive function, and children with certain forms of muscular dystrophy may have deterioration limited to motor skills.

V. Causes of degenerative disorders
   - **A. Isolated involvement of the CNS**
      1. **Disorders predominantly involving white matter** manifest as spasticity and motor regression. There may be visual loss and polyneuropathy. Cognitive slowing occurs later. There is prominent demyelination on magnetic resonance (MR) images and there may be slowing of peripheral nerve conduction velocities. Examples include metachromatic leukodystrophy, globoid cell leukodystrophy, Alexander's disease, Canavan's disease, Pelizaeus–Merzbacher disease, and adrenoleukodystrophy.
      2. **Disorders predominantly involving gray matter** start with seizures or loss of cognitive function. In this category are found aminoaciduria, organic aciduria, Tay–Sachs disease, ceroid lipofuscinosis, and Rett's disorder. Acquired immunodeficiency syndrome encephalopathy may manifest as cognitive decline.
      3. **Disorders with prominent abnormalities of posture or movement.** Disorders that involve dystonia include torsion dystonia, Wilson's disease,

Hallervorden–Spatz syndrome, and Niemann–Pick disease type C. With juvenile Huntington's disease and juvenile parkinsonism, there may be rigidity and chorea or tremor. Chorea is a prominent component of Lesch–Nyhan syndrome.

   4. **Disorders with prominent ataxia.** Ataxia can be a component of many degenerative and metabolic disorders. It is most pronounced in ataxia-telangiectasia, Refsum's disease, abetalipoproteinemia, Friedreich's ataxia, and the many other familial ataxia syndromes.

   5. **Disorders with prominent peripheral nervous system involvement.** In globoid cell and metachromatic leukodystrophy, there is a demyelinating neuropathy. With neuroaxonal dystrophy, there is a combination of dementia, hypotonia, and areflexia. A child with Fabry's disease has an angiectatic rash and a painful sensory neuropathy.

B. **Disorders involving both the CNS and other organs**
   1. **Disorders with prominent dysmorphic features** all have coarse facial features in common. In this category are mucopolysaccharidosis, mucolipidosis, the sialidosis, and GM_1 gangliosidosis.
   2. **Disorders with both organomegaly and CNS involvement.** Hepatomegaly is a major feature in most forms of mucopolysaccharidosis, galactosemia, Pompe's disease, Zellweger syndrome, GM_1 gangliosidosis, and Niemann–Pick disease. Splenomegaly is more prominent in type 2 Gaucher's disease.

VI. **Evaluation**
A. **History.** The history involves a careful review of complications of pregnancy, labor, and delivery, subsequent injuries and illnesses, and a detailed family history. The developmental history documents both when milestones were met and when symptoms and signs began. By means of the history, one can usually assign the child to a progressive or nonprogressive category. For a child with static encephalopathy, the history and examination may be all that is needed for the appropriate diagnosis. An example is a child who was a very premature infant and had multiple complications, including intraventricular hemorrhage, and now has spastic quadriparesis and cognitive delay. Difficulties arise when the child has a severe metabolic disorder that manifests acutely in the neonatal period, has an insidiously progressive disorder, and is seen when there is a falling away from the normal developmental curve but no loss of milestones. In the first case, the diagnosis is suspected when there is no clear cause of the encephalopathy that occurred in the neonatal period. In the second case, repeated evaluations may be necessary.

B. **Examination.** A standard pediatric and neurologic examination helps place the condition into a category that makes laboratory assessment more efficient. Dysmorphic features may be seen with chromosomal disorders and storage diseases. Skin lesions are seen with the neurocutaneous disorders, Fabry's disease, and adrenoleukodystrophy. Neurologic signs and organomegaly are outlined in **V.** as a means of categorizing the causes of degenerative disorders. Referral to an ophthalmologist is helpful. Optic atrophy is observed in many forms of leukodystrophy. Macular or retinal pigmentary degeneration occurs in ceroid lipofuscinosis, abetalipoproteinemia, Refsum's disease, and certain forms of mucopolysaccharidosis. Cherry red spots are present in Tay–Sachs disease, sialidosis, and some cases of Niemann–Pick disease and GM_1 gangliosidosis. Lens opacities occur in galactosemia, Wilson's disease, Marinesco–Sjögren syndrome, and homocystinuria. Corneal opacities accompany certain storage diseases. The presence of a Kayser–Fleischer ring helps in the diagnosis of Wilson's disease.

C. **Diagnostic studies**
   1. **Nonprogressive encephalopathy** should not require extensive evaluation. Neuroimaging helps define brain malformations and is important for ruling out hydrocephalus and mass lesions. Chromosomal studies are necessary if the cause is not obvious from the history. Audiologic evaluation is essential if there is absence of or delay in acquiring language. Assessment of vision and hearing is essential for appropriate developmental and educational planning.

2. **Progressive encephalopathy.** Appropriate studies are determined by the history and examination findings.
   a. Computed tomography (CT) or MR imaging (MRI) may be necessary to rule out hydrocephalus or mass lesion. MRI also depicts the demyelination that accompanies leukodystrophy.
   b. Electroencephalography (EEG) is necessary for evaluation of seizures.
   c. Thyroid function studies should be performed if there are coarse facial features.
   d. Urine should be checked for amino acids and organic acids if the child has seizures and cognitive delay. Urine is checked for reducing substances when the presence of hepatomegaly or cataracts suggests galactosemia. A urine screen for mucopolysaccharides should be performed if there are coarse facial features or organomegaly.
   e. Slowing of nerve conduction and delays in evoked response tests are observed in association with leukodystrophy.
   f. Abnormal or no response on electroretinograms are characteristic of retinitis pigmentosa and tapetoretinal degenerative disorders.
   g. The definitive diagnosis of many of these disorders requires demonstration of enzyme deficiencies in leukocytes or cultured fibroblasts.
   h. Identification and cloning of genes and mutations associated with inherited neurologic disorders has lead to changes in diagnostic evaluations. A steadily increasing number of specific DNA tests are available for progressive encephalopathy. Consultation with a geneticist may be helpful for remaining informed about newer diagnostic studies. Updated information also can be found at *www.genetests.org*

Nonepileptiform Paroxysmal Events

This section reviews intermittent, transient, and recurrent episodes of neurologic dysfunction. Between episodes, the child is usually normal. The most common disorders are headaches, seizures, and syncope. Headaches are discussed in Chapters 20 and 21 and seizures in Chapter 6.

I. **Evaluation**
   A. **History.** The description should be obtained from the child and from witnesses to the event. Review the situation immediately before the episode, asking specifically about any potential trigger. Ask the child to describe how he or she felt before and after the episode. Witnesses can provide detailed descriptions of the episode. Review the history for predisposing conditions and any family history of paroxysmal disorders.
   B. **Examination.** Between episodes, examination findings usually are normal. For possible syncopal episodes, blood pressure is measured with the child both supine and standing. If it seems that there was a trigger for the event, repeating this precipitant may help with the diagnosis. Families may be able to videotape the episode and give the physician a chance to see the event.
   C. **Diagnostic studies.** If there is a possibility of epilepsy, serum glucose and calcium tests and EEG are necessary. If the initial EEG does not provide enough information for a diagnosis, consider prolonged video EEG if the episodes occur frequently enough to be captured in the EEG laboratory. Electrocardiography, Holter monitoring, and cardiac ultrasonography are parts of the evaluation for syncope. Neuroimaging is essential if headaches and loss of function occur during the same episode.
II. **Diagnostic approach based on major symptom**
   A. **Episodic loss of function with a clear-cut precipitant**
      1. **Breath-holding spells.** The triggers for breath-holding spells are pain, anger, frustration, surprise, and fright. In the **cyanotic form,** the child cries, holds the cry in expiration, becomes cyanotic, and loses consciousness. The child may become rigid and may exhibit a few clonic movements. The entire episode is brief, usually less than 60 seconds. In the **pallid form,** the child does not cry, becomes pale and apneic, and loses consciousness. In both forms, there can be urinary incontinence and profound bradycardia. These

episodes are most common between 6 months and 3 years of age and are not associated with increased risk of epilepsy or learning disability. They usually cease within 2 to 3 years. The family history is often positive for similar episodes among first-degree relatives.

2. **Syncope** is the result of a sudden decrease in brain perfusion, most commonly from a vasovagal reflex. Syncope is more frequent among adolescents than among younger children. It typically occurs after prolonged standing or sudden standing. It rarely occurs while the child is sitting and does not happen when the child is lying down. The trigger may be emotional situations, embarrassment, a Valsalva maneuver, or a sudden change in position. The child first notes light-headedness or dizziness or may fall without warning. Loss of muscle tone and loss of consciousness occur simultaneously. The child may have a few clonic jerks during the period of decreased consciousness. The period of alteration in consciousness is usually less than 1 minute.

3. **Reflex epilepsy** (see Chapter 6). Potential triggers are flashing lights, startling events, and in rare instances, somatosensory or auditory stimuli or complex activities such as reading.

B. **Episodic movement disorders**

1. **Weakness.** Periods of weakness with recovery between episodes may occur in association with myasthenia gravis. Periods of weakness also are characteristic of periodic paralysis. This type of paralysis is a group of autosomal dominant disorders in which weakness is triggered by rest after exertion, carbohydrate loads, cold exposure, or stress. The serum potassium level may be low, mildly elevated, or normal.

2. **Ataxia.** Intermittent ataxia occurs with seizures, migraine, and several X-linked or autosomal recessive metabolic disorders, including Hartnup disease, a form of maple syrup urine disease, and certain urea cycle abnormalities. Autosomal dominant episodic forms of ataxia may be responsive to acetazolamide. Episodic ataxia type 1 is caused by a mutation in the potassium channel gene on chromosome 12p. Episodic ataxia type 2 is associated with a mutation in the calcium channel gene (CACNA1A) on chromosome 19.

3. **Chorea.** There are both kinesigenic and dystonic forms of chorea. The kinesigenic form is precipitated by movement or a startling event and lasts less than 5 minutes. The dystonic form can be precipitated by fatigue, caffeine, or alcohol and last as long as 4 hours. Both forms are familial.

4. **Other movements.** Three disorders that occur only among children are spasmus nutans, shuddering attacks, and paroxysmal torticollis.
   a. Spasmus nutans begins at 3 to 30 months of age and consists of episodes of monocular nystagmus, head tilt, and head bobbing. The episodes last for seconds to a few minutes.
   b. Shuddering attacks are brief shaking spells usually experienced by infants. The infant remains alert throughout the episode. Shuddering attacks may be associated with later onset of essential tremor.
   c. Paroxysmal torticollis occurs during the first 2 to 3 years of life. The episodes may last for a few minutes or as long as several weeks. The child may vomit but remains alert during the episode. This condition can evolve into benign paroxysmal vertigo.

C. **Episodic sensory disturbances**

1. **Transient visual loss** is an uncommon symptom in childhood. With epilepsy, there are almost invariably other symptoms at the time of the visual loss or a history of seizure immediately before the loss. Transient visual loss can be the aura of childhood migraine, although this aura is more common among older persons. Transient visual loss during headache should raise the possibility of a mass lesion causing increased intracranial pressure. A graying-out of vision can be part of a hyperventilation syndrome or presyncope.

2. **Episodic numbness or paresthesia.** Episodes of numbness may be the sole manifestation of a partial complex seizure and can occur as an aura in childhood migraine. Tingling of the hands or, less often, the feet, along with shortness of breath, suggests a hyperventilation syndrome.

3. **Vertigo** is differentiated from incipient syncope by rotational symptoms. An acute onset of vertigo that persists for more than 1 hour suggests the following: labyrinthitis; otitis media; drug exposure, including aminoglycosides, alcohol, anticonvulsants, hypnotics, tranquilizers, and aspirin; trauma causing an inner ear fistula; or tumors of the inner ear or the vestibular portion of the eighth cranial nerve. Recurrent episodes of vertigo suggest motion sickness, migraine, and epilepsy. Basilar artery migraine can cause vertigo and a throbbing occipital headache. Benign paroxysmal vertigo affects preschool children and causes brief episodes of vertigo not associated with alteration of consciousness or headache. Some of these children later have migraines. Partial complex seizures may start with vertigo as an aura followed by a brief alteration of consciousness. Paroxysmal positional vertigo following head trauma and Ménière's disease may be the cause of recurrent vertigo among adolescents but are rare among children.

Headache
I. Differential diagnosis
A. Acute headache
1. **Febrile children.** Headaches are commonly associated with systemic febrile illnesses and infectious processes involving the head and neck. With uveitis, the pain is periorbital, and with otitis media, the pain is in the temporal region. The pain of sinusitis may be localized directly over the sinus or may be more diffuse, usually in the frontal or retroorbital region. The pain should resolve within 3 days of starting appropriate antibiotic therapy. The combination of fever, headache, nuchal rigidity, and alteration in level of consciousness suggests meningitis. Other causes include cervical adenopathy and retropharyngeal abscess.
2. **Afebrile children.** In an afebrile child with normal findings at neurologic examination, an acute onset of headaches could be the beginning of childhood migraine or tension-type headache, but the diagnosis cannot be made without follow-up evaluation. Other possibilities include hypertensive headache, hydrocephalus, leukemic meningitis, and drug use. The drugs most often associated with headache are diet pills containing phenylpropanolamine and CNS stimulants such as amphetamines. Headache plus neurologic abnormalities suggests a mass lesion or subarachnoid hemorrhage. In children, subarachnoid hemorrhage usually is a result of head trauma, arteriovenous malformations and aneurysms being much less common causes.

B. Chronic headache
1. **Abnormal findings at neurologic examination.** Headache may be the first symptom experienced by children with increased intracranial pressure from mass lesions. Within 4 months of the onset of headaches, 90% of children with mass lesions have definite abnormalities at neurologic examination. If CT or MRI is normal, possibilities are chronic meningitis and pseudotumor cerebri (also called *idiopathic intracranial hypertension*). At lumbar puncture, the opening pressure is elevated in both chronic meningitis and pseudotumor cerebri; an abnormal cerebrospinal fluid cell count is present only in chronic meningitis. The usual symptoms of pseudotumor cerebri in children are headache, vomiting, diplopia, and blurred vision. Although this condition has been associated with several disorders, the most frequently encountered are cerebral venous thrombosis, otitis media or mastoiditis, corticosteroid use, thyroid dysfunction, vitamin A excess, and tetracycline use. Treatment is essential to prevent potential visual loss.
2. **Normal findings at neurologic examination.** The most common causes of chronic headache in children are migraine and tension-type headaches. Throbbing vascular-type headaches can be caused by hypertension and arteriovenous malformations. Nonvascular headaches can be caused by disorders of the nasal sinuses, the muscles of the head and neck, the cranial periosteum, or the cervical or cranial nerves. With acute sinusitis,

there may be frontal headaches or facial pain. With temporomandibular joint dysfunction, there may be temporal headaches, especially after eating. Occipital neuralgia causes lancinating pains starting in the neck and spreading to the top of the head. Ocular problems are relatively uncommon causes of frontal or temporal headaches. Increasingly severe headaches should prompt reevaluation of the diagnosis and consideration of a mass lesion as a possible cause.

II. **Classification and clinical manifestations of the most common chronic headaches**

   A. **Migraine** affects 2% to 5% of elementary school children and 5% to 10% of teenagers. Initially, the sex ratio is equal, but by the teenage years, twice as many girls are affected. More than 75% of children with migraine have a family history of this disorder. Common triggering factors are stress or excitement, sleep deprivation or excess, exercise, menstrual periods, upper respiratory tract infections, and skipping of meals. Migraine attacks can follow minor head trauma. Chocolate, nitrates or nitrites, monosodium glutamate, or dairy products occasionally trigger migraine headaches. In comparison with adults, children are less likely to have classic auras or unilateral headaches. They more commonly have bilateral throbbing frontal headaches with associated nausea and vomiting. Most children try to find a quiet, dark room and go to sleep to get rid of the headache. Cyclic vomiting and benign paroxysmal vertigo may be migraine equivalents in children. Younger children may have ophthalmoplegic migraine with ptosis and complete third-nerve palsy, including on occasion pupillary dilatation. Acute confusional migraine, a confusional state followed by throbbing headaches, is more common among teenagers. Adolescents may have basilar migraine with ataxia or other brainstem signs, including alterations in consciousness, followed by throbbing occipital headaches.

   B. **Tension-type headache**
      1. **Episodic tension-type headache** is probably the most common type of headache. The childhood form is similar to the adult form. Such headaches occur more often in the afternoon or evening and are associated with stress or with excessive exertion or fatigue. They can be occipital or frontal or involve the entire head and are described as a steady ache or sensation of pressure. They generally respond well to mild analgesics or rest.
      2. **Chronic tension-type headache** is similar in character to the episodic form but occurs daily for more than 180 days per year. Such headaches are not responsive to standard medications. They can be disabling and can cause excessive school absence. These headaches have been called *psychogenic headaches* in the past and are best considered a somatoform disorder. The "sick role" should be discouraged, and the child should be pushed to take part in normal activities. Instead of medication, self-relaxation techniques and behavioral therapies are used to help the child cope with these headaches.
      3. **Chronic daily headache** is not one of the classifications listed by the International Headache Society. The prevalence among children ranges from 0.5% to 1%. It can evolve from migraine or follow overuse of analgesics. As is found with chronic tension-type headache, there is a significant association with anxiety, depression, school phobia, and conduct disorders.

III. **Evaluation**
   A. **History.** Assessment of headaches involves a history of the headaches over time and a description of a typical individual headache. Important factors include changes in frequency or intensity, triggers, time of occurrence both seasonally and during the day, and factors that cause worsening or improvement during the headaches. The description of an individual headache includes prodrome, auras, location and quality of the pain, associated symptoms, and the postheadache period. If the child has more than one type of headache, a description of a typical headache should be solicited for each type.
   B. **Examination.** A complete neurologic examination is essential. In addition, tenderness over the sinuses, clicks in or misalignment of the temporomandibular joint, decreased visual acuity, and cervical lymphadenopathy are important eti-

ologic clues. Blood pressure must be recorded and auscultation of the skull performed for cranial bruits.
  C. **Diagnostic studies.** For typical headaches, little is needed. If the child has fever and a headache, studies are obtained to determine the source of the fever.
    1. Lumbar puncture should be performed if meningitis cannot be confidently excluded on the basis of the history and examination findings.
    2. For a child with an acute headache but no fever, MRI of the brain may be necessary. If imaging is not performed, follow-up evaluation is necessary to ensure that no signs of increased intracranial pressure are present. If the child has chronic headaches, neuroimaging is needed if the headaches worsen, if there are atypical features, if the child has complicated migraine, or if abnormal neurologic signs appear.
    3. EEG may be indicated for a child with confusional migraine or hemiplegic migraine.
    4. For the child with chronic tension-type headaches, eye and ear, nose and throat evaluations may be necessary. MRI of the brain may be needed to help assure the family that there is no life-threatening illness. Psychological testing may be helpful to determine appropriate therapy.

Enuresis
  I. Clinical description. Urinary continence usually is attained by 2 to 3 years of age. Occasional wetting during the first few years after toilet training is considered a normal variant. Nocturnal enuresis is a common problem that affects boys more than it does girls. Approximately 10% of 6-year-olds and 1% of 18-year-olds have nocturnal enuresis at least once per month.
  II. Evaluation
    A. **History.** A history of pain on urination, past urinary tract infections, trouble initiating or maintaining a forceful urinary stream, or chronic dribbling suggests disorders of the urinary tract. Back pain or difficulty walking may indicate a spinal cord or cauda equina lesion. Symptoms that can represent frontal cerebral dysfunction or nocturnal seizures include lethargy, apathy, or confusion the morning after the episode of enuresis. Headaches, visual loss, and growth disturbances suggest a frontal lobe lesion with a neurogenic bladder. A developmental evaluation is essential. A child with significant delays might be expected to be incontinent if the developmental level is less than $2\frac{1}{2}$ years of age.
    B. **Examination.** At physical examination, the presence of a fatty mass, tuft of hair, or hemangioma in the midline overlying the lower spine or a sacral dimple often signals the presence of a tethered cord or a lipoma involving the cauda equina. In addition, absence of ankle jerks or weakness in the muscles of the feet suggests cord lesions. Observing the urinary stream may help diagnose anomalies of the urinary system.
    C. **Diagnostic studies**
      1. Urinalysis and urine culture are necessary.
      2. MRI of the lumbosacral spine should be performed if there is any indication of cord problems. MRI of the head should be performed if there is a suggestion of hydrocephalus or mass lesion involving the frontal lobe.
      3. EEG should be performed if there are additional symptoms or signs of nocturnal seizures.
      4. Intravenous pyelography and cystoscopy should be performed if there has been a history of urinary tract infection or if there are signs or symptoms of anomalies involving the urinary tract.
  III. Differential diagnosis. In most cases, enuresis is best considered a developmental problem and not a true illness. Fewer than 5% of children with enuresis have organic lesions. Enuresis sometimes is associated with transient regression following hospitalization, the absence of a parent, or the birth of a new sibling or with excess rigidity or battles between parent and child over the establishment of toilet control.

Motor Disorders
Many motor disorders that occur among children are similar to those that occur among adults. This section discusses disorders that occurring only or predominantly among children.

I. Motor development. The following are the average ages for reaching motor milestones.

2 months: lifts head for several seconds while prone, hands usually fisted
4 months: head steady while in sitting position, reaches and grasps objects
6 months: rolls prone to supine, transfers objects hand to hand
10 months: sits without support, thumb and two finger grasp
12 months: walks, pincher grasp
18 months: climbs stairs with help, feeds self and throws toys
24 months: runs, balances on one foot for 1 second, builds tower of 4 to 6 blocks
3 years: walks on toes and heels, balances for 5 seconds, alternating movements performed slowly
4 years: walks with arms still at side, smooth finger-to-nose movement, draws square
5 years: walks with limited arm swing, smooth and accurate finger-to-nose movement, balances for 10 seconds
6 years: balances for 13 to 16 seconds, unsteady heel-to-knee movement, awkward, rapid alternating movements
8 years: balances more than 20 seconds, smooth rapid alternating movements
9 years: no mirror movements

II. Weakness. The causes of weakness are similar for children and adults. The differential of weakness among adults is presented in Chapter 30. A major area of difference is in children younger than 1 year. A child with hypotonia and weakness often is called a *floppy infant.* The causative lesion may be located anywhere from brain to muscle.

    A. Evaluation

        1. History. The diagnosis may be suggested by the presence of similar neuromuscular disorders in other family members, by known asphyxia or seizures at birth, or by complications of delivery. Lethargy or poor responsiveness indicates CNS dysfunction. Variations in the degree of weakness may occur in neuromuscular junction disorders.

        2. Examination. The presence of brisk or normal reflexes and fisting are clues to CNS damage. Dysmorphic features and organomegaly also indicate possible CNS dysfunction. A level with normal function proximally and weakness distally occurs with spinal cord damage. Disorders of the lower motor unit cause depressed to absent reflexes. Fasciculations may be seen in the tongue but are harder to find in the extremities. Joint contractures (arthrogryposis) can accompany both upper and lower motor unit lesions. Examination of the mother can be helpful. A diagnosis of myotonic muscular dystrophy or myasthenia gravis can be made easier in the mother.

        3. Diagnostic studies

            a. Creatine kinase level is elevated in inflammatory and rapidly progressive muscular dystrophy.

            b. Electromyography and nerve conduction studies help differentiate neuropathy, neuromuscular junction disorders, and myopathy. With myasthenia gravis, there is an improvement in strength after administration of neostigmine (0.02 to 0.04 mg/kg per dose) or edrophonium chloride (0.1 to 0.2 mg/kg per dose).

            c. Muscle biopsy is necessary for adequate diagnosis of myopathy.

            d. Specific DNA probes can be used for many disorders. Current examples include Duchenne and Becker muscular dystrophy, myotonic dystropy, spinal muscular atrophy, and Prader–Willi syndrome. Additional specific DNA tests are becoming available regularly.

    B. Causes of floppy infant syndrome

        1. Central hypotonia

            a. Acquired central hypotonia. Infants who have ischemic or hypoxic damage in the perinatal period and who are destined to have cerebral palsy may be hypotonic and weak. Increased tone first appears distally and may cause persistent fisting of the hands. At the same time, there is decreased truncal tone, causing poor head control. There are steady increases in reflexes, tone, and strength. Spinal cord lesions may be associated with complicated breech delivery.

   b. **Chromosomal anomalies and metabolic–degenerative disorders.**
   Hypotonia with mild weakness is a feature of Down syndrome and of
   Prader–Willi syndrome. Weakness and hypotonia may be prominent in
   early-onset disorders such as GM_1 gangliosidosis and Zellweger syndrome (cerebrohepatorenal syndrome).
2. **Lower motor unit disorders**
   a. **Anterior horn cell disorders.** Acute infantile spinal muscular atrophy
   (Werdnig–Hoffmann disease) and chronic infantile spinal muscular atrophy are degenerative disorders that manifest as profound weakness, areflexia, and fasciculations in the tongue. Both are progressive. The acute
   form leads to death in 1 year. The chronic form often stabilizes for long
   periods, allowing some children to live into the young adult years. A neurogenic form of arthrogryposis manifests as weakness, areflexia, and joint
   contractures and usually is not associated with progressive weakness.
   b. **Neuropathy** is rare among young children. Neuropathy can be a component of diffuse leukodystrophy or result from Guillain–Barré syndrome. Familial dysautonomia (Riley–Day syndrome) causes failure to
   thrive, hypotonia, decreased reflexes, and absence of tears. The diagnosis can be confirmed by the absence of the flare response to intradermal
   administration of histamine.
   c. **Neuromuscular junction disorders.** Transient neonatal myasthenia
   occurs among infants whose mothers have myasthenia gravis. The
   infant's weakness resolves over 4 to 6 weeks. There are several congenital myasthenic syndromes in which ptosis, ophthalmoplegia, breathing
   or feeding trouble, and generalized weakness begin in the first 2 years
   of life. Referral to a research center is necessary for exact diagnosis.
   Infant botulism causes a similar signs and symptoms with the additional
   findings of nonreactive or poorly reactive pupils, constipation, poor feeding, and hypotonia. The diagnosis is confirmed with identification of
   Clostridium botulinum organisms and botulinus toxin in the feces.
   d. **Myopathy.** Many different disorders of the muscles occur among children, and referral to a specialized clinic is often warranted. Duchenne
   muscular dystrophy begins by 2 to 3 years of age with hip weakness,
   enlarged calves, and marked elevation of serum level of creatine kinase.
   Congenital myopathy, diagnosed on the basis of changes found at muscle biopsy (e.g., nemaline rod, central core, and myotubular myopathy),
   may manifest as pronounced weakness in the neonatal period or with
   very slowly progressive hip and shoulder weakness. Pompe's disease, a
   glycogen storage disease, starts in the first few months of life with both
   weakness and cardiac failure. Some forms of mitochondrial myopathy
   are associated with cardiac disease. A severe form of myotonic muscular
   dystrophy can begin in the neonatal period in an infant who has the gene
   for this disorder and whose mother is affected. The infant has both weakness and mental retardation.
   e. **Connective tissue disorders.** Children with Ehlers–Danlos syndrome
   and those with Marfan syndrome have hypotonia with normal reflexes
   and normal or only mildly diminished strength.
III. **Ataxia**
   A. **Definition.** Ataxia is impairment of balance and incoordination of volitional
   movement. Sensory ataxia involves disruption of the vestibular connections to
   the caudal vermis of the cerebellum or sensory pathways in the spinal cord con-
   necting to the brainstem and cerebellum. Motor ataxia is observed in association
   with cerebellar damage or damage to the frontopontocerebellar fibers.
   B. **Evaluation**
      1. **History.** The first step is assessment of the course of the ataxia. Ataxia can
      be initially divided into acute onset, chronic progressive, chronic nonprogres-
      sive, and intermittent forms. A history of recent infection or exposure to tox-
      ins is helpful in evaluating acute ataxia. Symptoms of increased intracranial
      pressure and a family history of ataxia may be found in chronic progressive

ataxia. Patients with chronic nonprogressive ataxia may have a history of trauma, meningitis, lead poisoning, or hypoglycemia. Intermittent ataxia can be caused by seizures, migraine, or metabolic disorders.

2. **Examination.** Damage to a cerebellar hemisphere produces ipsilateral limb ataxia and nystagmus. Damage to the rostral vermis causes gait and truncal ataxia. Involvement of sensory pathways in the spinal cord is indicated by a Romberg sign.

3. **Diagnostic studies.** CT or MRI should be performed in most cases of acute ataxia and all cases of chronic ataxia. Patients with acute ataxia need toxicology screens, lumbar puncture, and tests for urinary catecholamines. Metabolic studies that can be helpful in evaluations of children with chronic ataxia include tests for urinary amino acids and serum levels of ammonia, vitamins A and E, cholesterol, triglycerides, lipoproteins, cholestanol, phytanic acid, and biotin. DNA testing is available for Friedreich's ataxia and many forms of spinocerebellar ataxia. Children with episodic ataxia need EEG and measurement of blood lactate and pyruvate and urinary amino acids during the attack if at all possible.

C. **Causes of ataxia among children**
   1. **Acute-onset ataxia**
      a. **Intoxication.** Ataxia can follow ingestion of alcohol, sedative drugs, or anticonvulsants.
      b. **Infection.** Ataxia can be acute or occur during recovery from bacterial meningitis. Viral cerebellitis has been associated with mumps and the enteric viruses. Postinfectious cerebellar ataxia may occur at the end of a course of chickenpox. The prognosis is excellent, most patients recovering completely. Ataxia also can be a prominent part of Fisher's syndrome, a variant of Guillain–Barré syndrome.
      c. **Paraneoplastic disorders.** Relatively acute ataxia can accompany neuroblastoma. The patient has a combination of ataxia, opsoclonus, and myoclonus. The tumor may be found in the abdomen or mediastinum.
   2. **Chronic progressive ataxia**
      a. **Tumors.** The posterior fossa is the most common location of brain tumors in children. A child with medulloblastoma has headaches, vomiting, and gait ataxia. A child with a cerebellar astrocytoma usually has ipsilateral limb ataxia and a good prognosis for cure. Brainstem glioma causes a combination of cranial nerve palsy, spasticity, and ataxia. Hydrocephalus can cause progressive gait unsteadiness.
      b. **Degenerative disorders.** A large number of hereditary forms of ataxia may necessitate referral to a specialty center for diagnosis. One of the more common is Friedreich's ataxia. It begins at the end of the first decade of life and causes scoliosis and pes cavus, truncal ataxia, decreased reflexes, and reduced vibratory and position senses in the legs. Ataxia–telangiectasia is an autosomal recessive disorder. Ataxia develops first, and by 3 to 6 years of age, the child has telangiectasia. The patient has frequent infections and low levels of immunoglobulins A and E.
      c. **Metabolic disorders.** Ataxia, abdominal pain, and failure to thrive as a result of fat malabsorption are symptoms of abetalipoproteinemia. Wilson's disease can cause ataxia, dystonia, learning and behavioral disturbances, and hepatic damage. Other metabolic disorders causing ataxia include vitamin E deficiency, biotin-responsive multiple carboxylase deficiency, and urea cycle defects.
   3. **Chronic nonprogressive ataxia**
      a. **Malformations** include the Dandy–Walker malformation (dilatation of the fourth ventricle and hypoplasia of the cerebellar vermis), Chiari type I malformation (downward displacement of the cerebellar tonsils), and Joubert's syndrome (vermal agenesis, hyperpnea, pendular eye movements, and delay).
      b. **Acquired cerebellar damage.** Ataxia can follow head trauma or meningitis. It has also been reported as a sequela of severe hypoglycemia

and lead poisoning. With ataxic cerebral palsy, there usually is spasticity or dystonia, and ataxia.

  c. **Clumsy child syndrome** is also called **developmental dyspraxia** or, in the *Diagnostic and Statistical Manual of Mental Disorders, 4th Edition (DSM-IV)*, **developmental coordination disorder.** These children have poor handwriting and trouble dressing. They run awkwardly and fall frequently. Their poor performance in sports may lead to a lowering of self-esteem.

 4. **Intermittent ataxia**

  a. **Migraine.** Basilar artery migraine occurs most often among adolescent girls. Ataxia, vertigo, and vomiting may last from minutes to several hours. There is usually a throbbing occipital headache associated with the ataxia.

  b. **Metabolic disorders** are rare. The intermittent form of maple syrup urine disease causes intermittent ataxia, is diagnosed by finding branched chain keto acids in the urine, and is managed with thiamine. Other examples include acetazolamide-responsive familial periodic ataxia associated with mutations in either potassium or calcium channel genes, urea cycle defects, and Hartnup disease, a disorder of amino acid transport.

  c. **Epilepsy.** In rare instances, either partial complex or generalized seizures have ataxia as a major sign, usually accompanied by clouding of consciousness or clonic movements.

IV. Chorea

 A. **Definition and evaluation.** See Chapter 28.

 B. **Causes of chorea among children**

 1. **Acute-onset chorea.** Intoxication with stimulants, anticonvulsants, oral contraceptives, antihistamines, lithium, and the phenothiazines can cause chorea. Chorea can occur after infarction of the basal ganglia and can follow surgical procedures in which deep hypothermia is used.

 2. **Subacute onset of chorea.** Sydenham's chorea follows streptococcal infections by several weeks. Chorea, hypotonia, and emotional lability develop slowly. Recovery can take months. Chorea can be a symptom of childhood lupus, endocrine disorders including hyperthyroidism and Addison's disease, and tumors involving the basal ganglia.

 3. **Chronic chorea.** Static chorea and athetosis following kernicterus are now relatively uncommon. Progressive chorea may be observed with Lesch–Nyhan syndrome, chorea acanthocytosis, juvenile Huntington's disease, and ataxia-telangiectasia.

V. Tics

 A. **Definition and evaluation.** See Chapter 28.

 B. **Etiology**

 1. **Isolated tics.** Tics are common among children. Approximately 25% of children have tics, usually involving facial muscles and lasting for more than 1 month but less than 1 year. Chronic motor tics, which last for more than 1 year, are uncommon, and are thought by some experts to be a variant of Tourette's disorder.

 2. **Tourette's disorder** is common, affecting 4 to 5 children per 10,000. It is an autosomal dominant disorder of varying severity and affects boys more often than it does girls. Tourette's disorder usually begins as a motor tic involving facial muscles. These first symptoms appear between 4 and 7 years of age. With time, the child has multiple motor tics and vocalizations consisting of throat-clearing sounds, coughing, snorting, barking, or multiple other odd sounds. Coprolalia, part of the original description, is relatively rare among children but can be debilitating when present. Behavioral problems often are more disruptive than tics. These children have a high incidence of attention-deficit problems, obsessive–compulsive disorder (OCD), and emotional lability. The tics change with time, reaching peak intensity at approximately 11 to 12 years of age. The severity of tics then progressively

decreases, two thirds becoming asymptomatic or much improved by the end of adolescence.

3. **Pediatric autoimmune neuropsychiatric disorders associated with streptococcal infection (PANDAS)** is a new diagnosis. The children have episodic tics or OCD with abrupt onset or exacerbations of symptoms associated with streptococcal infection.

VI. Dystonia

A. **Definition and evaluation.** See Chapter 28.

B. **Causes of childhood dystonia**

1. **Acute dystonia.** Phenothiazine exposure is the most common cause of acute dystonia, although cases have been associated with exposure to lithium, antihistamines, and anticonvulsants. Acute torticollis may follow trauma to muscles in the neck and may accompany cervical adenitis or retropharyngeal abscess.

2. **Chronic dystonia**

   a. **Isolated torticollis.** Congenital torticollis suggests an anomaly of the cervical spinal column or fibrosis following hematoma in the sternocleidomastoid muscle. Acquired torticollis may result from bone abnormalities including tumor, infection, subluxation, and basilar impression, from superior oblique muscle palsy, or from tumors of the cerebellum or spinal cord.

   b. **Generalized dystonia.** Torsion dystonia is a familial disorder that most often begins in the feet and progresses over months or years to involve the rest of the body. A child with hemiplegia may have dystonia in the involved extremity. Dystonia can be a part of Wilson's disease, Hallervorden–Spatz syndrome, and Niemann–Pick disease type C.

   c. **Paroxysmal dystonic choreoathetosis** is an autosomal dominant disorder with abnormal movements lasting up to a few hours.

Abnormal Head Size, Scoliosis, and Neurocutaneous Disorders

I. **Abnormal head size**

A. **Definition.** Macrocephaly is defined as a head size greater than the ninety-eighth percentile and microcephaly as a head size less than the second percentile.

B. **Etiology**

1. **Macrocephaly.** In familial macrocephaly, one parent has a head size greater than the ninety-eighth percentile. In these cases, the child's development and neurologic examination usually are normal. In rare instances, bone overgrowth in chronic anemia or cranioskeletal dysplasia can cause macrocephaly. Chronic subdural effusion following trauma or meningitis causes enlargement of the head, as do all forms of progressive hydrocephalus. The most common forms of hydrocephalus are communicating hydrocephalus from obstruction of the arachnoid villi, obstruction at the fourth ventricle in Dandy–Walker malformation, and lateral and third ventricular enlargement from aqueductal stenosis. Megalencephaly results from storage diseases that cause progressive retardation and macrocephaly. In the first year of life, large supratentorial tumors can cause macrocephaly from the bulk of the tumor.

2. **Microcephaly.** If the small head size is proportional to the body size, endocrine disorders or syndromes (see Jones KL, *Smith's Recognizable Patterns of Human Malformation*) should be suspected. Premature closure of the sutures, craniosynostosis, may prevent appropriate brain growth and, when multiple sutures are involved, necessitates surgical correction. Primary failure of brain growth can be familial, either autosomal dominant with mild delay or autosomal recessive with more severe delay, or can be the result of a chromosomal anomaly. Acquired brain damage with subsequent microcephaly can follow intrauterine infection, hypoxia or ischemia, trauma, or postnatal CNS infection.

C. **Evaluation**

1. **History.** Developmental delay is expected with congenital and static problems, and progressive loss of milestones is characteristic of storage disorders

and evolving mass lesions. Symptoms of increased intracranial pressure, headache, irritability, vomiting, and lethargy can accompany pancraniosynostosis, hydrocephalus, and tumors.

2. **Examination.** Both the child's and the parents' head sizes are measured. Serial measurement can be helpful. A head size that continues to parallel the normal curve is less worrisome, whereas a head size that crosses percentiles is of more concern. A bulging fontanel, widened sutures, failure of upgaze, and hyperactive reflexes are signs of increased intracranial pressure. Areas of abnormal retinal pigmentation on funduscopic examination suggest intrauterine infection as a cause of microcephaly.

3. **Diagnostic studies.** CT or MRI should be performed on almost all children with abnormal head size to assess brain structure. CT with bone windows can be used to evaluate sutures in a child with microcephaly. Chromosomal studies are performed if there are dysmorphic features or brain malformations. Metabolic studies are needed if there are megalencephaly and progressive loss of milestones.

II. Scoliosis

A. **Definition.** Scoliosis is defined as abnormal curvature of the spine. In children, it is idiopathic in approximately 70% of cases.

B. **Clinical manifestations.** In practice, scoliosis may first be found during a routine screening examination, often performed in schools or as a part of well child care, or may be detected during regular examinations of children at risk of scoliosis. Examples of the latter are children with cerebral palsy, various neuromuscular disorders, and neurofibromatosis.

C. **Etiology**

1. **Abnormalities of bone.** Congenital anomalies such as hemivertebra or fused ribs can cause early-onset scoliosis. Diastematomyelia is a congenital midline bone spur that can cause both scoliosis and spinal cord dysfunction below the level of the lesion. Sharp angulation of the spinal column resulting from bone anomaly may be associated with neurofibromatosis.

2. **Lower motor unit disorders.** Scoliosis can be a complication of myopathy. The diagnosis is suggested by associated weakness and can be confirmed with muscle biopsy. Progressive scoliosis can contribute to increasing respiratory insufficiency. Scoliosis also can accompany neuropathy such as peroneal muscular atrophy (Charcot–Marie–Tooth disease) or postpolio syndrome.

3. **CNS disorders.** Scoliosis is a frequent finding among children with spastic quadriparetic, athetoid, or dystonic cerebral palsy. It can become a fixed deficit in children with torsion dystonia, and it is observed in spinocerebellar ataxia. Spinal cord tumors and syringomyelia can manifest as scoliosis, lower motor unit signs at the level of the lesion, and spasticity below the level of the lesion.

4. **Idiopathic scoliosis** most often affects adolescent girls, with a girl-to-boy ratio of approximately 8:1. The findings at neurologic examination are otherwise normal, and patients can be observed with regular examinations.

D. **Evaluation**

1. **History.** Back pain, bowel or bladder problems, and leg or foot weakness suggest spinal cord involvement and necessitate immediate evaluation. Progressive weakness or clumsiness indicates a neuromuscular disorder or spinocerebellar degeneration.

2. **Examination.** The screening examination starts with the child standing straight. Scoliosis can cause tilting of the hips or unequal heights of the shoulders. With the child bending forward to touch the toes, there may be a hump over the ribs on one side. A midline patch of hair or a mass over the spinal column suggests diastematomyelia. Café-au-lait spots are a sign of neurofibromatosis. A complete neurologic examination is essential because of the multiple levels of involvement that can be associated with scoliosis.

3. **Diagnostic studies.** The basic screening tool is a posteroanterior radiograph of the spine. Any suggestion of a spinal cord lesion at neurologic examination or the presence of bowel or bladder dysfunction should lead

to MRI of the spine. If the child has diffuse weakness or decreased tendon reflexes, electromyography, nerve conduction studies, and muscle biopsy may be needed.

III. **Neurocutaneous disorders.** In neurocutaneous disorders, there is both skin and brain involvement. The two most common disorders are neurofibromatosis, with a prevalence of 1 case per 5,000 persons, and tuberous sclerosis, with a prevalence of 1 case per 25,000 persons.

A. **Neurofibromatosis type 1 (NF1)**

1. **Definition.** NF1 (von Recklinghausen's disease) is an autosomal dominant disorder with a gene locus on chromosome 17. Approximately 50% of cases are new mutations. Using the National Institutes of Health criteria, one can make a diagnosis of NF1 if there are two or more of the following seven items: café-au-lait spots, neurofibromas, axillary freckling, characteristic bone anomalies, optic nerve glioma, iris (Lisch) nodules, and a definite diagnosis of NF1 in a first-degree relative.

2. **Evaluation**

   a. **History.** In one half of cases, there is a family history of NF1, although determining such a history may require asking about birthmarks and tumors as well as neurofibromatosis. Approximately one half of children with NF1 have mild delay or learning disabilities. A history of constipation and headaches is common. A history of decreased vision or growth problems suggests optic nerve glioma.

   b. **Examination.** Isolated café-au-lait spots are common in the normal population. Children with NF1 have six or more spots at least 5 mm in diameter. The café-au-lait spots are found most often on the trunk. The freckling in NF1 is in the axillary and inguinal regions. Plexiform neurofibromas are ropy cords of tumor that can lead to distortion of involved structures. Dermal neurofibromas are soft tumors with purplish or red discoloration of the overlying skin. Kyphoscoliosis occurs in 2% of patients with NF1, and pseudoarthrosis occurs in 0.5% to 1%. Hypertension can result from renal arterial stenosis or pheochromocytoma. Repeated neurologic examinations are needed to watch for CNS tumors. A slit-lamp examination by an ophthalmologist is needed to find iris hamartomas (Lisch nodules).

   c. **Diagnostic studies.** If there is a family history of neurofibromatosis, chromosomal studies can be used for early diagnosis. MRI is performed if there is any suggestion of CNS dysfunction or any change in visual acuity that suggests optic nerve glioma. Areas of increased signal intensity often are found in the basal ganglion at MRI of the brain in children with NF1. If there is evidence of developmental delay or academic underachievement, the child needs psychological assessment for learning disability.

3. **Natural history.** A child with NF1 may have café-au-lait spots, plexiform neurofibroma, or glaucoma in infancy; increased head size, pseudoarthrosis, and growth delay in the toddler years; iris nodules, freckling, learning disabilities, headaches, and constipation in the elementary school years; and neurofibromas, scoliosis, and hypertension in the adolescent years.

4. **Differential diagnosis.** Four or fewer café-au-lait spots may be a normal variant. Café-au-lait spots may be seen in children with Noonan syndrome or Watson syndrome. Single neurofibroma and optic nerve glioma may be observed in children without other evidence of NF1. If a child comes to medical attention during infancy with more than café-au-lait spots, there is a 50% to 60% chance that additional signs of NF1 will develop.

B. **Neurofibromatosis type 2 (NF2)** is an autosomal dominant disorder with a gene locus on chromosome 22. It is much less common than NF1. The primary features are schwannomas involving the vestibular portion of the eighth cranial nerve and meningiomas and gliomas in the CNS. Café-au-lait spots are fewer in NF2 than in NF1. Symptoms develop more often in the adolescent or young adult years.

C. Tuberous sclerosis
  1. **Definition.** Primary features of tuberous sclerosis are facial angiofibromas, ungual fibromas, hypomelanotic macules, shagreen patch, cortical tubers, subependymal nodules, subependymal giant cell astrocytoma, cardiac rhabdomyoma, renal angiomyolipomas, lymphangiomyomatosis, and retinal hamartomas. Gene loci are found on chromosomes 9q34 and 16p13.3.
  2. **Evaluation**
      a. **History.** Children with tuberous sclerosis are at increased risk of seizures, autism, or developmental delay. Delay is most common among children with tuberous sclerosis who have infantile spasms or partial seizures with an onset before the child is 2 years of age.
      b. **Examination.** The skin lesion of tuberous sclerosis are hypopigmented macules, angiofibromas over the bridge of the nose, and shagreen patches, which are raised, thickened, leathery lesions found most often on the trunk. Signs of increased intracranial pressure suggest giant cell astrocytoma at the intraventricular foramen (foramen of Monro). Cardiac failure is observed in association with cardiac rhabdomyoma. An abdominal mass or hypertension may accompany angiomyolipoma of the kidney and renal cysts.
      c. **Diagnostic studies.** CT scan is effective in depicting the calcified periventricular nodules of tuberous sclerosis and can show the giant cell astrocytoma that can cause hydrocephalus. MRI is more effective than is CT in delineating cortical tubers. Renal function studies and renal ultrasonography are used for detecting the possible renal tumors or polycystic changes of tuberous sclerosis. Echocardiographic findings establish the diagnosis of cardiac rhabdomyoma. DNA probes are available at research centers and can be found through the Tuberous Sclerosis Alliance (*www.tsalliance.org*).
  3. **Natural history.** Cardiac tumors, hypopigmented macules, infantile spasms, and delay can occur in the first year of life. Hydrocephalus from giant cell astrocytoma can occur at any time. Renal complications occur more often in the adolescent years. The facial angiofibromas usually are present by the elementary school years.
  4. **Differential diagnosis.** Band heterotopia can be differentiated from subependymal nodules by the continuous nature of the band heterotopia and the more isolated nodules of tuberous sclerosis. Familial polycystic kidneys occur in families with no other signs of tuberous sclerosis.
D. Other neurocutaneous disorders
  1. **Vascular skin lesions.** Sturge–Weber syndrome consists of a port-wine-colored stain involving the upper eyelid and other areas of the face and a hemangioma of the ipsilateral surface of the brain that causes seizures and contralateral hemiplegia. In Klippel–Trénaunay–Weber syndrome, there are cavernous hemangiomas and hypertrophy of the extremity under the hemangiomas. Telangiectasis starting first on the conjunctiva and later involving the face, neck, elbows, and knees is a sign of ataxia–telangiectasia.
  2. **Pigmentary changes.** Incontinentia pigmenti manifests as linear, whorled, hyperpigmented skin lesions, and, in 20% to 30% of affected children, alopecia and seizures, delay, and spasticity. In hypomelanosis of Ito, there are linear streaks of hypopigmentation and, in 75% of cases, seizures and delay. A linear hyperkeratotic, verrucous, hyperpigmented nevus appears on the forehead in the linear sebaceous nevus sequence. These children often have seizures, delay, and ipsilateral brain malformation.
  3. **Neurotrichosis (hair anomalies).** Menkes syndrome is an X-linked recessive disorder with seizures, hypertonia, brain infarcts, and short, coarse, easily broken hair. Serum levels of copper and ceruloplasmin are low. Other disorders with hair abnormalities include biotin deficiency, argininosuccinicaciduria, and Pollitt syndrome. All three are characterized by seizures, delay, and alopecia or easily broken hair.

Behavioral Disorders
 I. Definitions. Behavioral disorders are common in the practice of child neurology. Children with the most common neurologic disorders are at increased risk of behavioral trouble. Approximately 25% to 35% of children with epilepsy may have problems such as attention deficit hyperactivity disorder, depression, and learning difficulties. Children with migraines and chronic tension-type headaches seem to have an increased prevalence of depression and anxiety. Some disorders, such as adrenoleukodystrophy, may manifest as learning and behavioral disorders. In other disorders, the behavioral component may seem to be the main problem. Examples include the case of a child with tuberous sclerosis and severe autism and that of a child with Tourette's disorder who has well-controlled tics but severe problems with attention and emotional lability.
 II. Autistic disorder
  A. Definition. In *DSM-IV,* autistic disorder is defined as a combination of impairment in social interaction, impairment in communication, and a restricted, repetitive, stereotyped pattern of behavior, interests, or activities that begins before 3 years of age and cannot be more appropriately classified as another pervasive developmental disorder.
  B. Clinical manifestations
   1. Social interaction. Autistic children do not develop normal awareness of others, empathy, and adequate peer interactions.
   2. Communication. Speech may be very delayed, or the child may be mute. Echolalia is common.
   3. Unusual behaviors. A child with autistic disorder has repetitive stereotypical behaviors, unusual preoccupations, and an inflexible adherence to routine.
  C. Evaluation
   1. History. After the various components of autistic disorder are delineated, the history should be reviewed for neurologic disorders, such as fragile X syndrome and tuberous sclerosis, that have been associated with autism and for complications such as mental retardation (observed in 75% of children with autism) and seizures (observed in 25%).
   2. Examination. Dysmorphic features, skin lesions, and CNS abnormalities may suggest an underlying brain disorder that might be the cause of autistic disorder. Children with autistic disorder on average have larger heads than do unaffected siblings. During the examination, a child with autistic disorder may have poor eye contact, trouble using speech for conversation, hyperactivity, and unusual play or interests.
   3. Diagnostic studies. If the child has delay in language, a hearing screen should be performed. Use of structured observation instruments such as the Childhood Autism Rating Scale is helpful in diagnosis. The child should be referred to a psychologist for cognitive evaluation. The basic laboratory studies should include complete blood cell count, thyroid function studies, measurement of glucose, electrolytes, and ammonia, urine studies for amino acids and organic acids, chromosomal analysis, neuroimaging, and EEG.
  D. Differential diagnosis. A child with mental retardation has communication and social skills commensurate with his or her level of development. Rett's disorder is differentiated from autism by regression beginning at 6 to 9 months of age. Rett's disorder affects only girls, causes loss of hand function, and leads to an acquired microcephaly. Asperger's disorder is thought by some to be a mild form of autism in which there is impaired social interaction and abnormal patterns of behavior with normal language and cognitive development. With disintegrative psychosis, there is a definite regression beginning after 2 years of age.
 III. Attention deficit hyperactivity disorder (ADHD)
  A. Definition. In *DSM-IV,* ADHD is defined as symptoms of inattention, hyperactivity, and impulsiveness that start before 7 years of age and are exhibited both at home and at school. The symptoms cause considerable impairment and are not caused by any other psychiatric disorder.
  B. Clinical description. Younger children with ADHD usually come to medical attention with hyperactivity. They fidget and squirm, have trouble remaining

seated, run instead of walk, and may be described as driven by a motor. They are noisy, talk excessively, and constantly interrupt parents and teachers. They alienate peers by their inability to wait their turn. During the elementary school years, problems with attention become obvious. The children have trouble paying attention in school, make frequent careless errors, and are easily distracted. They have poor organization and difficulty finishing tasks. They are forgetful and often lose books, homework, and clothes. Some children have only inattention and not hyperactivity. Oppositional defiant disorder, conduct disorder, and learning disorders often are comorbid conditions.

C. **Evaluation**
1. **History.** The time of onset of the disorder is important. Problems of temperament begin in the first months of life, and ADHD more often begins around 3 to 4 years of age. Barbiturates, benzodiazepines, and theophylline can cause symptoms of hyperactivity. Symptoms of sadness, fearfulness, or anxiety suggest other psychiatric causes of the attention deficit. A developmental assessment is needed, because children with mental retardation and pervasive developmental disorders may have inattention and hyperactivity as a component of the disorders.
2. **Examination.** The findings at neurologic examination may be normal or may show "soft signs." Soft signs are developmental findings that are normal at one age but abnormal at a later stage of development. They are often inconsistent and are of concern only if they fit an overall pattern of delay.
3. **Diagnostic studies.** Basic chemistries are seldom helpful. Some researchers have noted changes in results of thyroid function studies in a few children with ADHD, and elevated lead levels have been found occasionally. EEG and neuroimaging are indicated only if additional abnormalities are found at examination. Standardized rating scales help with diagnosis and monitoring of response to medication. Computerized continuous performance tasks can help the assessing response to medication.

D. **Differential diagnosis.** A normally active child may appear hyperactive to an excessively strict, controlled parent or to an overly rigid school system. This is particularly true for children with an active temperament—a congenital style of behavior that is a source of distress when the child's fit with the environment is poor. Symptoms of ADHD that are present only in one setting should suggest problems in that area. The child with symptoms only at school may be incorrectly placed, being either too advanced for the class or too far behind to keep up. If the ADHD is present only at home, a chaotic home environment or stresses within the family should be considered. Other psychiatric disorders to consider in the differential diagnosis include anxiety disorders, depression, pervasive developmental disorders, and substance abuse.

IV. **Anxiety disorders**
A. **Definition.** The anxiety disorders most often seen by a child neurologist are OCD and posttraumatic stress disorder (PTSD). OCD is defined by recurrent obsession and compulsions that cause distress or impairment. In PTSD, a child who has been exposed to an event involving injury or death, begins reexperiencing the event, avoids reminders of the episode or becomes withdrawn, and has chronically increased arousal.

B. **Clinical manifestations**
1. **OCD.** A child neurologist usually diagnoses OCD when assessing a child with Tourette's disorder. Common obsessions include a need to have things exactly right, a demand for sameness, and intrusive aggressive or sexual thoughts. Common compulsions include touching or tapping, arranging objects symmetrically, counting, and repeating acts.
2. **PTSD.** A child with PTSD may have vivid recurring nightmares or intrusive memories that occur during the daytime and may be mistaken for seizures or dissociation. The avoidant behavior may consist of an inability to recall the traumatic event, a decreased interest in people or activities, and emotional numbing. Increased arousal causes an exaggerated startle, poor sleep, and trouble concentrating.

    C. Examination. Both OCD and PTSD are found during a mental status examination. Children seldom volunteer information about obsessions and compulsions. Ask about thoughts they cannot get rid of and things they have to do to prevent becoming anxious. Compulsions can be difficult to differentiate from complex motor tics. If suppression of the act results in increasing anxiety, the behavior is more likely a compulsion. Children with PTSD may describe the nightmares, trouble sleeping, and frightening memories. Parents are more likely to describe the array of compulsions seen in OCD and the change in behavior seen in PTSD.

V. Depression
    A. Definition. In *DSM-IV,* a major depressive episode is defined by at least five of the following symptoms: depressed or irritable mood, decreased interest or pleasure in usual activities, weight loss or gain, sleep disturbance, agitation or retardation, fatigue, feeling of guilt or worthlessness, trouble concentrating, and suicidal thoughts. The symptoms must be present for at least 2 weeks and cause distress or impairment.

    B. Clinical manifestations. Children with epilepsy, migraine or chronic tension-type headaches, and newly acquired neurologic deficits are at risk of depression. Irritability, withdrawal, school failure, and sleep disturbance are common among children with depression. Suicidal ideation and guilt are more common among adolescents.

Referrals

Much of the assessment and follow-up care of children with delayed development can be performed by a family practitioner or pediatrician. It is often necessary to refer the patient to a psychologist for specific intellectual and achievement testing and to have vision and hearing screening performed. If a progressive form of retardation develops, we suggest referral to a child neurologist or a geneticist, because many of these disorders are rare and difficult to diagnose. A child neurologist or geneticist also may have new information about possible therapies for these disorders.

A child with nonepileptiform paroxysmal events (such as headaches) or enuresis can undergo evaluation and follow-up care with the primary physician. We refer such a patient to a child neurologist only if the diagnosis is unclear or the child does not respond to conventional treatment.

Because of the multitude of disorders that can cause motor problems in childhood, we suggest referral for an initial evaluation in all cases of progressive motor disorders and for most cases of static disorders. Many disorders of acute onset can be rapidly diagnosed and do not have to be evaluated by a child neurologist. For chronic and progressive conditions, a child neurologist may be able to make beneficial suggestions for treatment.

For children with microcephaly or macrocephaly, an initial evaluation should provide clues to directions for referral. Children with hydrocephalus or craniosynostosis need referral to a neurosurgeon. If there are dysmorphic features, evaluation by a geneticist may be helpful. If the child has progressive scoliosis, orthopedic evaluation is important to monitor for appropriate surgical corrections. A child with neurofibromatosis may benefit from evaluation and periodic follow-up visits in a specialty clinic, where counseling and follow-up care can be obtained for the variety of complications of this illness. A child who has tuberous sclerosis may benefit from evaluation in a specialty clinic or by a child neurologist.

In cases of behavioral disturbance, many of the developmental problems can be managed on an outpatient basis without referral to a specialist. Children with autism present many difficult behavioral problems and usually benefit from evaluation by a specialist in child psychiatry or child neurology. We refer children with ADHD only if they do not respond to initial treatment or if they have complicating factors such as severe learning disabilities or oppositional defiant disorder. A child psychiatrist or child neurologist can help with ongoing therapy. Patients with OCD, PTSD, or depression often need psychotherapy and psychotropic medication.

Recommended Readings

Aicardi J. *Epilepsy in children,* 2nd ed. New York: Raven Press, 1994.
Cohen DJ, Leckman JF. Developmental psychopathology and neurobiology of Tourette's syndrome. *J Am Acad Child Adolesc Psychiatry* 1994;33:2–15.

Diagnostic and statistical manual of mental disorders, 4th ed. Washington, DC: American Psychiatric Association, 1994.

Fenichel GM. *Clinical pediatric neurology: a signs and symptoms approach,* 3rd ed. Philadelphia: WB Saunders, 1997.

Filipek PA, Accardo PJ, Ashwal S, et al. Practice parameter: screening and diagnosis of autism. *Neurology* 2000;55:468–479.

Fink JK. Approach to patients with inherited neurologic disorders. *Semin Neurol* 1998;18: 211–219.

Gay CT, Bodensteiner JB. The floppy infant: recent advances in the understanding of disorders affecting the neuromuscular junction. *Neurol Clin* 1990;8:715–726.

Gutmann DH, Aylsworth A, Carey JC, et al. The diagnostic evaluation and multidisciplinary management of neurofibromatosis 1 and neurofibromatosis 2. *JAMA* 1997;278:51–57.

Jones KL. *Smith's recognizable patterns of human malformation,* 5th ed. Philadelphia: WB Saunders, 1997.

Lyon G, Adams RD, Kolodny EH. *Neurology of hereditary metabolic diseases of children,* 2nd ed. New York: McGraw–Hill, 1996.

Menkes JH, Sarnat HB, eds. *Child neurology,* 6th ed. Philadelphia: Lippincott Williams & Wilkins, 2000.

Percy AK. The inherited neurodegenerative disorders of childhood: clinical assessment. *J Child Neurol* 1987;2:82–97.

Roach ES, DiMario FJ, Kandt RS, et al. Tuberous sclerosis consensus conference: recommendations for diagnostic evaluation. *J Child Neurol* 1999;14:401–407.

Rothner AD. Headaches in children: a review. *Headache* 1979;18:156–162.

Tusa RJ, Saada AA, Niparko JK. Dizziness in childhood. *J Child Neurol* 1994;9:261–274.

Helpful Websites

www.ninds.nih.gov / health_and_medical / disorder_index.htm (provides a brief description of disorders, selected references, organizations, and NINDS publications).

www.genetests.org (provides up to date information on available genetic tests and clinics).

35. APPROACH TO ETHICAL ISSUES IN NEUROLOGY

Michael P. McQuillen

Clinical ethics—the business of being human in the interchange between physician and patient—has been an integral part of that interchange for as long as there has been a profession of medicine. Until the past few decades, however, it was assumed that being a physician meant being ethical; that everyone's ethics were the same (or at least of equivalent worth); and that there was no underlying theory or set of standards necessary for ethical decision-making. In part, this state of affairs was a reflection of the simplicity of life in general and of medicine in particular. With advances in technology, more options became possible—options to evaluate new forms of treatment (research) as well as to utilize proven diagnostic and therapeutic modalities (with their inherent risk-benefit calculus). Questions of *who* should make *which* decisions in *what* circumstances began to be asked. Particular judgments no longer stood in isolation but led to the formulation of **rules** that could govern in similar situations; a recognition of the **principles** upon which such rules might be based; and the development of **theories** underlying the principles—much as an understanding of anatomy, biochemistry, pathophysiology, and other basic sciences made it possible to clarify approaches to the complicated problem of stroke (for example). Some theorists appealed directly to **conscience**, developed and refined in reflection on individual cases without the formality of the process just described. Underlying it all, however, was the realization that ethical problems arise in almost any clinical situation and that such problems should be addressed as systematically as any dimension of the given clinical situation. This realization called forth a new academic discipline (biomedical or clinical ethics) out of what previously had been purely philosophical, and in a sense impractical, thought (ethics).

From the start, this discipline found fertile ground in neurology, where ethical theory met real-life problems such as "brain death," the "vegetative state" and other conditions of incapacity; neurogenetic diseases, and a gamut of issues at the end of life. Early on, this meeting generated encounters with the law and the recognition that what is ethical may not be legal and vice versa. To plow the field, one must first understand the background of ethical theories, develop a structured approach to the recognition and solution of ethical problems, and understand how that approach helps to deal with particular problems and how an effective interface can be developed with the law.

    I. Ethical theories. Before accepting any ethical theory as a basis upon which practical judgments can ultimately and validly be made, one should inquire whether the theory is adequate to the task by virtue of its satisfying certain criteria and then look to the basis of the theory to determine its usefulness and applicability. No one theory satisfies every clinical situation. Some are better adapted to one circumstance and others to another, while yet additional circumstances demand a hybrid of complementing theories.

        A. Criteria of an adequate theory. Beauchamp and Childress set forth a series of questions that should be answered in the affirmative with regard to any particular theory, if that theory is to be regarded as adequate and helpful with clinical conundra. Their questions are as follows:

            1. Is it clear? Or is the language by which the theory is formulated so complex as to muddle the situation?

            2. Is it coherent? Coherence is a necessary (although not sufficient) criterion of an adequate theory. It is missing when theory elements are in contradiction, one with another.

            3. Is it complete, or at least comprehensive? Does the theory deal with *all* of the *major* questions raised in diverse clinical circumstances, or are there serious concerns on which the theory is silent?

            4. Is it simple? Are there enough norms so that the theory can be used without confusion by clinicians, or are there so many that the answer becomes lost in practice?

            5. Can it explain and justify the conclusions reached with its help? Or does it simply set forth in other words a preexistent, intuitive belief?

            6. Does use of it yield new insights? Or does it only serve to repeat old convictions?

            7. Is it practical? In short, does it provide a useful answer to the clinical problem or one that is attractive in theory only?

B. Types of ethical theory

  1. **Utilitarianism.** This theory looks at the consequences of acts, and holds that an action is good if it produces more benefit than harm. Problems come when one looks for definitions of *benefit* and *harm*; to the relation between the individual acting and the society in which that individual acts; and at single actions each in isolation or at classes of actions governed by rules that appeal to the principle of utility.

  2. **Obligation-based theory.** The test of this theory is the **categorical imperative** of Immanuel Kant: the reason for an action should apply to everyone, and in all situations; moral rules are absolute. Problems arise when such rules—often abstract and legalistic, rather than relational—are found to be in conflict with each other in a particular circumstance.

  3. **Virtue-based, or character, ethics.** This approach looks to the person acting and to the motives and desires that propel the person's action. Because even the most virtuous person can act wrongly—even for the best of reasons—a viable ethical theory cannot rest on character alone.

  4. **Rights-based ethics, or liberal individualism.** Rights are justified claims that an individual or group is entitled to make upon a society at large. Such claims, while protecting the interests of an individual, at the same time may impose a corresponding obligation upon others. Rights may be *positive* (requiring an action by others) or *negative* (precluding such action). Overemphasis on rights may neglect the legitimate demands of the society at large.

  5. **Communitarian ethics.** Rather than the rights of the individual, communitarians look to the needs of society at large. Prescinding from *how* such needs may be articulated *by whom,* an overemphasis on this aspect of morality may neglect the legitimate interests of the individual.

  6. **An ethics of care.** Sometimes referred to as *feminist ethics,* the focus of this approach is on a caring, attached relationship between persons and on the implications of such a relationship. Impartiality and balance may suffer as a consequence, the result being a less complete and practical system than obtains with other theories.

  7. **Casuistry.** This term evokes an image of Jesuitical sophistry but really refers to the need to make decisions according to the particulars of any given situation. In reality, it was St. Thomas Aquinas who first described "situational ethics," a much (and properly) maligned theory when reduced to the proposition that all morality is relative, dependent *solely* on the circumstances of an action. Every detail of the case is examined and weighed, and a judgment reached often by analogy to similar cases. The connection between cases provides a maxim to rule the case—but which maxim is given most credence in any particular situation, and why?

  8. **Ethics based on principles, or "common morality."** A "bottom up" approach to validating particular judgments looks to rules that govern such judgments, and from rules to the principles from which they are derived. Four such principles are woven into "common sense" morality—an ethics that grows out of the nature of human beings, one that is simply put as "do good and avoid evil." The principles in question are as follows:

   a. Respect for the autonomous choices of other persons (autonomy)
   b. The obligation not to inflict harm intentionally (nonmaleficence)
   c. Actions taken for the benefit of others (beneficence)
   d. A fair, equitable, and appropriate distribution of goods in society (justice)

   Critics of the principlist approach refer to its elements as a mantra without substance, one that does not offer a schema for resolving conflict when more than one principle applies, a ritualistic incantation without a unifying, overriding theory to govern its use. When all is said and done, similar objections can be leveled against *any* ethical theory. The heart of the matter is to recognize the (ethical) problem and to admit with honesty which approach to solving it is used, and why. In today's medical climate, however—when *physicians* have become *providers, patients* are now *clients,* and any cost is a *medical loss* to the insurance company (or governmental agency) that funds a *managed care* plan (see **III.A.3.**)—any of these theories, meant to guide ethical decision-making in the practice of medicine, comes in conflict with the principles of business ethics. Those who are guided by the principles of business ethics have a primary fiduciary duty to the providers of capital—taxpayers, investors, society at large—whose goals may be vastly different than those of traditional medicine. In a certain sense, the principle of justice comes to the fore in resolving these conflicts. Practical solutions (see **III.A.3.**) that preserve the essentials of the theory on which the physician's judgment and actions are based in any particular situation must be sought as a way out of such dilemmas.

  II. Case method approach to clinical ethics. Fletcher et al. have developed a case method approach to the recognition and solution of ethical dilemmas that mimics standard decision-making in medicine. The elements of the method are as follows.

   A. Assessment. What are the nature of the medical problem and the relevant context in which it occurs? What are the options for therapy, their foreseeable risks and benefits, their short- and long-term prognoses, and the costs and resources or mechanisms for payment? What do the patient, family, and surrogate decision-makers *want*? What does the patient *need,* and what other needs may compete with that need? Are there any institutional, societal, or legal factors impinging on the patient or problem? What are the ethnic, cultural, and religious backgrounds from which the problems have arisen?

   B. Identification of ethical problem(s). Which ethical problems, ranked in order of importance, are self-evident and which are hidden? Which ethical theories are most relevant to such problems? Are there analogous cases in medicine or law, and if so, how do they apply? Which guidelines are most appropriate?

   C. Decision-making and implementation. What are the ethically acceptable options for solving the problems, and which are most acceptable? What justifications can be given for the preferred resolution of the problems? How can the preferred resolutions of the problems be accomplished? Is ethics consultation necessary or desirable? Is judicial review necessary or desirable?

   D. Evaluation. This is an ongoing process that seeks to recognize missed opportunities and correct unworkable solutions. The process carries a preventive dimension that may propose changes in policy or provide educational opportunities to minimize the chance that similar problems will occur.

 III. Approach to particular problems

   A. Decision-making (in general). At the heart of any interaction between physician and patient is the matter of *who* decides *what* shall be done *when*. The physician brings to this interaction experience, knowledge, skill—and a set of personal values that may or may not be the same as, or even compatible with, those of the patient. In years past, the physician's judgment ruled supreme. Today that judgment is tempered not only by a primacy of respect for the wishes of the patient but also by the rules and regulations of various health care plans as well as by statutory and case law.

   1. The primacy of the patient. A competent patient with the capacity for decision-making can and should decide—even before the fact, anticipating the future through advance directives (e.g., "living will" and durable power of attorney for health care decisions—"health care proxies"). Because many neurologic illnesses are chronic and inexorably disabling, often leaving the patient without the capacity to decide, it is wise to introduce discussion of advance directives early in the course of care of such a patient. (Indeed, federal regulations now *require* patients to be asked, on admission to the hospital, whether they have, or wish to, execute an advance directive.) A bond of trust should first be established, so that the patient does not interpret such discussions as a plan to abandon them at the end of life. (This element is missing in the federal requirement just mentioned.) It is important to emphasize that minds may change as a situation evolves.

   2. Surrogate decision-making. When capacity is lost, surrogates may be called upon to decide for the patient. Unless previously identified (in a health care proxy), the appropriate surrogate may be selected according to a hierarchy spelled out in state law. In extreme circumstances, a court-appointed surrogate may be necessary. Surrogates may strive to determine what it is the patient would have wanted (**substituted judgment standard**) or may try to decide what is best for the patient (**best interests standard**). The former standard is generally thought to be better, avoiding as it does conclusions made by one person (the surrogate) about another's "quality of life." Courts may require "clear and convincing evidence" of what it is the patient would have wanted in the circumstance in question. However, because such a scenario rarely exists in fact, and people often change their minds, requirements of this sort are most impractical. In all instances, it is wise to seek consensus, and to continue to act in favor of life until that consensus is reached. It may take time to develop consensus, even when a surrogate has previously been appointed, especially when capacity is lost suddenly and without warning (e.g., after stroke).

   3. **"Managed care" plans.** The spiraling cost of health care, among many contributing factors, has fueled a process of "health care reform"—much of which is basically about money. Because an immediate effect of physician decisions is the expenditure of money, a feature common to many proposals for such reform is a process requiring approval before such decisions can be implemented. Sometimes the process has at its center a "gatekeeper"—often a primary care physician, who may be guided by situation-specific protocols. The rewards built in to the system are key to its ethical dimension. Under traditional fee-for-service medicine, the more a physician did, the more that physician was paid. Under "managed care," the less a physician does, the more that physician is paid. The concept of "managed care" emphasizes the physician's obligation to *all* patients covered by a given plan—indeed, to society at large. Nevertheless, *any* decision made by a physician should be made in the particular *patient's* best interest. No test should be done, no treatment instituted, without that interest in the forefront of the physician's mind. If the system stands in the way of such decisions, physicians should oppose the system on behalf of their patients, vigorously—but fairly as well, not "gaming" the system with fabrications and the like. "Managed care" plans that reward physicians with incentives that limit or compromise care (e.g., by restricting the time that can be spent with a patient, denying access to appropriate consultants, and requiring the use of generic drugs) should be avoided.

   To guide the physician through this narrow maze of ever-diminishing resources at a time of ever more complex and expensive options for diagnosis and therapy, the field of **evidence-based medicine** has developed. **Practice guidelines, critical pathways,** and similar approaches are being articulated from a wide range of sources. Physicians are well-advised to listen to and follow such approaches *unless* the approach is of the *gobsat* ("good old boys sitting around a table") variety.

B. **"Brain death."** An unwanted consequence of the development of more effective intensive care was the recognition that patients whose brains had suffered complete and irreversible loss of all brain function could continue to manifest adequate cardiovascular, renal, and gastrointestinal functions, as long as pulmonary function was supported by a ventilator. The *presence* of death—previously identified by the absence of heart action and breathing—could no longer be affirmed in such patients. This state of affairs called for the development of a new set of *criteria* by which the presence of death could be recognized—*not* for a new *definition* of death. Once those criteria are satisfied, the patient *is dead*—an unsettling conclusion for many to whom a warm body with a strong pulse and a chest moving in rhythm with a machine *cannot* be dead, *must* be asleep.

   1. **"Whole brain" criteria.** Death of the *whole* brain is recognized in a normothermic body when loss of brain function results from an identifiable, irreversible, structural lesion, in the absence of sedative–hypnotic drugs or other, potentially reversible, metabolic conditions. Clinical examination for death of the whole brain requires the absence of brainstem reflexes (e.g., oculocephalic

and ice water caloric stimulation evokes no eye movement, pupils are dilated and fixed to light, corneal responses are not present) and no ventilatory movement when the ventilator is stopped after a period of ventilation with 100% oxygen, even though the PCO_2 increases above 60 torr without ventilation. Recognition must be affirmed with a second examination, separated in time from the first by a variable interval, dependent on factors such as age and clinical cause. The interval may be specified by local statute or hospital policy. As with the use of cardiorespiratory criteria to recognize the presence of death, the patient is dead when the criteria are satisfied—that is, when the second examination affirms the findings of the first. A number of **confirmatory tests** are helpful when the clinical condition is compromised (e.g., when a patient has been in barbiturate coma after head injury) and may be required in certain circumstances (e.g., the patient is a child younger than 1 year). However, such tests are neither necessary nor sufficient to affirm the presence of death by themselves.

2. **"Brainstem" criteria.** In the United Kingdom (UK), emphasis has been placed on the fact that the clinical examination on which the criterion of "brain death" is based looks only at the function of the brainstem and not at whole-brain function. Higher cortical function is irrelevant in UK practice. This means that a person whose brainstem has irreversibly ceased to function but whose cerebral hemispheres are still working—a person with the so-called "locked-in syndrome"—can be declared dead in the UK even though their cerebral hemispheres are still functioning. In part for this reason, many "brain death" policies and procedures in the United States require a confirmatory test to demonstrate that higher brain function is or must be absent (e.g., isoelectric electroencephalography or cerebral angiography showing no flow within the cranium).

3. **"Higher brain" death.** Certain philosophers (e.g., Robert Veatch) have called for a new *definition* of death, one that holds that death is the permanent loss of that which is essential to the nature of a human being—consciousness and cognition. Prescinding from the difficulty of establishing the *criteria* by which death, so defined, might be recognized, certain practical problems arise when one considers the implementation of such a definition (e.g., can someone in the end stages of Alzheimer's disease, still breathing with normal vegetative function, be buried?).

4. **Ethical considerations**
   a. **Telling the family.** Once the physician has recognized the presence of death using "brain death" criteria, the fact of that recognition should be conveyed to the family and others with ethical standing in the case. The physician should be aware that statutory law (as in New Jersey) or department of health regulations (as in New York) may make allowance for the family to reject the use of "brain death" criteria on religious grounds—in which case the physician may be required to rely on traditional (cardiorespiratory) criteria in identifying the fact that death has occurred. As in every interchange between physician and patient (including the extended patient—family and others), the physician should convey the fact gently, with compassion, and repeatedly until the fact is understood and accepted, if necessary. Although the family and others should not be burdened by being asked for permission to discontinue the ventilator (and thus to allow cardiovascular death to ensue within a short time), the physician should be sensitive to reactions of denial and the like. The family should be given time to assimilate and accept the sorrowful fact of death. The physician should be sensitive to different ethnic and cultural heritages and to unresolved issues from the past, which can determine how long it will take for acceptance of that fact to occur. Terms such as *brain death* and *life support* should be avoided, because they convey erroneous information. When someone *is* dead, *the person* is dead—not just the brain—and there is no longer any *human* life to support.

b. **After "brain death."** In addition to solving the problem of inappropriate and theoretically interminable use of a scarce resource (the intensive care bed), recognizing the death of a person whose body can continue to be kept "alive" permits a utilitarian calculus for the benefit of others. This is true in two instances—organ donation and the continued nurturing of an unborn child beyond the point of viability inside the body of a mother who has died. Permission for either action must be sought in the standard manner (see **III.A.1.,2.**). Considerations of justice weigh heavily in these situations. Different ethical theories come to different conclusions with regard to either action.

C. **The "vegetative state."** Although the condition is regarded by some as a fate worse than death, a certain proportion of patients who have incurred overwhelming damage to their cerebral hemispheres (from anoxia after cardiac arrest or from massive brain trauma or stroke) may—after a period of coma—evolve into a state of "wakefulness without awareness" accompanied by sleep–wake cycles and essentially intact brainstem and autonomic functions. Other patients may reach this state at the end of a chronic degenerative process. A multisociety task force published its consensus on the clinical, diagnostic, and prognostic features of this condition—a consensus with the particulars of which some physicians disagree, particularly because the task force did not acknowledge the concept of a "minimally conscious state" or deal with implications of the "locked-in" syndrome and other stations along the way to full consciousness. At the heart of the matter is the issue of whether a patient in a "vegetative (or any related) state" is *truly unaware* of all stimuli and has *no conscious* thought, *when* the condition can be regarded as *persistent* and *permanent,* and what, if any, impact may be had by a variety of therapeutic efforts and at what cost. Some regard these issues as incapable of anything but an arbitrary resolution. The task force deemed that any motor response in a patient in a "vegetative state" was primitive, random or reflex and as such could not be interpreted as evidence of cognition. Further, the task force relied on imaging and pathologic studies as excluding any anatomic substrate for consciousness.

1. **Withholding/withdrawing.** It is generally accepted that patients with the capacity to decide for themselves are *not* obliged to accept *all* treatments, diagnostic studies, and the like, and may reject these even if one of the results of such rejection is death. With patients in the "vegetative state," such decisions devolve upon surrogates, duly identified (see **III.A.2.**). Most commonly, a burdens–benefits calculus is used to make a decision to reject. Such decisions never should be made with the *intent* of *causing* death but may be made even when the probability is that death will ensue. The obligations of the physician in this process are threefold: to reach medical certainty, as far as that is possible; to convey that certainty to the decision-makers as gently and as often as is necessary to ensure understanding and acceptance; and to respect and implement the decision, as long as that does not violate the conscience of the physician. From an ethical point of view, *withholding* is more problematic than *withdrawing.* Withholding does not give the patient the benefit of a therapeutic trial. The physician does not know whether what might have been proposed would have helped the patient if it is not tried. It is imperative that all involved recognize (and behave accordingly with such recognition) that it is *not care* that is being withheld or withdrawn but rather a burdensome treatment or diagnostic study without sufficient benefit for the patient. The natural tendency to avoid such patients, visit them less often, even not to speak as though they might understand, should be steadfastly eschewed.

2. **Nutrition and hydration.** Given the deep meaning of food and water in human society, it is no wonder that some have balked at the withholding or withdrawing of these as symbolic of abandonment of the patient. Others have equated the nutrition and hydration given to a patient in the "vegetative state"—generally through a gastrostomy tube, with all of its attendant paraphernalia and cost—with any other therapy that may be rejected (for

reasons previously given). Clearly, it is licit to reject nutrition and hydration for the *benefit* of the patient—as when the *intent* is to minimize excess gastric or pulmonary secretions, incontinence, and the like. However, when the *intent* is to *cause* death, some regard that not as a benefit for the patient but rather as the beginning of a "slippery slope" that would lead inexorably to the elimination of "absolutely worthless human beings."

3. **Other considerations.** In making judgments about *level of care* of patients in the "vegetative state" or with other devastating, irremediable neurologic conditions, the physician is increasingly called upon to consider questions of **distributive justice.** These arise in such matters as access to intensive care, "managed care" decisions, and even conservation of individual and group resources. Ethical physicians owe primary responsibility to their patients, unless both have knowingly entered into a contract with each other that permits limitation of care on such bases. That is not to demean the need to be in constant dialogue with the patient or surrogate, in a gentle yet persistent effort to convince them of the wisdom of a considered position that may differ from theirs.

D. **Neurogenetic diseases.** There has been an explosion in the understanding of heritable neurologic disorders since in 1983, when a marker for the gene for Huntington's disease was identified on chromosome 4.

1. **Diagnostic testing.** Research and commercial laboratories can provide the physician with DNA and non-DNA information helpful in the diagnosis of more than two dozen disorders of the central and peripheral nervous system (including various genetic forms of myopathy) with the likelihood that information about more diseases—and even such considerations as behavioral traits—will be available in the near future. Such testing may yield information pertinent not only to the diagnosis of an existing condition but also in the presymptomatic—even prenatal—situation as well as with regard to carrier detection. Some—but by no means all—institutions use an extensive counseling system before and after testing to ensure thorough, informed decision-making for testing and appropriate support after results are made known to the patient or the guardian or surrogate.

2. **Ethical considerations.** Because the information garnered through diagnostic testing for neurogenetic disease in essence belongs to the persons being tested, it is important to their decision-making that they understand all of the implications of testing and are prepared—with support from the physician—to deal with those implications. For example, knowledge that one is a carrier of a neurogenetic disease may allow more responsible parenthood. Prenatal recognition that a neurogenetic disease is present in a developing infant may allow that infant's parents to prepare to shoulder the burden of that disease or to elect termination of the pregnancy. Because certain neurogenetic diseases (e.g., Huntington's disease) are associated with a higher rate of suicide than obtained in the population at large, presymptomatic diagnosis may enhance the risk of suicide, especially in a person who has experienced the ravages of the disease in an affected family member. Confirmation of the diagnosis of a neurogenetic disease may help the patient to cope with that disease, because certainty is always easier to deal with than uncertainty. Caution must be expressed over the misuse of information from diagnostic testing—by employers and insurers (especially health care insurers), who might arbitrarily exclude persons with proven neurogenetic disease without reference to the impact (present or future) of the particular disease on specific job performance or to its call on pooled health care resources. With regard to the latter issue, competing considerations of justice enter in and may require the person being tested to disclose the results of testing. In the last analysis, the physician requesting the test as well as the person being tested should be aware of and informed about the various aspects of testing before proceeding with it. Genetic testing should never be done as part of the "routine" evaluation of a patient without such considerations first being taken into account and explored.

3. Gene therapy. A promise for the future in neurogenetic disease is the hoped-for ability to insert or replace missing or defective genes in the cells of persons affected by such diseases. When the manipulation is directed at the affected cells, the procedure is termed **somatic cell therapy;** when it is directed at the initial fusion of sperm and ovum (or at those precursors of new human life themselves), it is termed **germ cell therapy.**

Somatic cell therapy raises issues common to research (see **III.G.**). Germ cell therapy, with its implications for future generations, raises other considerations beyond the scope of this chapter. Mention should be made, however, of the proposed role of **stem cells** in this line of research. Stem cells, as the name implies, have the capacity of developing into any tissue (*totipotential*), many but not all tissues (*pluripotential*), or only some tissues (*unipotential*). They differ in *source* of derivation. Totipotential cells come from an embryo at the very earliest stage of development, pluripotential cells come from fetal tissue, and unipotential cells from adult tissue (e.g., bone marrow). The embryo and fetus do not survive harvesting of stem cells, so although the goal of stem cell development (e.g., cure of neurodegenerative diseases, repair of traumatic brain and spinal cord injury, and cure of stroke) may be understandably laudable, the moral status of the source of stem cells cannot be ignored.

E. Static or progressive disorders with intact cognition. A spectrum of neuromuscular or spinal cord diseases have in common absence or loss of varying degrees of motor function (and hence—basically—of independence) with intact higher cortical function. Examples include spinal muscular atrophy, muscular dystrophy, and spinal cord dysraphisms (e.g., meningomyelocele), injuries, and other illnesses (e.g., multiple sclerosis).

1. Truth-telling. Truth-telling becomes exceptionally painful for a physician when confronted with a healthy mind in a body now or predictably about-to-be robbed of its normal function. Maintaining hope and thwarting inevitable depression without making false and empty promises is an art not easily learned—and yet one whose reward is one-hundred-fold from the patient and family, for whom life does, indeed, go on. Truth—though painful for physician and patient alike—is a reliable ally in the practice of this art. Physicians must be exceedingly sensitive to, and take time to care for, the emotional dimensions of the state in which their patients find themselves. As difficult as it may be not to do so, one must never abandon patients in this state. This is especially true in circumstances in which breathing becomes progressively more difficult.

2. Problems at the end of life. Despite all attempts at describing life on a ventilator, the patient may not be able to decide what that life might be like unless a trial of assisted ventilation is undertaken. After this point, the problem of withdrawing such assistance enters the scene. Minimizing suffering during withdrawal (e.g., with sedative–analgesic medications) runs the risk of suppressing what ventilatory function the patient still has. However, as long as the intent is the relief of that suffering and not to cause a more rapid demise, the use of such medication is appropriate (see **III.H.**). In all such circumstances, physicians should call upon colleagues with complementing skills, such as nurses, social workers, physiotherapists, hospice workers, to carry out the health care decisions reached by their patients, properly informed.

F. Static or progressive disorders with impaired cognition. Absence or loss of that which makes us uniquely human—consciousness and related higher neurologic functions—poses a number of dilemmas for the physician, who must deal with surrogates or even the courts in attempting to resolve those dilemmas. The paradigm clinical conditions range from anencephaly at one end of life to end-stage Alzheimer's disease at the other, with varying degrees of mental retardation and behavioral disorders—all of diverse causation—in between.

1. Limiting care. Until a new definition of death (see **III.B.3.**) is accepted, persons with these conditions remain human beings—as difficult as it may be to recognize that fact at any given clinical moment. One may argue whether some human beings have more of a right to use health care resources than others, but that is a societal decision that must not be invoked at the bedside of a particular patient by that patient's physician, absent agreement by the decision-maker for the patient. On the other hand, the focus of decision-making should properly be on compassionate *care,* not high-technology *cure,* once it is clear that one is dealing with a definitive, irreversible process.

2. **Making decisions.** Surrogate decision-making according to a **substituted judgment** standard (see **III.A.2.**) is particularly problematic when the person has never had the capacity for independent judgment (e.g., an infant with anencephaly or a person of any age with severe mental retardation). A sorry chapter in U.S. jurisprudence in this regard deals with involuntary sterilization—justified by the alternate, more subjective **best interests** standard. The latter standard often is used in dealing with unwanted, sometimes self-injurious, behavior by means of medication, restraints, institutionalization, and the like—even "psychosurgery." Extreme caution must be the rule and compassion the guide. The use of **advance directives**— particularly the appointment of someone to hold a **durable power of attorney for health care decisions**—is critical in making decisions when patients can no longer articulate their own decisions. Physicians who care for patients with neurodegenerative disorders (in particular) are well-advised to encourage their patients to consider and implement advance directives earlier rather than later, involving friends and family in discussions that will make possible valid substituted judgments, when and if those become necessary, well *before* their patients lose the capacity for truly informed decision-making.

3. **Involvement of family.** Family members, and others bearing responsibility for the care of persons without the capacity to decide for themselves, should be intimately involved with decision-making for persons in this category, unless there is a valid reason for them not to be involved. When capacity has been present and is now lost (as in the end stages of Alzheimer's disease), attention should be paid to health care proxies if previously executed. It must be borne in mind that people change their minds, even as circumstances change. Few of us can *truly* be aware of what it is like to become demented, nor can we *truly* know what it is we would decide for ourselves if and when we were to reach such a state. The burden of dementia is on those who care for the demented, not on the demented themselves.

G. **Research in neurology.** Dr. Labe Scheinberg once described the practice of neurology with the aphorism, "diagnose—then adios!" The last decade of the twentieth century was deemed the "Decade of the Brain" because of the remarkable advances in the understanding and management of neurologic disease. The move from Scheinberg's aphorism to a brave and wonderful new world occurred in large measure because of research—often involving human subjects early (because no appropriate animal models existed), often with great risk (in searching for an elusive benefit), and often raising the specter of a conflict of interest (between physicians caring for patients and conducting meaningful research by enrolling patients in controlled clinical trials).

1. **Valid versus invalid research.** The *sine qua non* of valid research is peer review—approval of a research proposal by a thoughtful, responsible, knowledgeable group of peers who judge the question as worthy of being asked, the answer as likely to be forthcoming, and the hoped-for benefit as worth the predicted risk. The availability of external funding makes it possible to conduct approved research honestly and openly, without employing the subterfuge of paying for research under the guise of accepted patient care. The process that effects valid research involves institutional review boards and other oversight bodies to ensure validity at every step along the way.

2. **Consent issues.** Persons with devastating illnesses are particularly vulnerable to any offer of hope, even when that offer wears the cloak of a research hypothesis. The offer of hope may come in the form of a controlled clinical

trial, in which the decision as to which treatment (e.g., active medication or placebo) the patient is to receive is made by the parameters of the trial, not by the physician. Physicians who refer patients for enrollment in such a trial must agree that the trial is necessary, that there is not, as yet, any proven approach that would guarantee benefit to the patient, and that the risks of the trial are balanced by the benefits the patient can expect. If there is no expected benefit to patients then, at the very least, society should benefit from the expected gain in knowledge that will come from the trial. Consent is especially problematic for children and for others without the capacity to give their own consent. Some have gone so far as to take the position that nontherapeutic research should not be done on patients, whereas others emphasize a broader debt to society that can be paid only by advancing knowledge through research.

H. **Chronic pain.** Diverse neurologic conditions are commonly associated with pain, often requiring hefty doses of potent analgesics for relief—doses of medications that may suppress respiration, lower blood pressure to dangerous levels, and have other unwanted effects. The ruling principle here is that of the "double effect"—the unwanted (indirect, merely permitted) effects (in this instance, possible aspiration or even death) are allowed as long as the primary (direct, intended) effect (in this instance, relief of pain) is desirable and cannot be achieved in any other way. It is important to remember that pain can be physical and identifiable or metaphysical and existential. Adequate relief of both kinds of pain is at the heart of "comfort care," which can be chosen by patients at any stage of their lives, especially at the end of a terminal illness. In this regard, **hospice** may be an ideal setting in which to provide such care (although the trajectory of neurologic illness often exceeds the arbitrary limits set by Medicare and other funding agencies for the provision of hospice care).

IV. Interface with the law. Many of the most notable, landmark cases in the recent history of biomedical or clinical ethics have dealt with patients with neurologic problems. In the matter of surrogate decision-making with regard to the withholding or withdrawal of medical treatment, *Quinlan* and *Saikewicz* set the standard of substituted judgment for once-competent and never-competent patients, respectively. *Conroy* affirmed the fact that autonomy remains intact, even when a person is no longer able to assert that right or even appreciate its effectuation. *Cruzan* acknowledged the right of states to require stringent ("clear and convincing") evidence of the prior wishes of a once-competent person as applicable to his or her current status. The physician should be aware of such cases and should try to discern their relevance to the situation at hand (see **II.B.**). The physician should recognize that the impact of such cases (in terms of setting precedent) is limited to the jurisdiction in which the decision was rendered but may (in terms of argument) be of probative value in other jurisdictions.

V. Referrals. Most ethical dilemmas can and should be dealt with by physicians with colleagues in the care of their patients (nurses, social workers, clergy, and the like)—perhaps with the help of ethics consultation and the awareness of hospital administration and attorneys. In solving such dilemmas, physicians should keep the general principles of decision-making, of truth telling, and of involvement of family (see **III.A.1., 2. and III.F.**, in particular) in mind at all times. Physicians should not hesitate to seek the guidance and assistance of senior, more experienced clinicians in dealing with these issues at a practical level. Generally, recourse to the courts should be a last resort, as the legal process takes interminable time and often is not sensitive to the important nuances of a particular clinical situation.

Recommended Readings

American Academy of Neurology Code of Professional Conduct. *Neurology* 1993;43:1257.
American Medical Association Council on Ethical and Judicial Affairs. *Code of medical ethics.* Chicago: American Medical Association, 1994.
Beauchamp TL, Childress JF. *Principles of biomedical ethics.* New York: Oxford University Press, 1994.
Bernat JL. *Ethical issues in neurology.* Boston: Butterworth–Heinemann, 2002.
Brody BA. *Life and death decision making.* New York: Oxford University Press, 1988.
Brody H. *The healer's power.* New Haven: Yale University Press, 1992.

Cassell EJ. *The nature of suffering and the goals of medicine.* New York: Oxford University Press, 1991.

In re Conroy, 98 N.J. 321, 486 A.2d 1209, 1985.

Cruzan v. Director, Missouri Department of Health, 497 U.S. 261, 1990.

Faden RR, Beauchamp TL. *A history and theory of informed consent.* New York: Oxford University Press, 1986.

Fletcher JC, Lombardo PA, Marshall MF, et al., eds. *Introduction to clinical ethics,* 2nd ed. Frederick, MD: University Publishing Group, 1997.

Holmes HB, Purdy LM, eds. *Feminist perspectives in medical ethics.* Bloomington, IN: Indiana University Press, 1992.

Jonsen AR, Siegler M, Winslade WJ. *Clinical ethics.* New York: Macmillan, 1998.

Lynn J, ed. *By no extraordinary means: the choice to forgo life-sustaining food and water.* Bloomington, IN: Indiana University Press, 1989.

Multi-Society Task Force on PVS. Medical aspects of the persistent vegetative state, I and II. *N Engl J Med* 1994;330:1499–1508, 1572–1579.

Pellegrino ED, Thomasma DC. *For the patient's good: the restoration of beneficence in health care.* New York: Oxford University Press, 1988.

President's Commission for the Study of Ethical Problems in Medicine and Biomedical and Behavioral Research. *Defining death: medical, ethical, and legal issues in the determination of death.* Washington, DC: US Government Printing Office, 1981.

President's Commission for the Study of Ethical Problems in Medicine and Biomedical and Behavioral Research. *Making health care decisions: the ethical and legal implications of informed consent in the patient-practitioner relationship.* Washington, DC: US Government Printing Office, 1982.

President's Commission for the Study of Ethical Problems in Medicine and Biomedical and Behavioral Research. *Deciding to forgo life-sustaining treatment: ethical, medical, and legal issues in treatment decisions.* Washington, DC: US Government Printing Office, 1983.

Quill TE. *Death and dignity: making choices and taking charge.* New York: WW Norton, 1993.

In re Quinlan, 70 N.J. 10, 355 A.2d 647, *cert. denied sub nom. Garger v. New Jersey,* 429 U.S. 922, 1976.

Rodwin, MA. Medicine, money, and morals: physicians' conflicts of interest. New York: Oxford University Press, 1993.

Superintendant of Belchertown State School v. Saikewicz, Mass. 370 N.E. 2d 417, 1977.

Veatch RM. The impending collapse of the whole-brain definition of death. *Hastings Cent Rep* 1993;23:18–24.

II. TREATMENT

36. ISCHEMIC CEREBROVASCULAR DISEASE

José Biller

Cerebrovascular disease comprises a heterogeneous group of diseases that herald their presence by producing symptoms and signs resulting from either ischemia or hemorrhage within the central nervous system. The term **stroke** is most commonly used by both physicians and the general public to refer to any one of this diverse group of disorders. It connotes the idea that the onset of symptoms is abrupt (seconds to hours) and leaves a lasting physical or cognitive disability. A stroke is a "brain attack," a sudden interruption of blood flow to the brain that causes brain damage and loss of function.

Cerebrovascular disease is the third leading cause of death, after cardiovascular disease and cancer, and a primary cause of long-term disability in much of the industrialized world. Cerebrovascular disease is a major cause of chronic disability and the most common neurologic condition necessitating hospitalization. There are two main types of strokes—ischemic and hemorrhagic. The focus of this chapter is to outline the general approach to the diagnosis and management of ischemic stroke.

Of the 700,000 new or recurrent strokes in the United States each year, approximately 80% to 85% result from **cerebral infarction.** Ischemic stroke may result from (1) large-artery stenosis or occlusion, (2) small-artery occlusion (lacunes), (3) cardioembolism, (4) hemodynamic (watershed) infarction, (5) nonatherosclerotic vasculopathy, (6) hypercoagulable disorders, or (7) infarction of undetermined causation.

Ischemia sets in motion a cascade of biochemical alterations leading to lactic acidosis, influx of calcium and sodium, and efflux of potassium that culminates in cell death. The pathogenesis of ischemic strokes can be conceptualized as a permanent lack of blood flow to a focal region of the brain, depriving it of needed glucose and oxygen. Normal cerebral blood flow (CBF) is 50 to 55 mL/100 g per minute. The threshold for synaptic transmission failure occurs when CBF decreases to approximately 8 to 10 mL/100 g per minute. At this level, neuronal death can occur. The brain region with a CBF level from 8 to 18 mL/100 g per minute sometimes is called the **ischemic penumbra.** Rational treatment of patients with ischemic cerebrovascular disease depends on accurate diagnosis. The cause of an ischemic stroke must first be established through careful history-taking, detailed physical examination, and paraclinical investigations.

A basic evaluation, to be performed for all patients with ischemic stroke, includes complete blood cell count with differential and platelet count, erythrocyte sedimentation rate, prothrombin time, activated partial thromboplastin time (aPTT), plasma glucose level, blood urea nitrogen, serum creatinine, lipid analysis, luetic serologic testing, urinalysis, chest radiography, and electrocardiography. Computed tomography should also be performed on all patients because it may depict hemorrhagic lesions that can mimic an ischemic stroke. Magnetic resonance imaging (MRI) is superior to CT in evaluation for cerebral ischemia, particularly assessment of ischemic areas in the posterior fossa. Magnetic resonance angiography (MRA) complements the information obtained with MRI and frequently delineates the pathoanatomic substrate of the stroke. Diffusion-weighted imaging can be complemented with information obtained from perfusion-weighted imaging to delineate fairly accurately areas of necrosis and surrounding ischemic and potentially salvageable tissue.

The emphasis in screening should be on noninvasive testing for evaluating carotid artery disease, including Duplex sonography, and transcranial Doppler imaging. Cardiac investigations to determine whether emboli have cardiac sources are advised in selected circumstances. Two-dimensional echocardiography for older patients with ischemic stroke should be limited to patients with clinical clues of heart disease. Two-dimensional echocardiography should be considered for all patients younger than 45 years with otherwise unexplained ischemic stroke. Transesophageal echocardiography should be used for selected individuals, particularly for evaluation of mitral and aortic prosthetic valves or vegetations, whenever there is a need for better visualization of the left atrial appendage or interatrial septum, or when a right-to-left shunt is suspected.

Most patients with ischemic stroke have cerebrovascular atherosclerosis. Therefore the mechanism of ischemia results from thrombotic vascular occlusion, embolization of atherosclerotic debris, or hemodynamic disturbances causing focal hypoperfusion in areas in which the circulation is inadequate. The results of the North American Symptomatic Carotid Endarterectomy

Trial (NASCET) and the European Carotid Surgery Trial have emphasized the need for accurate quantification of the degree of extracranial internal carotid stenosis. Although MRA complements the information obtained with MRI and frequently delineates the pathoanatomic substrate of the stroke, the standard for establishing the extent of vascular disease remains conventional angiography or intraarterial digital subtraction angiography.

I. **Natural history and prognosis**
   A. **Ischemic stroke resulting from large-artery atherosclerotic disease**. Large-artery atherothrombotic infarctions almost always occur in patients who already have significant risk factors for cerebrovascular atherosclerosis, such as arterial hypertension, cigarette smoking, diabetes, asymptomatic carotid bruits, asymptomatic carotid stenosis, and transient ischemic attacks (TIAs).
      1. A **TIA** is defined as a temporary focal neurologic deficit, presumably related to ischemia of the brain or retina, that lasts less than 24 hours. Yet most TIAs last only a few minutes. TIAs involving the anterior or carotid circulation should be distinguished from those involving the posterior or vertebrobasilar circulation.
         a. The following symptoms are considered typical of TIAs in the **carotid circulation:** ipsilateral amaurosis fugax, contralateral sensory or motor dysfunction limited to one side of the body, aphasia, contralateral homonymous hemianopia, or any combination thereof.
         b. The following symptoms represent typical TIAs in the **vertebrobasilar system:** bilateral or shifting motor or sensory dysfunction, complete or partial loss of vision in both homonymous fields, or any combination of these symptoms. Isolated diplopia, vertigo, dysarthria, and dysphagia should not be considered TIAs, but in combination with one another or with any of the symptoms just listed, they should be considered vertebrobasilar TIAs.
         c. Preceding TIAs occur in approximately 50% of patients with atherothrombotic brain infarction.
         d. A TIA is a risk factor for stroke. The independent risk of a subsequent stroke is at least three times greater for patients with histories of TIAs than for those who have not had TIAs.
      2. **Atherosclerosis** tends to occur in areas of reduced shear, such as the lateral aspect of the carotid artery bulb. It primarily affects the larger extracranial and intracranial vessels. Approximately 80% of ischemic strokes occur in the **carotid or anterior circulation** and 20% in the **vertebrobasilar or posterior circulation** (Fig. 36.1).
      3. The mechanism of large-artery atherothrombotic infarction is either **artery-to-artery embolization** or **in situ formation of a thrombus** in the setting of preexisting arterial stenosis. Artery-to-artery embolism is a common mechanism of cerebral ischemic events. Embolism from ulcerated carotid atherosclerotic plaques is the most common cause of cerebral infarction. In situ thrombosis occurs in the proximal carotid, distal vertebral, and basilar arteries. Such a circumstance may arise in association with hypercoagulable states. Episodes of dehydration also can trigger these events.
   B. **Ischemic strokes resulting from small-vessel or penetrating artery disease (lacunes)**. Long-standing arterial hypertension affects primarily the smaller penetrating intracranial vessels. It induces hypertrophy of the media and deposition of fibrinoid material into the vessel wall (fibrinoid necrosis), which eventually leads to occlusion. **Lacunes** are small ischemic infarcts in the deep regions of the brain or brainstem that range in diameter from 0.5 to 15.0 mm and result from lipohyalinosis of penetrating arteries or branches related to long-standing arterial hypertension—chiefly the anterior choroidal, middle cerebral, posterior cerebral, and basilar arteries. Diabetes mellitus and extracranial arterial and cardiac sources of embolism are found less frequently.
   C. **Ischemic stroke resulting from cardioembolism.** Embolic occlusion of intracranial vessels can be caused by material arising proximally—most commonly from the heart, from the aorta, from the carotid or vertebral arteries and

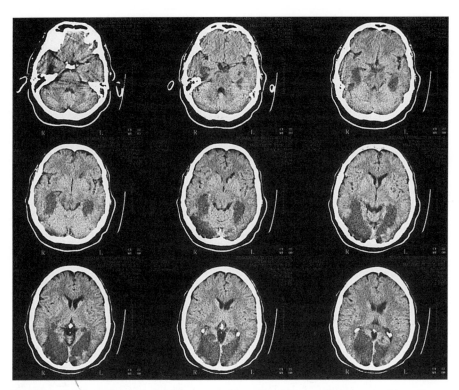

FIG. 36.1 Axial unenhanced cranial computed tomographic scan shows areas of low attenuation involving the medial aspects of both temporal lobes, both occipital lobes, the midbrain, and the pons in a patient with a diagnosis of basilar arterial occlusion.

rarely from systemic veins. Embolism of cardiac origin accounts for approximately 15% of all ischemic strokes. Emboli from cardiac sources frequently lodge in the middle cerebral artery territory, often are large, and often have the worst outcomes. Although most types of heart disease can produce cerebral embolism, certain cardiac disorders are more likely to be associated with emboli (Table 36.1). Identification of a cardiac source of potential embolism is helpful for management. However, finding a potential cardiac embolic source is not by itself sufficient to diagnose embolic cerebral infarction, because many cardiac problems can coexist with cerebrovascular atherosclerosis.

D. **Ischemic stroke resulting from hemodynamic mechanisms.** Another mechanism of ischemic central nervous system damage is decreased systemic perfusion pressure, which causes diminished blood flow to the brain in a diffuse manner. This occurs most commonly in the setting of cardiac pump failure, or systemic hypotension. Border-zone ischemia often is explained by the combination of two frequently interrelated processes—hypoperfusion and embolization. This type of insult is most critical in border-zone territories, or so-called watershed areas, in the most distal regions of supply of the major arterial territories. Border-zone ischemia can result in several characteristic syndromes, depending on whether the ischemia is in the border-zone territory of all three major arterial systems (anterior, middle, and posterior cerebral arteries), the territory between the anterior and middle cerebral arteries, or the territory between the middle and posterior cerebral arteries. Watershed infarcts often are bilateral but can be unilateral when preexisting ipsilateral vascular disease causes focal

Table 36.1 Common sources of cardiac emboli

Acute myocardial infarction	Mitral valve prolapse
Left ventricular aneurysm	Infective and nonbacterial thrombotic endocarditis
Dilated cardiomyopathy	Prosthetic heart valve
Cardiac arrhythmia	Intracardiac tumor
Atrial fibrillation	
Bradytachyarrhythmia	Intracardiac defect with paradoxic embolism
Valvular heart disease	Atrial septal defect
Rheumatic mitral valve disease	Patent foramen ovale
Calcific aortic stenosis	Atrial septal aneurysm

hypoperfusion in the most distal territory. Other mechanisms whereby watershed infarcts develop include microemboli and hematologic abnormalities.

E. Ischemic stroke resulting from nonatherosclerotic vasculopathy. Several nonatherosclerotic forms of vasculopathy are predisposing factors for ischemic stroke. These vasculopathies include, among others, cervicocephalic arterial dissection, moyamoya, fibromuscular dysplasia, and cerebral vasculitis. Together these uncommon conditions represent 5% of all ischemic strokes. They are relatively more common among children and young adults.

F. Ischemic stroke resulting from hypercoagulable disorders. Alterations in hemostasis have been associated with an increased risk of ischemic stroke. These conditions include deficiencies in the anticoagulant proteins such as antithrombin III, protein C, protein S, activated protein C resistance, factor V Leiden mutation, prothrombin G20210 mutation, and heparin cofactor II; disorders of fibrinogen or of the fibrinolytic system; and secondary hypercoagulable states encountered in the nephrotic syndrome, polycythemia vera, sickle cell disease, thrombotic thrombocytopenic purpura (TTP), and paroxysmal nocturnal hemoglobinuria. A hypercoagulable state may also may be present in patients with antiphospholipid antibody syndrome. These disorders account for 1% of all strokes, and for 2% to 7% of ischemic strokes in young patients.

G. Ischemic stroke of undetermined causation. Despite extensive evaluation, in as many as one third of ischemic strokes, a cause cannot be determined. This percentage is possibly higher among patients younger than 45 years. It is possible that some of these strokes are caused by cardioembolic or hematologic events not demonstrable with present means of investigation. The risk of recurrence of these strokes appears to be slightly less than that of ischemic strokes of other types.

II. Prevention. The prevention of strokes follows three main avenues—control of modifiable risk factors, pharmacologic therapy, and surgical intervention. Knowledge and control of modifiable risk factors are paramount in prevention of primary and secondary strokes. Treatable or modifiable risk factors include hypertension, diabetes mellitus, cigarette smoking, hyperlipidemia, excessive alcohol intake, obesity, and physical inactivity. Other risk factors include age and gender, cardiac disease, TIAs, previous strokes, asymptomatic carotid bruit or stenosis, high hemoglobin level or hematocrit, increased fibrinogen level, use of oral contraceptives, and possibly race and ethnicity.

A. Hypertension predisposes to ischemic stroke by aggravating atherosclerosis and accelerating heart disease. Arterial hypertension is the most important modifiable risk factor for stroke, increasing the relative risk threefold to fourfold. Blood pressure treatment resulting in a decrease in mean diastolic blood pressure of 5 mm Hg over 2 to 3 years is associated with a 40% reduction in risk of stroke.

B. Diabetes mellitus increases the risk of ischemic cerebrovascular disease twofold to fourfold compared with the risk among persons without diabetes. In addition, diabetes increases morbidity and mortality after stroke. There is presently no evidence to suggest that tighter diabetic control decreases the risk of stroke or recurrent stroke.

C. Cigarette smoking is an independent risk factor for ischemic stroke among men and women of all ages. More than 5 years may be required before a reduction in stroke risk is observed after cessation of smoking.

D. **Hyperlipidemia.** Some studies have shown a significant positive relation between serum cholesterol level and death resulting from nonhemorrhagic stroke. This relation has not been consistent, however, possibly because different risks are associated with different lipoprotein subtypes. Persons with high serum lipoprotein(a) levels have a higher risk of ischemic stroke. Additional studies may hold clues to the potential value of lipid-lowering agents in reducing the risk of ischemic stroke.

E. **Excessive alcohol use.** There is a J-shaped association between alcohol consumption and ischemic stroke. Lower doses (up to two drinks a day) offer reduced risk and higher doses elevate the risk. Moderate alcohol intake may elevate high-density lipoprotein concentration.

F. **Obesity and physical inactivity.** Obesity exerts an independent increase in risk of stroke among men younger than 63 years. This increase is greater among cigarette smokers and patients with hypertension, elevated blood glucose, or hyperlipidemia. There is some evidence that physical activity can reduce the risk of stroke.

III. **Treatment.** Ischemic stroke is approached as a medical emergency. Any patient with acute ischemic stroke should be admitted to a hospital for evaluation and treatment. This is best accomplished in an intensive care unit or stroke unit. Management must be individualized according to the pathophysiologic process.

    A. **General measures.** Particular attention should be paid to the following parameters (Table 36.2).

        1. **Medical measures**

            a. **Respiratory tract protection and infection.** The airway of an obtunded patient should be protected. Some critically ill patients need ventilatory assistance. Aspiration and atelectasis should be prevented. Nosocomial pneumonia frequently complicates stroke and is a leading cause of mortality in the second to fourth weeks following cerebral infarction. Risk factors for nosocomial pneumonia in stroke patients include advanced age, prolonged hospitalization, serious medical comorbidity, immunosuppression, and endotracheal intubation. Dysphagia is common after stroke. Failure of the swallowing process increases the risks of aspiration, malnutrition, and dehydration. The risk of pneumonia is increased by aspiration, which occurs in as many as 25% of unilateral hemispheric strokes and 70% of bilateral hemispheric or brainstem strokes. A meticulous history and examination of the oral, pharyngeal, and esophageal stages with a modified barium swallow using videofluorography are often recommended. Oral ingestion of food or liquids often is precluded in the first 24 to 48 hours. Nasogastric feedings often are necessary. Some patients may need a gastrostomy to maintain adequate nutritional intake.

            b. **Urinary tract infections.** Urinary bladder dysfunction can complicate stroke, particularly basal ganglia, frontoparietal, and bilateral hemispheric strokes. There are three major mechanisms of occurrence of urinary incontinence after an acute ischemic stroke: (1) disruption of the neuromicturition pathway, which results in bladder hyperreflexia and urgency incontinence; (2) stroke-related cognitive and language deficits with normal bladder function; and (3) concurrent neuropathy or medication use that result in bladder hyporeflexia and overflow incontinence.

Table 36.2 Areas of emphasis in general medical measures

Respiration	Hospital-acquired infection
Blood pressure	Venous thromboembolism
Fluids and electrolytes	Seizures
Skin care	Spasticity
Dysphagia, aspiration	Depression
Urinary dysfunction	

Urinary tract infections are an important cause of hyperpyrexia following stroke. They contribute to almost one third of stroke-related deaths and are present in almost one half of patients in autopsy series. Incontinent or comatose patients should be catheterized, preferably with a condom catheter for men or a closed Foley catheter for women. Many patients need an indwelling catheter, which is associated with a risk of infection. In addition, even continent patients can have postvoiding residuals, which also increase the likelihood of urinary tract infections.

  c. Electrolytic and metabolic disturbances
    (1) **Electrolytic disturbances.** Stroke patients are at risk of electrolyte disturbances resulting from reduced oral intake, potentially increased gastric and skin losses, and derangements in secretion of antidiuretic hormone (ADH). Levels of ADH increase after stroke. In some cases, inappropriate secretion of ADH places the patient at risk of hyponatremia. Possible mechanisms include damage to the anterior hypothalamus and a prolonged recumbent position. In most cases, these alterations do not persist beyond the first week after a stroke.
    (2) **Hyperglycemia** in acute stroke is a common phenomenon and correlates with a poor outcome. Experimental studies with animals indicate that hyperglycemia increases the extent of ischemic brain damage. High serum glucose levels increase anaerobic metabolism, increase lactic acid production in ischemic brain tissue, and cause cellular acidosis. Despite current controversy, hypotonic solutions or fluids containing glucose should be avoided.
  d. Venous thromboembolism is a common complication among patients with acute ischemic stroke. The risk is highest in the early weeks after ictus but remains significant in the chronic phase. In the absence of prophylactic measures, deep venous thrombosis develops in approximately 60% to 75% of patients with hemiplegia, and lethal pulmonary embolism occurs among fewer than 3%. Prevention includes the use of pressure gradient stockings, pneumatic compression stockings, low-dosage subcutaneous heparin (5,000 units every 8 to 12 hours), adjusted-dosage heparin, low-molecular-weight heparin (LMWH) and low-molecular-weight heparinoids.
  e. Cardiac events constitute an important cause of death after acute stroke, because 40% to 70% of these patients have baseline **coronary artery disease.** Approximately 15% of the deaths following ischemic stroke are from fatal arrhythmia or myocardial infarction (MI). As many as 30% of patients have ST segment depression on an electrocardiogram in the first 48 hours after the event, and 35% have ventricular couplets or tachycardia. Other changes include QT interval prolongation, T-wave inversion, or increases in duration and amplitude of T waves. Patients with lesions of the left cerebral hemisphere, especially the insular area, tend to have more cardiac disturbances.
  f. Cerebral autoregulation is lost during acute ischemic stroke. The blood pressure should be measured frequently during the first few days after ischemic stroke. Transient blood pressure elevation following acute cerebral infarction and normalization over days without treatment are common. Mild to moderate hypertension may be compensatory, and rapid lowering of the blood pressure is generally not recommended. Exceptions to this rule include patients with hypertensive encephalopathy and cerebral ischemia secondary to aortic dissection.
  g. Pressure sores. Results of surveys suggest that 3% to 10% of patients in acute care hospitals have pressure sores. Stroke patients, like other patients with reduced mobility, are at increased risk. Altered level of consciousness, peripheral vascular disease, and malnourishment are contributing factors. Pressure sores develop most often over bony prominences—sacrum, ischium, trochanters, and the areas around the

ankles and heels. The patient's position should be changed frequently to reduce pressure and shear forces. Flotation beds help reduce the risk. Treatment includes debridement and moist dressing. Surgical treatment sometimes is necessary. Cellulitis in the surrounding skin and systemic infection necessitate antibiotic therapy.

    h. Depression can be an aggravating factor causing increased disability. Depression affects one half of all stroke patients, and it often fulfills the criteria for major depression. Depression occurs in the first few weeks after stroke but is maximal between 6 and 24 months afterward. Patients with left frontal strokes appear to be more susceptible than are those with right hemisphere or brainstem strokes. Depression also correlates with severity of neurologic deficit and quality of available social support. Finally, although depressed patients gain some benefit from rehabilitation, the effects are not sustained. Therapy for poststroke depression is the same as that for endogenous depression.

  2. Neurologic measures. The condition of approximately 30% of patients with acute ischemic strokes worsens after the initial event, but deterioration after stroke or "stroke in evolution" does not necessarily indicate propagating thrombus or recurrent embolism (Table 36.3).

    a. Brain edema is the most common cause of deterioration and early death during the first week after acute cerebral infarction. Young patients and patients with large infarcts are most affected. Massive cerebral edema complicates approximately 10% of large hemispheric strokes. Edema develops within several hours after an acute ischemic insult to the brain and peaks after 24 to 96 hours. Ischemic brain edema is initially cytotoxic and later vasogenic. Cytotoxic edema involves predominantly the gray matter, whereas vasogenic edema involves predominantly the white matter. No specific pharmacologic agent has been proved effective against ischemic cerebral edema. Physicians often make the erroneous assumption that depressed consciousness in patients with large cerebral infarcts is caused solely by increased intracranial pressure. They inappropriately begin "conventional" intracranial hypertension therapies such as hyperventilation to maintain a PCO_2 at 30 to 35 mm Hg (possibly useful in the first 24 hours), and osmotherapy with mannitol supplemented by nonosmotic diuretics. Corticosteroids have not been proved useful in the management of ischemic cerebral edema and may even be detrimental. Mannitol does not cross the blood–brain barrier and may accentuate compartmentalized pressure gradients between abnormal and normal brain regions. Hypernatremia, hypokalemia, and hypocalcemia can result from excessive osmotherapy. Excessive osmotherapy also can result in intravascular volume depletion and arterial hypotension. Normal saline solution is administered to prevent intravascular depletion. In appreciation of the role of brain tissue shifts, surgical evacuation of life-threatening supratentorial infarctions by means of hemicraniectomy may have to be considered. In cases of cerebellar infarction with mass effect, when fourth ventricular compression and hydrocephalus are the primary concerns, some neurosurgeons prefer to perform ventriculostomy; however, this procedure is

Table 36.3 Causes of "stroke in evolution"

Thrombosis of a stenotic artery	Brain edema
Thrombus propagation	Seizures
Recurrent embolism	Metabolic evolution of ischemic insult
Collateral failure	Pneumonia
Hypoperfusion resulting from	Urosepsis
hypovolemia, decreased systemic	Medication effects
pressure, or decreased cardiac output	Herniation syndromes
Hypoxia	Hemorrhagic transformation

associated with a risk of upward cerebellar herniation through the free edge of the tentorial incisura (Fig. 36.2). For this reason, other neurosurgeons favor posterior fossa decompressive surgery for such patients.

b. **Hemorrhagic transformation** occurs in approximately 40% of all ischemic infarcts, and of these, 10% show secondary clinical deterioration. Hemorrhagic transformation often occurs in the first few weeks following stroke, most often in the first 2 weeks. Risk factors for hemorrhagic transformation include large strokes with mass effect, enhancement on contrast CT scans, and severe initial neurologic deficits.

c. **Seizures** occur in 4% to 6% of cases of ischemic infarction, mostly in carotid territory cortical infarcts. Infarcts in the posterior circulation are infrequently associated with seizures. Cardioembolic strokes have been found more epileptogenic than atherothrombotic strokes, but several studies have found no significant difference. Seizures associated with lacunar infarcts are extremely rare. Partial seizures are more common than are generalized tonic–clonic seizures. Many seizures occur within

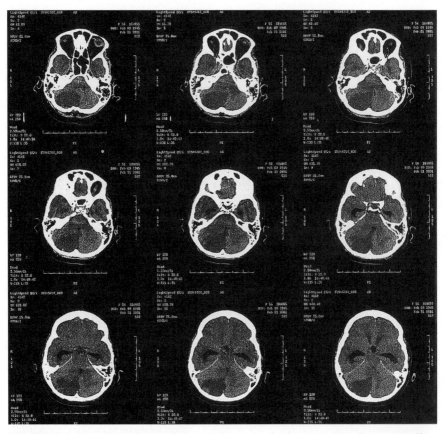

FIG. 36.2 Axial unenhanced cranial computed tomography demonstrates a large area of low attenuation involving the inferior and posterior aspects of the right cerebellar hemisphere (territory of the posterior–inferior cerebellar artery) causing effacement of the brainstem cisterns and compression of the fourth ventricle, causing acute obstructive hydrocephalus. The patient required a right occipital craniectomy secondary to her large edematous cerebellar infarction.

48 hours of the onset of symptoms. In general, seizures are self-limited and respond well to medication. Patients with seizures that occur in the first few days after the ischemic event do not have increased mortality. Status epilepticus is unusual.

3. **Rehabilitation**. Prevention of complications is the first stage of rehabilitation. Patients who need inpatient rehabilitation are transferred to the appropriate rehabilitation facility. The long-term prognosis for stroke depends on severity and type of neurologic deficit, the cause of the stroke, medical comorbidity, premorbid personality, family constellation, home environment, type of community and available services, and the rehabilitation team. Approximately 50% to 85% of long-term survivors of stroke are able to walk independently, most of the recovery taking place in the first 3 months. Approximately two thirds of long-term survivors eventually become independent for activities of daily living, and approximately 85% of surviving patients eventually return home.

B. **Specific measures**

1. **Medical therapy.** General measures and use of antithrombotic agents (antiplatelet agents or anticoagulants) and thrombolytic agents remain the mainstays of medical therapy for acute ischemic stroke.

a. **Antiplatelet agents** that are beneficial include aspirin, clopidogrel, ticlopidine, and slow release dipyridamole in combination with aspirin. These agents are indicated for secondary prevention of stroke.

(1) **Aspirin** is the standard medical therapy for prevention of stroke and recurrent stroke. The mechanism of action of aspirin is irreversible inhibition of platelet function through inactivation of cyclooxygenase. Metaanalyses have shown that aspirin reduces the combined risk of stroke, MI, and vascular death by approximately 25%. Studies proving the effectiveness of aspirin in the secondary prevention of stroke were performed with doses ranging from 30 to 1500 mg/d. Some authors have advocated higher doses of aspirin given that these doses may have useful effects unrelated to cyclooxygenase inhibition. In the Aspirin in Carotid Endarterectomy Trial (ACE), 2,804 patients who had undergone carotid endarterectomy were randomly assigned to compare the benefits of low-dose aspirin (81 to 325 mg/d) with the effects of high-dose aspirin (650 to 1300 mg/d). The primary end points in the ACE trial were stroke, MI, or death. Three months after surgery, the risk of stroke, MI, or death was 6.2% in the low-dose aspirin group versus 8.4% in the high-dose aspirin group. The difference was less apparent when only stroke or death was evaluated as the end point. In 1998, the U.S. Food and Drug Administration recommended a dose of 50 to 325 mg/d of aspirin for stroke patients. The main side effect is gastric discomfort. Gastrointestinal hemorrhage occurs in 1% to 5% of cases. Enteric-coated preparations are generally best tolerated by patients.

(2) **Clopidogrel.** In a study enrolling more than 19,000 patients with atherosclerotic vascular disease manifested as either recent ischemic stroke, recent MI, or symptomatic peripheral arterial disease, 75 mg of clopidogrel was more effective than 325 mg of aspirin in reducing the combined risk of ischemic stroke, MI, or vascular death. After nearly 2 years of follow-up study, the absolute risk reduction was modest (annual risk of end points among clopidogrel-treated patients was 5.32% versus 5.83% among aspirin-treated patients), although it was statistically significant. In the group of more than 6,400 patients who entered the study with a stroke, there was an insignificant relative risk reduction of 7.3% in favor of clopidogrel. Most of these patients had a reoccurrence of stroke as the first outcome measure. The side-effect profile was thought to be relatively benign, with no increased incidence of neutropenia. However, a more recent report associated the use of clopidogrel

with TTP in 11 patients. In the treatment of most patients, clopidogrel had been used for less than 14 days before the onset of TTP. Several patients were taking concomitant medications—five were taking "statins," three were taking atenolol, and one was taking cyclosporine.

(3) **Ticlopidine.** Compared with placebo, ticlopidine has been proved to reduce the risk of stroke, MI, and vascular death among patients with recent noncardioembolic stroke. Ticlopidine (500 mg/d) was compared with aspirin (1,300 mg/d) in the treatment of patients with TIAs and mild stroke. The 3-year rate for nonfatal stroke or death was lower in the ticlopidine group than in the aspirin group (17% versus 19%). Rates of fatal and nonfatal stroke also were lower in the ticlopidine group (10% versus 13%). The recommended dose of ticlopidine is 250 mg two times per day. Ticlopidine has more side effects than does aspirin, including diarrhea, nausea, dyspepsia, and rash. However, its use has been limited by marked hematologic side effects, including a reversible neutropenia and agranulocytosis, aplastic anemia, pancytopenia, and thrombocytopenia. Fatal cases of TTP also have occurred among patients taking ticlopidine. The estimated incidence of ticlopidine-associated TTP is 1 case per 1,600 to 5,000 patients treated.

(4) **Dipyridamole plus aspirin.** The Second European Stroke Prevention Study (ESPS-2) randomized 6,602 patients with previous TIA or stroke to treatment with aspirin alone (25 mg twice per day), modified-release dipyridamole (200 mg twice per day), the two agents in combination, or placebo. The investigators reported an additive effect of dipyridamole (37%) when coprescribed with aspirin. There was a decrease in stroke rate with combined treatment versus either agent alone (aspirin, 18%; dipyridamole, 16%). Both low-dose aspirin and high-dose dipyridamole in a modified release form alone were better than placebo. Among the 25% of patients who withdrew from the study, most were in the dipyridamole and the combination groups. The main side effects of dipyridamole are gastrointestinal distress and headache. The combination of aspirin and dipyridamole was effective in reducing the rate of nonfatal stroke, but had little effect on the rate of MI or fatal stroke.

(5) **Other agents.** There is no persuasive evidence from current or past trials that patients benefit from the use of sulfinpyrazone or suloctidil.

(6) **Summary.** Aspirin at doses of 50 to 325 mg/day (or higher) often is recommended. Extended-release dipyridamole 200 mg plus aspirin 25 mg twice daily, clopidogrel 75 mg/day, and ticlopidine 250 mg twice daily all are acceptable alternatives for initial therapy.

b. **Anticoagulants**

(1) **Prevention.** Oral anticoagulation with warfarin is indicated for primary and secondary prevention of stroke among patients with nonvalvular atrial fibrillation. Results of several multicenter studies suggest that in this clinical situation, warfarin is the most effective drug for stroke prevention unless the patient has lone atrial fibrillation. Warfarin is also indicated for prevention of stroke in the care of patients with rheumatic atrial fibrillation or mechanical heart valves. Less clear, but accepted, indications are secondary prevention of stroke in patients with other high-risk cardiac sources of embolism, those with high-grade intracranial stenosis, or those with documented atherothrombotic TIAs or minor strokes who continue to have symptoms despite antiplatelet therapy.

(2) **Treatment**

(a) **Anticoagulants** (unfractionated heparin, LMWH, heparinoids) sometimes are initiated during the acute phase of infarction with the intention to (1) reduce the risk of stroke progression or recurrent cerebral thromboembolism and (2) prevent other thromboembolic complications, such as deep venous thrombosis and pulmonary embolism. These goals have to be achieved while the risk of hemorrhagic transformation of the infarct is minimized. There is still considerable debate regarding the use of these agents in acute ischemic stroke, and such use is not accepted by all physicians. Although convincing statistical proof is still lacking, anecdotal evidence supports early initiation of intravenous unfractionated heparin to prevent stroke recurrence in several uncommon situations. These indications include cerebral infarction in the setting of inherited or acquired hypercoagulable states, intraluminal arterial thrombus, extracranial cervicocephalic arterial dissection, and cerebral venous thrombosis. Aggregate data from randomized and nonrandomized studies on the use of anticoagulants in "stroke in evolution" suggest that intravenous heparin may reduce the rate of progression of cerebral infarction. However, some studies have not shown a beneficial effect of intravenous heparin in the care of these patients. Despite such controversy, many physicians have attested to having observed improvement during the time heparin is administered and continue to use intravenous heparin to treat selected patients with "stroke in evolution" caused by large-vessel atherothrombosis. When heparin is administered, many neurologists do not use a bolus and aim to keep the activated partial thromboplastin time between 1.5 and 2 times the control level. However, no cause-and-effect relation between heparin administration and clinical improvement can be established.

LMWH and heparinoids have been evaluated for prophylaxis or management of venous thrombosis and as alternatives to heparin in cases of heparin-induced thrombocytopenia. The potential advantages of these agents over conventional heparin include increased bioavailability and longer half-lives. They also have better antithrombotic activity through more efficient inhibition of coagulation factor X and fewer bleeding side effects because of better preservation of platelet function. One randomized, double-blind, placebo-controlled trial of subcutaneous nadroparin calcium (Fraxiparine; Sanofi-Synthelabo, Paris, France) as therapy for acute ischemic stroke (FISS) has been completed with 312 patients at four centers. The primary end point was poor outcome, defined as the total of all-cause mortality and dependency with respect to activities of daily living during the 6 months after randomization. Poor outcome at 3 months was a secondary end point. The study showed no significant difference in poor outcome at 3 months. At 6 months, there was a significant dose-dependent reduction in the rate of poor outcome in favor of nadroparin. A second randomized double-blind study involving 750 patients in 120 centers (FISS bis) failed to confirm these initial observations. The International Stroke Trial (IST) evaluated the value of unfractionated heparin (5,000 IU or 12,500 IU) administered subcutaneously twice a day for 14 days. Patient outcome at 6 months among those who received heparin (n = 9,641) was not different form that among those who did not receive heparin (n = 9,644). The heparinoid agent ORG 10172 has been evaluated in phase I and II trials of the treatment of patients with ischemic stroke given the agent within 24 hours of presentation. Few bleeding episodes were reported, and the compound appeared safe overall. Encouraging functional outcomes were observed at 3 months. However, a large, prospective, double-blind, multi-center trial (ORG 10172, n = 641; placebo, n = 634) showed no difference in favorable outcome at 3 months between patients receiving ORG 10172 and those treated with placebo.

On the basis of available results of the most recent random-ized trials of unfractionated heparin, LMWH, or heparinoids, inadequate data are available to support a recommendation for use of any of these agents for stroke treatment.

(b) **Thrombolytics**. In the last 4 years, the results of eight national and international trials of thrombolytic therapy for ischemic stroke have become available. Three of these trials—the Multi-center Acute Stroke Trial-Italy (MAST-I), the Multicenter Stroke Trial-Europe (MAST-E), and the Australian Streptoki-nase (ASK) trials—were conducted with intravenous adminis-tration of streptokinase within 4 to 6 hours of acute ischemic stroke. The results achieved were poor, with demonstration of increased morbidity and mortality among patients treated with **streptokinase.**

Of four studies in which **recombinant tissue plasminogen activator (rt-PA)** was used—National Institute of Neurologi-cal Disorders and Stroke (NINDS), European Cooperative Acute Stroke Study (ECASS), ECASS-II, and the Alteplase Thrombolysis for Acute Noninterventional Therapy in Ischemic Stroke (ATLANTIS) trial—only one (NINDS) showed signifi-cant improvement in clinical outcome at 3 months without a dif-ference in mortality in the treated group. The ECASS and ECASS-II trials applied 6-hour windows for administration of treatment and showed comparable results, but neither was sta-tistically positive for the predefined primary end point. The ATLANTIS trial was terminated early because of lack of statis-tically significant efficacy at interim analysis among patients treated between 3 and 5 hours after the event.

Recombinant prourokinase (r-pro-UK) is another throm-bolytic agent that has been tested in the last 4 years in the Prourokinase in Acute Cerebral Thromboembolism (PROACT II) trial. In this multicenter, phase III, randomized, controlled trial, 180 patients with angiographically proven occlusion of the middle cerebral artery were given local intraarterial pro-UK within 6 hours of symptom onset. Forty percent of the treated patients were functionally independent, compared with 25% of the placebo group patients 3 months after treatment. The effi-cacy of treatment seemed to fall off after approximately 5 hours. Treated patients, however, also encountered a higher risk of intracranial hemorrhage with neurologic deterioration with 24 hours of treatment (10%, versus 2% in the placebo group). Currently, intraarterial treatment remains experimental and requires a dedicated team, which is most likely to be found at a tertiary stroke care center.

(c) **Defibrinogenating agents. Ancrod,** an enzyme extracted from the venom of the Malayan pit viper, lowers fibrinogen and blood viscosity, inhibits erythrocyte aggregation, indi-rectly stimulates thrombolysis by t-PA up-regulation and pos-sibly causes local vasodilation by acting on the prostacyclin-stimulating factor. It also has a weak anticoagulant effect at high dosages. Its effect was tested in the Stroke Treatment with Ancrod Trial (STAT), in which 500 patients with acute ischemic stroke were randomized to receive either ancrod (n = 248) or placebo (n = 252) within 3 hours of stroke onset. Results of this trial were favorable.

2. **Experimental medical therapies** consist mainly of neuroprotective agents aimed at salvaging neurons around the area of infarction subject to the so-called penumbral ischemia and interrupting programmed cell death (**apoptosis**). Almost 120 controlled clinical trials involving more than 21,000 subjects and investigating more than 50 neuroprotective interventions have yielded negative results. New agents [spin trap agents, oxygenated fluorocarbon nutrient emulsions, α-amino-3-hydroxy-5-methyl-4-isoxazole propionic acid (AMPA) antagonists, and potassium channel openers] have been proposed. The combination of low-dose thrombolytic therapy with a neuroprotective agent may be useful in ischemic stroke therapy by attenuating infarct size, improving neurologic recovery, and reducing the risk of intracranial hemorrhage.

   a. **Inhibitors of neutrophil adhesion and migration.** Intracellular adhesion molecules (ICAMs) are molecules to which leukocytes adhere and which facilitate migration of leukocytes through the endothelium. Some of these molecules are expressed in the cerebral vasculature during ischemia. Neutrophils in particular can contribute to tissue injury by obstructing capillaries and possibly by liberating cytotoxic products. Prevention of neutrophil adhesion by infusion of monoclonal antibodies directed at ICAMs improved neurologic outcome in animal models of transient ischemia. Clinical trials yielded negative results.

   b. **Cytoprotective agents.** The sudden decrease in blood flow after ischemia provokes a cascade of events eventually leading to cell death. These events include the release of excitatory amino acids (EAAs) with secondary opening of ion channels, which leads to an increase in intracellular calcium concentration, activation of enzymes, and generation of free radicals. Several agents have been shown in vitro and in animal studies to interfere at one step or another with this cascade, thus potentially protecting the cells from ischemia.

      (1) **Calcium channel blockers.** Cerebroselective calcium channel blockers such as nimodipine have been tested in acute stroke. The benefits of nimodipine administration for patients with acute ischemic stroke remain unproved.

      (2) **EAA antagonists.** In the last few decades, several observations have provided support for the hypothesis that endogenous EAA neurotransmitters play a major role in the pathogenesis of cerebral ischemia. In animals, EAA antagonists have been shown to reduce the size of an infarct after occlusion of a major artery. From preliminary studies, some of these compounds appear to be safe in humans, but their efficacy has not been demonstrated. Several clinical trials yielded negative results. Optimal protective regimens may necessitate blockading of both (NMDA) and non-NMDA receptors.

      (3) **Free radical scavengers.** Free radicals produced during ischemia can degrade polyunsaturated lipids, which are building blocks of cellular membranes, by means of lipid peroxidation. The central nervous system appears particularly susceptible to free radical injury. The 21-aminosteroid compounds inhibit lipid peroxidation by scavenging free radicals. Tirilazad is one such compound and has been shown in experimental animal models to decrease damage secondary to global ischemia. Its clinical application in the treatment of patients with ischemic stroke has not been established.

      (4) **Neurotrophins** are factors known to promote cell growth in certain neuronal populations. Studies have shown that some of these factors given intraventricularly to animals during ischemia reduce infarct size. The mechanism of action is still unknown but could be related to interaction with EAAs.

      (5) **Calpain inhibitors.** Calpains are cytosomal enzymes that are normally quiescent but become activated by increases in intracellular calcium concentration. These enzymes have many proteins as

Table 36.4 Current status of medical management
of cerebral ischemia: results of selected therapies

Therapy	Conclusion
Antithrombotic Agents	
Aspirin	Positive
Clopidogrel	Positive
Ticlopidine	Positive
Slow release dipyridamole and aspirin	Positive
Sulfinpyrazone	Negative
Suloctidil	Negative
Warfarin	Positive[a]
Warfarin	Negative[b]
Heparin	Negative
LMWH (Fraxiparin)	Negative
LMWH, heparinoid ORG 10172	Negative
Thrombolytic Therapy	
Streptokinase	Negative
t-PA	Positive (within 3 h of stroke onset; intravenous use)
r-pro-Urokinase	Positive (within 6 h of stroke onset; intraarterial use)[c]
Hemorheologic Therapy	
Hemodilution	Negative
Pentoxifylline	Negative
Ancrod	Positive (within 3 h of stroke onset; intravenous use)[c]
Cerebral Protection (Partial List)	
Nimodipine	Negative
Tirilazad	Negative
Excitatory aminoacid antagonists	Negative
Neurotrophins	Negative
Calpain inhibitors	Negative
Other Agents	
Gangliosides	Negative
Barbiturates	Negative
Prostacyclins	Negative
Opiate antagonists	Negative
Aminophylline	Negative
β-Adrenergic receptor blockers	Negative
Vasopressor therapy	Negative
Anti-ICAM antibodies	Negative
Lubeluzole	Negative
Fosphenytoin	Negative
Enlimomab	Negative
Basic fibroblast growth factor	Negative
Naftidrofuryl	Negative
Magnesium (intravenous)	Under investigation
Glyceryl trinitrate	Under investigation
Astrocyte inhibitors (ONO-2506)	Under investigation
Serotonin agonists (repinotan)	Under investigation

[a] For primary and secondary prevention in care of patients with nonvalvular atrial fibrillation.
[b] No additional benefit (INR = 1.4–2.8) in preventing recurrent ischemic stroke in patients with noncardioembolic infarcts.
[c] Currently, neither r-pro-urokinase nor ancrod is available or approved by the U.S. Food and Drug Administration for use in acute ischemic stroke.
LMWH, low-molecular-weight heparin; t-PA, tissue plasminogen activator; ICAM, intracellular adhesion molecule.

their targets, and thus their activation can cause considerable damage. In experimental models of stroke in animals, intraarterial infusion of calpain inhibitors given after onset of ischemia significantly reduced infarct size compared with controls. The value of calpain inhibitors in humans has not been established.

(6) **Other agents.** The value of intravenous magnesium (NMDA antagonist) is under investigation. Treatments with gangliosides, barbiturates, prostacyclins, opiate antagonists, aminophylline, β-adrenergic receptor blockers, vasopressor therapy, naftidrofuryl, clomethiazole, inhibitors of leukocyte adhesion, citicoline, fosphenytoin, lubeluzole, basic fibroblast growth factor, and isovolemic, hypovolemic, and hypervolemic hemodilution have ineffective (Table 36.4).

3. **Surgical therapy.** Precise determination of vessel stenosis has significant potential in the routine clinical assessment of ischemic cerebrovascular disease. Carotid endarterectomy is recommended for secondary prevention in the care of selected patients and is indicated for patients with symptomatic carotid territory TIAs or minor strokes with 70% to 99% stenosis at angiography (as measured by reduction in lumen diameter). The results of the NASCET for symptomatic moderate stenosis (50% to 69%) revealed a reduced stroke rate with endarterectomy versus medical treatment. However, the absolute benefit of surgery was less than that for patients with >70% stenosis and among women and patients with retinal TIAs. The decision to perform carotid endarterectomy on this subgroup of patients with symptoms should be based on age, sex, comorbid status, and surgical complications at each institution. Patients with <50% carotid artery stenosis should undergo medical therapy. Patients with symptomatic moderate to severe stenosis (50% to 99%) who are at high risk of perioperative morbidity and mortality should undergo detailed preoperative medical and anesthetic consultations to optimize management.

The issue is far from settled with regard to asymptomatic carotid artery stenosis of 60% or more. Investigators in the Asymptomatic Carotid Arteriosclerosis Study found carotid endarterectomy combined with aspirin and medical risk factor management of benefit in the treatment of patients with asymptomatic carotid artery stenosis of more than 60% and whose general health makes them good candidates for elective surgery, provided the arteriographic and surgical complication rates are low. However, some experts recommend surgery only when the degree of stenosis is more than 80%. Emergency carotid endarterectomy for acute stroke is highly controversial.

Carotid angioplasty and stenting is an ongoing experimental intervention being developed and tested in a greater number of centers for its effectiveness. Vertebrobasilar and intracranial vessel angioplasty also have been attempted with a good degree of technical safety and with promising results in selected cases.

Recommended Readings

Adams HP Jr, Woolson RF, Biller J, et al. Studies of Org 10172 in patients with acute ischemic stroke. *Haemostasis* 1992;22:99–103.

Albers GW, Hart RG, Lutsep HL, et al. Supplement to the guidelines for the management of transient ischemic attacks: a statement from the Ad Hoc Committee on Guidelines for the Management of Transient Ischemic Attacks, Stroke Council, American Heart Association. *Stroke* 1999;30:2502–2511.

Antiplatelet Trialists' Collaboration. Collaborative overview of randomised trials of antiplatelet therapy, I: prevention of death, myocardial infarction, and stroke by prolonged antiplatelet therapy in various categories of patients. *Br Med J* 1994;308:81–106.

Atrial Fibrillation Investigators. Risk factors for stroke and efficacy of antithrombotic therapy in atrial fibrillation: analysis of pooled data from five randomized controlled trials. *Arch Intern Med* 1994;154:1449–1457.

Barnett HJM, Eliasziw M, Meldrum HE. Drugs and surgery in the prevention of ischemic stroke. *N Engl J Med* 1995;332:238–248.

Bennett CL, Connors JM, Carwile JM, et al. Thrombotic thrombocytopenic purpura associated with clopidogrel. *N Engl J Med* 2000;342:1773–1777.

Biller J, Love BB, Gordon DL. Antithrombotic therapy for ischemic cerebrovascular disease. *Semin Neurol* 1991;4:353–367.

Brandstater ME, Roth EJ, Siebens HC. Venous thromboembolism in stroke: literature review and implications for clinical practice. *Arch Phys Med Rehabil* 1992;73:S379–S391.

CAPRIE Steering Committee. A randomised, blinded, trial of clopidogrel versus aspirin in patients at risk of ischaemic events (CAPRIE). *Lancet* 1996;348:1329–1339.

Cerebral Embolism Study Group. Immediate anticoagulation of embolic stroke: a randomized trial. *Stroke* 1983;14:668–676.

Chimowitz MI, Mancini JGB. Asymptomatic coronary artery disease in patients with stroke: prevalence, prognosis, diagnosis and treatment. *Stroke* 1992;23:433–436.

Donnan GA, Davis SM, Chambers BR, et al. Streptokinase for acute ischemic stroke with relationship to time of administration. *JAMA* 1996;276:961–966.

Dyken ML, Barnett HJ, Easton JD, et al. Low-dose aspirin and stroke. "It ain't necessarily so." *Stroke* 1992;23:1395–1399.

European Atrial Fibrillation Trial Study Group. Secondary prevention in non-rheumatic atrial fibrillation after transient ischaemic attack or minor stroke. *Lancet* 1993;342:1255–1262.

European Carotid Surgery Trialists' Collaborative Group. MRC European Carotid Surgery Trial: Interim results for symptomatic patients with severe (70–99%) or with mild (0–29%) stenosis. *Lancet* 1991;337:1235–1243.

European Stroke Prevention Study (ESPS-2) Working Group. ASA/dipyridamole is superior to either agent alone and to placebo. *Stroke* 1996;27:195.

Executive Committee for the Asymptomatic Carotid Atherosclerosis Study. Endarterectomy for asymptomatic carotid artery stenosis. *JAMA* 1995;273:1421–1428.

Fisher M. Potentially effective therapies for acute ischemic stroke. *Eur Neurol* 1995;35:3–7.

Fleck JD, Biller J. Choices in medical management for prevention of acute ischemic stroke. *Curr Neurol Neurosci Rep* 2001; 1:33–38.

Food and Drug Administration, Department of Health and Human Services. Internal analgesic, antipyretic, and antirheumatic drug products for over-the-counter human use: final rule for professional labeling of aspirin, buffered aspirin, and aspirin in combination with antacid drug products. *Federal Register* 1998 Oct 23 63:56802–56819.

Furlan A, Higashida M, Wechsler L, et al. Intra-arterial prourokinase for acute ischemic stroke: the PROACT II study: a randomized controlled trial. *JAMA* 1999; 282:2003–2011.

Gent M, Blakely JA, Easton JD, et al. The Canadian American Ticlopidine Study (CATS) in thromboembolic stroke. *Lancet* 1989;1:1215–1220.

Hankey GJ, Sudlow CLM, Dunbabin DW. Thienopyridine derivatives (ticlopidine, clopidogrel) versus aspirin for preventing stroke and other serious vascular events in high vascular risk patients (Cochrane Review) [abstract]. Available at: http://www.cochrane.org/cochrane/revabstr/ab001246.htm. Oxford, UK: Update Software, 2001.

Hass WK, Easton JD, Adams HP, Jr, et al. A randomized trial comparing ticlopidine hydrochloride with aspirin for the prevention of stroke in high-risk patients. Ticlopidine Aspirin Stroke Study Group. *N Engl J Med* 1989, 321:501–507.

Hobson RW, Weiss DG, Fields WS, et al. Efficacy of carotid endarterectomy for asymptomatic carotid stenosis. *N Engl J Med* 1993;328:221–227.

International Stroke Trial Collaborative Group. The International Stroke Trial (IST): a randomised trial of aspirin, subcutaneous heparin, both, or neither among 19435 patients with acute ischaemic stroke. *Lancet* 1997;349:1569–1581.

Johnson ES, Lanes SF, Wentworth CE III, et al. A metaregression analysis of the dose-response effect of aspirin on stroke. *Arch Intern Med* 1999;159:1248–1253.

Kay R, Wong KS, Yu YL, et al. Low molecular-weight heparin for the treatment of acute ischemic stroke. *N Engl J Med* 1995;333:1588–1593.

Loftus CM, Biller J. Acute cerebral ischemia, I: pathophysiology and medical treatment. *Contemp Neurosurg* 1994;16:1–6.

Lutsep HL, Clark WM. Current status of neuroprotective agents in the treatment of acute ischemic stroke. *Curr Neurol Neurosci Rep* 2001;1:13–18.

Marsh EE 3rd, Adams HP Jr, Biller J, et al. Use of antithrombotic drugs in the treatment of acute ischemic stroke: a survey of neurologists in practice in the United States. *Neurology* 1989;39:1631–1634.

Meschia JF, Brott TG. New insights on thrombolytic treatment of acute ischemic stroke. *Curr Neurol Neurosci Rep* 2001;1:19–25.

Mohr JP, Thompson JLP, Lazar RM, et al. Comparison of warfarin and aspirin in the prevention of recurrent ischemic stroke. *N Engl J Med* 2001;345:1444–1451.

Multicenter Acute Stroke Trial–Italy (MAST-I) Group. Randomized controlled trial of streptokinase, aspirin, and combination of both in treatment of acute ischemic stroke. *Lancet* 1995;346:1509–1514.

National Institute of Neurological Disorders and Stroke rt-PA Stroke Study Group. Tissue plasminogen activator for acute ischemic stroke. *N Engl J Med* 1995;333:1581–1587.

North American Symptomatic Carotid Endarterectomy Trial Collaborators. Beneficial effect of carotid endarterectomy in symptomatic patients with high-grade carotid stenosis. *N Engl J Med* 1991;325:445–453.

Powers WJ. Acute hypertension after stroke: the scientific basis for treatment decisions. *Neurology* 1993;43:461–467.

Publication Committee for the Trial of ORG 10172 in Acute Stroke Treatment (TOAST) Investigators. Low molecular weight heparinoid ORG 10172 (danaparoid), and outcome after acute ischemic stroke: a randomized controlled trial. *JAMA* 1998;279:1265–1272.

Robinson RG, Lipsey JR, Price TR. Diagnosis and clinical management of post-stroke depression. *Psychosomatics* 1985;26:769–778.

Sandercock P. Is there still a role for intravenous heparin in acute stroke? No. *Arch Neurol* 1999;56:1160–1161.

Sherman DG. Heparin and heparinoids in stroke. *Neurology* 1998;51:556–558.

Sherman DG, Atkinson RP, Chippendale T, et al. Intravenous ancrod for treatment of acute ischemic stroke: the STAT study; a randomized controlled trial. *JAMA* 2000;283:2395–2403.

Siesjo BK. Pathophysiology and treatment of focal cerebral ischemia, I: pathophysiology. *J Neurosurg* 1992;77:169–184.

Siesjo BK. Pathophysiology and treatment of focal cerebral ischemia, II: mechanisms of damage and treatment. *J Neurosurg* 1992;77:337–354.

Taylor DW, Barnett HJ, Haynes RB, et al. Low-dose and high-dose acetylsalicylic acid for patients undergoing carotid endarterectomy: a randomized controlled trial. ASA and Carotid Endarterectomy (ACE) Trial Collaborators. *Lancet* 1999;353:2179–2184.

Wardlaw JM, Warlow CP. Thrombolysis in acute ischemic stroke: does it work? *Stroke* 1992;23:1826–1839.

Wysowksi DK, Bacsanyi J: Blood dycrasias and hematologic reactions in ticlopidine users [letter]. *JAMA* 1996;276:952.

Zeiler K, Kollegger H. Risk factors associated with ischaemic stroke: implications for disease prevention. *CNS Drugs* 1994;1:132–145.

37. HEMORRHAGIC CEREBROVASCULAR DISEASE

Harold P. Adams, Jr.
Muhammad A. Shoaib

Hemorrhagic stroke (hemorrhagic cerebrovascular disease or intracranial hemorrhage) is a life-threatening condition that is second only to acute heart disease as a medical cause of sudden death (death that happens within 24 hours of onset of symptoms). The 1-month mortality of hemorrhagic stroke is estimated to be 25% to 52%. Despite advances in diagnosis and treatment of intracranial hemorrhage, no major decline in mortality has occurred during the last two decades. Approximately one half of deaths occur during the first 48 to 72 hours after the bleeding. Approximately 10% of patients do not survive long enough to reach a hospital, or they die soon after arriving in the emergency department. Mortality is highest among patients older than 60, those with intraventricular extension (intraventricular hemorrhage [IVH]), and those with severe neurologic impairments. Many survivors of hemorrhagic stroke have major disabilities and only 20% of patients will be independent.

Although head injury is the most common cause of intracranial bleeding, it usually is not included in this group. Hemorrhagic strokes include nontraumatic bleeding that occurs primarily in the brain (intraparenchymal or intracerebral hemorrhage), the ventricles (IVH), the subarachnoid space (subarachnoid hemorrhage [SAH]), or the subdural space (subdural hematoma). Bleeding often simultaneously involves the brain, ventricles, and subarachnoid space.

Hemorrhage accounts for approximately 15% to 20% of the 750,000 strokes that occur annually in the United States. Although the incidence of stroke, including hypertensive hemorrhage, has declined since the 1970s, the rate of SAH, largely as the result of ruptured aneurysms, has not dropped. The frequency of hemorrhagic stroke may increase in the future as the result of the aging of the population and an increase in the prevalence of cerebral amyloid angiopathy, increased abuse of drugs associated with increased risk of bleeding, and the more widespread administration of medications that may affect coagulation. Although the risk of hemorrhagic stroke increases with advancing age, children and young adults also are affected. Because ischemic strokes are relatively uncommon among children and young adults, the relative proportion of hemorrhagic strokes is very prominent in these groups. The patient's age also influences the diagnosis of the cause of hemorrhagic stroke. For example, cerebral amyloid angiopathy and hypertension are important causes of bleeding among the elderly, whereas the average age of a patient with a ruptured vascular malformation is approximately 30 years. Even when trauma is excluded, hemorrhagic stroke is more frequent among men than among women. The incidence of hemorrhagic stroke is higher among Americans of African or Asian ancestry than among those with European heritage. Intracranial hemorrhage is an especially important cause of death among African Americans.

I. **Causes of hemorrhagic stroke.** Intracranial hemorrhage is a manifestation of an underlying disease (Table 37.1). In most cases, the most likely cause of hemorrhagic stroke can be identified.

    A. **Occult craniocerebral trauma.** Trauma is a potential cause of intracranial bleeding—typically subdural or epidural hematoma or parenchymal contusions. A history of injury may be lacking when a patient is found unconscious and other clues must be sought, such as lacerations or soft-tissue swelling. Conversely, a patient who has a primary hemorrhage may suffer secondary trauma. For example, a patient with SAH may have a secondary seizure and fall. In such circumstances, observers and the patient should be carefully quizzed about the course of the illness and whether the neurologic symptoms preceded the injury.

    B. **Hypertension.** Either acute or chronic hypertension is a predisposing factor for bleeding. Chronic arterial hypertension leads to degenerative changes in the penetrating arteries of the brain. Sudden severe hypertension presumably overwhelms the autoregulatory responses of the brain, and a vessel ruptures. Situations that can lead to severe, acute arterial hypertension include acute glomerulonephritis, eclampsia, severe emotional stress, or use of a sympathomimetic agent. The most common locations of hypertensive hemorrhage are the basal ganglia (putamen), thalamus, brainstem, and cerebellum. Hypertension should be considered as the likely cause of a hematoma located in the deep gray matter structures of the cere-

Table 37.1 Causes of hemorrhagic stroke

Occult craniocerebral trauma	Arterial hypertension
Saccular aneurysm	Sustained
Nonsaccular aneurysm	Acute
Infective	Stress
Neoplastic	Eclampsia
Traumatic	Cerebral amyloid angiopathy
Dolichoectatic	Vasculitis
Dissection	Multisystem
Vascular malformation	Isolated
Arteriovenous malformation	Bleeding disorders
Venous malformation	Hemophilia
Cavernous malformation	Sickle cell disease
Telangiectasis	Thrombocytopenia
Moyamoya	Leukemia
Drug abuse	Thrombolytic agents
Amphetamines	Anticoagulants
Cocaine	Antiplatelet agents
Phenylpropanolamine	Venous thrombosis
Tumors	Hemorrhagic transformation of ischemic
Primary	stroke
Metastatic	

bral hemisphere if a patient has a history of hypertension. Other features of chronic hypertension, such as retinopathy, renal dysfunction, or left ventricular hypertrophy support the diagnosis. Hemorrhagic stroke frequently is attributed to arterial hypertension because of the presence of a markedly elevated blood pressure measured on arrival to an emergency department. However, arterial hypertension is common among acutely ill patients with intracranial bleeding, and the finding should not automatically lead to the diagnosis of hypertensive hemorrhage. Although hypertension can be the cause of primary IVH, it is not a common cause of primary SAH.

C. **Saccular aneurysm.** Rupture of a saccular aneurysm is the most common cause of nontraumatic SAH, and it is an important cause of intracerebral hemorrhage. Approximately 1% to 5% of adults harbor intracranial aneurysms, but a minority of these lesions actually rupture during life. These patients have a higher-than-expected frequency of coarctation of the aorta, fibromuscular dysplasia, and polycystic kidney disease. Approximately 10% of patients have a family history of cerebral aneurysm. Approximately 85% of saccular aneurysms are in the carotid circulation, and they arise at vascular bifurcations. The most common sites are the junction of the anterior cerebral and anterior communicating arteries, the origin of the posterior communicating artery from the internal carotid artery, and the bifurcation of the middle cerebral artery. The most common locations in the posterior circulation are the bifurcation of the basilar artery and the origin of the posterior inferior cerebellar artery.

D. **Other aneurysms.** Infective, neoplastic, and traumatic aneurysms are rare causes of intracranial bleeding. These lesions usually are located in peripheral branch arteries on the cortical surface of the cerebral hemispheres, and they are smaller than saccular aneurysms. Dolichoectatic (fusiform) aneurysms are tortuous, elongated arterial enlargements most commonly found in the basilar arteries of patients with extensive atherosclerosis in other vascular beds. They usually cause ischemic stroke or compression of brainstem structures or cranial nerves. Hemorrhage is an uncommon complication. Spontaneous or traumatic dissecting aneurysms of intracranial arteries, particularly of the basilar or distal vertebral arteries, are potential causes of atypical SAH.

E. Vascular malformations. These lesions are a leading cause of hemorrhagic stroke, particularly among children and young adults. Vascular malformations are classified as arteriovenous malformation (AVM), venous malformations, cavernous malformations, and telangiectasias. They can arise in any part of the brain. Although familial cases, as with hereditary hemorrhagic telangiectasia, are reported, most are sporadic. Hemorrhage is the symptom when the patient comes to medical attention in approximately 50% of cases. Nonhemorrhagic symptoms, which typically antedate hemorrhage, include seizures, recurrent headaches, and progressive neurologic impairment. Patients with large malformations leading to turbulent blood flow can have a cranial bruit auscultated. The patient also may report hearing the sound.

F. Amyloid angiopathy. Cerebral amyloid angiopathy (congophilic angiopathy) is an important cause of lobar hemorrhage among the elderly. With aging, amyloid is deposited in the walls of leptomeningeal and cortical arterioles, and presumably the protein accumulation leads to fragility of the vessel. The hemorrhages are typically located at the junction of the white matter and cerebral cortex in the cerebral hemispheres. Most hemorrhages are in the frontal or parietal lobes. Multiple hemorrhages or recurrent hemorrhages are common. Cerebellar hemorrhages also can occur. The presence of concomitant cerebral amyloid angiopathy may be a factor for some cases of cerebral hemorrhage that occur in elderly patients receiving thrombolytic therapy for either acute myocardial infarction or ischemic stroke. Cerebral amyloid angiopathy should be considered as the likely cause of lobar hemorrhage among persons older than 75 years. Because approximately 70% of these patients have a history of Alzheimer's disease, a history of dementia or cognitive impairments increases the likelihood that a hemorrhage in an elderly patient is due to cerebral amyloid angiopathy.

G. Vasculitis. Multisystem or isolated central nervous system vasculitis rarely causes hemorrhage. Bleeding is most commonly associated with necrotizing arteritis, such as polyarteritis. Vasculitis may be the cause of bleeding among some young patients who have hemorrhagic stroke after use of a sympathomimetic drug.

H. Bleeding disorders. Intracranial hemorrhage complicates several inherited or acquired disorders of coagulation, including hemophilia, sickle cell disease, thrombocytopenia, and leukemia. Intracranial bleeding also can complicate the use of thrombolytic agents, anticoagulants, or antiplatelet agents. In general, the severity of bleeding is greater and the prognosis is poorer among patients with coagulopathy than they are among patients who have spontaneous hematoma. Approximately 0.5% of patients who receive thrombolytic agents for management of acute myocardial infarction can have complicating intracranial hemorrhages, and the risk of bleeding is much higher among patients who receive the medications for treatment of acute ischemic stroke. Concomitant administration of an anticoagulant or antiplatelet agent increases the likelihood of intracranial hemorrhage.

Bleeding can complicate treatment with heparin, particularly among patients who have had large ischemic strokes. Although the risk is lower than that of thrombolytic therapy, both traditional heparin and low-molecular-weight heparins are associated with an increase in brain hemorrhage. No specific dosage or treatment regimen is associated with a higher or lower risk of bleeding. Intracranial bleeding is a side effect of treatment with oral anticoagulants, and this complication should be considered whenever a patient has acute neurologic symptoms while taking oral anticoagulants even if there is no other evidence of bleeding. The risk of intracranial hemorrhage is especially high among the elderly and persons who have leukoaraiosis present on brain imaging studies. In addition, those with a history of stroke or poorly controlled hypertension have a high risk of serious bleeding complications from oral anticoagulants. The risk of intracranial bleeding increases when the prothrombin time–international normalized ratio (INR) is excessively prolonged. The risk of bleeding increases rapidly when the INR exceeds 3 to 4. Although the frequency of hemorrhagic stroke is lower with antiplatelet agents than with oral anticoagulants, use of aspirin has been associated with the complication. The combination of warfarin and aspirin has a higher risk of bleeding than does administration of either agent alone.

I. **Drug abuse.** Intracranial hemorrhage has been attributed to abuse of sympathomimetic agents, including cocaine and methamphetamine. Another agent, phenylpropanolamine, which is used as a diet suppressant or therapy for upper respiratory infections, was withdrawn from the U.S. market because of an apparent relation to hemorrhagic stroke. These agents may lead to bleeding because of sudden increases in blood pressure or because of the development of a vasculitis. Intracranial hemorrhage also has been associated with heavy alcohol use.

J. **Moyamoya disease** is an uncommon cause of intracranial hemorrhage among young adults and children. The arteriographic hallmark of moyamoya is occlusions of the major arteries of the anterior circulation and the appearance of a mesh of fine blood vessels at the base of the cerebral hemispheres. Moyamoya disease is inherited on an autosomal dominant basis and is most common in northeastern Asia. Moyamoya disease is diagnosed when the arteriographic findings occur among patients with a number of acquired disorders. Hemorrhages can be secondary to rupture of the small collateral channels or aneurysms.

K. **Venous thrombosis.** Occlusion of a cortical vein (cortical venous thrombosis) or sinus (sinus thrombosis) is an uncommon cause of hemorrhagic stroke. Bleeding is most common among patients with sagittal sinus thrombosis; in this situation, the areas of bleeding are located parasagittally in a thumbprint pattern. The clinical course of venous thrombosis differs from that of most other hemorrhagic strokes. Most patients have worsening headaches, seizures, altered consciousness, and focal neurologic signs that evolve over a few days. Venous thrombosis often develops in the peripartum period but it also occurs among persons who are dehydrated, who have malignant disease, have undergone a recent cranial operation, or have an otolaryngologic infection.

L. **Brain tumors.** Hemorrhage can be the initial symptom of a highly vascular primary or metastatic brain tumor. Leading metastatic tumors associated with hemorrhage are choriocarcinoma, melanoma, and carcinoma of the kidney, thyroid, liver, lung, or breast. The chief primary brain tumors are glioblastoma and pilocytic astrocytoma. Patients often have a history of evolving neurologic symptoms such as headaches or personality changes before the bleeding event. The presence of extensive brain edema in the first few hours after hemorrhage or multiple hemorrhagic lesions should prompt consideration of an underlying brain tumor.

M. **Hemorrhagic transformation of an ischemic stroke.** Modern brain imaging has allowed detection of asymptomatic hemorrhagic changes in the ischemic lesions in a sizable proportion of patients with recent stroke. A smaller percentage of patients have neurologic worsening secondary to hemorrhagic transformation of the infarction. The risk of this complication increases with administration of thrombolytic agents, anticoagulants, or antiplatelet agents in the first hours after stroke.

II. **Manifestations of hemorrhagic stroke.** The manifestations of hemorrhagic stroke generally are similar for adults and children. However, the symptoms of SAH and IVH differ slightly from those of intracerebral hemorrhage in that focal neurologic impairment often is not prominent. Because of the absence of focal impairment, errors in diagnosis are more likely to occur among patients with SAH than among patients with bleeding primarily in the brain.

A. **History**

1. Hemorrhagic stroke usually is a sudden, dramatic event. The patient or observers often relate the circumstances surrounding the onset of symptoms. The headache, of any quality and location, usually is described as intense. A headache accompanied by transient loss of consciousness or one that is of cataclysmic onset is the premier symptom of SAH; it is often described as the "the worst headache of my life." Approximately 40% of patients with intracerebral hemorrhage have headache. Accompanying symptoms include nausea, vomiting, prostration, photophobia, phonophobia, and nuchal rigidity. The presence of nausea and vomiting and focal

signs suggestive of a stroke in the cerebral hemisphere are predictive of a hemorrhagic event.

2. Disturbed consciousness is common. Prolonged unresponsiveness (coma) occurs among patients who have major bleeding. Transient alteration in alertness at the time of bleeding (syncope) may be secondary to a temporary increase in intracranial pressure (ICP). Disorientation, confusion, or delirium can occur. Although focal or generalized seizures can happen, recurrent seizures or status epilepticus are uncommon.

3. Focal neurologic signs reflect the location of the hematoma inside the brain. The most common pattern is a hemiparesis and hemisensory loss secondary to a hematoma in the basal ganglia. Patients with cerebellar hemorrhage often have a subacute course. They report headache, dizziness (vertigo), disturbed balance, nausea, and vomiting. Signs of increased ICP or brainstem compression subsequently appear, including cranial nerve palsy, motor impairment, and disturbed consciousness. Although most patients with SAH or primary IVH do not have focal neurologic symptoms, some patients with aneurysms have focal findings. The most common symptoms are diplopia or ptosis secondary to third cranial nerve palsy.

B. Examination

1. Assessment of the vital signs and the ABCs of emergency care (airway, breathing, circulation) are the first steps in the examination (Table 37.2). Vital signs are measured frequently, and close neurologic monitoring is required. The airway should be secured for patients with altered consciousness, seizures, vomiting, or prominent weakness. Patients with severe hemorrhage often have respiratory abnormalities that lead to hypoxia, hypercapnia, or acidosis. Fever is relatively common, and it is especially prominent among patients with IVH. Electrocardiographic abnormalities and cardiac arrhythmias can be detected. Arterial hypertension is frequent.

2. A bruit auscultated over the head or neck suggests an AVM. Multiple sites of ecchymosis or petechiae point to infective endocarditis, recent trauma, or an underlying coagulation disorder. Evidence of cervical spinal, facial, or cranial injury, such as Battle's sign (basilar skull fracture) should be sought. Neck pain or tenderness can represent an associated spinal fracture. The neck should not be flexed to check for signs of meningeal irritation until the possibility of cervical spinal fracture is eliminated.

3. Meningeal irritation is caused by blood in the subarachnoid space. Nuchal rigidity (Brudzinski's sign) may not be present in patients with hematoma

Table 37.2 Examination of patients with suspected intracerebral hemorrhage

Vital signs	Signs of meningeal irritation
Airway	Brudzinski's sign
Breathing and respiratory pattern	Kernig's sign
Heart rate	Ocular signs
Temperature	Subhyaloid hemorrhage
Blood pressure	Papilledema
Cardiovascular examination	Level of consciousness
Screening for bleeding elsewhere	Glasgow Coma Scale
Petechiae	Other neurologic findings
Ecchymosis	Language or cognitive
Signs of craniocerebral trauma	Articulation
Battle's sign	Motor
Raccoon eye	Sensory
Ocular hemorrhage	Cranial nerves
Scalp laceration	
Skull tenderness	

restricted to the parenchyma or in comatose patients. A stiff neck is prominent among most patients with SAH, but it may take several hours to appear. Ocular bleeding (subhyaloid, conjunctival, or retinal) develops in approximately 20% of patients, but the presence is highly specific for serious hemorrhage. Because the course of the illness usually is short, papilledema is not commonly observed.

4. **Assessment of consciousness** is the most important component of the neurologic examination because the level of consciousness correlates strongly with the severity of hemorrhage. Although the easily calculated Glasgow Coma Scale score was originally developed to assess head injuries, it is directly applicable to persons with acute nontraumatic brain diseases, including hemorrhage. In general, a score of 6 or less on the Glasgow Coma Scale correlates with a very poor prognosis. The rest of the neurologic examination is aimed at detecting abnormalities specific for different locations of the hemorrhage within the brain.

III. Differential diagnosis of hemorrhagic stroke. Imaging of the brain—computed tomography (CT) in particular—greatly expedites the diagnosis of hemorrhagic stroke. The differential diagnosis is not extensive. The brief duration, clinical severity, and prominent focal neurologic signs are relatively specific.

A. **Ischemic stroke.** The leading alternative diagnosis is acute ischemic stroke. Although there are no unique features, patients with hemorrhagic stroke generally are more seriously ill than are those with ischemic stroke. The symptoms usually are more severe than those of occlusion of a single artery, as in ischemic stroke. Headaches, alterations in consciousness, nausea, vomiting, and photophobia and phonophobia also are more prominent in hemorrhagic stroke.

B. **Craniocerebral trauma.** Differentiation of traumatic from spontaneous bleeding can be difficult when a patient is comatose and no history is available. In general, hemorrhage deep in the brain is not the result of trauma. Conversely, multiple small cortical petechiae in the frontal, temporal, and occipital poles usually are caused by injuries.

C. In contradistinction to that of intracerebral hemorrhage, the differential diagnosis of SAH is broad (Table 37.3). Although patients with SAH usually seek medical attention because of the severity of their symptoms, physicians can be misled. The diagnosis of SAH is missed in approximately 25% of cases, most commonly among the least seriously ill patients. Failure to recognize a ruptured aneurysm has serious implications because of the risk of potentially fatal recurrent hemorrhage and the availability of therapies that are effective when administered early. The only way to avoid missing SAH is to maintain a high index of suspicion. Patients who have the sudden onset of an exceptionally severe headache or a headache associated with loss of consciousness should be evaluated for SAH. The absence of focal neurologic signs or meningeal irritation does not preclude the diagnosis. Atypical symptoms include severe neck, face, shoulder, eye, and ear pain. A ruptured aneurysm in the posterior fossa occasionally can manifest as neck or back pain as the primary symptom.

IV. Diagnostic studies. The goals of the emergency evaluation are to confirm hemorrhagic stroke as the cause of the neurologic symptoms and to look for acute complications (Table 37.4). These critically ill persons are at high risk of a variety of serious neurologic or medical side effects. The most frequent neurologic problems are brain edema, hydrocephalus,

Table 37.3 Differential diagnosis of subarachnoid hemorrhage

Migraine headache	Tension headache
Sinusitis	Viral meningitis
Influenza	Hypertensive crisis
Eclampsia	Head injury
Cervical spinal injury	Cervical herniated disk
Alcohol intoxication	Drug intoxication

Table 37.4 Diagnostic studies for patients with hemorrahgic stroke

Emergency
  CT of the brain
  Chest radiograph
  Lateral cervical spine radiograph (if a neck injury is suspected)
  Electrocardiogram
  Arterial blood gases (if hypoxia or respiratory failure is suspected)
  Complete blood cell count
  Platelet count
  Serum electrolytes
  Blood glucose
  Prothrombin time, international normalized ratio
  Activated partial thromboplastin time
  Cerebrospinal fluid examination (if subarachnoid hemorrhage is suspected
    and no blood seen on CT scans)

Subsequent
  CT with contrast enhancement
  CT angiography
  MR imaging of the brain
  MR angiography
  Arteriography
  Transcranial Doppler ultrasonography
  Fibrinogen
  Blood cultures (if infective endocarditis is suspected)
  Sickle cell screen
  Erythrocyte sedimentation rate
  Urine and blood screens for illicit drugs
  Brain and meningeal biopsy

CT, computed tomography; MR, magnetic resonance.

increased ICP, and seizures. The most serious early medical complications are myocardial ischemia, cardiac arrhythmia, gastrointestinal bleeding, respiratory abnormalities, and fluid and electrolyte disturbances. Before they are moved, obtunded patients with possible craniocerebral trauma need radiography of the cervical spine to eliminate occult fracture.

  A. **CT of the brain** is the single most important diagnostic test. It is available in most medical centers, is relatively inexpensive, is noninvasive, and can be performed quickly. The yield of unenhanced CT among patients with hemorrhagic stroke is extraordinarily high. When CT is performed within 24 hours of onset, blood density can be detected in almost 100% of patients with intraparenchymal hematoma and approximately 95% of those with SAH. Sequential CT studies during the first hours after the ictus can depict enlargement of a hematoma presumably as the result of continued bleeding. CT can miss a small collection of subarachnoid blood in a patient with mild hemorrhage or if the bleeding is restricted to the posterior fossa. If CT is performed several days after the onset, the yield decreases because the collection of blood may have been reabsorbed. CT also helps detect early complications, including brain edema and hydrocephalus. The location of blood also is used to guide further diagnostic studies and provides clues to the likely cause of hemorrhage. For example, the presence of subarachnoid blood restricted to the perimesencephalic cisterns usually is not due to an aneurysm. CT also provides prognostic information; for example, large amounts of subarachnoid blood are predictive of vasospasm and ischemic stroke after SAH. The presence of intraventricular extension also forecasts a poor prognosis.

  B. **Magnetic resonance imaging (MRI)** depicts intracranial bleeding and provides additional data about the likely cause. Multisequence MRI can be as sensitive as CT in the detection of intracranial bleeding. Although it is more expensive and not as widely available as CT, MRI does have advantages. Because of changes in the responses of iron in hematomas of different ages, MRI can provide information about the age of the hemorrhagic lesion. It can depict microhemorrhage in patients with small-vessel disease such as cerebral amyloid angiopathy or lipohyalinosis. Abnormalities in flow voids can be found in patients with vascular malformations. Thus, MRI is an important ancillary diagnostic study.

C. **Cerebrospinal fluid (CSF) examination.** Although examination of the CSF helps identify bleeding within the subarachnoid space, its importance has declined with the advent of modern brain imaging. There is no reason to do a lumbar puncture to search for blood if CT shows a hemorrhage. Conversely, CSF examination is important if SAH is suspected and CT does not show blood. CSF examination can help detect bleeding among alert patients who have mild signs. The risk of neurologic complications, including herniation, is low in an alert patient who has no focal impairment and no mass detected at CT. Determining whether the source of bloody CSF is an intracranial hemorrhage or a traumatic lumbar puncture (bloody tap) can be difficult. Bloody CSF from SAH generally does not clear in sequentially collected tubes. Xanthochromia (yellowing) of the CSF supernatant after centrifugation is the most reliable sign, but it can take up to 12 hours after SAH to develop. A physician should immediately centrifuge a bloody CSF specimen to check for xanthochromia because a delay of several hours can give a false-positive result. The CSF findings evolve, and if the lumbar puncture is delayed several days, only slightly yellow fluid, an elevated CSF protein level, or an inflammatory response that suggests viral meningitis may be detected.

D. **Additional screening studies.** Additional tests for determining the cause of hemorrhage are ordered on a case-by-case basis after the patient's status has been stabilized. Contrast-enhanced CT or MRI may help detect an AVM or aneurysm. CT angiography is becoming a valuable method to image the vasculature at the base of the brain and, in particular, to examine the anatomic relations of saccular aneurysms. Magnetic resonance angiography (MRA) also is an effective screening tool to detect aneurysms or vascular malformations. MRA is the best method to screen for a venous thrombosis. Electrocardiography, chest radiography, and hematologic, coagulation, and biochemical studies also should be performed.

E. **Arteriography.** Arteriography remains a key component of evaluation, especially in cases of SAH. This study usually is not needed for examination of older patients with a history of hypertension who have a hemorrhage in the basal ganglion or thalamus. Although it is invasive and has some risk, arteriography generally is safe for patients with hemorrhagic stroke. Arteriography remains the best means of detecting a saccular or small peripheral aneurysm or a vascular malformation. Besides depicting the aneurysm, arteriography provides information about the anatomic features of the adjacent blood vessels and the presence of vasospasm—findings that influence decisions about surgery. Arteriography also provides information about the presence, location, and extent of cerebral vasculitis.

V. **Treatment**

A. **Prevention.** Hemorrhagic stroke is an expensive illness. Not only are health care costs high, but also the secondary economic consequences, including lost productivity, are considerable. The most cost-effective therapy is prevention. Several treatments, selected on the basis of potential causes, can decrease the risk of hemorrhagic stroke. Either acute or chronic sustained elevations of blood pressure can lead to intracranial bleeding, but antihypertensive agents can decrease the risk of this complication. Care in the use of thrombolytic, antithrombotic, and antiplatelet aggregating agents should decrease the likelihood of intracranial bleeding. Management of inherited or acquired disorders of coagulation also prevents hemorrhage. Surgical management of an unruptured aneurysm or AVM can be a potential prophylactic measure. The benefits of prophylactic clipping of unruptured saccular aneurysms seem to be limited to patients with large lesions. Endovascular therapies and focused radiation also are potential therapies.

B. **Referral and admission.** Patients with hemorrhagic stroke are critically ill. Inpatient care is warranted because intracranial hemorrhage is life threatening and is accompanied by many serious medical and neurologic complications. The facilities and personnel required for successful care of these patients may not be available at many hospitals. Admission to a specialized treatment facility that has monitoring capabilities or an intensive care unit usually is needed. The high-risk nature of hemorrhagic stroke means that most patients should be transferred to centers that have neurologic and neurosurgical expertise. Primary care physicians should not attempt to treat these patients but should refer them to specialized treatment centers as soon as possible.

C. **Management**

1. **General management.** Measures for control of acute medical and neurologic complications are part of emergency treatment (Table 37.5). Endotracheal intubation and ventilatory assistance may be needed. Hypoxic patients should receive supplemental oxygen. Fever should be controlled. Access for intravenous administration of medications and fluids is needed and normal saline solution is infused slowly. Hypotonic solutions generally are avoided because of their potential effects on formation of edema. Hypoglycemia or a markedly elevated blood sugar level should be managed. Cardiac monitoring to detect arrhythmia and frequent assessment of vital signs and neurologic status are performed. Medications to control arrhythmia are selected on a case-by-case basis. Symptoms such as headache, agitation, and vomiting warrant treatment. Patients who have had seizures are given anticonvulsants, but prophylactic administration of anticonvulsants to patients who have not had seizures is controversial. Because of fears that the stress of a seizure may cause rebleeding, many physicians give anticonvulsants to patients who have ruptured aneurysms.

   a. **Arterial hypertension.** Markedly elevated blood pressure can worsen intracranial bleeding, and the blood pressure often is volatile during the first few hours. It usually declines as pain, agitation, seizures, and vomiting are controlled. The level of blood pressure that mandates medical treatment is not known, and the choice of initial treatment is affected by the severity of arterial hypertension. The goal should be cautious lowering of the blood pressure. Responses to antihypertensive agents are exaggerated. Short-acting parenteral medications are preferred because the dosages can be titrated in response to the patient's blood pressure and neurologic status. The best medications for this setting include labetalol, esmolol, nitroprusside, hydralazine, or enalapril (Table 37.6).

   b. **ICP and brain edema.** Management of increased ICP is important. Impaired venous return, agitation, fever, hypoxia, hypercapnia, and hypoventilation aggravate increased ICP and should be managed. Early measures are elevation of the patient's head, control of pain and agitation, modest fluid restriction, and avoidance of potentially hypoosmolar fluids, such as 5% dextrose in water. Neither conventional nor large doses of corticosteroids are helpful. Intubation and hyperventilation are prescribed when a patient's condition is deteriorating and are comple-

Table 37.5 Emergency management of hemorrhagic stroke

ABC of life support
Frequent measurement of vital signs and blood pressure
Frequent neurologic assessment
Cardiac monitoring
Control of fever
Supplemental oxygen if hypoxia is present
Intravenous access with slow infusion of normal saline solution
Control of pain, nausea, vomiting, and seizures

ABC, airway, breathing, circulation.

Table 37.6 Emergency management of hypertension for patients with hemorrhagic stroke

Blood pressure	Treatment
Systolic blood pressure >230 mm Hg or diastolic blood pressure >140 mm Hg on two readings, 5 min apart	Institute nitroprusside
Systolic blood pressure 180–230 mm Hg or diastolic blood pressure 105–140 mm Hg, or mean arterial blood pressure >130 mm Hg on two readings, 20 minutes apart	Institute treatment with intravenous labetalol, esmolol, or enalapril
Systolic blood pressure <180 mm Hg and diastolic blood pressure <105 mm Hg	Defer antihypertensive therapy

mented by infusion of 20% mannitol, in a dosage of 0.5 to 1 g/kg. The effects of mannitol appear within a few minutes and last up to 4 to 6 hours. Recurrent doses of mannitol may be needed to prevent rebound increases in ICP, although a hyperosmolar state is possible. Monitoring of ICP is used frequently to guide treatments in such a critical situation. Furosemide also may be helpful.

2. **Emergency surgical management.** A critical early decision involves the need for surgical evacuation of the hematoma. A ventricular catheter can be used to drain CSF if the patient has secondary hydrocephalus. This measure can lower ICP and forestall craniotomy. Removal of a large hematoma can be life saving when a patient's condition is deteriorating. However, the overall utility of surgery in improving outcome has not been established, especially among patients with large hematomas deep in the cerebral hemisphere. Several different surgical strategies have been used, including direct surgical exploration, endoscopic removal, and stereotactic placement of a catheter to withdraw the clot. Installation of a thrombolytic agent is used to facilitate aspiration of the hematoma. The location and size of the hematoma and the patient's neurologic status, course, and general health affect such a decision (Table 37.7). Surgery is recommended for management of a large cerebellar hematoma that is compressing the brainstem or obstructing CSF outflow. Patients with small to moderate-sized hematomas of the cerebral hemispheres who do not have mass-related signs usually do not need surgery. Patients with large superficial hemispheric hematoma can be treated operatively.

3. **General inpatient care.** Emergency management is continued after admission. The patient is kept at bed rest until the situation has stabilized. Careful nursing care, monitoring. and regular assessments of the patient's neurologic

Table 37.7 Indications for emergency surgical evacuation of intracerebral hematoma

Surgery Indicated
    Cerebellar hematoma >3 cm in diameter with compression of brainstem or development of hydrocephalus
    Hemorrhage with a structural lesion (aneurysm or vascular malformation) that can be managed surgically
    Patient young with moderate to large lobar hemorrhage and whose condition is becoming worse

Surgery not Indicated
    Patient with small hematoma or minimal impairment
    Patient with very severe impairment (coma)

status and vital signs are continued. Patients not admitted to an intensive care unit often are housed in a quiet environment. To decrease the risk of aspiration and pneumonia, liquids and food are not given by mouth until the patient's ability to swallow safely has been confirmed. Care in avoiding pulmonary complications is part of general management. Modest fluid restriction is continued for patients who have a large hematoma. Other patients, including most of those with SAH, usually do not need this limitation. Management with intravenous fluids should emphasize maintaining normal electrolyte status. Incontinence or the need for accurate measurement of urine output often mandates placement of an indwelling bladder catheter. Because of the risk of urinary tract infection, the catheter should be removed as soon as possible. Because bedridden patients have a high risk of deep venous thrombosis that can lead to pulmonary embolism, they are treated with alternating pressure devices and antiembolism stockings. Because heparin can worsen bleeding, it usually is not prescribed. When the patient's condition has stabilized, increased activity, mobilization, and rehabilitation begin.

4. **Cause-specific treatment.** Management of the cause of the bleeding is key. For example, underlying coagulopathy should be corrected, and the effects of an antithrombotic agent should be reversed.

   a. **Vascular malformations.** Patients with ruptured vascular malformations usually undergo definitive therapy to prevent recurrent hemorrhage. Because the risk of early rebleeding is relatively low, treatment usually is delayed until the hematoma has been reabsorbed. The decision whether to perform a surgical procedure is influenced by the size and location of the malformation and the number and caliber of the feeding arteries. Lesions in neurologically eloquent areas and those that are deep in the brain may not be surgically approachable. A high-flow malformation also is a problem because a postoperative state of hyperperfusion leading to hemorrhage or severe brain edema can follow resection. A staged procedure with endovascular therapies may precede surgical excision. Endovascular placement of microemboli or a sclerosing agent also can be used as monotherapy. Small and deep vascular malformations can be managed with focused, high-intensity radiation that leads to secondary fibrosis and gradual occlusion of the vessels. Patients with very large malformations may not be treatable with any of the currently available modalities.

   b. **Aneurysms.** Patients with ruptured aneurysms are vulnerable to recurrent hemorrhage and ischemic stroke (Table 37.8).

   Recurrent aneurysmal rupture is a largely fatal event that peaks during the first 24 hours, when the risk is approximately 4%. The overall risk of recurrent hemorrhage during the first 10 days approaches 20%. The symptoms of rebleeding are similar to those of the initial hemorrhage, and CT shows more blood. Several therapies are aimed at avoiding recurrent hemorrhage, but the most effective is direct surgical obliteration of the aneurysm. The timing of surgery is influenced by the patient's condition, the location of the aneurysm, the presence of serious comorbid diseases, the presence of vasospasm, and the preference of the surgeon. Most surgeons favor early surgery. The condition of very seriously ill patients and of those with relatively inaccessible aneurysms is stabilized before surgery is undertaken. Endovascular placement of a coil or balloon can be prescribed as an alternative. Antifibrinolytic agents are effective in preventing rebleeding, but they are associated with increased risk of brain ischemia. As a result, these medications have been largely abandoned.

   Vasospasm is a localized or generalized arterial process that occurs almost exclusively in association with aneurysmal SAH. Vasospasm is most likely to occur when CT shows extensive subarachnoid blood. Thick collections of blood in the subarachnoid space trigger the progressive arterial narrowing that peaks at 7 to 10 days after the SAH. Thereafter, vasospasm gradually abates. Arterial narrowing causes hypoperfusion,

Table 37.8 Management of hemorrhage secondary to ruptured aneurysm

Prevention of Recurrent Hemorrhage
Surgical treatment—clipping, wrapping, trapping
Endovascular placement of coil or balloon
Antihypertensive agent
Antifibrinolytic agent

Prevention of Vasospasm and Ischemic Stroke
Avoidance of dehydration, hyponatremia, and hypotension
Avoidance of use of antifibrinolytic agents
Reduction of increased intracranial pressure
Surgical lavage of subarachnoid space with installation of thrombolytic agents
Nimodipine
Hypervolemic hemodilution and drug-induced hypertension
Angioplasty

which causes ischemia that progresses to infarction. The symptoms of vasospasm are worsening headache, altered consciousness, and focal neurologic signs that wax and wane. Transcranial Doppler ultrasonography is used to detect alterations in flow velocity in major arteries before the clinical signs appear. These studies often are performed at regular intervals during the period of highest risk. Arteriography is the most definitive means of diagnosing the arterial narrowing.

Avoiding administration of antifibrinolytic or antihypertensive agents, controlling increased ICP, and correcting hyponatremia and dehydration can decrease the risk of ischemia secondary to vasospasm. Nimodipine is efficacious in improving outcomes after SAH, but it is unclear whether the medication has any effect on vasospasm. Nimodipine presumably protects the brain from the consequences of ischemia because it can be given before the ischemia begins. Nimodipine is relatively safe, although it can cause hypotension. No other medication has been found as effective in reversing arterial narrowing. Surgical evacuation of the blood in the subarachnoid space, possibly with administration of a thrombolytic agent to promote aspiration, shows promise in preventing the development of vasospasm.

Hypervolemic hemodilution and drug-induced hypertension are prescribed frequently to patients in whom ischemic symptoms develop. Although no controlled trials have shown the efficacy of this regimen, several studies have shown improvement. The regimen is vigorous, and monitoring is critical because myocardial ischemia, congestive heart failure, and pulmonary edema are possible adverse experiences. The regimen also can promote recurrent rupture of an aneurysm that has not been operatively treated. Angioplasty has been performed to treat patients with vasospasm who have not responded to medical interventions.

Recommended Readings
Adams HP Jr, Jergenson DD, Kassell NF, et al. Pitfalls in the recognition of subarachnoid hemorrhage. *JAMA* 1980;244:794–796.
Al-Jarallah A, Al-Rifai MT, Riela AR, et al. Non-traumatic brain hemorrhage in children: etiology and presentation. *J Child Neurol* 2000;15:284–289.
Broderick J, Brott T, Tomsick T, et al. Lobar hemorrhage in the elderly. The undiminishing importance of hypertension. *Stroke* 1993;24:49–51.
Broderick J, Adams HP Jr, Barsan W, et al. Guidelines for the management of spontaneous intracerebral hemorrhage: a statement for healthcare professionals from a special writing group of the Stroke Council, American Heart Association. *Stroke* 1999;30:905–915.
Fisher CM. Clinical syndromes in cerebral thrombosis, hypertensive hemorrhage, and ruptured saccular aneurysm. *Clin Neurosurg* 1995;22:117–147.

Gebel JM, Broderick JP. Intracerebral hemorrhage. *Neurol Clin* 2000;18:419–438.

Hofmeister C, Stapf C, Hartmann A, et al. Demographic, morphological, and clinical characteristics of 1289 patients with brain arteriovenous malformations. *Stroke* 2000;31:1307–1310.

Kase CS. Intracerebral hemorrhage: non-hypertensive causes. *Stroke* 1986;17:590–594.

Kassell NF, Torner JC, Haley EC Jr, et al. The International Cooperative Study on the Timing of Aneurysm Surgery, II: surgical results. *J Neurosurg* 1990;73:18–36.

Martin NA, Saver J. Intensive care management of subarachnoid hemorrhage, ischemic stroke and hemorrhagic stroke. *Clin Neurosurg* 1999;45:101–112.

Mayberg MR, Batjer HH, Dacey R, et al. Guidelines for the management of aneurysmal subarachnoid hemorrhage: a statement for health care professionals from a special writing group of the Stroke Council, American Heart Association. *Stroke* 1994;25:2315–2328.

Nieuwkamp DJ, de Gans K, Rinkel GJ, et al. Treatment and outcome of severe intraventricular extension in patients with subarachnoid or intracerebral hemorrhage: a systemic review of the literature. *J Neurol* 2000;247:117–121.

Prasad K, Shrivastava A. Surgery for primary supratentorial intracerebral haemorrhage (Cochrane Review) [abstract]. Available at: http://www.cochrane.org/cochrane/revabstr/ab000200.htm. Oxford, UK: Update Software, 2001.

Roob G, Fazekas F. Magnetic resonance imaging of cerebral microbleeds. *Curr Opin Neurol* 2000;13:69–73.

Schellinger PD, Jansen O, Fiebach JB, et al. A standardized MRI stroke protocol: comparison with CT in hyperacute intracerebral hemorrhage. *Stroke* 1999;30:765–768.

Vermeulen M, van Gijn J. The diagnosis of subarachnoid hemorrhage. *J Neurol Neurosurg Psychiatry* 1990;50:365–372.

38. EPILEPSIES IN CHILDREN

Hema Patel
David W. Dunn

Approximately 3% of the population of the United States can be expected to have epilepsy at some time during their lives. Among children, 3% to 4% have a febrile seizure during the first 6 years of life, 2% have a single afebrile seizure, and 0.5% have recurrent afebrile seizures.

I. Classification. Accurate characterization of epilepsy has practical significance. The differentiation between partial and generalized seizures is important for the correct choice of antiepileptic drug (AED) therapy, determination of the etiologic factor, and prognosis. The most widely used classification describes epilepsies and epileptic syndromes with particular reference to age at onset, etiologic factor, site of seizure onset, and prognosis. Chapter 39 provides clinical descriptions of the different types of seizures.

    A. Localization-related epilepsies and syndromes are characterized by partial seizures arising from a focal cortical area with occasional progression to a generalized seizure. If this progression is rapid, the initial focal nature may be masked. A simple partial seizure is associated with intact consciousness, whereas during a complex partial seizure, consciousness is impaired. Electroencephalography (EEG) shows focal epileptiform discharges overlying the epileptogenic region. A simple partial seizure can progress to a complex partial seizure. During any focal seizure (simple or complex partial), the focal epileptic excitation can spread diffusely, resulting in a secondarily generalized tonic–clonic seizure (GTCS).

        1. Idiopathic epilepsy with age-related onset is a group of common epileptic syndromes that constitute approximately one fourth of all cases of epilepsy with onset before 13 years of age. Idiopathic epilepsy is characterized by genetic predisposition; focal (localization-related) seizures and EEG abnormalities; normal intellect and normal findings at neurologic examination and neuroimaging and laboratory studies; and an excellent prognosis. At present, the following syndromes are established, but more maybe identified in future.

            a. Benign focal epilepsy of childhood with centrotemporal spikes (BFECTS). This disorder was previously known as *benign rolandic epilepsy.*

                (1) BFECTS accounts for 75% of cases of benign focal childhood epilepsy.

                (2) Age at onset is between 3 and 13 years, peak age 8 to 9 years.

                (3) Clinical features include unilateral paresthesia of the tongue, lip, and cheek, unilateral motor seizures mainly involving facial grimacing and twitching, inability to speak, salivation, and occasional progression to a GTCS. Seizures usually are nocturnal, during sleep.

                (4) EEG shows frequent, unilateral or bilateral, high-amplitude centrotemporal spikes with a horizontal dipole that are activated by sleep. If initial EEG findings are normal, a sleep-deprived EEG to include sleep should be obtained.

                (5) Treatment usually is unnecessary after the first or even the second seizure. AED therapy can be initiated if the seizures are frequent, or if they are sufficiently disturbing to the patient or family. All major AEDs have been reported to be successful even in small doses. Carbamazepine is the drug of choice. Valproic acid also is effective. Phenobarbital and phenytoin, although effective, have the disadvantages of sedative and cosmetic side effects. It may be preferable to maintain AED therapy up to 14 to 16 years of age. Seizures spontaneously resolve by that time.

                (6) Prognosis is excellent. Approximately 13% to 20% of patients have only a single seizure. Seizures usually resolve within 1 to 3 years of onset and no later than 16 years of age. Approximately 1% to 2% persist into adult life.

b. Benign childhood epilepsy with occipital paroxysms (BEOP)

   (1) BEOP accounts for 25% of the benign focal childhood epilepsy.

   (2) Age at onset is 4 to 5 years, girls being affected more frequently than boys.

   (3) Clinical features include frequent, brief (a few seconds to 2 to 3 minutes) diurnal seizures characterized by visual illusions (multicolored circles or spots) or blindness, followed by postictal headaches. Consciousness may be preserved, but it is impaired if the seizure secondarily generalizes. BEOP often is misinterpreted as basilar (Bickerstaff's) migraine.

   (4) EEG shows occipital paroxysms of high amplitude, often bilateral sharp or spike slow-wave complexes attenuating with eye opening. Generalized or centrotemporal spike waves are found in one third of all cases.

   (5) Treatment is similar to that of patients with BFECTS.

   (6) Prognosis. BEOP carries a good prognosis, although it is not as benign as BFECTS. Clinical remission rates vary from 60% to 90%.

c. Primary reading epilepsy. Onset is typically in late puberty, manifesting as simple motor seizures characterized by jaw jerks or clicks triggered by reading, with little tendency to spontaneous seizures. GTCS may occur if the reading is not interrupted. During reading, paroxysmal activity is recorded over the parietotemporal regions, especially on the dominant side. The course is benign.

   Apart from these types of idiopathic localization-related epilepsy of childhood, partial seizures that may have a genetic predisposition may occur among adult patients. Two syndromes have been recognized—autosomal dominant nocturnal frontal lobe epilepsy (ADNFLE) and benign familial temporal lobe epilepsy (BFTLE).

2. Symptomatic partial (localization-related) epilepsy. Most forms of localization-related epilepsy are symptomatic or acquired. The clinical manifestation of the seizure depends on the anatomic location of the epileptogenic focus. Temporal lobe seizures (complex partial seizures) are the most common type of symptomatic partial seizures.

B. Generalized epilepsy and syndromes are characterized by seizures that are generalized from onset with initial involvement of both hemispheres. These seizures usually are associated with impairment of consciousness, and the EEG patterns are generalized and bilateral, reflecting involvement of both hemispheres. They include absence seizures, atypical absence seizures, myoclonic seizures, atonic seizures, GTCS, tonic seizures, clonic seizures, and infantile spasms.

1. Idiopathic epilepsy with age-related onset. In these disorders, which are listed in order of age of appearance, the seizures and EEG abnormalities are generalized from the onset. Intellect and findings at neurologic examination, neuroimaging, and laboratory studies other than EEG are normal (idiopathic). There is a genetic predisposition with no other identifiable etiologic factor.

   a. Benign familial neonatal convulsions. This is a rare, autosomal dominant form of epilepsy with a genetic defect localized to chromosome 20q. Seizures occur on the second or third day of life and are relatively refractory to AED therapy. Other causes of neonatal seizures, such as infection or metabolic, toxic, or structural abnormalities, should be excluded. Approximately 10% of infants experience subsequent nonfebrile seizures.

   b. Benign idiopathic neonatal seizures (fifth-day fits). Seizures occur on the fifth day of life without known cause and generally cease within 15 days. The prognosis is good with no seizure recurrence, and there is normal subsequent psychomotor development.

   c. Benign myoclonic epilepsy in infancy

   (1) Age at onset is 1 to 2 years.

(2) **Clinical features** are brief, generalized myoclonic seizures in an otherwise normal child, usually with a family history of epilepsy.

(3) **EEG** shows brief, generalized bursts of spike–polyspike wave activity.

(4) **Treatment.** Valproic acid is the drug of choice. Clonazepam can be used if valproic acid is ineffective. Seizures are exacerbated by phenytoin and carbamazepine.

(5) **Prognosis.** Response to treatment is good. Occasionally, some psychomotor delay and behavioral abnormalities may persist.

d. **Childhood absence epilepsy (pyknolepsy).** See Chapter 6.

e. **Juvenile absence epilepsy.** See Chapter 6.

f. **Juvenile myoclonic epilepsy (impulsive petit mal) of Janz.** See Chapter 6.

g. **Epilepsy with GTCS on awakening.** See Chapter 6.

2. **Symptomatic or cryptogenic epilepsy.** These disorders, which are listed in order of age of appearance, include generalized epilepsy syndromes secondary to known or suspected disorders of the central nervous system (CNS) (symptomatic) or to disorders the causes of which are hidden or occult (cryptogenic).

a. **West syndrome (infantile spasms), salaam convulsions**

(1) **Etiology.** Approximately 30% to 40% of cases are cryptogenic. In symptomatic cases, there is evidence of previous brain damage (mental retardation, neurologic and radiologic evidence, or a known etiologic factor) (Table 38.1.)

(2) **Age at onset.** Onset occurs in infancy (peak 4 to 8 months).

(3) **Clinical features** compose the triad of infantile spasms, mental retardation, and hypsarrhythmia. Several infantile spasms occur in clusters, frequently during drowsiness and on awakening. They are characterized by brief nodding of the head associated with extension or flexion of the trunk, and often of the extremities, and they occur rapidly, suggestive of a startle reaction. They can be flexor (salaam attacks), extensor, or most commonly, mixed spasms. They almost always are associated with arrested development.

(4) **EEG** shows hypsarrhythmia—chaotic, high-amplitude, disorganized background with multifocal spikes. Intravenous (i.v.) pyridoxine (vitamin B_6) should be administered in a dose of 100 mg during the EEG to exclude pyridoxine-dependent infantile spasms.

Table 38.1 Causes of secondary generalized epilepsy syndromes (infantile spasms and Lennox–Gastaut syndrome)

Idiopathic, Cryptogenic

Symptomatic
Perinatal factors: hypoxic–ischemic encephalopathy, hypoglycemia, hypocalcemia
Infection: intrauterine infection (toxoplasmosis, rubella, cytomegalovirus, herpes), meningoencephalitis
Cerebral malformation: holoprosencephaly, lissencephaly, Aicardi's syndrome
Vascular: infarction, hemorrhage, porencephaly
Neurocutaneous syndromes: tuberous sclerosis, Sturge–Weber syndrome, incontinentia pigmenti, others (e.g., neurofibromatosis)
Metabolic disease: nonketotic hyperglycinemia, pyridoxine deficiency, aminoacidopathy (phenylketonuria, maple syrup urine disease)
Degenerative disorder: neuronal ceroid lipofuscinosis (Batten disease)
Chromosomal disorders: Down syndrome, Angelman's syndrome (happy puppet syndrome: abnormality in chromosome 15q11–13, seizures, developmental delay, dysmorphic features, paroxysms of inappropriate laughter)

(5) Treatment

    (a) Underlying conditions are managed as identified.

    (b) Adrenocorticotropic hormone (ACTH). Opinions vary regarding dosage and duration of ACTH therapy, ranging from high-dose therapy (160 units/m^2 per day) to low-dose therapy (20 to 40 units/day). We recommend starting at 40 to 80 units/day administered intramuscularly and continuing for 3 to 4 weeks, or for a shorter period if an early positive clinical response is observed. The dosage is slowly decreased approximately 20% per week over 6 to 9 weeks. If seizures recur during withdrawal, the dosage should be increased to the previous effective level. ACTH therapy is initiated in the hospital under the guidance of a pediatric neurologist. Parents should be taught the injection technique with systematic rotation of the injection site.

    (c) Side effects of ACTH therapy are irritability, hyperglycemia, hypertension, sodium and water retention, potassium depletion, weight gain, gastric ulcers, occult gastrointestinal bleeding, suppression of the immune system, cardiomegaly, and diabetic ketoacidosis.

    (d) Laboratory tests before initiation of ACTH therapy include baseline EEG, serum electrolytes, blood urea nitrogen, serum creatinine, glucose, urinalysis, complete blood cell count (CBC), chest radiograph, and tuberculin skin test.

    (e) Laboratory tests performed weekly during ACTH therapy include serum electrolytes, blood glucose, stool guaiac, and monitoring of weight and blood pressure.

    (f) Concomitant management. An antacid or the histamine H$_2$ receptor antagonist (cimetidine) should be administered during ACTH therapy.

(6) Alternative treatment

    (a) Prednisone may be substituted when ACTH cannot be administered because parents cannot or will not learn to give injections. Prednisone is administered orally at 2 to 3 mg/kg per day for 3 to 4 weeks and gradually withdrawn in a schedule similar to ACTH withdrawal.

    (b) Valproic acid is initiated at 10 to 15 mg/kg per day in three divided doses and is increased according to the clinical response. Usually, high therapeutic levels of 75 to 125 µg/mL are needed to achieve seizure control.

    (c) Benzodiazepines. Clonazepam at 0.03 mg/kg per day is administered in two or three divided doses and gradually increased to 0.1 mg/kg per day. Common side effects include extreme somnolence and excessive oral secretions. Nitrazepam at a dosage of 0.5 to 1.5 mg/kg per day also has been tried but is not commercially available in the United States. Clobazam also has been used.

    (d) Ketogenic diet requires hospitalization for initiation under the expertise of a pediatric neurologist and an experienced dietitian. To be effective, the diet should be maintained for at least 1 year. Hypoglycemia, vomiting, and dehydration are common associated problems.

    (e) Vigabatrin 60 to 150 mg/kg per day has been used in Europe with some success, the best response rates occurring among patients with tuberous sclerosis. This drug is not yet approved in the United States.

    (f) Vitamin B$_6$. The efficacy of this vitamin has not been confirmed.

    (g) Excisional surgery of the region of cortical abnormality defined at EEG, magnetic resonance imaging (MRI), and positron emission tomography (PET) is being performed on children with infantile spasms intractable to medical therapy, but only in specialized centers. Further studies are needed to determine which patients may benefit from surgery and whether long-term development is significantly improved after surgical intervention.

(7) **Prognosis.** West's syndrome has a high morbidity, with a 90% incidence of mental retardation. From 25% to 50% of cases evolve into Lennox–Gastaut syndrome, infantile spasms transforming to other seizure types (GTCS, myoclonic, and tonic seizures) over subsequent years. Favorable prognostic indicators are as follows.

   (a) Cryptogenic spasms, which have a better prognosis than cases in which there are preexisting neurologic conditions

   (b) Normal development and neurologic examination before the onset of spasms

   (c) Short duration of seizures before control

b. **Lennox–Gastaut syndrome**

   (1) **Etiology.** A large number of patients have a history of infantile spasms. From 10% to 40% of cases are cryptogenic. In 60% to 90% of symptomatic cases, a specific cause, usually perinatal insult, is found (Table 38.1).

   (2) **Age at onset** is 1 to 8 years.

   (3) **Clinical features** are seizures of multiple types that often are frequent and intractable to medical treatment—commonly tonic, atonic, or atypical absence seizures but also myoclonic, GTCS, and partial seizures. Seizures usually are associated with severe psychomotor retardation.

   (4) **EEG** shows slow background activity, generalized, bisynchronous, arrhythmic, sharp-and-slow-wave discharges (1 to 2 Hz) activated by sleep, generalized paroxysmal fast spike activity (10 Hz), and other multifocal abnormalities.

   (5) **Treatment.** *Sedative AED therapy should be avoided* if possible, because these AEDs can increase seizure frequency by decreasing alertness in patients.

      (a) **Valproic acid monotherapy** is effective against all the different types of seizures associated with Lennox–Gastaut syndrome. However, these seizures often are intractable, and valproic acid may have to be used in combination with phenytoin, ethosuximide, phenobarbital, primidone, carbamazepine, or even benzodiazepines (clonazepam, nitrazepam, clobazam), depending on the types of seizures. Carbamazepine can exacerbate absence seizures.

      (b) **Ketogenic diet** may be effective for occasional patients with otherwise intractable seizures. Benefits include fewer seizures, less drowsiness, and fewer concomitant AEDs.

      (c) **Lamotrigine and topiramate** have successfully demonstrated efficacy as adjunctive therapy in the care of children with Lennox–Gastaut syndrome. Clobazam is not currently approved in the United States, but like other benzodiazepines has been occasionally effective. Felbamate also has been found effective but is infrequently used because of reported severe side effects such as aplastic anemia and acute liver failure.

      (d) **ACTH** has been found to be effective in the treatment of some patients.

      (e) **Psychological support** for the child and family often are helpful.

      (f) **Referral to occupational therapy** for protective helmets to prevent head injuries in patients with drop attacks is helpful.

      (g) **Surgical procedures** such as corpus callostomy, hemispherectomy, and rarely resection of a localized lesion have been tried with variable results. Vagal nerve stimulation also has been reported to be effective with at least 50% reduction in seizure frequency in follow-up periods as long as 5 years.

   c. **Symptomatic seizures.** Myoclonic seizures are difficult to differentiate from nonepileptic myoclonus. However, characteristic epileptiform discharges associated with myoclonic jerks in myoclonic epilepsy help differentiate the two. Valproic acid in high doses may be effective. It may have to be used in combination with clonazepam, lorazepam, nitrazepam, or the ketogenic diet.

   (1) **Early myoclonic encephalopathy.** The cause of this disorder is not known. Other causes of symptomatic myoclonic epilepsy, including inborn errors of metabolism (particularly nonketotic hyperglycinemia), hypoxic ischemic encephalopathy, and dysgenetic brain disorders, should be excluded. Early myoclonic encephalopathy is characterized by onset of medically intractable myoclonic seizures in early infancy before 3 months of age, burst suppression on EEG seen predominantly in sleep, and very poor prognosis, including death in the first year of life, or profound neurologic impairment.

   (2) **Early infantile epileptic encephalopathy (Ohtahara's syndrome)** is characterized by an early onset of tonic spasms within the first few months of life, but myoclonic seizures are rare. The suppression–burst pattern on the EEG is present during waking and sleep states. Seizures are intractable, and the prognosis is poor.

   (3) **Symptomatic myoclonic epilepsy** is associated with specific progressive neurologic diseases such as Lafora's disease, Baltic myoclonus (Unverricht–Lundborg disease), neuronal ceroid lipofuscinosis (Batten disease), sialidosis, mitochondrial encephalomyopathy, and Ramsay Hunt syndrome.

C. Epilepsy and syndromes undetermined as to being focal or generalized
   1. **Neonatal seizures.** Seizures occur most frequently in the neonatal period than at any other time in childhood, with an incidence of 1.5 per 1,000 to 5.5 per 1,000 live births.

   a. **Clinical features.** Neonatal seizures are more fragmentary than are seizures among older children. GTCS do not occur in neonates. Common causes are outlined in Table 38.2. Some types of seizures are almost always associated with electrographic changes. Neonatal seizures can be classified as follows.

   (1) **Seizures associated with electrographic signatures** include focal and multifocal clonic seizures, focal tonic seizures, generalized myoclonic seizures, and, rarely, apnea. These seizures usually

Table 38.2 Common causes of neonatal seizures

Hypoxic–ischemic encephalopathy
Trauma: subdural hematoma, intracerebral hemorrhage
Congenital abnormalities: lissencephaly, holoprosencephaly and other migrational disorders
Metabolic: hypocalcemia, hypomagnesemia, hypoglycemia, hyponatremia, hypernatremia
Infection: meningitis, abscess, TORCH (toxoplasmosis, other such as HIV, rubella,
   cytomegalovirus, herpes)
Drug withdrawal: heroin, barbiturate, methadone
Pyridoxine dependency
Amino acid disturbances: urea cycle disorder, nonketotic hyperglycinemia
Neurocutaneous and genetic syndromes: tuberous sclerosis, phenylketonuria, galactosemia
Benign familial epilepsy

HIV, human immunodeficiency virus.

are associated with focal structural lesions (infarction or hemorrhage), infection, or metabolic abnormalities (hypoglycemia or hypocalcemia).

(2) Seizures not associated with electrographic signatures include generalized tonic seizures, focal and multifocal myoclonic seizures, and subtle seizures (oral–buccal–lingual movements, bicycling movements, and some rhythmic ocular movements such as horizontal eye deviation). These seizures usually are observed among lethargic, comatose neonates with poor prognoses, such as those with severe hypoxic ischemic encephalopathy.

b. Evaluation. Neonatal seizures should be managed in a neonatal intensive care unit by experienced personnel, including a pediatric neurologist and a neonatologist.

(1) History and examination. A detailed history, including illness during pregnancy, maternal drug and alcohol abuse, perinatal history, and family history, should be obtained. A general physical examination, including evaluation of the skin and the anterior fontanel, and neurologic and ophthalmologic examinations, should be performed.

(2) Laboratory data. The following tests usually are indicated: serum glucose, electrolytes, magnesium, calcium, phosphate, blood urea nitrogen, serum creatinine, ammonia, arterial blood gases, CBC, lumbar puncture (LP) to rule out infection and subarachnoid hemorrhage, urinalysis for amino acids, organic acids, and ketones, maternal and infant titers for toxoplasmosis, rubella, cytomegalovirus, herpes, and human immunodeficiency virus (TORCH), and Venereal Disease Research Laboratory. Additional studies, such as cerebrospinal fluid lactate, plasma amino acids and very-long-chain fatty acids, and leukocyte and fibroblast enzyme studies, may be indicated if metabolic disorders are suspected. Ultrasonography of the head at bedside to rule out intracranial hemorrhage and a non–contrast-enhanced computed tomography (CT) of the head when the neonate's condition is stable, can be performed. EEG is especially useful for the diagnosis of subclinical seizures and for assessment of prognosis.

c. Treatment

(1) Management of underlying cause. Treatment begins with the underlying cause of the seizures, such as CNS infection or specific metabolic abnormality (hypoglycemia, hypocalcemia, or hypomagnesemia).

(2) Phenobarbital is the initial drug of choice. A loading dose of 20 mg/kg is given i.v. Additional 5 to 10 mg/kg boluses are given as needed to control clinical seizures and attain therapeutic serum levels of 20 to 40 mg/mL. Maintenance doses of 3 to 4 mg/kg per day given in twice-a-day dosing are sufficient because phenobarbital has a relatively long half-life in neonates. Close cardiorespiratory monitoring is important because i.v. administration of phenobarbital can be associated with respiratory depression and hypotension.

(3) Phenytoin is added if a phenobarbital level of 40 mg/mL is not sufficient to control seizures. An i.v. loading dose of 20 mg/kg results in serum levels ranging from 15 to 20 mg/mL. Thereafter a maintenance dose of 3 to 4 mg/kg per day is administered in twice-a-day dosing. Phenytoin is infused slowly with cardiac monitoring, because it can cause cardiac arrhythmias and prolonged QT intervals.

(4) Lorazepam 0.05 to 0.1 mg/kg administered i.v. can be used for seizures that do not respond to the sequential use of phenobarbital and phenytoin. Lorazepam enters the brain rapidly, being effective in less than 5 minutes. It is does not redistribute from the brain as rapidly as does diazepam, because it is less lipophilic, the duration of action being 6 to 24 hours. Lorazepam is less likely to produce respiratory depression or hypotension. Diazepam has been effective administered by means of i.v. infusion in isotonic saline solution at 0.1 to 0.3 mg/kg per hour. However, diazepam is not used because of increased risk of cardiorespiratory collapse when used with barbiturates and rapid clearance from the brain, making it a poor drug for maintenance. In addition, the vehicle for i.v. preparations contains sodium benzoate, which is an effective uncoupler of the bilirubin–albumin complex and can increase the risk of kernicterus.

(5) **Pyridoxine** (100 mg i.v.) administered during EEG monitoring stops seizures and normalizes the EEG within minutes in the rare patient with pyridoxine-dependent seizures.

2. **Acquired epileptic aphasia (Landau–Kleffner syndrome)** is characterized by acquired aphasia, including verbal auditory agnosia, rapid reduction of spontaneous speech, and behavioral and psychomotor disturbances. Seizures (generalized and focal) and EEG abnormalities including multifocal spikes and spike–wave discharges are rare and usually remit before the age of 15 years. However, the ultimate outcome is still unclear.

D. **Special syndromes**
  1. **Situation-related seizures**
     a. **Febrile seizures**
        (1) **Incidence.** Febrile seizures occur in 2% to 5% of young children.
        (2) **Age at onset** ranges from 3 months to 5 years (peak 6 months to 2 years). The disorder is familial.
        (3) **Clinical features**, which usually manifest within the first few hours of acute infection, include upper respiratory infection, otitis media, and gastrointestinal infection. Intracranial infection and other defined causes such as dehydration and electrolyte imbalance should be excluded.
           (a) **Simple febrile seizures** present as single, brief GTCS without associated evidence of intracranial infection or defined cause.
           (b) **Complex febrile seizures** are prolonged (more than 15 minutes), have focal features (postictal focal onset or Todd's paralysis) and occur at a rate of more than one seizure within 24 hours.
        (4) **Evaluation.** LP is indicated unless the possibility of meningitis can be confidently eliminated clinically. LP should be performed for all children younger than 18 months, because they may not always have meningeal signs in the face of meningitis. If in doubt, err on the side of performing LP. It should be strongly considered in the evaluation of infants and children who have received antibiotic treatment, because such treatment can mask evidence of meningitis. Serum electrolyte and glucose tests should be performed.
        (5) **Acute management of seizure**
           (a) The patient should be admitted overnight for observation if the seizure was prolonged or multiple.
           (b) Phenobarbital in an i.v. loading dose of 15 to 20 mg/kg is administered slowly at the rate of 1 mg/kg per minute, followed the next day by a maintenance dose of 3 to 5 mg/kg per day in twice-a-day dosing. Lorazepam, 0.05 to 0.1 mg/kg i.v., with a maximum total dose of 4 mg can be used.
           (c) Some pediatric neurologists use oral or rectal diazepam (0.1 to 0.3 mg/kg) only when fever is present and have found it effective in reducing the risk of recurrent febrile seizures. Possible side effects include lethargy, irritability, and ataxia.
           (d) Any underlying infection or fever should be controlled.
        (6) **Long-term management of seizure.** No treatment is necessary if the patient has isolated simple febrile seizures without major risk factors for recurrence.

> > > **(a)** Daily phenobarbital treatment reduces the risk of recurrent febrile seizures and may be indicated in the care of patients with a substantially increased risk of later epilepsy. These include complex febrile seizures, abnormal findings at neurologic examination, family history of nonfebrile seizures, recurrent febrile seizures, or febrile seizures before 1 year of age. Because 90% of febrile seizures recur within 2 years, treatment should be continued for at least 2 years or for 1 year after the last seizure, whichever is longer.
> > > **(b)** Valproic acid is the second choice because of an increased incidence of side effects, including liver toxicity, in this age group. Carbamazepine and phenytoin are ineffective in the management of febrile seizures.
> > **(7) Prognosis.** Approximately 33% of children with febrile seizures have at least one recurrence, and 9% have three or more seizures. Remission occurs by 6 years of age in approximately 90% of children.
> > > **(a)** Risk factors for recurrence include young age (less than 1 year) at initial seizure and family history of febrile seizures.
> > > **(b)** Risk factors for the development of epilepsy include complex febrile seizures, underlying developmental or neurologic abnormalities, and family history of nonfebrile seizures.
> **b. Seizures related to identifiable situations.** Such situations include stress, hormonal changes, use of drugs (theophylline, stimulants, or neuroleptics), use of alcohol, and sleep deprivation.
> **2. Isolated, apparently unprovoked epileptic events.** Treatment is not indicated unless there are significant risk factors for recurrence.
> **3. Epilepsy characterized by specific modes of seizure precipitation** include seizures occurring in response to discrete or specific stimuli (reflex epilepsy), such as reading epilepsy, hot water epilepsy, and arithmetic epilepsy.
> **4. Chronic progressive epilepsia partialis continua of childhood (Kojewnikoff's syndrome)** is thought to be a result of chronic encephalitis (Rasmussen's encephalitis). The cause is unknown. It is characterized by partial motor seizures, often associated with myoclonus, that are resistant to treatment. This condition results in progressive hemiplegia with unilateral brain atrophy and mental retardation.

II. Evaluation. Details regarding histories, physical examinations, and studies such as EEG and neuroimaging are discussed in Chapter 6. Important aspects of the evaluation with respect to children are as follows.

> **A.** It is important to determine whether the paroxysmal events in question are in fact epileptic. They should be differentiated from nonepileptic paroxysmal events in children (see Chapter 34).
> **B.** Specific predisposing factors for childhood seizures
> > **1. Birth history**
> > > **a. Prenatal.** Duration of pregnancy, complications (e.g., toxemia or premature labor), medications, and smoking, alcohol and drug abuse
> > > **b. Perinatal.** Complications of labor and delivery, use of vacuum or forceps, birth weight, and Apgar scores
> > > **c. Postnatal.** Care received in nursery (including intensive respiratory care) and problems such as intraventricular hemorrhage and exchange transfusions
> > **2. Developmental history.** Learning disabilities, attention deficit, and developmental regression (loss of previously attained developmental milestones) that may be associated with a degenerative disease
> **C. Physical examination** is an extension of the information obtained in the history. In addition to the physical examination described in Chapter 6, specific aspects in children include the following.
> > **1. Head circumference.** Microcephaly and macrocephaly are associated with various neurologic disorders.

2. **Height and weight** abnormalities may be secondary to endocrine disorders related to midline CNS tumors.
3. **Dysmorphic features** associated with storage diseases or brain malformations
4. **Skin.** Neurocutaneous disorders: café-au-lait spots suggest neurofibromatosis, hypopigmented macules and adenoma sebaceum are observed in tuberous sclerosis, and facial hemangiomas are seen in Sturge–Weber syndrome.
5. **Hair.** Broken hair and alopecia suggest metabolic disorders (biotinidase deficiency, Menkes syndrome, and argininosuccinic aciduria).
6. **Mental status and behavioral pattern.** Evaluate development. Loss of previously attained milestones may be indicative of a neurodegenerative disease, whereas delays in achieving developmental milestones reflect static encephalopathies (e.g., cerebral palsy). Presence of anxiety, depression, and family conflict may lead to the possible diagnosis of psychogenic seizures.
7. **Systemic exam.** Organomegaly may suggest a storage disease or an inborn error of metabolism.

D. **Laboratory testing.** In addition to EEG and MRI of the head, other important studies in children include the following.

1. **Chemical and metabolic screening.** Electrolytes, glucose, calcium, magnesium, hepatic and renal function tests, and toxic screening for possible drug ingestion. Elevation of serum prolactin and serum creatine kinase levels is seen with GTCS and may be normal with focal seizures. These levels can help differentiate seizures from nonepileptiform paroxysmal disorders. However, they must be measured within 30 minutes after an episode and then be compared with baseline values. Thyroid function tests should be performed because seizures are rarely associated with thyrotoxicosis. Specific metabolic or neurodegenerative disorders may be diagnosed with tests such as urinalysis for amino acids, organic acids, lysosomal enzymes (mucopolysaccharidosis and Batten disease), and very-long-chain fatty acids (peroxisomal disorders such as adrenoleukodystrophy).
2. **LP** is indicated if there are signs of acute CNS infection or inflammation (e.g., fever or stiff neck). LP is indicated for all children younger than 18 months with a history of fever and seizures, because clinical signs of CNS infection may be absent. LP should be performed on all febrile patients with new-onset seizures.
3. **Chromosomal analysis** is indicated if dysmorphic features suggest chromosomal abnormalities.
4. **Skin biopsy** is performed to diagnose certain metabolic diseases such as Batten disease.
5. **Simultaneous prolonged video EEG monitoring** in an epilepsy unit can help determine the exact nature of paroxysmal events if they cannot be defined with routine EEG.

III. **Treatment**
A. **Single seizure.** Approximately 9% of the population has a seizure sometime during their lives, and approximately 3% have more than one seizure. The risk of recurrence is highest in the first year after a single seizure. It is low if the patient has normal findings at neurologic examination, a single GTCS with a negative family history, normal findings at neuroimaging, and a normal or mildly slow EEG.
1. **Indications for treatment**
   a. Clear-cut epileptiform abnormalities at EEG
   b. Lesions on CT scans or MR images
   c. Abnormal findings at neurologic examination that suggest previous brain damage
   d. Active CNS infection (encephalitis, meningitis, or abscess)
   e. Status epilepticus as the first seizure
   f. Certain types of seizures, including infantile spasms, Lennox–Gastaut syndrome, and focal seizures

    g. Unprovoked or asymptomatic single seizure with history suggesting that one may have occurred earlier

  2. Treatment is not indicated when seizures are provoked by a correctable metabolic disturbance (glucose or electrolyte abnormalities), sleep deprivation, exposure to drugs or alcohol, febrile illness, or physical or emotional stress. In such cases the underlying disturbance should be corrected.

B. General principles of treatment

  1. Choice of appropriate drug should be based on the clinical description of the seizures (Table 38.3). This choice may be influenced by other factors, such as the patient's age, economic circumstances, and child-bearing potential (e.g., phenytoin is preferred in the child-bearing age group because it has the least teratogenic side effects).

  2. Monotherapy. Start with one drug beginning at one-third to one-half the recommended dose and gradually increase it until seizures are controlled or intolerable side effects appear. Approximately 75% to 80% of children should respond to monotherapy. If the first drug is ineffective, start a second AED with a different mechanism of action and low potential for adverse effects and drug interactions. After therapeutic levels are achieved, gradually withdraw the first drug.

  3. Polypharmacy is indicated only if monotherapy with at least two first-line AEDs fails. Polypharmacy should be initiated only after consultation with a pediatric neurologist. Problems with polypharmacy include drug interactions, difficulties in acquiring therapeutic levels of either drug despite use of very high doses, increased risks of toxicity, increased cost, and reduced compliance.

  4. Simplify medication schedule. Decreasing the number of doses improves compliance. For older children, phenobarbital and phenytoin can be given in single nighttime doses. However, carbamazepine and valproic acid have shorter half-lives and should be given in at least two or three divided daily doses.

  5. Avoid sedative anticonvulsants such as benzodiazepines, especially for patients with secondarily generalized epilepsy syndrome, because increased sedation can increase seizure frequency.

  6. Maintain a seizure diary. Record seizure frequency, medication dosages and levels, and occurrence of side effects, if any.

Table 38.3 Drugs for the management of epilepsy

Seizure type	First-line drug	Second-line drug
Partial		
Simple partial, complex partial, secondary generalized tonic–clonic seizure	Carbamazepine, phenytoin, valproic acid	Lamotrigine, topiramate, oxcarbazepine, phenobarbital, primidone, zonisamide, levetiracetam, tiagabine, gabapentin
Generalized		
Absence (typical, atypical)	Ethosuximide, valproic acid	Lamotrigine, clonazepam, acetazolamide
Myoclonic	Valproic acid	Clonazepam, lamotrigine, phenobarbital, primidone, acetazolamide, clorazepate
Tonic–clonic	Valproic acid, phenytoin	Lamotrigine, topiramate, carbamazepine, phenobarbital, primidone
Atonic	Valproic acid	Clonazepam, clorazepate, phenobarbital

7. **Anticonvulsant level** should be checked just before a dose, preferably the morning dose to obtain the lowest (trough) level. It is helpful to monitor the level at a consistent time to avoid misinterpretation of fluctuations. CBC and aspartate aminotransferase (AST) levels are checked every 1 to 2 months initially and then every 6 months after a steady dosage has been established. AED blood level should be checked.

   a. After starting a medication, to aid in initial titration of dose to achieve a therapeutic level.

   b. After making a major change in drug dosage.

   c. If seizures recur with the usual dosage of AED.

   d. If seizures persist despite "correct therapy."

   e. If symptoms of toxicity develop.

   f. If noncompliance is suspected.

8. **Repeat EEG** during therapy if there is a change in the character of the seizures or if the child has been seizure-free for a considerable period to help decide whether medications can be withdrawn.

C. **Drug therapy.** The following information serves as a broad guideline for AEDs commonly used to treat children. Details regarding their metabolism, side effects, and interactions are discussed in detail in Chapter 39.

   1. **Phenytoin (Dilantin; Pfizer, New York, NY, U.S.A.)**

      a. **Indications.** Focal seizures (simple and complex partial seizures, partial seizures with secondary generalization), status epilepticus, and generalized epilepsy manifested by GTCS

      b. **Dosage.** 3 to 8 mg/kg per day in a single dose or two divided doses

      c. **Serum half-life.** 24 ± 12 hours

      d. **Metabolism.** Hydroxylated by liver. Phenytoin has nonlinear elimination kinetics. Therefore, small increases in dose after therapeutic levels of 10 to 20 mg/mL have been achieved result in large increases in plasma levels and toxicity.

      e. **Therapeutic blood level.** 10 to 20 mg/mL

      f. **Formulation.** Capsules: 30 and 100 mg; Infatabs: 50 mg; suspension: 125 mg/5 mL and 30 mg/5 mL. Dilantin suspension is not recommended for routine use because it is unreliable. Parenteral preparation: injectable sodium phenytoin (Dilantin and generic 50 mg/mL), fosphenytoin (Cerebyx [Pfizer] 50 mg phenytoin equivalent per milliliter).

      g. **Side effects.** Dose-related side effects are nystagmus, ataxia, and drowsiness. Gingival hypertrophy (20% to 50% of patients) requiring more frequent dental cleaning, hirsutism, coarsening of features, blood dyscrasias, Stevens–Johnson syndrome, lymphadenopathy, and megaloblastic anemia also can occur. Fetal hydantoin syndrome is characterized by craniofacial anomalies, hypoplasia of distal phalanges, intrauterine growth retardation, and mental deficiency. It occurs not only in children exposed to phenytoin in utero but also in those exposed to other AEDs such as phenobarbital, primidone, mephobarbital, and phensuximide.

      h. **Fosphenytoin (Cerebyx)** is a water-soluble disodium ester prescribed as equimolar amounts of phenytoin called *phenytoin equivalents* (PE). This prodrug is rapidly converted to phenytoin by phosphatase in the blood stream, reaching peak brain levels 15 minutes after administration. The loading and maintenance doses of fosphenytoin in phenytoin equivalents are identical to those of phenytoin. Fosphenytoin can be administered i.v. and intramuscularly with minimal local tissue damage and at faster rates of administration with fewer adverse effects than with phenytoin. Pruritus and paresthesia can occur.

   2. **Carbamazepine (Tegretol; Novartis, East Hanover, NJ, U.S.A.)**

      a. **Indications.** Focal seizures (simple and complex partial seizures, partial seizures with secondary generalization) and generalized epilepsy manifested by GTCS (in which it may exacerbate absence, atypical absence, and myoclonic seizures).

      b. **Dosage.** Start at 5 mg/kg per day and increase by 5 mg/kg per day every 3 to 4 days to a maximum of 10 to 30 mg/kg per day in two or three divided doses. Check levels at that time and titrate the dosage further if needed to achieve therapeutic blood levels.

   c. **Serum half-life.** 12 ± 6 hours
   d. **Metabolism.** Hepatic conversion to epoxide and other metabolites
   e. **Therapeutic blood level.** 4 to 12 mg/mL
   f. **Formulation.** Tablets: 200 mg; chewable tablets: 100 mg; elixir: 100 mg/5 mL; Tegretol XR: 100 mg, 200 mg, 400 mg; Carbatrol extended-release capsules (Shire-Richwood) 200 mg, 300 mg. If oral administration is contraindicated, Tegretol elixir (100 mg/5 mL) can be given rectally, diluted 1:1 with water in an enema at a dose of 10 to 30 mg/kg to attain therapeutic levels.
   g. **Side effects.** Dose-related side effects are sedation, blurred vision, and leukopenia. Agranulocytosis, aplastic anemia, and syndrome of inappropriate antidiuretic hormone secretion (SIADH) also may occur. There is a 0.5% risk of spina bifida with first-trimester exposure to carbamazepine. Developmental delay also can occur.

3. **Oxcarbazepine (Trileptal; Novartis)**
   a. **Indications.** Adjunct for partial seizures in care of children 4 to 16 years of age; adjunct and monotherapy for partial seizures in adults.
   b. **Dosage.** 10 mg/kg per day, to be increased by the same amount weekly to 20 to 30 mg/kg per day two or three times a day.
   c. **Serum half-life.** 8 to 10 hours
   d. **Metabolism.** Oxcarbazepine, a 10-keto analogue of carbamazepine, is rapidly metabolized to an active metabolite 10 monohydroxy derivative in the liver. It has less potential for drug interactions because of lack of autoinduction.
   e. **Therapeutic blood level.** 20 to 200 µg/mL.
   f. **Formulation.** Tablets: 150 mg, 300 mg, 600 mg
   g. **Side effects.** Somnolence, dizziness, headaches. Cross allergy between carbamazepine and oxcarbazepine occurs in 35% of cases. Hyponatremia is more frequent than with carbamazepine.

4. **Phenobarbital**
   a. **Indications.** Focal seizures (simple and complex partial seizures, partial seizures with secondary generalization), GTCS of generalized epilepsy (in which it can exacerbate absence, atypical absence, and myoclonic seizures), febrile seizures, and status epilepticus
   b. **Dosage.** 3 to 8 mg/kg per day in a single daily dose or two divided doses
   c. **Serum half-life** increases with age. It is 20 to 65 hours for patients younger than 10 years and 64 to 140 hours for those older than 15 years. Therefore, children need higher maintenance dosages of 4 to 8 mg/kg par day; adults need only 1 to 2 mg/kg per day.
   d. **Metabolism.** Hydroxylation by the liver
   e. **Therapeutic blood level.** 15 to 40 mg/mL
   f. **Formulation.** Tablets: 15, 30, 60, and 100 mg; elixir: 20 mg/5 mL
   g. **Side effects.** Paradoxic hyperactivity, sedation, learning disabilities, personality changes, and Stevens–Johnson syndrome

5. **Valproic acid (Depakene, Depakote; Abbott, Abbott Park, IL, U.S.A.)**
   a. **Indications.** Primary generalized epilepsy (absence, myoclonic, GTCS), secondarily generalized epilepsy syndrome (infantile spasms, Lennox–Gastaut syndrome), complex partial seizures, and febrile seizures
   b. **Dosage.** Start at 10 to 15 mg/kg per day and gradually increase to a maximum of 60 mg/kg per day in three divided doses.
   c. **Serum half-life.** 5 to 15 hours
   d. **Metabolism.** Hepatic
   e. **Therapeutic blood level.** 40 to 100 mg/mL
   f. **Formulation.** Depakote (divalproex sodium): enteric-coated tablets, 125, 250, and 500 mg; sprinkles, 125 mg. Depakene (valproic acid): capsules, 250 mg; elixir, 250 mg/mL. Also available as i.v. preparation: Depacon (100 mg/mL) starting at 10 to 15 mg/kg per day increased 5 to 10 mg/kg per week to a maximum of 60 mg/kg per day infused over

60 minutes at a rate not to exceed 20 mg per minute. If oral administration is contraindicated (e.g., paralytic ileus), Depakene elixir (250 mg/5 mL) can be given rectally, diluted 1:1 with water in an enema at a dose of 20 mg/kg to attain therapeutic levels of 40 to 50 mg/mL.

g. Side effects. Dose-related side effects are nausea, vomiting, and gastric irritation, which can be minimized with the use of the sprinkle or enteric-coated preparation or administration after meals. Other side effects include weight gain, alopecia, tremor, thrombocytopenia, and liver failure. Liver failure is more common among children younger than 2 years. It can be a fulminant progressive failure or a subacute. gradually progressive failure. Valproic acid is therefore contraindicated in the treatment of children with preexisting hepatic damage, organic aciduria, or carnitine deficiency. A 10% solution of carnitine (Carnitor; Sigma-Tau, Gaithersburg, MD, U.S.A.) should be administered 50 mg/kg per day in two or three divided doses in conjunction with valproic acid to children undergoing long-term, high-dose therapy with poor nutrition (e.g., cerebral palsy). Baseline liver function and serum ammonia should be checked before starting valproic acid and at least monthly for the first 4 to 6 months while this medication is being given. There is a 1.5% risk of neural tube defects such as spina bifida and, less commonly, myelomeningocele in the fetus when valproic acid is used during pregnancy.

6. **Lamotrigine (Lamictal; Glaxo Wellcome, Research Triangle Park, NC, U.S.A.)**
   a. **Indication.** Adjunct for partial seizures in children older than 16 years and in management of Lennox–Gastaut syndrome for children older than 2 years.
   b. **Dosage.** Children not taking valproic acid: initial dose of 0.6 mg/kg per day for 2 weeks, increased to 1 mg/kg per day for 2 weeks and thereafter, slowly titrated to a maximum of 5 to 15 mg/kg per day twice a day. Children taking valproic acid: initial dose of 0.15 mg/kg per day for 2 weeks, increased to 0.3 mg/kg per day for 2 weeks and slowly titrated to a maximum of 1 to 5 mg/kg per day twice a day.
   c. **Serum half-life.** 24 hours. It is shortened when the drug is used concomitantly with enzyme-inducing AEDs (phenobarbital, phenytoin, carbamazepine) to 13.5 hours and increased when used with enzyme inhibitors (valproic acid) to 50 hours.
   d. **Metabolism.** Negligible first-pass effect so that its bioavailability is almost 100%.
   e. **Therapeutic blood level.** 4 to 20 µg/mL
   f. **Formulation.** Chewable dispersible tablet: 5 mg, 25 mg; tablets: 25 mg, 100 mg, 150 mg, 200 mg
   g. **Side effects.** Common adverse effects among children include somnolence, rash, vomiting, laryngitis, ataxia, and headache. The incidence of rash increases with higher initial doses and faster rates of dose escalation, especially among children receiving valproic acid.

7. **Topiramate (Topamax; Ortho-McNeil, Raritan, NJ, U.S.A.)**
   a. **Indications.** Adjunct for partial seizures, primary generalized tonic–clonic seizures and Lennox–Gastaut syndrome in adults and children older than 2 years.
   b. **Dosage.** Initiated at 0.5 to 1 mg/kg per day increased slowly to 4 to 9 mg/kg per day twice a day. Faster titration schedules have resulted in increased CNS side effects.
   c. **Serum half-life.** 12 to 15 hours in children
   d. **Metabolism.** Most of the drug is excreted in the urine unchanged with some of the drug being metabolized by the liver.
   e. **Therapeutic blood level.** 20 to 50 µg/mL.
   f. **Formulation.** Tablets: 25 mg, 100 mg, 200 mg; sprinkle capsule: 15 mg, 25 mg

    g. Side effects. Somnolence, dizziness, ataxia, psychomotor slowing, speech disorder, paresthesia, kidney stones (1% to 2% of patients)

8. Zonisamide (Zonegran; Elan, South San Francisco, CA, U.S.A.)

    a. Indications. Adjunct for partial seizures in adults and children older than 12 years. May be effective in myoclonic seizures as in Unverricht–Lundborg syndrome (Baltic myoclonus). It has ben available in Japan for more than 10 years.

    b. Dosage. 4 to 8 mg/kg per day divided twice a day

    c. Serum half-life. 24 to 60 hours

    d. Metabolism. Principally hepatic

    e. Therapeutic blood levels. 10-40 µg/mL

    f. Formulation. Capsule: 100 mg

    g. Side effects. Somnolence, dizziness, anorexia, headaches, confusion, renal calculi (1.5 to 2.5% of patients). Contraindicated in care of patients with hypersensitivity to sulfonamides (zonisamide is a sulfonamide).

9. Felbamate

    a. Indications. Complex partial seizures, Lennox–Gastaut syndrome (atypical absences, tonic seizures, drop attacks) in children older than 2 years.

    b. Dosage. Begin at 15 mg/kg per day for 1 week, 30 mg/kg per day for the second week and 45 mg/kg per day divided three times a day from the third week (maximum 3,600 mg/day)

    c. Formulation. Tablets: 400 mg, 600 mg; suspension 600 mg/5 mL

    d. Metabolism. Hydroxylation and conjugation in the liver

    e. Serum half-life. 16 to 22 hours in adults

    f. Therapeutic blood level. 30 to 100 µg/mL

    g. Adverse effects. Gastrointestinal side effects, including weight loss and anorexia, have been most prominent. Insomnia, somnolence, and fatigue also have occurred. Rash may occur if the patient is also taking Depakote. Unfortunately, on August 1, 1994, 1 year after felbamate was approved, several cases of aplastic anemia and hepatotoxicity were reported. Physicians should restrict use of this drug only to children with severe epilepsy, especially Lennox—Gastaut syndrome, that is refractory to other therapies.

10. Ethosuximide (Zarontin; Pfizer)

    a. Indication. Absence seizures

    b. Dosage. 20 to 40 mg/kg per day in two or three divided doses

    c. Serum half-life. 30 to 66 hours

    d. Metabolism. Hepatic

    e. Therapeutic blood level. 40 to 80 mg/mL

    f. Formulation. Capsules: 250 mg; elixir: 250 mg/5 mL

    g. Side effects. Anorexia, nausea, vomiting, hiccups, and hallucinations

11. Primidone (Mysoline; Elan)

    a. Indications. GTCS and focal seizures (simple and complex partial seizures, partial seizures with secondary generalization)

    b. Dosage. 10 to 25 mg/kg per day in two divided doses

    c. Serum half-life. 12 to 66 hours

    d. Metabolism. Hepatic conversion to phenobarbital and phenylethyl-malonamide (PEMA)

    e. Therapeutic blood levels. Primidone, 5 to 12 µg/mL; phenobarbital, 15 to 40 µg/mL

    f. Formulation. Tablets: 50 and 250 mg; suspension: 250 mg/5 mL

    g. Side effects. Sedation, tremor, behavioral changes, and rash

12. Clonazepam (Klonopin; Roche, Nutley, NJ, U.S.A.)

    a. Indications. Myoclonic, focal (simple and complex partial), absence, and atonic seizures

    b. Dosage. 0.03 to 0.10 mg/kg per day in two or three divided doses

    c. Serum half-life. 22 to 33 hours

    d. Metabolism. Hepatic

    e. Therapeutic blood level. 40 to 70 ng/mL

       f. Formulation. Tablets: 0.5, 1, and 2 mg

       g. Side effects. Drowsiness, blurred vision, ataxia, and drooling

    13. Clorazepate (Tranxene; Abbott)

       a. Indications. GTCS, focal seizures, and secondarily generalized epilepsy syndrome

       b. Dosage. 0.3 to 3.0 mg/kg per day, increased to a maximum of 60 mg/day

       c. Serum half-life. 50 to 150 hours (prolonged in obesity)

       d. Metabolism. Converted to N-desmethyldiazepam (active form) in stomach within 20 minutes of oral administration, extensively metabolized by the liver

       e. Therapeutic blood level. Not established

       f. Formulation. Tablets: 7.5 mg

       g. Side effects. Drowsiness, dizziness, ataxia, and drooling

    14. Other antiepileptic medications available in the United States include levetiracetam (Keppra; UCB, Smyrna, GA, U.S.A.), tiagabine (Gabitril; Abbott), and gabapentin (Neurontin; Pfizer). Vigabatrin (Sabril; Hoechst Marion Roussel, Laval, Quebec, Canada) is not approved in the United States.

    15. Newer antiepileptic drugs still under evaluation include stiripentol, ganaxolone, remacemide, losigamone, pregabalin and rufinamide.

  D. Psychosocial issues. The patient's family should be advised in regard to the following concerns.

    1. Risk factors to be avoided are fatigue, sleep deprivation, and medications that may lower the seizure threshold. Seat belts and bicycle helmets should be worn to prevent head injuries that may lead to seizures.

    2. Febrile illness must be controlled promptly.

    3. Bathtubs should be avoided; only showers should be taken. Activities such as climbing of heights, swimming without supervision, driving, contact with heavy machinery and fire, and other activities that could be dangerous in the event of a seizure should be avoided.

    4. Parents should guard against overprotection, which can develop out of fear and anxiety. Unnecessary limitations prevent the child from taking the risks necessary for him or her to become an independent person and develop self-confidence.

    5. Parents must inform schoolteachers (as well as baby-sitters) about the child's seizures. This allows teachers to be prepared to deal with seizures in the classroom and the reactions of classmates.

    6. Participation in activities such as sports and exercise should be permitted. If certain activities must be restricted because of poor seizure control, substitute exercise programs must be found.

    7. A medication schedule that avoids school hours should be planned, because it often is inconvenient and embarrassing for a child to take AEDs at school.

    8. Teachers should be expected to provide information about frequency of seizures during school hours, changes in the child's behavior that may indicate side effects, unexplained changes in school performance that may reflect increases in frequency or severity of seizures, and abnormal behavioral and social problems that may require referral for counseling.

    9. Referral to services such as the Epilepsy Foundation of America or local support groups for counseling should be recommended.

IV. Status epilepticus

  A. Definition. One or more seizures lasting for more than 30 minutes without full recovery of consciousness between seizures

  B. Types

    1. Generalized convulsive status epilepticus is characterized by persistent GTCS. In children, it is associated with a higher morbidity and mortality than in adults. We therefore focus on the management of this type of status epilepticus.

    2. Nonconvulsive status epilepticus includes cases of absence status and complex partial status and often is described as "twilight state."

  C. Precipitating factors. Status epilepticus can be an initial unproved event or can occur as a result of the following:

1. Abrupt discontinuation of or changes in anticonvulsant therapy (noncompliance).
2. Acute intercurrent infections such as meningitis and encephalitis
3. Acute metabolic or toxic disturbances, such as electrolyte disturbances, hypoglycemia, hyperpyrexia, and lead intoxication.
4. Acute cerebral insult such as subarachnoid hemorrhage, subdural hematoma, anoxia, hypoxia–ischemia, and depressed skull fractures

D. **Prognosis.** Approximately 15% of all patients with epilepsy have an episode of status epilepticus at some time in their lives. Morbidity is higher among children than among adults (approximately 10% to 25%), including most commonly hemiplegia and mental retardation. Recurrent status epilepticus is more common among children.

E. **Treatment**
1. **Confirmation of diagnosis of status epilepticus.** The longer the seizure continues, the more difficult it is to control and the greater the possibility of permanent brain damage. One should be certain that the patient is in status epilepticus and is not merely postictal.
2. **General measures**
    a. Position the child's head on one side to allow drainage of secretions. Loosen clothing and place a soft object (e.g., a pillow) under the head to avoid injuries during seizures.
    b. Establish airway patency and ventilation by means of gentle suctioning to avoid enhancing seizure activity by overstimulation. A plastic airway should be inserted and taped securely. *Wooden tongue blades and hard objects should not be used,* because they can cause injuries to the mouth and teeth.
    c. Be prepared to administer oxygen through a nasal cannula and to quickly initiate general anesthesia with endotracheal intubation if needed
    d. Monitor vital signs, including heart rate, blood pressure, and temperature (fever may be indicative of an infective process).
    e. Place an i.v. line (preferably two, one with normal saline solution). Blood should be obtained at this time for CBC, electrolytes, calcium, magnesium, glucose, liver function tests, AED levels, toxicology screening, and blood cultures.
    f. Administer i.v. glucose (50% solution) at 2 mL/kg.
    g. Consider LP later for any child with a fever, especially if younger than 18 months, because meningitis can occur without clinical signs of neck stiffness.
    h. Obtain a history surrounding the status epilepticus and perform general and neurologic examinations. Subsequent evaluation and treatment often are determined by the history. For a patient with known seizures in whom status epilepticus may have been caused by AED withdrawal, the treatment of choice is reinstatement of the same drug.
3. **Drug treatment** involves administration of a drug for immediate termination of the seizure and a second drug for maintenance therapy. The initial treatment is similar regardless of the type of seizure. Maintenance treatment varies depending on the type of epilepsy. The protocol is presented in Table 38.4.
    a. **Benzodiazepines**
        (1) **Lorazepam (Ativan; Wyeth-Ayerst, Philadelphia, PA, U.S.A.)** is recommended as a first-line treatment in a dosage of 0.05 to 0.10 mg/kg at a rate of 1 to 2 mg/min to a maximum of 5 mg and can be repeated after 10 minutes. The advantages are rapid onset of action, prolonged antiepileptic activity compared with diazepam, and less respiratory depression after previous administration of anticonvulsants such as phenobarbital.
        (2) **IV diazepam** (0.2 to 0.5 mg/kg per dose, maximum of 5 mg administered over 2 to 5 minutes) also can be used. The disadvantages include short duration of action (less than 30 minutes), high incidence

Table 38.4 Management of generalized tonic–clonic status epilepticus in children

Time from start of treatment	Procedure
0 minutes	Verify diagnosis of status epilepticus. Monitor cardiorespiratory function. ECG, pulse oximetry, and stabilize. EEG if possible. Insert oral airway, administer oxygen if needed. Insert i.v. catheter with normal saline solution. Draw AED levels, glucose, electrolytes, calcium, magnesium, BUN, CBC, arterial blood gas.
5 minutes	Start i.v. normal saline solution. Administer 50% glucose at 2 mL/kg.
10–30 minutes	i.v. lorazepam, 0.1 mg/kg, at 1–2 mg/min to maximum of 5 mg. Start i.v. fosphenytoin 20 mg PE/kg infused at 150 mg/min (or i.v. phenytoin 18–20 mg/kg, at a rate not to exceed 1 mg/kg per minute or 50 mg/min) with ECG and blood pressure monitoring; additional 10 mg/kg may be given after ward monitoring.
31–60 minutes	If seizures persist, administer i.v. phenobarbital at a rate not to exceed 50 mg/min until seizures stop or to a loading dose of 20 mg/kg.
>60 minutes	If seizures persist, options include: (1) i.v. diazepam—continuous infusion, 50 mg diluted in 250 mL normal saline solution or D5W at 1 ml/kg per hour (2 mg/kg per hour) to achieve blood levels of 0.2–0.8 mg/mL. (2) i.v. pentobarbital—initial loading dose of 5 mg/kg followed by maintenance infusion of 1–3 mg/kg per hour (with EEG monitoring) to produce burst suppression pattern on EEG. Decrease infusion rate 4–6 h later to check for reappearance of seizures. If seen, repeat procedure. If not, taper over 12–24 h. If seizures are not controlled, ask an anesthesiologist to institute general anesthesia with halothane and neuromuscular blockade.

ECG, electrocardiogram; EEG, electroencephalography; i.v., intravenous; AED, antiepileptic drug; BUN, blood urea nitrogen; CBC, complete blood cell count; PE, phenytoin equivalent; D5W, 5% dextrose in water.

of respiratory depression, and tendency to precipitate tonic status in patients with Lennox–Gastaut syndrome.

  b. After i.v. lorazepam has been administered, **IV fosphenytoin** 20 mg PE per kilogram is given at a rate not to exceed 150 mg PE per minute (IV phenytoin 18 to 20 mg/kg, not to exceed 1 mg/kg per minute or a total of 50 mg/min also can be used). This results in therapeutic levels of 18 to 20 mg/mL. Disadvantages of phenytoin include cardiac arrhythmias and hypotension requiring close electrocardiographic and blood pressure monitoring. Intramuscular administration is avoided because of unpredictable absorption and muscle irritation. Intravenous extravasation can result in phlebitis and tissue necrosis. Poor absorption occurs in children, resulting in difficulty in maintaining steady therapeutic levels, especially when the patient is switched to the oral form for maintenance. Phenytoin should be administered in normal saline solution, because it precipitates in glucose solutions.

  c. If seizures persist, 15 to 20 mg/kg **IV phenobarbital** is administered at a rate of 50 mg/min. In the treatment of neonates, this may be administered as a single dose. In the care of older children, it may be divided into aliquots of 10 mg/kg to avoid respiratory depression until seizures stop or a maximum loading dose of 20 mg/kg has been administered. Disadvantages of phenobarbital include hypotension and respiratory depression.

  d. **A more detailed history interview and neurologic examination** should be performed at this time. Evaluate the initial blood work. Before initiating additional therapies, it is preferable to obtain CT scans without contrast enhancement and to perform LP to look for causes such as intracranial structural lesions or infections.

  e. **Refractory status epilepticus.** If seizures persist for 60 minutes and the patient does not respond to loading doses of phenytoin and phenobarbital, the following drugs can be administered.

  (1) **Diazepam drip** (50 mg) diluted in 250 mL of normal saline solution or 5% dextrose in water (D5W) in continuous infusion at a rate of 1 mL/kg per hour to achieve blood levels of 0. 2 to 0.8 mg/mL.

  (2) **Pentobarbital coma.** Initial i.v. loading dose of 5 mg/kg followed by a maintenance dose of 1 to 3 mg/kg per hour, titrating dosage to achieve a burst suppression pattern on the EEG.

  (3) **Phenobarbital** can be used in additional i.v. boluses of 5 to 10 mg/kg with EEG monitoring until seizures stop and a burst suppression pattern is obtained on the EEG. The disadvantage of phenobarbital coma is that because of a longer half-life, the effect takes longer to wear off. The recommended duration of coma is 48 to 72 hours. During this time, the patient is rechecked for seizures by means of decreasing the infusion rate. If seizures persist, the procedure is repeated. If seizures are adequately controlled, medication is slowly withdrawn. Administration of coma requires an intensive care unit setting with controlled mechanical ventilation and close cardiac monitoring.

  (4) **Midazolam** has been used effectively for management of convulsive status epilepticus, but the dosing is not yet established for children.

  f. If seizures are still not controlled, general anesthesia with halothane and neuromuscular blockade is recommended.

V. Medication withdrawal. Although there is no consensus on how long a patient should remain seizure free before drug withdrawal is considered, a seizure-free period of 2 to 4 years is recommended. Relapse rates are higher among adults than among children. Children with febrile seizures have a 97% chance of outgrowing them by 6 years of age. There is an 80% to 85% chance of remission among children with absence seizures.

  A. **Favorable factors associated with lower relapse rate**
    1. Reasonable ease of seizure control
    2. Normal neurologic examination findings and developmental milestones
    3. Normal EEG findings at time of withdrawal
    4. Early onset (before 8 years of age)
    5. Certain seizure types—febrile seizures, absence seizures, GTCS

  B. **Unfavorable factors associated with increased chance of recurrence**
    1. Seizures of long duration before successful establishment of control
    2. Abnormal EEG findings at time of medication withdrawal
    3. Abnormal neurologic examination findings
    4. Later age at onset (after 9 years)
    5. Certain seizure types—focal seizures, jacksonian epilepsy, infantile spasms, Lennox–Gastaut syndrome

VI. Vagal nerve stimulation. Indications in open and compassionate trials have included refractory complex partial epilepsy, Lennox–Gastaut syndrome, generalized tonic–clonic seizures and epileptic encephalopathy in children. In the United States, Food and Drug Administration approval indicates use as adjunctive therapy for refractory partial seizures in the care of adults and children older than 12 years. Indications for consideration of the device include medically refractory seizures, adequate trial of at least three AEDs, exclusion of nonepileptic events, and lack of surgery candidacy. Children who have undergone vagotomy (unilateral or bilateral) should not be given implants. Cervical masses should be excluded because cervical MRI may not be performed once the device is implanted. Cardiac arrhythmias, conduction abnormalities, and chronic obstructive pulmonary diseases also are considered as risk factors.

VII. Surgical therapy. Procedures that resect or disconnect epileptogenic areas can reduce or eliminate seizures in patients with medically intractable epilepsy. These procedures are performed in specialized epilepsy centers. Extensive preoperative evaluation includes video EEG monitoring to identify seizure focus, neuropsychiatric evaluation, neuroimaging studies (MRI, SPECT, and PET), intracarotid amobarbital test (Wada's test), and even invasive studies (subdural and depth electrodes) if indicated. The most common types of epilepsy surgery in the care of children are as follows.

    A. Resective surgery. Removal of the epileptogenic area (e.g., temporal lobectomy)

    B. Corpus callosotomy. Interruption of the anterior two thirds of the corpus callosum, effective for atonic seizures, tonic seizures, and GTCS

    C. Hemispherectomy. One cerebral hemisphere is disconnected from the rest of the brain, and a limited area is resected. It is performed for early-onset or congenital hemiplegia in which seizures arise from one side of the brain.

Recommended Readings

Aicardi J. Epilepsy in children, 2nd ed. New York: Raven Press, 1994.

Commission on Classification and Terminology of the International League Against Epilepsy. Proposal for revised classification of epilepsies and epileptic syndromes. *Epilepsia* 1989;30: 389–399.

Levy RH, Mattson RH, Meldrum BS, et al., eds. *Antiepileptic drugs,* 4th ed. New York: Raven Press, 1995.

Pellock JM, Dodson WE, Bourgeoise B, eds. Pediatric epilepsy: diagnosis and therapy, 2nd ed. New York: Demos, 2001.

Wilmore JL, ed. New antiepileptic drugs: basic science and clinical use in children and adults. *Epilepsia* 1999;40[Suppl 5].

Wolf P, ed. Epileptic seizures and syndromes. London, UK: John Libbey, 1994.

Wyllie E, ed. The treatment of epilepsy: principles and practice, 2nd ed. Baltimore: Williams & Wilkins, 1997.

Omkar N. Markand

I. **Definitions**
   A. An epileptic seizure is a transient and reversible alteration of behavior caused by a paroxysmal, abnormal, and excessive neuronal discharge.
   B. Epilepsy usually is defined as two or more recurring seizures not directly provoked by intracranial infection, drug withdrawal, acute metabolic changes, or fever. Antiepileptic drug (AED) therapy usually is initiated after at least two epileptic seizures have occurred, that is, when a diagnosis of epilepsy has been made.
II. **Classifications.** There are two classifications—one of seizure types and one of epilepsy or epileptic syndromes. Accurate diagnosis of the type of epileptic seizure and the categorization of epilepsy (or epileptic syndrome) for each patient are essential for proper selection of AED therapy and for prognosis.
   A. **Classification of epileptic seizures** is based on the patient's behavior during seizures and on the associated electroencephalographic (EEG) characteristics. Epileptic seizures are classified into two main types—partial and generalized.
      1. **Partial (focal) seizures** arise at specific loci in the cerebral cortex and are associated with focal interictal and ictal EEG changes. Clinically, a partial seizure can range in intensity from a disorder of sensation without loss of consciousness to a generalized convulsion.
         a. **Simple partial seizures.** Consciousness remains intact. Such seizures can be motor seizures (focal motor twitching or jacksonian seizures), sensory seizures (numbness or tingling involving parts of the body), autonomic seizures, or seizures with psychic symptoms.
         b. **Complex partial seizures.** Consciousness is impaired during complex partial seizures. Previously, these seizures were called *psychomotor seizures.* They constitute the most common type of seizure in adults. Approximately 85% have an epileptogenic focus in the temporal lobe, whereas the remaining 15% are of extratemporal origin, usually frontal.
         c. **Secondarily generalized (tonic–clonic) seizures.** During any focal seizure (simple or complex partial), the epileptic excitation can spread widely to the entire brain, resulting in a generalized tonic–clonic convulsion.
      2. **Generalized seizures** are characterized by generalized involvement of the brain from the outset and have no consistent focal areas of ictal onset. There are of many subtypes.
         a. **Absence seizures** were formerly known as *petit mal seizures.* The dominant feature is a brief loss of consciousness with no or minimal motor manifestations (e.g., twitching of the eyelids). During the seizure, EEG shows 3-Hz generalized spike–wave discharges.
         b. **Myoclonic seizures** are brief jerks involving part of the body or the entire body.
         c. **Clonic seizures** are rhythmic twitching of the body.
         d. **Tonic seizures** are brief attacks of stiffness in part of the body or the entire body.
         e. **Atonic seizures** are losses of posture with resultant drop attacks.
         f. **Tonic–clonic seizures** are generalized convulsions or grand mal seizures. It is important to emphasize that some tonic–clonic (grand mal) seizures are generalized from the outset and some are secondarily generalized (they start as focal seizures and then become generalized). The second type is the most common among adults. The presence of an aura, focal manifestations during the seizure, and postictal focal deficits favor a secondarily generalized tonic–clonic seizure.
         Confusion can arise in differentiating absence seizures and complex partial seizures. Both can present with a brief loss of awareness or altered responsiveness, and in both there may be automatic activities of various kinds. Diagnosis is aided by EEG findings (generalized spike–wave

discharges in absence seizures and focal epileptiform abnormalities in complex partial seizures). Correct diagnosis is critical for instituting proper AED therapy.

B. **Classification of epilepsy or epileptic syndromes.** Classifying the seizure type, although useful, is of limited value because seizures usually appear as part of a cluster of other symptoms and signs that include etiologic factor, site of seizure onset, age, precipitating factors, response to medication, and prognosis. Hence, in diagnosing epilepsy or an epileptic syndrome, it is critical that all these features be taken into account.

1. **Localization-related (focal, or partial) epilepsy or epileptic syndromes** are disorders in which a localized origin of the seizures can be established. The patient has focal or secondarily generalized tonic–clonic seizures. EEG shows focal epileptiform discharges overlying the epileptogenic focus.

    a. Most localization-related forms of epilepsy are **acquired** or **symptomatic.** Temporal lobe epilepsy is the common localization-related epilepsy among adults.

    b. There are age-related **idiopathic** or **primary** localization-related epileptic syndromes. The best known is benign rolandic epilepsy of childhood.

2. **Generalized epilepsy or epileptic syndromes** are disorders that involve one or more types of generalized seizures. EEG shows generalized epileptiform abnormalities.

    a. **Primary generalized epilepsy** is characterized by generalized seizures without any identifiable etiologic factor. Genetic factors predominate in these forms of epilepsy. Common syndromes include absence epilepsy, juvenile myoclonic epilepsy, and tonic–clonic seizures occurring in the early morning (awakening grand mal).

    b. **Secondarily generalized epilepsy** is characterized by various types of generalized seizures resulting from acquired cerebral diseases (e.g., seizures secondary to ischemic–hypoxic encephalopathy or following severe cerebral trauma or intracranial infection) or from inborn errors of metabolism (e.g., lipidosis, progressive myoclonus epilepsy). Patients usually have varying degrees of cognitive and neurologic deficits, and the seizures are often drug resistant. Within this category are two commonly recognized age-related syndromes—**West's syndrome** (infancy) and **Lennox–Gastaut syndrome** (childhood).

III. **Evaluation.** It is essential to establish that the spells or episodes are indeed epileptic seizures. Nonepileptic physiologic disorders that result in transient, reversible alterations of behavior or function, such as syncope, migraine, breath-holding spells, anxiety episodes, transient ischemic attacks, hypoglycemic episodes, and narcoleptic–cataplectic attacks, must be differentiated from epileptic seizures. Moreover, there are nonepileptic psychogenic seizures or pseudoseizures that are conversion reactions characterized by episodes of motor activity and loss of consciousness but not associated with ictal EEG patterns and without an underlying physiologic basis.

A. A **history** of the episodes, obtained not only from the patient but also from one or more observers, is perhaps the most essential element in making the diagnosis of epileptic seizures and differentiating them from nonepileptic disorders. The history can aid in ascertaining the type of epileptic seizures.

B. **Physical and neurologic examinations** can help detect the underlying cause of the brain disorder responsible for the epilepsy by uncovering evidence of a focal cerebral lesion or another organic disorder, such as tuberous sclerosis or neurofibromatosis.

C. **Neuroimaging.** Although computed tomography of the head with and without contrast enhancement is performed on most patients believed to have epilepsy, magnetic resonance imaging of the head is the imaging procedure of choice. Magnetic resonance imaging is particularly sensitive in detecting hamartoma, cavernous malformation, and low-grade glioma and in providing evidence of mesial temporal sclerosis in patients with temporal lobe epilepsy.

D. EEG is the most informative test for confirmation of the diagnosis of epilepsy and proper classification of the seizure type and even the epileptic syndrome. It also aids in initiation, selection, and discontinuation of antiepileptic therapy. It is uncommon for an actual seizure to occur during an EEG study unless the patient has absence or myoclonic seizures. Hyperventilation can help precipitate an absence seizure. In the event that an actual seizure is recorded during an EEG study, the type of ictal EEG pattern accompanying the seizure establishes the diagnosis of epilepsy beyond a doubt and provides critical information necessary to classify the type of seizure.

The usefulness of EEG depends largely on the interictal epileptiform abnormalities (spikes, sharp waves, or spike–wave discharges). These abnormalities constitute interval discharges that certainly have a high correlation with clinical seizures but do not automatically imply epilepsy. Generalized epileptiform abnormalities occur in generalized epilepsy, whereas focal abnormalities suggest focal or localization-related epilepsy.

Not all patients with epilepsy have interictal epileptiform abnormalities; approximately 50% have such abnormalities in a routine awake-and-asleep EEG study that includes hyperventilation and intermittent photic stimulation. The yield increases with repeated EEG studies with sleep deprivation and extra recording electrodes. On the other hand, 1% to 2% of healthy persons without clinical seizures have epileptiform abnormalities in EEG studies. Hence, an interictal EEG alone can neither prove nor exclude a diagnosis of epilepsy. Similarly, the presence of interictal epileptiform EEG abnormalities does not automatically warrant AED therapy, and the absence of such abnormalities is not sufficient grounds for discontinuing AED treatment.

E. Intensive video EEG monitoring. Patients with drug-resistant epilepsy or poorly characterized episodes may need intensive monitoring that consists of simultaneous monitoring of the patient's behavior and EEG to provide detailed clinical and EEG correlation of episodic events. This is an expensive and time-consuming technique and thus is left to the discretion of a consulting neurologist specialized in epilepsy. Only 5% to 10% of patients believed to have epilepsy need this technique to characterize and classify the epileptic episodes. Video EEG monitoring is most helpful in the evaluation of patients who have frequent episodes that are suspected to be of the nonepileptic type. These episodes are not accompanied by the characteristic ictal pattern in the simultaneously recorded EEG.

IV. Basic principles in treating patients with epilepsy

A. AED therapy should be initiated only when the diagnosis of epileptic seizures is well established. If the patient's episodes are yet to be clearly defined and there is reasonable doubt of their being epileptic in nature, it is prudent to wait until the diagnosis of epilepsy can be confirmed.

B. AED therapy usually is not initiated after the first tonic–clonic seizure. There is broad agreement that treatment is postponed until a second seizure occurs and the diagnosis of recurrent seizures or epilepsy is made. The first seizure can be an isolated episode and not necessarily the onset of epilepsy. This is particularly true if a single tonic–clonic seizure was related to sleep deprivation, physical or mental stress, drug or alcohol withdrawal, or use of psychotropic drugs (e.g., cocaine). In a large series, approximately 50% of patients had recurrence after the first tonic–clonic seizure. The range was less than 25% among subjects with low-risk factor profiles to 65% or more for those with two or more of the following risk factors: strong family history, focal-onset seizure, postictal paralysis, abnormal findings at cognitive and neurologic examinations, evidence of a structural cerebral lesion at neuroimaging, and the presence of epileptiform abnormalities at EEG. Patients with two or more of these risk factor therefore may need prompt initiation of therapy after the first tonic–clonic seizure.

C. Monotherapy is preferable to the use of several drugs because it has fewer toxic side effects, less likelihood of drug interactions, and better compliance. The chosen AED (Table 39.1) should be slowly increased until seizures are controlled or until clinical signs of toxicity develop. If seizures are not adequately controlled at the maximum tolerable dosage, a second AED is slowly introduced. After the

Table 39.1 Antiepileptic drugs (AEDs) of choice for specific type of seizures and epilepsy syndromes

Type of seizure or syndrome	Recommended AED		
	First choice	Second choice	Possibly useful
Partial (Focal) Epilepsy			
Simple partial, complex partial; secondary generalized tonic–clonic seizures	CBZ/OXC/PHT	TPM/LTG/LTC/TOP/VPA/ZNS	GBP/PB/PRM/TGB
Primary Generalized Epilepsy			
Primary generalized tonic–clonic seizures	VPA/PHT	TPM/LTG[a]	CBZ/OXC/PB/PRM
Absence epilepsy without motor seizures	ESM	VPA/LTG[a]	CLZ
Absence epilepsy with generalized tonic–clonic seizures	VPA	LTG[a]	CLZ
Myoclonic seizures	VPA	LTG[a]/TPM/ZNS[b]	CLZ
Myoclonic seizures with absence or generalized tonic–clonic seizures	VPA	LTG[a]/TPM	
Secondary Generalized Epilepsy			
Usually multiple seizure types, e.g., tonic, absence, myoclonic, clonic, atonic, tonic–clonic	VPA	LTG/TPM	FBM[c], PHT/CBZ/OXC, ketogenic diet

AEDs separated by virgules are roughly equal in efficacy. The choice of specific AED for a given patient should be based on factors such as toxicity and cost. Sedative AEDs are generally considered second-line drugs.
[a] Because of the risk of neural tube defect with VPA, LTG may be the drug of first choice in treatment of women considering pregnancy.
[b] Particularly useful for progressive myoclonic epilepsy.
[c] High incidence of serious side effects.
CBZ, carbamazepine; OXC, oxcarbazepine; PHT, phenytoin; TPM, topiramate; LTG, lamotrigine; LTC, levetiracetam; VPA, valproic acid; ZNS, zonisamide; GBP, gabapentin; PB, phenobarbital; PRM, primidone; TGB, tiagabine; ESM, ethosuximide; CLZ, clonazepam; FBM, felbamate.

second drug attains therapeutic levels, the first drug is gradually withdrawn. Monotherapy adequately controls new-onset epilepsy in 50% to 75% of patients.

D. Only if monotherapy with two or more first-line AEDs has been unsuccessful does **polytherapy** with a combination of two AEDs (usually one traditional and one newer AED) become necessary. This decision should be made in consultation with a neurologist. One should avoid using more than two AEDs simultaneously. If a combination of two AEDs in the treatment of a compliant patient with blood levels in the therapeutic range fails to provide adequate control of epileptic seizures, **referral to an epileptologist or epilepsy center** is indicated for further evaluation and management.

E. Avoid using AEDs with sedative or hypnotic side effects unless first-choice AED does not work. Drugs with these effects include phenobarbital, primidone, and clonazepam. Often a patient undergoing polytherapy that includes one of the aforementioned sedative AEDs is best served by very gradual withdrawal of the sedative AED while the dosage of the other AED is maximized. Such changes in medication must be made in consultation with a neurologist. Discontinuation of sedative–hypnotic AEDs is followed not only by a reduction in side effects but also by better control of seizures in many instances.

F. Avoid using less well-known AEDs. Acquire experience with the use of a few major traditional AEDs, such as phenytoin, carbamazepine, valproic acid, and ethosuximide. Use of new AEDs may be entrusted to a neurologic consultant with experience in treating patients with epilepsy refractory to traditional AEDs.

G. Avoid complicated drug schedules. Most AEDs have long elimination half-lives (Table 39.2) and thus can be prescribed in a single daily dose or two divided daily doses. Exceptions include the traditional AEDs, such as valproic acid and carbamazepine, and the new AEDs such as gabapentin and tiagabine, which have to be given in two or three divided daily doses. With multiple AEDs, half-lives of some AEDs are shorter than when the same drug is given in monotherapy. Thus larger doses and multiple dosing are required.

H. Any change in the drug schedule should be made gradually, and the effects of the change should be assessed over a long period. Because of the long biologic half-lives of many AEDs, it takes several days to several weeks before a steady state is reached after any change in schedule.

I. After a properly chosen AED is started, it should not be discarded unless a hypersensitivity reaction occurs or there is inadequate benefit with the maximum tolerable dose, not just with the dosage that produces blood levels within a so-called therapeutic range.

J. Regularity in taking the daily doses must be emphasized. Medication is best taken at the time of meals for easy remembrance. For most AEDs, an occasional missed dose can be made up by taking an additional dose within the same 24-hour period. It is also convenient for the patient to put the medication in a plastic pillbox with divided compartments and to ensure at bedtime that the entire day's medication has been taken.

K. Advise the patient to maintain a **seizure diary.** Such a diary provides an accurate record of the frequency of seizures and assists in evaluating the effectiveness of the therapy.

L. Emphasize to the patient the need for constant **medical follow-up care.** Once AED therapy is well established and the seizures have been brought under satisfactory control, the patient should be examined every 6 to 12 months. During the follow-up visits, evaluate the patient for evidence of drug toxicity or development of a progressive neurologic disorder. Complete blood cell count (CBC), liver function tests, and serum calcium measurement are performed every 6 to 12 months to detect untoward effects of AEDs on the bone marrow and liver. A patient who achieves good control with drug therapy may have a **"breakthrough" seizure** during periods of physical or mental stress, sleep deprivation, or infection. Appropriate management of such precipitants rather than increases in dose or changes in the AED is indicated.

M. Generic substitution for brand-name AEDs can reduce the cost of medication, but the bioavailabilities of generic and proprietary AEDs are not the same. Generic

Table 39.2 Pharmacokinetics and adult dosages of traditional antiepileptic drugs (AEDS)

AED	Bio-availability (%)	Peak plasma level (h)	Volume of distribution (L/kg)	Protein binding (%)	Elimination half-life (h)	Time to steady state (d)	Elimination route	Starting adult dose (mg/d)	Usual adult maintenance dose (mg/d)	Maintenance dose (mg/kg)	Dosing regimen (times per day)	Therapeutic level (µg/mL)
Phenytoin	>90	2–12	0.8	90	10–50[a]	7–21	H	300	300–400	4–10	1–3	10–20
Carbamazepine	75–85	4–12	0.8	75	10–50[b]	20–30[c] 3–7[d]	H	200	600–2,000	10–30	3	4–12
Ethosuximide	>90	1–4	0.65	0	30–60	7–14	H 75, R 25	500	500–1,500	15–30	2	40–100
Valproic acid	>90	1–8	0.2	70–95[e]	5–20	2–5	H	500	750–3,000	15–60	2, 3	40–120
Phenobarbital	>90	1–4	0.8	40–50	50–120	14–21	H 75, R 25	60	60–180	1–5	1	15–40
Primidone[f]	>90	2–4	0.75	0	6–12	—	H	125	750–1,500	10–20	3	5–12
Clonazepam	>90	1–4	3.0	85	20–40	7–14	H	1.0	1.5–10	0.03–0.1	1–3	0.02–0.08

[a] Elimination half-life is concentration dependent; at higher levels the half-life is long.
[b] Elimination half-life is longer in the initial 2–4 wk of therapy before self-induction becomes significant.
[c] Before autoinduction is complete.
[d] After autoinduction is complete.
[e] Concentration dependent, higher binding at low total levels.
[f] Primidone therapy produces three active metabolites; primidone, phenobarbital and phenylethylmalonamide (PEMA).
H, hepatic; R, renal; numbers are approximate percentages for each route.

preparations are required by the U.S. Food and Drug Administration (FDA) to provide bioavailabilities within ±20% of those of the corresponding proprietary formulations, but some patients may be sufficiently sensitive to these fluctuations that replacing one with the other leads to either loss of seizure control or signs of neurotoxicity. This problem applies primarily to phenytoin and carbamazepine. The proprietary phenytoin (Dilantin; Pfizer, New York, NY, U.S.A.) is more slowly absorbed than is generic phenytoin, so blood levels are maintained with less fluctuation, and no more than one or two daily doses are required. Similarly, brand-name carbamazepine (Tegretol; Novartis, East Hanover, NJ, U.S.A.) is absorbed more slowly than is the generic formulation. The patient should avoid switching between formulations of AEDs. When a generic AED is used, the formulation by the same manufacturer should be refilled.

N. Therapeutic drug levels are rough guides to the ranges that in most patients provide best seizure control while avoiding dose-related side effects. They are not to be followed rigidly for a given patient with epilepsy. Some patients may attain complete seizure control at low "therapeutic" levels, and increasing the dose to attain idealized levels is not indicated. On the other hand, there are patients who need higher than "therapeutic" levels for control of their seizures and tolerate such levels without significant untoward side effects. In such patients, it is fully justified to maintain phenytoin level as high as 20 to 30 µg/mL, valproic acid level as high as 100 to 150 µg/mL, and carbamazepine level as high as 12 to 15 µg/mL. Anticonvulsant blood levels are indicated under the following circumstances:

1. To determine the baseline plasma dose level
2. When the patient is believed to be noncompliant
3. When the patient does not respond adequately to the usual dosage of an AED
4. When symptoms and signs of clinical toxicity are suspected
5. When there is a question of drug interaction
6. To establish the correct dosage of an AED for a patient with diseases affecting absorption, metabolism, or excretion (hepatic, renal, or gastrointestinal disorders)

Total serum levels of AEDs usually are obtained. When metabolism of AEDs may be altered or serum protein levels are likely to the low (e.g., hepatic or renal disorders, pregnancy), free levels of highly protein-bound AEDs may become necessary.

O. Most AEDs have linear or first-order elimination kinetics. This means that progressive increases in dose are associated with proportional increases in blood levels. Major exceptions are phenytoin and valproic acid. Phenytoin has nonlinear kinetics, particularly after a blood level of 12 to 15 µg/mL has been attained. With further dose increments, a disproportionately higher level occurs. It is therefore very important that increases in phenytoin dose be made in smaller steps (30 mg/d or so) when the blood levels are higher than 15 µg/mL. This is also true when the dose of phenytoin is reduced because of high levels or clinical toxicity.

Binding of valproic acid to serum protein is nonlinear, and higher concentrations of valproic acid exceed the capacities of binding sites. Hence, at high blood levels, free valproic acid is disproportionately higher than is the bound fraction. It is the free fraction that relates to drug effectiveness and the presence of drug toxicity.

V. General management

A. Educate the patient and family members regarding epilepsy, its causes, its significance, and the necessity of continuing medication for several years despite prompt control of seizures with AEDs, taking the medication regularly, and not discontinuing it suddenly without medical advice.

B. Emphasize the need to regularize the time and duration of sleep, because sleep deprivation tends to potentiate seizures.

C. Inform the patient that alcohol in any form is best avoided or used in small amounts (e.g., one drink) because of possible interactions with most AEDs.

D. Be aware drugs that lower the seizure threshold (e.g., tricyclic antidepressants and phenothiazines) or those that can cause drug interactions (increasing or decreasing the levels of AEDs) should be used with caution. Some AEDs affect the elimination kinetics of many drugs metabolized in the liver (e.g. birth control pills, corticosteroids, anticoagulants, and cyclosporine), necessitating proper dose adjustment of these comedications.

E. Encourage the patient to make the adjustments necessary for leading a normal life as much as possible. Moderate exercise does not affect seizure frequency. Encourage a regular exercise program. Participation in highly competitive sports increases the risk of physical injury. Individualize instructions to the patient by considering the risk of a particular sport against the patient's needs. Swimming may be permitted under supervision for a patient with good control of seizures. Bathing in a bathtub is to be avoided; taking a shower is recommended instead.

F. Most adults who have epilepsy are able to maintain competitive employment and should be encouraged to do so. This improves their self-esteem and their acceptance in the mainstream of society. There are, however, some realistic limitations on the types of work a patient with epilepsy can be permitted to do. Certain occupations, such as working with heavy machines, working above ground level, working close to water or fire, driving trucks or buses, and flying planes, may be off limits for reasons of personal and public safety. There are still scores of jobs, such as secretary, lawyer, physician, accountant, and stockbroker that are acceptable.

G. Some women have increased frequency of seizures just before or during **menstruation,** probably related to hormonal changes and water retention. These patients may benefit from intermittent use of acetazolamide at 250 to 500 mg/d, starting 2 to 4 days before the onset and then continuing during menstruation. An alternative is to cover this period with additional doses of the AED or to use a benzodiazepine such as lorazepam for a few days.

H. Family members or caregivers should be educated regarding proper care of the patient when a seizure occurs. During a grand mal seizure, the patient should be helped to lie on the ground, a bed, or a couch and should be turned on one side or placed in the prone position to avoid aspiration. An object such as a spoon or a finger should *never be thrust into the patient's mouth.* It is a myth that the tongue can be swallowed during a seizure. Pushing a hard object into the mouth often results in broken teeth. The patient must be closely watched and the sequence of events observed during the seizure, which can help determine the type of seizure.

I. For a patient with a known history of seizures, an isolated self-limiting seizure does not constitute a need to call for an ambulance and have the patient rushed to an emergency department. However, if the seizure lasts longer than 15 minutes or if the patient has repeated seizures without regaining consciousness between them, prompt transfer to a nearby hospital becomes essential.

J. **Driving.** Most states have laws denying driving privileges to patients with uncontrolled epilepsy but permit driving once the seizures have been brought under control with AEDs. In a few states, doctors are required to report cases of epilepsy. The period of time that the patient must remain seizure-free before being permitted to drive varies from 3 months to 2 years, depending on the state. Rare patients who have only nocturnal seizures or who have only simple partial seizures (no loss of consciousness) may be exempted from driving restrictions. Reinstitution of driving privileges may require reapplication, a letter from the treating physician, or a determination made by a state-appointed board. Some states require the treating physician to certify at regular intervals that the patient has continued to remain seizure-free before reissuing the driving permit. Because the laws regarding driving vary widely among different states and are frequently changing, physicians are best advised to obtain their current state registration.

In general, patients with frequent seizures with altered consciousness must be advised to refrain from driving until seizures can be satisfactorily controlled. That the patient has been properly advised must be documented in the patient's record.

There is no consensus as to how long the patient should be advised not to drive after having a breakthrough seizure after a long seizure-free period. If such a seizure follows a known precipitant such as infection, mental or physical stress, prolonged sleep deprivation, or poor compliance, observation for at least 3 to 6 months is required before driving is again permitted.

VI. Selection of AED. Table 39.1 lists AEDs effective for managing various forms of epilepsy and epileptic syndromes.

   A. Symptomatic partial (localization-related) epilepsy. For simple partial, complex partial, and secondarily generalized tonic–clonic seizures, several AEDs, including phenytoin, carbamazepine, phenobarbital, and primidone have very similar antiepileptic potencies but differ greatly in toxicity. **Carbamazepine** and **phenytoin** are the first-line drugs because they have fewer side effects. Several newer AEDs have been approved as adjunctive therapy. Primidone and phenobarbital are more often associated with neurotoxicity and are usually avoided. There are very small differences in overall effectiveness and basic mechanism of action between carbamazepine and phenytoin.

   Phenytoin is relatively inexpensive, is better tolerated in the initial period of therapy, and can be used in a single daily dose or two divided daily doses. However, it has a high incidence of chronic dysmorphic side effects, such as hirsutism, coarsening of facial features, and acneiform eruptions. **Carbamazepine** has side effects that are most bothersome at the start of therapy, but these effects can be minimized by starting the therapy at a low dose and increasing it slowly over 3 to 4 weeks. Carbamazepine has no dysmorphic effects and hence is better accepted by adolescent and young adult female patients. Its short half-life usually necessitates using carbamazepine in three or four divided doses. Cognitive side effects with long-term use of phenytoin or carbamazepine have been found to be equally frequent in recent studies. Oxcarbazepine, which has lesser side effects, rapid titration, and no requirement for monitoring, may become a more favored alternative to carbamazepine in the future.

   Most physicians recommend that carbamazepine be used initially, especially in the treatment of young women. If carbamazepine is ineffective, it can be replaced with phenytoin. If monotherapy with carbamazepine or phenytoin fails to achieve satisfactory control, combination therapy with valproic acid is tried—carbamazepine plus valproic acid, phenytoin plus valproic acid. If traditional AEDs are ineffective, adjunctive therapy with newer AEDs should be strongly considered by adding topiramate, lamotrigine, or levetiracetam to phenytoin or carbamazepine. Combination therapy is more likely to produce cognitive and other side effects.

   Even with adequate AED therapy, only 40% to 60% of patients with symptomatic partial epilepsy, particularly those with complex partial seizures (the most common type of seizures among adults) attain full control of seizures.

   B. Primary generalized epilepsy (PGE). Most patients with PGE have either absence, myoclonic, or tonic–clonic seizures and most have more than one type of seizure, although one type may dominate. Depending on seizure type, several epileptic syndromes are identified under the heading PGE. The best example is juvenile myoclonic epilepsy, which is characterized by myoclonic seizures in the early hours after waking, but most patients also have occasional tonic–clonic seizures. Less often, even absence seizures may occur. Other syndromes include primary tonic–clonic seizures (contrasted to secondarily generalized tonic–clonic seizures, which are part of focal epilepsy), which also tend to occur in the morning hours and hence are called *awakening grand mal* seizures. Absence seizures as the dominant manifestation of PGE commonly occur in childhood, but in rare cases start in adolescence or early adulthood (juvenile absence epilepsy syndrome).

      1. **Valproic acid** is the drug of choice for PGE manifesting as primary grand mal seizures, juvenile myoclonic epilepsy, photosensitive seizures, or combined absence–grand mal epilepsy. The advantage of valproic acid is that it is effective against many seizure types comprising PGE.

      2. Rare juvenile or adult patients who have absence seizures unaccompanied by myoclonic or tonic–clonic seizures can be treated with either ethosuximide or valproic acid. **Ethosuximide** is preferred because of its lesser toxicity. The longer half-life of ethosuximide allows it to be taken in only one or two divided daily doses.

      3. Appropriate AED therapy is generally more effective in various syndromes of PGE. Good seizure control is possible for as many as 70% to 90% of patients with PGE.

4. If valproic acid fails, carbamazepine or phenytoin can be tried for primary tonic–clonic seizures as monotherapy or in combination with valproic acid. Carbamazepine, phenobarbital, primidone, and phenytoin not only are ineffective for absence seizures but also may even exacerbate them.

5. **Clonazepam** is an effective AED for myoclonic and absence seizures but has certain disadvantages. It has a high incidence of sedative and cognitive side effects, and patients develop a tolerance to its antiepileptic potency after several months of therapy. Clonazepam therefore is used less often since the introduction of newer AEDs. If used for myoclonic or absence seizures, clonazepam can be added to valproic acid if the latter by itself fails to be fully effective.

6. Of the newer AEDs, lamotrigine is becoming well established as adjunctive therapy (with valproic acid) or as monotherapy for the management of all types of seizures among patients with PGE. Topiramate alone or with valproic acid may be another alternative.

C. **Secondarily generalized epilepsy,** which is secondary to multifocal or diffuse cerebral disorders (static or progressive), occurs mostly among children and less often among adults. Patients have multiple seizure types, including atypical absence seizures, myoclonic seizures, tonic seizures, tonic–clonic seizures, and drop attacks.

In general, response to any AED is poor, only 20% to 40% of patients attaining acceptable seizure control. Such patients commonly end up being treated with polypharmacy, which not only fails to provide better seizure control than do one or two AEDs but also may even exacerbate certain types of seizures (absence seizures, myoclonic seizures, and drop attacks).

Valproic acid is the AED of first choice for secondarily generalized epilepsy and may be started as monotherapy. However, most patients need an addition of newer AEDs. Of these, lamotrigine and felbamate are particularly effective, but the later has potentially serious hepatic and bone marrow toxicity. Topiramate and zonisamide have been found useful in clinical trials. When drug combinations are prescribed, appropriate dosages should be used to avoid sedation, which tends to exacerbate minor seizures in such patients.

VII. **Traditional AEDs.** Selected pharmacokinetic characteristics and adult dosages of the seven most commonly used traditional AEDs are listed in Table 39.2.

A. **Phenytoin** was introduced in 1938. Its antiepileptic activity is to reduce the frequency of repetitive firing of action potentials through use-dependent blockage of Na^+ channels.

1. **Indications.** Phenytoin is effective for all types of focal epilepsy (simple partial, complex partial, and secondarily generalized tonic–clonic seizures) and for primary and secondarily generalized epilepsy manifesting as tonic–clonic seizures. It also is one of the major AEDs used for controlling generalized convulsive status epilepticus.

2. **Pharmacokinetics.** Phenytoin is heavily bound (>90%) to plasma proteins and eliminated primarily through hepatic metabolism, through microsomal cytochrome P-450 enzymes. A unique characteristic of phenytoin is its nonlinear kinetics resulting from saturation of hepatic microsomal enzymes. Increases in dosage in the therapeutic window of 10 to 20 μg/mL should be made with 30-mg capsules. Giving a 100-mg capsule to a patient with a blood level of 15 μg/mL for a daily dose of 300 mg can lead to levels of more than 20 or even 30 μg/mL and introduce a risk of toxicity.

3. **Preparations.** Proprietary 100-mg and 30-mg capsules (Dilantin) are sustained-release preparations. The proprietary 50-mg preparation (Infatab; Pfizer) and generic phenytoin are both prompt-release preparations. Because of different bioavailabilities, switching from one formulation to another is to be avoided. Phenytoin is also available for parenteral use during status epilepticus.

4. **Administration.** Phenytoin usually is started at a daily dose of 300 mg. A long elimination half-life allows either a single daily dose or at the most two divided daily doses. After 1 to 2 weeks, when the steady state has reached

the trough level, plasma levels should be obtained for further manipulation of the dosage.

When promptness is needed, an oral loading dose of 15 mg/kg can be used, followed by 300 mg/d. An alternative is to give the patient 300 mg three times on the first day, 300 mg twice on the second day, and 300 mg/d thereafter. With such loading treatment, adequate therapeutic levels can be established in 2 to 3 days. Phenytoin is not recommended for intramuscular (i.m.) use because of its slow and erratic absorption when administered by this route.

5. **Side effects.** Frequent side effects include **coarsening of the facies** caused by thickening of the subcutaneous tissue around the eyes and nose, **facial and body hirsutism** in women (30%), and **gum hyperplasia** (30%). These cosmetic effects are particularly concerning to young women and require consideration of an alternative therapy, such as carbamazepine. Phenytoin is also associated with **idiosyncratic reactions,** including rash (2% to 5% of patients) and, in rare cases, even **Stevens–Johnson syndrome.** Other rare reactions include **lupus-like syndrome** (positive results of an antinuclear antibody test), **blood dyscrasia, pseudolymphoma,** and **hepatitis.**

Several dose-related side effects also occur. Higher doses result in neurotoxicity characterized by **nystagmus, ataxia, drowsiness,** and **behavioral disturbances.** Other side effects include megaloblastic anemia resulting from folic acid deficiency, low level of protein-bound thyroxine, hypocalcemia, osteoporosis, and mild elevation in serum alkaline phosphatase level. Many of these side effects do not require discontinuation of phenytoin. Neurotoxicity is managed by means of reductions in dose, and other side effects are countered by supplements of folic acid (1 mg/d), vitamin D, and calcium.

6. **Drug interactions.** Certain drugs use the same hepatic microsomal enzymes used for degradation of phenytoin. Such drugs increase phenytoin levels by means of **competitive inhibition.** These drugs include sulthiame, para-amino-salicylic acid, cycloserine, isoniazid (INH), dicumarol, disulfiram (Antabuse; Wyeth-Ayerst, Philadelphia, PA, U.S.A.), chloramphenicol (Chloromycetin; Monarch, Bristol, TN, U.S.A.), methylphenidate (Ritalin; Novartis, East Hanover, NJ, U.S.A.), cimetidine, phenothiazine, phenylbutazone, propoxyphene, salicylates, and valproic acid. Starting any one of these drugs can increase phenytoin levels and cause toxicity.

Phenytoin induces microsomal hepatic enzymes and increases biotransformation of certain drugs, reducing their levels and effectiveness. Phenytoin decreases the effectiveness of estrogens, dicumarol, cycloserine, corticosteroids, digitalis, and other drugs.

B. **Carbamazepine.** This AED was introduced in the management of epilepsy in 1974. Its basic mechanism of action is on voltage-dependent Na$^+$ channels, similar to that of phenytoin.

1. **Indications** are similar to those of phenytoin, that is, all types of partial (focal) epilepsy and generalized tonic–clonic seizures.

2. **Pharmacokinetics.** Carbamazepine has less protein binding than phenytoin. It is metabolized in the liver and induces its own metabolism, called **autoinduction.** The elimination half-life is initially 20 to 40 hours, but elimination increases 2 to 4 weeks after initiation of therapy, and the half-life decreases to 10 to 20 hours. The elimination half-life of carbamazepine decreases further to 8 to 12 hours with concomitant therapy with enzyme-inducing AEDs (phenobarbital, phenytoin, or primidone).

3. **Administration.** Carbamazepine is available only for oral use. Slow release forms are now available to ensure more steady levels with two divided daily doses. Because of autoinduction and to avoid untoward neurotoxicity, it is very important to start with a small dosage, usually 100 mg twice a day in an adult. The dose is gradually increased over 3 to 4 weeks, and most adults ultimately need a daily dose of 600 to 1,000 mg given in three divided doses. Blood levels are measured after 3 to 4 weeks of the start of therapy for further dosage adjustments. Large doses, given in 3 or 4 divided doses are required when carbamazepine is used with enzyme-inducing AEDs.

   4. **Side effects.** Common dose-related side effects, which are more bothersome in the initial period of therapy, include **sedation, blurred or double vision,** and **dizziness.** These side effects are most apparent when therapy is begun with higher doses or if the dose is increased too rapidly at the start of therapy. Other side effects of carbamazepine include **allergic rashes, hyponatremia,** and **hematologic alterations.**
      The hematologic side effects of carbamazepine have received inordinate publicity. Severe complications such as aplastic anemia and agranulocytosis are extremely uncommon. On the other hand, usually benign leukopenia occurs in 10% to 20% of patients. A total white blood cell count of 3,000/mL and an absolute granulocyte count of 1,000/mL are well tolerated and do not indicate reduction or discontinuation of carbamazepine.
      Hyponatremia is most likely to occur after several weeks or months of carbamazepine therapy. It is considered a result of inappropriate secretion of antidiuretic hormone, but this is controversial. Asymptomatic hyponatremia in the range of 125 to 135 mEq/L may be followed with periodic electrolyte determination. If the condition becomes symptomatic or if serum sodium concentration decreases to less than 125 mEq/L, fluid restriction is instituted. If this fails, dose reduction or a trial of another AED may be needed.
   5. **Drug interactions.** Carbamazepine, like phenytoin, is an inducer of hepatic microsomal enzymes. Several drug interactions of carbamazepine are similar to those of phenytoin.
      Enzyme inducers—phenobarbital, phenytoin, and primidone—tend to stimulate biotransformation of carbamazepine and to lower carbamazepine level, requiring higher doses of carbamazepine to be given in more daily divided doses. On the other hand, the intermediary metabolite, carbamazepine-10-11-epoxide, increases in proportion and may contribute to additional neurotoxic side effects.
      Erythromycin markedly inhibits metabolism of carbamazepine. **Cimetidine** and **propoxyphene** have similar but lesser effects. These drugs should be avoided, because carbamazepine levels may rise and cause clinical toxicity.
C. **Valproic acid.** Introduction of this AED in 1978 was a major breakthrough in the treatment of epilepsy. It prevents repetitive neuronal firing by blocking Na^+ channels, similar to the action of phenytoin and carbamazepine. It also reduces T-type Ca^{2+} currents and enhances γ-aminobutyric-acid (GABA)–mediated inhibitory neurotransmission in the central nervous system.
   1. **Indications.** Valproic acid has a broad antiepileptic range.
      a. Valproic acid has antiabsence efficacy similar to that of ethosuximide. Patients who have absence seizures and suffer from generalized tonic–clonic attacks are best treated with valproic acid.
      b. Valproic acid is the drug of choice for PGE, including juvenile myoclonic epilepsy, PGE manifesting as grand mal seizures, and photosensitive epilepsy.
      c. Valproic acid also is the drug of choice for secondarily generalized epilepsy syndromes, although satisfactory seizure control is attainable in only one third of patients with these syndromes.
      d. Valproic acid is effective for managing focal or partial epilepsy, although probably less effective than carbamazepine, phenytoin, and primidone. Valproic acid is indicated as an add-on agent for complex partial or secondarily generalized seizures.
      e. Valproic acid is now available for intravenous (i.v.) use (Depacon; Abbott, Abbott Park, IL, U.S.A.) to control absence status.
   2. **Pharmacokinetics.** Valproic acid is strongly bound (70% to 95%) to plasma proteins, and the proportion is concentration dependent. At higher levels, the proportion of protein-bound drug is less, and more is present in free or unbound form. Elimination is primarily by the hepatic route. Valproic acid acts as a strong competitive inhibitor of certain hepatic enzymes, increasing levels of many AEDs, such as phenobarbital and lamotrigine.

3. **Preparations.** Depakene (Abbott) is the form of valproic acid that is available in tablets and syrup. It has more rapid absorption and a higher incidence of gastric disturbances than does Depakote (Abbott). Divalproex sodium (Depakote) is a stable coordination compound composed of sodium valproate and valproic acid in a 1 : 1 molar relation. It is available in the form of delayed-release tablets (Depakote tablets) and sprinkle capsules. Depakote tablets cause less gastric disturbance and have slower gastrointestinal absorption than does Depakene and therefore are the forms preferred for adults.

4. **Administration.** In adults, valproic acid usually is started as a dose of 250-mg Depakote tablets given once or twice a day. The dosage is gradually increased 250 mg every week until seizures are controlled or side effects occur. The usual adult dose is 750 to 3,000 mg/d, which should be given in three or four divided daily doses because of a relatively short elimination half-life.

Smaller daily doses (blood levels of 40 to 60 µg/mL) usually are needed for patients with PGE (absence epilepsy, juvenile myoclonic epilepsy, or primary tonic–clonic seizures) than for patients with secondarily generalized epilepsy. The latter patients may need doses up to 4.0 g or 60 mg/kg and blood levels of 100 to 120 µg/mL for adequate seizure control.

When used with such enzyme-inducing AEDs as phenytoin, carbamazepine, phenobarbital, and primidone, valproic acid must be given in much larger doses because increased metabolism results in shortening of elimination half-life.

5. **Side effects.** Nausea and vomiting are common initial side effects, particularly if a large starting dose is given or if the dose is increased too rapidly. Gastric irritation can be reduced by taking valproic acid immediately after meals. A common dose-related side effect is **tremor** associated with high blood levels. Valproic acid is relatively free of cognitive and behavioral side effects. Some patients have excessive **hair loss** or **weight gain** as a result of increased appetite.

The risk that valproic acid causes hepatic toxicity has been overstated. The incidence of serious hepatic toxicity is of concern only among very young children (younger than 2 years) who have metabolic defects or intellectual deficits and are undergoing polytherapy. Adult patients without underlying liver disease and not taking any other hepatotoxic drug rarely have serious toxic hepatitis (1 in 10,000 to 20,000 patients). Another idiosyncratic effect is **pancreatitis,** which is more common than is hepatic toxicity. Mild **hyperammonemia** is common, particularly with high doses. Hyperammonemia is renal rather than hepatic in origin and is not a reason to discontinue therapy unless lethargy occurs.

Valproic acid is reported to produce **thrombocytopenia,** interference in the platelet aggregation, and an increased tendency toward bleeding.

Baseline CBC, platelet count, and liver function tests (aspartate aminotransferase) should be performed. These tests are repeated after 2 to 4 weeks of therapy and then every 6 to 12 months. If the patient is to undergo surgery, these tests are repeated before the operation. Routine ammonia levels do not predict rarely occurring serious hepatic complications and thus serve no purpose.

6. **Drug interactions** are common. Valproic acid inhibits metabolism of many AEDs. It consistently increases phenobarbital levels, resulting in toxicity. Phenobarbital doses should be reduced by 20% to 40% when valproic acid is added. Valproic acid decreases the total (free plus bound) phenytoin level without changing the free level owing to competition for protein binding sites. These changes do not necessitate changes in phenytoin dosage.

D. **Ethosuximide** has a limited spectrum of antiepileptic activity, being effective only against absence seizures. The mechanism of action is to reduce the low threshold, T-type Ca^{2+} currents in the thalamic neurons.

1. **Indication.** Ethosuximide continues to be the drug of choice for PGE of the pure absence type, which is more common in children than in adults. (Remember that absence-like seizures in adults often are brief complex partial

seizures that are not helped by ethosuximide.) Ethosuximide also is ineffective against convulsive seizures.

    2. Administration. Ethosuximide can be started at a dosage of 250 mg twice a day and gradually increased every 1 to 2 weeks until the seizures are controlled or side effects occur. Although the elimination half-life is long enough to allow a single daily dose, it is better to use two divided daily doses to reduce gastrointestinal toxicity.

    3. Side effects. Serious side effects are rare with ethosuximide. Gastrointestinal upset, hiccups, and hallucinations may occur when high doses are used.

E. Phenobarbital is the oldest and the least expensive of the traditional AEDs. The principal antiepileptic effect is its enhancement of the GABA-ergic inhibitory neurotransmission by allosterically modulating the GABA$_A$ inotropic receptor and increasing chloride conductance.

    1. Indications. Phenobarbital is effective in managing simple partial, complex partial, and secondarily generalized tonic–clonic seizures. It is also used to control generalized convulsive status epilepticus. Although often used to treat patients with secondarily generalized epilepsy syndromes, phenobarbital can exacerbate certain types of seizures (e.g., absence, tonic–clonic, and myoclonic seizures) in such patients.

    2. Administration. Because of its very long elimination half-life, phenobarbital can be used in a single daily dose. The usual adult dose is 1 to 3 mg/kg. Patients should be warned not to terminate phenobarbital abruptly, because such termination often produces withdrawal convulsions even in patients without seizure disorders and does so more frequently in patients with epilepsy.

    3. Side effects. The undesirable chronic side effects limiting the use of phenobarbital are its **sedative effects** and the **paradoxical hyperactivity** it produces in children. Idiosyncratic reactions such as rash are uncommon.

F. Primidone is converted to three active antiepileptic blood metabolites— primidone, phenobarbital, and phenylethylmalonamide—but only the first two usually are measured.

    1. Indications. Primidone monotherapy is as effective as phenytoin or carbamazepine against all types of partial seizures, but primidone is less well tolerated by patients because of its clinical toxicity, especially during the initial period of therapy.

    2. Administration. Primidone can only be given orally. It appears to be better tolerated by adults when started at a very small dosage of 50 mg at night for 3 days. Larger initial doses have resulted in hypersomnolence in some patients. The dosage is then increased to 125 mg/d and is further increased in steps of 125 mg at weekly intervals up to an initial target daily dose of 750 to 1,000 mg. Although the elimination half-life of its major metabolite, phenobarbital, is long, that of primidone itself may be as short as 6 to 8 hours, which requires that it be given in three divided doses.

    3. Side effects. The major side effect is **sedation,** which initially may be severe but can be avoided if the drug is introduced in small doses and if increments are made very slowly. Other side effects are similar to those of phenobarbital and include **dizziness, allergic rash, behavioral and cognitive changes, ataxia, respiratory depression,** and **erectile dysfunction.**

G. Clonazepam is a benzodiazepine that has antiepileptic action primarily by enhancing GABA-ergic inhibitory neurotransmission through allosterically modulating GABA receptor complex and thereby increasing the chloride conductance of this ligand-gated channel.

    1. Indications. This benzodiazepine is useful in the management of primary and secondarily generalized epilepsy manifesting as absence, myoclonic, and other minor motor seizures. Because of its sedative side effects and because tolerance develops to the antiepileptic effectiveness after several months of therapy, clonazepam is a second-line drug that usually is used in combination with other AEDs for difficult-to-treat patients.

    2. Administration. Clonazepam is administered once daily starting with a small dose of 0.01 to 0.03 mg/kg (usually 0.5 to 1.0 mg for adults), which is gradually increased 0.5 mg every 5 to 7 days to a maximum daily dose of 0.2 mg/kg given in 1 to 3 divided doses.

3. **Side effects** include **drowsiness, dizziness, blurred vision, ataxia,** and **personality changes.**

VIII. **Newer AEDs.** Approximately 60% to 80% of patients with newly diagnosed epilepsy become seizure free when treated with traditional AEDs (see **VI.**) as monotherapy. The remaining 20% to 40% are either unresponsive to traditional AEDs or obtain satisfactory seizure control only with polytherapy, but at a price of side effects and drug interactions. Furthermore, many of these AEDs are associated with cognitive side effects, teratogenic effects in 5% to 10% of pregnancies, and drug–drug interaction, especially for those metabolized in the liver. Hence, newer AEDs are needed that may have a better side effect profile, work through novel basic mechanisms to control epileptogenesis, and have more desirable pharmacokinetics, including fewer or no serious drug interactions.

After a lapse of more than a decade, a number of new AEDs have been introduced in the United States, starting in 1993. Most of these, with few exceptions, are approved as add-on therapy to manage localization-related or partial epilepsy refractory to traditional AEDs. Some of these are now being used as monotherapy, especially gabapentin, lamotrigine, and topiramate. Use of the newer AEDs may be entrusted to a neurologist with expertise in treating patients with medically refractory epilepsy. They are briefly discussed, and the pharmacokinetics and dosages for adults are summarized in Table 39.3. Because many of the new AEDs are used in combined therapy with the traditional AEDs, knowledge of pharmacokinetic interactions between these two groups of AEDs is essential. These drug interactions are summarized in Table 39.4.

A. **Felbamate (Felbatol; Wallace, Cranbury, NJ, U.S.A.).** Introduced in 1993, felbamate fell in repute in a couple of years because of the relatively high risk rates for aplastic anemia and liver toxicity besides its common side effects of weight loss, insomnia, and gastrointestinal symptoms. Although it has a broad spectrum of effectiveness against partial-onset seizures and generalized seizures, it has many significant drug interactions. The drug is indicated in the care of children or adults with severe refractory epilepsy, especially for patients with secondarily generalized epilepsy of Lennox–Gastaut type.

B. **Gabapentin (Neurontin; Pfizer).** A cyclic GABA analogue originally synthesized to mimic GABA action, gabapentin was introduced in the United States in 1993. Despite chemical similarity to GABA, it does not affect GABA transmission in therapeutic doses. The mechanism of action remains to be fully established.

1. **Indications.** Gabapentin is indicated as adjunctive therapy for partial or secondarily generalized seizures not adequately controlled with traditional AEDs such as carbamazepine, phenytoin, and valproic acid.

2. **Pharmacokinetics.** Gabapentin has dose-dependent absorption and bioavailability of approximately 60% with oral doses up to 1,200 mg/d. Bioavailability decreases further with higher doses. Gabapentin has many ideal pharmacologic characteristics, including absence of plasma protein binding, renal elimination as unchanged gabapentin, only minimal dose-dependent toxicity, no drug interactions, and no requirement for periodic laboratory monitoring.

3. **Side effects.** Dose-related side effects include **drowsiness, tiredness, dizziness, incoordination, double vision, tremor,** and **weight gain.**

4. **Administration.** The optimal daily dose of gabapentin has not been established. It is increasingly recognized that doses of 3,600 to 4,800 mg/d are well tolerated and may be more effective. Gabapentin is started at 300 mg/d. The dose can be rapidly increased 300 mg every other day to a target dose. Although less effective than other newer AEDs, gabapentin appears to be a particularly good drug in treatment of the elderly because of its low incidence of neurotoxic side effects and absence of drug interaction. Renal elimination requires the dose to be adjusted downward in patients with compromised renal function.

C. **Lamotrigine (Lamictal; Glaxo Wellcome, Research Triangle Park, NC, U.S.A.).** This new broad-spectrum AED was introduced in the United States in

Table 39.3 Pharmacokinetics and adult dosages of newer antiepileptic drugs (AEDs)

AED	Bioavailability (%)	Peak plasma level (h)	Volume of distribution (L/kg)	Protein binding (%)	Elimination halflife (h)	Time to steady state (d)	Elimination route	Starting adult dosage (mg/d)	Usual adult maintenance dose (mg/d)	Maintenance dose (mg/kg)	Dosing regimen (times per day)	Target serum level[a] (µg/mL)
Felbamate	>90	1–4	0.75	25	15–25[b] 11–15[c]	3–6	H 50 R 50	1,200	1,200–3,600	40–80	2, 3	40–100
Gabapentin	30–60	1–4	0.8	0	5–9	1–2	R	300	900–3,600	30–40	3, 4	5–25
Lamotrigine	>90	1–4	0.9–1.4	55	24[b] 15[c] 60[d]	3–15	H 90 R 10	50[b,c] 12.5[d]	200–600[b,c] 100–200[d]	1–15	1, 2	5–20
Topiramate	>80	1–2	0.6–0.8	15	20–30[b] 12–15[c]	3–5	H 40 R 60	25–50	200–600	5–9	2	5–25
Tiagabine	>90	1–2	1.0	96	6–9[b] 4–6[c]	1–2	H	4	32–56	0.1–1.0	2–4	5–70
Levetiracetam	100	1–2	0.5–0.7	<10	6–8	2	R 66	1,000	1,000–3,000	20–60	2	20–40
Zonisamide	>50	1–4	1.5	40	50–70[b] 25–40[c]	7–15	H 65 R 35	100	200–600	4–8	1, 2	10–30
Oxcarbazepine[e]	>95	5–8	0.75	40	7–11	2	H	600	1,200–2,400	15–30	2	12–35

[a] These are not therapeutic ranges, but levels commonly encountered in treated patients.
[b] When administered alone.
[c] When administered with enzyme-inducer AEDs (e.g., phenobarbital, phenytoin, carbamazepine, primidone).
[d] When administered with valproic acid.
[e] Kinetic parameters refer to monohydroxy derivative, for which oxcarbazepine is a prodrug.
H, hepatic; R, renal; numbers are approximate percentage for each route.

Table 39.4 Pharmacokinetic interactions among antiepileptic drugs (AEDs)

A. Effects of Traditional AEDs on Serum Levels of Newer AEDs

	FBM	GBP	LTG	TPM	TGB	LTC	ZNS	OXC
PHT	↓	–	↓	↓	↓	–	↓	↓
CBZ	↓	–	↓	↓	↓	–	↓	↓
PB	↓	–	↓	↓	↓	–	↓	↓
PRM	↓	–	↓	↓	↓	–	↓	↓
VPA	↑	–	↑	–	–	–	–	–
ESM	–	–	–	–	–	–	–	–

B. Effects of Newer AEDs on Serum Levels of Traditional AEDs

	PHT	CBZ	PB	PRM	VPA	ESM
FBM	↑ >30%	↑ E	↑ 25%	–	↑ >30%	–
GBP	–	–	–	–	–	–
LTG	–	–	–	–	↓ 25%	–
TPM	May ↑	–	–	–	–	–
TGB	–	–	–	–	Slight ↓	–
LTC	–	–	–	–	–	–
ZNS	–	–	–	–	–	–
OXC	May ↑	↑ E	Slight ↑	–	–	–

See Table 39.1 for abbreviations.
↓, decrease; –, no change; ↑, increase; ↑ E, CBZ-epoxide only elevated, CBZ may be decreased.

1994. The basic mechanism of action is on voltage-dependent Na^+ channels, similar to that of phenytoin, carbamazepine, and valproic acid. In addition, lamotrigine preferentially reduces presynaptic release of the excitatory neurotransmitter glutamate, thereby reducing glutamatergic excitation.

1. **Indications.** Lamotrigine is approved for adjunctive treatment of adults with partial seizures not adequately controlled with traditional AEDs. It is also effective against primary generalized epilepsy, particularly absence and myoclonic seizures, and secondarily generalized epilepsy of Lennox–Gastaut syndrome in children and adults.

2. **Pharmacokinetics.** When lamotrigine is given as monotherapy, the elimination half-life is long (approximately 24 hours) but shortens to approximately one-half that in patients receiving hepatic enzyme–inducing AEDs such as phenobarbital, carbamazepine, phenytoin, or primidone. Valproic acid, on the other hand, prolongs the half-life twofold to threefold by means of inhibiting hepatic metabolism of lamotrigine.

3. **Side effects.** In adjunctive therapy, lamotrigine is well tolerated with few side effects, which include **somnolence, dizziness, incoordination,** and **double vision. Rash** is of concern, occurring in 5% to 15% of patients but serious enough to necessitate discontinuation of treatment in only 2% to 5%. Stevens–Johnson syndrome also may occur, although rarely. Rashes usually occur within 6 weeks of initiation of lamotrigine therapy and are more likely to occur among children, with fast titration, and with valproic acid comedication.

4. **Administration.** Lamotrigine is started in low doses and titrated upward slowly. In a patient on an enzyme inducer AED, lamotrigine is started at a dosage of 50 mg/d for the first 2 weeks followed by 100 mg/d for the next 2 weeks. Thereafter, titration is upward in doses of 100 mg/d at weekly intervals to a maximum dosage of 500 to 600 mg/d given in two divided doses.

If the patient is taking valproic acid, the starting dosage of lamotrigine is 25 mg every other day for the first 2 weeks, followed by 25 mg/d for the next 2 weeks. The drug is then titrated upward 25 mg per day every 1 to 2 weeks to a maximum dosage of 100 to 200 mg/d in two divided doses.

D. Topiramate (Topamax; Ortho-McNeil, Raritan, NJ, U.S.A.) became available in 1997 in the United States. It is a broad-spectrum AED with the following antiepileptic effects: blocking of Na⁺ channels, blocking of glutamate-mediated excitatory neurotransmission, enhancement of GABA-mediated inhibition, and weak inhibition of carbonic anhydrase activity.

   1. **Indication.** Topiramate is approved for adjunctive therapy for partial seizures refractory to traditional AEDs. The drug is also effective against primary generalized epilepsy and secondarily generalized epilepsy of the Lennox–Gastaut type.

   2. **Pharmacokinetics.** Topiramate has a long half-life, has few drug interactions (slight increase in phenytoin levels), and may be given in two divided daily doses. The drug is primarily excreted unchanged in the urine.

   3. **Side effects.** Adverse effects are generally mild and reversible. These include **sedation, dizziness, incoordination, decreased appetite, weight loss, paresthesia,** and **cognitive dysfunction** (e.g., slow mentation, word-finding difficulties, problem in concentration, thinking abnormalities, impaired memory, and encephalopathy).

   Renal stones are reported in 1.5% of patients, mostly adults, and may be related to individual susceptibility rather than the dose or duration of therapy. A family history of kidney stones may be a relative contraindication to use of topiramate.

   4. **Administration.** Topiramate is initiated at a dosage of 25 to 50 mg/d in adults with weekly increases by the same amount up to an initial target dosage of 200 to 400 mg/d. Slower titration (weekly increments of 25 mg/d) may reduce neurotoxicity in patients on polytherapy. In adults, there appears to be a plateau therapeutic effect with dosages more than 600 mg/d.

E. Tiagabine (Gabitril; Abbott). Introduced in the United States in 1997, tiagabine is a designer drug composed of a GABA uptake inhibitor that potentiates GABA inhibition in the central nervous system.

   1. **Indications.** Tiagabine is indicated for adjunctive therapy for partial or secondarily generalized seizures not controlled with traditional AEDs.

   2. **Pharmacokinetics and side effects.** Tiagabine not only has lower effectiveness in comparison with other newer AEDs but also has a higher rate of untoward side effects (**somnolence, dizziness, tremor, abnormal thinking, depression,** and de novo **nonconvulsive status**) and a requirement for more divided daily doses (2 to 4 times a day) because of a short elimination half-life. Tiagabine is heavily bound to serum proteins (96%), and elimination is predominantly hepatic, both undesirable because of increased potential for drug interactions.

   3. **Administration.** The average daily dose is 32 to 56 mg divided in three or four divided daily doses for adults taking enzyme-inducing drugs. The recommended initial dosage is 4 to 8 mg/d with weekly increases of 8 mg/d.

F. Levetiracetam (Keppra; UCB, Smyrna, GA, U.S.A.), introduced in the United States in 1999, has favorable pharmacokinetics, efficacy, and safety profiles. The mechanism of action is not yet fully understood but does not involve inhibitory or excitatory neurotransmission.

   1. **Indication.** Levetiracetam is indicated in the treatment of adults with focal onset seizures refractory to traditional AEDs.

   2. **Pharmacokinetics.** Levetiracetam has rapid and complete absorption, linear pharmacokinetics, minimal (<10%) protein binding, no hepatic metabolism, predominantly renal excretion, and no known drug interactions.

   3. **Side effects.** The drug is generally well tolerated. The most common adverse events when levetiracetam is used with other AEDs are **somnolence, asthenia,** and **dizziness** occurring mainly during the first month of treatment.

4. **Administration.** The starting dosage is 1,000 mg given in two divided doses and is effective in many patients. If necessary, the dose can be increased an additional 1,000 mg/d at 2-week intervals up to a maximum daily dose of 3,000 mg given in two divided doses.

G. **Zonisamide (Zonegran; Elan, South San Francisco, CA, U.S.A.),** a sulfonamide, was introduced in 2000 for the treatment of adults with partial seizures refractory to traditional AEDs. Zonisamide has the following antiepileptic effects: blocking of Na^+ channels, reduction of low-threshold T-type Ca^{2+} currents, and weak inhibition of carbonic anhydrase activity.

1. **Indications.** Zonisamide may prove to be a broad-spectrum AED. It is indicated in the treatment of adults with focal-onset seizures refractory to traditional AEDs. It is also effective in the management of primary generalized epilepsy and progressive myoclonic epilepsy.

2. **Pharmacokinetics.** Zonisamide has modest (40%) binding to plasma protein and has linear kinetics in doses up to 400 mg/d. One third of the dose is excreted as unchanged drug, and the remaining is metabolized in the liver by hepatic microsomal enzymes. The long elimination half-life allows the daily dose to be given once or in two divided doses. It does not affect the levels of other AEDs.

3. **Side effects.** The side effects are mild to moderate and include **somnolence, fatigue, dizziness, anorexia, headaches, double vision, incoordination, insomnia, cognitive difficulties,** and **tremor. Rashes** develop in 5% of patients and in some may be severe or even life threatening. **Renal stones** occur with an incidence of approximately 1%, so a history of renal stones may constitute a relative contraindication. Because it is a sulfonamide, zonisamide is contraindicated in the care of persons with a history of allergy to sulfonamides.

4. **Administration.** The initial dosage of zonisamide is 100 mg once a day with titration upward 100 mg/d every 2 weeks up to 400 mg/d, administered once or twice daily. Doses of 600 to 800 mg have been well tolerated by some patients.

H. **Oxcarbazepine (Trileptal; Novartis),** introduced in 2000 in the United States, is a derivative of carbamazepine with similar indications and mechanism of action.

1. **Pharmacokinetics.** The antiepileptic activity is exerted primarily by the almost complete conversion of the drug to an active 10-monohydroxy metabolite (MHD). The latter is metabolized in the liver by means of glucuronide conjugation, and 80% of the administered dose is excreted as MHD or MHD glucuronide. Unlike carbamazepine, oxcarbazepine is not subject to autoinduction. Hepatic enzyme–inducing AEDs decrease MHD plasma concentration, whereas oxcarbazepine can increase plasma concentration of phenytoin and phenobarbital and decrease plasma concentration of the active hormonal components of oral contraceptive drugs.

2. **Side effects.** The untoward side effects of oxcarbazepine are similar to those of carbamazepine, including **somnolence, dizziness, fatigue, headache, incoordination,** and **nausea.** The incidence of **rash** is approximately one-half of that encountered with carbamazepine. Oxcarbazepine is associated with marked **hyponatremia** in 3% of patients. A minor decreases in red blood cell, white blood cell, or platelet count also may occur. The overall the risk of side effects and drug interactions is likely to be less with oxcarbazepine than with carbamazepine.

3. **Administration.** Oxcarbazepine is started at a dosage of 600 mg/d, given in two divided doses. If needed, the dose can be increased the same amount at weekly intervals to a maximum dose of 2,400 mg/d. In patients with impaired renal function, oxcarbazepine should be started at 300 mg/d and increased slowly. Because hematologic and hepatic parameters are rarely affected, no specific monitoring is recommended.

IX. **Status epilepticus**

A. **Definition.** Status epilepticus is defined as continuous seizure activity persisting for at least 30 minutes or two or more sequential seizures repeating within 30 minutes without full recovery of consciousness between seizures.

B. Types. Any type of seizure can manifest as status epilepticus, but the common forms include the following.

   1. **Generalized convulsive status epilepticus (GCSE)** manifests as repeated major motor convulsions without full recovery of consciousness between seizures. In the past, the term *status epilepticus* implied essentially this form of status.

   2. **Nonconvulsive status epilepticus** produces a continuous or fluctuating "epileptic twilight" state. This includes absence status and complex partial status.

   3. **Simple partial status epilepticus** is characterized by repeated focal motor seizures, epilepsia partialis continua, and focal impairment of function (e.g., aphasia) without accompanying alteration of consciousness.

C. Cause of GCSE. GCSE is the most common and most serious type of status epilepticus. Unconsciousness associated with convulsive major motor seizures is the cardinal feature. The motor activity varies in symmetry and form depending on the history of seizures, duration of status, duration of treatment, and associated pathologic processes in the brain. GCSE occurs mainly in the following settings.

   1. **Acute cerebral insult** or **acute encephalopathy** accounts for one half of cases of GCSE. These disorders include meningitis, encephalitis, head trauma, hypoxia, hypoglycemia, drug intoxication (e.g., cocaine), drug withdrawal, and strokes or metabolic encephalopathy.

   2. GCSE can occur in patients with a **history of epilepsy** due to remote neurologic insults. Common precipitants of GCSE include changes in AEDs, sudden discontinuation or reduction in AEDs, systemic infection, physical and emotional stress, and sleep deprivation.

   3. GCSE can occur as an **initial unprovoked epileptic event** in an otherwise healthy person. Such "idiopathic" cases may account for one third of all cases of GCSE.

D. Prognosis. GCSE is an emergency associated with substantial morbidity and mortality. The overall mortality may be as high as 30% among adults. GCSE associated with acute neurologic insults has the poorest prognosis, which essentially depends on the underlying cerebral etiologic factor.

   When GCSE is the first epileptic event for an otherwise neurologically intact patient, or when it occurs in a patient with a previously known history of epilepsy but has a benign or reversible cause (e.g., hypoglycemia or drug or alcohol withdrawal), the prognosis is good if therapy is instituted promptly.

   Without adequate and prompt treatment, GCSE can progress to a state of electromechanical dissociation in which the patient becomes increasingly unconscious or encephalopathic from the ongoing status but the convulsive activity becomes increasingly subtle although EEG continues to show an ictal pattern. Patients with this condition, which is often called *subtle status epilepticus,* are considered to be candidates for an aggressive therapy, as are those with overt GCSE.

E. Management of GCSE. The treatment protocol outlined in Table 39.5 is useful in the management of GCSE.

   1. Diagnose status epilepticus by observing either continued seizure activity or one additional generalized convulsion in a patient who has a history of GCSE.

   2. **Assess vital functions** and systemic abnormalities and stabilize the vital functions as much as possible.

      a. **Maintain an adequate airway and oxygenation.** This usually can be accomplished with an oral airway. The airway should be suctioned periodically to maintain patency. Oxygen should be administered through a nasal cannula or with a mask and a bag-valve-mask ventilator. If, after bagging, respiratory assistance is still needed, endotracheal intubation should be considered.

      b. **Assess blood pressure** and maintain it at a normal or high-normal level during prolonged GCSE. Use vasopressors if necessary.

      c. **Establish an i.v. infusion line** using normal saline solution. Blood should be drawn initially for CBC, blood sugar, blood urea nitrogen,

Table 39.5 Treatment protocol for status epilepticus (generalized tonic–clonic) in adults

Time (min)	Treatment
0–5	Diagnose status epilepticus by observing either continued seizure activity or one additional seizure. Assess vital functions, insert oral airway, and give oxygen.
6–10	Establish i.v. infusion line with normal saline solution. Monitor temperature and BP. Draw blood for electrolytes, glucose, Ca, Mg, AED levels, CBC, BUN, and AST. Administer 100 mg of thiamine followed by 50 mL of 50% glucose i.v. push.
11–20	Give lorazepam 0.1 mg/kg i.v. push at a rate of <2 mg/min, or give diazepam 0.2 mg/kg i.v. at a rate of <5 mg/min. Diazepam can be repeated until seizures stop or a total of 20 mg has been given.
21–60	Whether or not lorazepam or diazepam stops the seizures, administer phenytoin 20 mg/kg i.v. no faster than 50 mg/min. Instead, fosphenytoin can be given i.v. in phenytoin equivalent doses. Monitor BP and ECG during phenytoin (or fosphenytoin) infusion, and if hypotension or ECG changes occur, slow the infusion or temporarily withhold the drug. If seizures continue, an additional 5–10 mg/kg of phenytoin (or fosphenytoin) can be given.
>60	If seizures continue, perform endotracheal intubation before giving phenobarbital 20 mg/kg i.v. at a rate of <100 mg/min. If status persists, start pentobarbital coma. Use a dose of 5 mg/kg i.v. to produce at least a suppression-burst pattern on EEG, and continue a maintenance dose of 0.5–3.0 mg/kg per hour to maintain seizure free state or at least suppression-burst pattern on EEG. Slow rate of infusion after 24–96 h periodically to determine whether seizures have stopped clinically and on EEG. Monitor EEG, BP, ECG, and respiratory function. If pentobarbital is not effective, change to continuous infusion of propofol or midazolam.

i.v., intravenous; BP, blood pressure; Ca, calcium; Mg, magnesium; AED, antiepileptic drug; CBC, complete blood cell count; BUN, blood urea nitrogen; AST, aspartate aminotransferase; ECG, electrocardiogram; EEG, electroencephalogram.

serum electrolytes (including calcium and magnesium), and AED levels, and both urine and blood should be obtained for toxicology screening.

    d. Assess oxygenation by means of oximetry or periodic arterial blood gas determination.

    e. Monitor rectal temperature. Body temperature can increase to a high level during prolonged status epilepticus as a result of increased motor activity.

    f. If hypoglycemia is documented or if it is impossible to obtain prompt blood sugar determination, **administer 50 mL of 50% glucose** by means of i.v. push. In adults, **thiamine** (100 mg) is always given before glucose to protect a thiamine-deficient patient from exacerbation of Wernicke's encephalopathy.

    g. Administer bicarbonate therapy only if serum pH is so low as to be immediately life threatening. Acidosis commonly develops during GCSE, but acidosis usually responds promptly once the seizure activity is controlled.

    h. For rare patients with GCSE resulting from hyponatremia (serum sodium concentration less than 120 mEq/L), hypocalcemia, or hypomagnesemia, administer appropriate electrolytes by means of i.v. drip.

  3. Drug therapy for control of GCSE. The goals of therapy are rapid termination of the clinical and EEG evidence of seizure activity and subsequent maintenance of a seizure-free state.

a. **Benzodiazepines.** If the patient is having active convulsions, administer either diazepam or lorazepam, which are effective in rapidly terminating GCSE. Followed with a long-acting AED such as phenytoin to prevent recurrence of convulsions.

Lorazepam is administered 0.1 mg/kg i.v. at a rate of less than 2 mg/min. **Diazepam** is given at 0.2 mg/kg at a rate less than 5 mg/min. The dose of diazepam can be repeated if the seizures do not stop after 5 minutes. Up to a total of 20 mg of diazepam may be administered.

Most experts prefer lorazepam to diazepam. Although diazepam can stop GCSE slightly faster than can lorazepam, lorazepam has a much longer duration of effectiveness. Diazepam enters the brain exceedingly rapidly and is very prompt in terminating GCSE. However, it is extremely lipid soluble and is quick to redistribute to body fat stores. The result is that the blood and brain concentrations decrease to as low as 20% of initial concentration within 20 minutes, allowing seizures to recur within 30 minutes of i.v. administration of the bolus. Lorazepam has relatively rapid effectiveness and yet has a prolonged duration of action against status epilepticus. Both diazepam and lorazepam can produce serious respiratory depression or hypotension, particularly when given in combination with barbiturates.

b. **Phenytoin or fosphenytoin.** If seizures are still continuing after administration of a benzodiazepine, i.v. administration of phenytoin (or fosphenytoin) should be initiated promptly. Even if the benzodiazepine has been successful in terminating the seizure activity, phenytoin (or fosphenytoin) usually is needed to prevent recurrence of convulsions, especially after the use of diazepam.

   (1) **Administration.** The usual loading dose of phenytoin is 20 mg/kg, given through a syringe into the i.v. port close to the patient at a rate less than 50 mg/min. Injection is preferably performed by a physician. Blood pressure and electrocardiogram (ECG) are continuously monitored throughout the infusion. The rate of infusion should be slowed or temporarily stopped if sufficient hypotension develops or if the ECG shows widening of the QT interval or development of arrhythmias. Some experts prefer diluting phenytoin in 100 mg of saline solution, but most recommend administering it undiluted because the drug can precipitate in i.v. solutions, particularly glucose.

   (2) There is a significant risk of **skin complications** when i.v. phenytoin is given. These include phlebitis, tissue sloughing after extravasation, and most serious, purple glove syndrome, a delayed soft tissue injury that can result in severe edema, arterial occlusion, and tissue necrosis that can necessitate amputation. These complications occur because for i.v. use, phenytoin has to be dissolved in 40% propylene glycol and 10% ethanol at a pH of 12.2.

   (3) Cutaneous complications are now avoidable because of the introduction of **fosphenytoin,** a phosphate ester of phenytoin that is enzymatically converted to phenytoin by serum phosphatases. It is available for parenteral use (i.v. or i.m.). Because it is dissolved in TRIS buffer at a pH of 8 to 9, fosphenytoin does not cause tissue injury as phenytoin does. Three parts of phenytoin are bioequivalent to two parts of phenytoin but the fosphenytoin dose is labeled in phenytoin equivalents (PE), so that 150 mg of fosphenytoin is labeled 100 mg PE. Although somewhat confusing, it apparently allows easy conversion of phenytoin to fosphenytoin dosing. Fosphenytoin can be administered more rapidly (up to 150 mg PE/min compared with up to 50 mg/min for phenytoin). The shorter infusion time compensates for the time needed for its conversion to active phenytoin. The result is that peak levels of phenytoin are attainable with i.v. fosphenytoin as rapidly as with phenytoin infu-

sion itself. Blood pressure and ECG monitoring are recommended during fosphenytoin infusion, as they are with i.v. phenytoin.

(4) If the standard loading dose of 20 mg/kg of phenytoin (or 20 mg PE/kg of fosphenytoin) fails to stop GCSE, an additional 5 to 10 mg/kg may be given. Some patients may need high blood levels (30 to 40 µg/mL) before the seizure terminates. Phenytoin or fosphenytoin is effective in the treatment of 40% to 90% of patients with GCSE.

(5) Phenytoin or fosphenytoin should be used cautiously in the care of elderly patients, patients with known cardiac abnormalities, and patients with low baseline blood pressure.

c. **Phenobarbital** is generally the next choice in the care of adults if the GCSE does not respond to phenytoin. Close attention to respiratory status is required, especially if the patient has already received a benzodiazepine. Respiratory assistance, including endotracheal intubation, usually becomes necessary at this stage, and the physician must be prepared for this eventuality.

The usual dose of phenobarbital is 20 mg/kg given intravenously at a rate less than 100 mg/min. Sedation, respiratory compromise, and hypotension are potential side effects requiring attention. There is little evidence that the use of a fixed dose of phenobarbital as the third drug provides significant additional improvement in the control of status. On the contrary, large doses of phenobarbital can substantially delay recovery of consciousness because of the long half-life of this drug (2 to 5 days). Therefore, some experts recommend going directly to i.v. infusion anesthesia if lorazepam followed by phenytoin (or fosphenytoin) fails to control the status.

4. **Management of refractory GCSE**

a. **Consultation with a neurologist** is recommended in managing GCSE if the patient continues to have altered consciousness and administration of a benzodiazepine and phenytoin fails to control seizures.

b. GCSE is successfully terminated with one to three drugs in approximately 75% of patients in whom lorazepam is the first drug, phenytoin (or fosphenytoin) the second, and phenobarbital the third.

c. If the triple therapy fails to control GCSE, the patient needs **general anesthesia** to eliminate not only clinical seizures but also electrical discharges indicative of continuing seizure activity. There is no randomized comparative study of the management of refractory GCSE on which to base the choice of the drug to induce general anesthesia. Continuous i.v. infusion of pentobarbital, propofol, midazolam, diazepam, and lorazepam has been reported to be effective. The choice of a drug is largely based on the clinical experience of the physician. If one agent in optimal dosages is unsuccessful in controlling status, another should be tried. Continuous EEG monitoring is mandatory. The rate of administration of the drug is adjusted to ensure at least suppression burst or, as some experts recommend, cessation of all epileptiform activity, which may require making the EEG pattern almost isoelectric. The anesthesia is continued for 1 to 4 days before an attempt is made to lighten it. If clinical seizures or ictal EEG patterns return, the infusion is appropriately increased.

Pentobarbital-induced anesthesia has been most commonly used for refractory GCSE. It is started intravenously with a loading dose of 5 mg/kg, followed by a maintenance dosage of 0.5 to 3.0 mg/kg per hour to maintain an EEG suppression-burst pattern or bring about cessation of all epileptiform discharges. Barbiturate coma is almost always associated with considerable hypotension, which requires the use of **pressor agents.**

5. **Additional diagnostic studies.** When the seizures have been stopped or sufficiently controlled and the patient's vital signs have been stabilized, additional diagnostic studies, such as **chest radiographs, lumbar puncture,**

brain imaging, and **EEG,** are performed to evaluate the cause of the GCSE and the effectiveness of the antiepileptic therapy.

6. **Long-term antiepileptic therapy.** After the episode of GCSE has been brought under control, most patients need continuation of some form of AED therapy. Long-term AED therapy is indicated when GCSE is caused by a structural brain lesion or when the patient has a history of epileptic seizures. When GCSE constitutes the patient's first seizure and no cause is found, the decision to initiate long-term AED therapy should be individualized, but most physicians initiate long-term treatment under such circumstances. If the GCSE was caused by acute central nervous system involvement, such as metabolic encephalopathy, meningoencephalitis, or cerebrovascular compromise, antiepileptic therapy is continued for a short period of 3 to 6 months.

F. **Management of other types of status epilepticus.** Other forms of status epilepticus do not pose the same emergency situation that GCSE poses. **Complex partial status epilepticus** has been reported to result in long-term neurologic deficits (e.g., permanent memory impairment) and should be controlled promptly with a benzodiazepine (e.g., lorazepam) followed by i.v. phenytoin (or fosphenytoin) and even phenobarbital. Barbiturate coma is rarely indicated.

Management of absence status or simple partial status (focal motor seizure or epilepsia partialis continua without loss of consciousness) is not standardized. **Absence status** is best managed with an i.v. benzodiazepine (diazepam or lorazepam), which is effective in most cases. If a benzodiazepine is not effective, valproic acid can be given intravenously, in a dose of 25 mg/kg to promptly achieve therapeutic blood levels. After the absence status is controlled, valproic acid therapy is continued orally. **Simple partial status** responds to phenytoin (or fosphenytoin), usually in large doses to maintain blood levels as high as 30 µg/mL. Benzodiazepines and phenobarbital are not desirable because of the sedative side effects, except when one or two doses of i.v. diazepam are used initially.

X. **Management of acute seizure cluster.** Some patients have repetitive series or clusters of epileptic seizures that occur within a short period, not meeting the definition criteria of status epilepticus. Such seizure clusters can be intermittently managed with either of the following two approaches.

A. Most physicians use benzodiazepine (lorazepam or diazepam) to manage a cluster. Lorazepam is given in doses of 2 to 4 mg orally (sublingually) or parenterally (i.m. or i.v.), usually becoming effective in approximately 30 minutes. Administration may be repeated in doses of 1 to 2 mg with a maximum dose of 6 to 8 mg in 24 hours.

Recently the FDA has approved diazepam gel for rectal administration in the management of repetitive seizures. It is as effective, if not better, than lorazepam. Diazepam gel is administered in doses of 0.2 to 0.5 mg/kg rectally and is effective in 15 minutes. If social or logistic reasons make the use of rectal administration difficult, sublingual or oral lorazepam is a better alternative.

B. Another approach is to use loading with fosphenytoin (up to 20 PE/kg) either i.m. or i.v. as described in **IX.E.3.b.(4).**

C. A relatively new option is parenteral administration of valproic acid in doses of 10 to 25 mg/kg infused over 30 to 60 minutes.

D. Once the cluster is controlled, it is not necessary to continue long-term treatment with the AED used to control the cluster of seizures.

XI. **Epilepsy and pregnancy**

A. **Major problems.** Pregnancy in a woman with epilepsy is considered to constitute a high risk for the following reasons.

1. **Increased frequency of seizures** occurs among more than one third of pregnant women, especially during the second and third trimesters.

2. A major factor for exacerbation of seizures is the **alteration of the pharmacokinetics of AEDs.** Marked decreases occur in the serum concentrations of phenytoin, carbamazepine, phenobarbital, valproic acid, and primidone.

3. The incidence of **fetal malformation** is two to three times higher among mothers with epilepsy than among women without epilepsy. Most of this effect is a result of fetal exposure to AEDs. The overall incidence of major birth

defects (oropalatal clefts, urogenital and congenital heart anomalies, and neural tube defects) among infants of epileptic mothers is approximately 7%.

All major AEDs have potential teratogenic effects, and there is no evidence that any one is safer than any other. Valproic acid and carbamazepine, however, are more likely to be associated with spina bifida and other neural tube defects. The incidence of birth anomalies has been higher among women undergoing polytherapy than among those using monotherapy.

   4. **Hemorrhagic disease** is reported among 7% of newborns delivered by women who have received hepatic enzyme-inducing AEDs (phenobarbital, primidone, phenytoin, and carbamazepine) because of their effect in decreasing the vitamin K–dependent clotting factors.

B. **Management guidelines.** Management of pregnancy for an epileptic woman is a therapeutic challenge that requires the physician to keep the patient free of seizures while minimizing the adverse effects of seizures and AEDs on the course of pregnancy and the fetus. The major guidelines, which preferably are initiated before the patient becomes pregnant, are as follows.

   1. Withdraw AEDs before pregnancy if the patient has remained free of seizures for several years.
   2. Counsel the patient about the higher incidence of fetal malformation but assure her that most pregnant women (more than 90%) exposed to AEDs still bear healthy offspring.
   3. For a woman who is longing to bear a child, select the best drug for the patient's seizure type and use monotherapy. Because of the relatively high incidence of neural tube defects with valproic acid (1% to 2%) and with carbamazepine (0.5% to 1.0%), avoid these AEDs if at all possible and replace them with other AEDs before the patient becomes pregnant.
   4. Do not stop AED therapy after the pregnancy has been diagnosed. The risk of fetal malformation is highest during the first 4 to 8 weeks of pregnancy. It usually is too late to protect the fetus by the time pregnancy is confirmed. Stopping or changing the drug can induce more frequent and more violent seizures with adverse consequences on both the mother and the fetus.
   5. Monitor the AED serum level (preferably free level) before conception, at each trimester, in the last month of pregnancy, and through 8 weeks postpartum, and adjust the dosage accordingly. Avoid both low and high blood levels during pregnancy.
   6. If the patient is taking valproic acid or carbamazepine, measure serum **α-fetoprotein** at 15 to 16 weeks of gestation to be followed by high-definition **ultrasound imaging** of the fetus at 16 to 20 weeks to detect spina bifida or neural tube defects. **Amniocentesis** is indicated only if the α-fetoprotein level is high and the ultrasound examination does not provide positive exclusion of a neural tube defect.
   7. Supplemental multivitamins and folic acid (to decrease incidence of neural tube defects) are prescribed during the entire pregnancy. Supplementation with 0.4 mg of folic acid a day is recommended during pregnancy for women without epilepsy. Women at risk of having a child with neural tube defect (previous child or family history) are advised to supplement with 4.0 mg/d. The precise dose for women with epilepsy has not been defined, but 1.0 mg/d is commonly used. Folic acid supplementation is recommended throughout childbearing age for sexually active women with epilepsy.
   8. Give oral vitamin K_1 (phytonadione) to the mother at 10 to 20 mg/d during the last month of pregnancy. Administer vitamin K_1 (1.0 mg i.m.) to the neonate immediately after birth. These measures help reduce the incidence of AED-related hemorrhagic disease of the newborn.
   9. Unless the infant has symptoms, breast-feeding is allowed. Most AEDs, with the possible exception of ethosuximide, do not reach sufficient concentrations in the breast milk to pose a serious concern for the infant.

C. **Prevention of pregnancy with oral contraceptives**
   1. Oral contraceptives do not exacerbate epilepsy despite the warnings on package inserts.

2. The major concern in using oral contraceptives is the higher failure rate (more than 6% per year) among women taking hepatic enzyme–inducing AEDs (e.g., phenytoin, carbamazepine, phenobarbital, primidone, felbamate, topiramate, oxcarbazepine). The commonly used "minipill" containing 35 μg or less of estrogen and similarly subdermal levonorgestrel rods (Norplant; Wyeth-Ayerst) may be less effective. Breakthrough bleeding can be a warning of decreased contraceptive efficiency. Patients taking inducing antiepileptic drugs may therefore need a medium-dose oral contraceptive containing at least 50 μg of ethinyl estradiol or mestranol.

3. Valproic acid, which is not an enzyme inducer, is unlikely to cause failure of oral contraception. Of the new antiepileptics, lamotrigine, gabapentin, levetiracetam, and zonisamide do not affect hormonal metabolism.

XII. AED treatment of the elderly. Common causes of seizures among the elderly are cerebrovascular disease, degenerative dementia, and neoplasms in that order of frequency. Seizures are nearly exclusively partial onset, being simple partial, complex partial, or secondarily generalized type.

A. **Major problems.** Elderly patients with epilepsy constitute a special patient population because of age-related changes in the pharmacokinetics of AEDs, comorbidity, and multiple drug therapy. There is an overall decrease in protein binding of AEDs, hence total concentration of highly bound AEDs becomes misleading. Hepatic drug metabolism is decreased, and there is a steady decline in glomerular filtration rate, decreased tubular secretory function, and decreased renal blood flow with normal aging. These changes lead to longer elimination half-life and reduced clearance. In addition, concomitant medical problems and, consequently, multiple comedication further affect the absorption, disposition, and metabolism of AEDs. Elderly patients also tend to experience more side effects of AEDs, especially somnolence, confusion, gait disturbances, and postural and other tremors.

B. **Management guidelines for using AEDs to treat the elderly**
1. AEDs should be prescribed only when the diagnosis of epileptic seizures is firmly established and there is a high probability of recurrence.
2. AED therapy should be initiated at lower doses and titrated more slowly to a daily dose that is on average lower than used to treat younger adults.
3. For high protein bound AEDs, measurement of free rather than total concentration may be more useful in evaluating seizure control or drug-related toxicity.
4. "Therapeutic ranges" of the traditional AEDs do not apply to the elderly mainly because of an overall decrease tolerability for drugs in this age group. Aim for a "low therapeutic" serum level, increasing the dose only if clinically necessary.
5. The AEDs metabolized in the liver are more likely to cause drug interactions than are those eliminated by kidney. Generally, many of the newer AEDs have fewer drug interactions and have predominant renal elimination (e.g. gabapentin, lamotrigine, or levetiracetam). However, the dose has to be adjusted downward in the presence of renal impairment.
6. Gabapentin has no drug interactions and has a favorable side-effect profile to be an ideal AED for elderly persons. Lamotrigine has only minor interactions, hence it is another alternative among newer AEDs.
7. If cost is an important issue, the traditional AEDs, which are less expensive, may be the first option. Phenytoin, carbamazepine, and valproic acid are equally efficacious against focal and secondarily generalized seizures. The choice depends on the side-effect profile. Carbamazepine may be tried first because of its efficacy, relatively good tolerability, and predictable pharmacokinetics. Titration must be slower; the aim is a smaller daily dose of 400 to 600 mg/d over 4 weeks.

XIII. Discontinuation of AEDs. The decision to discontinue AEDs in the care of a patient who has been seizure free for several years depends on many prognostic factors. The relapse rate after AED withdrawal is approximately 30% to 40% among adults with chronic epilepsy.

A. **Prognostic factors**
1. **Types of epilepsy**
a. Some childhood forms of epilepsy (e.g., benign rolandic epilepsy and childhood absence epilepsy) usually remit during adolescence.

    b. Patients **PGE** with onset in adolescence or adulthood have a good prognosis. Many have remission, but many need lifelong therapy.

    c. Patients with localization-related epilepsy (simple partial seizures, complex partial seizures, and secondarily generalized tonic–clonic seizures) have a high recurrence rate (40% to 50%) after discontinuing AEDs. This is especially true of adults with complex partial seizures, for which the relapse rate can approach or exceed 50%.

    d. Patients in whom seizures occur in the setting of an acute cerebral insult (e.g., trauma, infection, or stroke) may not have chronic epilepsy. Such patients should be considered for withdrawal of AED after a seizure-free period of 3 to 6 months.

  2. **EEG findings** obtained just before discontinuation of AED therapy are useful predictors of the outcome. If EEG shows epileptiform abnormalities, the relapse rate is four to five times higher than if EEG findings are normal or minimally abnormal. Hence, most physicians consider continuing AEDs if EEG continues to show paroxysmal abnormalities.

  3. **Other predictors of outcome.** A high frequency of seizures, a long duration before seizures are controlled with AEDs, and multiple seizure types in a patient carry a less favorable prognosis. Similarly, patients who have structural abnormalities responsible for seizures or who have mental retardation or neurologic deficits are more likely to have recurrence of seizures after discontinuation of AEDs.

  4. **Duration of seizure-free period.** There is no consensus on how long a patient should remain seizure free before drug withdrawal is considered. Most physicians recommend a seizure-free period of 2 to 5 years, but such recommendations must be individualized because of the serious socioeconomic effect of recurrence of seizures.

B. General guidelines for withdrawing AEDs

  1. After assessing the risks and benefits, discontinuation of AEDs may be considered by the physician and the informed patient (or parent) if the patient has been seizure free for 2 to 5 years while taking AEDs, has had a single type of seizure, has normal neurologic examination findings and normal intelligence quotient, and normalized EEG with treatment.

  2. Adult patients with PGE who have remained seizure free for 2 to 5 years and whose EEGs show no paroxysmal abnormalities are good candidates for withdrawal of therapy.

  3. Women who want to bear children and who have been seizure free for several years should be considered for withdrawal of medication to avoid possible ill-effects of AEDs on their fetuses.

  4. On the other hand, most adults with focal epilepsy or PGE manifesting as multiple seizure types probably need long-term, if not lifelong, AED therapy unless continuation of the medication and the seizure-free state are possible only at the cost of unpleasant side effects.

C. AED withdrawal mode and precautions

  1. AEDs must be withdrawn slowly, typically over 3 to 6 months or even longer, especially barbiturates and benzodiazepines.

  2. Patients taking more than one AED should have the less or least effective drug withdrawn before the first-line drug. Only after the patient has remained seizure free taking only one drug for several months is the final drug withdrawn.

  3. During the withdrawal period, the patient is advised to follow a restricted lifestyle (no driving or hazardous occupational or recreational activities) to minimize the consequences should the seizures recur.

  4. If the seizures recur, the patient is promptly placed on an adequate dosage of an appropriate AED, which then probably has to be continued on a lifelong basis.

  5. During the withdrawal period, attention has to be paid to such lifestyle issues as getting adequate sleep, avoiding alcohol, and avoiding anxiety that can cause recurrence.

XIV. Counseling for psychosocial problems. Patients with epilepsy face many personal and psychosocial difficulties that require counseling. Driving restrictions, concerns regarding pregnancy, and possible transmission of epilepsy to the offspring are some of the concerns that have to be addressed. Employers usually regard employees with epilepsy as at high risk of accidents and often terminate their jobs when seizures occur at work. Persons with epilepsy have difficulty in obtaining automobile and life insurance. All these adversities lead to economic hardships, emotional problems, dependence, and poor self-esteem. It is important to detect these problems, respond to them promptly, and refer patients to appropriate specialists for further therapy and counseling. Patients should also be put in touch with local support groups, state epilepsy associations, and the Epilepsy Foundation of America.

XV. Referrals. Patients who need comprehensive care can be referred to local epilepsy clinics or centers equipped with multidisciplinary teams capable of providing psychosocial and vocational counseling in addition to the appropriate medical therapy.

  A. Epilepsy centers for comprehensive care and experimental AEDs. Approximately 15% to 25% of patients with epilepsy who have medically intractable seizures may be helped by referral to regional epilepsy centers, which can conduct ongoing clinical trials of new AEDs. Such patients often need combination therapy with two or more AEDs, which is best handled by an epileptologist in a comprehensive epilepsy center.

  B. Surgical treatment

   1. Resective surgery. Patients who have medically refractory complex partial or secondarily generalized tonic–clonic seizures should be referred, at least after 2 years, to a comprehensive epilepsy center for presurgical evaluation to determine whether they are suitable candidates for surgical treatment. After multimodality presurgical evaluation, if found to have a single epileptogenic focus that does not involve eloquent cortex, these patients may be candidates for resective surgery (anterior temporal lobectomy, selective amygdalohippocampectomy or corticectomy).

   2. Vagal nerve stimulation. The FDA has approved vagal nerve stimulation (VNS) with a neurocybernetic prosthesis as adjunctive therapy for medically refractory seizures in adults and children. VNS is considered in the care of patients with focal or generalized epilepsy who have undergone unsuccessful polytherapy trials of several AEDs, including newer AEDs, and who are not candidates for resective surgery or have undergone unsuccessful resective surgery.

   VNS requires implantation of a programmable signal generator subcutaneously in the chest. This device is capable of delivering intermittent stimulation to the left vagus nerve in the neck (by means of bipolar electrodes) at the desired settings. In addition, the patient or a companion can activate the generator by placing the accompanying magnet over the generator for several seconds to interrupt a seizure or reduce its severity if administered at seizure onset.

   The mechanism of action of VNS is unknown, but several large trials showed that approximately 30% to 40% of patients with refractory partial-onset seizures had a 50% or greater reduction in seizure frequency. Only a few had complete control of seizures. Overall, VNS has the same efficacy as many of the newer AEDs. Would this degree of improvement justify surgical treatment with potential surgical complications and cost considerably higher than trying a newer AED? The final answer remains to be provided. The common side effects include hoarseness, throat pain, coughing, dyspnea, and muscle pain. Possible surgical complications of hematoma, wound infection, and injury to the vagus nerve and carotid sheath are rare when the procedure is performed by an experienced surgeon.

Recommended Readings

Bourgeois BFD. Pharmacokinetic properties of current antiepileptic drugs. What improvements are needed? *Neurology* 2000;55[Suppl 3]:S11–S16.

Browne TR. The pharmacokinetics of antiepileptic drugs. *Neurology* 1998;51[Suppl 4]:2–7.

Browne TR, Holmes GL. *Handbook of epilepsy,* 2nd ed. Philadelphia: Lippincott Williams & Wilkins, 2000.

Commission on Classification and Terminology of the International League against Epilepsy. Proposal for revised clinical and electroencephalographic classification of epileptic seizures. *Epilepsia* 1981;22:489–501.

Commission on Classification and Terminology of the International League against Epilepsy. Proposal for revised classification of epilepsies and epileptic syndromes. *Epilepsia* 1989;30: 389–399.

DeLorenzo RJ, Towne AR, Pellock JM, et al. Status epilepticus in children, adults, and the elderly. *Epilepsia* 1992;33[Suppl 4]:S15–S25.

Engle J, Pedley TA, eds. *Epilepsy: a comprehensive textbook,* vol. 2. Philadelphia: Lippincott–Raven, 1997.

Levy RH, Mattson RH, Meldrum BS, eds. *Antiepileptic drugs,* 4th ed. New York: Raven Press, 1995.

Lowenstein DH, Alldredge BK. Status epilepticus. *N Engl J Med* 1998;338:970–976.

Mattson RH. Efficacy and adverse effects of established and new antiepileptic drugs. *Epilepsia* 1995;36[Suppl 2]:S12–S26.

Mattson RH, Cramer JA, Collins JF. A comparison of valproate with carbamazepine for the treatment of complex partial seizures and secondarily generalized tonic–clonic seizures in adults. *N Engl J Med* 1992;27:765–771.

Mattson RH, Cramer JA, Collins JF, et al. Comparison of carbamazepine, phenobarbital, phenytoin, and primidone in partial and secondarily generalized tonic–clonic seizures. *N Engl J Med* 1985;313:145–151.

Quality Standards Subcommittee of the American Academy of Neurology. Practice parameter: a guideline for discontinuing antiepileptic drugs in seizure free patients [summary statement]. *Neurology* 1996;47:600–602.

Ramsay RE, DeToledo J. Intravenous administration of fosphenytoin: option for the management of seizures. *Neurology* 1996;46[Suppl 1]:S17–S19.

Report of the Quality Standards Subcommittee of the American Academy of Neurology. Practice parameter: management issues for women with epilepsy [summary statement]. *Neurology* 1998;51:944–948.

Rowan AJ. Reflections on the treatment of seizures in the elderly population. *Neurology* 1998;51(suppl 4):28–33.

Therapeutics and Technology Assessment Subcommittee of the American Academy of Neurology. Assessment: generic substitution for antiepileptic medication. *Neurology* 1990; 40:1641–1643.

Therapeutic and Technology Assessment Subcommittee of the American Academy of Neurology. Reassessment: vagus nerve stimulation for epilepsy. *Neurology* 1999;53:666–669.

Treiman DM, Meyers PD, Walton NY, et al. A comparison of four treatments for generalized convulsive status epilepticus. *N Engl J Med* 1998;339:792–798.

Wilder BJ. Management of epilepsy: consensus conference on current clinical practice. *Neurology* 1998;51[Suppl 4]:1–43.

Working Group on Status Epilepticus. Treatment of status epilepticus. *JAMA* 1993;270: 854–859.

Zahn CA, Morrell MJ, Collins SD, et al. Management issues for women with epilepsy: a review of the literature. *Neurology* 1998;51:949–956.

40. MULTIPLE SCLEROSIS

Galen W. Mitchell

Multiple sclerosis (MS) is a primary demyelinating disease of the central nervous system (CNS). The disorder appears to be immune mediated, although the actual development of the disease and the subsequent clinical course are probably influenced by genetic and environmental factors along with many factors that have not yet been determined. MS is an important neurologic disorder because of its prevalence, chronicity, induced disability, and tendency to affect young adults. The goal of this chapter is to provide an overview of MS with general information for patient counseling and insights into diagnosis, disease forms, clinical course, and therapy.

    I. Epidemiology. The estimated number of patients with MS in the United States is between 250,000 and 350,000. MS is a disorder of young adults, the onset of disease most frequently between the ages of 20 and 35 years among women and 35 and 45 years among men. The prevalence of MS is approximately four times higher among women than among men, and the disease is much more common among white persons than among other races. Although there are no definite mendelian patterns of inheritance with MS, first-degree relatives of the person with the index case have a 10- to 20-fold increased risk of the disorder. This genetic risk has been borne out in twin studies, in which the monozygotic concordance rate is approximately 30%, compared with 5% for dizygotic twins. HLA studies have shown a subtle but significant correlation between MS and different HLA antigens within various ethnic groups. Together, these suggest that there is a genetic predisposition toward development of the disorder but that noninherited factors play a more dominant role.

    II. Pathogenesis. The exact pathogenesis of MS remains elusive, but substantial clinical and laboratory data suggest an autoimmune process. Although patients with MS have significant abnormalities in humoral immune function, the disorder appears to be primarily mediated through T cells. The target of the autoimmune disorder is the myelin sheath that surrounds axons in the CNS. This myelin is important for saltatory conduction along the axon. Demyelination frequently occurs in localized areas. The result is a pathologic lesion called a **plaque.** These plaques usually are located deep in the cerebral white matter, near the ventricles, but they can occur anywhere, including gray matter, cerebellum, brainstem, spinal cord, and proximal nerve roots. This almost limitless variation of distribution is responsible for the variety of clinical presentations. The pathologic appearance of the plaque changes with repeated episodes of demyelination and chronicity. In an early active plaque, there is breakdown of the blood–brain barrier with demyelination but with relative sparing of the axons. Perivascular infiltrates of lymphocytes, macrophages, and occasionally plasma cells are present in small veins and venules. Demyelination may spread outward from the plaque, especially along these vessels. Perivascular and interstitial edema may be prominent. At the edge of the plaque, there is hyperplasia of oligodendrocytes and activated astrocytes. These hyperplastic oligodendrocytes are probably involved in remyelination, but thin myelin sheaths found at electron microscopic examination suggest this remyelination often is suboptimal and incomplete. In older plaques, oligodendroglia disappear, astrocytes show hypertrophy and hyperplasia ("sclerosis"), and axonal loss occurs.

    III. Clinical features. Areas of CNS demyelination or plaques can produce conduction abnormalities with delayed or blocked conduction, impaired response to repetitive stimulation, or ephaptic conduction. The first three conduction defects can result in negative signs or symptoms. Depending on the extent of the conduction defect and location of the lesion in the CNS, the patient may have visual loss, numbness, weakness, ataxia, or nearly any loss of function attributable to a CNS lesion. Often the lesion comes and goes in a clinically silent area of the brain, the patient is not aware of any symptoms. Ephaptic conduction may result in positive signs and symptoms, including pain, seizures and paroxysmal syndromes. The variations of positive and negative signs and symptoms that may develop further contribute to the complexity of the clinical disorder.

        A. Presenting symptoms. Patients with MS may come to medical attention with a variety of neurologic symptoms. The most common symptoms at onset are visual or oculomotor, accounting for 49% of the cases. Next are weakness or a sensory disturbance of one or more limbs, accounting for 43% and 41% of cases. Twenty-three percent of patients come to medical attention with incoordination. Ten percent of patients have genitourinary or bowel dysfunction. Four percent have cerebral dysfunction. These percentages vary between reports. It is common for patients to have multiple symptoms, accounting for a total percentage greater than 100.

B. Clinical course. Approximately 20% to 30% of patients with MS have a benign disorder. Some of these patients have only a few exacerbations; then the disorder appears to resolve. Others, typically with predominately sensory exacerbations, have recurrent events over years, without significant residual defects. More characteristically, all exacerbations do not fully resolve, and neurologic dysfunction accumulates gradually. Approximately 10% of patients have a highly malignant course with severe disability within months to a few years and in some cases, even within weeks or days.

C. Disease forms. There are several forms of MS.

   1. The most common form at presentation is **relapsing–remitting MS,** in which neurologic dysfunction builds over days to weeks, reaches a plateau, and resolves over weeks to months. In some cases, the exacerbation is maximal within minutes to hours.

   2. A smaller group of patients have only partial or no recovery from the exacerbations, and disability accumulates in a stepwise manner. This disease is called **progressive-relapsing MS.**

   3. More frequently, patients have relapsing–remitting disease that later becomes linear in progression. This disease form is classified as **secondary progressive MS** and accounts for most cases of MS later in the disease course.

   4. The last subset accounts for a small number of cases of near linear progression from onset and is called **primary progressive MS.** The patients are typically older at disease onset, and the dysfunction manifest mainly as insidiously progressive spastic paraparesis with ataxia and bladder dysfunction. Even in the primary progressive form of the disorder, the condition of a substantial number of patients stabilizes after several years. Regrettably, there may be severe residual disability before stabilization.

D. Prognosis is difficult in the care of patients with newly diagnosed MS. The most reliable prognostic factor is disease form. Patients with discrete exacerbations with significant recovery have the best prognosis. In this group, there is a trend toward better outcome when the onset of disease is at a younger age and the symptoms are restricted to one region of the CNS. This is especially true if the symptoms are predominantly sensory. Patients who begin with the primary progressive disorder usually have a much more severe course. These patients usually have disease onset later in life and are more frequently men. Overall, the Kurtzke 5-year rule is reasonably reliable. This states that the absence of significant motor or cerebellar dysfunction at 5 years correlates with limited disability at 15 years.

IV. Diagnosis. An accurate diagnosis of MS is extremely important because the disorder mimics many diseases of the CNS. Unfortunately, the diagnosis cannot be achieved reliably through any single paraclinical study. Rather, the entire clinical syndrome must be evaluated with a careful clinical history and examination. Those findings direct further laboratory studies to eliminate other disorders or to support the diagnosis of MS wth paraclinical studies such as magnetic resonance imaging (MRI), evoked potentials, and examination of the cerebrospinal fluid (CSF). Optimally, the clinician should understand the relative importance, specificity, and sensitivity of each symptom, sign, and paraclinical study for each clinical form of MS at varying points of time in the clinical course. Evaluation by means of this approach allows an experienced clinician to obtain a diagnosis of greater than 95% accuracy in many cases.

A. Clinical aspects of diagnostic importance

   1. Age. The peak age at disease onset is between 20 and 45 years. It is rare for the disease to start before 14 years of age or after 60 years. Careful consideration must be given to other disorders in patients who have MS-like symptoms in an atypical age group.

   2. Character of signs and symptoms

      a. Lesion localization. Symptoms should suggest a CNS origin. Examples of exceptions include infranuclear cranial nerve palsy or monoradiculopathy due to plaque formation over the exit of the cranial nerve or nerve root within the CNS.

      b. Onset features and course. Most symptoms develop over hours to days, plateau, and then begin to decline. On occasion, the symptoms are maximal within seconds or minutes. Consideration should be given to infarction in these cases, especially if localization suggests a vascular territory. For all but patients with primary progressive MS, the most consistent history is relapses and remissions involving various areas of the CNS at different points in time. The diagnosis of primary progressive disease is more difficult. These patients usually have an insidiously progressive spinal cerebellar syndrome that may mimic several disorders, including mass or compressive lesions, infectious agents, metabolic disorders, inherited spinal cerebellar syndromes and degenerative disease. Presentation with aphasia, dementia, psychosis, acute anxiety, movement disorders, and intense pain is unusual in MS.

    3. Differential diagnosis. Early on, a subset of patients with many CNS disorders have symptoms suggestive of the various disease forms of MS. A partial list of these disorders includes systemic lupus erythematosus, antiphospholipid antibody syndrome, Sjögren's syndrome, primary CNS vasculitis, polyarteritis nodosa, Behçet's disease, sarcoidosis, Lyme disease, tropical spastic paraparesis, progressive multifocal leukoencephalopathy, subacute sclerosing panencephalitis, acute disseminated encephalomyelitis, postinfectious demyelination, vitamin B_{12} deficiency, adrenomyeloneuropathy, idiopathic and inherited spinocerebellar syndromes, CNS mass lesions, and paraneoplastic syndromes. Because of the potential overlapping symptoms and findings, a clinician must always pursue a complete evaluation of patients with suspected MS and never force a diagnosis of MS in the setting of atypical features or findings.

B. MRI. Overall, cranial MRI is the most sensitive paraclinical study in the diagnosis of MS. Lesions are most frequently detected with proton density–weighted images (first echo of a T2-weighted sequence) and the fluid attenuated inversion recovery (FLAIR) sequence.

    1. Frequency of MRI abnormalities in MS

      a. Definite MS: 85% to 97%

      b. Suspected MS: 60% to 85%

    2. MRI abnormalities

      a. Images typically reveal multiple focal periventricular areas of increased T2-weighted and FLAIR signals that are irregular in shape and less than 2.5 cm long. Unfortunately, none of these characteristics is specific to lesions secondary to MS. For example, in older normal control populations, it is common for MRI to reveal multiple, punctate, nonspecific areas of increased T2-weighted signal in the deep white matter.

        (1) Abnormalities more suggestive of demyelination are multiple lesions, some of which are larger than 6 mm in diameter, ovoid, or abut the body of the lateral ventricle or have a combination of these features. In MS, it is also common to find lesions involving the corpus callosum or that are infratentorial.

      b. Gadolinium-enhancing lesions are transient and reflect local temporary breakdown of the blood–brain barrier, as occurs in active plaque. These contrast-enhanced MR images reflect acute disease more accurately than do nonenhanced studies.

      c. T1-weighted sequence lesions correlate well with tissue destruction and subsequent disability.

      d. Atrophy is common in long-standing disease.

C. Spinal fluid examination. The CSF examination is frequently performed in evaluation for MS. Certain patterns of CSF abnormalities are highly suggestive of the disorder. These patterns are not specific to MS and can be seen with other inflammatory or infectious disorders.

    1. The appearance of the CSF and the opening pressure are normal.

    2. Cell count. The red blood cell count is normal. Mild lymphocytosis is typical; more than one third of patients have more than 5 cells/mm³. In the unusual event that more than 50 cells/mm^3 are found, consideration should be given to an infectious process.

3. **Protein.** The CSF protein level usually is mildly elevated. More than one fourth of patients have a protein level greater than 54 mg/dL. A protein of greater than 100 mg/dL is rare.

4. **Myelin basic protein.** Myelin is destroyed in MS plaque. Approximately 30% of CNS myelin is myelin basic protein (MBP). MBP is released with the destruction of myelin, and its presence in the CSF is one of the most reliable indicators of current demyelination; the level is proportional to the extent of myelin destruction. This elevated level is seen during the first 2 weeks after a substantial exacerbation in 50% to 90% of patients then disappears with time. MBP is not disease specific and can be seen in any process with myelin destruction, such as infarction or CNS infection.

5. **Immunoglobulin.** CSF immunoglobulin levels (primarily IgG, but also IgM and to a lesser extent IgA) are elevated (>12% of total protein) in 60% to 80% of patients with MS. The increase occurs because is abundant plasma cells produce immunoglobulin in the brain and spinal cord. A smaller component of immunoglobulin arises from normal transfer from the serum and increased entry through a disturbed blood–brain barrier.

   a. **IgG synthesis rate** is a calculated estimate of the rate of synthesis of IgG within the intrathecal space. It increases to more than 3 mg/d in 80% to 90% of patients with MS, but rarely more than 130 mg/d. This rate correlates with MRI plaque burden and decreases with corticotropin or glucocorticoid therapy. The rate is increases in 12% of healthy persons and in 30% to 50% of patients with CNS infection.

   b. The **IgG index** is a calculation—(CSF IgG/serum IgG)/(CSF albumin/serum albumin)—that reflects the increased amount of IgG in the intrathecal space. The index is increased (>0.7) in 86% to 94% of patients with MS and often is the first CSF abnormality found in early disease.

6. **CSF oligoclonal bands (OCB)** are discrete bands frequently detected in the CSF of patients with MS. Most data indicate that OCBs are not directed against a specific antigen and are not involved in pathogenesis of disease. They are present in 30% to 40% of possible and 90% to 97% of definite cases of MS. OCBs also are present in other chronic inflammatory diseases of the CNS, infectious disorders, and 7% of healthy controls. Although the prevalence of OCBs increases when CSF is sampled later in the course of the disease, these bands are not related to current disease activity or therapy. The pattern of bands varies among different patients. In a single patient, the pattern tends to be relatively stable with some minor changes and addition of bands over a period of time. The bands in MS usually are seen only in the CSF when paired CSF and sera samples are evaluated simultaneously. This differs from the typically paired OCBs found in many other conditions such as inflammatory neuropathy, neoplasms, or systemic immune response.

D. **Evoked potentials** provide electrophysiologic evidence of conduction blocks or delays caused by demyelination. Before the availability of MRI, these studies were important to document widespread lesions. They still play an important role in the diagnosis of MS for some patients.

   1. **Visual evoked potential (VEP).** Demyelination frequently occurs in the optic nerves and chiasm in patients with MS. Although some patients have symptoms consistent with optic neuritis, others have no associated visual symptoms. VEPs are obtained to evaluate conduction defects in the visual pathways. In most patients with previous demyelination of the optic nerve, VEPs remain abnormal. VEPs are abnormal in approximately 40%, 60%, and 85% of possible, probable, and definite cases of MS.

   2. **Somatosensory evoked potentials (SSEPs)** are obtained to detect conduction defects in the somatosensory pathways. The study involves stimulation of the large myelinated fibers of the peroneal, tibial, or median peripheral

nerve and recording over the contralateral sensorimotor cortex. SSEPs are abnormal in approximately 50%, 70% and 80% of possible, probable and definite patients with MS.

   3. **Brainstem auditory evoked potentials (BAEPs)** are obtained to evaluate conduction disturbances in the auditory pathways after auditory stimulation. BAEPs are abnormal in approximately 30%, 40% and 70% of possible, probable, and definite cases of MS.

V. Therapy. The complex, highly variable signs and symptoms of MS result in a clinical disorder that often is a challenge to manage. Therapy for MS is both symptomatic and immune modulating. Symptomatic therapy involves management of fatigue, spasticity, neurobehavioral disorders, paroxysmal disorders, pain, bladder dysfunction, and cerebellar dysfunction. Immune-modulating therapies are directed at altering the clinical course. This may involve management of acute exacerbations or the overall progression of the disease.

   A. **Symptomatic therapy.** Patients with mild or early disease may have limited neurologic dysfunction and need minimal therapy. Among these patients, the main therapy is limited to counseling and education. Patients with more severe disease or later in the clinical course often have many symptoms that respond to treatment.

   1. **Spasticity** is common with severe or long-standing MS. Patients describe tightness or stiffness of the affected limbs or trunk and reflex spasms. These spasms can be provoked by a variety of stimuli or occur spontaneously. Spasticity also can increase after initiation of interferon beta therapy. Spasticity makes walking difficult, causes fatigue, makes transfer arduous, may interfere with sleep, and causes pain. During an exacerbation or with otherwise asymptomatic urinary tract infection, there may be a significant increase in spasticity. Management of the underlying disorder often returns the spasticity to baseline. Range of motion exercises around each joint in the spastic limb may decrease spasticity and prevent fibrosis of the muscle. Pharmacologic agents usually are needed when a substantial amount of strength is wasted to overcome the spastic component to walk or when the patient is too weak yet spasticity causes discomfort and difficulty with transfers. Overmedication should be avoided in the care of ambulatory patients because a small amount of extensor spasticity is beneficial for weight bearing in weak lower limbs.

      a. **Baclofen** is an effective agent for reducing spasticity, especially of spinal cord origin. The medication may be started at a low dose of either 10 mg at bedtime or 10 mg twice daily and slowly increased weekly or biweekly by 10 mg/d as tolerated or needed. When the dosage is too high, patients notice a decline in strength. At that point, decreasing the dose by 10 mg/d usually offers the optimal level of function with spasticity maximally treated but without significant induction of weakness. Higher doses often are tolerated and needed by patients with spastic paraplegia, for whom ambulation is not an issue. The maximal dosage recommended by the manufacturer is 80 mg/d day in four divided doses; however, many physicians prescribe higher doses. The most common side effects are the dose-related weakness, sedation, dizziness, and confusion. When the drug is discontinued, the dosage should be gently tapered because abrupt withdrawal can cause confusion and seizures.

      b. **Tizanidine** is effective in reducing spasticity by increasing presynaptic inhibition of motor neurons. Although related to clonidine, tizanidine has less potential for lowering blood pressure. However, care must be exercised when starting this medication because orthostatic hypotension can be induced. Consideration should be given to discontinuing all antihypertensive agents before initiating the therapy because the effect can be profound. Tizanidine is started at 2 mg at bedtime and gradually increased to as high as 36 mg a day in three divided doses as needed or tolerated. The major side effects are somnolence, dry mouth, and asthenia. Tizanidine should be used with care to treat the elderly, who clear the drug slowly, and to treat patients with renal impairment. Oral contraceptives decrease the clearance of tizanidine by 50%. Finally, the medication is primarily metabolized in the liver and induces liver toxicity in some patients. It should be used carefully or not at all in the treatment of patients with impaired hepatic function or in patients taking other hepatotoxic medications. Liver function should be monitored before initiation of therapy and especially for the first several months of administration. Tizanidine and baclofen work together in a synergistic manner. Baclofen typically is administered first because there are fewer complications. If the patient does not respond adequately to the baclofen, tizanidine is slowly added. Often, both the tizanidine and baclofen can be given at lower doses, yet with increased control of spasticity.

   c. **Benzodiazepines** provide benefit to a subset of patients with severe spasticity refractory to baclofen and tizanidine. The addition of small doses of diazepam to baclofen or tizanidine can result in a synergistic effect. Usual doses are 0.5 to 1 mg two to three times a day. If patients are intolerant of baclofen, diazepam may be used alone. The dosage may be started at 1 to 2 mg two to three times daily, gradual increasing to a maximum of 20 to 30 mg/d. Dependence can develop, so the drug is tapered slowly when discontinued.

   d. **Dantrolene** may be used for spasticity when baclofen, tizanidine, and benzodiazepines are ineffective. Weakness induced by the drug limits its usefulness in many patients already compromised with motor impairment. In the rare patient whose strength is preserved in the presence of severe spasticity, the drug may provide benefit. Other patients who are good candidates for this therapy have severe weakness with no useful function of the legs and spasticity that contributes to flexion contracture, discomfort, and difficulty with transfer and activities of daily living. In this situation, the loss of strength is of less consequence. The dosage is usually started at 25 mg/d and gently increased to 100 mg four times a day if needed. Liver function must be monitored because liver toxicity is a rare but potentially fatal complication of this medication. The risk is highest among women, patients older than 35 years, and those taking a dosage greater than 200 mg/d. Other side effects include diarrhea at higher doses and occasionally pericarditis or pleuritis. Although the drug usually has little effect on cardiac or smooth muscle, it should be used with care to treat patients with myocardial disease.

   e. **Botulinum toxin type A** may be used for isolated spastic muscle groups.

   f. When these pharmacologic agents are contraindicated because of complications or do not control spasticity, **surgical intervention** may be considered. The procedures include percutaneous radiofrequency foraminal rhizotomy, sciatic neurectomy, intramuscular neurolysis, tenotomy, neurectomy, and myelotomy. Intrathecal baclofen delivered with a subcutaneous pump is an effective alternative for some patients. Again, this therapy should be reserved for patients with severe spasticity unresponsive to oral therapy or patients in whom oral agents caused severe complications. The pump is expensive, requires frequent dosage adjustments, especially during the first several months, and requires refilling every 1 to 3 months. The battery has a limited life and requires replacement along with the pump (not the catheter) every few years.

2. **Fatigue and heat sensitivity.** Most patients with MS report fatigue that varies from mild to severely disabling. This symptom can be potentiated by spasticity, depression, current infection, sleep disorders, or interruption of sleep due to nocturia from bladder dysfunction. After these causes are controlled, patients should be instructed to conserve energy through time management, economy of effort, and work simplification. A subset of patients report extreme fatigue and even exacerbation of focal neurologic symptoms in hot environments and increased body temperature during exertion or with a febrile illness. Heat-sensitive patients should be advised to decrease ambient temperature to comfortable levels, dress lightly to enhance heat dispersion, and aggressively control fevers.

    a. Amantadine provides a modest reduction in fatigue for most patients. The dosage is 100 mg twice a day, and the medication is discontinued if there is no benefit after 1 month.

    b. Modafinil is effective in decreasing fatigue in many patients with MS without affecting memory, concentration, or learning. Unfortunately, the medication has been approved only for narcolepsy. Before using the medication, patients must be informed that it is being prescribed in a non-approved manner, and insurance companies may not provide coverage. Patients typically respond to 200 to 400 mg given in the morning. Higher doses are associated with increased side effects. The abuse potential for the drug is low, and patients have not had withdrawal symptoms when it is discontinued. Oral clearance of modafinil is reduced in the elderly, especially in patients with hepatic impairment, in which the serum concentration of modafinil can double. The most commonly observed adverse events in clinical trials included headache, nausea and vomiting, nervousness, anxiety, and insomnia. Modafinil can cause failure of oral contraceptives or hormonal contraceptive-containing implants or devices owing to induction of the CYP3A4 isoenzyme metabolism of ethinyl estradiol or the progestins in these products.

    c. Pemoline may be used for patients undertaking a short-term project or activity in which fatigue causes considerable dysfunction. The stimulant effect and abuse potential of this medication preclude long-term use. The initial dose of 18.75 mg every morning and may be increased to 37.5 mg or higher.

    d. Selective serotonin reuptake inhibitors often give an energy boost, even when the patient says there are no depressive symptoms. These drugs are typically quite safe. A trial may be merited in the care of a patient with severe fatigue.

    e. Experimental medications. Preliminary trials with the potassium channel blockers 4-aminopyridine and 3,4-diaminopyrimidine have shown promise with improved level of function and decreased fatigue and heat sensitivity. These medications have the potential for several complications and need further evaluation to establish efficacy and safety for long-term use.

3. Neurobehavioral disorders. Patients with MS may have several neurobehavioral disorders, including depression, euphoria, emotional lability, dementia or cognitive impairment, and in rare instances, bipolar disease, extreme anxiety, and psychosis. Recognition of these disorders is important because some are amenable to therapy, thereby decreasing disability and improving quality of life.

    a. Depression is common in MS. The reported prevalence varies considerably with a reasonable range probably between 25% and 50%. The cause of the depression is most likely multifactorial, having biologic, psychological, and social elements. All factors should be considered with therapy tailored to each patient. When the depression appears to be a reaction to the illness, the patient may benefit from counseling and management of the MS. Although actual investigation of drug efficacy in MS is limited, for many patients, a trial of antidepressants should be considered.

       (1) Selective serotonin reuptake inhibitors are the medication of choice for depressive symptoms in patients with MS. These medications usually have few anticholinergic side effects to enhance several types of bladder dysfunction, and they often give an energy boost to help alleviate the fatigue that accompanies the disease as well as the depression.

       (2) Tricyclic antidepressants may be used as a second-line choice when the anticholinergic side effects are of less detriment then is control of pain or when they actually control the type of bladder dysfunction that the patient exhibits.

(3) **Electroconvulsive therapy** may have a limited role in the care of patients with MS. It has been complicated by exacerbations in anecdotal cases.

b. **Other neurobehavioral disorders** include euphoria, pathologic laughing and crying, anxiety, and psychosis.

   (1) **Euphoria** is defined as a persistent change in mood consisting of cheerfulness and optimism. This mood may persist in spite of the patient's awareness of very suboptimal circumstances, including severe disability. No treatment is required.

   (2) **Emotional lability** is common among patients with MS. This ranges from mild giggling or tearing to pathologic laughing and crying or, in severe cases, complete emotional incontinence. Usually the patient is aware of the lability, and these emotional outbursts are socially distressing. Amitriptyline improves emotional control for many patients. The drug may be given at bedtime, starting at 25 mg and increased as needed. Most patients respond to less than 100 mg. If amitriptyline is ineffective, a trial of levodopa or bromocriptine is merited.

   (3) Extreme **anxiety** is rare in MS. Alprazolam given at a dosage of 0.25 to 0.50 mg two to three times a day may decrease the symptoms. An alternative medication is diazepam. Both medications have abuse potential and should be prescribed with care and tapered gently when discontinued.

   (4) Although rare, **psychosis** does occur among patients with MS. This is typically associated with agitated depression or a complication of steroid therapy rather than an isolated phenomenon. Antipsychotic drugs are used as they are in the care of persons with psychiatric illnesses.

4. **Paroxysmal disorders** are typically intense ephaptic events that last seconds to minutes with a tendency to reoccur in a stereotypic manner. These occur in 1% to 4% of patients with MS without associated epileptiform activity on an electroencephalogram. Some are unique to MS and on occasion are the initial symptom. They may occur during an exacerbation or in isolation and frequently last weeks to months then spontaneously resolve. A careful inquiry for the presence of these disorders is important because they can cause the patient considerable discomfort or dysfunction.

   a. **Management of paroxysmal disorders.** Most paroxysmal disorders respond to anticonvulsant agents. The drug of choice is carbamazepine or oxcarbazepine.

      (1) **Carbamazepine** often provides relief, even at low doses such as 200 mg each day or twice a day.

      (2) **Oxcarbazepine** is less likely than carbamazepine in inducing CNS side effects such as truncal ataxia or hematologic abnormalities such as leukopenia. Drug levels are rarely monitored. However, hyponatremia may occur and the physician must consider periodic checks of sodium, especially during the first 3 months. The dosage of oxcarbazepine should be started at 300 mg PO each day and increased as indicated by 300 mg/day every third day or 600 mg/day at weekly intervals up to 2400 mg/day in two divided doses.

      (3) If these therapies are ineffective consideration may be given to phenytoin, acetazolamide or phenobarbital.

      (4) Therapy should be tapered and discontinued after two to three months since the disorder may have resolved.

      (5) Additional information is included under trigeminal neuralgia because that disorder often is more difficult to manage.

   b. **Trigeminal neuralgia** is characterized by triggered and nontriggered paroxysmal episodes of facial pain in the trigeminal distribution. It occurs in 1% to 2% of patients with MS. In MS, the pain is similar to that in the general population except that it occurs at a higher incidence, at a younger age, and is more often bilateral. Also, there is an increased incidence of atypical trigeminal neuralgia with longer episodes of intense pain superimposed on persistent facial discomfort. Carbamazepine or oxcarbazepine, used alone or in combination with baclofen or phenytoin, gives complete relief in some patients and reduces the pain in most. When trigeminal neuralgia is refractory to these medications, the orally active antipsychotic agent pimozide may be considered. This medication should be used with care because most patients with MS have adverse effects, including lethargy, impaired concentration, hand tremors, involuntary movements during sleep, and slight parkinsonian features. Other medications that may offer relief are clonazepam, amitriptyline, or misoprostol. When there are serious drug complications or a lack of pain control with conservative management, surgical intervention such as percutaneous stereotactic thermal rhizotomy or glycerol rhizotomy often is effective. The patient may need two to three treatments before complete control is obtained.

c. **Other paroxysmal sensory or painful symptoms** include a variety of sensations, including burning paresthesia, severe or aching pain, unpleasant quivering sensations, spontaneous Lhermitte's-like phenomena, and itching. Most of these episodes last seconds to a few minutes and most frequently involve the extremities, although they can affect any part of the body. Paroxysmal itching varies from the other sensations. The episodes last as long as 30 minutes, sometimes occurring in a dermatomal distribution, especially over the shoulders and neck.

d. **Tonic spasms** are severe spasms that last seconds to minutes. They begin in the limbs or trunk and spread upward or downward, sometimes crossing the midline. Many times, an intense pain or unpleasant sensation starts at a trigger zone and precedes or accompanies the spasm. In other patients, the spasms occur without discomfort. These spasms can be provoked by movement, tactile stimulation of a trigger zone, or hyperventilation, or they can occur spontaneously. In an individual patient, the tonic spasm, with or without the pain, reoccurs in a stereotypic pattern. These episodes can occur as part of an exacerbation or when the patient's condition is stable. Tonic spasms should be differentiated from flexor spasms. With tonic spasms, the spasms are more intense, usually are associated with severe pain, spread in a stereotypic manner, and are not correlated with the degree of underlying spasticity. Although flexor spasms are best managed with baclofen, tonic seizures usually respond to the anticonvulsants previously mentioned.

e. **Paroxysmal dysarthria and ataxia.** These episodes usually last less than 1 minute but can reoccur several times in one day. In some patients, anxiety or hyperventilation precipitates the episodes. Ataxia can result in falls, and dysarthria can be so severe that speech cannot be interpreted. Although dysarthria and ataxia are always present, other symptoms can be associated, including diplopia, numbness, and weakness.

f. **Diplopia** can occur with dysarthria and ataxia or occur in isolation. Isolated episodes of diplopia last seconds to a few minutes and can occur as often as 100 times a day.

g. **Other paroxysmal disorders** include akinesia in one or more limbs that lasts a few seconds and frequently reoccurring several times a day, weakness usually of a leg or hand lasting 10 to 20 seconds to a few minutes with resultant unexpected falls or dropping of objects, and paroxysmal hemiataxia and crossed paraesthesia.

5. **Pain.** Although pain rarely is an initial symptom of MS, it commonly develops during the course of the disease and affects more than 50% of the patient population. The paroxysmal pain syndromes that respond best to anticonvulsant medications have already been discussed. More commonly, patients have chronic pain that includes dysesthetic pain, back pain, and painful leg spasms. The typical burning or aching dysesthetic pain responds best to the

anticonvulsant gabapentin. Therapy usually is started at 100 to 300 mg at bedtime and increased as needed or tolerated to 2,400 mg/d in three divided doses. Patients frequently respond by the time they have taken 1,500 mg in a day. The typical main side effect is fatigue. If gabapentin is ineffective or if side effects preclude its use, antidepressant drugs such as amitriptyline and imipramine may be used. Patients may need doses up to 100 mg/d. Other medications that may offer benefit are capsaicin cream applied to the skin or topiramate, which has provided benefit to a subset of patients. A combination of aggressive physical therapy and nonsteroidal antiinflammatory agents provides partial relief to most patients with chronic back pain. Addition of gabapentin or antidepressant medications may be necessary. Patients resistant to therapy and debilitated with severe pain may need intrathecal morphine, intrathecal phenol, or a neurolytic procedure such as dorsal rhizotomy.

6. **Bladder dysfunction.** Patients with MS frequently have neurogenic bladder at some point during the illness. In many, bladder dysfunction persists and causes major social concerns. This dysfunction may be caused by an uninhibited small capacity or a flaccid neurogenic bladder, a combination of these dysfunctions or detrusor–sphincter dyssynergia. The symptoms of uninhibited neurogenic bladder are primarily irritative, whereas those of a flaccid neurogenic bladder are primarily obstructive. There is a substantial amount of overlap between the symptoms, and a clinical history frequently is insufficient for diagnosis. Because several conditions are associated with MS, the optimal approach is for the patient to undergo a urologic evaluation to determine the exact bladder dysfunction. This is especially true because the therapies for these disorders are frequently directly antagonistic.

Mechanical dysfunction often leads to urinary tract infections. These can result in pseudoexacerbation with increased lower extremity sensory loss and weakness of tone that resolve when the infection is appropriately managed. One should avoid prescribing empiric antibiotics because resistant strains of bacteria often develop. Allow the therapy to be directed by the culture and sensitivity results.

7. **Sexual dysfunction.** Erectile dysfunction is common among men with MS. It can be caused by demyelination in the spinal cord from lesions of the motor and sensory pathways or decreased testosterone levels that can complicate the disorder. A variety of other issues, such as medications, fatigue, spasticity, paraparesis, and psychological issues, such as poor self-esteem and self-image, fear of rejection, fear of incontinence, or depression, can lead to erectile dysfunction. The cause of dysfunction should be sought vigorously. If the dysfunction appears to have a nonhormonal physiologic cause, sildenafil may be tried at 25 to 100 mg 1 hour before sexual intercourse. The side effects typically are minimal and include headache, flushing, dyspepsia, and musculoskeletal pain. Reports suggest caution in the treatment of patients with cardiovascular disease. Older traditional approaches may include intracavernous papaverine, prostaglandin E, phentolamine, vacuum devices, and a penile prosthesis.

Sexual dysfunction in women has not been as well studied as it has in men but also may be caused by several of the previously mentioned causes with the exception of decreased testosterone levels and the addition of pelvic floor weakness. When nonphysiologic issues have been excluded, sildenafil also may be effective for women.

8. **Cerebellar dysfunction**
   a. Cerebellar dysfunction is common, especially in the primary progressive form of the disease. Upper extremity ataxia and tremors may be so severe that activities of daily living are impossible, and nursing home care is required. This dysfunction is especially resistant to therapy. Despite of reported benefit in small trials, isoniazid, carbamazepine, primidone, and glutethimide all provide only marginal control in most patients. Other medications that have been used with little success are baclofen, clonazepam, propranolol, choline, and lecithin. In summary, there is no

effective medical therapy to date. Surgical intervention is controversial and has included stereotaxic thalamotomy and deep brain stimulation. Exacerbations have occurred after surgery, and it is difficult to predict the response of tremors to surgical procedures. When a patient begins to have significant cerebellar dysfunction, consideration should be given to more aggressive immune-modulating therapy.

B. **Immune modulating therapy.** Although the exact pathogenesis of MS is unknown, it appears to be multifactorial with a substantial autoimmune contribution. This has prompted numerous clinical trials of immune-modulating agents in an attempt to alter the course of the disease. Available therapies remain inadequate and have the potential for substantial complications.

1. **Management of exacerbations**

   a. **Indications for therapy.** Exacerbations are common among patients with active relapsing–remitting or relapsing–progressive MS. There are few data to support changes in long-term clinical course or disability with management of exacerbations. The advantage of therapy is to expedite recovery from an exacerbation to allow a person to return to a higher level of function more quickly than if the exacerbation had been allowed to run its natural course. My colleagues and I have found that many patients initially have an excellent response to treatment, but the benefit is lost after several interventions. In light of these factors, not all patients with exacerbations should be treated. We typically reserve therapy for patients with a definite change in functional status, usually related to a significant decline in vision, motor, or cerebellar function.

   b. **Therapy.** Acute exacerbations usually are managed with methylprednisolone or corticotropin. There are no definitive data to indicate which drug is more effective. Methylprednisolone is probably superior because it usually is given over a shorter time. The cortisol response to corticotropin is not consistent or may be delayed, and the endogenous steroid production may never reach the range generally recommended for inflammatory autoimmune diseases. The optimal doses and treatment schedules are not well studied. Most treatment protocols for acute exacerbation call for 25 to 60 units of corticotropin given intramuscularly or infused over 8 hours and tapered gradually over 2 to 4 weeks. Intravenous methylprednisolone may be given in doses of 500 to 1,000 mg each morning for 5 days. This may be followed by prednisone, 60 mg every morning for 3 days, then decreased every 3 days by 10 mg on a relatively rapid taper. The prednisone appears to help prevent immediate relapses after discontinuation of the methylprednisolone.

   Exacerbations may be managed with oral prednisone without the preceding methylprednisolone. My colleagues and I are now more reluctant to treat patients in this manner because an optic neuritis trial showed benefit from methylprednisolone followed by oral prednisone but increased relapse rates for optic neuritis after treatment with oral prednisone alone. Treatment with glucocorticoids is avoided in the care of pregnant patients. Severe exacerbations in these patients have been managed successfully with plasma exchange in isolated cases. Finally, consideration may be given to intravenous immune globulin, plasma exchange, and intravenous bolus cyclophosphamide in the care of patients with fulminate disease for which where glucocorticoids have provided no benefit.

2. **Management of relapsing–remitting disease.** Three agents are frequently used in the United States to manage relapsing–remitting disease. These medications are very expensive and have generated substantial controversy as to the most efficacious agent. The medications cannot objectively compared because each was tested against placebo and not directly compared with the other. Furthermore, comparisons between studies are difficult because each trial entailed different clinical, laboratory, statistical, and MRI measures. Overall, glatiramer acetate (Copaxone; Teva Marion, Kansas City, MO, U.S.A.) typically has the fewest side effects, and interferon β-1b (Betaseron; Berlex, Richmond, CA, U.S.A.) has the most.

   a. Interferon-beta (INF-β) has been shown to reduce the number and severity of exacerbations as well as the number of enhancing lesions as detected at cranial MRI. These interferons are INF β-1a (Avonex; Biogen, Cambridge, MA, U.S.A.) and INF β-1b (Betaseron). They have generally been well tolerated. The most common side effects are a flulike syndrome of fever and myalgia during the first weeks to months of therapy. Interferon β-1b also causes injection site reactions that can last weeks and usually reoccur as long as the drug is administered. Other side effects include mild lymphopenia and elevation of serum transaminase levels that rarely necessitate withdrawal of treatment. Interferon β-1a requires weekly intramuscular injections, and interferon β-1b subcutaneous injections every other day. These medications are most efficacious when started early in the management of relapsing–remitting disease. The hope is that they will prevent disease progression as well as exacerbations. Rebif (Serono, Geneva, Switzerland) is a formulation of interferon β-1a very similar to Avonex but administered subcutaneously at a higher dosage. Rebif has been studied in Europe with good results and is being studied in a head to head trial with Avonex in the United States.

   b. Glatiramer acetate copolymer 1 (Copaxone) is composed of a random assortment of four amino acids constituting a synthetic polymer. As with interferon β, glatiramer acetate is more efficacious administered early in the disease. It is injected daily in a subcutaneous manner. This medication has decreased the exacerbation rate on essentially the same order as interferon β-1a and interferon β-1b. MRI data were not available from the original study. Extended studies, however, have shown MRI evidence of decreased lesions with use of glatiramer acetate, although the effect seems to be more delayed than with the interferons. Side effects include local injection site reactions and rare transient systemic postinjection reactions, including chest pain, flushing, dyspnea, palpitations, and anxiety. No laboratory monitoring is necessary.

3. **Management of progressive disease.** Medications used to manage primary and secondary progressive disease are even more controversial than are those for the management of relapsing–remitting disease and often have worse side effects. With the establishment of progressive disease, patients frequently are more difficult to treat. Clinicians must carefully evaluate whether they are using immune-modulating agents to control fixed lesions with substantial gliosis and scarring or actual active plaques. Because it often is the former, patients typically have little response. Furthermore, the agents used often are so harsh that they may be employed only a short while; however, the disease may still progress for years. In each case, both clinician and patient must carefully weigh the risk-to-benefit ratio and reach full agreement after the patient has been completely informed. The complex nature of choosing these medications for particular disease forms and patients makes it difficult to make prudent decisions without substantial background information and expertise. A clinician specializing in the treatment of patients with MS more optimally makes these decisions.

   a. Agents under investigation. Several agents have been evaluated for the management of progressive disease. Azathioprine, cyclophosphamide, and cyclosporine provide benefit to individual patients, but the adverse effects of these agents preclude their use to treat the patient population at large. Methotrexate has shown some promise in the management of primary and secondary progressive MS, and further investigation is merited. Interferon β-1b has been studied in the management of secondary progressive disease in Europe with excellent results. However, the results were suboptimal when the trial was attempted in the United States. Glatiramer acetate is currently being studied in the United States in the management of primary progressive MS, and interferon β-1a (Avonex) is being studied in the management of secondary progressive disease. Other agents or approaches are being considered or are under investigation.

b. **Mitoxantrone** has been approved for the management of worsening relapsing–remitting and of primary and secondary progressive disease. It has been shown in trials to reduce relapses and disability as well as development of new enhancing lesions at MRI. The medication is dose limited by cardiac toxicity, which is its main adverse affect. This cumulative toxicity limits usage to less than 3 years. Consequently, this drug is reserved for patients with severe disease that has not resolved with other medications who agree to accept the risk. There is also concern about leukemia that will have to be resolved over time. Because of toxicity, before administration of the first dose, left ventricular ejection fraction is measured by means of echocardiography or multiple gated acquisition (MUGA) scanning. The ejection fraction is then reassessed if symptoms of congestive heart failure develop or if at least 100 mg/m^2 of the drug is administered. Mitoxantrone is typically not given to patients who have received at least 140 mg/m^2, patients with an ejection fraction of less than 50%, or those in whom a significant reduction in ejection fraction has occurred throughout the course of administration. Mitoxantrone is given as a 5 to 15 minute IV infusion of 12 mg/m^2 every 3 months. Before each administration, a complete blood cell count and metabolic profile are obtained. Patients with elevated results of liver function tests or an absolute neutrophil count less than 1,500 cells/mm^3 are excluded. Finally, women of childbearing potential should have negative results of a pregnancy test before each dose.

4. Future therapies for MS. There is currently a substantial amount of research involving immune system modifications as therapy for MS. Some of these areas include modification of adhesion molecules, costimulating factors, the trimolecular complex, interferons, phosphodiesterase inhibitors, matrix metalloproteinase inhibitors, and nitric oxidase inhibitors. There is also interest in growth factors, oligodendroglia transplantation, and bone marrow transplantation. It is beyond the scope of this chapter to discuss this research in detail. Through the tremendous efforts by many investigators and participation in clinical trials by many patients, there has been substantial progress in the understanding and management of MS in the last few years. The development of optimal immune-modulating therapies for the future will require the continued collaboration of clinical and laboratory scientists. This is a very exciting and hopeful time in the treatment of patients with MS.

Recommended Readings

Andrews KL, Husmann DA. Bladder dysfunction and management in multiple sclerosis. *Mayo Clin Proc* 1997;72:1176–1183.

Canadian Coop MSS. The Canadian cooperative trial of cyclophosphamide and plasma exchange in progressive multiple sclerosis. *Lancet* 1991;337:441–446.

European Study Group on Interferon β-1b in Secondary Progressive MS. Placebo-controlled multicenter randomised trial of interferon β-1b in treatment of secondary progressive multiple sclerosis. *Lancet* 1998;352:1491–1497.

Fazekas F, Deisenhammer F, Strausser-Fuchs S. Randomized placebo-controlled trial of monthly intravenous immunoglobulin therapy in relapsing-remitting multiple sclerosis. Austrian Immunoglobin in Multiple Sclerosis Study Group. *Lancet* 1997;349:586–587.

Goodkin DE, Rudick RA, Medendorp SV, et al. Low-dose (7.5 mg) oral methotrexate reduces the rate of progression in chronic progressive multiple sclerosis. *Ann Neurol* 1995;37:30–40.

IFNβ Multiple Sclerosis Study Group. Interferon beta-1b is effective in relapsing-remitting multiple sclerosis: clinical results of a multicenter, randomized, double-blind, placebo-controlled trial. *Neurology* 1993;43:655–661.

IFNβ Multiple Sclerosis Study Group, University of British Columbia MS/MRI Analysis Group. Interferon beta-1b in the treatment of multiple sclerosis: final outcome of the randomized controlled trial. *Neurology* 1995;45:1277–1285.

Jacobs LD, Cookfair DL, Rudick RA, et al. Intramuscular interferon beta-1a for disease progression in relapsing multiple sclerosis. *Ann Neurol* 1996;39:285–294.

Johnson KP, Brooks BR, Cohen JA, et al. Copolymer 1 reduces relapse rate and improves disability in relapsing-remitting multiple sclerosis: results of a phase III multicentre double-blind, placebo-controlled trial. *Neurology* 1995;45:1268–1276.

Johnson KP, Brooks BR, Cohen JA, et al. Extended use of glatiramer acetate (Copaxone) is well tolerated and maintains its clinical effect on multiple sclerosis relapse rate and degree of disability. Copolymer 1 Multiple Sclerosis Study Group. *Neurology* 1998;50:701–708.

Lublin FD, Reingold SC, The National Multiple Sclerosis Society USA Advisory Committee on Clinical Trials of New Agents in Multiple Sclerosis. Defining the clinical course of multiple sclerosis: results of an international survey. *Neurology* 1996;46:907–911.

Minden SL, Schiffer RB. Affective disorders in multiple sclerosis: review and recommendations for clinical research. *Arch Neurol* 1990;47:98–104.

Mitchell GW, Whitaker JN. Immunotherapy for neuroimmunologic disorders. In: Appel SH, ed. *Current neurology.* St Louis: Mosby, 1994:73–109.

Moulin DE, Foley KM, Ebers GC. Pain syndromes in multiple sclerosis. *Neurology* 1988;38: 1830–1834.

Offenbacher H, Fazekas F, Schmidt R, et al. Assessment of MRI criteria for a diagnosis of MS. *Neurology* 1993;43:905–909.

Optic Neuritis Study Group. The 5-year risk of MS after optic neuritis: experience of the Optic Neuritis Treatment Trial. *Neurology* 1997;49:1404–1413.

Paty DW, Li DKB, Duquette P, et al. Interferon beta-1b is effective in relapsing-remitting multiple sclerosis, 2: MRI analysis results of a multicenter, randomized, double–blind, placebo-controlled trial. *Neurology* 1993;43:662–667.

Poser CM. The epidemiology of multiple sclerosis: a general overview. *Ann Neurol* 1994;36: S180–S193.

Prineas JW, Barnard RO, Kwon EE, et al. Multiple sclerosis: remyelination of nascent lesions. *Ann Neurol* 1993;33:137–151.

Prineas JW, Barnard RO, Revesz T, et al. Multiple sclerosis: pathology of recurrent lesions. *Brain* 1993; 116:681–693.

PRISMS Study Group. Randomised double-blind placebo controlled study of interferon beta-1a in relapsing/remitting multiple sclerosis. *Lancet* 1998;352:1498–1504.

Rao SM, Reingold SC, Ron MA, et al. Workshop on neurobehavioural disorders in multiple sclerosis. *Arch Neurol* 1993;50: 658–662.

Rudick RA, Cohen JA, Weinstock-Guttman B, et al. Management of multiple sclerosis. *N Engl J Med* 1997;337:1604–1611.

Runmarker B, Andersen O. Prognostic factors in a multiple sclerosis incidence cohort with 25 years of follow-up. *Brain* 1993;116:117–134.

Sadovnick AD, Ebers GC. Epidemiology in multiple sclerosis: a critical overview. *Can J Neurol Sci* 1993;20:17–29.

Tourtellotte WW, Baumhefner RW, Syndulko K, et al. The long march of the cerebrospinal fluid profile indicative of clinical definite multiple sclerosis; and still marching. *J Neuroimmunol* 1988;20:217–227.

Trapp BD, Peterson J, Ransohoff RM, et al. Axonal transection in the lesions of multiple sclerosis. *N Engl J Med* 1998;338: 278–285.

Yudkin PL, Ellison GW, Ghezzi A, et al. Overview of azathioprine treatment in multiple sclerosis. *Lancet* 1991;338:1051–1055.

41. MOVEMENT DISORDERS

Xabier Beristain
Joanne M. Wojcieszek

Movement disorders can be classified into two major groups—**hypokinetic** and **hyperkinetic**. The clinical features of hypokinetic and hyperkinetic movement disorders are outlined in Chapters 28 and 29. The primary **hypokinetic movement disorder** is parkinsonism, which consists of bradykinesia, rigidity, tremor, and postural instability. The **hyperkinetic movement disorders** include chorea, tics, myoclonus, tardive dyskinesia syndromes, dystonia, and tremor.

I. **Hypokinetic movement disorders**
   A. **Parkinson's disease (PD)** is the most common cause of degenerative parkinsonism, accounting for approximately 80% of all cases. The other 20% represent what have been called **Parkinson-plus syndromes.** PD symptoms usually respond well to antiparkinsonian medications to the extent that a robust and persistent response to levodopa is considered to confirm the diagnosis of PD. However, patients with Parkinson-plus syndromes may have an initial transient response to antiparkinsonian medications, making the differential diagnosis more challenging early in the course of the disease. Management of PD includes nonpharmacologic, pharmacologic, and surgical options.
      1. **Nonpharmacologic management** of PD includes education about the disease, support of patient and family, appropriate nutrition, and exercise. Several support organizations in North America (Table 41.1) can provide informational materials and updates in ongoing research. Exercise can improve stamina, maximize flexibility, and increase the patient's sense of well-being. An appropriate, well-balanced diet is essential because patients with PD are at increased risk of malnutrition and weight loss. As the disease advances, patients taking levodopa become more sensitive to fluctuations in serum levodopa level. Because dietary protein interferes with absorption of levodopa in the gastrointestinal tract and with the penetration through the blood–brain barrier, redistribution of dietary protein can be beneficial in the care of patients with advanced PD.
      2. **Pharmacologic therapy** for PD should include measures directed at preventing or minimizing neuronal damage and thus slowing progression of the disease (**neuroprotection**) and symptomatic treatment.
         a. **Neuroprotection.** The ideal situation would be to identify and eliminate the causes of PD. However, because the cause of PD is unknown, measures directed at slowing or stopping neuronal degeneration are a more realistic approach. In a large prospective study known as Deprenyl and Tocopherol Antioxidative Therapy of Parkinsonism (DATATOP), two drugs with antioxidant effects were studied as potential neuroprotective agents in PD. Tocopherol was not beneficial for patients with PD. On the other hand, selegiline (deprenyl) was shown to delay the need for initiation of levodopa. Whether this finding was a result of a protective effect of selegiline or simply a therapeutic effect of the drug has become a focus of some controversy. There is indirect evidence that dopamine agonists also may be neuroprotective. On the other hand, there is concern that the use of levodopa for management of PD may cause increased oxidative stress and therefore accelerate disease progression. The potential neurotoxicity of levodopa is a highly controversial topic, and there is no clear clinical evidence that levodopa is toxic to striatal neurons in PD.
            (1) **Selegiline** (Eldepryl; Somerset, Tampa, FL, U.S.A.) is a selective inhibitor of monoamine oxidase B (MAO-B) at prescribed dosages of up to 10 mg/d. It is most frequently used as an initial treatment because of its potential protective effects. It has a very modest symptomatic therapeutic effect, which is often imperceptible for

Table 41.1 Support organizations for Parkinson's disease

The American Parkinson Disease Association, Inc. 1250 Hylan Blvd, Suite 4B Staten Island, NY 10305-1946 Phone: (718) 981-8001 Toll free: (800) 223-2732 Fax: (718) 981-4399 Website: http://apdaparkinson.org	National Parkinson Foundation, Inc. Bob Hope Parkinson Research Center 1501 NW 9th Ave, Bob Hope Rd Miami, FL 33136-1494 Phone: (305) 547-6666 Toll Free: (800) 327-4545 Fax: (305) 243-4403 E-mail: mailbox@parkinson.org Website: http://www.parkinson.org
The Parkinson Foundation of Canada 4211 Yonge St, Suite 316 Toronto, Ontario, Canada, M2P 2A9 Phone: (416) 227-9700 Toll Free: (800) 565-3000 Fax: (416) 227-9600 E-mail: General.info@parkinson.ca Website: http://www.parkinson.ca	The Parkinson's Disease Foundation, Inc. William Black Medical Building Columbia–Presbyterian Medical Center 710 West 168th St New York, NY 10032-9982 Phone: (212) 923-4700 Toll free: (800) 457-6676 Fax: (212) 923-4778 E-mail: info@pdf.org Website: http://www.pdf.org

most patients when the drug is used as monotherapy. Sometimes the symptomatic effect is evident only when the drug is stopped and the patient feels a worsening of PD symptoms, which usually occurs 2 to 4 weeks after drug discontinuation. Selegiline is effective as an adjunct to levodopa to reduce "wearing off." The addition of selegiline often allows the levodopa dosage to be lowered 25%.

(2) The currently recommended dose of selegiline is 5 to 10 mg/d; however, smaller doses can have neuroprotective effects independent from MAO-B inhibition. Doses as low as 2.5 mg every other day have been suggested for potential neuroprotection.

(3) **Adverse effects** of selegiline are relatively infrequent when the drug is used early in the disease. Occasional patients report insomnia related to its amphetamine-like (N-propynyl-methamphetamine) structure. Using the recommended regimen of one tablet in the morning and one at noon can minimize insomnia. Any of the other "dopaminergic" adverse effects that can occur with other antiparkinsonian medications can be associated with selegiline (gastrointestinal upset, orthostatic hypotension, worsening or onset of dyskinetic movements, and development of mental status changes such as visual hallucinations and agitation).

(4) The emergence of dyskinetic movements (see **I.A.2.b.4.**) after the addition of selegiline to levodopa frequently can be managed most effectively by lowering of the dose of levodopa or of selegiline. The tyramine or "wine and cheese" reaction mediated by inhibition of MAO-A has not been associated with the use of selegiline given at the recommended dosage.

(5) **Patients taking selegiline should not be given meperidine** (Demerol; Sanofi, New York, NY, U.S.A.) for pain control. There have been reports of "serotonin syndrome" in patients taking selegiline with specific serotonin reuptake inhibitors (SSRIs) for depression. However, this risk is minimal, and patients with PD taking selegiline commonly take SSRIs without serious problems.

b. **Symptomatic management of PD.** Many drugs are useful for improving parkinsonian symptoms. Initiation of PD treatment should be tailored to the needs of a particular patient. Age of the patient, employment status, predominant PD symptoms, severity of illness, intercurrent medical problems, side-effect profile of previous medications, and cost should be taken into account when initiating treatment. In many instances, it is appropriate to withhold medication until symptoms interfere with activities of daily living or become bothersome for the patient.

(1) **Amantadine** (Symmetrel; Endo Pharmaceuticals, Chadds Ford, PA, U.S.A.) has been used for many years in the management of mild to moderate Parkinson's disease and has recently been found to help those with advanced disease. The mechanism of action, although not well understood, is related to its weak glutamine N-methyl-D-aspartate (NMDA) receptor antagonism that may decrease the release of striatal acetylcholine. Amantadine also promotes dopamine release, blocks dopamine reuptake, and stimulates dopamine receptors.

   (a) Amantadine can be used as initial therapy for PD, particularly for patients who have mild to moderate bradykinesia, rigidity, and tremor. The half-life of amantadine is between 10 and 28 hours, and the drug is excreted unchanged in the urine. Patients with **renal failure** should have their doses adjusted to prevent toxicity. The use of amantadine with selegiline or dopamine agonists in the care of patients with early disease can provide quite acceptable control of symptoms. Amantadine also can be used for adjunctive treatment of patients taking levodopa. It can be useful in advanced disease to help reduce or suppress dyskinesia. The usual dosage range for amantadine is 100 mg two or three times a day (Table 41.2). Elderly patients and those sensitive to the effects of medications should probably start with 25 mg/d for a few days. The dosage can be titrated upward to twice a day dosing with the suspension preparation of amantadine (50 mg/5 mL).

   (b) **Adverse effects** of amantadine are generally mild; however, a large number of patients cannot tolerate it. The most important potential dopaminergic effects are changes in mental status, nightmares, insomnia, and hallucinations that are more common in older patients, especially if they are taking other antiparkinsonian medications. Patients also may have anticholinergic side effects such as dry mouth, blurred vision, poor short-term memory, and urinary hesitation or obstruction. A macular rash of the lower extremities, known as **livedo reticularis,** is common, although this rash is of primarily cosmetic importance. The common lower extremity edema caused by

Table 41.2 Antiparkinsonian medications

Drug	Total daily dose (mg)	Frequency
Selegiline	5–10	b.i.d. (morning and noon)
Amantadine	200–400	b.i.d.–q.i.d.
Trihexyphenidyl	4–8	b.i.d.–q.i.d.
Benztropine	2–4	b.i.d.–q.i.d.
Levodopa	300–2,500	t.i.d. initially
Levodopa CR	400–1,600	b.i.d. initially
Bromocriptine	7.5–60	t.i.d.
Cabergoline	1–10	q.d.
Pergolide	0.75–8.0	t.i.d.
Pramipexole	1–4.5	t.i.d.
Ropinirole	3–24	t.i.d.

b.i.d., twice a day; q.i.d., four times a day; t.i.d., three times a day; q.d., every day.

amantadine can be so severe as to necessitate discontinuation of the drug.

(2) **Anticholinergic drugs** have been used for many years in the management of PD and were used before the discovery of levodopa. Dopamine depletion in the striatum causes a relative "hypercholinergic" state that responds to the use of anticholinergic drugs. Many centrally acting anticholinergic drugs are available, but the two most commonly used in the United States are **trihexyphenidyl** (Artane; Lederle, Pearl River, NY, U.S.A.) and **benztropine** (Cogentin; Merck, West Point, PA, U.S.A.). **Diphenhydramine** (Benadryl; Pfizer, New York, NY, U.S.A.) is only infrequently used in PD because of its sedative side effects. **Biperiden** (Akineton; Knoll, Mount Olive, NJ, U.S.A.), **orphenadrine** (Norflex; 3M Pharmaceuticals, St. Paul, MN, U.S.A.), and **procyclidine** (Kemadrin; GlaxoSmithKline, Thoerismaus, Switzerland) are used in Europe.

   (a) Anticholinergics may be used early in the course of PD and seem to be particularly effective in controlling tremor with lesser effects on bradykinesia and balance problems. Anticholinergics also may be effective for patients with more advanced disease, but their use may be limited by adverse effects (see **I.A.2.b.2.b**). Typically, **trihexyphenidyl** is started at doses of 1 mg/d and increased weekly up to 2 mg three times per day until symptomatic control is obtained or until the development of side effects. **Benztropine** usually is started at 0.5 mg/d and titrated up to 4 mg/d. **Table 41.2** shows dosage ranges used for trihexyphenidyl and benztropine. If anticholinergics are to be discontinued, this should be done gradually to avoid withdrawal effects.

   (b) **Adverse effects** of anticholinergic medications include both peripheral and central side effects. **Peripheral antimuscarinic side effects** include dry mouth, impaired visual accommodation, urinary retention, constipation, tachycardia, and impaired sweating. These side effects are especially troublesome to patients with closed-angle glaucoma and prostatic hypertrophy. **Central effects** include sedation, dysphoria, memory difficulties, confusion, and hallucinations. Central side effects are more common among older patients with more advanced PD and limit the use of anticholinergics in this population.

(3) **Dopamine receptor agonists** are medications that directly stimulate dopamine receptors. Five dopamine agonists are available in the United States—**bromocriptine** (Parlodel; Novartis, East Hanover, NJ, U.S.A.), **pergolide** (Permax; Elan Pharmaceuticals, South San Francisco, CA, U.S.A.), **pramipexole** (Mirapex; Pharmacia & Upjohn, Kalamazoo, MI, U.S.A.), **ropinirole** (Requip; GlaxoSmithKline, Research Triangle Park, NC, U.S.A.), and **cabergoline** (Dostinex; Pharmacia & Upjohn, Peapack, NJ, U.S.A.). Apomorphine is available in other countries.

   (a) Dopamine receptor agonists may relieve all of the cardinal manifestations of PD. These drugs have several theoretical advantages over levodopa. They act on striatal dopamine receptors independently of the degenerating dopaminergic neurons. They cause less **dyskinesia** and **motor fluctuation** because of their longer duration of action. They have a levodopa "sparing" effect. Finally, they may be neuroprotective. Agonists are useful in the management of **early PD** both as monotherapy and as adjuncts to levodopa. To minimize side effects, the dosage of a dopamine agonist should be started at a very small dose and gradually increased every few days until the desired effect is obtained. **Bromocriptine** usually is started at 1.25 mg twice a day and increased slowly to at least 2.5 mg three times a day. **Cabergoline** is started at 0.25 mg/d and increased to an average dose of 4 mg/d. **Pergolide** usually is started at 0.025 mg/d for 3 days and slowly titrated every 3 days. **Pramipexole** usually is started at 0.125 mg three times a day for 1 week and titrated up in weekly increments. **Ropinirole** usually is started at 0.25 mg three times a day and titrated up weekly. The therapeutic dosage ranges for the agonists are listed in Table 41.2. **Apomorphine** is a short-acting dopamine agonist that usually is administered subcutaneously for patients with advance PD as a "rescue" agent for severe "off" periods. An apomorphine challenge is required to determine the correct dose of the drug. This challenge should be carried out after pretreatment with **domperidone** for 3 days and after an electrocardiogram has been obtained to rule out serious cardiac arrhythmia.

(b) Adverse effects of dopamine receptor agonists are generally similar to the dopaminergic effects discussed in **I.A.2.b.4.d.** They include **nausea, vomiting, postural hypotension,** and **psychiatric manifestations.** These side effects usually abate over days to weeks. However, some patients occasionally have difficulty with gastrointestinal upset despite a gradual increase in dosage. In such cases, the dosage can be increased even more slowly, or adjunctive treatment with **domperidone** (Motilium; Janssen-Ortho, North York, Ontario, Canada) can be given. Elderly and cognitively impaired patients are more prone to psychiatric side effects. With the agonists, this may be related to the high limbic dopamine D3 receptor affinity of some of these agonists. Changes in mental status can be managed as discussed in **sec. I.A.2.b.8.** Dopamine agonists also can cause considerable **ankle edema.** Daytime **hypersomnia** with episodes of falling asleep at inappropriate times has been described in patients taking dopamine agonists. This excessive sleepiness may resolve with dose reduction or with the addition of a stimulant such as modafinil (Provigil; Cephalon, West Chester, PA, U.S.A.). In addition, **ergot-derivative dopamine agonists** such as bromocriptine, cabergoline, and pergolide in rare instances cause **pulmonary** and **retroperitoneal fibrosis, vasospasm,** and **erythromelalgia** and can exacerbate **angina** and **peptic ulcer disease.**

(4) **Levodopa** is the most effective antiparkinsonian medication and is the standard with which other drugs are compared. Levodopa is the precursor of dopamine. It is absorbed mainly in the proximal small intestine by a carrier-mediated process for neutral amino acids and is similarly transported across the blood–brain barrier. Once in the brain, it is converted to dopamine by the enzyme dopa decarboxylase. Levodopa is routinely administered in combination with a peripheral **dopa decarboxylase inhibitor** (carbidopa or benserazide) that does not cross the blood–brain barrier. Inhibition of peripheral dopa decarboxylase markedly reduces the required total daily dose of levodopa and minimizes the gastrointestinal upset and hypotension caused by peripheral conversion of levodopa to dopamine. Early in the course of the disease, levodopa can provide almost complete relief of symptoms. Unfortunately, in more advanced disease, the use of levodopa can be complicated by **response fluctuations** and **dyskinesia** (see **I.A.2.b.4.c.**).

(a) Available preparations of levodopa include **regular** (also known as "immediate-release") **carbidopa-levodopa** (Sinemet; Bristol-Myers Squibb, Princeton, NJ, U.S.A.) and a

controlled-release preparation (Sinemet CR). A minimum of 75 mg/d of carbidopa is required for appropriate peripheral dopa decarboxylase inhibition. In Europe, **benserazide-levodopa preparations** (Madopar; Roche Pharma, Basel, Switzerland) are also available. Carbidopa-levodopa preparations are available as 10/100, 25/100, and 25/250 tablets (milligrams carbidopa/milligrams levodopa) and as 25/100 and 50/200 tablets in the controlled-release preparation. Benserazide-levodopa preparations are available as 25/100 and 50/200 tablets (milligrams benserazide/milligrams levodopa). Sustained-release benserazide-levodopa is also available (Madopar HBS). Sustained release preparations are 30% less bioavailable than are immediate release forms (e.g., 500 mg of sustained release levodopa is equivalent to approximately 350 mg of immediate release formulation).

(b) Levodopa generally relieves all of the cardinal signs of PD—bradykinesia, tremor, and rigidity. Other associated symptoms, such as hypophonia, dysphagia, and loss of postural reflexes, are less reliably relieved. A lack of response to levodopa suggests a possible diagnosis of one of the Parkinson-plus syndromes. An adequate trial of carbidopa-levodopa with doses up to 1,500 mg of levodopa should be tried for approximately 4 weeks before it is concluded that the patient is a nonresponder. Treatment with carbidopa-levodopa usually is initiated using one 25/100 standard-release tablet three times a day or one 50/200 controlled-release tablet twice a day. Some physicians prefer to start at smaller doses and titrate upward over several days to minimize acute side effects. The dose used should be the lowest effective dose that will provide good control of PD symptoms. Some patients may have acute side effects such as **nausea, vomiting,** and **hypotension.** This may reflect insufficient inhibition of the peripheral dopa decarboxylase and can be managed by means of adding extra carbidopa 25 to 50 mg (Lodosyn; Bristol-Myers Squibb, New York, NY, U.S.A.) or benserazide 20 minutes before each levodopa dose. Another option is to use a peripheral dopamine receptor blocker such as **domperidone** in doses of 10 to 20 mg 20 minutes before each dose of levodopa. Domperidone is not currently available in the United States but is widely used in many countries.

(c) During the first few years of levodopa therapy, patients experience continuous clinical benefit regardless of when they take the medication (the so-called **levodopa honeymoon period**). As the disease progresses and with long-term use of levodopa, patients begin to notice **wearing off** of benefit before the next scheduled dose, or they have new choreiform or dystonic movements (dyskinesia). The motor fluctuation and dyskinesia usually occur in patients with moderate to advanced disease after 2 to 10 years of levodopa therapy. Patients younger than 40 years are more prone to dyskinesia and motor fluctuations. Despite a levodopa plasma half-life of 1 to 2 hours, the effect of the medication lasts much longer in patients with mild disease, perhaps as a result of the storage of dopamine by the remaining dopaminergic neurons. Later in the disease, the control of PD symptoms depends on the minute-to-minute availability of levodopa from the blood.

The short half-life of immediate-release levodopa is believed to be a major factor in the development of motor complications. The incidence of fluctuation and dyskinesia has been significantly lower in both human and animal studies of the use of long-acting agents such as dopamine agonists. Sustained-release formulations should theoretically limit the pulsatile delivery of levodopa and therefore reduce the incidence of motor complications, although this has not been proved in controlled clinical trials.

Wearing off is a gradual loss of medication effectiveness before the next dose; however, with time patients may have more dramatic and abrupt changes between **on states** when PO symptoms are minimal and **off states** when PO symptoms are prominent. There is also potential for **rebound worsening,** in which PD symptoms are more severe at the end of a dose of levodopa than at baseline before levodopa is taken.

Higher blood levels of levodopa can cause **dyskinetic movements** in patients with moderate to advanced disease. Dyskinetic movements usually are choreatic and most commonly involve the head and neck. The movements can, however, be quite diverse and involve feet, legs, trunk, and the oral–buccal–lingual muscles. They can appear when levodopa is controlling PD symptoms (**peak dose dyskinesia**) or occur at the beginning of or at the end of a dose of levodopa (**diphasic dyskinesia**). These diphasic forms of dyskinesia often are severe and debilitating. Other potential forms of dyskinesia in PD include **off-period dystonia,** which usually is quite painful. This can occur in the morning before the first dose of levodopa or at the end of a dose (**end of dose dystonia**). Mild dyskinetic movements usually are well tolerated by patients because they occur when medications are effectively controlling PD symptoms. Patients often prefer to be dyskinetic and mobile rather than akinetic and rigid. Management of response fluctuations is discussed in **I.A.2.b.7.**

- **(d)** **Adverse effects** of levodopa are representative of those of dopaminergic excess. When carbidopa-levodopa is initiated, **gastrointestinal upset** can occur, even with typically sufficient dosages of carbidopa. Gastrointestinal upset usually resolves gradually with continued use of the drug. This effect can be minimized by having patients take carbidopa-levodopa after meals or take **supplemental carbidopa** or **domperidone** as discussed in **I.A.2.b.(4)(b). Changes in mental status** can occur, especially in patients with moderate to advanced disease. These changes can take the form of overt psychosis, paranoia, sexual preoccupation, mania, or agitation. **Visual hallucinations** can be quite vivid and frequently occur in the form of people or animals. Usually the patient retains insight into the nature of these hallucinations, and they are not menacing for them. However, later in the course of the disease, the hallucinations and delusions can become quite bothersome and frightening. Nightmares, vivid dreams, and night terrors often precede the development of hallucinations. Mental status changes usually are dose dependent and typically lessen with medication reduction. Anecdotal reports of accelerated melanoma growth prompt us to use levodopa with caution in the care of patients with a history of such malignant tumors.
- **(5)** **Catechol-O-methyl-transferase (COMT) inhibitors** are used as adjuncts to levodopa. They block the peripheral conversion of levodopa to 3-O-methyldopa and increase the bioavailability of levodopa. Two COMT inhibitors are available—tolcapone (Tasmar; Roche, Nutley, NJ, U.S.A.) and entacapone (Comtan; Novartis, East Hanover, NJ, U.S.A.). Tolcapone is used in doses of 100 to 200 mg three times a day, and 200 mg entacapone is given with each dose of levodopa up to 2,000 mg/d. Use of tolcapone is greatly

restricted because of a few reported cases of **liver failure** and **death** among patients taking this drug. If tolcapone is used, liver function tests should be performed biweekly. Entacapone does not have liver toxicity, so no monitoring is indicated. Side effects of COMT inhibitors are related to increased bioavailability of levodopa (dyskinesia and neuropsychiatric side effects). In addition, **diarrhea** and a **brownish-orange discoloration of the urine** may occur. These drugs are mainly used to treat patients with wearing off to prolong the levodopa response.

(6) It is now recommended that initiation of levodopa treatment of patients younger than 70 years be delayed to prevent long-term complications. For young patients, dopamine agonists can be used in monotherapy or in combination with anticholinergics, selegiline, or amantadine. For **young patients with PD with tremor-predominant disease,** sole use of an anticholinergic agent can be considered. For **patients older than 70 years,** and those with **cognitive problems,** consider starting with levodopa to avoid the cognitive side effects of other antiparkinsonian medications. If levodopa is started, the **sustained-release formulation** can be considered. This agent has the theoretical advantage of a more continuous stimulation of the striatum compared with the immediate-release formulation. Another alternative is to use a COMT inhibitor with carbidopa-levodopa to obtain more constant, nonpulsatile stimulation of dopamine receptors. The COMT inhibitors are currently reserved for late PD; however, they may have a role in earlier stages of the disease.

(7) **Management of response fluctuations** can be complex. Response fluctuations include **peak-dose choreoathetoid dyskinetic movements, diphasic dyskinesia or dystonia, gradual loss of medication effect (wearing off),** or the **sudden random loss of medication effect (on-off phenomenon).** Management response fluctuations frequently require combination therapy. **Peak-dose dyskinetic movements** often lessen with reduction of the levodopa dose or discontinuation of selegiline. **Diphasic dyskinesia** can be managed by means of increasing dopamine agonists or increasing the dose of levodopa.

Early morning dystonia can be managed with nocturnal doses of sustained release levodopa, nocturnal dopamine agonists, taking levodopa earlier in the morning, adding a COMT inhibitor to the evening dose of levodopa, or with botulinum toxin injections. If dystonia appears during wearing off, management of the wearing off relieves the dystonia. **Peak-dose dystonia** can be managed in a manner similar to that for peak-dose dyskinesia. As in other forms of dystonia, peak-dose dystonia may be relieved with benzodiazepines, baclofen, muscle relaxants, or botulinum toxin injections.

Wearing off can be improved with the use of sustained-release levodopa, adding or increasing dopamine agonists, increasing the frequency of administration or the dose of levodopa, adding selegiline or adding a COMT inhibitor. **Unpredictable on-off episodes** are extremely difficult to manage. One can begin by changing from controlled-release levodopa to immediate-release preparation, by adding or increasing dopamine agonists, adding a COMT inhibitor, modifying the distribution of dietary protein, or using apomorphine. Patients with complex patterns of response fluctuations are best treated by a physician experienced in the use of combination therapy for PD. When medical management does not achieve appropriate control of dyskinesia and complex motor fluctuation, surgical options become a consideration (see **I.A.3.**).

(8) **Visual hallucinations** and **psychosis** are adverse effects that can occur in association with almost any antiparkinsonian medication.

These effects usually are improved simply by lowering the doses of antiparkinsonian medications, if possible. The initial approach is trying to identify and control the triggering event, such as infection or metabolic derangement. If no other cause can be identified, it may be assumed that the psychosis is due to dopaminergic excess or anticholinergic toxicity. The order in which antiparkinsonian agents should be decreased or discontinued should be as follows: anticholinergics, amantadine, selegiline, and dopamine agonists. If worsening of motor symptoms make such a reduction impossible, the judicious use of an atypical neuroleptic medication may be necessary. To avoid exacerbation of the parkinsonism, neuroleptic agents with the least possible extrapyramidal side effects should be chosen. **Clozapine** (Clozaril; Novartis) is an atypical neuroleptic drug that does not worsen PD but can actually relieve dyskinesia and tremor and control hallucinations and psychosis. The beginning dose is usually 6.25 mg at bedtime. Doses of 50 mg often are sufficient to control hallucinations. One percent to 2% of patients taking clozapine experience **agranulocytosis.** Weekly blood counts are needed during the first 6 months of therapy and biweekly thereafter. Another atypical neuroleptic, quetiapine (Seroquel; Astra-Zeneca, Wilmington, DE, U.S.A.), is effective in the management of dopaminergic psychosis at doses of 12.5 mg to 50 mg at night. **Ondansetron** (Zofran; GlaxoSmithKline, Research Triangle Park, NC, U.S.A.), a serotonin ($5\text{-}HT_3$) antagonist used to manage nausea and vomiting can control hallucinations without interfering with PD symptoms (doses of 12 to 24 mg/d). Among the classic neuroleptics, thioridazine (Mellaril; Novartis) probably has the fewest extrapyramidal side effects and could be used if atypical agents are unavailable.

(9) **Constipation** is a common problem among patients with PD. Management should include dietary modifications, increasing fluid and fiber intake, and exercise. Psyllium (Metamucil; Procter & Gamble, Cincinnati, OH, U.S.A.) 1 tsp (5 mL) two to four times a day may be added. Anticholinergics, if in use, should be stopped. Osmotic agents such as sorbitol and lactulose (10 to 20 g/d) often are helpful. Agents that stimulate intestinal motility, such as bisacodyl (Dulcolax; Novartis), can be added if necessary. Metoclopramide (Reglan; Robins, Richmond, VA, U.S.A.) should not be given, because it worsens parkinsonism. Some patients may need enemas.

(10) Other potential problems of patients with PD include **nocturia, urinary urgency and frequency, erectile dysfunction, dysphagia, orthostatic hypotension,** and **sleep problems** (see Chapters 7, 9, 18, 31). **Depression** requires special mention because it is very common (present in 40% of patients with PD) and responds well to antidepressant medications such as SSRIs, bupropion (Wellbutrin; GlaxoSmithKline), and tricyclic antidepressants. Bupropion has the theoretical advantage of relieving PD symptoms owing to its enhancement of dopaminergic neurotransmission.

(11) **Contraindicated medications** for patients with PD generally are those with antidopaminergic activity, such as neuroleptics and some antiemetics—promethazine, prochlorperazine, and metoclopramide. Meperidine and SSRIs are discussed in I.A.2.a.

3. **Surgery.** The stereotactic surgical options for treatment of patients with PD are ablative procedures and **chronic stimulation** at different targets—ventral intermediate nucleus of the thalamus (Vim), globus pallidus interna (Gpi), and subthalamic nucleus (STN). The success of surgical treatment of patients with PD depends on a careful selection of the appropriate candidates. First, only patients with idiopathic PD should be considered. Patients with advanced disease and poor response to levodopa, dementia, uncontrolled depression, uncontrolled hallucinations, unstable medical problems,

or a cardiac pacemaker or defibrillator are poor candidates for these operations, especially for **deep brain stimulation (DBS).** Patients undergoing surgery should need a presurgical neuropsychological evaluation to rule out significant cognitive dysfunction. Finding the optimal DBS parameters (voltage amplitude, pulse width, rate, polarity, and electrode configuration) for a particular patient can be time consuming and requires frequent visits for adjustments, especially in the first few months.

   a. Thalamotomy and **thalamic DBS** are procedures directed at managing contralateral medically intractable **tremor.** Neither of these two procedures improves other features of PD. During thalamotomy, an ablative radiofrequency lesion is applied in the **Vim** with stereotactic guidance. For DBS, an electrode is stereotactically placed in the Vim and connected to the stimulator unit, which is implanted subcutaneously under the homolateral clavicle. Tremor reduction occurs in approximately 80% of patients. Thalamic ablation and DBS seem to be equally efficacious. However, bilateral thalamotomy is associated with a high incidence of dysarthria and for this reason is not performed. The potential benefit of thalamic DBS is that interruption of bilateral thalamic output can be achieved with fewer side effects. The procedure also allows manipulation of stimulation parameters to maximize tremor control over the course of years. Complications can occur with either treatment modality. With DBS, transient paresthesia, paresis, dysarthria, dystonia, and chorea have been described when the stimulator is on. Local infection and lead fractures are not infrequent.

   b. Pallidotomy and **pallidal DBS** targeting the posteroventral Gpi are useful treatments of patients with PD with severe dyskinesia and motor fluctuations. These operations are performed on the Gpi contralateral to the more symptomatic side. Bilateral ablative procedures are associated with a high incidence of speech complications and usually are not recommended. Improvement in motor function can be striking in patients who still respond well to levodopa, mainly by decreasing dyskinesia. PD symptoms that persist during the on state (e.g., freezing, dysarthria) do not respond well to pallidotomy. Improvement in the off state is approximately 30% for pallidotomy and 40% for pallidal DBS. The ideal candidate for unilateral pallidotomy is an old, cognitively intact patient with PD who has asymmetric disease with marked dyskinesia and excellent response to levodopa. However, given the ablative nature of pallidotomy, DBS is becoming the favored mode of treatment of such patients.

   c. STN DBS is currently the preferred surgical procedure for advanced PD with motor fluctuations and dyskinesia. This operation can be performed on both sides at the same time or serially and can improve tremor, akinesia, postural stability, and gait. The improvement is mainly during the off state with 60% improvement in motor scores. DBS may improve the quality of the on state approximately 10%. For this reason, a poor response to levodopa before surgery precludes good results of STN DBS. STN stimulation allows greater reduction of antiparkinsonian medication compared with that possible with pallidal operations. Side effects include intracranial hematoma during surgery, local infection, transient changes in mental status, and dystonia, among others. In general, placement of intraparenchymatous electrodes is associated with a complication rate between 1% and 3%. The ideal candidate for bilateral STN DBS is a patient younger than 70 years with excellent response to levodopa and no cognitive problems who has a good social support system and realistic expectations of the procedure. Patients should be aware that it can take months to determine optimal stimulation parameters in conjunction with medication changes.

B. Parkinson-plus syndromes are a group of uncommon degenerative conditions that share some features with idiopathic PD, mainly the rigid-akinetic syndrome.

   1. Multiple system atrophy (MSA) is a progressive, adult-onset degenerative disease characterized by various proportions of **parkinsonism, cerebellar**

dysfunction, and **autonomic failure.** (When parkinsonism predominates, this is **striatonigral degeneration;** when cerebellar features predominate, this is **olivopontocerebellar degeneration;** and when autonomic failure predominates, this is **Shy–Drager syndrome.**). The parkinsonism usually is more symmetric than in PD and with a lower incidence of resting tremor. The presence of pyramidal features, severe early orthostatic hypotension, urinary incontinence, early erectile dysfunction, Raynaud's phenomenon, inspiratory stridor, anterocollis, and cerebellar signs should suggest the diagnosis of MSA.

a. Dopaminergic therapy with levodopa usually provides modest improvement of parkinsonism but approximately one fourth to one third of patients may have a transient good to excellent response.

b. Orthostatic hypotension is frequently of greatest concern and can be worsened by most antiparkinsonian medications. Treatment may include nonpharmacologic measures such as liberalizing salt and water intake, using waist-high elastic stockings, and elevating the legs several times per day. Raising the head of the bed 8 inches (20 cm) at night may help prevent supine hypertension and excessive nocturnal diuresis. Patients should be careful rising from the sitting or supine positions and should avoid heavy meals. Caffeine in the morning and after meals often is effective. Treatment with **fludrocortisone** (Florinef; Bristol-Myers Squibb, Princeton, NJ, U.S.A.), usually at doses of 0.1 to 0.3 mg/d, may be needed. Pedal edema and supine hypertension can become troublesome as a result. The α-adrenergic agonist **midodrine** (ProAmatine; Roberts, Eatontown, NJ, U.S.A.) is a short-acting drug useful for orthostatic hypotension. Doses up to 30 mg/d can be used, but doses in the evening should be avoided to prevent hypertension when recumbent. Should this occur, the use of a short-acting antihypertensive medication at bedtime may be necessary. **Indomethacin,** 25 mg three times a day, also can improve orthostasis for some patients. Other potentially useful drugs are erythropoietin, ergots, and desmopressin.

c. **Urinary frequency** or **incontinence** should be evaluated with the assistance of a urologist, because other causes of urologic dysfunction, such as prostate enlargement or frequent urinary tract infections, are common in this age group. Treatment such as **oxybutynin** (Ditropan; ALZA, Mountain View, CA, U.S.A.) or **tolterodine** (Detrol; Pharmacia & Upjohn) for a spastic bladder or **bethanechol** (Urecholine; Odyssey, East Hanover, NJ, U.S.A.) for a hypotonic bladder may provide relief. Some patients need intermittent or continuous catheterization. **Sildenafil** (Viagra; Pfizer) may be useful for management of erectile dysfunction. Surgical management of impotence may be necessary in some cases.

d. Patient with other problems of MSA, such as dysarthria and dysphagia, may benefit from evaluation by a speech therapist. Some patients with severe dysphagia need tube feeding. Gait difficulties and instability may necessitate use of supportive devices and physical therapy. Many patients with MSA who have daytime stridor should undergo a sleep study to determine whether they have sleep apnea.

2. **Progressive supranuclear palsy (PSP)** is a Parkinson-plus syndrome characterized by early postural instability, neck rigidity, supranuclear vertical gaze abnormalities, pseudobulbar palsy, subcortical or frontal dementia, and apathy. One of the primary sources of disability for these patients is profound loss of balance, dysphagia, and dysarthria.

a. **Management** of PSP is extremely limited. Antiparkinsonian medications may have a transient or mild effect. In general, it may be worthwhile to introduce a brief trial of levodopa, amitriptyline, or amantadine. However, these agents are not typically helpful in the long term.

b. Symptomatic palliative therapies for PSP include management of dysarthria and dysphagia with the assistance of a speech therapist and may include the use of a gastrostomy tube among other measures. Because of the significantly decreased blinking rate, patients with PSP are at increased risk of keratitis and should use artificial tears. Blepharospasm and neck dystonia can be managed with botulinum toxin injections. Depression and emotional incontinence can be managed with antidepressants. Gait instability can be managed with physical therapy and supportive devices (e.g., weighted walkers).

II. **Hyperkinetic movement disorders**

   A. **Chorea** is an involuntary movement disorder characterized by irregular, unpredictable, brief, jerky movements that flit from one part of the body to another in a random sequence. Chorea can result from a variety of disorders of the basal ganglia, including neurodegenerative diseases, drugs, toxic and metabolic abnormalities, vascular insults, and autoimmune diseases. Management of chorea is uniform regardless of the underlying cause.

   1. **Huntington's disease (HD)** is an autosomal-dominant degenerative brain disorder characterized by the insidious development of motor, cognitive, and psychiatric symptoms progressing toward death an average of 21 years after onset of symptoms. The underlying genetic defect is the expansion of a CAG trinucleotide repeats in the first exon of the HD gene, the product of which is a protein called **huntingtin.** Pathologically, there is early and selective neuronal loss of **medium-sized spiny neurons** in the striatum. Symptomatic treatment is directed at the major clinical features of the disease. Many clinical trials of drugs with putative neuroprotective effect have been conducted, including use of baclofen, dextromethorphan, lamotrigine, tocopherol, and idebenone, among others. The results of these studies have been largely negative. **Coenzyme Q-10** has been shown to significantly decrease cortical lactate levels in patients with HD and to be well tolerated in doses up to 1,200 mg/d. There is evidence that creatine can delay brain atrophy in transgenic HD mouse models. Caspases, the proteases responsible for apoptotic mechanisms, appear to be involved in the molecular pathologic mechanism of HD by directly cleaving huntingtin and generating toxic protein fragments containing polyglutamine tracts. Inhibition of caspases may be a potential therapeutic strategy for management of HD.

      a. Choreiform movements can be reliably controlled with **neuroleptics** that have potent postsynaptic dopamine blocking effects. Anxiolytics such as lorazepam and clonazepam also may decrease chorea. Although chorea is the hallmark of HD, it can be one of the least disabling features of the disease and does not necessitate treatment unless it is troublesome to the patient. Among the neuroleptics, haloperidol (Haldol; Ortho-McNeil, Raritan, NJ, U.S.A.) is one of the most commonly prescribed for management of chorea, but others may be equally effective. Relatively low dosages, typically 1 to 2 mg two or three times a day, starting with 0.5 mg at bedtime, usually are required. There is no added benefit for management of chorea with more than 10 mg of haloperidol. Neuroleptics must be used judiciously in the care of patients with HD because these agents can worsen postural reflexes, depressive symptoms, and the parkinsonism that accompanies juvenile and advanced adult HD. Neuroleptics also can cause tardive syndromes and worsen the overall functional status of the patient. Tetrabenazine, a reversible dopamine depleter and postsynaptic dopamine blocker, is effective in reducing chorea but is not commercially available in the United States.

      b. **Depression** affects at least 30% to 50% of patients with HD and can precede the motor manifestations by an average of 5 years. In HD, the suicide rate is 4 to 8 times greater than in the general population. Depression is more common among patients with late-onset HD than those with earlier onset disease. Depression can be managed with all standard agents used for the management of major depression. **SSRIs** typically are the drug of choice for HD, but use of **tricyclic antidepressants** with low anticholinergic effects also can be considered. **Mirtazapine** (Remeron; Organon, West Orange, NJ, U.S.A.) can be helpful in the care of HD patients with cachexia, and anxiety and insomnia as it can increase body weight and assist in sleep induction.

  c. **Irritability** may be the most common psychiatric disorder in HD. Patients may overreact or exhibit explosive behavior. **Nonpharmacologic strategies** such as identification and avoidance of triggers should be implemented. However, **SSRIs** are commonly needed to manage irritability.

  d. **Aggressive behavior** in HD most commonly accompanies irritability. Patients with HD may have a low threshold for anger, and their responses may be disproportionate to the provocative stimulus. Violent behaviors of all type are more frequent in the early stages of the disease rather than in the middle and late stages. Treatment is based on the predominant cause of the behavior; neuroleptics for delusion-based violence, antidepressants for depressive suicidal behavior, and propranolol for aggression associated with frustration and impatience.

  e. **Mania** and **hypomania** can occur in HD. Approximately 10% of HD patients may exhibit hypomanic behavior that can last for several days to several months. Mania in HD responds better to carbamazepine than to lithium. Other therapeutic alternatives are valproic acid and clonazepam.

  f. **Psychosis** has an estimated frequency of 3% to 25% among patients with HD and is more common among patients with early-onset disease than with disease that begins in midlife or old age. Neuroleptics usually are more useful to control delusions than they are hallucinations. Atypical antipsychotic agents such as **clozapine, quetiapine, olanzapine,** and **risperidone** are effective in controlling psychotic symptoms with a lower risk of extrapyramidal side effects or of tardive dyskinesia.

  2. Other causes of chorea include neurodegenerative disorders (e.g., neuro-acanthocytosis, Wilson's disease, dentatorubropallidoluysian atrophy), Sydenham's chorea, systemic lupus erythematosus, hyperthyroidism, and drug-induced chorea (e.g., from phenytoin, oral contraceptives, stimulants, or antiparkinsonian drugs). Regardless of the underlying cause, the movements can be improved with the use of neuroleptics. The risk of tardive dyskinesia should be discussed with the patient and documented in the chart if prolonged treatment is anticipated. The main point of concern in these cases is identification of the underlying diagnosis because symptomatic treatment is relatively straightforward.

  3. **Hemiballismus** is a rare condition of violent, flailing motion of the proximal portion of limbs on one side of the body. It usually is caused by lesions in the **contralateral subthalamic nucleus.** Treatment includes supportive care, prevention of self-injury, and pharmacologic agents such as benzodiazepines, neuroleptics, and catecholamine-depleting agents like reserpine and tetrabenazine. γAminobutyric acid–ergic drugs such as valproic acid may be another therapeutic option. Surgical alternatives exist for patients who do not appropriately respond to medical therapy.

B. **Tics** are common movement disorders, affecting as many as 20% of children. Tics are brief, usually rapid, purposeless, repetitive movements involving one or more muscular groups. They are differentiated from other movement disorders by their suppressibility, premonitory "urge," and stereotypic appearance.

  1. **Tourette's syndrome (TS)** is a childhood-onset neuropsychiatric disorder characterized by motor and vocal tics. Tics range from simple head movements or vocalizations to complex ritualistic behaviors. Slow, sustained tics are possible and referred to as **dystonic tics.** Tics wax and wane and tend to improve considerably during adulthood. **Obsessive–compulsive behavior** and **attention deficit disorder (ADD)** are comorbid conditions frequently associated with TS and are typically more disabling than tics themselves.

  a. **Tics** do not require treatment unless they are troublesome to the patient. The first step in treatment is education and reassurance. If further intervention is needed, clonidine (Catapres; Boehringer Ingelheim, Ridgefield, CT, U.S.A.) starting at 0.05 mg at bedtime and increased 0.05 mg every few days can be considered (most patients respond to 0.1 mg three or four times a day). Once the initial titration is completed, the patch preparation can be used once per week instead of the oral preparation. There are anecdotal reports that brand-name Catapres may be more efficacious than the generic preparation. However, the efficacy of clonidine for tic control is modest at best. Guanfacine (Tenex; Robins) starting at 0.5 to 1 mg at bedtime is another option that may be less sedating than clonidine.

Neuroleptics are the most efficacious agents for tic suppression. Haloperidol is probably the most common neuroleptic used for tics. Pimozide (Orap; Gate, Sellersville, PA, U.S.A.) was developed specifically for use in TS and may cause less sedation than does haloperidol. Pimozide may prolong the QT interval, and it is contraindicated in the care of patients with long-QT syndrome or arrhythmias or those patients taking other drugs that prolong the QT interval. There are dietary restrictions with pimozide; for example, grapefruit juice should not be ingested. Other neuroleptics such as trifluoperazine (Stelazine; GlaxoSmithKline) and thiothixene (Navane; Pfizer) also can be helpful. Atypical antipsychotics such as risperidone (Risperdal; Janssen, Titusville, NJ, U.S.A.) are starting to be used with increasing frequency. However, risperidone causes significant weight gain, which limits its usefulness. The new atypical agent, ziprasidone (Geodon; Pfizer), has the advantage of not causing weight gain, but it can prolong the QT interval.

A given neuroleptic used to manage TS may become ineffective over time, in which case substitution for a different neuroleptic can improve tic control. Low dosages of these medications (e.g., less than 6 mg/d haloperidol) usually are required, although the necessary dosage can vary widely among patients and at different times for a given patient. The usual adverse effects of neuroleptics can occur; in particular, sedation or depression may be troublesome. Although the risk of tardive dyskinesia appears to be low among patients with TS, this potential long-term adverse effect must be discussed with patients and documented in the medical record. The usual order of agents used to manage tics typically is clonidine (or guanfacine), risperidone, and haloperidol. Pimozide is becoming a fourth-line agent because of its potential drug interactions and rare reports of sudden death due to prolonged QT syndrome. Clonazepam (Klonopin; Roche) and baclofen may be helpful to some patients. Botulinum toxin injections may be helpful for some tics, such as blinking and blepharospasm.

  b. **Management** of obsessive–compulsive behavior associated with TS is identical to that of the purely psychiatric condition. SSRIs such as sertraline (Zoloft; Pfizer) or fluoxetine (Prozac; Lilly, Indianapolis, IN, U.S.A.) and clomipramine (Anafranil; Novartis) may be used in this regard. The major adverse effects of clomipramine are sedation and anticholinergic effects.

  c. **ADD** and other behavioral disorders of children may be difficult to control. Clonidine, tricyclic antidepressants, or selegiline may be effective. Use of central nervous system (CNS) stimulants such as methylphenidate (Ritalin; Novartis) may ease ADD, but may worsen motor tics. Motor tics occasionally occur first during a trial of medication for ADD. The diverse behavioral abnormalities sometimes exhibited by children with TS not infrequently necessitate family counseling and other nonpharmacologic approaches.

C. **Myoclonus** is shocklike, brief, involuntary movement caused by muscular contraction (positive myoclonus) or inhibition (negative myoclonus). Myoclonus can originate from the cortex, subcortical areas, brainstem, or spinal cord. Quite often an individual patient may have multiple neuroanatomic generators of the myoclonus. Common causes of myoclonus include metabolic derangements, such as renal and hepatic failure, and epileptiform disorders.

  1. **Diagnosis** should include at least the following tests if the diagnosis is not evident after a thorough history and physical examination: blood glucose

and electrolytes, drug and toxin screen, renal and hepatic function tests, brain imaging, and electroencephalography. If this evaluation does not yield to a clear diagnosis, a search for inborn errors of metabolism and paraneoplastic antibodies is indicated.

2. The ideal therapy for myoclonus is to manage the underlying condition. However, symptomatic treatment should be used if treatment is likely to make a significant clinical difference (Table 41.3). Clonazepam at 2 to 6 mg/d, valproic acid 250 to 1,500 mg/d, and piracetam up to 24 g/d (not available in the United States) are first-line drugs for the management of myoclonus. Newly approved anticonvulsants such as zonisamide and levetiracetam are extremely promising therapies for myoclonus. Acetazolamide, anticholinergics, 5-hydroxytryptophan, and tetrabenazine also can be helpful. Many patients need polytherapy to control myoclonus, and sometimes more than four agents are necessary.

D. **Tardive dyskinesia (TD)** is a generic term used to describe persistent involuntary movements that occur as a consequence of long-term treatment with dopamine receptor antagonists. Antipsychotics are the main cause of this disorder, but antiemetics such as metoclopramide and prochlorperazine (Compazine; GlaxoSmithKline), and promethazine (Phenergan; Wyeth-Ayerst, Philadelphia, PA, U.S.A.) also can cause TD. The risk factors for development of classic TD include old age, female sex, mood disorder, and "organic" brain dysfunction. Classic TD usually consists of oral–buccal–lingual dyskinesia that may be associated with a variety of repetitive limb or trunk stereotyped movements.

1. The pathophysiologic mechanism of tardive dyskinesia is not completely understood, but it is thought to be related to an increased number and affinity of postsynaptic D2 dopamine receptors in the striatum. Thus the involuntary movements characteristically worsen, or may first appear, just after the neuroleptic agent is discontinued or after the dose is decreased. Because of the masking of the underlying receptor abnormality, the patient's condition may initially improve after the neuroleptic agent is restarted or after the dosage is increased. Unfortunately, restarting a dopamine receptor antagonist or increasing the dosage is likely to perpetuate the problem.

2. Ideal management of TD would be prevention of this condition by avoiding unnecessary use of dopamine blocking agents and using the minimally effective dose. As a rule, anticholinergic medications can worsen TD. Amantadine and dopamine receptor agonists have been suggested as means of

Table 41.3 Medications used in the management of myoclonus

Drug	Total daily dose (mg)	Frequency
USUALLY HELPFUL DRUGS		
Clonazepam	0.5–20	b.i.d.–t.i.d.
Valproic acid	250–2,500	b.i.d.–q.i.d.
Piracetam	1,000–24,000	t.i.d.
Levetiracetam	500–3,000	b.i.d.–t.i.d.
Zonisamide	100–600	qd, b.i.d.
Primidone	125–1,500	b.i.d.–t.i.d.
5-Hydroxytryptophan with carbidopa	100–3,000	q.i.d.
SOMETIMES HELPFUL DRUGS		
Trihexyphenidyl	1–60	t.i.d.
Methysergide	1–8	q.d.
Propranolol	40–240	b.i.d.–t.i.d.
Fluoxetine	20–60	q.d.
Tetrabenazine	25–200	t.i.d.

b.i.d., twice a day; t.i.d., three times a day; q.i.d., four times a day; q.d., every day.

"down-regulating" dopamine receptors, but a clear demonstration of clinical benefit from this pharmacologic manipulation is lacking.

   a. Drugs that presynaptically suppress dopaminergic neurotransmission have the greatest degree of effectiveness with the least likelihood of worsening the underlying condition. Reserpine or tetrabenazine (not available in the United States) have been most widely used in this regard. Dosages of reserpine usually are started at 0.10 to 0.25 mg three times a day and may be gradually increased to 3 to 5 mg/d. Reserpine has several possible adverse effects, including parkinsonism, depression, orthostatic hypotension, and peptic ulcer disease. Tetrabenazine can be started at 25 mg/d and gradually increased up to 150 mg/d in divided doses. Oral absorption is erratic, and the most common limiting side effects are sedation, depression, and parkinsonism. These side effects are dose related and are relieved with dose reduction. Despite these limitations, these drugs can provide substantial relief of symptoms.

   b. Benzodiazepines may prove useful for patients with mild symptoms. Studies have shown a loss of γ-aminobutyric acid receptors in animal models of TD. Long-acting agents such as clonazepam (usually 1.5 to 3 mg/d) provide the most consistent relief of symptoms. The usual potential adverse effects include sedation and depression.

   c. Neuroleptics, used in the lowest possible dosages, may be necessary if symptoms markedly interfere with activities of daily living. Dosages of haloperidol as low as 0.25 mg/d can provide some relief of symptoms. When withdrawn, the neuroleptic should be reduced gradually over as long a time as 2 years. Once the neuroleptic has been withdrawn, every attempt should be made to avoid the future use of medications that can cause TD.

   d. Vitamin E has been reported to modestly improve symptoms in several studies. It can be given at a dosage of 400 IU three times a day with meals.

   e. Tardive dystonia is a subtype of TD that typically affects young persons. Tardive dystonia involves the neck and trunk muscles and unlike classic TD is painful and routinely disabling. Management of tardive dystonia differs from that of classic TD in that anticholinergics are beneficial and botulinum toxin can be used in focal or segmental forms. Clozapine is extremely helpful to control psychiatric symptoms while allowing TD symptoms to abate over the course of months or years. Dopamine depleters, such as reserpine and tetrabenazine, also are useful.

   f. A long-term strategy is important in the management of TD. For many patients, combination therapy is most effective. The use of a benzodiazepine with either a dopamine depleter or a low dosage of an atypical neuroleptic may be necessary. Gradual improvement after a neuroleptic has been discontinued can occur for as long as 2 years. The eventual rate of remission is approximately 60%. For some elderly patients, the decision can be made simply to continue to suppress the movements with the neuroleptic, but this strategy is reliably effective for only several months.

E. Dystonia is a syndrome of sustained muscle contraction causing abnormal repetitive movements, twisting, or abnormal postures. At least 12 different types of dystonia can be differentiated genetically and are designated dystonia (DYT) 1 to 12. Idiopathic dystonia can be generalized or restricted to a particular muscle group. In patients with idiopathic dystonia, the basal ganglia have no gross or microscopic abnormalities. DYT1 and DYT7 have abnormalities in the **torsin A gene.** Secondary dystonia includes several inherited inborn errors of metabolism such as **dopa-responsive dystonia** (also known as dystonia with diurnal variation, or the Segawa variant) and Wilson's disease. Trauma, vascular disease, space-occupying lesions, and drugs and toxins are other causes of secondary dystonia. As might be expected, given to the lack of understanding of the relevant neurochemistry, a variety of medications have been used and reported to be effective for reducing the severity of dystonia. The use of botulinum toxin injections for focal and segmental dystonia has greatly improved the quality of life of patients with this condition.

1. **Dopa-responsive dystonia (DRD)** or **DYT5** is an autosomal dominant disorder caused by a mutation in the GTP cyclohydrolase I (GCHI) gene. It usually becomes apparent during childhood with a gait disorder, foot cramping, or toe walking. DRD can involve the trunk and arms and can be misdiagnosed as cerebral palsy. Symptoms of parkinsonism (rigidity, postural instability, and bradykinesia) usually are present but can be subtle. Approximately 10% of patients with childhood-onset dystonia have DRD. Patients with this form of dystonia have few symptoms after first awakening; the symptoms progress throughout the day. The importance of this disorder is that it is exquisitely sensitive to small doses of levodopa (50 to 200 mg). Prolonged treatment is only rarely complicated by the response fluctuations that accompany Parkinson's disease. A brief trial of levodopa for childhood-onset dystonia is frequently recommended to exclude DRD.

2. Medical management of dystonia of any cause can be attempted with the medications listed in Table 41.4. None of these medications provides complete relief of symptoms. Combinations of medications can be beneficial. Extremely high doses of anticholinergic drugs such as trihexyphenidyl have been reported to benefit more than 50% of patients in some trials (sometimes at doses greater than 100 mg/d). Therapy usually is started with 1 mg/d and increased 1 to 2 mg per week divided on a three times a day schedule until control of symptoms is achieved or intolerable adverse effects appear. The usual adverse effects of anticholinergic medications can be minimized with very gradual increases in dosage. Children tolerate high doses of anticholinergics much better than do adults. Clinical improvement may continue to increase even after the highest tolerated dose of anticholinergics is reached. A second agent may be added after few months once the highest tolerated dose of anticholinergic has been reached. In addition to the usual anticholinergic adverse effects such as urinary retention, dry mouth and blurred vision, high doses of these medications can cause memory loss, difficulties with concentration, and confusion, especially among adults. For severe cases of dystonia, consultation with a neurologist with expertise in movement disorders is advisable. The combination of a dopamine depleter such as reserpine, an anticholinergic, and a postsynaptic dopamine blocker may be beneficial to

Table 41.4 Medications used in the management of dystonia

Class	Example	Dosage
Anticholinergics	Trihexyphenidyl	6–100 mg/d
Dopaminergics	Levodopa	50–300 mg/d
	Bromocriptine	7.5–40 mg/d
Antidopaminergics	Haloperidol	2–20 mg/d
Benzodiazepines	Diazepam	5–20 mg/d
	Clonazepam	1–10 mg/d
GABA agonists	Baclofen	15–240 mg/d
Antidepressants	Amitriptyline	25–150 mg/d
Anticonvulsants	Carbamazepine	300–1,200 mg/d
	Valproic acid	500–1,500 mg/d
Dopamine depleters	Reserpine	0.5–5 mg/d
	Tetrabenazine	50–300 mg/d
Toxins	Botulinum toxin type A	Up to 400 MU
	Botulinum toxin type B	5,000 to 25,000 MU

GABA, γ-aminobutyric acid; MU, mouse units.

patients with severe dystonia. There is increasing interest in the use of stereotactic surgery targeting the globus pallidus to manage pharmacologically
intractable and disabling dystonia.

3. Injection of **botulinum toxin** is the first line of treatment of many patients
with focal and segmental dystonia. This agent can be used locally in the
treatment of some patients with generalized dystonia. There are seven botulinum toxin serotypes, but only types A and B are available in the United
States—**botulinum toxin type A (Botox; Allergan, Irvine, CA, U.S.A.)
and botulinum toxin type B** (MyoBloc; Elan, South San Francisco, CA,
U.S.A.). In Europe, a different preparation of toxin type A is available (Dys-
port; Ipsen, Maidenhead, UK), and in Japan toxin type F is used clinically.
The toxin is injected directly into the affected muscle, producing reversible
pharmacologic denervation. Injections usually are repeated at an average
interval of 12 to 16 weeks when toxin type A or B is used. Guidance with electromyography is suggested for some muscle groups, especially in the limbs
and neck. Side effects include excessive transient weakness of the injected
and adjacent muscles, dry mouth, and local hematoma. Over time, there
may be loss of effectiveness due to development of antibodies against botulinum toxin. Doses greater than 400 U or 6 MU/kg of botulinum toxin type
A should not be used. Although toxin type B has been shown effective in the
treatment of patients naive to other toxin serotypes, current use of toxin type
B is reserved for patients with loss of effect to toxin type A. Botulinum toxin
injections should be performed by clinicians experienced in identification of
the appropriate muscles and who are familiar with dosing.

F. **Tremor** is probably the most common movement disorder. It is involuntary,
rhythmic oscillation of a body part. It can have a variety of causes, and identification of the underlying cause is of primary importance in determining the
appropriate treatment regimen.

1. **Essential tremor (ET)** typically includes both postural and kinetic tremor.
Rest tremor can be seen in elderly patients with advanced ET. Tremor typically improves with small amounts of alcohol. Approximately 50% of patients
have an autosomal dominant inheritance pattern. The underlying cause is
unknown, although recent studies have suggested abnormalities of the inferior olive and the cerebellum. Generally, it is not possible to eliminate the
tremor, and the goal of therapy should be to normalize activities of daily living. One half to three fourths of patients with ET benefit from some of the
following drugs. In some cases, the tremor may be quite resistant to any
pharmacologic management, and surgical treatment should be considered.

a. **β-Adrenergic receptor antagonists** have been used most extensively
to manage essential tremor. The clinical response to β-blockers is variable and usually incomplete. These drugs reduce tremor amplitude but
not tremor frequency and appear to be less effective in managing voice
and head tremor. These drugs are thought to act through a peripheral
β_2 mechanism on muscle spindles. For this reason, nonselective β-blockers
such as propranolol (Inderal; Wyeth-Ayerst) are preferred. Both the immediate release and the sustained release formulations have been shown
effective. Propranolol should be started at small doses (e.g., 10 mg three
times a day) and titrated upward as needed to obtain satisfactory control of tremor. Doses larger than 320 mg/d usually do not confer additional benefit. Potential side effects of β-blockers include congestive
heart failure, second- or third-degree atrioventricular block, worsening
of obstructive lung disease, masking of signs of hypoglycemia among
persons with diabetes, and worsening of distal perfusion in patients with
peripheral vascular disease. β-Blockers also can cause fatigue, nausea,
diarrhea, rash, erectile dysfunction, and depression. Monitoring of pulse
rate and blood pressure is recommended. If adverse central nervous system effects such as depression or nightmares occur with propranolol,
switching to nadolol (Corgard; Bristol-Myers Squibb) can be an option as
this drug does not readily cross the blood–brain barrier. Nadolol has a

24-hour half-life and can be taken once a day. Metoprolol (Lopressor; Novartis) and timolol (Blocadren; Merck) also have been found effective in the management of ET.

b. **Primidone** (Mysoline; Elan) is an anticonvulsant that may improve ET. When primidone is used to manage ET, it is given in a much lower dosage than when it is used as an anticonvulsant. Treatment usually is started at 25 mg at bedtime, and a good response usually is observed at doses between 50 and 350 mg/d. Doses higher than these do not usually offer additional benefit. The mechanism of action of primidone for management of tremor is unknown. Primidone decreases the amplitude of a tremor but does not alter its frequency. Primidone is converted into two active metabolites, phenylethylmalonamide (PEMA) and phenobarbital. PEMA has no effect on tremor, and the effect of phenobarbital is very modest for management of ET. Acute side effects occur in approximately 20% to 30% of patients and include vertigo, nausea, unsteadiness, and drowsiness.

c. **Carbonic anhydrase inhibitors** such as methazolamide (Neptazane; Lederle) and acetazolamide (Diamox; Lederle) have been shown in open label studies to have some effectiveness in the management of ET. Methazolamide was found to relieve head and voice tremor. Adverse reactions were common, including sedation, nausea, epigastric distress, anorexia, and paresthesia. However, these results were not replicated in a double-blind, placebo-controlled study.

d. **Benzodiazepines** may be used if other forms of therapy do not provide sufficient control of symptoms. Only partial improvement can be expected because it is thought that the main effect of these drugs is reduction of tension and anxiety, which can enhance tremor. Long-acting agents such as clonazepam can be used, but many patients prefer to use shorter-acting agents such as alprazolam (Xanax; Pharmacia & Upjohn). Clonazepam 1 to 3 mg/d can be very effective in kinetic-predominant tremor as well as in orthostatic truncal tremor. Potential adverse effects include sedation, ataxia, and tolerance.

e. **Botulinum toxin injections** have been shown effective in reducing dystonic tremor and have been tested in other tremor disorders. A randomized, double-blind, placebo-controlled study of botulinum toxin for ET showed improvement of tremor in 75% of patients. This improvement was mild to moderate. However, no significant improvement in functional scales was observed. Transient weakness was the most common side effect.

f. **Other drugs** that may have minimal efficacy for the management of ET are gabapentin (Neurontin; Parke-Davis, Morris Plains, NJ, U.S.A.), **calcium channel blockers, clonidine** (Catapres), and **theophylline. Clozapine** (Clozaril; Novartis) may also improve ET; however the potential risk of idiosyncratic agranulocytosis makes this option unappealing. There is increasing interest in the potential role of the anticonvulsant **topiramate (Topamax; Ortho-McNeil)** (25 mg twice a day to 200 twice a day), which showed benefit in a small open-label study of ET.

g. **Surgery** can be used in selected cases when activities of daily living are severely affected despite medical management. Stereotactic thalamotomy targeting the **Vim** has been demonstrated to improve contralateral tremor from several different causes (see **I.A.3.a.**). Thalamotomy of the second side has a good chance of decreasing tremor but a high incidence of speech problems. For this reason, when both sides are to be treated, bilateral implantation of a DBS on the Vim nucleus is the preferred treatment option. Overall, ablative thalamotomy and chronic stimulation have comparable effectiveness, but adverse cerebral events are less frequent with DBS because of the ability to adjust stimulation parameters.

2. **Other causes** of tremor include PD and dystonia. Management of tremor associated with PD is discussed in **I.A.2.b.**). β-Blockers can be effective if the

tremor has a substantial postural component. The hand tremor associated with dystonia typically has a postural component and may respond to therapy for essential tremor. Clonazepam, anticholinergics such as trihexyphenidyl and botulinum toxin may be useful for management of dystonic tremor (see **II.E.**). **Rubral tremor** is a wide-amplitude proximal tremor that can be seen at rest but is accentuated with action and posture holding. Lesions of the cerebellar outflow pathways in the brainstem cause rubral tremor. Ataxia also is frequently present. Management of this type of tremor usually is disappointing, but β-blockers and benzodiazepines can be attempted. Other drugs have been tried with anecdotal benefit in some cases (isoniazid, glutethimide, levodopa, anticholinergics, baclofen, sodium valproate, and L-5-hydroxytryptophan).

G. **Wilson's disease (WD)** is an autosomal recessive disorder of copper accumulation caused by a defect in copper excretion into the bile. Low plasma levels of ceruloplasmin characterize WD. Loss of the binding protein causes deposition of copper in the liver, iris, and basal ganglia. The clinical presentation typically occurs between the ages of 10 and 40 years. Patients may come to medical attention with hepatic, neurologic, or psychiatric disease. Systemic involvement with renal, hematologic, or rheumatologic problems is not uncommon. A variety of movement disorders can accompany WD, including tremor, dystonia, chorea, and parkinsonism. Symptomatic management of the movement disorder is as discussed in above. More important is recognition of WD and prevention of additional copper deposition and worsening of end-organ damage. Once a diagnosis of WD is made, it is highly recommended that a clinician with expertise in WD be consulted to guide treatment, even if the consultation is by telephone.

1. **Recommended screening** methods for patients with a neurologic signs and symptoms of WD:
   a. **Serum ceruloplasmin** and **slit-lamp examinaiton** for **Kayser–Fleischer (KF) rings.** Approximately 90% of WD patients who have neurologic symptoms have a low ceruloplasmin level. This test should be used to increase or decrease the index of suspicion. It can be only used for screening when combined with a slit-lamp examination. KF rings are present in 99.9% of WD patients who have neurologic symptoms but in only approximately 50% of WD patients who have hepatic symptoms. Patients with obstructive liver disease such as primary biliary cirrhosis also may have KF rings. KF rings typically begin superiorly in the iris and disappear with chelation therapy.
   b. **24-Hour urine copper.** In patients with neurologic WD, the 24-hour urine copper level is always more than 100 μg before chelation treatment. This value may be falsely elevated in patients with long-standing liver disease.
2. **Zinc** blocks mucosal absorption of copper by inducing intestinal cell metallothionein. Dosages of 50 mg three times a day between meals are used. It is important to take zinc separate from food, waiting at least 1 hour before having a meal. The toxicity of zinc is negligible, although it can cause abdominal discomfort and overtreatment may cause microcytic anemia. Zinc is too slow acting to be used for initial management of WD with neurologic symptoms; however, it is the drug of choice for maintenance therapy and in presymptomatic or pregnant patients.
3. **Penicillamine** (Cuprimine; Merck) acts by means of reductive chelation of copper. It mobilizes large amounts of copper, mainly from the liver. During initial penicillamine treatment, quantities of copper are excreted in the urine up to 10 to 15 mg per 24 hours. Over time, these values fall as total body stores of copper are mobilized. Total daily dosages of 750 to 1,500 mg usually are used. The standard dosage is approximately 250 mg four times a day, each dose separated from food. The dose can usually be decreased to 500 to 750 mg/d during the maintenance phase. Several potentially serious adverse effects are associated with penicillamine. Approximately 50% of patients treated with penicillamine have marked neurologic deterioration,

and half of these patients do not recover to the pre-penicillamine level of function. For this reason, an alternative treatment (such as trientine or other agents) should be considered for initial therapy of WD. **Induction therapy with trientine leads to less neurologic deterioration** (in 25% of patients) than does induction with penicillamine. Approximately one third of patients who start taking penicillamine have an **acute hypersensitivity reaction.** Other subacute potential toxicities include **bone marrow suppression,** membranous glomerulopathy, Goodpasture's syndrome, myasthenia gravis, reduced immune response, hepatitis, pemphigus vulgaris or foliaceus, collagen disorders, and a lupus erythematosus–like syndrome with a positive antinuclear antibody result and teratogenicity. Because of the potential hematologic and renal adverse reactions, a complete blood cell cont, platelet count, and urinalysis are recommended every 2 weeks for the first 6 months of therapy and monthly thereafter. When safer alternative medications are available, penicillamine should be avoided in the initial management of WD with neurologic symptoms.

4. **Trientine** (Syprine; Merck) is a U.S. Food and Drug Administration–approved chelating agent that induces urinary excretion of copper and has a more favorable side-effect profile than does penicillamine. Dosage and administration are identical to those of penicillamine. Although trientine promotes less copper excretion than does penicillamine, it does not cause a hypersensitivity reaction. The other toxicities are somewhat similar to those of penicillamine but less frequent.

5. **Tetrathiolmolybdate** is an experimental drug that prevents absorption of copper from the intestine and is absorbed into the blood, where it binds to copper to form nontoxic complexes. It has been used successfully at a dose of 120 mg/d to manage acute WD with neurologic manifestations.

6. **A low-copper diet** is important for patients with Wilson's disease. Foods containing large amounts of copper include lobster, liver, and chocolate.

7. **Liver transplantation** is curative of WD.

Recommended Readings

Bannister R. Multiple-system atrophy and pure autonomic failure. In: Low PA, ed. *Autonomic nervous disorders.* Boston: Little, Brown, 1993.

Brewer GJ, et al. Diagnosis and treatment of Wilson's disease. *Semin Neurol* 1999;19:261–270.

Ferrante RJ, Andreassen OA, Jenkins BG, et al. Neuroprotective effects of creatine in a transgenic mouse model of Huntington's disease. *J Neurosci* 2000;20:4389–4397.

Hallett M. Classification and treatment of tremor. *JAMA* 1991;266:1115–1117.

Hallett M, Litvan I. Evaluation of surgery for Parkinson's disease: a report of the therapeutic and technology subcommittee of the American Academy of Neurology. *Neurology* 1999;53:1910–1921.

Hutton JT, Morris JL. Long-acting carbidopa-levodopa in the management of moderate and advanced Parkinson's disease. *Neurology* 1992;42:51–56.

Jankovic J. New and emerging therapies for Parkinson disease. *Arch Neurol* 1999;56:785–790.

Jankovic J, Beach J. Long-term effects of tetrabenazine in hyperkinetic movement disorders. *Neurology* 1997;48:358–362.

Jankovic J, Brin MF. Therapeutic uses of botulinum toxin *N Engl J Med* 1991;324:1186–1194.

Jankovic J, Marsden D. Therapeutic strategies in Parkinson's disease. In: Jankovic J, Tolosa E, eds. Parkinson's disease and movement disorders. Baltimore: Williams & Wilkins: 1998:191–220.

Klein C Breakefield XO, Ozelius LJ. Genetics of primary dystonia. *Semin Neurol* 1999;19:271–280.

Koller WC, Hristova A, Brin M. Pharmacologic treatment of essential tremor. *Neurology* 2000;54[Suppl 4]:S30–S38.

Koroshetz WJ, Jenkins BG, Rosen BR, et al. Energy metabolism defects in Huntington's disease and effects of coenzyme Q_{10}. *Ann Neurol* 1997;41:160–165.

Lewitt PA. Therapeutics of Tourette syndrome: new medication approaches. *Adv Neurol* 1992;58:263–270.

Litvan I, Agid Y, Jankovic J, et al. Accuracy of clinical criteria for the diagnosis of progressive supranuclear palsy (Steele-Richardson-Olszewski syndrome). *Neurology* 1996;46:922–930.

Nygaard TG. Dopa-responsive dystonia: delineation of the clinical syndrome and clues to pathogenesis. *Adv Neurol* 1993;60:577–585.

Olanow CW, et al. Cell death and neuroprotection in Parkinson's disease. *Ann Neurol* 1998;44 [Suppl 1]:S1—S196.

Olanow CW, et al. Levodopa-induced dyskinesias. *Ann Neurol* 2000;47[Suppl 1]:S1–S203.

Olanow CW, Koller WC. Management of Parkinson's disease. *Neurology* 1998;50[Suppl 3]: S2–S57.

Parkinson Study Group. Effects of tocopherol and deprenyl on the progression of disability in early Parkinson's disease. *N Engl J Med* 1993;328:176–183.

Quinn N. Multiple system atrophy. In: Marsden DC, Fahn S, eds. *Movement disorders 3.* Oxford, UK: Butterworth–Heinemann, 1994:262–281.

Rinne UK, Bracco F, Chouza C, et al. Early treatment of Parkinson's disease with cabergoline delays the onset of motor complications: results of a double-blind levodopa controlled trial. The PKDS009 Study Group. *Drugs* 1998;55[Suppl 1]:23–30.

Siemers E. Movement disorders. In: Biller J, ed. *Practical neurology.* Philadelphia: Lippincott–Raven, 1997:449–460.

Simpson GM. The treatment of tardive dyskinesia and tardive dystonia. *J Clin Psychiatry* 2000;61[Suppl 4]:39–44.

Weiner WJ, Lang AE. *Behavioral neurology of movement disorders.* New York: Raven Press, 1995.

Wellington CL, Hayden MR. Caspases and neurodegeneration: on the cutting edge of new therapeutic approaches. *Clin Genet* 2000;57:1–10.

42. DEMENTIA

Martin R. Farlow
Ann Marie Hake

Dementia is defined as a decline in memory and at least one other cognitive deficit that impairs the patient's ability to function in the activities of daily living. Behavioral abnormalities are common and contribute to the impairment of function. Neurodegenerative processes, particularly Alzheimer's disease (AD), account for more than 90% of dementia cases. Therapeutic approaches have until recently concentrated on identifying the few patients with reversible etiologic factors and on palliating disabling symptoms for as long as possible in the care of patients with progressive disease.

I. **Dementia (reversible causes).** The current percentage of patients with dementia whose disorders have reversible underlying etiologic factors is relatively small (approximately 5%). However, as many as 40% of elderly patients with no reversible underlying etiologic factors have modifiable abnormalities, the correction of which can slow progression or temporarily improve the patient's ability to function.

    A. **Structural lesions causing dementia.** Space-occupying masses or abnormalities in brain structure for which the patient can be treated may be identified with brain imaging studies, including computed tomography (CT), magnetic resonance imaging, single photon emission computed tomography, and positron emission tomography. Unfortunately, neurosurgical intervention in many of these patients can halt deterioration but not greatly improve clinical symptoms.

        1. **Normal pressure hydrocephalus (NPH).** Patients with ataxia, urinary incontinence, dementia, and ventricular enlargement out of proportion to sulci on computed tomographic scans or magnetic resonance images should be referred for neurosurgical evaluation and possible placement of a ventriculoperitoneal shunt. Patients whose symptoms improve after lumbar puncture are particularly likely to improve after shunting. Ataxia and incontinence are more likely to improve than is memory. Overall, one third of patients improve, one third remain unchanged, and one third continue to have progressive symptoms.

        2. **Subdural hematoma and hygroma.** Chronic subdural hematoma and hygroma can be asymptomatic, cause cognitive impairment, or cause frank dementia in the elderly. Neurosurgical evaluation is required. Increases in the size of the fluid collection and progressive clinical impairment are indications for surgical intervention. Surgery often does not improve cognition but stops progression of cognitive impairment.

        3. **Frontal, temporal, and parietal lobe tumors.** Large meningiomas, gliomas, and metastatic lesions to the brain that occupy substantial space or cause marked edema in the adjacent frontal, temporal, or parietal lobe can cause dementia. Patients with such tumors should be treated by means of neurosurgical excision or by means of biopsy and radiation therapy or chemotherapy, as appropriate for the tumor type and location. Among patients older than 65 years, the prognosis for meaningful recovery from cognitive impairment and clinical dysfunction after such treatments is guarded.

    B. **Metabolic abnormalities associated with dementia.** Relatively subtle deviations from the normal ranges for metabolic parameters can cause or significantly exacerbate mental impairment in elderly patients. A history of fluctuating deficits suggests a metabolic cause of dementia. Changes in mental status often are reversible with correction of the underlying cause of the metabolic disturbance.

        1. **Hypokalemia and hyperkalemia.** Hypokalemia in elderly patients most commonly occurs during antihypertensive therapy with diuretic drugs. It can be managed by means of stopping the diuretic, supplementing potassium, or switching to a potassium-sparing diuretic such as spironolactone. Steroids also can cause hypokalemia in the elderly, and potassium supplements should be supplied if necessary. Hyperkalemia can result from oversupplementation of potassium and use of potassium-sparing antihypertensive agents. The offending agents should be discontinued.

2. **Hyponatremia and hypernatremia.** Hypernatremia is most common in association with dehydration and often is found in physically impaired patients who are dependent on caregivers for their oral intake. For dehydrated patients, both free water and electrolytic deficits should be calculated and corrected, and body weight and electrolytes should be measured frequently and adjusted as necessary. Relatively minor hyponatremia with serum sodium (Na$^+$) at 120 to 130 mg/dL can significantly impair cognition in the elderly. Management of hyponatremia can totally reverse mental impairment. Hyponatremia with Na$^+$ less than 120 mg/dL should be corrected over 3 or more days, because overrapid normalization can precipitate central nervous system (CNS) demyelination.

3. **Hypocalcemia and hypercalcemia.** Abnormalities in serum calcium levels can be associated with hypoparathyroidism or hyperparathyroidism, antihypertensive therapy, cancer, and renal disease. The underlying cause should be determined and controlled when possible.

4. **Hypoglycemia and hyperglycemia.** Many patients with diabetes mellitus have dementia with varying degrees of reversibility. The long-term effects of diabetes mellitus can contribute to microvascular ischemic changes in the brain and accelerate atherosclerosis in the major vessels supplying the brain. Both can cause irreversible vascular dementia. Many patients with diabetes have very high blood glucose levels (greater than 300 to 400 mg/dL) and variable changes in mental status during the day. These subtle cognitive deficits can be difficult to recognize, and rapid changes in blood glucose levels difficult to control. Similarly, some patients may have periods of confusion associated with unrecognized hypoglycemia. Management of glucose abnormalities requires careful monitoring of blood glucose levels and correction by means of adjustments in diet and in dosages of oral hypoglycemic agents, or by means of insulin injections as necessary to achieve normalization of blood glucose level.

C. **Endocrine abnormalities that cause dementia.** Chronic endocrine diseases can cause cognitive impairment and dementia in elderly persons with few, if any, of the other physical findings associated with deficiency or excess hormonal state. Detection and correction of these conditions can lead to complete reversal of dementia, including return to normal activities of daily living.

1. **Thyroid disease**
   a. **Hypothyroidism.** In the elderly, hypothyroidism should be managed initially with levothyroxine (T$_4$) at a dosage of 0.025 mg/d. The dosage may be increased in 0.025-mg increments at monthly intervals, with routine monitoring of T$_4$ and thyroid-stimulating hormone levels. The dose should be increased until symptoms improve and until T$_4$ levels are in the therapeutic range. If the initial T$_4$ thyroid level is very low in an elderly patient, supplemental steroids, such as prednisone (Deltasone; Pharmacia & Upjohn, Kalamazoo, MI, U.S.A.) at 5.0 to 7.5 mg/d, may be given for the first 2 weeks after levothyroxine is initiated.
   b. **Hyperthyroidism.** An endocrinologist should generally be consulted and appropriate therapy begun, including propranolol to decrease pulse rate and anxiety, medical therapy with methimazole or with radioactive iodine, or surgical excision of the thyroid gland. Most mental status changes associated with thyroid disease are highly reversible.

2. **Diabetes mellitus.** See I.B.4.

3. **Hypoparathyroidism and hyperparathyroidism.** See sec. I.B.3.

D. **Dementia secondary to systemic organ failure.** The CNS depends on the functions of all of the major organ systems. Mild abnormalities in systemic organ functions in an elderly patient can cause mental status changes including confusion, disorientation, and memory loss.

1. **Pulmonary disease.** Both acute illnesses (such as pneumonia) and chronic obstructive lung disease can cause hypoxemia resulting in dementia. Supplemental oxygen administered by nasal cannula or face mask can improve cognitive function. Various diseases of the lungs, particularly small-cell

cancer, can metastasize or have distant effects on the brain and cause dementia. The underlying tumor should be the focus of treatment.

2. **Hepatic disease.** Diseases of the liver, such as the various forms of hepatitis and cirrhosis (hereditary and alcoholic), can cause dementia. Dementia
in such cases often is associated with elevated blood ammonia levels. The
underlying liver disease is the focus of treatment. Cognitive improvement
results from lowering ammonia levels with lactulose, neomycin, or both.

3. **Cardiac disease.** Cardiac dysfunction can contribute to the process of dementia in different ways. Congestive heart failure can decrease the blood supply
to the brain. Enlarged heart chambers and valvular disease can promote formation of thrombi that can embolize to the brain. Arrhythmias may decrease
blood flow to the brain. Management of the underlying cardiac disease should
be the focus.

4. **Renal disease.** Chronic or acute renal failure can cause uremic encephalopathy. Dialysis and transplantation have decreased the frequency of this illness. Patients with renal disease are more prone to fluctuating changes in
mental status resulting from a variety of metabolic abnormalities. Aluminum occasionally accumulates in some patients, causing dialysis dementia. Chelation with deferoxamine can reverse some symptoms associated
with cognitive decline.

E. **Chronic CNS infection.** Infectious diseases that cause systemic illness often
directly or indirectly affect CNS function. In elderly patients, urinary tract infections and upper respiratory infections can secondarily cause declines in cognitive
function that clear after effective antibiotic treatment. In the elderly, chronic
meningitis or encephalitis can be caused by syphilis, tuberculosis, cryptococcus
and other fungal infections, or Whipple's disease. Symptoms include intermittent
fevers, night sweats, headache, stiff neck, papilledema, nuchal rigidity, rapidly
progressive dementia, ataxia, and urinary incontinence (see Chapter 2). Therapy
should be appropriate to the identified causative organism. Dementia occurs relatively frequently among persons with human immunodeficiency virus infection.
These patients also are at higher risk of contracting chronic meningitis or other
opportunistic infections, including progressive multifocal leukoencephalopathy
(caused by the JC virus), toxoplasmosis, or cytomegalovirus, which can cause cognitive decline. Dementia also occurs among patients who have had herpes simplex encephalitis. These deficits may gradually be ameliorated, although some
patients may have permanent cognitive deficits. Creutzfeldt–Jakob disease,
although not reversible, also is a transmissible form of dementia caused by exposure to prions, usually through contact with nervous system tissue or fluid from
an infected person. The typical clinical course is rapid cognitive decline with myoclonus, ataxia, or cerebellar signs that progresses to death in 3 to 6 months.

F. **Epilepsy (partial complex status epilepticus).** Symptoms or signs of intermittent confusion, staring spells, lip smacking, and automatisms suggest the
possibility of intermittent partial status epilepticus. Ictal activity should be demonstrated at electroencephalography. Diazepam or lorazepam should be given for
acute suppression of seizures. Phenytoin, carbamazepine, or valproic acid can be
given for longer-term management of the seizure disorder.

G. **Side effects of medications taken by the elderly for chronic illnesses.** As
many as 75% of elderly patients take three or more medications, several of which
have the potential to cause side effects of chronic confusion and deficits in cognition and memory. The worst offenders are anticholinergic drugs such as
bethanecol and oxybutynin, antihypertensives, antidepressants, and antianxiety
and antipsychotic medications. Anticonvulsants, sleep medications, and analgesics also frequently cause impairment in mental function. Excessive dosages and
numbers of medications are probably the most common reversible causes of
dementia among the elderly. Medications should be titrated to the lowest dosage
levels sufficient for control of symptoms. Medications that are not clearly effective
should be eliminated.

II. **Dementia (irreversible causes).** Most patients with dementia have underlying
etiologic factors that are not reversible (e.g., AD, diffuse Lewy body disease, vascular demen-

tia, or frontotemporal dementia). Therapeutic strategies for neurodegenerative dementia have focused on the use of cholinesterase inhibitors and other drugs to improve symptoms of memory loss, other deficits in cognition, mood disorders, and behavioral disturbances and on development of neuroprotective and neurotrophic agents to slow progression of the disease.

A. **Symptomatic therapy for AD**

  1. **Treatment of cognitive deficits.** AD is characterized by deficits in the brain of several neurotransmitters, particularly acetylcholine. Several cholinesterase inhibitor drugs are now approved in the United States for managing the primary symptoms of AD. These drugs increase the available levels of acetylcholine at the synapse by slowing the hydrolysis of acetylcholine, and they produce modest improvements in cognition and behavioral and psychiatric abnormalities in some patients with mild to moderately severe AD. Peripheral and central cholinergic side effects are common with treatment with this class of drugs. The most common adverse symptoms are nausea, vomiting, dyspepsia, and diarrhea, although facial flushing, dizziness, headache, and nasal discharge occur among some patients. These effects most commonly occur when therapy is initiated and dosages of these drugs are being increased. Tolerability can be improved by means of administration with food or by slowing the rate of titration.

     a. **Tacrine,** the first cholinesterase inhibitor developed to manage AD, became available in the United States in 1993. It is dosed four times a day with an initial total daily dose of 40 mg. The daily dose is increased 40 mg every 6 weeks as tolerated to a maximum total daily dose of 160 mg (40 mg four times a day). Because of potential hepatotoxicity, liver function tests must be performed every 2 weeks and the dose reduced or discontinued if the alanine aminotransferase level is elevated more than three or five times the upper limit of normal, respectively. The drug has been mostly supplanted by the newer drugs, which have more favorable safety and tolerability profiles and more convenient dosing.

     b. **Donepezil,** a selective acetylcholinesterase inhibitor approved in the United States in 1997, is dosed once a day, usually at bedtime. The initial dose is 5 mg/d. This is increased to 10 mg/d after 6 weeks. The most common side effect is diarrhea. There is no hepatotoxicity, and laboratory monitoring is not needed.

     c. **Rivastigmine,** an acetyl-butyrylcholinesterase inhibitor, was approved in 2000. It is administered twice a day after meals with an initial total daily dose of 3 mg. The dose should be flexibly titrated upward every 4 weeks, as tolerated, in 3 mg/d increments to a maximum total daily dose of 12 mg (6 mg twice a day). The therapeutic range is 6 to 12 mg/d. The most common side effects, particularly during titration, are nausea or vomiting. Laboratory monitoring is not required.

     d. **Galantamine,** an acetylcholinesterase inhibitor that also modulates nicotinic receptors and became available in 2001, is given twice a day, beginning with a total daily dose of 8 mg. This is titrated to 16 mg/d (8 mg twice a day) after 4 weeks and can be further increased to 12 mg twice a day in another 4 weeks, as tolerated. Adverse effects such as nausea, vomiting, and diarrhea, which occur in some patients with dosage increases during up-titration, can be minimized by giving with food or lengthening titration intervals. Laboratory monitoring is not necessary.

  2. **Management of behavioral symptoms.** The management of agitation, depression, anxiety, and sleep disorders for patients with dementia can be challenging. Drugs that improve behavioral symptoms can worsen dementia. Some drugs that improve behavioral symptoms in younger patients without dementia may have paradoxic effects, worsening behavioral disturbances. However, dosage ranges that provide effective control of behavioral symptoms vary widely in individual patients, so frequent adjustments in therapy may be necessary to control such symptoms. In general, dosage should be started low, and the rate of increase should be slow.

     a. **Agitation, hallucinations, delusions, and bizarre or violent behavior.** Precipitants of the abnormal behaviors, such as changes in the patient's environment, pain, or infection, should be identified and modified, if possible. The atypical neuroleptic agents may be useful in small doses. Target behavioral symptoms for potential improvement should be identified before therapy is begun. Therapy can start with risperidone 0.5 mg, olanzapine 2.5 mg, or quetiapine 12.5 mg, as necessary, with frequency from once per day at night up to three or four times a day. The dosages can be adjusted upward as necessary to control behavior and downward as necessary to minimize side effects. Behavior can actually worsen if the doses are too high. Trazodone at a dosage of 50 to 200 mg before bedtime and, if necessary, an additional 50 mg twice a day, can be used for agitation, but daytime dosing can be excessively sedating for some patients. Abnormal behavior becomes progressively more common as disease worsens, occurring in most patients with AD. Cholinesterase inhibitors have been shown to reduce new occurrence of abnormal behavior, especially in the moderate to severe stages of AD, but are not useful for managing acute psychiatric symptoms.

   b. Depression. Symptoms of depression are present in at least 25% of patients with AD, often in the early stages of the illness. Therapy for depression can improve cognitive function; therefore, aggressive management is warranted. The selective serotonin reuptake inhibitors (SSRIs) such as sertraline, citalopram, fluoxetine, fluvoxamine, or paroxetine are useful in treatment of the elderly population because they carry relatively low risk of side effects. These drugs often are effective in lower dosages than those used to treat younger adults. For this reason, treatment should be initiated at one-half the usual starting dose. Some of the newer atypical antidepressants such as venlafaxine or bupropion may also give good results, especially if the response to SSRIs is not adequate.

   c. Anxiety, phobias, and excessive motor activities. When caregivers of patients with dementia describe symptoms suggestive of anxiety, phobias, or excessive motor activities (e.g., constant pacing, hand washing), several questions should be asked. Is this behavior disturbing to the patient? Is it interfering with the patient's function in activities of daily living? Are these behavioral symptoms making it difficult for the caregiver to manage the patient? Small doses of atypical neuroleptics given either as needed or at the time of day that the behavior usually occurs are generally effective. Small doses of a benzodiazepine such as lorazepam at a dose of 0.5 to 1.0 mg or alprazolam at a dose of 0.25 to 0.5 mg may be used to control these symptoms. In the care of patients with dementia, however, these drugs can be excessively sedating, and there is an increased risk of falling. SSRIs also can be helpful, especially for irritability or obsessive–compulsive behaviors.

   d. Insomnia. Disturbances in the sleep–wake cycle can contribute to depression, anxiety, and agitation in a patient with dementia. A patient with dementia who is active in the middle of the night puts extraordinary stress on the caregiver. Daytime napping should be discouraged. If the patient is taking donepezil at bedtime, dosing should be moved to the morning. Atypical neuroleptics given at bedtime often are helpful. Some patients have responded to melatonin. Diphenhydramine (25 to 50 mg) also can be useful.

B. Disease-modifying management of AD (neuroprotective approach). Currently there is no approved therapy that delays the degenerative processes of AD. However, several promising approaches to keeping neurons in the brain alive and retarding the clinical progression of the disease are being investigated.

   1. Free radical generation may cause neuronal death in AD. A study of therapy with vitamin E 2,000 IU/d and selegiline showed that both agents delayed progression to severe-stage AD or to nursing home placement. Unfortunately, cognitive deterioration was not delayed. Both were approximately equally effective and there was no additional benefit to combining the two drugs. A study is underway to determine whether vitamin E delays the onset of AD among persons with isolated memory loss (mild cognitive impairment).

2. **Inflammation in AD.** Results of retrospective epidemiologic studies have suggested that patients with rheumatoid arthritis taking nonsteroidal antiinflammatory drugs have a decreased prevalence of AD. Results of a preliminary double-blind, placebo-controlled pilot trial of indomethacin suggested that disease progression was significantly retarded. However, subsequent large double-blind, placebo-controlled trials of cyclooxygenase-2 inhibitors and prednisone did not show benefit. The role of antiinflammatory drugs in the prevention of AD needs further investigation.

3. **Estrogens may improve cognition in some elderly women.** Epidemiologic studies have shown a reduced incidence of AD among women taking postmenopausal hormone replacement therapy. Although double-blind, placebo-controlled trials have not shown significant benefits among women already affected by AD, anecdotal evidence shows some individual women with AD have benefited from estrogen. For this reason, hormone replacement therapy is not recommended routinely as primary therapy for AD, but it should be considered in the care of women with other symptoms of estrogen deficiency.

4. **Vascular risk factors.** It has been found in several studies that among patients with AD who have concomitant vascular risk factors or vascular disease dementia begins at an earlier age and progresses more rapidly than among those without vascular risk factors. Vigorous control of hypertension, hyperlipidemia, and hyperglycemia, supplementation with folic acid to reduce homocysteine levels, and administration of prostaglandin inhibitors, if indicated, may slow the progression of the dementia.

C. **Therapies for other irreversible forms of dementia.** Few double-blind, placebo-controlled trials have been conducted for management of other types of dementia. Preliminary evidence suggests, however, that cholinesterase inhibitors may be useful to patients with some of these other forms of dementia.

1. **Diffuse Lewy body dementia** may be the primary cause of or contribute markedly to the symptoms of 10% to 15% of all patients with irreversible dementia. There is considerable overlap of this entity with AD. Results of trials of cholinesterase inhibitors suggest that these agents may actually be more effective in the treatment of patients with diffuse Lewy body disease than of those with AD. The approach to evaluating and treating patients with this entity is the same as that for AD.

2. **Frontotemporal dementia (including Pick's disease).** Frontotemporal dementias are diagnosed in approximately 2% to 5 % of patients with dementia and clinical symptoms often overlapping those of AD. Early symptoms often are behavioral abnormalities and language problems. Memory deficits typically occur during the later stages of the illness. Behavioral disorders should be managed as described in **II.A.** Because of the overlap with AD, it is reasonable to treat patients with cholinesterase inhibitors as a trial, particularly if there are significant deficits in memory and cognition. Cognitive symptoms in some patients anecdotally have improved with dopaminergic agents such as amantadine, pergolide, or carbidopa–levodopa.

3. **Vascular dementia.** No drugs have been approved for management of vascular dementia. Accurate diagnosis is important for determining the cause and preventing or delaying progression of the disease.

   a. **Ischemic vascular dementia** may be the principal cause of symptoms in 5% to 15% of patients with dementia and may occur jointly with AD in another 10%. Control of hypertension and use of antiplatelet aggregating agents may help prevent progression of dementia in patients with multiple infarctions. In patients with elevated levels of cholesterol and triglycerides, reduction should be encouraged by changes in diet and administration of either a statin, niacin, or gemfibrozil. Cholinesterase inhibitor therapy may be useful because most patients with clinically diagnosed vascular disease are found at autopsy to also have coexistent AD.

b. Multiple infarctions secondary to emboli. Occasionally, dementia occurs after repeated embolic strokes. Treatment involves stopping or decreasing new infarctions by means of identification of the embolic source and instituting appropriate therapy. Carotid source emboli can be managed medically with antiplatelet agents or, if there is more than 70% stenosis, surgically with carotid endarterectomy. Cardiac source emboli usually necessitate full anticoagulation with heparin and then long-term therapy with warfarin. If the cause is infective endocarditis, the patient should not be given anticoagulants, but antimicrobial therapy should target the underlying infection.

c. Amyloid angiopathy is suggested by intermittent parenchymal hemorrhage of the brain. Angiography shows no evidence of aneurysm or arteriovenous malformation. In a small number of these cases with a positive family history, the cause is hereditary cerebral hemorrhage with amyloidosis of the Dutch type (HCHWA-D) or hereditary cerebral hemorrhage with amyloidosis in Icelandic kindred (HCHWA-I). There is no treatment but aspirin, and *nonsteroidal therapy should be specifically avoided.*

d. Vasculitis. The diagnosis of vasculitis is suggested in patients with dementia with diffuse brain disease when there is elevation of the Westergren sedimentation rate to greater than 75 mm/h without another identified cause and elevation of cerebrospinal fluid protein level to greater than 75 mg/dL with fewer than 10 cells/mm^3. Angiography shows characteristic areas of narrowing in the small vessels, which confirms the diagnosis. Patients with vasculitis should be treated aggressively with high-dose intravenous steroids followed by tapering oral steroid therapy. Steroid therapy may improve memory and cognitive deficits dramatically.

e. Emotional incontinence in vascular dementia. Many patients with multiple infarcts in the frontal lobes interrupting frontal lobe tracts may exhibit characteristic verbal outbursts triggered by even the most minor emotional stimulus. These emotional verbal outbursts may have characteristics of both crying and laughter. They are involuntary and can be very disturbing to patients and their families, often leading to avoidance of social activities. SSRIs or low doses of tricyclic antidepressants often are effective in controlling these symptoms.

Acknowledgment

This work was supported by NIA grant AG10133-04.

Recommended Readings

American Psychiatric Association. Dementia of the Alzheimer's type. In: *Diagnostic and Statistical Manual of Mental Disorders,* 4th ed. Washington, DC: American Psychiatric Association, 1994.

Arnold SE, Kumar A. Contemporary clinical neurology: reversible dementias. *Med Clin North Am* 1993;77:215–230.

Borson S, Raskind MA. Clinical features and pharmacologic treatment of behavioral symptoms of Alzheimer's disease. *Neurology* 1997;48[Suppl 6]:S17–S24.

Corey-Bloom J, Anand R, Veach J, et al. A randomized trial evaluating the efficacy and safety of ENA 713 (rivastigmine tartrate), a new acetylcholinesterase inhibitor, in patients with mild to moderately severe Alzheimer's disease. *Int J Geriatr Psychopharmacol* 1998;1:55–65.

Cummings J, Anand R, Koumaras B, et al. Rivastigmine provides behavioral benefits to Alzheimer's disease patients residing in a nursing home: findings from a 26-week trial. *Neurology* 2000;54[Suppl 3]:A468–A469.

Farlow M, Gracon SI, Hershey LA, et al. A controlled trial of tacrine in Alzheimer's disease. *JAMA* 1992;268:2523–2529.

Farlow MR, Hake AM. Drug-induced cognitive impairment. In Biller J, ed. *Iatrogenic neurology.* Boston: Butterworth–Heinemann, 1998;203–214.

Geldmacher D, Whitehouse PJ Jr. Differential diagnosis of Alzheimer's disease. *Neurology* 1997;48[Suppl 6]:S2–S9.

Henderson VW, Paganini-Hill A, Emanuel CK, et al. Estrogen replacement therapy in older women. *Arch Neurol* 1994;51:896–900.

Henderson VW, Paganini-Hill A, Miller BL, et al. Estrogen for Alzheimer's disease in women: randomized double-blind, placebo-controlled trial. *Neurology* 2000;54:295–301.

Katz IR, Jeste DV, Mintzer JE, et al. Comparison of risperidone and placebo for psychosis and behavioral disturbances associated with dementia: a randomized, double-blind trial. *J Clin Psychiatry* 1999;60:107–115.

Lebowitz B, Pearson JL, Schneider LS, et al. Diagnosis and treatment of depression in late life: consensus statement update. *JAMA* 1997;278:1186–1190.

Levy R. Alzheimer's disease and Lewy body dementia. *Br J Psychiatry* 1994;164:268.

Levy R, Eagger S, Griffiths M, et al. Lewy bodies and response to tacrine in Alzheimer's disease. *Lancet* 1994;343:176.

McKeith I, Del Ser T, Spano P, et al. Efficacy of rivastigmine in dementia with Lewy bodies: a randomised, double-blind, placebo-controlled international study. *Lancet* 2000;356: 2031–2036.

Mulnard RA, Cotman CW, Kawas C, et al. Estrogen replacement therapy for treatment of mild to moderate Alzheimer's disease: a randomized controlled trial. *JAMA* 2000;283:1007–1015.

Paganini-Hill A, Henderson VW. Estrogen deficiency and risk of Alzheimer's disease in women. *Am J Epidemiol* 1994;140:256–261.

Rogers SL, Farlow MR, Doody RS, et al. A 24-week, double-blind placebo-controlled trial of donepezil in patients with Alzheimer's disease. *Neurology* 1998;50:136–145.

Sano M, Ernesto C, Thomas RG, et al. A controlled trial of selegiline, alpha-tocopherol, or both as treatment for Alzheimer's disease. *N Engl J Med* 1997;336:1216–1222.

Stewart WF, Kawas C, Corrada M, et al. Risk of Alzheimer's disease and duration of NSAID use. *Neurology* 1997;48:626–632.

Street JS, Clark WS, Gannon KS, et al. Olanzapine treatment of psychotic and behavioral symptoms in patients with Alzheimer disease in nursing care facilities: a double-blind, randomized, placebo-controlled trial: the HGEU study group. *Arch Gen Psychiatry* 2000;57: 968–976.

Tariot P, Solomon PR, Morris JC, et al. A 5-month, randomized, placebo-controlled trial of galantamine in AD. *Neurology* 2000;54:2269–2276.

Wilcock GK, Scott MI. Tacrine for senile dementia of Alzheimer's or Lewy body type. *Lancet* 1994;344:544.

World Health Organization. *Tenth Revision of the International Statistical Classification of Diseases and Related Health Problems (ICD-10)*. Geneva, Switzerland: World Health Organization, 1992.

43. CENTRAL NERVOUS SYSTEM INFECTIONS

Karen L. Roos

I. Bacterial meningitis. The initial signs and symptoms of bacterial meningitis are fever, stiff neck, headache, lethargy, confusion or coma, nausea and vomiting, and photophobia. Examination of the cerebrospinal fluid (CSF) shows an elevated opening pressure (>180 mm water), a decreased glucose concentration (<40 mg/dL), polymorphonuclear pleocytosis, and an elevated protein concentration. The diagnosis is made by demonstrating the organism with Gram's stain or in culture. *Bacterial meningitis is a neurologic emergency,* and initial treatment is empiric until a specific organism is identified.

   A. Therapeutic approach

   1. **Dexamethasone therapy.** The American Academy of Pediatrics recommends consideration of dexamethasone in the treatment of infants and children 2 months of age and older with proven or suspected bacterial meningitis on the basis of findings at CSF examination, a Gram's-stained smear of the CSF, or antigen test results. In clinical trials, dexamethasone improves the outcome of meningitis. For infants and children with *Haemophilus influenzae* type b (Hib) meningitis, dexamethasone therapy reduces the incidence of moderate or more severe sensorineural hearing loss and reduces meningeal inflammation. In experimental models of bacterial meningitis, dexamethasone inhibits synthesis of the inflammatory cytokines, decreases leakage of serum proteins into the CSF, minimizes damage to the blood–brain barrier, and decreases CSF outflow resistance. Dexamethasone also decreases brain edema and intracranial pressure (ICP). There are ongoing clinical trials of dexamethasone in the treatment of adults with bacterial meningitis. Despite the paucity of clinical data for adults, current understanding of the molecular basis of brain injury in bacterial meningitis supports the use of dexamethasone.

   The recommended dosage of dexamethasone is 0.15 mg/kg i.v. every 6 hours for the first 4 days of therapy. The initial dose of dexamethasone should be given before or at least with the initial dose of antimicrobial therapy for maximum benefit. Dexamethasone is not likely to be of much benefit if started 24 hours or more after antimicrobial therapy has been initiated. The concomitant use of an intravenous (i.v.) histamine-2 receptor antagonist is recommended with dexamethasone to avoid gastrointestinal bleeding.

   2. **Antimicrobial therapy.** If bacterial meningitis is suspected, antimicrobial therapy must be initiated immediately. This should be done before the performance of computed tomography (CT) or lumbar puncture. Initial antimicrobial therapy is empiric and is determined by the most likely meningeal pathogen according to the patient's age and underlying condition or predisposing factors.

      a. The most likely etiologic organisms of bacterial meningitis in **neonates** are group B streptococci, enteric gram-negative bacilli (*Escherichia coli*), and *Listeria monocytogenes*. Empiric therapy for bacterial meningitis in a neonate should include a combination of ampicillin and cefotaxime and an aminoglycoside.

      b. Empiric therapy for community-acquired bacterial meningitis in **infants and children** should include coverage for *Streptococcus pneumoniae* and *Neisseria meningitidis*. A third-generation cephalosporin (ceftriaxone or cefotaxime) and vancomycin are recommended as initial therapy for bacterial meningitis in children in whom the etiologic agent has not been identified. Cefuroxime, also a third-generation cephalosporin, is not recommended for therapy for bacterial meningitis in children because of reports of delayed sterilization of CSF cultures associated with hearing loss in children treated with cefuroxime.

      c. Empiric therapy for community-acquired bacterial meningitis in **adults** (15 to 50 years of age) should include coverage for *S. pneumoniae* and *N. meningitidis*. A third-generation cephalosporin (ceftriaxone or cefotaxime) or a fourth-generation cephalosporin (cefepime) plus vancomycin is recommended for empiric therapy. All CSF isolates of pneumococci and meningococci should be tested for antimicrobial susceptibility. Cefotaxime or ceftriaxone is recommended for relatively resistant strains of pneumococci (penicillin minimal inhibitory concentrations [MIC], 0.1 to 1.0 µg/mL). For highly penicillin-resistant pneumococcal meningitis (MIC greater than 1.0 µg/mL), a combination of vancomycin and a third-generation or fourth-generation cephalosporin is recommended. Penicillin G or ampicillin can be used for meningococcal meningitis.

   d. Initial therapy for meningitis in **postneurosurgical patients** should be directed against gram-negative bacilli, *Pseudomonas aeruginosa,* and *Staphylococcus aureus.* A third-generation cephalosporin is recommended for management of gram-negative bacillary meningitis. Ceftazidime is the only cephalosporin with sufficient activity against *P. aeruginosa* in the central nervous system (CNS). Vancomycin should be added until infection with staphylococci is excluded.

   e. In infants, children, and adults with **CSF ventriculoperitoneal shunt infections,** initial therapy for meningitis should include coverage for coagulase-negative staphylococci and *S. aureus.* The assumption can be made that the organism will be resistant to methicillin; therefore, initial therapy for a shunt infection should include i.v. vancomycin. Intrashunt or intraventricular vancomycin also may be needed to eradicate the infection.

   f. In **immunocompromised patients,** the infecting organism can be predicted on the basis of the type of immune abnormality. In patients with neutropenia, initial therapy for bacterial meningitis should include coverage for *L. monocytogenes,* staphylococci, and enteric gram-negative bacilli. Patients with defective humoral immunity and those who have undergone splenectomy are unable to mount an antibody response to a bacterial infection or to control an infection caused by encapsulated bacteria. These patients are at particular risk of meningitis caused by *S. pneumoniae,* Hib, and *N. meningitidis.*

   g. The most common organisms causing meningitis in **older adult** (50 years or older) are *S. pneumoniae* and enteric gram-negative bacilli; however, meningitis caused by *Listeria* organisms and Hib are increasingly recognized. The recommended initial therapy for meningitis in the older adult is either ceftriaxone or cefotaxime in combination with vancomycin and ampicillin. Table 43.1 lists empiric antimicrobial therapy for bacterial meningitis by age group. Tables 43.2 and 43.3 list the recommended antimicrobial therapy for bacterial meningitis in neonates, infants and children, and adults by meningeal pathogen.

3. **Management of increased ICP.** Increased ICP is an expected complication of bacterial meningitis and should be anticipated.

   a. **Elevation of the head of the bed** 30 degrees
   b. **Hyperventilation** to maintain $PaCO_2$ between 27 and 30 mm Hg
   c. **Mannitol**

Table 43.1 Empiric antimicrobial therapy for bacterial meningitis

Age group	Antimicrobial agent
Neonates	Ampicillin plus cefotaxime with or without aminoglycoside
Infants and children	Ceftriaxone or cefotaxime plus vancomycin
Adults (15–50 years)	
Community acquired	Ceftriaxone or cefotaxime plus vancomycin
Postneurosurgical	Ceftazidime plus vancomycin
Immunocompromised	Ceftazidime plus ampicillin
Older adults	Third-generation cephalosporin plus vancomycin plus ampicillin

Table 43.2 Recommended antimicrobial therapy for bacterial meningitis in neonates, infants, and children by organism

Organism	Total daily dose		
	Neonates (<1 wk)	Neonates (1–4 wk)	Infants and children (>4 wk)
Haemophilus influenzae type b (Hib)	Cefotaxime 100 mg/kg a day q12h	Cefotaxime 150 mg/kg a day q8h	Ceftriaxone 100 mg/kg a day i.v. in a once or twice daily dosing regimen, or cefotaxime 225 mg/kg a day i.v. in divided doses q6h
Streptococcus pneumoniae[a]	Cefotaxime	Cefotaxime	Ceftriaxone or cefotaxime
Group B streptococci	Ampicillin 100–150 mg/kg a day q12h plus amikacin 15 mg/kg a day q12h, or gentamicin 5 mg/kg a day q8h	Ampicillin 200 mg/kg a day q8h plus amikacin 30 mg/kg a day q8h, or gentamicin 7.5 mg/kg a day q8h	Ampicillin 150–200 mg/kg a day q4–6h plus amikacin 20 mg/kg a day q8h, or gentamicin 5 mg/kg a day q8h
Listeria monocytogenes[b]	Ampicillin with or without gentamicin	Ampicillin with or without gentamicin	Ampicillin with or without gentamicin
Neisseria meningitidis	Penicillin G 50,000–150,000 U/kg a day q8h, or ampicillin 100–150 mg/kg a day q12h	Penicillin G 150,000–200,000 U/kg a day q6h, or ampicillin 200 mg/kg a day q8h	Penicillin G 250,000–400,000 U/kg a day q4h, or ampicillin i.v. in divided doses q4–6h
Enteric gram-negative bacilli[a]	Cefotaxime	Cefotaxime	Ceftriaxone or cefotaxime
Staphylococcus aureus	Oxacillin 50–100 mg/kg a day q6h	Oxacillin 100–200 mg/kg a day q6h	Oxacillin 200–300 mg/kg a day q4h
Methicillin-resistant staphylococci	Vancomycin 20–30 mg/kg a day q12h	Vancomycin 40 mg/kg a day q6h	Vancomycin 40 mg/kg a day q6h, may also add intrashunt or intraventricular vancomycin 10 mg once a day

[a] Dosages are the same as for Hib.
[b] Dosages are the same as for group B streptococci.

Table 43.3 Recommended antimicrobial therapy for bacterial meningitis in adults by organism

Organism	Antimicrobial agent
Streptococcus pneumoniae	Ceftriaxone 4 g/d (q12h) or cefotaxime 12 g/d (q4h) or cefepime 4 g/day (q12h) plus vancomycin 2 g/day (q6–12h)
Neisseria meningitidis	Penicillin G 20–24 million U/kg a day (q4h) or ampicillin 12 g/d (q4h)
Gram-negative bacilli (except *P. aeruginosa*)	Ceftriaxone 4 g/d (q12h) or cefotaxime 12 g/d (q4h)
Pseudomonas aeruginosa	Ceftazidime 8 g/d (q8h)
Haemophilus influenzae type b	Ceftriaxone or cefotaxime
Staphylococcus aureus (methicillin-sensitive)	Oxacillin 9–12 g/d (q4h) or nafcillin 12 g/d (q4h)
Staphylococcus aureus (methicillin-resistant)	Vancomycin 2 g/d (q6–12h)
Listeria monocytogenes	Ampicillin 12 g/d (q4h) with or without gentamicin
Enterobacteriaceae	Ceftriaxone or cefotaxime

(1) **Children.** 0.5 to 2.0 g/kg infused over 30 minutes and repeated as necessary

(2) **Adults.** 1.0 g/kg bolus injection and then 0.25 g/kg every 2 to 3 hours. A dose of 0.25 g/kg appears as effective as a dose of 1.0 g/kg in lowering ICP. The main exception is that the higher dose has a longer duration of action. Serum osmolarity should not be allowed to rise above 320 mOsm/kg.

d. **Pentobarbital**

(1) **Loading dose.** 10 mg/kg over 30 minutes

(2) 5 mg/kg per hour for 3 hours, supplemented with 200-mg i.v. boluses until a burst–suppression pattern is obtained on an electroencephalogram (EEG)

(3) **Maintenance dosage.** 1 mg/kg per hour by constant intravenous infusion

4. **Seizure activity** is such a common complication of bacterial meningitis in adults, especially pneumococcal meningitis, that prophylactic anticonvulsant therapy is not unreasonable.

a. **Prophylactic therapy.** Phenytoin is administered at a dosage of 18 to 20 mg/kg at a rate no faster than 50 mg/min. Fosphenytoin is administered at a dosage of 18 to 20 mg PE/kg at a rate no faster than 150 mg/min. Phenytoin can prolong the QT interval or lead to hypotension and therefore should be administered intravenously while the electrocardiogram and blood pressure are monitored. If either of these side effects is observed, the rate of administration should be decreased. It is recommended that phenytoin be administered no faster than 25 mg/min in the elderly. A standard maintenance dosage is 100 mg every 8 hours. A serum concentration of 10 to 20 µg/mL should be maintained.

b. **Status epilepticus**

(1) **Lorazepam** (0.1 mg/kg for adults; 0.05 mg/kg per dose for children) or diazepam (5 to 10 mg for adults; 0.2 to 0.3 mg/kg per dose for children) is administered i.v.

(2) **Phenytoin** is administered in a dose of 18 to 20 mg/kg as described in **I.A.4.a.** Fosphenytoin is administered in a dose of 20 mg PE/kg

as described in **I.A.4.a.** If seizures are not controlled, a repeat bolus of fosphenytoin of 10 mg PE/kg can be given.

(3) If a dose of 18 to 20 mg/kg of phenytoin fails to control seizure activity, an additional 500 mg of phenytoin should be given.

(4) If phenytoin fails to control seizure activity, phenobarbital is administered intravenously at a rate of 100 mg/min to a loading dose of 20 mg/kg. The loading dose of phenobarbital for children also is 20 mg/kg. The most common adverse effects of phenobarbital loading are hypotension and respiratory depression. Before phenobarbital loading, an endotracheal tube has been placed and mechanical ventilation begun. The primary reason for failure to control seizure activity is that either anticonvulsants are administered in subtherapeutic dosages or, as is the case for phenobarbital, the rate of administration is too slow.

(5) For more information on the management of refractory status epilepticus see Chapters 38, 39, and 58.

5. **Fluid management.** Most children with bacterial meningitis have hyponatremia (serum sodium concentration less than 135 mEq/L) at the time of admission. For this reason, fluid restriction to correct serum sodium level is important. The initial rate of intravenous fluid administration is limited to approximately one-half normal maintenance requirements, or approximately 800 to 1000 mL/m^2 per day. A 5% dextrose solution with one-fourth to one-half normal saline solution and 20 to 40 mEq/L potassium is recommended. The volume of fluids administered can be gradually increased when serum sodium concentration increases to greater than 135 mEq/L.

B. **Expected outcome.** Despite appropriate antimicrobial therapy, patients with bacterial meningitis are very sick. Prognosis depends on age, underlying or associated conditions, time from onset of illness to institution of appropriate antimicrobial therapy, and the infecting organism. Pneumococcal meningitis has the worst prognosis, and a poor prognosis is associated with the extremes of age. The very young and the very old have significantly higher rates of morbidity and mortality than do older children and younger adults.

C. **Referrals.** Patients who are comatose should be seen by a neurologist.

D. **Prevention**

1. Rifampin is recommended for all close contacts with a patient who has **meningococcal meningitis.** It is given in divided doses at 12-hour intervals for 2 days as follows: adults, 600 mg; children, 10 mg/kg; neonates (younger than 1 month), 5 mg/kg. A single oral dose of ciprofloxacin (750 mg) also has been found efficacious in adults in the eradication of the carrier state of meningococcal infection.

   The Advisory Committee on Immunization Practices recommends that college freshmen be vaccinated against meningococcal meningitis with the tetravalent (Men A,C,W135,Y) meningococcal polysaccharide vaccine. Men C polysaccharide vaccine would also be effective.

2. For prophylaxis of **Hib meningitis,** rifampin is recommended not only for all close contacts with the patient but also for the patient, because the organism usually is not eradicated from the nasopharynx with systemic antimicrobial therapy. Rifampin in the following dosages is recommended: adults, 20 mg/kg a day orally for 4 days; children, 20 mg/kg a day orally (maximum 600 mg/d) for 4 days; and neonates (younger than 1 month), 10 mg/kg a day for 4 days. Rifampin is not recommended for pregnant women.

   The FDA has approved only the Hib conjugate vaccines HbOC and PRP-OMP for administration to children younger than 15 months. Patients should be vaccinated with Hib conjugate vaccine as follows.

   a. All infants should be vaccinated at ages 2, 4, and 6 months.

   b. Unvaccinated children 12 to 14 months of age should receive one dose plus a booster dose after 15 months of age.

   c. Unvaccinated children 15 to 60 months of age should receive a single dose and do not need a booster.

      d. Children older than 5 years should be vaccinated on the basis of disease risk.

      e. Rifampin prophylaxis should be given to children—whether or not they have been vaccinated with the Hib vaccine—who come in contact with patients who have Hib meningitis.

  II. Herpes encephalitis. Encephalitis is inflammation of the brain parenchyma. Herpes simplex virus (HSV-1) is the principal cause of herpes encephalitis. Initial infection occurs either after exposure to infected saliva or respiratory secretions, the virus gaining access to the CNS along the olfactory nerve and tract into the limbic lobe, or as a result of reactivation of latent virus from the trigeminal ganglion. Virus is transmitted from infected persons to other persons only through close personal contact. The typical clinical presentation is a several-day history of fever and headache followed by memory loss, confusion, olfactory hallucinations, and seizures. The hallmark sign is a focal neurologic deficit suggestive of a structural lesion in the frontotemporal area. The EEG often is abnormal, demonstrating periodic sharp-wave complexes from one or both temporal regions on a background of low-amplitude activity. The abnormalities on the EEG arise from one temporal lobe initially but typically spread to the contralateral temporal lobe over a period of 6 to 10 days. On CT scans, there is a low-density lesion within the temporal lobe with mass effect. On MR images, the infection appears as an area of high signal intensity on T2-weighted (Fig. 43.1) and fluid-attenuated inversion recovery (FLAIR) images. Examination of the CSF shows lymphocytic pleocytosis (with an average white blood cell count of 50 to 500 cells/mm^3), elevation in protein concentration, and normal

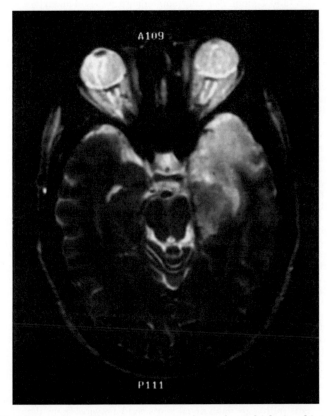

FIG. 43.1 T2-weighted magnetic resonance image shows classic high signal intensity lesion in left temporal lobe in herpes encephalitis.

or mildly decreased glucose concentration. The polymerase chain reaction technique used to detect HSV DNA in CSF has become the standard for the diagnosis of HSV encephalitis. CSF also should be evaluated for HSV immunoglobulin G antibody titers. Because this infection produces areas of hemorrhagic necrosis, the CSF may contain red blood cells or xanthochromia. Red blood cells in the CSF may inhibit the PCR, giving a false-negative result.

   A. Therapeutic approach

      1. Antiviral activity. Acyclovir is the antiviral drug of choice for HSV-1 encephalitis. It is given at a dosage of 10 mg/kg every 8 hours (30 mg/kg a day) i.v., each infusion lasting more than 1 hour, for a period of 3 weeks. Intravenous acyclovir can cause transient renal insufficiency secondary to crystallization of the drug in renal epithelial cells. For this reason, it is recommended that acyclovir be infused slowly over a period of 1 hour and that attention be paid to adequate intravenous hydration of the patient.

      2. Anticonvulsant therapy. Seizure activity, either focal or focal with secondary generalization, occurs in two thirds of patients with HSV-1 encephalitis. Anticonvulsant therapy is indicated if seizure activity develops, and the following drugs are recommended.

         a. Lorazepam at dosages of 0.1 mg/kg for adults and 0.05 mg/kg for children, or diazepam at 5 to 10 mg for adults and 0.2 to 0.3 mg/kg per dose for children

         b. Phenytoin at a dosage of 18 to 20 mg/kg at a rate no faster than 50 mg/min, or fosphenytoin at a dose of 18 to 20 mg PE/kg no faster than 150 mg/min. The daily maintenance dosage of phenytoin should be determined by serum levels.

      3. Therapy for increased ICP. Increased ICP is a common complication of herpes encephalitis and is associated with a poor outcome. Increased ICP should be aggressively managed as outlined in **I.A.3.**

   B. Expected outcome. Among untreated patients with HSV-1 encephalitis, the mortality is higher than 70%, and only 2.5% of patients return to normal function after recovery. Patients treated with acyclovir have a significantly lower mortality of 19%, and 38% of these patients return to normal function.

   C. Referrals. A patient who comes to medical attention with an altered level of consciousness or in a coma has a poor prognosis. Because the clinical diagnosis of herpes encephalitis typically requires interpretation of the neurologic presentation, the EEG, neuroimaging studies, and CSF, the diagnosis of this severe and devastating neurologic illness should be made in consultation with a neurologist or a neurosurgeon and an infectious disease specialist.

III. Herpes zoster (shingles)

   A. Therapeutic approach. Oral valacyclovir 1,000 mg three times a day has been found superior to acyclovir in reducing zoster-associated pain. Oral acyclovir 800 mg five times a day and valacyclovir accelerate the rate of cutaneous healing and reduce the severity of acute neuritis. Neither valacyclovir nor acyclovir reduces the incidence or severity of postherpetic neuralgia. Valacyclovir and acyclovir are most beneficial if treatment is initiated within 48 hours after the onset of the zoster.

   B. Side effects. Oral acyclovir therapy has not been associated with renal dysfunction. This is an uncommon and reversible side effect of intravenous administration of acyclovir. Oral acyclovir and valacyclovir can cause dizziness, nausea, and headaches.

IV. Lyme disease is caused by the spirochete ***Borrelia burgdorferi,*** which is transmitted by the bite of an infected tick. Lyme disease is endemic in the coastal northeast from Massachusetts to Maryland (particularly in New York), in the upper midwest in Minnesota and Wisconsin, and on the Pacific coast in California and southern Oregon.

Lyme disease is typically classified into three stages. **Early local infection** is characterized by the classic appearance of erythema migrans, an annular erythematous cutaneous lesion with central clearing. This lesion appears within 3 days to 1 month after a tick bite. **Early disseminated Lyme disease** is characterized by cardiac conduction abnormalities, large-joint arthritis (although small distal joints can be involved), myalgia, fatigue, fever, meningitis, and cranial and peripheral neuropathy and radiculopathy. The most common neurologic abnormality during early disseminated Lyme disease is meningitis. The clinical features are typical of viral meningitis with symptoms of headache, mild neck stiffness, nausea, vomiting, low-grade fever, and photophobia. These symptoms may be associated with a unilateral or bilateral facial nerve palsy or with symptoms of radiculitis (paresthesia and hyperesthesia) with or without focal weakness, transverse myelitis or cognitive difficulties. **Late Lyme disease** is associated with progressive encephalopathy characterized by impaired memory, impaired concentration, and fatigue. There may also be sensorimotor axonal polyradiculoneuropathy. A rare and late CNS manifestation of Lyme disease is **progressive encephalomyelitis.**

The only distinct clinical marker of Lyme disease is the typical erythema migrans lesion. Unfortunately, not all patients have this lesion, and in some cases, it goes unrecognized. It is standard practice to run a serologic test for antibodies against *B. burgdorferi* when Lyme disease is suspected. Most laboratories use an enzyme-linked immunosorbent assay technique. False-positive serologic results are a problem with this test for two reasons:

1. Tests can be performed on identical sera in several different laboratories with several different results. Because these tests are not well standardized, it is recommended that the physician use a laboratory that is reliable in performing this test. A positive test result may indicate only exposure to *B. burgdorferi* rather than active infection. Persons who live in high-risk areas may have measurable antibodies without having Lyme disease.
2. False-positive serologic results can occur with rheumatoid arthritis, Rocky Mountain spotted fever, infectious mononucleosis, syphilis, tuberculous meningitis, and leptospirosis.

The CSF is generally abnormal in neurologic Lyme disease. The typical spinal fluid abnormalities include lymphocytic pleocytosis (100 to 200 cells/mm^3), an elevated protein concentration, and a normal glucose concentration. The CSF should be examined for intrathecal production of anti–*B. burgdorferi* antibodies. The Centers for Disease Control and Prevention requires the following for a diagnosis of Lyme disease: erythema migrans at least 5 cm in diameter or one or more late disease features (neurologic, rheumatologic, or cardiac) with laboratory isolation of the spirochete, detection of *B. burgdorferi* antibodies in serum or CSF, or a rising antibody titer in acute and convalescent serum samples. Most physicians, however, would opt to treat any patient with a clinical presentation or course suggestive of Lyme disease and possible exposure to a tick in an endemic area.

   A. **Therapeutic approach**
      1. Patients with facial nerve palsy without other neurologic manifestations can be treated with doxycycline 100 mg by mouth twice a day for 4 weeks. *Doxycycline should not be given to pregnant women.*
      2. Parenteral antibiotics are indicated for patients with neurologic complications of Lyme disease, as follows: Ceftriaxone is the drug of choice for neurologic Lyme disease. The adult dosage is 2 g/d, which may be given in a single daily dose, and the dosage for children is 75 to 100 mg/kg a day (up to 2 g/d). Treatment is given for at least 2 weeks and should be continued for an additional 2 weeks if the response to treatment is slow or there is severe infection. The major side effects of ceftriaxone are gastrointestinal disturbance (including *Clostridium difficile* colitis), hypersensitivity reaction, and cholelithiasis.
      3. Alternatives to ceftriaxone are penicillin G and cefotaxime. Penicillin G is administered at an adult dosage of 3 to 4 million units (miU) every 4 hours for 10 to 14 days or at a child dosage of 250,000 U/kg a day in divided doses. The major side effect of penicillin G is hypersensitivity reaction. Cefotaxime is given at dosages of 2 g three times a day for adults and 120 to 200 mg/kg a day (every 6 hours) for children. The major side effects of cefotaxime are hypersensitivity reaction and gastrointestinal disturbance as well as inflammation at the injection site.
   B. **Expected outcome.** The condition of patients with neurologic complications of early disseminated Lyme disease (meningitis, cranial neuropathy, and peripheral neuropathy) should improve clinically within days, although improvement of facial weakness and radicular symptoms can take weeks. The condition of patients with encephalopathy associated with late Lyme disease may not improve, and the patient continues to have fatigue and memory impairment. The longer the neurologic symptoms go untreated before initiation of parenteral antibiotic therapy, the greater is the risk they will persist.

   C. **Prevention.** The deer tick is the usual vector of Lyme disease in the northeastern and the midwestern United States. Persons who pursue outdoor occupational or recreational activities should be able to recognize the deer tick. Wearing protective clothing can help decrease the risk of infection. Transmission of infection is unlikely if the tick has been attached for less than 24 hours. Pets allowed to roam in tick-infested areas should be fitted with tick-repellant collars and inspected for ticks.

V. **Cryptococcal meningitis.** The diagnosis of cryptococcal meningitis is made when examination of the CSF shows lymphocytic pleocytosis, a decreased glucose concentration, and a positive result of a CSF cryptococcal antigen assay, fungal smear, or culture.

   A. **Therapeutic approach.** The standard therapeutic regimen for cryptococcal meningitis has developed into a three-stage strategy. Induction therapy includes amphotericin B 0.7 mg/kg a day in combination with flucytosine 100 mg/kg a day divided into four daily doses for 2 weeks. Treatment then is switched to fluconazole 400 to 800 mg/d or to itraconazole 400 mg/d for 8 to 10 weeks. In the treatment of patients with human immunodeficiency virus (HIV) infection, fluconazole 200 mg/d is continued for lifelong suppressive therapy. In the care of patients without HIV infection, the length of maintenance therapy with fluconazole is less clear, but it should be continued for at least 6 months to 1 year.

   B. **Side effects.** The most important adverse effect of amphotericin B is renal dysfunction, which occurs in 80% of patients. Renal function should be monitored closely. Serum creatinine, blood urea nitrogen, serum potassium, sodium and magnesium, bicarbonate, and hemoglobin concentrations should be monitored. Renal toxicity appears to be reduced or prevented by means of careful attention to serum sodium concentration at the time of administration of amphotericin B. If renal insufficiency develops, AmBisome (Fujisawa, Deerfield, IL, U.S.A.) 4 mg/kg a day or amphotericin B lipid complex (ABLC) 5 mg/kg a day can be substituted for amphotericin B. Flucytosine is generally well tolerated; however, bone marrow suppression with anemia, leukopenia, or thrombocytopenia can develop. These hematologic abnormalities occur more often when serum concentrations of the drug exceed 100 mg/mL; therefore serum concentrations of flucytosine should be monitored and the peak serum concentration kept well below 100 mg/mL. Gastrointestinal symptoms, including nausea, vomiting, diarrhea, and severe enterocolitis as well as drug-induced hepatitis, have been reported in association with the use of flucytosine.

VI. **Neurosyphilis in immunocompetent patients.** In immunocompetent patients, the clinical presentation of neurosyphilis falls into one or more of the following categories: (1) asymptomatic neurosyphilis, (2) meningitis, (3) meningovascular syphilis, (4) dementia paralytica, and (5) tabes dorsalis. The diagnosis of neurosyphilis is based on a reactive serum treponemal test and CSF abnormalities. In neurosyphilis, there is often mild CSF mononuclear pleocytosis with a mild elevation in the CSF protein concentration or a reactive CSF Venereal Disease Research Laboratory (VDRL) test. A nonreactive CSF VDRL result does not exclude neurosyphilis. The CSF VDRL test is nonreactive in 30% to 57% of patients with neurosyphilis.

   A. **Therapeutic approach.** The regimen recommended by the CDC for management of neurosyphilis is intravenous aqueous penicillin G at 12 to 24 million U/d (2 to 4 million U every 4 hours) for 10 to 14 days. An alternative regimen is intramuscular procaine penicillin at 2.4 million U/d and oral probenecid at 500 mg four times a day, both for 10 to 14 days.

   B. **Expected outcome.** The serum VDRL titer should decrease after successful therapy for neurosyphilis. The serum fluorescent treponemal antibody absorption test and the microhemagglutination–*Treponema pallidum* test remain reactive for life. The CSF white blood cell count should be normal 6 months after therapy is completed. If on reexamination of the CSF, the white blood cell count remains elevated, repetition of treatment is indicated.

VII. **Tuberculous meningitis**

   A. **Clinical presentation.** Tuberculous meningitis manifests as either subacute or chronic meningitis, as a slowly progressive dementing illness, or as fulminant meningoencephalitis. The intradermal tuberculin skin test is helpful when the result is positive. Radiographic evidence of pulmonary tuberculosis is found more often in children with tuberculous meningitis than in adults with tuberculous meningitis. The classic abnormalities at CSF examination are decreased glucose concentration, elevated protein concentration, and polymorphonuclear or lymphocytic pleocytosis. The CSF pleocytosis is typically neutrophilic initially but then becomes mononuclear or lymphocytic within several weeks. Acid-fast bacilli are difficult to find in smears of CSF. Culture of CSF is the standard for diagnosis but is insensitive. Cultures are reported to be positive in 25% to 75% of cases of tuberculous meningitis, requiring 3 to 6 weeks for growth to be detectable. The CSF tuberculostearic acid assay has high sensitivity and high specificity, but it is difficult if not impossible to find a laboratory to do this assay. PCR on CSF for detection of *Mycobacterium tuberculosis* DNA holds promise but has not been perfected yet.

B. **Therapeutic approach.** Current recommendations for the management of tuberculous meningitis in children and adults include a combination of isoniazid (5 to 10 mg/kg a day up to 300 mg/d), rifampin (10 to 20 mg/kg a day up to 600 mg/d), and pyrazinamide (25 to 35 mg/kg a day up to 2 g/d). If the clinical response is good, pyrazinamide is discontinued after 8 weeks, and isoniazid and rifampin are continued for an additional 10 months. Ethambutol is added, and the course of treatment is extended to 1 to 2 years for immunocompromised patients. The American Academy of Pediatrics recommends addition of streptomycin at 20 to 40 mg/kg a day to the foregoing regimen for the first 2 months. Pyridoxine may be administered at a dosage of 25 to 50 mg/d to prevent the peripheral neuropathy that can result from use of isoniazid. Corticosteroid therapy is recommended when clinical deterioration occurs after treatment has begun. Dexamethasone can be administered at a dosage of 0.3 to 0.5 mg/kg a day for the first week of treatment and followed by oral prednisone.

VIII. **Neurocysticercosis.** A diagnosis of neurocysticercosis should be considered when a patient has seizures and neuroimaging evidence of cystic brain lesions. Cysticercosis is acquired by ingesting the eggs of the *Taenia solium* tapeworm shed in human feces. This occurs most often in areas where drinking water is contaminated with human feces.

A. **Principal forms.** The lesions of neurocysticercosis can be found in the brain parenchyma, the ventricles, the subarachnoid space, or in the basilar cisterns (racemose forms). In the parenchymal form, single or multiple cysts are found in the gray matter in the cerebrum and cerebellum. The most common clinical manifestation of parenchymal neurocysticercosis is new-onset seizure activity. In the ventricular form, single or multiple cysts are adherent to the ventricular wall or free in the CSF. Cysts are most common in the area of the fourth ventricle. In subarachnoid neurocysticercosis, cysts are found in the subarachnoid space or fixed under the pia and burrowed into the cortex. In the racemose form, cysts grow, often in clusters, in the basilar cisterns and obstruct the flow of CSF. Hydrocephalus and cysticercotic encephalitis, a severe form of neurocysticercosis due to intense inflammation around cysticerci and cerebral edema, are the most common cause of increased ICP.

B. **Diagnosis.** The diagnosis of neurocysticercosis depends on either histologic demonstration of the parasite in a biopsy specimen, evidence of cystic lesions demonstrating the scolex at CT or MRI, or clinical features and neuroimaging abnormalities (Fig. 43.2) suggestive of neurocysticercosis in addition to a positive result of a serologic assay for the detection of antibodies to *T. solium*.

C. **Therapeutic approach**
   1. **Cysticidal therapy** consists of praziquantel at a dose of 100 mg/kg in three divided doses at 2-hour intervals (single-day course) or albendazole at a dosage of 15 mg/kg a day for 8 days.
   2. **Corticosteroids.** Cysticidal therapy frequently causes an inflammatory response with an increase in CSF protein concentration and CSF pleocytosis. This may result in an exacerbation of signs and symptoms. The incidence of an inflammatory response is reduced by the concomitant use of corticosteroids. Plasma levels of albendazole are increased by dexamethasone; plasma levels of praziquantel are decreased by dexamethasone therapy. This should

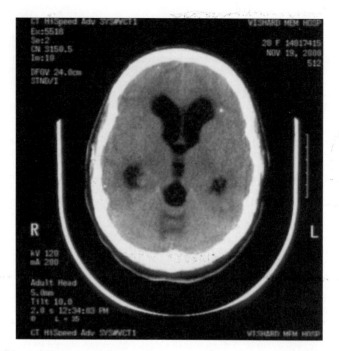

FIG. 43.2 Computed tomographic scan shows parenchymal brain calcification and hydrocephalus due to neurocysticercosis.

be taken into consideration when corticosteroid therapy is used to decrease the headaches and vomiting induced by the destruction of parasites in cysticidal therapy. Dexamethasone 24 to 32 mg/d is recommended for patients with subarachnoid cysts, encephalitis, angiitis, or arachnoiditis.

3. **Side effects.** Phenytoin and carbamazepine decrease serum praziquantel levels. If one of these anticonvulsants is used with praziquantel, it is recommended that oral cimetidine be added at a dosage of 800 mg twice a day. Phenytoin and carbamazepine decrease serum praziquantel levels by inducing the cytochrome P-450 liver enzyme system. Cimetidine inhibits the cytochrome P-450 enzyme system, and in this way increases serum levels of praziquantel.

4. **Surgical therapy.** Intraventricular cysts necessitate surgical therapy, and when they obstruct the flow of CSF with resulting hydrocephalus, an intraventricular shunting device is indicated.

D. **Expected outcome.** The prognosis among patients with parenchymal neurocysticercosis is very good with cysticidal therapy. Cystic lesions should disappear within 3 months of treatment. The mortality is higher among patients with increased ICP, hydrocephalus, or the racemose form of the disease.

E. **Prevention.** Humans can acquire cysticercosis by eating food handled and contaminated by *T. solium* tapeworm carriers. Persons at high risk of tapeworm infestation who are employed as food handlers should be screened for intestinal parasites. Improved sanitation can decrease the incidence of cysticercosis from contaminated food or drinking water.

Recommended Readings
Barry M, Kaldjian LC. Neurocysticercosis. *Semin Neurol* 1993;13:131–143.

Corona T, Lugo M, Medina R, et al. Single day praziquantel therapy for neurocysticercosis. *N Engl J Med* 1996;334:125.

Coyle PK. Neurologic Lyme disease. *Semin Neurol* 1992;12:200–208.

Del Brutto OH, Wadia NH, Dumas M, et al. Proposal of diagnostic criteria for human cysticercosis and neurocysticercosis. *J Neurol Sci* 1996;142:1–6.

Gottfredsson M, Perfect JR. Fungal meningitis. *Semin Neurol* 2000;20:307–322.

Kent SJ, Crowe SM, Yung A, et al. Tuberculous meningitis: a 30-year review. *Clin Infect Dis* 1993;17:987–994.

Lebel MH, Freij BJ, Syrogiannopoulos GA, et al. Dexamethasone treatment for bacterial meningitis: results of two double-blind, placebo-controlled trials. *N Engl J Med* 1988;319: 964–971.

Marra CM. Syphilis and human immunodeficiency virus infection. *Semin Neurol* 1992;12: 43–50.

Meyding-Lamade U, Hanley DF, Skoldenberg B. Herpesvirus encephalitis. In: Hacke W, ed. *Neurocritical care.* Berlin: Springer–Verlag, 1994:455–467.

Newton RW. Tuberculous meningitis. *Arch Dis Child* 1994;70:364–366.

Pfister HW, Roos KL. Bacterial meningitis. In: Hacke W, ed. *Neurocritical care.* Berlin: Springer–Verlag, 1994:377–397.

Reik L, Steere AC, Bartenhagen NH, et al. Neurologic abnormalities of Lyme disease. *Medicine (Baltimore)* 1979;58:281–294.

Roos KL, Tunkel AR, Scheld WM. Acute bacterial meningitis in children and adults. In: Scheld WM, Whitley RJ, Durack DT, eds. *Infections of the central nervous system.* New York: Raven, 1991:335–409.

Skoldenberg B. Herpes simplex encephalitis. *Scand J Infect Dis* 1991;78:40–46.

Sotelo J, Guerrero V, Rubio F. Neurocysticercosis: a new classification based on active and inactive forms—a study of 753 cases. *Arch Intern Med* 1985;45:442–445.

Whitley RJ, Gnann JW. Drug therapy: acyclovir—a decade later. *N Engl J Med* 1992;327: 782–789.

Wood MJ, Shukla S, Fiddian AP, et al. Treatment of acute herpes zoster: effect of early (<48h) versus late (48–72h) therapy with acyclovir and valacyclovir on prolonged pain. *J Infect Dis* 1998;178[Suppl 1]:S81–S84.

44. NEUROLOGIC COMPLICATIONS IN AIDS

Bruce A. Cohen

I. General considerations. The nervous system is involved early in the course of human immunodeficiency virus (HIV) infection and may produce the presenting clinical manifestations. Data from natural history studies indicate that neurologic symptoms and signs occur in 40% to 70% of patients with HIV infection during the course of the disease. Autopsy series show neuropathologic changes in 90% to 100% of persons with acquired immunodeficiency syndrome (AIDS), at any level of the neuraxis. These neurologic manifestations can result from effects of the HIV itself or from opportunistic processes. Acute meningitis, meningoencephalitis, or polyneuritis can mark HIV seroconversion. Later in the course of infection, neuropathy, encephalopathy, myelopathy, and myopathy can occur. Opportunistic illnesses of the central nervous system (CNS) occur in conjunction with marked immune suppression after the development of AIDS. Current therapeutic advances with combinations of antiretroviral agents known as **highly active antiretroviral therapy (HAART)** and primary prophylactic agents for opportunistic illnesses among those known to be at risk have had a profound effect on the frequency of both primary and opportunistic CNS disease in the United States and Europe. Neurologic complications still occur, however, as manifestations among persons not already known to have HIV infection, among those who are noncompliant with or lack access to expensive combination therapy regimens, or among those who do not have success with current combination therapies because of the emergence of resistant HIV strains.

Because of the variety of neurologic pathologic conditions that can occur in association with AIDS and the frequency with which they occur, the physician must be vigilant and thoughtful in approaching neurologic diagnosis and the treatment of these patients. Several postulates may be helpful to keep in mind in approaching neurologic syndromes in a patient with HIV infection.

   A. The imaging modality of choice in most instances of HIV-related CNS disease is magnetic resonance imaging (MRI); however, imaging patterns often are nonspecific.

   B. Multiple concurrent pathologic conditions in the nervous system are common and are found in one third or more of patients in autopsy series. Vigilance during therapy therefore is important, and reevaluation to detect concurrent or alternative conditions should be considered when abrupt or atypical changes in condition occur or the anticipated responses are not observed.

   C. Most opportunistic complications appear after marked immunosuppression has occurred, as reflected by CD4 lymphocyte counts of $100/mm^3$ or less.

   D. Neurologic manifestations of opportunistic infections in patients with AIDS can be subtle and lack classic features.

   E. Opportunistic processes can develop rapidly, with changes in imaging, laboratory, and clinical values over brief temporal intervals.

   F. Specific diagnosis of opportunistic illnesses requires confirmation through demonstration of immunologic or genetic markers in cerebrospinal fluid (CSF) or neuropathologic sampling. Empiric therapy is appropriate in some settings; however, thresholds for biopsy should be low in the care of patients with AIDS and localized parenchymal neurologic lesions and either atypical clinical features or lack of response to empiric therapy.

   G. Not all neurologic symptoms occurring in patients with HIV infection are the result of neurologic complications of the viral infection, particularly when immune competence is present. These patients are subject to all of the common neurologic conditions that affect the general population.

   H. Treatment strategies in AIDS are continuously and rapidly evolving. The National Institutes of Health (NIH) sponsors AIDS Clinical Trials Units (ACTU) through the Division of AIDS of the National Institute of Allergy and Infectious Diseases (NIAID). In the care of patients with neurologic conditions for which satisfactory therapies have not yet been established, referral to neurologic protocols available at ACTUs should be considered when feasible. Entities causing neurologic complications in AIDS are summarized in Table 44.1.

Table 44.1 Entities causing neurologic complications in AIDS

Encephalopathy	**Myelopathy** (*continued*)
Diffuse	Tuberculosis
HIV	Toxoplasmosis
PML	Vitamin B_{12} deficiency
CMV	*Nocardia asteroides*
VZV	Pyogenic abscess
Syphilis	
Toxoplasmosis	**Meningitis**
Aspergillosis	HIV
Toxic (medications)	Cryptococci
Metabolic (e.g., hypoxia, sepsis)	Syphilis
Focal	Tuberculosis
Toxoplasmosis	Lymphoma
PML	CMV
Lymphoma	HSV
Cryptococci	VZV
CMV	Other fungi
HSV	
VZV	**Neuropathy**
Syphilis	HIV
Tuberculosis	Toxic (e.g., dideoxynucleosides)
Fungal abscess	CMV
Nocardia asteroides	Lymphoma
Pyogenic abscess	Syphilis
	Vitamin B_{12} deficiency
Myelopathy	
HIV	**Myopathy**
CMV	HIV
HSV	Toxic (zidovudine)
VZV	Toxoplasmosis
Syphilis	Pyogenic
Lymphoma	CMV

HIV, human immunodeficiency virus; PML, progressive multifocal leukoencephalopathy; CMV, cytomegalovirus; VZV, varicella–zoster virus; HSV, herpes simplex virus.

II. Conditions attributed to HIV infection
A. HIV-associated dementia (HIVD)
1. Natural history. HIVD (HIV dementia, AIDS dementia complex, HIV encephalopathy) develops in approximately 15% of patients with AIDS, usually appearing after marked immunosuppression has developed. On occasion (3% of cases), it may be the initial manifestation of AIDS. HIVD is most often gradually progressive, evolving over months, although some cases emerge subacutely within weeks. The course is variable, sometimes deteriorating rapidly within 6 months, at other times stabilizing with only modest deterioration over years. Although about 30% of patients with AIDS eventually have measurable cognitive changes, not all of these patients go on to frank dementia. Those with impairment not severe enough to qualify as dementia are considered to have HIV-associated minor cognitive–motor disorder.

    The pathogenesis of HIVD is not understood. Clinical impairment is disproportionate to the degree of cytolytic destruction found at autopsy; however, significant reductions in both neuronal populations and synaptic complexity have been found in patients with AIDS. Multinucleated giant cells derived from macrophages and containing HIV genetic material have been correlated with the severity of HIVD; however, the syndrome has been shown to occur in their absence. Currently, perturbations of neuronal function due to toxic products of productive infection, loss of necessary trophic factors, and loss of regulatory factors are postulated as putative pathophysiologic mechanisms.

2. **Clinical features.** A clinical triad of cognitive impairment, behavioral changes, and motor impairment characterizes HIVD. Cognitive features include slowness of thought, perseveration, and impaired recall of acquired memories with relative preservation of recognition. Behavioral features include apathy and withdrawal from social interaction resembling depression. Uncommonly, mania or atypical psychoses occur. Motor features include hyperreflexia, hypertonia, and ataxia, typically affecting the legs initially. Extrapyramidal features of bradykinesia, facial masking, and postural instability may be observed. Tremors occur, and frontal release signs such as grasp and snout reflexes may be found.

3. **Diagnosis.** Progressive cognitive impairment with clear sensorium and typical behavioral and motor features in an AIDS patient with low CD4 counts suggests the diagnosis. Opportunistic processes must be excluded with MRI and CSF analysis. MRI may show atrophy or symmetric leukoencephalopathy. CSF analysis usually shows only protein elevation or normal fluid.

4. **Therapy**

   a. **Antiviral agents.** At the time of this writing, zidovudine, which inhibits HIV reverse transcriptase and penetrates into CSF reasonably well, is the only antiretroviral agent shown in a controlled prospective trial to have efficacy in HIVD, as measured by means of serial neuropsychometric testing. Higher doses of zidovudine were more effective. Other agents that have shown beneficial trends in less rigorous or statistically definitive studies include stavudine, abacavir, and nevirapine. Current HAART therapy with combinations of antinucleosides and protease inhibiting agents has been associated with a marked reduction in the frequency of HIVD in natural history studies, despite the fact that many of the newer protease inhibitors do not penetrate well into the CSF. Current strategies in which agents are selected for their CNS penetration are being pursued but as of this writing have not been shown to have superior efficacy in the management of HIVD.

   Studies have correlated measures of viral load in CSF with HIVD independently from plasma and shown differences in viral strains recovered from blood and CSF. The results suggest that independent viral evolution may occur in the CNS. Emergence of resistant virus during HAART may necessitate adjustment in therapy. This requires the introduction of several new agents. Current studies are evaluating the relation of CSF viral loads to manifestations of both neurologic and neuropsychologic disease and their response to HAART.

   b. **Adjunctive therapy.** Clinical trials are currently evaluating a number of agents proposed to counteract HIV-induced damage through in vitro effects on cytokine levels or HIV toxicity in cell cultures. Such agents, combined with antiretroviral therapy, may influence intermediate steps to achieve favorable modification of HIV neuropathogenesis. At the time of this writing, agents under evaluation include memantine, an N-methyl-D-aspartate antagonist, selegiline, an antioxidant, and tumor necrosis factor antagonists for their potential neuroprotective properties.

   c. **Supportive therapy**

      (1) **Apathy and withdrawal** can be managed with methylphenidate at 5 to 10 mg two or three times a day. Side effects include hepatotoxicity and gastrointestinal intolerance, delirium, seizures, anxiety, and sleep disturbances.

      (2) **Depression** can be managed with tricyclic antidepressants such as amitriptyline at initial dosages of 25 mg at bedtime, increasing in 25-mg increments every 1 to 2 weeks or with selective serotonin reuptake inhibitors (SSRIs) such as fluoxetine starting at 10 to 20 mg/d and increasing in 10-mg increments (or equivalent alternative SSRI regimens). Adverse reactions to amitriptyline and other

tricyclic agents include anticholinergic effects (such as urinary retention, constipation, dry mouth, and ileus), cardiac conduction abnormalities and arrhythmias, hypotension, sedation (which is often transient), toxic delirium, seizures, tremors, paresthesia, sleep disturbances, gastrointestinal intolerance, changes in appetite and increased weight, and alteration of taste. Uncommon effects, such as myelosuppression, hepatic toxicity, and movement disorders also can occur. Adverse reactions to SSRIs include chills, fever, nausea, headache, cardiac conduction abnormalities and arrhythmias, angina, blood pressure elevation or depression, arthralgia, gastrointestinal intolerance, hepatotoxicity, tremors, ataxia, hypomania, agitation and restlessness, respiratory tract irritation, menstrual irregularities, and seizures. Uncommonly, movement disorders, syncope, and myelosuppression occur.

(3) Seizures can occur in HIVD and can be managed with any currently available anticonvulsant; however, it is best to avoid agents that can accentuate the myelosuppression common in this population. An important consideration in patients using HAART is the risk that anticonvulsants metabolized by microsomal enzymes can alter the metabolism and thus the viral suppressive effect of some protease inhibitors, possibly increasing the risk of emergence of resistant organisms.

(4) Supervision. Progression of HIVD results in loss of ability to manage personal business and financial affairs. Provisions for legal transfer of decision-making powers for both financial and health care decisions, and advance health care directives, should be made. Assistance in the home is eventually needed for maintenance, provision of meals, and assistance with personal care. Residence in a sheltered facility can be considered when the need for assistance precludes independent living. Hospice programs can provide valuable support as the disease progresses.

5. Outcome. Although HAART has reduced the frequency of HIVD, its value in the management of established cases is less clearly established at this time. No definitive combination regimen with superior efficacy in HIVD has been identified, nor is it yet clear what disease markers in CSF might be useful for guiding therapy. Rational choices at the time of this writing in the care of a therapeutically naive patient include agents with good CSF penetration such as zidovudine, stavudine, nevirapine, and abacavir. However, for a patient with previous exposure to any of these agents, the risk of evolution of resistant strains of HIV may favor other choices. Progression of HIVD despite therapy should prompt reconsideration of the therapeutic regimen. Changes should introduce several new agents to hinder rapid emergence of resistance to the new regimen. Abrupt changes in neurologic function in the setting of AIDS should prompt evaluation for a superimposed opportunistic process.

B. HIV myelopathy

1. Natural history. Neuropathologic evidence of myelopathy is found at autopsy in as many as 40% of patients with AIDS although it affects fewer patients clinically. The most common pattern is a vacuolar demyelinating myelopathy. Pathologic changes are found predominantly in the dorsal and lateral columns of the thoracic spinal cord. Concurrent encephalopathy may or may not be present. Symptoms typically appear gradually over months and may progress or plateau over years. The specific etiologic factor is unknown. Active HIV infection is not usually found in the spinal cord. In rare instances, acute self-limited myelitis has been reported as a seroconversion reaction to HIV; however, this has not been associated with subsequent vacuolar myelopathy.

2. Clinical features. Gradually progressive spastic paraparesis and sensory ataxia evolving over months in a patient AIDS with immunosuppression are typical of vacuolar myelopathy. Disturbances of urinary bladder function commonly occur, and sensory deficits reflect dorsal column involvement with impairment of vibration and position sensation.

3. **Diagnosis** can be made on the clinical features once other causes of chronic myelopathy have been excluded, particularly vitamin B_{12} (cobalamin) deficiency, syphilis, human T-cell lymphotropic virus type I (HTLV-I) infection, and indolent opportunistic infections. Toxic myelopathy resulting from recurrent inhalation of nitrous oxide or toluene also can mimic vacuolar myelopathy. MRI findings most often are normal, or the images show atrophic changes. CSF analysis reveals nonspecific protein elevation, but the findings are otherwise unremarkable.

4. **Therapy.** No specific therapy has been shown to prevent progression of myelopathy. Although optimizing HIV HAART therapy is generally recommended, no favorable effect on the course of the myelopathy has been shown to date. Supportive therapy is beneficial. Spasticity can be managed with baclofen at 5 to 20 mg three or four times a day. Anticholinergic agents such as oxybutynin at 2.5 to 5.0 mg three or four times a day may relieve urinary frequency, urgency, and incontinence. Adverse reactions to baclofen include gastrointestinal intolerance, hepatotoxicity, and, at higher dosages, lethargy or weakness. High doses of baclofen cannot be stopped abruptly; the dosage should be gradually tapered to prevent withdrawal-related seizures and encephalopathy. Oxybutynin can produce anticholinergic side effects such as decreased gastrointestinal motility, dry mouth, abdominal cramping and nausea, urinary hesitation or retention, and decreased sweating. Lethargy or delirium can occur, and tachycardia or vasodilatation may be observed. Anticholinergics cause mydriasis and can increase intraocular pressure. External supports enhance safety and mobility in patients with sufficient leg strength. Motorized wheelchairs can maintain mobility in weaker patients who are otherwise capable of independent activity.

5. **Outcome.** Most patients with HIV myelopathy follow a slowly progressive course. Long survival times with current HAART regimens result in need for managing chronic disability. Patients need periodic neurologic examinations to adjust supportive therapy. Abrupt changes should prompt evaluation for a superimposed opportunistic process.

C. **HIV distal sensory neuropathy (DSN)**
1. **Natural history.** DSN is the most common neuropathy among patients with AIDS. It produces clinical symptoms in about one third of patients late in the disease course. Small pathologic series have shown neuropathic changes in as many as 100% of subjects. The cause is unknown, but progressive axonal degeneration with endoneurial and epineurial inflammation may be found at nerve biopsy.

2. **Clinical features.** DSN is characterized by symmetric burning or shooting pain, beginning in the feet, and gradually ascending up the legs. The distal parts of the upper extremities are involved later and to a lesser degree, usually with paresthesia. Examination reveals distal impairment of vibration and pinprick perception, absent or diminished ankle reflexes with variable depression of other reflexes, and sensory ataxia. Motor weakness in distal muscles may be present but is overshadowed by the sensory symptoms.

3. **Diagnosis.** The principal differential consideration often is the toxic effects of dideoxynucleoside antiretroviral agents (didanosine, stavudine), which can mimic or exacerbate DSN. Other potentially neurotoxic agents are used to treat HIV patients, including hydroxyurea, dapsone, isoniazid, and vincristine. Vitamin B_{12} deficiency is common in this population. Lymphoma can produce neuralgia by direct invasion of nerves or by paraneoplastic effects. Alcohol, diabetes, and other conventional causes of neuropathy should be excluded. Electrophysiologic studies reveal diminished amplitude and conduction in sural nerves and variable-amplitude decrements in other nerves with relatively preserved conduction. Distal denervation changes may be detected by means of electromyography.

4. Therapy

    a. Direct HIV therapy has not been convincingly shown to relieve DSN. Current treatment is directed at disabling sensory symptoms. Potential neurotoxic agents should be discontinued to the extent possible, particularly dideoxynucleosides. Toxic symptoms may persist for 6 to 8 weeks after discontinuation. Any metabolic deficiency should be corrected.

    b. Neuralgic pain may be treated with combinations of anticonvulsants, such as gabapentin, carbamazepine, or diphenylhydantoin, and tricyclic agents such as amitriptyline. Gabapentin often is used initially because it is less likely to cause myelosuppression or interact with other medications such as protease inhibitors. Typical dosages range from 300 to 600 mg three or four times a day. In the absence of leukopenia, carbamazepine can be initiated at dosages of 100 mg three or four times a day and increased 200 mg weekly to 800 to 1,200 mg/d as tolerated. Diphenylhydantoin is an additional alternative in dosages of 100 mg three or four times a day. Amitriptyline is begun at 25 mg at bedtime and increased 25 mg every 1 to 2 weeks as required up to 100 mg at bedtime. Patients who do not respond may be given a trial of mexiletine at 150 mg twice a day, increased to 300 mg twice a day as needed after anticonvulsants and tricyclics have been discontinued. Patients who do not obtain relief may need narcotic analgesia.

        (1) Adverse reactions to gabapentin include dizziness, ataxia, sedation, and fatigue. Diplopia, nystagmus, and tremor also may occur. Carbamazepine may cause drowsiness, ataxia, and gastrointestinal intolerance, particularly when dosages are increased rapidly. Confusion, visual blurring, diplopia, headache, leukopenia, and thrombocytopenia may occur, and aplastic anemia, cardiac arrhythmias, inappropriate secretion of antidiuretic hormone, hepatotoxicity, and Stevens–Johnson syndrome occur in rare cases.

        (2) Diphenylhydantoin can produce thrombocytopenia, hepatotoxicity, hirsutism, gingival hyperplasia, nystagmus, and, at higher serum levels, ataxia, drowsiness, and confusion. A rash indicates common hypersensitivity and should prompt discontinuation to prevent progression to Stevens–Johnson syndrome. Less common side effects include fever, lymphadenopathy, lupoid or pseudolymphoma syndromes, and pulmonary infiltrates. Osteomalacia and peripheral neuropathy can occur after long-term use. Adverse reactions to amitriptyline are listed in **II.A.4.d.** Mexiletine can produce cardiovascular toxicity with conduction block, arrhythmia, hypotension, or syncope; gastrointestinal intolerance including ulceration, hemorrhage, and dysphagia; hepatotoxicity; and, rarely, Stevens–Johnson syndrome.

5. Outcome. Symptomatic management can be helpful in alleviating discomfort, but reversal of DSN is unlikely. Abrupt changes in severity of DSN sometimes occur in association with active cytomegalovirus (CMV) infection, and screening for CMV may be indicated when compatible systemic symptoms are present.

D. Inflammatory demyelinating polyneuropathy (IDP)

    1. Natural history. Acute IDP usually occurs early in the course of HIV infection and may represent a reaction to seroconversion. The natural history is similar to that of Guillain–Barré syndrome in the population without HIV infection and is presumed to result from an immune reaction that results in peripheral demyelination. Chronic IDP also can be caused by immune mediated demyelination. Neurologic symptoms of chronic IDP may be relapsing or progressive.

    2. Clinical features. Acute IDP manifests as progressive motor weakness, areflexia, and variable sensory and autonomic symptoms that evolve over days and usually begin in the lower extremities and ascend. Some cases progress to respiratory insufficiency necessitating mechanical ventilatory support. Chronic IDP may follow a progressive or relapsing course over months with similar motor weakness and areflexia but with more prominent sensory impairment.

3. **Diagnosis.** Typical clinical features are suggestive of IDP. Electrophysiologic studies reveal prominent slowing and motor nerve conduction blocks, prolonged or absent F-wave responses, and variable degrees of axonal damage and denervation. CSF typically shows prominent protein elevation. Unlike the situation in the population without HIV infection, acute IDP can be associated with moderate lymphocytic pleocytosis. Such a finding should prompt serologic testing for HIV infection in a patient not previously known to have HIV infection.

4. **Therapy**
    a. Patients with IDP may recover spontaneously, but those with considerable motor impairment need treatment with plasma exchange totaling 200 to 250 mL/kg divided into five exchanges over a 2-week period with 5% albumin replacement. An alternative therapeutic option is the use of pooled human immune globulin in dosages of 0.4 g/kg daily for 5 days given as an intravenous (i.v.) infusion at 0.05 to 4.0 mL/kg per hour as tolerated. Patients with chronic IDP need maintenance therapy with one treatment every 2 to 4 weeks. Intervals can be gradually extended as response occurs. Additional benefit may result from combining the two methods. Because of the risk of facilitating opportunistic infections, corticosteroid therapy for chronic IDP is less often used in the treatment of the population with HIV infection. Patients with impending respiratory failure in acute IDP (vital capacity <1,000 mL) need elective intubation until adequate respiratory function returns.
    b. Adjunctive therapy is important to prevent complications of immobility and maintain function in anticipation of neuromuscular recovery. Nonambulatory patients should be given subcutaneous heparin at 5,000 U every 12 hours and intermittent calf compression to prevent deep venous thrombosis. Physical therapy should be initiated at the bedside for passive range of motion to prevent contracture formation and should be advanced with improvement in strength. Occupational therapy should be started early for patients with upper-extremity weakness. Neuralgic pain can be treated in the same manner as in DSN (see **II.C.4.b.**). As strength improves, mobilization may require support devices or orthotics, particularly for patients with chronic IDP.
    c. Adverse reactions to plasmapheresis include complications of hypervolemia or hypovolemia, hemolytic anemia, infection, allergic reactions, hypoglycemia, hemorrhage, and complications of catheter placement. Side effects of therapy with human immune globulin include risk of transmissible disease, myalgia, arthralgia, headache, light-headedness, chills, tremors, gastrointestinal intolerance, and, in patients with immunoglobulin (Ig) A deficiency, hypotension, and dyspnea. Many of these reactions can be ameliorated by slowing the infusion rate.

5. **Outcome.** Acute IDP usually resolves with complete recovery in most patients. Chronic IDP has a more variable outcome, and residual neurologic impairment often persists.

E. **HIV myopathy**
    1. **Natural history.** Myopathy may develop in patients with HIV infection as a result of zidovudine toxicity, HIV-related polymyositis, or, rarely, infection with opportunistic pathogens. Zidovudine myopathy usually appears after at least 6 months of treatment and is thought to result from mitochondrial toxicity. The pathogenesis of HIV myopathy is unknown, and the disorder occurs at any stage of infection. Uncommonly, opportunistic myositis due to toxoplasmosis or other agents can occur in immunocompromised patients.
    2. **Clinical features.** Symmetric progressive proximal weakness with elevation of serum creatine kinase levels is typical of both HIV and zidovudine myopathy. Myalgia is variable.

3. **Diagnosis.** The clinical pattern and elevated creatine kinase levels are suggestive. Electromyography shows small myopathic motor unit potentials with increased recruitment, fibrillation, and complex discharges. Concurrent neuropathy is not uncommon. Muscle biopsy shows scattered muscle fiber degeneration. Mitochondrial abnormalities and inclusions such as nemaline rod bodies may be present. Scattered inflammatory infiltrates may be seen.

4. **Therapy.** Patients taking zidovudine who experience myopathy should discontinue the therapy. If no improvement occurs after 1 to 2 months, muscle biopsy should be considered. For patients with acute severe myalgia and immune compromise, biopsy should be pursued earlier to exclude opportunistic myositis. Antiretroviral therapy may produce clinical improvement. Progressive myositis can be managed with corticosteroids. Prednisone may be started at 40 to 60 mg/d and tapered to lower, alternate-day dosages as response allows. Some risk of facilitating opportunistic infections may occur. Human immune globulin may be considered in accordance with the regimens described for IDP (see **II.D.4.a.**). In addition to opportunistic infections, adverse effects from corticosteroid therapy include hyperglycemia, hypertension, hyperlipidemia, weight gain, osteoporosis, gastrointestinal ulceration and hemorrhage, myopathy, psychosis, mood changes, cataracts, and impaired healing of wounds.

5. **Outcome.** Most patients respond to either withdrawal of zidovudine or institution of antiretroviral or steroid therapy. Lack of response to empiric measures should prompt muscle biopsy to establish the presence of inflammation and exclude opportunistic myositis before corticosteroids are started.

F. **Aseptic meningitis** may appear with HIV seroconversion. It typically manifests as headache, fever, neck stiffness, and occasionally cranial neuropathy and confusion or lethargy. This condition is self-limited and necessitates no therapy other than analgesia. Chronic, subclinical, aseptic meningitis occurs in many patients with HIV infection who have moderate protein elevation, modest lymphocytic pleocytosis, elevated gamma globulin index, and occasionally oligoclonal banding. The importance of this condition lies primarily in its potential for causing diagnostic confusion during evaluation for possible neurosyphilis or opportunistic disease. In patients with significant immunosuppression, aseptic meningitis should prompt investigation for opportunistic infection.

III. **Opportunistic diseases.** Neurologic opportunistic diseases in patients with AIDS are currently seen less frequently than in recent years as a result of advances in primary HIV therapeutics (HAART) and the use of primary prophylaxis for a number of the more common pathogens in patients known to be at risk. These conditions are still seen, however, as presenting manifestations of AIDS and in patients who have no response to or lack access to current therapeutic regimens.

A. **Cryptococcus**

1. **Natural history.** *Cryptococcus neoformans* is the most common opportunistic organism causing meningitis among patients with AIDS. This disease affected as many as 10% of patients in studies conducted before HAART and routine use of primary prophylaxis became available. Extraneurologic cryptococcal infection can be found in lung, bone marrow, liver, and skin. Localized cryptococcomas may be found in brain parenchyma. The fungus is acquired through inhalation and spreads to the CNS hematogenously. The infection becomes symptomatic with immune suppression.

2. **Clinical features.** The most common presentation is meningitis, and symptoms may be subtle with only headache, malaise, and fever. Nausea and emesis occur in approximately one half of patients. Meningismus occurs in approximately one third. Cranial neuropathy is the most common focal impairment. Seizures and focal CNS signs may be observed with parenchymal involvement, which in rare instances occurs in the absence of meningitis.

3. **Diagnosis.** Findings at imaging studies may be normal or show meningeal enhancement in patients with meningitis. Parenchymal cryptococcoma has variable enhancement patterns. Cystic lesions caused by extension of organisms into Virchow–Robin spaces in basal ganglia and other sites do not

become enhanced. On lumbar puncture, the CSF is usually under increased pressure. CSF pleocytosis is often modest and may be absent in one half of cases. Depressed glucose levels and modest protein elevations are more common, but nonspecific. Results of cryptococcal antigen titers usually are positive, and cultures always yield cryptococci in patients with meningitis, however, results of both tests may be negative when isolated parenchymal disease is present. Cryptococcal antigen can be measured in serum, where it is highly sensitive, to indicate initial exposure to the pathogen. Definitive diagnosis of isolated parenchymal lesions typically is made at biopsy.

4. **Therapy**

   a. Initial therapy for cryptococcal meningitis may be undertaken with amphotericin B at 0.7 to 1.0 mg/kg a day with or without flucytosine at 25.0 mg/kg four times a day in the treatment of patients with normal renal function. Fluconazole at a dosage of 200 mg twice a day was shown to produce similar response rates in one large study but produced less rapid CSF sterilization. Fluconazole has been used to treat patients with less severe infections who had normal mentation and CSF cryptococcal antigen titers less than 1:1000. Because mortality is highest within the first 2 weeks of infection, most authorities recommend induction regimens with high-dose amphotericin (0.7 to 1.0 mg/kg a day) with or without flucytosine at 100 mg/kg a day initially followed by a reduction in amphotericin dosage or a switch to fluconazole when successful sterilization of CSF has been accomplished. Amphotericin is now available in liposomal and lipid complexed formulations, which are less toxic although more expensive formulations.

   b. **Adjunctive therapy.** Patients with significant elevations of intracranial pressure should be treated with acetazolamide at 250 mg four times a day, mechanical drainage by means of serial lumbar puncture or CSF shunt, or both acetazolamide and drainage.

   c. **Maintenance therapy.** Successful sterilization of CSF with induction therapy should be followed by lifetime maintenance with fluconazole at 200 mg/d, because relapse rates greater than 50% have been reported among patients with AIDS not undergoing secondary prophylaxis.

   d. **Adverse effects of amphotericin B are common.** Fever and chills occur with administration and can be suppressed with ibuprofen, aspirin, or small doses of hydrocortisone. Nausea, emesis, headache, tachypnea, and hypotension also occur after infusion. Renal toxicity is considerable, and hydration and dosage reduction for signs of renal insufficiency may prevent more serious impairment. Pain at the infusion site, arthralgia, myalgia, phlebitis, and electrolyte disturbances with hypocalcemia, hypokalemia or hyperkalemia, and hypomagnesemia are observed. Hepatotoxicity, thrombocytopenia, leukopenia and granulocytopenia, coagulopathy, seizures, ototoxicity, encephalopathy, neuropathy, and anaphylactoid reactions can occur. Cardiac arrest, arrhythmia or congestive heart failure, dyspnea, pulmonary edema, and hypersensitivity pneumonitis have been reported.

   e. Flucytosine commonly causes gastrointestinal intolerance and myelosuppression. Nephrotoxicity, delirium or confusion, ataxia, ototoxicity, headache, paresthesia, neuropathy, hypoglycemia, hypokalemia, hepatotoxicity, and colitis can occur. Fluconazole can produce gastrointestinal intolerance, headache, hepatotoxicity, anaphylactic reactions, seizures, and leukopenia. Stevens–Johnson syndrome, hypokalemia, hypercholesterolemia, and hypertriglyceridemia have been reported. In patients undergoing concurrent therapy with warfarin or diphenylhydantoin, the effect of the latter agents may be potentiated, necessitating dosage adjustments.

5. **Outcome.** The acute mortality for cryptococcal meningitis in retrospective series of patients with AIDS ranges from 20% to 37%, two thirds of deaths occurring during the first 2 weeks. The most important prognostic factor is

the clarity of mentation and sensorium at presentation. Other factors thought to negatively affect prognosis are CSF cryptococcal antigen titers greater than 1:1,024, the presence of extraneurologic cryptococcal infection, elevated intracranial pressure, and hyponatremia. CSF should be sampled after completion of induction therapy. Persistently positive cryptococcal cultures should be managed with continued higher doses of antibiotics. Serum cryptococcal antigen cannot be used to monitor CSF response.

6. **Prevention.** Studies have shown a decreased incidence of cryptococcal meningitis among patients with AIDS taking fluconazole at dosages of 100 to 200 mg/d.

B. **CNS toxoplasmosis**

1. **Natural history.** *Toxoplasma gondii* is an intracellular parasite that typically is acquired by ingestion, usually remaining dormant unless immunosuppression allows reactivation. It is uncertain whether CNS toxoplasmosis in AIDS results from local reactivation or from hematogenous spread to the CNS after reactivation elsewhere. CNS toxoplasmosis is the most common opportunistic encephalitis among patients with AIDS.

2. **Clinical features.** The most common presentation is a subacute illness beginning with headache and fever followed by progressive focal or diffuse neurologic deficits appearing over several days. Some patients have an acute presentation with seizures.

3. **Diagnosis.** Imaging studies show multiple enhancing lesions in 85% of patients. MRI is more sensitive than is computed tomography. Most lesions appear as masses, but nonenhancing infarction-like patterns may be observed. Approximately 15% of patients have single lesions at MRI. The appearance of the lesions is nonspecific in most instances, although a signet ring sign has been suggested to be more specific when it is seen. Results of serologic studies for IgG antibodies to *Toxoplasma* organisms are positive in 97% of cases; however, IgM antibodies or convalescent increases in IgG titers are not often seen. Specific antibodies to *T. gondii* and *Toxoplasma* DNA amplified by polymerase chain reaction (PCR) techniques can be detected in CSF when the fluid can be obtained safely. Definitive diagnosis requires pathologic demonstration of organisms.

4. **Therapy**

a. Because of the rapidity of the response to therapy, empiric treatment of patients with HIV infection with multiple lesions typical of toxoplasmosis and positive serologic results is warranted for 2 to 3 weeks before brain biopsy is considered. Biopsy should be performed on single lesions with negative serologic results for toxoplasmosis. Optimal therapy combines sulfadiazine at 1.5 g by mouth every 6 hours and pyrimethamine by mouth in an initial dose of 100 mg followed by 50 mg/d. Folinic acid at 10 mg/d by mouth is added to counteract myelosuppression from the pyrimethamine. Patients unable to take sulfa can substitute clindamycin at 800 to 1,200 mg four times a day with similar efficacy for acute infection, although subsequent relapse rates may be slightly higher. Corticosteroids should be avoided to prevent diagnostic confusion when treatment is empiric. Seizures should be managed with anticonvulsants.

b. Successful initial therapy is continued for 6 weeks or until stable regression of all lesions. It is followed by lifetime maintenance therapy with sulfadiazine at 500 mg four times a day or clindamycin at 300 mg four times a day, combined with pyrimethamine at 50 mg/d and continuation of folinic acid. Patients unable to take either sulfa or clindamycin can be treated with atovaquone or azithromycin; however, efficacy may not be equivalent.

c. Adverse effects of sulfa include allergy, nephrotoxicity, gastrointestinal intolerance, pancreatic and hepatic toxicity, and, less frequently, hemolytic anemia resulting from glucose-6-phosphate dehydrogenase deficiency, toxic encephalopathy, neuritis, and dizziness. Adverse effects of clindamycin include gastrointestinal intolerance with diarrhea, pain, nausea, and emesis; hepatotoxicity; polyarthritis; and allergic reactions. Hypotension may occur after rapid intravenous infusion. Pyrimethamine produces thrombocytopenia, anemia, and leukopenia by causing folate deficiency and rare CNS toxicity with headache, confusion, seizures, tremor, ataxia, depression, or insomnia. Atovaquone can cause gastrointestinal intolerance, fever, insomnia, headache, dizziness, and allergic reactions. Rare CNS toxicity, nephrotoxicity, and myelosuppression also are reported with quinones.

5. **Outcome.** Therapeutic monitoring is particularly important for patients treated empirically for CNS toxoplasmosis. Imaging should be repeated 2 to 3 weeks after initiation of antibiotic therapy. Failure of lesions to respond should prompt brain biopsy. Biopsy should be performed on any lesion that enlarges despite therapy to exclude a concurrent process, irrespective of the behavior of other lesions. Most patients who respond can maintain control of the infection by taking suppressive antibiotic therapy. Approximately 10% of patients have relapses, usually because of discontinuation of maintenance therapy. Recurrence despite adequate maintenance therapy should prompt biopsy to exclude another process.

6. **Prevention.** Evidence from studies with patients taking sulfa to prevent *Pneumocystis* pneumonia suggests that toxoplasmosis can be prevented with daily trimethoprim–sulfamethoxazole double strength or dapsone at 50 mg/d and pyrimethamine 50 mg/wk.

C. **CNS lymphoma**

1. **Natural history.** Primary CNS lymphoma (PCNSL) affects 2% to 4% of patients with AIDS. The prognosis is poor even with therapy. Most patients die of the tumor or of another AIDS-related illness within 3 to 6 months of diagnosis.

2. **Clinical features.** Subacutely progressive headache, lethargy, cognitive impairment, and focal neurologic deficits related to tumor location, such as hemiparesis, aphasia, ataxia, or visual field deficits, are common manifestations. Cranial nerve palsy may be present. Presentations that are more acute include seizures, which can produce symptoms resembling transient ischemic attacks. Patients with AIDS also may have leptomeningeal lymphoma attributable to either seeding from a cerebral tumor or to metastasis of a systemic lymphoma. Manifestations include features of meningitis, meningoencephalitis, or meningoradiculitis.

3. **Diagnosis.** PCNSL typically produces enhancing mass lesions on cerebral imaging studies after infusion of contrast medium. Single or multiple lesions can be present, and most lesions cannot be differentiated from CNS toxoplasmosis or other cerebral abscesses during MRI. Radionuclide imaging with thallium single photon emission computed tomography (SPECT) often shows increased activity in a lymphomatous mass, unlike an abscess, which shows decreased activity. Such a finding supports early biopsy over empiric therapy. Leptomeningeal lymphoma may show meningeal enhancement on gadolinium-infused MR images. CSF may yield lymphoma cells in patients with leptomeningeal seeding. Diagnosis is generally made by brain biopsy in patients with mass lesions. Detection of Epstein–Barr virus (EBV) DNA in CSF is suggestive of lymphoma because almost all HIV-associated PCNSLs contain EBV DNA. Some authorities consider a typical SPECT scan and demonstration of EBV DNA in CSF sufficient for diagnosis in a patient with AIDS.

4. **Therapy.** PCNSL is radiosensitive, and referral for radiation therapy is appropriate for improvement in function and quality of life. Unfortunately, the therapy is palliative. Currently, clinical trials are evaluating the effect of chemotherapy and radiation on duration and quality of survival. There are reports of extended survival of patients treated with high doses of methotrexate or combination regimens. Patients with AIDS with leptomeningeal lymphoma have a poor prognosis. They can be treated with intrathecal cytosine arabinoside (ara-C) at a dosage of 50 mg/m^2 per week. Adverse effects of

intrathecal ara-C include headache; nausea; myelosuppression that may require support with erythropoietin, granulocyte colony-stimulating factor, or transfusions; encephalopathy; and hepatotoxicity.

5. **Outcome.** The prognosis for patients with AIDS with PCNSL is currently poor. Untreated persons usually die of the tumor within 3 months. Patients treated with radiation therapy alone generally survive for approximately 6 months, usually dying of opportunistic infection. Longer survival periods after therapy occur on occasion with chemotherapy. For patients who are treated, imaging studies are obtained serially during therapy to evaluate tumor response. Patients with leptomeningeal lymphoma also have a poor prognosis and are evaluated with serial CSF cytologic studies on samples obtained before each intrathecal treatment.

D. **Progressive multifocal leukoencephalopathy (PML)**

1. **Natural history.** PML may affect as many as 5% of patients with AIDS and among these represents the initial illness in as many as 25%. This disease results from reactivation of a polyoma virus, called JC virus acquired earlier in life but suppressed by normal immune function. Once symptoms appear, progression usually follows over months, usually resulting in death within 1 year. Some cases follow a more protracted course, with arrested or slowed progression and, rarely, improvement.

2. **Clinical features.** Subacute progressive cognitive impairment, visual field defects, hemiparesis, ataxia, and speech or language disturbances evolving over weeks to months are typical presentations. Some patients come to medical attention with seizures or stroke-like acute neurologic impairment.

3. **Diagnosis.** MRI typically reveals several asymmetric lesions in cerebral white matter that are best seen with T2-weighted sequences. The lesions usually do not become enhanced, although some may show marginal enhancement, and rarely exhibit mass effect. CT is less sensitive but may show areas of attenuation resembling infarcts. Single lesions are not uncommon when patients are seen early in the course. Definitive diagnosis requires pathologic confirmation of JC virus infection of CNS tissue. Studies with PCR amplification techniques can help detect JC virus DNA in both brain tissue and CSF. The specificity of JCV DNA from CSF for PML in a patient with typical brain lesions is high and currently is considered sufficient for diagnosis. The sensitivity of the assays, however, varies between laboratories, ranging from approximately 70% to 90%.

4. **Therapy.** No therapy has been proved effective in the management of PML. Anecdotal reports have described cases appearing to respond to HAART, cidofovir, and ara-C. A clinical trial conducted by the AIDS Clinical Trials Group comparing high-dose combination antiretroviral therapy with ara-C given intravenously or intrathecally failed to show prolonged survival for any of these treatment regimens compared with the others. Natural history studies have shown prolonged survival periods for patients with AIDS with PML treated with HAART, probably reflecting some recovery of immune competence. Persons with longer survival periods are more likely to have PML as the first AIDS-related illness and to have higher CD4 lymphocyte counts compared with those who die sooner. Available results of studies of the added value of cidofovir are conflicting and are reminiscent of the ara-C experience. Future controlled trials are needed to determine whether cidofovir or future candidate therapies offer any benefit beyond effective antiretroviral therapy.

5. **Outcome.** Current median survival periods among persons with AIDS-associated PML treated with HAART are approximately 12 months; however, some patients appear to abort disease progression and survive for many years after definitive diagnosis.

E. **Cytomegalovirus**

1. **Natural history.** CMV is commonly acquired early in life, and serologic evidence of infection is present in most U.S. adults. Although a transient systemic illness may occur on acquisition, normal immune function prevents

further manifestations. CMV is transmitted in body fluids, and almost all persons with HIV infection have serologic evidence of exposure. The most common symptomatic CMV infections in patients with AIDS occur in the retina and gastrointestinal tract. Autopsy studies have shown CMV in the brains of 10% to 40% of patients with AIDS.

2. **Clinical features.** CMV affects all levels of the neuroaxis in patients with AIDS but most commonly causes three syndromes. CMV encephalitis (CMVE) is characterized by subacute confusion, disorientation, or delirium; impaired attention, memory, and cognitive processing; and varying focal signs, including cranial neuropathy, nystagmus, weakness, spasticity, and ataxia. Focal encephalitis with mass lesions and aseptic meningitis also can occur. Clinical symptoms evolve over weeks. CMV polyradiculomyelitis (CMV-PRAM) manifests as subacute hypotonic motor weakness with areflexia and sphincter dysfunction (usually urinary retention) evolving over 1 to 3 weeks. Variable sensory features, including painful paresthesia in perineal and lower-extremity regions and indications of myelopathy such as a sensory level and Babinski signs, may be found at examination. Symptoms involve the lower extremities and may ascend, superficially resembling Guillain-Barré syndrome. CMV multifocal neuropathy is a subacute process evolving over weeks to months and characterized by motor weakness, depressed reflexes, and sensory deficits involving nerves of both upper and lower extremities in an asymmetric pattern. Motor features generally overshadow the sensory findings, although paresthesia may be the initial symptom. Less commonly, CMV can cause meningomyelitis or myositis.

3. **Diagnosis.** The clinical syndromes are suggestive of but not pathognomonic for CMV infection of the nervous system in AIDS. MRI with gadolinium may reveal enhancement of ventricular ependyma in approximately 10% of patients with CMVE, of meninges in some patients with meningoencephalitis or meningomyelitis, and of lumbar nerve roots and conus medullaris in some patients with CMV-PRAM. Imaging studies often have normal findings or show nonspecific atrophic changes. CSF studies characteristically reveal polymorphonuclear pleocytosis, hypoglycorrhachia, elevated protein level, and, approximately one half of the time, positive cultures for CMV in patients with CMV-PRAM. With CMVE, pleocytosis is less common, and CMV cultures are almost never positive. CSF is normal or reveals nonspecific protein elevation in patients with multifocal mononeuropathy. Demonstration of CMV DNA in CSF using PCR amplification techniques is both a sensitive and a specific indicator of active CMV infection. Almost all patients with AIDS and CMV infection of the nervous system have systemic infection as well, and ophthalmologic screening or evaluation of gastrointestinal symptoms may be revealing. CMV infection is also frequently found in the lungs and adrenal glands.

4. **Therapy.** Three agents are available for management of active CMV infection in AIDS. All are virustatic. Some authors recommend combination therapy in the treatment of patients with CNS CMV disease; however, there are no results of controlled clinical trials to guide choice of agents.

   a. Foscarnet has better CSF penetration than does ganciclovir and modest antiretroviral activity in addition to its efficacy against CMV. An induction dosage of 90 mg/kg i.v. twice a day for patients with normal renal function is given for 14 to 21 days and followed by reduction to a maintenance dosage of 90 to 120 mg/d. An indwelling catheter suitable for long-term use is placed to provide access. Doses must be reduced for patients with renal insufficiency. In addition to nephrotoxicity, adverse effects include fever, gastrointestinal intolerance, electrolyte imbalance, headache, paresthesia, seizures, and toxic encephalopathy. At times it may be difficult to differentiate adverse effects of foscarnet from the symptoms of CMV infection.

   b. Ganciclovir has been shown to have efficacy against CMV infection of the nervous system in patients with AIDS. Responses have been reported for

CMVE, CMV-PRAM, and multifocal neuropathy. Ganciclovir is given in an induction dosage of 5 mg/kg i.v. twice a day for 14 to 21 days followed by a maintenance dosage of 5 mg/kg a day. Myelosuppression, particularly neutropenia, is common with ganciclovir, especially when it is given concurrently with antiretroviral agents; doses of antiretroviral agents usually must be reduced. Other potential adverse effects of ganciclovir include hepatotoxicity, gastrointestinal intolerance, headaches, seizures, lethargy, paresthesia, toxic encephalopathy, and nephrotoxicity. As with foscarnet, it may be difficult to differentiate adverse effects of ganciclovir from disease manifestations of CMV.

    c. Cidofovir has been reported anecdotally to be associated with responses of neurologic CMV infections to therapy. Dosage in the setting of normal renal function is 5 mg/kg as an intravenous infusion in 1 L of fluid once a week for 2 successive weeks and then every 2 weeks. The dose must be decreased for impaired renal function, and additional hydration with a second liter of fluid is recommended if tolerable. Probenecid 2 g orally is given 3 hours before the infusion, and then 1 g is given 2 and 8 hours after completion of the infusion. Possible adverse effects include renal toxicity necessitating regular monitoring of blood urea nitrogen and creatinine levels, ocular hypotony necessitating regular monitoring of ocular pressure, uveitis, neutropenia, and metabolic acidosis. The renal toxicity of cidofovir and foscarnet may be additive, and patients previously treated with foscarnet may be at increased risk of cidofovir nephrotoxicity.

    d. Viral resistance may develop to any of these agents during prolonged therapy, and neurologic symptoms emerging during maintenance therapy for CMV retinitis or enteritis should be managed with induction dosages of alternate agents. Even when drugs have failed individually, patients may respond to combined therapy.

  5. Outcome. No prospective studies are available to guide therapy for CMV neurologic disease in AIDS, partly because of difficulties in premortem diagnosis. Responses to therapy for CMVE, CMV-PRAM, and multifocal neuropathy are reported anecdotally. Successfully treated patients should continue maintenance therapy, although the optimal regimen is yet to be devised. CSF studies appear to be the best markers of disease activity and should be performed on completion of induction therapy and for any progressive neurologic symptoms that occur during maintenance therapy. Recurrent inflammation and possibly persistent evidence of CMV DNA by PCR amplification may suggest active viral replication and imply resistance to the regimen used.

F. Herpes simplex virus (HSV)

  1. Natural history. HSV is ubiquitous in the general population, and patients with HIV infection have a high frequency of HSV-2 genital–rectal infection. Many episodes of HSV-2 aseptic meningitis are self-limited, but symptomatic meningoradiculitis, encephalitis, or myelitis may be severe enough to necessitate therapy. HSV-1 encephalitis has been reported among patients with HIV infection and may produce subtle and atypical pathologic changes in immunosuppressed patients.

  2. Clinical features. HSV-1 produces focal encephalitis with a predilection for the deep frontal and temporal lobes. Seizures, headaches, personality changes, and focal language disturbances may progress over days to confusion, obtundation, and coma. Some patients with HIV infection have a lesser degree of clinical progression. HSV-2 produces aseptic meningitis with fever and headache; meningoradiculitis, which can involve sacral roots and produce urinary retention; and meningoencephalitis. Patients with meningomyelitis have progressive weakness, spasticity, sensory impairment, and ataxia, typically affecting the lower extremities, associated with variable sphincter disturbances. Patients with HSV-2 meningoencephalitis appear with confusion, seizures, headaches, and fever with variable motor impairment. Neurologic manifestations of HSV-2 may be observed concurrently with or after genital–rectal eruptions or may occur independently.

3. **Diagnosis.** HSV-1 encephalitis may be suspected when focal enhancing lesions are detected in the inferior frontal or temporal lobes at MRI with gadolinium contrast infusion. Electroencephalograms may show characteristic periodic spike discharges. Patients with focal encephalitis caused by HSV-1 in other locations have no characteristic features. CSF studies typically show mixed pleocytosis, erythrocytes in some cases, modestly depressed or normal glucose levels, and elevated protein levels. Viral culture may yield HSV-1 on occasion. PCR amplification of HSV DNA in CSF is now available. When such confirmation to support diagnosis is lacking, patients with HIV infection with isolated temporal or frontal lesions should undergo biopsy because of the range of possible pathologic conditions. Patients with HSV-2 meningitis, meningomyelitis, or meningoencephalitis may have meningeal enhancement or have normal findings at MRI studies. CSF reveals lymphocytic pleocytosis or normal cell counts, normal or modestly depressed glucose levels, and variable protein levels. The result of a viral culture may be positive, and PCR amplification of HSV-2 DNA can support CSF diagnosis.
4. **Therapy**
   a. Acyclovir is a virustatic agent with efficacy against herpes viruses possessing thymidine kinase activity. This enzyme initiates formation of acyclovir triphosphate, which inhibits viral replication. Acyclovir in a dosage of 10 to 12 mg/kg i.v. three times a day should be started immediately on suspicion of HSV CNS disease while other diagnostic studies are pending. Patients with confirmed cases are treated for 14 to 21 days. Maintenance therapy sometimes is given for recurrent genital–rectal infections at a dosage of 200 mg by mouth five times a day. Resistant strains of HSV-2 are starting to appear, and patients with persistent or progressive neurologic manifestations of HSV should be treated with foscarnet at 60 mg/kg twice a day for 14 to 21 days.
   b. Adverse effects of acyclovir include nephrotoxicity, hepatotoxicity, gastrointestinal intolerance, and infusion-site irritation. The dose must be reduced for patients with renal insufficiency. Patients may have headaches and dizziness, and in rare instances toxic delirium with confusion, disorientation, hallucinations or delusions, and seizures may occur, usually with elevated serum acyclovir levels. Hypotension and myelosuppression have been reported.
5. **Outcome.** Results of few studies are available on the course of HSV meningitis or related CNS disease in AIDS. Many patients respond to therapy with acyclovir, but others do not because of either HSV resistance or inadequate immune function. Serial CSF studies are currently the best means of detecting resistance and should be performed after completion of antiviral therapy and for recurrent neurologic symptoms.

G. **Varicella–zoster virus (VZV)**
   1. **Natural history.** VZV commonly occurs in patients with HIV infection at multiple stages of the disease and may produce encephalitis or myelitis in addition to radiculitis. The virus, which causes chickenpox, is acquired early in life and resides latently in sensory ganglia, where it can intermittently produce recurrent radiculitis. Retrograde extension to the CNS along contiguous sensory roots and fiber tracts has been shown to occur. Patients with radiculitis often have self-limited dermatologic eruptions, which may be accompanied by prolonged neuralgia. CNS extension may be marked by vasculitis, particularly after ophthalmic zoster, resulting in cerebral infarction. CNS extension can result in necrotizing myelitis and brainstem encephalitis. Focal or diffuse cerebral encephalitis also can occur.
   2. **Clinical features.** VZV radiculitis usually is heralded by painful paresthesia in a restricted dermatomal distribution of a thoracic or trigeminal root. A vesicular rash usually follows, but cases of VZV occur in the absence of dermatomal eruptions. The rash typically heals over weeks, the vesicles crusting and then fading. Pain may persist. VZV myelitis usually is marked by weakness referable to the region of eruption and sometimes by associated

myoclonus. Myelitis may be limited or may be progressive, resulting in spastic weakness, sensory impairment, and sphincter dysfunction. Meningitis marked by lymphocytic pleocytosis, increased protein level, and depressed or normal glucose level often is associated. VZV myelitis can occur in the absence of dermatomal eruption. Polyradiculitis, which is clinically indistinguishable from CMV-PRAM can occur as a result of VZV. VZV encephalitis can be focal or diffuse in patients with AIDS, manifesting as seizures, confusion, progressive language and cognitive impairment, and sensory or motor abnormalities. Progression can be gradual and the level of immunosuppression modest. The CSF profile is similar to that of myelitis. VZV vasculitis can cause acute focal features resulting from cerebral or spinal infarction.

   3. **Diagnosis.** When the characteristic dermatologic eruption occurs, diagnosis is not difficult. For patients with isolated encephalitis or myelitis, however, the diagnosis can be elusive. CSF is nonspecific and rarely yields virus on culture. PCR amplification for identification of VZV DNA in CSF is available for diagnosis of CNS VZV infection. Immunohistochemical analysis of pathologic specimens obtained by means of biopsy of progressive cerebral lesions may be needed, but even histochemical techniques lack sensitivity. Imaged lesions may initially appear as focal areas of attenuation on CT scans or of high signal intensity on T2-weighted MR images. More diffuse leukoencephalopathy or enhancing focal lesions may be observed.

   4. **Therapy.** Patients with HIV infection and VZV radiculitis should be treated with acyclovir at 800 mg by mouth five times a day until all lesions have crusted. If more than one dermatome is involved, some authorities recommend intravenous therapy with 10 to 12 mg/kg i.v. every 8 hours. Neuralgia is best managed with gabapentin 300 to 600 mg three or four times a day, carbamazepine 100 to 200 mg four times a day to every 4 hours or with diphenylhydantoin 100 mg three or four times a day. Amitriptyline 25 mg at bedtime may be added and increased by 25 mg/d at weekly intervals to 100 mg at bedtime. Some patients who do not respond to these agents may benefit from the addition of baclofen 5 to 10 mg three or four times a day or topical application of capsaicin to the involved cutaneous area three or four times a day. Patients with encephalitis or myelitis should be treated with intravenous acyclovir for 14 to 21 days 10 to 12 mg/kg three times a day. The role of maintenance therapy to prevent recurrent eruptions is unclear, because resistance of VZV to acyclovir has begun to emerge. VZV CNS disease refractory to acyclovir should be assumed to reflect resistance and should be managed with foscarnet 60 to 90 mg i.v. twice a day for 10 to 21 days. Supportive therapy for myelitis is similar to that described for HIV myelopathy, including antispasticity agents, physical therapy, and orthotics as required and anticholinergic agents for hypertonic neurogenic bladder. Anticonvulsants are used to treat patients with seizures. Adverse effects of these medications are discussed in **II.B.4.**

   5. **Outcome.** Most patients with VZV radiculitis achieve resolution of the acute symptoms, although recurrences are common and may not involve the same distribution each time. The prognosis for progressive myelitis and encephalitis is variable, although only limited anecdotal data are available. The extent to which this reflects VZV resistance to acyclovir is unknown.

H. **Tuberculosis**
   1. **Natural history.** *Mycobacterium tuberculosis* (MTB) in a patient with HIV infection can cause tuberculous meningitis or cerebral mass lesions. The epidemiologic frequency of MTB infection in association varies widely within the United States and in other parts of the world. Mortality from tuberculous meningitis associated with AIDS appears to be related to immune competence as reflected by CD4 lymphocyte count and has been found to be higher than in the population without HIV infection.
   2. **Clinical features.** Patients with AIDS with MTB infection most commonly come to medical attention with meningitis or meningoencephalitis marked by headaches, fever, myalgia, confusion, lethargy, cranial neuropathy, ataxia,

seizures, or hemiparesis evolving over weeks. Contiguous extension of basal meningitis to blood vessels of the circle of Willis can result in vasculitis and cerebral infarction. Cerebral abscess formation results in focal symptoms, seizures, headaches, and signs of increased intracranial pressure. Tuberculous meningitis also can cause meningoradiculitis, myelitis, anterior spinal artery infarction, and epidural or intramedullary abscess formation. Tuberculous spondylitis can result in vertebral collapse with fever, back pain, and radiculopathy or compressive myelopathy.

3. **Diagnosis.** Imaging studies may reveal focal abscesses in the brain that are indistinguishable from lesions of toxoplasmosis or CNS lymphoma. Areas of attenuation typical of infarction, meningeal thickening and enhancement, exudate in basilar cisterns, and hydrocephalus are present in patients with MTB meningitis. CSF is usually under increased pressure and reveals mixed or lymphocytic pleocytosis, depressed glucose, and prominently elevated protein levels. Smears for acid-fast bacteria are uncommonly positive, and CSF cultures also may be negative in one third of cases, taking weeks to grow when they do yield organisms. PCR amplification of MTB DNA and MTB antigen assays provide more rapid detection in CSF. Diagnosis of mass lesions generally is made by means of histopathologic examination of biopsy material. Spinal MRI may reveal abscess formation and vertebral collapse.

4. **Therapy**
   a. Combined therapies with combinations of isoniazid at 300 mg by mouth, rifampin at 600 mg by mouth, and ethambutol at 15 to 25 mg/kg a day by mouth with pyrazinamide at 15 to 25 mg/kg by mouth daily added for the first 2 months, are commonly used. Pyridoxine (50 mg/d) is added for patients taking isoniazid. Resistance of MTB to these agents is now observed particularly in urban areas, and lack of response to treatment should prompt infectious disease consultation to modify therapy. Therapy should be continued for at least 6 months. Corticosteroids are added for arachnoiditis and basal meningitis, cerebral edema, and vasculitis.
   b. Adverse effects of isoniazid include hepatotoxicity, which is more likely after 35 years of age, gastrointestinal intolerance, hypersensitivity, and peripheral neuropathy resulting from vitamin B_6 deficiency. Other, uncommon effects are optic neuropathy; toxic encephalopathy with seizures, delirium, obtundation, and myoclonus; myelosuppression; lupoid reactions; and hyperglycemia. Rifampin imparts an orange color to urine and secretions. Adverse effects of rifampin include headaches, hepatotoxicity, gastrointestinal intolerance, interstitial nephritis, fatigue, lethargy, and myalgia, myelosuppression, hemolytic anemia, myopathy, delirium or confusion, and hypersensitivity reactions. Ethambutol can produce optic neuropathy, gastrointestinal intolerance, peripheral neuropathy with paresthesias, headaches, toxic encephalopathy, thrombocytopenia, hyperuricemia, and hypersensitivity reactions. Pyrazinamide can cause polyarthralgia, myalgia, hyperuricemia, hepatotoxicity, gastrointestinal intolerance, anemia, and coagulopathy.

5. **Outcome.** The mortality of AIDS-associated tuberculous meningitis has been reported to be as high as 33% and to be related to the degree of immune suppression as reflected by CD4 lymphocyte count. Patients with MTB meningitis need follow-up CSF studies 1 to 2 months after initiation of treatment and at completion of primary therapy to detect persistent infection from resistant organisms. Mass lesions suspected to be tuberculomas can be followed with serial imaging studies in the absence of life-threatening mass effects. Such lesions that enlarge despite therapy should be subjected to biopsy to detect resistant organisms or concurrent opportunistic processes. Potential drug toxicity should be monitored with serial complete blood count and chemistry profiles and ophthalmologic examinations every 6 months. Use of alcohol while taking isoniazid should be avoided.

I. **Neurosyphilis**
   1. **Natural history.** Although it is not an opportunistic infection, overlapping risk factors and atypical response to therapy make *Treponema pallidum*

infection a frequent concern among patients with HIV infection. Failure of conventional therapy, particularly benzathine penicillin, to prevent neurosyphilis and recurrence of neurosyphilis despite intravenous administration of penicillin has been reported.

2. **Clinical features.** Meningitis, meningoradiculitis, meningovasculitis with infarctions of small vessels, meningomyelitis, and encephalitis can occur in patients with AIDS. Mass lesions resulting from gumma formation may manifest with seizures, focal signs, and increased intracranial pressure. Cranial neuropathy, headache, and fever may mark syphilitic meningitis, and polyradiculitis may result in a cauda equina syndrome similar to CMV-PRAM. Luetic encephalitis and myelitis can be gradually or subacutely progressive.

3. **Diagnosis.** Meningitis is nonspecific with variable lymphocytic pleocytosis and elevated protein. The result of a Venereal Disease Research Laboratory (VDRL) test is often but not always positive in CSF. Specific treponemal antibody assays such as the *T. pallidum* hemagglutination assay and fluorescent treponemal antibody (FTA) indexes are more sensitive and are exclusionary when negative. Imaging studies may reveal infarcts or enhancing masses in patients with gummas; however, results of such studies do not confirm the diagnosis. Mass lesions usually are diagnosed at biopsy. Serum FTA testing should be performed for all patients with HIV infection and with neurologic disease, and CSF should be obtained for all patients with positive FTA results.

4. **Therapy.** Neurosyphilis should be managed with intravenous aqueous penicillin at a dosage of 2 to 4 million U every 4 hours for 14 to 21 days. Patients with asymptomatic CNS syphilis may be offered 2.4 million U/d of procaine penicillin intramuscularly plus probenecid at 500 mg by mouth twice a day for a similar duration. No other therapy has proven efficacy, although ceftriaxone at 2 g/d i.v. for 10 to 14 days may be tried in the treatment of patients allergic to penicillin who do not have cross-sensitivity to cephalosporins. Patients with neurosyphilis who are allergic to both agents should be evaluated by an allergist and infectious disease specialist for desensitization therapy to allow treatment with penicillin.

5. **Outcome.** Although the initial response often is good, recurrent neurosyphilis is common enough to warrant vigilance. Patients with luetic meningitis need CSF studies after completion of therapy and at 6-month intervals until the CSF VDRL result stabilizes or becomes nonreactive. Subsequent neurologic symptoms should prompt evaluation for recurrence.

J. *Nocardia asteroides*

1. **Natural history.** *N. asteroides* is a gram-positive intracellular bacterium found in soil and decaying organic matter and acquired by inhalation. In patients with immunosuppression, hematogenous spread to the CNS may result in meningitis or abscess formation.

2. **Clinical features.** In patients with AIDS, *Nocardia* abscesses manifest as subacutely progressive mass lesions with headaches, fever, focal signs related to localization, obtundation, confusion, and lethargy.

3. **Diagnosis.** Imaging studies typically show contrast-enhancing mass lesions that often are multiloculated in appearance. CSF, when obtainable, shows depressed glucose and elevated protein levels with variable polymorphonuclear pleocytosis. The diagnosis usually is made from smears or cultures of abscess fluid.

4. **Therapy.** Optimal therapy combines abscess excision and antibiotics. Sulfisoxazole at a dosage of 2 g by mouth four times a day or trimethoprim/sulfamethoxazole double strength twice a day may produce a clinical response, but recurrences are observed despite maintenance therapy. Treatment should be continued indefinitely. Recurrences despite therapy can be managed with minocycline at 100 to 200 mg by mouth twice a day, which is an alternative for patients allergic to sulfa. Ceftriaxone at 2 g i.v. twice a day may be used with minocycline. Adverse effects of sulfa are listed in **III.B.4.c.** Minocycline can produce gastrointestinal intolerance, pancre-

atic toxicity, hepatotoxicity, nephrotoxicity, photosensitivity, pseudotumor cerebri, hemolytic anemia, thrombocytopenia, neutropenia, eosinophilia, and hypersensitivity reactions, including Stevens–Johnson syndrome.

5. **Outcome.** Relapses occur despite maintenance therapy, and vigilance is required to detect concurrent opportunistic infections. Lesion size should be followed by means of serial imaging studies. New lesions that do not respond to brief trials of therapy directed at *Nocardia* should be subjected to biopsy.

K. **Other fungal opportunistic infections**

1. **Natural history.** Several other CNS fungal infections, including aspergillosis, blastomycosis, coccidioidomycosis, histoplasmosis, and mucormycosis, are reported in small numbers of patients with AIDS, usually in association with disseminated infection. Prognosis is generally poor despite therapy, although patients may respond occasionally.

2. **Clinical features.** Aspergillosis can manifest as multiple cerebral infarctions resulting from colonization of blood vessels, abscess formation, or meningitis. The presence of sinus or airway disease should prompt consideration of the diagnosis. Mucormycosis also invades blood vessels and may occur in intravenous drug users or persons with diabetes. Blastomycosis, coccidioidomycosis, and histoplasmosis can manifest as meningitis or cerebral abscesses. Meningomyelitis also can occur.

3. **Diagnosis.** Findings at CNS imaging are nonspecific. Diagnosis of these infections usually rests on examination of abscess fluid or culture of CSF when the result is positive. Culture of respiratory tract material obtained at biopsy may yield a diagnosis if the patient has meningitis and sinusitis or bronchitis.

4. **Therapy.** Amphotericin B at dosages of 0.5 to 1.0 mg/kg a day for at least 8 weeks is used initially. Maintenance therapy with itraconazole at 200 mg by mouth twice a day may be used for responders with aspergillosis, coccidioidomycosis, or histoplasmosis. Fluconazole at 200 mg by mouth twice a day may be used for coccidioidomycosis. Ketoconazole at 400 mg by mouth each day may be started with amphotericin B and continued as maintenance therapy for blastomycosis. Adverse effects of amphotericin B and fluconazole are described in **III.A.4.d.** Itraconazole and ketoconazole can produce gastrointestinal intolerance, hepatotoxicity, hypertension, lethargy, headaches, dizziness, and pruritus. Ketoconazole also can cause impotence, gynecomastia, and menstrual irregularities. Thrombocytopenia, leukopenia, hemolytic anemia, and depression occur uncommonly.

5. **Outcome.** The response is generally poor because of disseminated infection at the time of CNS manifestations, immunosuppression, and delays and difficulties in diagnosis. Occasional responders should continue maintenance therapy indefinitely. New lesions should prompt aggressive evaluation to differentiate recurrence from other CNS opportunistic pathogens.

Recommended Readings

American Academy of Neurology. The neurologic complications of AIDS. CONTINUUM. 2000;6:number 5.

Berger JR, ed. Neurological Complications of AIDS. Seminars in Neurology 1999;19:101–233

Berger JR, Cohen BA. Opportunistic infections of the nervous system in AIDS. In: Vinken PJ, Bruyn GW, Aminoff M, Goetz CG, eds. *Handbook of clinical neurology, III: systemic diseases.* Vol. 71. Amsterdam, The Netherlands: Elsevier Science, 1998:261–333.

Berger JR, Levy RM, eds. *AIDS and the nervous system,* 2nd ed. New York: Lippincott–Raven, 1997.

Evaluation and management of intracranial mass lesions in AIDS: report of the quality standards subcommittee of the American Academy of Neurology. *Neurology* 1998;50:21–26.

Gendelman H, Lipton S, Epstein L, et al., eds. *The neurological and neuropsychological manifestations of HIV-1 infection.* New York: Chapman-Hall, 1998.

45. SPINAL CORD DISORDERS

Edward C. Daly

I. **Developmental disorders** occasionally cause pain or progressive neurologic dysfunction in adults. Others are found incidentally. Results of studies have suggested that maternal folate supplementation during pregnancy prevents neural tube defects in offspring.

A. **Chiari malformations** are characterized by extension of the cerebellar tonsils through the foramen magnum with downward displacement of the medulla and kinking of the cervical spinal cord. Hydrocephalus, bony abnormalities of the skull base, and syringomyelia in the cervical cord are frequently found. Chiari I malformations (not associated with meningomyelocele) frequently do not manifest themselves until adulthood. Approximately 80% of patients will have syringomyelia.

1. No treatment is warranted if the patient has no symptoms. Cranial nerve signs, a history of sleep apnea, and radiologic evidence of syringomyelia should be sought. Baseline pulmonary function tests should be considered. Neurologic and radiologic follow-up evaluation is warranted, especially for children and young adults.

2. If the patient has symptoms, decompressive suboccipital craniectomy and upper cervical laminectomy with or without ventricular shunting are required.

   a. Respiratory depression is the most common postoperative complication necessitating close monitoring.

   b. Approximately 50% of patients benefit, 25% have no change, and 25% deteriorate.

B. **Spina bifida occulta** is the anomalous development of the posterior neural arch without an extraspinal cyst. The condition is found in 5% of the population. Cutaneous anomalies often overlie the bony defect. Evidence of other lumbosacral anomalies may be found by means of ultrasonography in infants younger than 3 months or by means of magnetic resonance imaging (MRI) in older patients. Dermal sinus tracts can cause recurrent meningitis. Lipomas and dermoids can impinge on the cord or the cauda equina.

1. Dermal sinus tracts are closed to prevent meningitis.

2. Biopsy is indicated for tissue diagnosis of mass lesions.

3. Surgery is indicated for progressive deficits.

C. **Tethering of the cord** by adhesions, lipomas, or a tight filum terminale is the most common finding associated with spina bifida occulta. The syndrome often manifests itself after growth spurts or minor trauma. Pain can be the predominant presentation in adults, whereas scoliosis is more common in children. Bladder and bowel symptoms are common in both.

1. Surgery is controversial in the care of children who have no symptoms. Arguments for early prophylactic surgery are strong because symptoms stabilize but rarely are relieved after surgery. Patients should undergo electromyography (EMG) and urodynamic evaluations before a final decision is made.

2. Surgical release stabilizes progression without a marked effect on bladder dysfunction. Results are mixed for the relief of pain. In follow-up care, the possibility of re-tethering of the spinal cord has to be monitored.

D. **Diastematomyelia** is splitting of the spinal cord by a bony or fibrous septum. The anomaly can become evident during growth spurts or minor trauma. Spina bifida occulta often is present. Pain is prominent in adults but not in children.

1. The septum is removed in children in response to expected progression.

2. Surgical treatment of adults is reserved for those with severe pain or progression.

E. **Platybasia** (upward displacement of the floor of the posterior fossa) and **basilar invagination** (protrusion of the odontoid through the foramen magnum) decrease the diameter of the foramen magnum. In adults, these conditions manifest as spastic tetraparesis or lower cranial nerve dysfunction.

1. Surgical options include decompressive suboccipital craniectomy with upper cervical laminectomy.

2. Counseling is indicated for the apparent genetic basis of skull base disorders.

F. Syringomyelia is a congenital pericentral cavity of the cervical spinal cord that may extend into the thoracic cord or upward into the medulla (syringobulbia). Chiari I malformation, arachnoiditis, or kyphoscoliosis may be present.

1. Syringomyelia usually manifests itself in adolescence or adulthood. The classic syndrome of upper-extremity weakness and atrophy (often asymmetric) with dissociated sensation in a "cape distribution" is found in 75% of cases. Enlargement of the syrinx can result in Horner's syndrome and myelopathy. Sleep-related respiratory disturbances are not uncommon, especially in syringobulbia.

2. Although this disorder often is slowly progressive, long periods of stabilization, as well as of acute deterioration, can occur. Neck or arm pain often is a prominent problem among older patients. Scoliosis may be prominent in younger patients.

   a. Surgery may not be indicated if symptoms are minimal or very severe, if symptoms have been present longer than 5 years, or if the cord is of normal size on MR images.

   b. Surgery may be indicated in the presence of mild deficits of short duration, enlargement of the cord on MR images, and predominant symptoms of pain or spasticity.

3. Surgery is indicated in progressive cases.

   a. Results of surgery: The condition of approximately one third of patients improves, of less than one half stabilizes, and of approximately one fourth deteriorates.

      (1) Pain and paraparesis show the best responses.

      (2) Sensory loss, lower motor neuron signs, and brainstem findings are the symptoms least likely to be relieved.

   b. Success is less likely in the presence of arachnoiditis.

   c. If no Chiari malformation is found, draining and shunting of the cavity are less satisfactory. Secondary cavitation into a tumor should be considered.

II. Vitamin deficiencies

A. Vitamin B$_{12}$ (cobalamin) deficiency is the most common disorder of the spinal cord for which specific medical therapy exists.

1. **Pernicious anemia** is the most common cause of vitamin B$_{12}$ deficiency and is thought to be an autoimmune disorder affecting all races and both sexes. Antibodies to parietal cells are found in almost 90% of patients, and antibodies to intrinsic factor are found in somewhat more than 60%. Increased clinical suspicion, automated red blood cell (RBC) indices, and insidious onset (it takes 5 to 10 years to deplete normal body stores of cobalamin) make the fully developed classic hematologic and neurologic manifestations clinical rarities today.

2. **Other causes** of vitamin B$_{12}$ deficiency include **gastrectomy, diseases of the terminal ileum** (Crohn's disease and diverticulosis), and less severe **gastric atrophy** (causing food-bound malabsorption). Dietary causes, once thought to be uncommon except in **vegans** and their breast-fed infants, may be an increasing problem among the elderly. **Nitrous oxide exposure** during anesthesia can result in precipitous neurologic manifestations in patients with "silent" deficiencies or marginal body stores. Nitrous oxide also can be the cause of an insidious myelopathy if abused.

3. **Clinical features**

   a. **Hematologic features.** The classic severe megaloblastic anemia of insidious onset is relatively rare. Approximately 25% of patients have normal hemoglobin values, 25% have normal RBC indices, and 10% to 20% have completely normal complete blood cell counts (CBCs).

   b. **Neurologic features.** Approximately 25% to 50% of patients with vitamin B$_{12}$ deficiency have neurologic symptoms or signs at diagnosis. One study showed that 27% of patients were without neurologic problems but had abnormal signs. Most patients experience leg dysesthesia as the first symptom. Neurologic presentations include the following:

      (1) **Polyneuropathy,** orthostasis, and decreased visual acuity

   (2) Subacute combined degeneration of the spinal cord affecting the posterior and lateral columns
   (3) Personality changes, dementia, and **psychiatric illness,** including psychosis.
4. **Diagnosis.** In large-scale screening of elderly persons without symptoms, between 10% and 20% may have cobalamin deficiency.
   a. **Serum vitamin B_{12}** (cobalamin). The sensitivity, specificity, and accuracy of this commonly used assay are controversial. Patients can have normal levels and cobalamin-responsive neurologic disorders; low levels and nonresponsive deficits; or low levels but no other evidence of deficiency. Despite these severe shortcomings, measurement of cobalamin in the serum is the screening test that is the most widely available. For most patients, serum folate should be measured at the same time. Cobalamin levels in blood are light and temperature sensitive.
   b. The **peripheral blood smear** should be examined for macroovalocytes and hypersegmentation of neutrophils. It may be abnormal in the absence of clinically significant anemia, although the sensitivity is low in mild vitamin B_{12} deficiency.
   c. **Methylmalonic acid (MMA)** (urine and serum) and serum **homocysteine** (HCYS) accumulate in vitamin B_{12} deficiency. HCYS level also is elevated in folate deficiency. Assays for these metabolites can be helpful in selected cases. In comparison with serum cobalamin measurement, these assays are characterized by the following:
      (1) Advantages include possibly better sensitivity and specificity.
         (a) These assays reflect the cellular status of cobalamin-dependent pathways.
      (2) Disadvantages are expense and limited availability.
         (a) Elevated MMA and HCYS levels are found in hypovolemia, renal failure, and inherited disorders.
         (b) HCYS level is elevated in hypothyroidism, pyridoxine deficiency, and psoriasis.
         (c) HCYS in unprocessed blood is relatively unstable
         (d) The implicit assumption is that all tissues have identical cobalamin requirements for optimal function.
5. Once a deficiency is suspected, a variety of tests can help determine the cause and appropriate treatment (Fig. 45.1).
   a. The **Schilling test** is used to measure absorption of radiolabeled crystalline vitamin B_{12} in the absence of exogenous intrinsic factor (stage I) and in its presence (stage II). The radioisotope in a 24-hour urine sample is used to measure absorption. An abnormal stage I with a normal stage II indicates deficiency of intrinsic factor; if both stages are abnormal, malabsorption is suggested. A persistently low result after a 7- to 10-day course of antibiotics (stage III) suggests bacterial overgrowth as the cause of malabsorption. Potential pitfalls are as follows.
      (1) Incomplete urine collection and renal insufficiency are serious problems for the elderly. Placement of an indwelling catheter for 24 hours often is considered.
      (2) Ileal mucosal injury in severe cobalamin or folate deficiency may prevent absorption of the cobalamin-intrinsic factor complex. Appropriate treatment for 1 to 3 months and repetition of the test clarifies the results.
      (3) A normal test result is found among patients with inadequate oral intake and those who absorb crystalline cobalamin but who may not be able to release the dietary vitamin bound to proteins. The latter scenario results in food-bound cobalamin malabsorption.
      (4) Bone marrow examination and measurement of MMA level, if ordered, should be performed before the Schilling test. The flushing dose (1 mg) of cobalamin given during the Schilling test may normalize results of these tests within 24 to 48 hours.

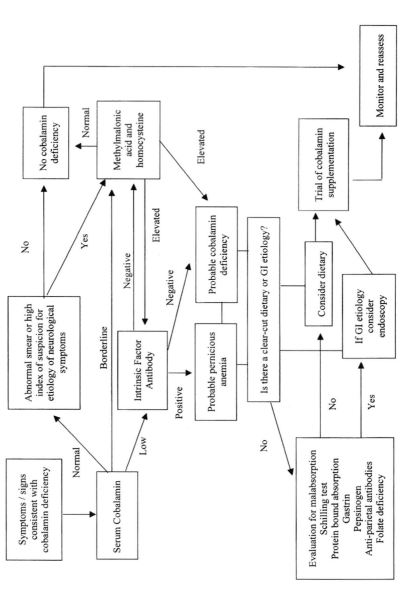

FIG. 45.1 Evaluation and diagnosis of a suspected cobalamin deficiency as a cause of neurologic disorders. *GI*, gastrointestinal.

    b. The **food-bound Schilling test** is used to measure absorption of cobalamin bound to protein (by mixing with egg yolks). Measurement of the administered dose is difficult, and the test is not widely available. Proton pump inhibitors may make food-bound malabsorption more likely but have not been implicated as the sole agent causing severe cobalamin deficiency.

    c. **Intrinsic factor antibody testing** is specific but suffers from low sensitivity (less than 60%). However, its low cost and simplicity make this test useful as an alternative confirmation of pernicious anemia.

    d. **Parietal cell antibody testing** is sensitive (more than 90%) but suffers from low specificity. A negative result makes pernicious anemia unlikely.

6. Treatment

    a. For patients with pernicious anemia, severe deficits, or poor compliance, the usual treatment is cyanocobalamin in the following dosages: 1 mg/d intramuscularly (i.m.) for 7 to 12 days, then 1 mg/wk i.m. for 3 weeks, and then 1 mg every 1 to 3 months i.m. for life. Less severe deficiencies can be initially treated with every other day injections for the first week, then weekly injections for the first month. Monthly injection is the standard maintenance regimen and provides the greatest ease of compliance. If longer intervals are used, MMA levels should document adequate treatment and compliance.

    b. The patient or caregiver should be taught to give the injections to avoid the costs of office visits. If self-injection is not feasible, a visiting nurse can be helpful with injections and compliance.

    c. The unusual patient with pernicious anemia and a strong aversion to injections may be offered **oral therapy** after initial cobalamin repletion. Large doses are needed, because only 1% to 3% of cobalamin is absorbed independently of intrinsic factor. Monitoring of cobalamin levels is needed until compliance is assured. The usual dosage is 1 to 2 mg/d by mouth for life. Recent evidence suggests oral therapy is at least as efficacious as parenteral therapy in reversing the clinical and biochemical indicators of vitamin B_{12} deficiency.

    d. For patients who are compliant, absorb oral vitamin B_{12} (the results of a standard Schilling test is normal and serum cobalamin level normalizes), have mild deficits, and want to avoid monthly injections, cyanocobalamin can be given at 50 to 1,000 μg/d by mouth for life. Cobalamin or MMA levels or both should document adequacy of the dosing schedule.

7. Prognosis. Degree of recovery depends on the severity and duration of deficits at diagnosis. Severe deficits or symptoms that have existed for more than 1 year often respond incompletely. Most improvement occurs within 6 to 12 months. If a patient has not shown some improvement after 3 months, a response is unlikely. Either the diagnosis was in error or a vitamin B_{12} deficiency was coexistent but not causal (commonly observed in dementia).

8. Therapeutic strategy. Predicting which neurologic deficits will respond to vitamin B_{12} is imprecise. I believe patients with symptoms or signs consistent with vitamin B_{12} deficiency and laboratory evidence of a possible vitamin B_{12} deficiency should be given a 6 to 12 month trial of vitamin B_{12} if other treatable disorders (including folic acid deficiency) have been eliminated. A less rigorous strategy, with no attempt to confirm the diagnosis or determine the cause, will miss treatable disorders. A more rigorous strategy, withholding treatment unless deficiency is "proved," may be based on an overestimation of our knowledge of cobalamin and one-carbon metabolism.

B. Folic acid deficiency is not generally appreciated as a cause of neurologic dysfunction similar to that found in vitamin B_{12} deficiency. As in vitamin B_{12} deficiency, the neurologic deficits can develop with normal or mildly abnormal hematologic values. The incidence of severe neurologic deficits is lower in folate deficiency than in cobalamin deficiency.

    1. Dietary inadequacy is the most common cause of folate deficiency, especially among the elderly. Pregnancy, alcoholism, generalized malabsorption, antiepileptic medication, chemotherapy, and congenital defects in absorption or one-carbon enzymes are other potential causes.

    2. Clinical features

       a. Instances of dementia, depression, psychosis, polyneuropathy, and subacute combined degeneration of the spinal cord all have been shown to be responsive to folate supplementation. Changes in mental status and higher cortical functions may be the most common presentations in adults.

       b. An association between maternal folate supplementation and prevention of neural tube defects in the offspring has been found. Folate appears to correct a subtle block in one-carbon metabolism rather than replenish a deficiency.

    3. Diagnosis. See Fig. 45.2.

       a. A low **serum folate** level indicates a negative balance and predicts the likelihood of folate deficiency if uncorrected. The serum level is a poor predictor of total body stores. Because RBC folate level is much greater than serum folate level, hemolyzed specimens should be rejected.

       b. RBC folate level indicates body stores during the lifetime of the RBC. The specificity, sensitivity, and usefulness of the value obtained by means of radioassay (the most common technique) is controversial. If both the serum and RBC folate levels are low, ongoing folate deficiency is suggested.

       c. Elevated **serum HCYS** level with a normal serum MMA level also is a marker of folate deficiency and can be helpful in equivocal cases. Because cobalamin deficiency also elevates homocysteine level, MMA has to be measured at the same time to differentiate the two deficiencies.

       d. A search for a gastrointestinal disorder should be undertaken when signs of malabsorption exist or if a dietary cause is not clear. Gastroenterologic referral and jejunal biopsy should be considered. Concurrent vitamin B_{12} deficiency can cause folate malabsorption and result in low serum and RBC folate levels. (Vitamin B_{12} deficiency is more likely to elevate serum folate levels consistent with the methylfolate trap hypothesis.)

    4. Treatment with folic acid at a dosage of 2.5 to 10.0 mg/d by mouth is sufficient in dietary deficiency. Parenteral (i.m.) doses are given in malabsorption syndromes. Treatment is for life or until body stores are replete and etiologic factors corrected. A multivitamin also should be taken. Compliance and adequacy of treatment can be monitored with HCYS levels.

    5. There is uncertainty concerning the possible **epileptogenic properties** of folic acid. Folate deficiency should be confirmed with serum HCYS measurement in the care of patients with seizures. Unless severe hematologic or neurologic deficits are present, less aggressive dosing (1 to 2 mg/d) may be best. Normalization of serum HCYS level is necessary to document compliance and to verify adequate treatment.

    6. Prognosis is generally good if treatment is started early. Poor responses in cases of dementia or depression with folate deficiency probably represent the concurrence of two common disorders in the elderly.

C. Vitamin E deficiency can cause polyneuropathy, myopathy, scotomata, and demyelination within the posterior columns and spinocerebellar tracts of the spinal cord. The ataxia and posterior column manifestations of abetalipoproteinemia, a rare autosomal recessive disorder of lipoprotein metabolism, are responsive to vitamin E supplementation. Rare cases of vitamin E deficiency usually manifest as long-standing malabsorption and steatorrhea. An isolated autosomal recessive defect in transport also exists. Reversal of neurologic deficits with vitamin E supplementation is variable but can be dramatic. Because prognosis appears related to duration of symptoms, a high index of symptoms is warranted. Large oral dosages of vitamin E (800 to 3,600 U/d) or semiweekly injections of α-tocopherol have been used.

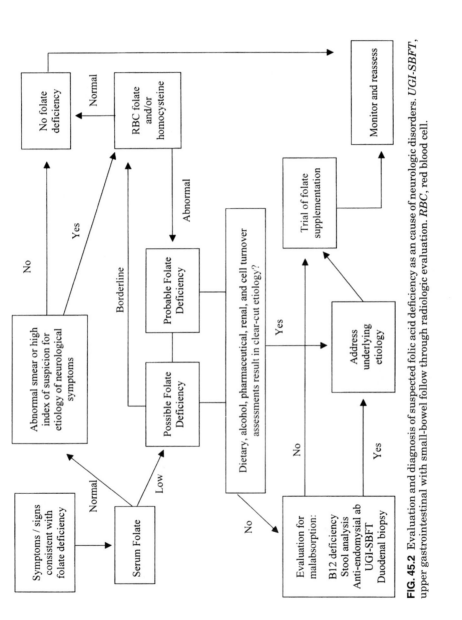

FIG. 45.2 Evaluation and diagnosis of suspected folic acid deficiency as an cause of neurologic disorders. *UGI-SBFT*, upper gastrointestinal with small-bowel follow through radiologic evaluation. *RBC*, red blood cell.

III. Acute spinal cord injury

A. Etiology. The major causes of acute spinal cord injury are motor vehicle accidents, falls, recreational injuries, and acts of violence. Fracture and compromise of the spinal cord (or cauda equina) occur most often at cervical and thoracolumbar levels. Although thoracic fractures are less common, neurologic injury is more common because of the narrowness of the spinal canal.

B. Natural history. Spinal cord injury occurs most often among young men. Neurologic impairment is approximately evenly divided among complete quadriplegia, complete paraplegia, incomplete quadriplegia, and incomplete paraplegia.

C. Prevention. Proper use of passive and active restraints in automobiles and use of helmets by motorcyclists and bicyclists prevent head and spinal injuries. For example, the Think First program, which addresses educational issues for youth in kindergarten through twelfth grade and is actively supported by the neurosurgical community, should be embraced by health care providers.

D. Prognosis. Improvement of even one level can have a dramatic effect on function, especially in cervical cord injuries (Table 45.1). Final neurologic function depends on severity of initial injury, prevention of secondary damage, and successful management of the complications and sequelae of the acute injury and intensive rehabilitation. Neurologic assessment 72 hours after injury according to American Spinal Injury Association guidelines is useful in estimating outcome.

  1. Features suggesting a possibility of neurologic improvement are as follows:
     a. Motor or sensory function below neurologic level ("incomplete lesion")
     b. Degree to which motor strength is preserved below neurologic level
     c. Preservation of pinprick response in addition to light touch below neurologic level
     d. Age younger than 30 years
     e. Residual anal sphincter tone
     f. Relatively well preserved vertebral alignment
  2. Features suggesting a poor prognosis are as follows:
     a. Absence of residual function ("complete lesion")
     b. Hemorrhage or multilevel edema on MR images

E. Principles of treatment

  1. **Immobilization of the spine** at the scene, in transport, and in the emergency department is critical in preventing further damage.
  2. **ABCs of trauma care;** supplemental oxygen should be provided
  3. **Primary survey** of associated damage
     a. Alteration of sensorium necessitates investigation for accompanying head injury.
     b. Neurologic level may mask the usual symptoms and signs of thoracic, abdominal, pelvic, or extremity injury. More reliance is placed on objective tests.
  4. **Radiologic evaluation** of level of skeletal injury
  5. **Skeletal traction** for stabilization and closed reduction if indicated
  6. Assessment of **neurologic level of injury**
     a. The neurologic level of injury is the most caudal segment at which both motor function and sensory function are intact bilaterally (Table 45.2).
     b. The completeness of the injury is defined by American Spinal Injury Association classes grades A through E, which describe function at least three levels below the neurologic level of injury. Grade A indicates a complete level, grade E indicates recovery, and grades B through D describe incomplete levels.
  7. **Secondary survey** and stabilization of patient's condition
  8. **Transport** to spinal cord injury center
  9. **Medications** to prevent secondary (oxidative) damage
     a. The National Acute Spinal Cord Injury Study 2 (NASCIS 2) showed a modest but significant benefit compared with placebo for high-dose methylprednisolone if started within 8 hours of injury. The initial dose of 30 mg/kg intravenous bolus is followed by 5.4 mg/kg per hour infusion

Table 45.1 Expected functional outcomes in spinal cord injury

Function	C1-4	C5	C6	C7-8	T1-9	T10-S5
Respiratory	Ventilator dependent[a]	Assisted cough	Assisted cough	Assisted cough	Decreased endurance	Intact
Bowel	Total assist	Total assist	Moderate assist	Moderate assist	Independent	Independent
Bladder	Total assist	Total assist	Moderate assist	Variable assist	Independent	Independent
Bed mobility	Total assist	Some assist	Some assist	Variable assist	Independent	Independent
Transfers	Total assist	Total assist	Variable assist	Variable assist	Independent	Independent
Pressure relief, positioning	Total assist	Independent with equipment	Independent with equipment	Independent	Independent	Independent
Eating	Total assist	Independent with equipment and setup	Variable assist	Independent	Independent	Independent
Dressing	Total assist	Near total assist	Moderate assist	Variable assist	Independent	Independent
Grooming	Total assist	Moderate assist	Independent with equipment	Independent	Independent	Independent
Bathing	Total assist	Total assist	Moderate assist	Variable assist	Independent	Independent
Wheelchair	Power with special controls	Near total assist or power	Moderate assist or power	Minimal assist	Independent	Independent
Ambulation	Not indicated	Not indicated	Not indicated	Not indicated	Typically not functional	Functional with variable assist
Communication	Moderate assist with equipment	Independent with equipment	Independent with equipment	Independent	Independent	Independent
Transportation	Total assist	Highly custom van with lift	Modified van with lift	Modified vehicle	Hand controls	Hand controls
Homemaking	Total assist	Total assist	Moderate assist	Variable assist	Independent, moderate assist	Independent, minimal assist
Assist required	24 h/d	16 h/d	10 h/d	8 h/d	3 h/d	0-2 h/d

[a] C4 level may be ventilator independent needing assisted cough.
Data from Consortium for Spinal Cord Medicine. Outcomes following traumatic spinal cord injury: clinical practice guidelines for health-care professionals. Paralyzed Veterans of America, 1999.

Table 45.2 Key muscles and sensory areas for determination of neurologic level of injury

Level	Muscle action	Key muscle	Key sensory area
C2	—	—	Occipital protuberance
C3	—	—	Supraclavicular fossa
C4	—	—	Top anterior shoulder
C5	Elbow flexion	Biceps brachialis	Lateral antecubital fossa
C6	Wrist extension	Extensor carpi radialis	Thumb
C7	Elbow extension	Triceps	Dorsal middle finger
C8	Finger flexion (third)	Extensor digitorum profundus	Dorsal little finger
T1	Finger abduction (fifth)	Abductor digiti minimi	Medial antecubital fossa
T2	—		Apex of axilla
T3	—		Third intercostal space
T4	—		Nipple line
T5	—		Midway between T4 and T6
T6	—		Xiphisternum
T7	—		Midway between T6 and T8
T8	—		Midway between T6 and T10
T9	—		Midway between T8 and T10
T10	—		Umbilicus
T11	—		Midway between T10 and T12
T12	—		Midpoint of inguinal ligament
L1	—		Midway between T12 and L2
L2	Hip flexion	Iliopsoas	Mid-anterior thigh
L3	Knee extension	Quadriceps	Medial femoral condyle
L4	Ankle dorsiflexion	Tibialis anterior	Medial malleolus
L5	Toe extension (first)	Extensor hallucis longus	Dorsum of foot at third metatarsophalangeal joint
S1	Ankle plantar fexion	Gastrocnemius, soleus	Lateral heel
S2	—		Mid popliteal fossa
S3	—		Ischial tuberosity
S4-5	—		Perianal sensation

Data from Maynard FM, Bracken MB, Creasey G, et al. International standards for neurological and functional classification of spinal cord injury. *Spinal Cord* 1997;35:266–274.

for 23 hours. Complications include pneumonia, sepsis, and gastrointestinal hemorrhage.

    b. NASCIS 3 showed an additional 24 hours of steroid infusion to be beneficial to patients who received the initial bolus between 3 and 8 hours after injury. In addition, treatment started at later than 8 hours after injury resulted in poorer outcomes than did placebo treatment.

    c. Concurrent use of GM-1 ganglioside has shown promise in preliminary trials.

  10. Restoration and maintenance of spinal alignment

IV. Sequelae of spinal cord injuries

  A. Pressure sores are the most preventable complication of spinal cord injury. They are classified according to depth, as follows:

Stage I: nonblanchable erythema of intact skin

Stage II: partial-thickness skin loss

Stage III: full-thickness skin loss

Stage IV: extension into muscle and bone

    1. Prevention. Patient and family education are important. Pressure is relieved by turning in bed every 2 hours and "wheelchair" lifts for 5 to 10 seconds every 15 to 30 minutes. Special mattresses and wheelchair cushions do not obviate proper positioning and frequent repositioning. The skin is kept clean, dry, and inspected daily. Attention is paid to nutritional requirements.

    2. Pressure relief. A repositioning schedule ensuring that the sore is always pressure free needs to be rigidly followed, because the reduced number of possible weight-bearing positions make another sore more likely. Simultaneous management of more than one pressure sore requires special frames or flotation beds.

    3. Débridement. Saline wet-to-dry gauze and whirlpool therapy are standard, but commercial enzyme preparations are less labor intensive. If the eschar is hard and blackened, necrotic tissue is removed surgically.

    4. Dressings. Shallow ulcers are covered with sterile gauze. Occlusive dressings may promote more rapid healing and have to be changed less often but are much more expensive. Deeper, pear-shaped ulcers are loosely packed with saline-soaked gauze to prevent abscess formation and to promote "bottom-up" healing. The goal is to keep the wound moist while the surrounding tissue is kept dry.

    5. Electrical stimulation may accelerate wound healing.

    6. Surgical excision with a myocutaneous flap to fill the cavity is usually required for deeper ulcers. Reduction of bony prominences may be necessary.

  B. Deep venous thrombosis is a serious concern after spinal cord injury. Pain may not be felt below a sensory level, and swelling may be masked by edema and vasomotor changes.

    1. Prophylaxis is needed for up to 3 months or until discharge from the rehabilitation unit. Intermittent pneumatic compression devices or compression stockings are used for the 2 weeks after injury. Anticoagulation with low-molecular-weight heparin or adjusted-dose unfractionated heparin should be started 48 to 72 hours after injury and continued 8 to 12 weeks depending on associated risk factors. Vena caval filters are placed in patients with contraindications to or who have undergone unsuccessful anticoagulation therapy. Filters also should be considered in addition to anticoagulation in the care of patients with complete C2 or C3 neurologic levels of injury.

    2. Treatment is the same as that of patients without spinal cord injury. Mobilization and exercise of the lower extremities should be withheld 48 to 72 hours until anticoagulation is adequate. Pain relief should be provided to lessen the possibility of autonomic dysreflexia.

  C. Autonomic dysreflexia. From 30% to 85% of patients with quadriplegia or high paraplegia have paroxysmal episodes of severe hypertension, sweating, flushing, and piloerection accompanied by headache, chest pain, and bradycardia or tachycardia in response to relatively benign stimuli below the level of injury. Pulmonary edema, intracranial hemorrhage, cerebral infarction, seizures, or death can result. Bladder and bowel distention, instrumentation, or irritation are the most common precipitating stimuli.

1. **Etiology.** In the setting of a spinal lesion above the major splanchnic outflow tract (T6-L2), reflex activation of sympathetic discharge occurs below the lesion unchecked by descending inhibitory pathways from supraspinal centers.
2. **Management.** Initial treatment entails removal of the precipitating stimulus and medication for the hypertensive crisis.
   a. **Removal of precipitating stimulus**
      (1) Stop procedure.
      (2) Check for urinary catheter blockage.
      (3) Remove tight clothing, shoes, straps, and other restrictive items.
      (4) Catheterize carefully with 2% lidocaine jelly.
      (5) Perform kidney, ureter, and bladder (KUB) and rectal examination with lidocaine jelly to check for impaction.
      (6) Check for sores, infection, trauma, and fractures.
      (7) Consider acute abdomen and deep venous thrombosis.
   b. **Management of hypertension**
      (1) Elevate head of bed or place patient in sitting position to induce postural changes in blood pressure.
      (2) Drug therapy
         (a) Nifedipine 10 mg by mouth (immediate release form—bite through capsule and swallow); monitor response *or*
         (b) Nitroglycerin 2% ointment—1 inch (2.5 cm) applied above neurologic site of injury; monitor response
      (3) If blood pressure remains critical, intravenous protocols (e.g., hydralazine, diazoxide, sodium nitroprusside) for hypertensive crisis must be initiated.
   c. **Management of profuse sweating without hypertension.** Give propantheline at 15 mg by mouth (may be repeated after 10 minutes) or oxybutynin at 5 mg by mouth (may be repeated after 10 minutes)
3. **Prophylactic medications**
   a. Nifedipine 10 mg by mouth 30 minutes before procedure
   b. Phenoxybenzamine 10 to 20 mg by mouth three times a day
   c. Scopolamine patch may help with reflex sweating
D. **Depression** must be continually assessed and managed.
E. **Central pain syndrome.** Development of chronic dysesthesia or central (neuropathic) pain above, at, or distal to the level of injury poses therapeutic challenges. Central pain is in addition to the musculoskeletal and visceral pain experienced by patients with spinal cord injuries.
   1. **Etiology**
      a. Above level of injury: compressive mononeuropathy (e.g., ulnar, median) and posttraumatic syringomyelia formation
      b. At level of injury: central pain from cord damage, radicular pain from root damage, and complex regional pain syndrome
      c. Below level of injury: central pain
   2. **Pharmacologic approach** is trial and error.
      a. **Tricyclic antidepressants** for nonlancinating pain
         (1) Amitriptyline (Elavil; AstraZeneca, Wilmington, DE, U.S.A.) or nortriptyline (Pamelor; Tyco Healthcare, Mansfield, MA, U.S.A.) 10 to 25 mg by mouth at bedtime; increase by 10 to 25 mg every 5 to 7 days as tolerated to 75 to 150 mg at bedtime
         (2) Side effects include sedation, anticholinergic effects, orthostatic hypotension, weight gain, and cardiac arrhythmia.
         (3) If side effects are not tolerable, a chemically unrelated compound, such as fluoxetine (Prozac; Lilly, Indianapolis, IN, U.S.A.) at 20 to 40 mg/d by mouth, may be tried.
      b. **Anticonvulsants** (frequently in combination with tricyclic antidepressants) for lancinating central pain

      (1) Carbamazepine (Tegretol; Novartis, Easy Hanover, NJ, U.S.A.) 100 mg twice a day increased 100 mg every 3 days as tolerated to a serum level of 8 to 10 mg/mL in three or four doses per day

        (a) Side effects include sedation, diplopia, gastrointestinal upset, ataxia, weakness, rash, and bone marrow suppression.

        (b) Monitor CBC with platelets every 2 weeks for 3 months, then CBC, platelets, and liver function every 3 to 6 months.

      (2) Gabapentin (Neurontin; Parke-Davis, Morris Plains, NJ, U.S.A., U.S.A.) 100 mg three times a day increased 100 to 300 mg every 3 days as tolerated up to 600 to 900 three or four times a day.

        (a) Side effects include drowsiness and dizziness.

        (b) Blood levels are not used clinically and no monitoring is needed. The major disadvantage is expense.

    c. Neuroleptics (with tricyclic antidepressant; stop anticonvulsant).

      (1) Must warn of the risk of tardive dyskinesia with the use of neuroleptics.

      (2) Fluphenazine (Prolixin; Apothecon, Princeton, NJ, U.S.A.): start at 1 mg/d, then slowly increase to 10 mg/d as tolerated.

        (a) Periodically attempt to wean or discontinue.

        (b) If no relief is obtained, discontinue.

  3. Physical methods may provide some temporary relief for central pain at the level of the injury.

    a. Transcutaneous electrical nerve stimulation (TENS)

    b. Warm or cool packs and ultrasound

  4. Surgical treatment should be considered only after conservative therapy has failed.

    a. Dorsal root entry zone (DREZ) surgery

      (1) Laminectomy and radiofrequency ablation of DREZ is performed two levels above and one level below the site of injury.

      (2) Improvement is realized in 60% to 90% of patients. Best results are achieved in patients with pain at or just below the level of injury.

      (3) Complications include loss of one or two sensory levels, cerebrospinal fluid leakage, hematoma, and bowel, bladder, and sexual dysfunction.

    b. Avoid sympathectomy, rhizotomy, and cordotomy.

  5. Narcotic therapy is indicated only after both conservative and surgical therapies have failed.

    a. Combination with tricyclic antidepressants may be synergistic.

    b. The patient must be carefully selected and carefully supervised.

    c. Methadone (Dolophine; Lilly, Indianapolis, IN, U.S.A.), sustained release oxycodone (Oxycontin; Purdue Pharma, Stamford, CT, U.S.A.), and an intrathecal morphine pump (if possible) are options for selected patients

      (1) A formal contract detailing expectations and criteria for termination of treatment is made with the patient.

      (2) Periodic attempts should be made to wean the medication.

      (3) Side effects include sedation and cognitive slowing, respiratory depression, constipation, and reduced sexual function.

F. Posttraumatic syringomyelia is recognized in 1% to 5% of spinal cord injury patients, but findings at MRI and autopsy studies suggest an incidence closer to 20%. Symptoms occur months to years after the original injury.

  1. Clinical symptoms are similar to those of autonomic dysreflexia.

    a. Onset or exacerbation of pain, especially if perceived above the level of original injury

    b. Change in level or completeness of neurologic deficits

    c. Increased spasticity

  2. Treatment

    a. Untethering the spinal cord at site of injury

    b. Surgical shunting of cavity

    c. Pain, spasticity, and autonomic dysreflexia respond best.

V. Spinal cord injury without radiologic abnormality (SCIWORA)

    A. This disorder is more common among children. Laxity of spinal ligaments allows transient, self-reducing subluxation of vertebrae. True SCIWORA is very rare among adults, but there may be no radiologic evidence of trauma in older patients with marked degenerative joint disease.

    B. Subtle or transient deficits may go unnoticed, especially in head or facial injuries. There is a high risk of delayed neurologic dysfunction if the syndrome is not recognized and managed appropriately.

    C. A full cervical spinal radiographic series (lateral, anteroposterior, oblique, and open mouth views), MRI, or both should be considered when there is a high index of suspicion for spinal cord injury.

    D. Treatment

        1. Rigid immobilization

        2. Avoidance of precipitating activities, especially sports

VI. Central cord syndrome

    A. Etiology. Hyperextension injuries (frequently falls of elderly persons with cervical spondylosis or athletic injuries among younger patients with congenital stenosis) without acute radiologic changes may produce spinal cord contusion primarily affecting the central gray matter. Lamination of tracks in the cervical cord (sacral fibers, lateral; cervical fibers, medial) explains the clinical signs and symptoms.

    B. Clinical features. Patients have "inverted quadriparesis," in which upper-extremity weakness exceeds lower-extremity weakness. Transient burning dysesthesia in the hands with little weakness, or urinary dysfunction also can occur. With recovery, the leg, bladder, and upper-extremity weaknesses improve. The fingers are last to recover.

    C. Prognosis. Almost all patients have improvement, but often to an incomplete degree among the elderly. Delayed progressive myelopathy can develop in approximately 25% of cases.

    D. Treatment

        1. Conservative therapy consists of rigid immobilization of the neck, physical therapy, and consideration of a course of corticosteroids.

        2. Surgical therapy. On the basis of neuroimaging findings, patients whose condition has not improved or has plateaued or who have instability of the spine are are considered for surgical decompression.

VII. Hyperextension–flexion injury (whiplash injury)

    A. Etiology. Automobile accidents account for approximately 85% of whiplash injuries. The cardinal symptoms of neck pain and headache are musculoskeletal. The roles of mild central nervous system injury and psychosocial factors are controversial and have led to biopsychosocial models of outcome in the disorder.

    B. Prevention. Automobile head restraints reduce flexion–hyperextension motion of the head in automobile accidents, especially during rear-end collisions. However, surveys have shown that the restraints frequently are adjusted incorrectly.

    C. Natural history. Rear-end collisions are involved in most whiplash injuries. Cynicism and controversy exist over the cause of chronic whiplash syndrome. Although figures vary widely, approximately 25% of patients continue to have symptoms 6 months after the injury. By 12 months, 80% of patients have no symptoms, whereas 5% of patients remain severely affected. Results of fluoroscopically guided nerve block studies suggest that zygapophyseal joint pain (usually C2-3) accounts for 50% of chronic neck pain after whiplash.

    D. Treatment. Compensation concerns hinder controlled clinical trials of treatment.

        1. Positive attitude and encouragement

        2. Ice for first 24 hours

        3. Muscle relaxants, nonsteroidal antiinflammatory drugs, and adequate pain relief in the first 7 to 14 days

        4. Resumption of most normal activities together with active therapy or home exercises results in better outcome than with conventional regimens of restricted activity, rest, and soft cervical collar.

        5. Heat, ultrasound, massage, and trigger-point injections often make patients more comfortable but remain unproven.

6. Percutaneous radiofrequency neurotomy for cervical zygapophysial joint pain may be considered, but the procedure is not widely available, and the pain frequently returns and necessitates repeated procedures.

VIII. Spasticity is one of the cardinal manifestations of chronic spinal cord disease. In acute spinal lesions, spasticity develops after a variable period of spinal shock, whereas in disorders with insidious onset, it may be the first symptom noticed.

A. The decision to treat a patient must be made on an individual basis. Treatment is indicated when the advantages of spasticity outweigh the disadvantages. Specific treatment goals need to be formulated.

1. Advantages

a. Bowel training maintains sphincter tone.

b. "Internal crutches" are available for ambulation.

c. Weight bearing is possible in transfers.

d. Osteopenia is reduced.

e. Muscle bulk is increased.

f. Venous tone is increased, and deep venous thrombosis may be decreased.

2. Disadvantages

a. Pain and falls result from paroxysmal spasms.

b. Hygiene is impaired owing to hip adductor spasticity.

c. Joint contractures occur.

d. Pressure sores form.

e. Renal damage occurs because of external sphincter spasticity.

f. Movements required for activities of daily living are impaired or interrupted.

B. Assessment of severity can be made with the modified Ashworth scale (Table 45.3).

C. A **changing pattern in a previously stable degree of spasticity** should alert the clinician to varying etiologic factors.

1. Medication: fluoxetine, sertraline, or trazodone

2. Anxiety

3. Tight clothing or shoes

4. Inadequate or prolonged postures

5. Formation of pressure sores

6. Development of deep venous thrombosis

7. Ingrown toenails

8. Spinal instability

9. Fractures

10. Posttraumatic syringomyelia

11. Gastrointestinal dysfunction: impaction, hemorrhoids, acute abdomen

12. Genitourinary dysfunction: infection, stones, blocked catheters, and disorders of testicle, prostate, vagina, uterus, or ovary

D. Management is based on a multidisciplinary approach with a rigorous program of both passive and active stretching.

Table 45.3 Modified Ashworth scale for measuring spasticity

Grade 0: Normal muscle tone
Grade 1: Slight increase in muscle tone; "catch" or minimal resistance at end of range of motion (ROM)
Grade 2: Slight increase; "catch" followed by minimal resistance for remainder of ROM
Grade 3: More marked increase in tone through most of ROM; parts moved easily
Grade 4: Considerable increase in tone; passive movement difficult
Grade 5: Affected part or parts rigid in flexion or extension
Total score is the average of bilateral hip flexion and abduction, knee flexion, and ankle dorsiflexion.

Adapted from McLean BN. Intrathecal baclofen in severe spasticity. *Br J Hosp Med* 1993;49:262–267.

1. **Physical modalities**
   a. Range of motion and stretching exercises
   b. Heat or cold
   c. Vibration (increases presynaptic spinal inhibition)
   d. Splints, casts, and orthotics to prevent contractures and increase mobility
2. **Useful medications** are summarized in Table 45.4. Muscle relaxants (antispasmodics) are not used in the long-term management of spasticity.
3. **Nerve blocks**
   a. **Alcohol** or **phenol** damages nerves nonselectively.
      (1) These agents are useful for relieving spasticity in a specific muscle, such as obturator nerve and hip adduction.
      (2) Test injections with a local anesthetic help determine whether this is a reasonable approach.
      (3) EMG-guided injection increases selectivity.
      (4) Parallel reductions occur in spasticity and strength.
      (5) The effect is not fully reversible; pain, scarring, and fibrosis at the site are potential complications.
   b. **Botulinum toxin type A** (Botox; Allergan, Irvine, CA, U.S.A.) injection has been found effective for focal spasticity at a variety of sites.
      (1) The discomfort and expense of numerous injections in large lower extremity muscles limit this technique to relatively small muscles.

Table 45.4 Drug management of spasticity

Drug	Daily dosage[a] (starting dosage)	Side effects and comments
Baclofen (Lioresal; Novartis, East Hanover, NJ)	10–160 mg (5 mg b.i.d.)	Drowsiness, weakness, tremor, ataxia, abrupt withdrawal with seizures, confusion, hallucinations
Tizanidine (Zanaflex; Athena Neurosciences, Inc., South San Francisco, CA)	8–32 mg (2 mg at bedtime)	Use with caution in liver disease Dry mouth, sedation, dizziness, risk of hypotension, insomnia, hallucinations, hepatotoxicity Liver monitoring at 1, 3, and 6 months Somewhat less weakness than with baclofen
Gabapentin (Neurontin; Parke-Davis, Morris Plains, NJ)	300–3,600 mg (100 mg t.i.d.)	Nausea, sedation, ataxia, dizziness
Diazepam (Valium; Roche Products, Nutley, NJ)	4–60 mg (2 mg at bedtime)	Sedation, cognitive changes, depression, weakness, dependence, abuse, withdrawal syndrome
Dantrolene[b] (Dantrium; Procter and Gamble Pharmaceuticals, Inc., Cincinnati, OH)	25–400 mg (25 mg once a day)	Weakness, hepatotoxicity, confusion, sedation, nausea, diarrhea Monitor liver function closely

[a] It is important to start with a low dosage and gradually build to a target dosage as tolerance of the sedation and most other side effects of the medication develops.
[b] The potentially fatal hepatotoxicity of dantrolene is more common among adults and those taking estrogens. This drug probably should be avoided by those with preexisting liver disease.
b.i.d., twice a day; t.i.d., three times a day.

       (2) Transient postinjection discomfort and side effects are generally well tolerated. Excessive weakness and flulike syndromes may be experienced at initiation of treatment. Botulinum injections should be avoided by patients receiving aminoglycosides. Neutralizing antibodies are more common with larger, more frequent doses.

       (3) Advantages are reversible block (2 to 6 months) and selectivity toward motor fibers.

       (4) Disadvantages are expense and need for repeated injections.

  4. Neurosurgical procedures

    a. An **intrathecal baclofen pump** is a safe alternative to ablative surgery for intractable spasticity at experienced centers.

      (1) Referral to an experienced center should be considered for patients with stable neurologic disorders accompanied by spasticity seriously interfering with quality of life. Oral agents should have been found ineffective or limited owing to intolerable side effects.

      (2) Patients are selected after a test dose of 50 to 75 µg baclofen administered by lumbar puncture. Spasticity is assessed 1, 2, 4, and 8 hours after injection with the modified Ashworth scale (Table 45.3). If two-point improvement is not documented and side effects are tolerable, a second larger test dose (75 to 100 µg) is given the next day.

      (3) During the first year after implantation, daily doses generally increase before stabilizing in the range of 300 to 800 µg per day.

      (4) Improvement is observed in muscle tone, mobility, and bladder function, and spasms and musculoskeletal pain are relieved. There is little or no relief of central pain.

      (5) Systemic side effects are less than with oral therapy. Drowsiness, nausea, hypotension, headache, and weakness may be experienced during the dose titration phase. Infections and catheter or pump complications are rare but potentially serious side effects.

      (6) Depletion of the pump battery in 5 to 7 years necessitates replacing the entire pump unit

      (7) Although life-threatening, all instances of drug overdose have been completely reversible. Experience and better pump design have decreased the complication rate to less than 5%. In early series of patients, surgical revision was needed in 20% of cases for catheter-related problems.

    b. Selective posterior rhizotomy with interoperative EMG selection of lumbosacral rootlets for sectioning is useful in the management of cerebral palsy. Two thirds of patients' conditions are improved with minimal sensory loss and few side effects. DREZ operations are functionally similar microsurgical procedures.

    c. Percutaneous posterior rhizotomy is technically more difficult, and recurrence may be more of a problem.

    d. Efficacy of spinal cord stimulators is controversial.

    e. Peripheral neurectomy is occasionally used to relieve specific joint contractures.

    f. Longitudinal myelotomy, nonselective posterior rhizotomy, and anterior rhizotomy are rarely performed.

  5. Orthopedic procedures are used most often performed in a supportive role to relieve pain, increase mobility, and decrease deformity in cerebral palsy.

    a. Tendon release, lengthening, and transfer

    b. Osteotomy and arthrodesis

IX. Amyotrophic lateral sclerosis (ALS) is a chronic degenerative disease involving motoneurons in the spinal cord and brain. Sensation and cognition are left intact. Eye movements and sphincters are affected very late, if at all. The cause remains unknown, and approximately 5% to 10% of the cases appear to be familial. A gene defect on chromosome 21 involving superoxide dismutase (SOD1) has been found in approximately 20% of familial cases.

  A. Prognosis. The course of the disorder is relentlessly progressive, leading to respiratory insufficiency secondary to weakness and death within an average of

3.5 years after the onset of symptoms. Approximately 20% of patients have a more benign course and survive for more than 5 years, but prognosis for an individual patient is generally not possible at the onset. Patients who have prominent involvement of the bulbar muscles at onset have a more rapid course, death occurring within 2.2 years on average.

B. Most physicians refer the patient to a neurologist for a second opinion when the diagnosis is suspected. Presentation of the diagnosis to the patient and family is always difficult. A prompt (2 to 3 weeks) and extended follow-up visit gives the patient and family an opportunity to ask questions and allows the physician to present a positive therapeutic strategy. This strategy should not be so detailed at this time as to overwhelm the patient. Patients must be given time before they can be expected to be active participants in such plans. However, advanced directives must be addressed while the patient is in relatively good health to maximize options.

C. The ALS C.A.R.E. (Clinical Assessment, Research, and Education) Project is a voluntary database of outcome among ALS patients. (www.umassmed.edu/outcomes/als/). It goals are to improve the care of patients and to identify the needs of caregivers.

D. Specific treatment

1. Although the clinical benefits are relatively modest and the expense great, riluzole (Rilutek; Aventis, Parsippany, NJ, U.S.A.), 50 mg by mouth twice a day on an empty stomach, is the first drug approved for management of ALS. Results of some studies suggest it improves survival time 3 to 9 months. No effect on sense of well-being, quality of life, or muscle strength has been demonstrated. Some physicians have recommended reserving riluzole for patients who have had symptoms less than 5 years, who have a forced vital capacity greater than 60% of predicted value, and who do not need a tracheostomy. Other investigators have found no subgroups of patients from whom treatment should be withheld.

   a. The side effects—nausea and dizziness—are generally tolerable.

   b. Mild elevation of liver function is common. Liver function tests should be performed monthly for the first 3 months after initiation of treatment, every 3 months for the rest of the first year, and then periodically. CBC with differential cell count and platelets is similarly monitored for neutropenia.

   c. Elevations of alanine aminotransferase level of up to three times normal are managed with more frequent monitoring, dosage reduction for several weeks, and reintroduction of full dosage.

   d. Higher elevations or jaundice lead to discontinuing riluzole and monitoring liver function until levels return to baseline.

2. Despite widespread use of gabapentin and antioxidant vitamins within the ALS community, clinical trials have shown no benefit.

E. Symptomatic treatment. Lacking curative therapy, the clinician offers supportive care to both patient and family.

1. Addresses of support groups should be offered to the patient and family. These associations coordinate local groups, provide patient and family education, and can notify patients of current research protocols that are open. Active electronic communities are beginning to form on the Internet. Two support groups are:

   The ALS Association
   27001 Agoura Rd, Suite 150
   Calabasas Hills, CA 91301-5104
   (800) 782-4747
   www.alsa.org
   Muscular Dystrophy Association
   3300 East Sunrise Dr
   Tucson, AZ 85718
   (800) 572-1717
   www.als.mdausa.org

2. A multidisciplinary team, with a leader readily identifiable by the patient and other team members, should consist of speech, dietary, and respiratory therapy, neurologic nursing, social service, rehabilitation medicine, psychology, pulmonary, otorhinolaryngology, and neurology professionals.

3. Maximizing familial, psychological, social, and religious support systems affects the quality of life to a great degree. Similarly, such support systems need to be made available to the caregiver, who is usually the spouse.

4. A program of aerobic exercise with the goals of maintaining conditioning and range of motion while maximizing endurance should be directed by a physical therapist familiar with the clinical course of ALS. Guidance in energy conservation techniques is as equally important.

5. The diagnosis and management of **dysphagia** and **dysarthria** are discussed in Chapters 18 and 19.

6. **Pseudobulbar palsy** is suggested by emotional lability and a brisk jaw jerk. It can frequently be helped with amitriptyline at 25 mg by mouth three times a day or amantadine at 100 mg by mouth twice a day.

7. A **feeding tube** often frees the patient and family from the burden that meals become. Tube feeding allows adequate nutrition as well as hydration to loosen secretions. Because of the dangers of general anesthesia, percutaneous placement is generally preferred.

8. A speech pathologist experienced in neurologic problems as well as communication aids should be employed early to maintain socialization of the patient.

9. Salivation
   a. **Drooling** can be helped with a portable suction machine and one of the following agents:
      (1) Amitriptyline 25 to 100 mg/d by mouth
      (2) Scopolamine (Transderm Scop; Novartis) patch every 3 days
      (3) Glycopyrrolate (Robinul; A.H.Robins, Richmond, VA, U.S.A.) 1 to 2 mg by mouth three times a day
      (4) Transtympanic neurectomy, salivary gland irradiation, or botulinum toxin may be helpful to selected patients.
   b. **Thickened secretions** are managed with hydration and expectorants.
      (1) Ensure adequate hydration.
      (2) Avoid caffeine beverages; stop diuretics if possible.
      (3) Dilute potassium iodide (SSKI; Upsher-Smith, Minneapolis, MN, U.S.A.) at 300 to 600 mg by mouth three or four times a day *or*
      (4) Guaifenesin (syrup or tablet) at 200 to 400 mg by mouth every 4 hours *or*
      (5) Gradual escalation of β-blockers (propranolol or metoprolol) while observing for fatigue or respiratory difficulties
      (6) Dried secretions within the oropharynx can be loosened with a cotton swab dipped in meat tenderizer.

10. **Respiratory care**
    a. **Pulmonary function** (forced vital capacity) is evaluated on a regular basis. Rate of decline in vital capacity correlates with prognosis.
    b. **Orthopnea** (resulting from diaphragmatic weakness) and sleep apnea (possibly a result of bulbar weakness) are frequent problems that can be helped by sleep posture (hospital bed) and assistive devices. Some physicians use low-dose theophylline for its possible stimulant effect on the diaphragm.
    c. **Assistive devices** such as bimodal positive airway pressure or intermittent positive-pressure ventilation can provide benefit when the forced vital capacity approaches 50% of predicted value. These devices are meant to affect quality of life and do not significantly prolong survival. The use of these assistive devices, as well as more invasive ventilatory support that can prolong life, should be discussed with the patient in advance of the anticipated need.
    d. The **anxiety** associated with dyspnea in patients not choosing mechanical ventilation should be managed with appropriate sedation. Specific

dosing schedules for opiates and anxiolytics are given in ALS treatment guidelines (Miller et al., 1999).

 e. Respiratory infection should be managed aggressively.

 f. Influenza and **pneumonia vaccination** should be kept up to date.

11. **Assistive devices** can help with activities of daily living.

 a. The patient can refer to a catalog or website of self-help aids, such as the following:

Sammons Preston
Ability One Corporation
4 Sammons Ct
Bolingbrook, IL 60440
(800) 323-5547
www.sammonspreston.com

 b. The home should be inspected for modifications that will improve mobility and quality of life.

 c. Microprocessor-controlled adaptive devices allow nearly complete control of the environment.

 d. Respite care should be available to the caregiver.

12. Hospice care should be discussed in advance with the patient and family.

Recommended Readings

Abalan F. Primer in folic acid: folates and neuropsychiatry. *Nutrition* 1999;15:595–598.

Albert SM, Murphy PL, Del Bene ML, et al. A prospective study of preferences and actual treatment choices in ALS. *Neurology* 1999;53:278–283.

Belanger E, Levi AD. The acute and chronic management of spinal cord injury. *J Am Coll Surg* 2000;190:603–618.

Bogduk N, Teasell R. Whiplash: the evidence for an organic etiology. *Arch Neurol* 2000; 57:590–591.

Bryce TN, Ragnarsson KT. Pain after spinal cord injury. *Phys Med Rehabil Clin N Am* 2000;11: 157–168.

Carmel R, Aurangzeb I, Qian D. Associations of food–cobalamin malabsorption with ethnic origin, age, *Helicobacter pylori* infection, and serum markers of gastritis. *Am J Gastroenterol* 2001;96:63–70.

Carter GT, Miller RG. Comprehensive management of amyotrophic lateral sclerosis. *Phys Med Rehabil Clin N Am* 1998;9:271–284.

Chanarin I, Metz J. Diagnosis of cobalamin deficiency: the old and the new. *Br J Haematol* 1997;97:695–700.

Colachis SC III. Autonomic hyperreflexia with spinal cord injury. *J Am Paraplegia Soc* 1992;15:171–186.

Davis EC, Barnes MP. Botulinum toxin and spasticity. *J Neurol Neurosurg Psychiatry* 2000;69:143–147.

Ditunno JF Jr, Formal CS. Chronic spinal cord injury. *N Engl J Med* 1994;330:550–556.

Drolet BA. Cutaneous signs of neural tube dysraphism. *Pediatr Clin North Am* 2000;47: 813–823.

Evans RW. Some observations on whiplash injuries. *Neurol Clin* 1992;10:975–997.

Green R, Kinsella LJ. Current concepts in the diagnosis of cobalamin deficiency. *Neurology* 1995;45:1435–1440.

Jackson CE, Bryan WW. Amyotrophic lateral sclerosis. *Semin Neurol* 1998;18:27–39.

Kita M, Goodkin DE. Drugs used to treat spasticity. *Drugs* 2000;59:487–495.

Kuzminski AM, Del Giacco EJ, Allen RH, et al. Effective treatment of cobalamin deficiency with oral cobalamin. *Blood* 1998;92:1191–1198.

Mariani C, Cislaghi MG, Barbieri S, et al. The natural history and results of surgery in 50 cases of syringomyelia. *J Neurol* 1991;238:433–438.

Maynard FM Jr, Bracken MB, Creasey G, et al. International Standards for Neurological and Functional Classification of Spinal Cord Injury. American Spinal Injury Association. *Spinal Cord* 1997;35:266–274.

McCarron MO, Russell AJ, Metcalfe RA, et al. Chronic vitamin E deficiency causing spinocerebellar degeneration, peripheral neuropathy, and centro-cecal scotomata. *Nutrition* 1999;15:217–219.

Meadows J, Kraut M, Guarnieri M, et al. Asymptomatic Chiari type I malformations identified on magnetic resonance imaging. *J Neurosurg* 2000;92:920–926.

Milhorat TH, Chou MW, Trinidad EM, et al. Chiari I malformation redefined: clinical and radiographic findings for 364 symptomatic patients. *Neurosurgery* 1999;44:1005–1017.

Miller RG, Rosenberg JA, Gelinas DF, et al. Practice parameter: the care of the patient with amyotrophic lateral sclerosis (an evidence-based review): report of the Quality Standards Subcommittee of the American Academy of Neurology: ALS Practice Parameters Task Force. *Neurology* 1999;52:1311–1323.

Newey ML, Sen PK, Fraser RD. The long-term outcome after central cord syndrome: a study of the natural history. *J Bone Joint Surg Br* 2000;82:851–855.

Nogues M, Gene R, Benarroch E, et al. Respiratory disturbances during sleep in syringomyelia and syringobulbia. *Neurology* 1999;52:1777–1783.

Peeters GG, Verhagen AP, de Bie RA, et al. The efficacy of conservative treatment in patients with whiplash injury: a systematic review of clinical trials. *Spine* 2001;26:E64–E73.

Quality Standards Subcommittee of the American Academy of Neurology. Practice advisory on the treatment of amyotrophic lateral sclerosis with riluzole: report of the Quality Standards Subcommittee of the American Academy of Neurology. *Neurology* 1997;49:657–659.

Ratliff J, Mahoney PS, Kline DG. Tethered cord syndrome in adults. *South Med J* 1999; 92:1199–1203.

Schmitt J, Midha M, McKenzie N. Medical complications of spinal cord disease. *Neurol Clin* 1991;9:779–795.

Smyth MD, Peacock WJ. The surgical treatment of spasticity. *Muscle Nerve* 2000;23:153–163.

Snow CF. Laboratory diagnosis of vitamin B_{12} and folate deficiency: a guide for the primary care physician. *Arch Intern Med* 1999;159:1289–1298.

Stabler SP, Lindenbaum J, Allen RH. Vitamin B-12 deficiency in the elderly: current dilemmas. *Am J Clin Nutr* 1997;66:741–749.

Woolsey RM, McGarry JD. The cause, prevention, and treatment of pressure sores. *Neurol Clin* 1991;9:797–808.

Zittoun J, Zittoun R. Modern clinical testing strategies in cobalamin and folate deficiency. *Semin Hematol* 1999;36:35–46.

46. NEUROPATHY

John C. Kincaid

Peripheral neuropathy is the general term for diseases that affect the peripheral nervous system. The primary sites of pathologic changes are the nerve cell bodies, the axons, and the myelin sheaths. Some terms used in describing the lesions are as follows.

neuronopathy: abnormality of the nerve cell body, usually producing motor or sensory dysfunction separately

radiculopathy: abnormality at the level of the nerve root, most often involving a single spinal level and resulting from compression by a herniated disk or osteophyte

polyradiculopathy: abnormality involving many spinal root levels caused by inflammation

polyradiculoneuropathy: same as polyradiculopathy, but involving the peripheral nerve trunks as well as the nerve roots

polyneuropathy: abnormality of multiple peripheral nerves, usually in a symmetric manner and affecting feet and legs before hands and arms

axonal neuropathy: pathologic changes primarily in the axon

demyelinating neuropathy: pathologic changes primarily in the myelin sheath

plexopathy, plexitis: abnormality at the level of the brachial plexus in the shoulder or lumbosacral plexus in the pelvis

mononeuropathy: abnormality of an individual peripheral nerve usually caused by entrapment or local trauma

mononeuritis multiplex: abnormality of multiple nerves independently, often spreading limb to limb in a patchy manner such that one nerve is affected but an adjacent one is initially spared, often caused by vasculitis affecting the vasa nervorum.

   I. Management based on symptoms. Whether or not the cause of neuropathy is known, the clinician, generalist or specialist, usually is presented with a group of symptoms that are similar from one patient to another. Adopting a standardized approach to the management of the symptoms is useful. Neuropathic symptoms consist of

Pain
Paresthesia
Sensory loss
Weakness
Unstable balance

   A. Pain often is the most bothersome symptom and can be the most difficult to satisfactorily manage. The pain may have several different characters.
      1. Fiery, burning pain (or cold, frostbite-like pain) often is felt in the toes, bottoms of the feet, and fingertips. This type of pain should first be managed with an antiepileptic medication, such as gabapentin or carbamazepine. If benefit is going to occur, at least some improvement often declares itself within a few days of beginning the medication. An initial dose of 100 mg twice a day for carbamazepine or 300 mg twice a day for gabapentin is reasonable. The dosage may then have to be increased at weekly intervals to optimize the response, but full antiepilepsy dosages are not often required. The complete blood cell count should be monitored for patients undergoing maintenance therapy with carbamazepine.
      Analgesics, which can be mild agents such as aspirin or acetaminophen, can help relieve low-level pain. Combination medications such as acetaminophen–propoxyphene napsylate are helpful for mild to moderate pain. There is no compelling evidence that nonsteroidal antiinflammatory drugs offer much relief for this type of pain, but these agents can be tried. If the pain is more severe, stronger analgesics such as tramadol or codeine, hydrocodone, or oxycodone in combination with acetaminophen may be needed. Longer-acting drugs such as sustained-release oxycodone or morphine and methadone may provide smoother pain control for patients with severe discomfort. Methadone is the least expensive of the three. It is important for the patient and physician to understand that analgesics will not usually pro-

vide complete pain relief. This knowledge may help limit the tendency toward overuse in search of complete relief. Moderate to good relief is a reasonable, usually achievable goal. Neuropathic pain often is worse when the patient retires for sleep, and if possible, the stronger analgesics should initially be reserved for this time.

Burning or freezing pain can be significantly lessened by tricyclic antidepressants. The medications likely act through brainstem pain-modulating pathways. Pain is reduced in intensity but not fully relieved. Medications such as amitriptyline, nortriptyline, desipramine, and doxepin are the preferred agents. Antidepressants of the selective serotonin reuptake inhibitor class do not seem to provide much pain-modulating benefit but can be tried. When starting one of these drugs, inform the patient that there may be some early side effects such as morning sedation, dry mouth, and blurred vision. These effects usually lessen within a few days. Start these medications at a low dosage, such as 25 mg 1 hour or so before bedtime. Pain benefit may begin within a few days but may take several weeks to become evident. Increase the dosage by 10 to 25 mg every 2 to 3 weeks if there has been no benefit at the initial dosage or if the pain intensity exacerbates after initial improvement. A dose of 35 to 75 mg usually is sufficient, but higher amounts can be used within the bounds of the particular drug. Monitoring and optimizing the serum drug level do not seem to help. If a medication is beneficial, it should be continued for at least 6 months. At that point, a taper of 10 to 25 mg should be tried to determine whether the drug is still providing benefit. If symptoms worsen, the agent is still effective and should be returned to the previous level. Long-term use may be needed.

Topical capsaicin creams also may be helpful for this type of pain. Depletion of neurotransmitters in pain-sensing neurons is the proposed mechanism of action. These preparations are applied to the painful areas three or four times a day. Several weeks are required for benefit to appear, and a short-term increase in the pain may occur before the benefit begins. These drugs are moderately expensive and somewhat cumbersome to use. Like the other interventions, they may lessen but will not eliminate the pain.

  2. **Short jabs of pain** are another form of neuropathic pain. These are often felt in the feet, lower legs, or fingers. Each lasts a second or two, and they move about from limb to limb. This pain often responds to anticonvulsant drugs such as phenytoin at 100 mg two or three times a day or carbamazepine at 100 mg twice a day up to 200 mg three times a day. The benefit often appears within a few days and is obvious to the patient. Monitoring of drug levels is probably not helpful in maximizing benefit but may be needed if higher doses are required. Complete blood cell count should be monitored for patients undergoing maintenance therapy with carbamazepine.

  3. **Tight or bandlike pressure pain** in the feet or lower parts of the legs is relatively resistant to treatment. This sensation usually occurs in combination with other types of pain that often are more bothersome. Encourage patients not to rely on medication to provide relief from this type of pain.

  4. **Painful hypersensitivity to nonnoxious stimuli** often is an accompaniment to spontaneous pain. The patient perceives light touch in the involved area as exquisitely uncomfortable during and a few seconds after the touch. Wearing light cotton socks or gloves can lessen these sensations, as can tents in the bed linens to keep the toes from being touched. Tricyclic antidepressants may improve these sensations to some degree.

B. Paresthesia is another form of sensory abnormality. This phenomenon takes the form of feelings of repetitive prickles, or "pins and needles" sensations. These sensations are felt in larger areas than the discrete jabs of pain discussed in **I.A.2.** and may, for example, be felt in the toes, the feet, or the hands. They occur spontaneously or may be produced by touching of the body part. These sensations may improve with antiepileptic medications such as phenytoin, carbamazepine, and gabapentin in the dosages mentioned for jabs of pain. Analgesics do not help these symptoms.

C. **Sensory loss** can produce feelings of the affected areas being "dead," or "like blocks of wood," or "leathery." Sensations such as these do not respond to symptomatic treatment, and reliance on medications such as analgesics for relief should be discouraged. Because of the sensory loss, it is important that body parts in these areas be visually inspected at least daily for local trauma such as blisters or cuts. The tips of the toes and bottoms of the feet are particularly important areas for such inspection. Unrecognized lesions may lead to more serious problems such as ulcers and infections. Properly fitting shoes are important.

D. **Weakness** can occur focally in mononeuropathy, plexopathy, or radiculopathy. Bracing with an orthosis, or support with a sling, may be required to partially compensate the deficit while recovery is awaited. Mobilization of the weak body part through a complete range of motion should be done at least daily to prevent ankylosis.

1. Patients with polyneuropathy tend to have **distal, symmetric weakness.** Minor weakness limited to the intrinsic foot muscles can be found in many patients but usually is not clinically significant. Progression to foot drop or weakness of hand grip usually is evident to the patient. Intervention by fitting ankle–foot orthotics may greatly improve walking and standing stability. Use of large-handled utensils may help compensate for finger and hand weakness.

2. The development of marked **proximal, symmetric weakness** that causes difficulty getting up from chairs or of arm weakness that produces lifting difficulties is relatively distinct and suggests inflammatory demyelinating neuropathy (Guillain–Barré syndrome or its chronic variants).

3. **Unilateral proximal leg weakness** can occur in lumbar plexopathy, such as diabetic amyotrophy. Knee weakness can predispose patients to falling. Patients compensate for such weakness by keeping the knee locked in extension. Minor dislodgment from that position, caused by a shift in body position or a slight bump from a passerby exposes the weakness and causes a fall. Compensation by bracing is more difficult for knee weakness than for weakness at the ankle. A lift chair may help with getting up from sitting.

4. Evaluation by a physical medicine rehabilitation physician can be very helpful in all of these situations.

E. **Unstable balance** can cause problems ranging from mild inconvenience in walking or standing still to substantial danger from falling. Balance difficulty can result from sensory loss, cerebellar dysfunction, or weakness in the legs at the ankles and knees. Mild imbalance may require no active management other than caution on the patient's part. More pronounced deficits require assistance. These can be informal such as another person's arm to hold, strategically placed pieces of furniture, or a shopping cart at the store. More formal aids include a cane, walker, wheelchair, or motorized scooter. Patients may have increased difficulty in darkness or in situations in which their eyes are closed, such as showering. A patient who has had several falls should be encouraged to use a wheelchair to avoid further injury. A physical medicine rehabilitation evaluation can be helpful.

II. **Management of specific conditions**

A. **Acute inflammatory demyelinating neuropathy** (Guillain–Barré syndrome)

1. **Clinical features.** This disorder manifests as weakness and sensory loss, which usually begins in the feet and then spreads proximally into the legs and arms. The onset may follow a viral or other infectious-type illness by a week or two, but the disorder also can appear spontaneously. The condition evolves over days to a few weeks before reaching a plateau. The deficits may remain mild or progress to a severe level, making the patient paretic and necessitating use of a ventilator. Weakness usually is the symptom that causes the patient to seek medical attention. Loss of muscle stretch reflexes is an expected finding.

2. **Laboratory findings** of increased spinal fluid protein concentration along with a normal or minimally elevated white blood cell count support the diagnosis. Nerve conduction studies that show marked slowing of conduction

velocity also support the diagnosis. Screening for arsenic intoxication and porphyria should be performed because these disorders can produce illnesses that appear similar to acute inflammatory demyelinating neuropathy. Tick bite paralysis also can mimic this condition.

3. **Treatment**

   a. Patients believed to have acute inflammatory demyelinating neuropathy need to be admitted to a hospital. Patients with mild cases may not need direct treatment but should be observed closely for several days to assure the weakness has stabilized. Weakness of a degree that impairs walking or use of the arms can be relieved with treatment. Treatment may lessen the duration or severity of the attack.

   b. Two treatments—plasmapheresis and intravenous gamma globulin infusion—have shown benefit. Both probably work by re-regulating the immune system.

      (1) **Plasmapheresis,** also called **plasma exchange,** is done by replacing a portion of the plasma to eliminate components, as yet undefined, that are the mediators of the attack. The treatment sequence usually involves a plasma exchange every other day for at total of four or five sessions. Vascular access through peripheral veins may be possible, but a central line usually is required. Treatments are generally well tolerated. Transient hypotension can occur, and therefore this mode may not be optimal for patients with labile cardiovascular systems.

      (2) **Intravenous gamma globulin infusion** on a regimen of 0.4 g/kg a day for 5 days has been shown to be equal in effectiveness to plasmapheresis. This treatment is logistically easier, because only peripheral venous access is required. Complications of this mode of treatment have been infrequent but have included vascular incidents presumably resulting from hyperviscosity due to the large protein infusion. Headache due to aseptic meningitis also can occur.

      (3) **With either treatment,** improvement may begin within a day or two of starting but may also appear only weeks later in the form of a shortened duration of the illness. Improvement is the natural course of the illness even without active treatment. Lack of improvement over the first week or so of treatment is not a valid reason to change treatment from the initially chosen method to another. A small percentage of the patients whose condition improves with treatment may have a relapse within a few weeks of the initial improvement. In such instances, another one or two plasma exchanges, or gamma globulin infusions, will reestablish the improvement. Major improvement occurs in a high percentage of patients, but even with these treatments, some patients have a prolonged, severe course necessitating weeks if not months of hospitalization. In the more severe cases, deficits of distal weakness, sensory loss, and paresthesia may show prolonged recovery over months to years or may become persistent.

   c. Corticosteroids do not benefit patients with the acute form of inflammatory neuropathy.

B. **Chronic inflammatory demyelinating neuropathy**

   1. **Clinical features.** The neuropathy is similar to the acute form but continues to worsen over a longer period, such as months. This form may not be relieved without treatment. The laboratory and nerve conduction results are similar to those of the acute form. Monoclonal gammopathy of the immunoglobulin M type can mimic this condition, and screening should be performed.

   2. **Treatment.** The **treatment** options are the same as for the acute form of the neuropathy with the exception that corticosteroids may benefit patients with the chronic type. Plasmapheresis or intravenous gamma globulin infusion is likely the more commonly chosen treatment. The schedule in **II.A.3.b.**

should be followed. If steroid treatment is chosen, prednisone 1 mg/kg a day should be used. Some signs of improvement should be evident within 1 month of initiation if the medication is going to work. Further improvement is likely over the next few months. After the first month, a tapering schedule of 10 mg per month reduction should be followed. If worsening occurs after a dose change, an increase back to the previous effective dose should be made. After a dose decrease, many patients report apparent worsening, which consists of general aching, stiffness, and listlessness. These symptoms do not represent a true exacerbation and are only nonspecific symptoms from the steroid dose decrease. They should clear within approximately 2 to 3 weeks of the dose decrease. If no true improvement has occurred within the first month of treatment, benefit is unlikely, and the medication should be tapered off completely off over the next month. Treatment with steroids can be much less expensive than plasmapheresis or gamma globulin infusion. Potential steroid side effects from long-term use and the relative benignity of the other treatments merit consideration in choosing the type of management.

3. In the care of some patients, one form of treatment may fail but another provide good benefit. Allow 1 to 2 months for any treatment to declare its benefit or lack thereof before deciding to change to another. Patients who show good initial response to gamma globulin infusion or plasmapheresis may need repeated treatments if relapse occurs after treatment. Worsening often appears within 3 to 8 weeks of initial treatment if it is going to. A single session of pheresis or intravenous immune globulin should be repeated and the patient observed for the next month. The need for further treatment is then dictated by the maintained remission or re-exacerbation. Repeated treatments may be needed for and an extended period every 1 to 3 months.

C. **Vasculitic neuropathy** occurs in the setting of inflammation of the vasa nervorum. The vasculitis usually is a component of a more generalized systemic disease but in rare cases may be limited to the vessels of the peripheral nerve alone.

1. **Clinical features.** The presentation and evolution of this type of neuropathy are unique. Progression occurs in a patchy manner such that a single nerve in a limb malfunctions and then a nerve in another location does the same. Individual deficits often appear rather suddenly, and then accumulate over days to weeks. This stepwise and cumulative pattern is termed **mononeuritis multiplex.** If left unchecked, the condition evolves into generalized, symmetric polyneuropathy. Careful history taking identifies the patchy pattern of progression.

   Vasculitic neuropathy can be extremely serious and continues to progress if left untreated. The neuropathy may occur in association with polyarteritis nodosa, rheumatoid arthritis, systemic lupus erythematosus, or Wegener's granulomatosis and may be the initial feature of these conditions.

2. The **diagnosis** is supported by results of laboratory studies that identify any of the aforementioned systemic illnesses. Electromyography can help by showing a patchy pattern of involvement suggestive of mononeuritis multiplex. Biopsy of a peripheral nerve in an area of clinical involvement, such as the sural nerve or a superficial radial nerve, can provide strong support if the results are positive.

3. **Treatment** requires **immunosuppressive therapy.** Prednisone at 1 mg/kg a day provides some improvement, but addition of **cyclophosphamide** usually is required for sustained benefit. *Cyclophosphamide should be given by physicians familiar with its use.* It can be administered by means of daily oral dosage or monthly intravenous pulse therapy. Recovery takes place over an extended period and declares itself first as a cessation of further worsening. Improvement appears over months and may continue for several years. Severely affected areas may show some degree of persistent deficit despite improvement.

D. **Alcoholic neuropathy** is sensorimotor neuropathy that affects the legs initially and may progress into the arms if the excess exposure continues.

1. **Clinical features and diagnosis.** The onset is insidious, and progression takes place over months or longer. Sensory symptoms include numbness, tingling paresthesia, and fiery pain. Motor abnormalities in the form of foot drop, hand weakness, and even proximal leg weakness can occur in more advanced cases. The neuropathy shows a pattern of axonal damage on an electromyogram. Supporting laboratory findings include liver enzyme abnormalities and macrocytosis.
2. **Therapy** consists of discontinuance of alcohol and supplementation of the diet with thiamine at 100 mg/d. Improvement takes place over months. Unstable walking as a result of alcoholic cerebellar disease shows much less recovery than the neuropathy and can limit overall improvement.
3. **Mononeuropathy** results from local compression of nerves during periods of alcoholic obtundation. Radial neuropathy at the spiral groove of the humerus, causing wrist drop, is the classic lesion. The deficit tends to recover over days to months as the pressure-injured internodal segments remyelinate. Other forms of **compressive mononeuropathy,** such as that affecting the peroneal nerve at the head of the fibula or the ulnar nerve in the area of the medial epicondyle, can also occur among persons with alcoholism. These lesions may not follow the course of spontaneous improvement as expected for the radial lesion. If deficits do not improve within 2 months of onset, electrodiagnostic testing and surgical treatment should be considered.
E. **Diabetic neuropathy** can appear in several different forms, which are not mutually exclusive. There is still no specific therapy for most forms of diabetic neuropathy, but knowledge of these several conditions can help the physician provide guidance for the patient. The principles of general symptom management outlined in **I.** should be followed.
   1. **Sensorimotor polyneuropathy** causing bilateral foot and hand numbness with or without a painful component is the most common type of diabetic neuropathy. Good blood sugar control is the foundation of management, but neuropathic symptoms may occur regardless.
   2. **Femoral neuropathy** or so-called diabetic amyotrophy is a distinctive syndrome among some patients with diabetes (see Chapter 25, **II.A.**). It often appears when blood sugar control goes from loose to better, as in a change from an oral agent to insulin, or in a period of considerable weight loss. The condition manifests as spontaneous onset of unilateral pain in the low back, hip, or proximal leg and can become quite severe over the next week or so. Days to a few weeks after onset of the pain, paresthesia, and sensory loss appear in the thigh and at times in the medial lower leg. Weakness of the quadriceps and hip flexor muscles appears about the same time. The weakness may be unappreciated until a fall occurs because the leg gives out under the patient. Notable atrophy of the quadriceps muscles can occur after the weakness has appeared. The pain often is poorly responsive to even major analgesics but begins to improve spontaneously within a month or so after onset. The long-term prognosis is good. Occasionally, as the initially involved side is improving the opposite side becomes involved. Reports in the literature suggest that a course of intravenous gamma globulin or oral steroids may shorten the course of this syndrome.
   3. **Thoracic radiculopathy** is somewhat similar to femoral neuropathy in circumstances of onset and time course. Unilateral bandlike pain that begins spontaneously in the chest or upper lumbar region is the main symptom. The pain can be severe. Cutaneous hypersensitivity that makes the touch of clothing uncomfortable in the involved area also may be reported. Localized weakness of the lateral or anterior abdominal muscles may produce localized bulging of the abdominal wall, particularly in the standing position. Analgesics provide mild relief at best. Tricyclic antidepressants may help ease the intensity of the pain and help the patient sleep. Local anesthetic nerve blocks of the involved dermatome may help to some degree, as can use of a transcutaneous electrical nerve stimulation (TENS) unit. The pain persists for some months but eventually resolves or is greatly relieved.
   4. **Diabetic polyradiculoneuropathy** is a distinctive syndrome but shares some features with femoral neuropathy and thoracic radiculopathy. This

condition often manifests at a time of change in the quality of blood sugar control. This change may be from loose to tight or may appear when previous good control becomes loose. Patients may report that they "just got sick." Symptoms appear over weeks to a few months. Patients often report loss of appetite and may lose notable amounts of weight. Neuropathic features can include back and flank pain, which can be bilateral, and leg weakness, which usually is proximal. The hip flexors, knee extensors, and adductors can be involved, at times severely, and the patient must use a wheelchair. This syndrome has a good long-term prognosis and tends to clear over months. Management is mainly symptomatic. Whether immunosuppression such as that used for the more typical diabetic amyotrophy syndrome can be helpful for this condition has not been established.

F. Lyme disease can produce several different types of peripheral neuropathy, as well as meningitis and chronic encephalopathy. The bites of certain ticks of the *Ixodes* genus (e.g., *I. dammini*, most often) transmit the infectious agent *Borrelia burgdorferi*. Endemic areas include southern New England and the Mid-Atlantic states, Michigan through Minnesota, and north coastal California and Oregon.

   1. **Clinical features.** The characteristic skin lesion erythema chronicum migrans develops 3 to 20 days after the bite, as does a general flulike syndrome of fever, malaise, and myalgia. The skin lesion occurs in approximately 80% of cases. Frank neurologic involvement occurs in approximately 15% of cases and tends to appear 1 to 3 months after the initial infection in the time frame termed the *early disseminated phase* of the illness. A positive serologic result for antibodies against the infectious agent is helpful for establishing the cause, but test results may be negative for a month or so after the initial infection.

   2. **Treatment.** Antibiotic treatment appears to relieve all of the manifestations, either by shortening the duration of episodes or by alleviating more persistent symptoms such as polyneuropathy. Oral antibiotics can be used to manage the rash and flulike phase of the initial stage of the infection. For adults, doxycycline 100 mg twice a day, amoxicillin 500 mg four times a day, or cefuroxime 500 mg twice a day for 2 to 3 weeks is acceptable. Peripheral and central nervous system manifestations are best managed with intravenous penicillin, 20 to 24 million U/d for 2 to 3 weeks, or ceftriaxone, 2 g daily for the same length of time.

   3. **Specific types of neuropathy of the early disseminated phase**
      a. **Facial nerve involvement** producing typical Bell's palsy, including pain in the ear region. Bilateral involvement occurs more frequently with Lyme disease than in the idiopathic form.
      b. **Thoracic radiculitis** producing a syndrome similar to that described for diabetic neuropathy (see **II.E.3.**) and consisting of dermatomal pain, which can reach a high level of intensity. Sensory loss may occur in the affected dermatomes.
      c. **Brachial plexitis** producing clinical features similar to those described in **II.H.**
      d. **Mononeuritis multiplex** producing clinical features similar to those described in **II.C.**
      These four types can occur in combination and appear sequentially rather than concurrently.

   4. The **late disseminated phase** of the infection occurs a year or longer after the initial infection. Polyneuropathy that produces mild distal paresthesia and minor abnormalities found at examination may be seen in this phase. Patients may have somewhat more impressive abnormalities at nerve conduction studies than the mild clinical features would suggest. Encephalopathy causing forgetfulness can occur in this phase of the illness. Antibiotic treatment may relieve these manifestations, if the patient has not previously received adequate dosages.

G. **Human immunodeficiency virus** infection can have several types of peripheral neuropathy within its clinical spectrum.
   1. Typical **acute inflammatory demyelinating neuropathy,** or Guillain–Barré syndrome, can occur early in the course of the infection. Cerebrospinal fluid pleocytosis is the only feature that usually differentiates this condition from the typical idiopathic variety. Therapy should be the same as for the idiopathic form of the disorder (see **II.A.3.**).
   2. More bothersome to both the patient and the physician is the **generalized neuropathy** with predominant painful sensory symptoms that occurs when acquired immunodeficiency syndrome (AIDS) is clinically full blown. Patients report painful paresthesia consisting of pressure- or burning-type sensations. The hands are involved to a lesser extent than the feet or are spared. Weakness is minimal. Cerebrospinal fluid tends to be normal to minimally abnormal. Nerve conduction studies show a pattern of axonal damage. Management of this type of neuropathy is symptomatic only and not particularly satisfactory. The general guidelines for painful neuropathy presented in **II.A.** should be followed.
   3. **Polyradiculitis** resulting from infection by **cytomegalovirus** is another distinctive forms of neuropathy that affects patients with AIDS in the advanced stage of the illness. This is a recognizable neuropathy. Patients report unilateral pain and weakness in lower extremities and the back. Within days to weeks, the opposite leg is involved. Sensory loss develops in the perineal area, as do bladder and bowel incontinence. Progression to arm involvement is infrequent. Spinal fluid shows pleocytosis and elevated protein level. Pathologic specimens show inflammation of the nerve roots of the lumbar and sacral areas. **Treatment** with ganciclovir may stabilize the condition, but in general this lesion is a poor prognostic indicator of survival.
H. **Brachial plexitis,** also known as **Parsonage–Turner syndrome** or neuralgic amyotrophy, is easily recognizable retrospectively but can be difficult to differentiate securely from cervical nerve-root compression or intrinsic shoulder disease at presentation or in the early stages of evolution. The upper trunk of the brachial plexus tends to be involved. Brachial plexitis can be idiopathic or may appear a few weeks after an infection, immunization, or surgery.

   The pain begins spontaneously in the neck, shoulder, or upper arm. It has a constant "deep in the bone" character and usually is unilateral. The pain intensifies over hours to a few days and can become excruciating. Neck movement tends to not worsen the pain, but arm or shoulder motion may. The patient often chooses to hold the arm quietly adducted to the side and flexed at the elbow. A week or longer after the onset of pain, symptoms of sensory loss and weakness appear. The sensory deficits occur in the radial forearm and thumb through middle fingers. The weakness tends to be in the deltoid, biceps, supraspinatus and infraspinatus, and serratus anterior muscles.

   Marked atrophy can occur in affected muscles. The pain is poorly responsive to even major analgesics but should be managed symptomatically the best possible way. The pain usually lessens within 3 to 6 weeks. The sensory loss and weakness improve over months, but long-term deficits may persist. Occasionally the contralateral side becomes symptomatic while the side initially involved improves. Maintaining range of motion in the affected joint during the period of pain can help enhance long-term outcome.

   Differentiating plexitis from intrinsic shoulder disease requires joint examination and radiography. Differentiation from a cervical disk syndrome may require imaging studies of the spine. Even though the plexus lesion is presumably inflammatory in nature, treatment with corticosteroids has shown no definite benefit.

Recommended Readings
Brown MR, Dyck PJ, McClearn GE, et al. Central and peripheral nervous system complications. *Diabetes* 1982;31[Suppl 1]:65–70.

Dyck PJ, ed. *Peripheral neuropathy,* 3rd ed. Philadelphia: Saunders, 1993.

Garcia-Monoco JC, Benach JL. Lyme neuroborreliosis. *Ann Neurol* 1995;37:691–702.

Krendel DA, Costigan DA, Hopkins LC. Successful treatment of neuropathies in patients with diabetes mellitus. *Arch Neurol* 1995;52:1053–1061.

McKahnn GM. Guillain-Barré syndrome: clinical and therapeutic observations. *Ann Neurol* 1990;27[Suppl]:S13–S16.

Miller RG, Parry GJ, Pfaeffl W, et al. The spectrum of peripheral neuropathy with ARC and AIDS. *Muscle Nerve* 1988;11:857–863.

Van Doorn PA, Vermeulen M, Brand A, et al. Intravenous gamma globulin in treatment of patients with chronic inflammatory demyelinating polyneuropathy. *Arch Neurol* 1991; 48:217–220.

47. MYOPATHY

Raúl N. Mandler

Myopathy is abnormality of the skeletal muscle in which striated muscle cells or connective tissue elements are affected. Myopathy can result from abnormalities of skeletal muscle proteins (Duchenne muscular dystrophy), alterations of the sarcolemmal sodium channels (hyperkalemic periodic paralysis), mitochondrial alterations (mitochondrial myopathy), or cell-mediated autoimmune mechanisms (polymyositis), to name a few examples. Because of the myriad abnormal mechanisms, treatments vary from one condition to the next. Progress in molecular biology, genetics, and immunology has considerably expanded our understanding of these complicated diseases. This chapter emphasizes current therapeutic approaches to the care of patients with relatively common forms of myopathy.

    I. Idiopathic inflammatory myopathy is autoimmune disease characterized by muscle weakness, pain, and fatigue. Inflammatory infiltrates are found at muscle biopsy. **Polymyositis,** the prototype of inflammatory myopathy, can occur in isolation, accompanying other connective tissue disorders or systemic autoimmune disorders, such as Crohn's disease, primary biliary cirrhosis, ankylosing spondylitis, Hashimoto's disease, and psoriasis. **Dermatomyositis, inclusion body myositis,** and **polymyalgia rheumatica** are the other three major categories of idiopathic inflammatory myopathy. The incidence of these diseases is approximately 1 case among 100,000 persons.
        A. Natural history and prognosis
            1. Polymyositis usually affects upper and lower girdle muscles in a rather symmetric manner after the second decade of life. Often, pharyngeal muscles and myocardium are affected. Patients with no family history of muscle weakness have subacute (weeks to months), progressive weakness of the deltoid, trapezius, neck flexor and extensor, biceps, triceps, iliopsoas, gluteus, quadriceps, and other muscles. In muscular dystrophy, however, there is a family history of the disease and progression of weakness usually is measured in years. Complete sparing of the distal musculature raises the suspicion of a limb-girdle type of muscular dystrophy.
                Patients characteristically have problems arising from a sitting position, shampooing their hair, or walking up or down stairs. Muscle pain often accompanies the weakness, especially early in the course. Fatigue, weight loss, and malaise are common. Often the syndrome is preceded by an upper respiratory infection. In some cases, the disease follows an acute course that can be complicated by myoglobinuria resulting from acute muscle necrosis. Pharyngeal muscle compromise can lead to dysphagia without dysarthria. The tongue usually is spared. Extraocular and facial muscles should not be impaired. Sensation is not affected. Cardiac involvement can occur in as many as 40% of cases and can lead to heart failure or arrhythmias. Pulmonary involvement can result from primary weakness of respiratory muscles or from pulmonary interstitial fibrosis.
                Polymyositis also occurs in association with connective tissue and systemic autoimmune disorders. Against popular belief, polymyositis is not associated with an increased incidence of malignant disease. An extensive evaluation for malignant disease is not justified simply because of a diagnosis of polymyositis. Inasmuch as tumors in patients with polymyositis have been diagnosed because of abnormal findings in medical histories and physical examinations, a complete annual physical with pelvic and rectal examinations, urinalysis, complete blood cell count, blood chemistry, and chest radiograph should suffice. On the other hand, it appears that dermatomyositis has a higher risk of being accompanied by malignant disease. T-cell-mediated immunity plays a prominent role in the pathogenesis of polymyositis.
            2. Dermatomyositis is characterized by a rash that accompanies or precedes muscle weakness. The characteristic skin abnormality is a heliotrope rash (purple discoloration of the eyelids) with a red rash on the rest of the face and upper trunk and erythema of the knuckles, unlike the erythema of systemic

lupus erythematosus, in which the phalanges are involved and the knuckles are spared. The erythematous rash also can affect the elbows, knees, neck, upper chest (V shape), or back and shoulders (shawl sign) and may be photosensitive. Subcutaneous nodular calcifications and dilated capillaries at the bases of the fingernails are rather characteristic.

In children, extramuscular manifestations are more frequent than they are in adults. Dermatomyositis usually occurs alone but may be associated with systemic sclerosis, mixed connective tissue disease, other autoimmune conditions, or malignant lesions. Fascitis and skin changes similar to those of dermatomyositis also may occur in patients with eosinophilia–myalgia syndrome secondary to ingestion of contaminated tryptophan. Dermatomyositis has a characteristic histologic pattern of perifascicular atrophy. It is mainly a humorally mediated microangiopathic disorder with vascular deposition of immunoglobulin G (IgG), C3, and membrane attack complex. This suggests that the primary immunologic event is generation of antibodies against antigens within the walls of intramuscular blood vessels. The microangiopathic change causes ischemic damage to the muscle fibers.

3. **Inclusion body myositis** characteristically involves distal muscles such as foot extensors and finger flexors, in addition to more proximal muscles. Weakness and atrophy can be asymmetric and selectively involve the quadriceps, simulating the femoral neuropathy or plexopathy that occurs among patients with diabetes. Often the diagnosis of inclusion body myositis is made retrospectively when a presumptive diagnosis of polymyositis has been made and the patient did not benefit from therapy. Inclusion body myositis may also be associated with autoimmune or connective tissue disorders. Familial forms have been described.

4. **Polymyalgia rheumatica** affects elderly men and women with a peak incidence at 74 years of age. Patients describe diffuse muscle aching with neck and shoulder stiffness. Pain predominates over weakness or atrophy. Low-grade fever and anemia are found. Approximately 15% of the patients also have temporal arteritis. The incidence of rheumatoid arthritis also is increased. The erythrocyte sedimentation rate is elevated to more than 40 mm/h. Despite the severity of the symptoms, muscle biopsy usually is noncontributory.

5. Noninfectious inflammatory myositis also occurs in the context of systemic lupus erythematosus, progressive systemic sclerosis, Sjögren's syndrome, rheumatoid arthritis, mixed connective tissue disease, sarcoidosis, hypereosinophilic syndromes, and other disorders.

B. **Diagnosis.** In addition to the clinical features, the diagnosis of inflammatory myopathy is supported by results of measurement of muscle enzymes, electromyography (EMG), and muscle biopsy.

1. **Muscle enzymes.** Creatine kinase (CK) is released from the sarcoplasm into the serum after muscle destruction, and the level may be elevated as much as 50-fold in polymyositis. Other muscle enzymes such as lactate dehydrogenase, aldolase, and aminotransferases are commonly elevated. Whereas CK levels often parallel disease activity, they can be normal in active polymyositis. In inclusion body myositis, CK level may be elevated as much as tenfold or remain normal. In some patients with active childhood dermatomyositis and in patients with associated connective tissue diseases, CK levels may be normal.

2. The main value of **EMG** resides in its ability to show that peripheral neuromuscular weakness originates from the muscle itself and not from denervation or from a defect in neuromuscular transmission. It can also help ascertain the presence of disease activity. The classic EMG findings include short-duration, small-amplitude motor unit potentials and increased membrane irritability signaled by increased insertional activity, fibrillations, and complex-repetitive potentials. These findings should not be considered specific for inflammatory myopathy, because they also can be found in acute toxic or metabolic myopathy and in dystrophy.

3. **Muscle biopsy** helps establish the diagnosis.

a. In **polymyositis,** light microscopic examination of paraffin-embedded sections displays inflammatory infiltrates, necrosis, atrophy and regeneration of muscle fibers, and increased amounts of connective tissue.

b. In **dermatomyositis,** the inflammatory infiltrates are present around the vessels or in the interfascicular septa, and perifascicular atrophy is characteristic. Small blood vessels with hyperplastic endothelia may be occluded. In polymyositis and inclusion body myositis, the infiltrates are inside the fascicles. Scattered atrophy prevails in polymyositis.

c. **Inclusion body myositis** is characterized by basophilic granular inclusions around the edges of vacuoles (rimmed vacuoles). Tissue should be prepared frozen and for electron microscopic biopsy, because paraffin processing can dissolve the granules.

d. Muscle biopsy has **limitations.** Certain drugs (penicillamine and zidovudine) and parasites (e.g., *Toxoplasma, Trypanosoma,* and *Cysticercus* organisms) also cause focal or generalized myopathy, which must be differentiated from idiopathic–autoimmune inflammatory myopathy. Because of sampling error, biopsy sometimes fails to disclose abnormalities expected from the clinical presentation.

C. Therapy

1. Prednisone

a. **Administration.** High-dose prednisone is the initial line of therapy for polymyositis and dermatomyositis. In severe cases, short courses of intravenous (i.v.) high doses of methylprednisolone (Solu-Medrol pulse; Pharmacia & Upjohn, Kalamazoo, MI, U.S.A.) 20 to 30 mg/kg a day for 3 to 5 days slowly over 2 hours with monitoring of electrocardiogram (ECG) and potassium level may be the preferable way to initiate therapy. In less acute cases and after the initial methylprednisolone pulse, the recommended dosage is 1.0 to 1.5 mg/kg a day in a single daily dose before breakfast for 3 to 4 weeks. The total dose should not exceed 100 mg. Daily administration should be used until there is unquestionable improvement muscle strength with recovery of ambulation. Then the dosage can be slowly reduced over 10 weeks to 1 mg/kg every other day. If no deterioration occurs, the dose is further reduced by 5 to 10 mg every 3 to 4 weeks until the lowest dose that controls the disease is reached. The dose should not be reduced if strength decreases. If treatment is effective, strength should improve within 3 months. However, most patients may need prednisone for at least 1 if not 2 years. A feeling of well-being and a decrease in muscle enzyme levels without an increase in muscle strength are not sufficient to decide that disease improvement has occurred. If after 3 months of therapy no improvement has been achieved, prednisone should be tapered off and another immunosuppressant medication begun.

b. **Side effects.** It is imperative that patients become acquainted with the numerous side effects of long-term prednisone treatment to better prevent them. Sodium chloride and fluid retention are prevented with a low sodium chloride diet. A low free sugar diet also is important to minimize weight gain. Potassium depletion may necessitate careful monitoring and sometimes replacement. Possible development of hypertension requires systematic monitoring. Aseptic necrosis of the hip, osteoporosis, and bone fractures are serious complications.

Prevention of osteoporosis requires supplemental calcium gluconate or carbonate (500 to 1,000 mg/d) and calcitriol (0.2 to 0.5 µg/d) as well as axial exercise and adequate passive range of motion maneuvers. Exercise also appears to reduce the risk of steroid myopathy. If there are no contraindications, estrogen and progesterone treatment of postmenopausal women should be considered. Alendronate (Fosamax; Merck, Whitehouse Station, NJ, U.S.A.) also can be used. Calcemia has to be monitored. A baseline dual energy x-ray absorption densitometry (DEXA) scan to measure bone density should be obtained for every patient before steroid treatment is started. The scan should be repeated every 6 months.

Flatulence, abdominal distention, and weight gain are common with prednisone. Antacids and histamine-2 blockers should be used to prevent peptic ulcers. Periodic eye examinations are needed for diagnosis of incipient cataracts or glaucoma. Impaired wound healing, hirsutism, acne, moon face, propensity to infection, insomnia, personality changes, headache, dizziness, and diabetes are other important side effects. Sometimes patients need separate therapy for the rash, preferably with topical steroids and sunscreen; as chloro- and hydroxychloroquine themselves can produce myopathy.

The use of prednisone might produce steroid myopathy, namely, increased muscle weakness with normal CK. Differentiating worsening of polymyositis and development of steroid myopathy can be difficult. The decision to raise or lower the prednisone dose has to be made after careful consideration of the patient's history of muscle strength, mobility, CK levels, and changes in medications in the preceding months.

2. **Azathioprine** is considered when serious complications preclude use of steroids, when the disease is not responding to adequate dosages of prednisone, or when it progresses rapidly and is accompanied by respiratory failure. A therapeutic response may take 3 to 6 months.

   a. **Administration.** Azathioprine typically is used in combination with prednisone at lower doses than those used in prednisone monotherapy. This approach may reduce prednisone-related side effects. Azathioprine can be administered at 2 (up to 3) mg/kg a day for 4 to 6 months. The initial dose should be approximately 50 mg/d with subsequent gradual increase. The total daily dose should be divided two or three times a day and given with meals.

   b. **Side effects.** Dose-independent side effects of azathioprine are fever, nausea, rash, and pancreatitis. Dose-dependent side effects are bone marrow suppression and liver toxicity. Complete blood cell count with differential and platelets and results of liver function tests should be performed weekly for the first month and monthly thereafter. Other side effects include anorexia, hair loss, possible development of cancer, and teratogenicity. *Concomitant administration of allopurinol is contraindicated.* Azathioprine should not be used to treat children.

   Mycophenylate mofetil (CellCept; Roche, Nutley, NJ, U.S.A.), a selective, noncompetitive, and reversible inhibitor of inosine monophosphate dehydrogenase inhibits proliferation of T and B lymphocytes and may bear promise in the management of inflammatory myopathy. For other immune disorders and prevention of transplant rejection, it is used at 2 g/d. Side effects include general immunosuppression, gastrointestinal side effects, hepatotoxicity and bone marrow inhibition, possible reactivation of chronic infection such as tuberculosis, and remote risk of malignant disease. Controlled studies will determine its safety and effectiveness.

3. **Methotrexate** (0.5 to 0.8 mg/kg per week intramuscularly or up to 15 to 25 mg/wk by mouth) is used as another method to spare use of prednisone or if prednisone has not been effective. Hepatotoxicity, leukopenia, alopecia, stomatitis, and risk of neoplasia can occur.

4. **High-dose intravenous gamma globulin** is effective in the management of polymyositis and in dermatomyositis but not of inclusion body myositis. The recommended dosage is 0.4 g/kg a day for 5 days. The initial rate of treatment should be slow, 0.01 to 0.02 mL/kg per minute, and then increased to 0.04 mL/kg per minute. Several preparations are available, not all of them biologically equal. Improvement after this therapy can be followed by relapses. Repeated monthly infusion may be needed. In some patients, high-dose immunoglobulin worsens the syndrome. Side effects include headaches, hypertension, and risk of acute renal failure and myocardial infarction owing to hyperviscosity. Aseptic meningitis due to treatment with high-dose gamma globulin may respond to prednisone treatment. IgA-depleted preparations reduce the risk of reactions related to anti-IgA antibodies. Solvent

detergent–treated, hepatitis B and C free, and human immunodeficiency virus (HIV)–free preparations are essential. Treatments are expensive. Despite these reservations, high-dosage intravenous gamma globulin might benefit patients who have been unresponsive to other medications. High-dose gamma globulin can be administered in outpatient facilities such as day treatment units and in home therapy.

5. In refractory cases, especially when interstitial lung disease occurs, cyclophosphamide (1 to 2 g/m² a month i.v.) may be needed. Side effects include nausea, vomiting, alopecia, hemorrhagic cystitis, teratogenicity, bone marrow suppression, carcinogenesis, and pulmonary fibrosis. Cyclophosphamide also can be used orally at doses of 1 to 2 mg/kg a day. Responses to cyclosporine and plasmapheresis have been disappointing.

6. **Physical therapy** and **adequate diet** should be emphasized.

7. In **polymyalgia rheumatica,** prednisone rapidly provides benefits, sometimes within hours. Duration of treatment and dosage have to be individualized and, because patients are elderly, monitored very carefully. In general, a starting dosage of 1 mg/kg a day should be appropriate. In mild cases, nonsteroidal antiinflammatory agents can be used. In patients suffering from temporal arteritis, corticosteroid treatment may prevent blindness.

D. **Prognosis.** Dermatomyositis and, to a lesser degree, polymyositis are responsive to treatment, whereas inclusion body myositis usually is resistant. Patients with interstitial lung disease may have a high mortality and need treatment with cyclophosphamide. When management of polymyositis is unsuccessful, the patient should be reevaluated and the muscle biopsy specimen reexamined to exclude inclusion body myositis or muscular dystrophy of the limb-girdle type. Finally, it is important to emphasize the need to evaluate the patient's strength and activities of daily living as measures of improvement, rather than simply adjusting treatment on the basis of CK levels alone.

II. **Viral inflammatory myopathy.** Viruses and retroviruses can cause acute or subacute inflammatory myopathy. Acute viral myopathy related to the influenza viruses and coxsackievirus are the most common. Viruses also can trigger subacute polymyositis, as in Reye's syndrome. Myopathy also can be associated with HIV infection and its management with zidovudine.

A. **Natural history, prognosis, and treatment**

1. **Influenza myositis** occurs among children and adults. Children have a brief, febrile illness characterized by myalgia with prodromic fever, malaise, sore throat, and rhinorrhea. Occasionally there is vomiting or myoglobinuria. Strength, which usually is normal, can be difficult to assess because of the pain. A similar syndrome may be related to infection with parainfluenza viruses, respiratory syncytial virus, herpes simplex virus, or *Mycoplasma pneumoniae.* Results of most laboratory studies are normal, but CK level may be elevated. The prognosis usually is favorable, especially among children. Among adults, weakness can be severe, CK level can be markedly elevated, cardiopulmonary complications can occur, and the prognosis may not be very favorable. There even is risk of death. In children, the culprit usually is influenza A; in adults, it usually is influenza B. Treatment consists of bed rest, fluids, and antipyretic agents other than aspirin. In adults, the syndrome can be more severe than it is in children. Myoglobinuria and renal failure may develop. In patients with myoglobinuria, intravenous hydration may be needed to prevent acute renal failure.

2. **Coxsackievirus B** produces pleurodynia (epidemic myalgia of Bornholm) accompanied by inflammatory myopathy. The disease occurs during the summer and fall, and it is contagious through the feces. The hallmark is abrupt onset of excruciating pain in the lower thorax or abdomen that is exacerbated by deep inspirations or coughing. The acute phase improves in a week, but fatigue and muscle pains may persist. Relapses may occur. Results of laboratory tests are negative, and treatment is symptomatic.

3. **Reye's syndrome** is acute encephalopathy with fatty degeneration of the liver that develops after varicella or influenza infections. This rare condition

that affects children and adolescents begins with repeated vomiting and continues with personality changes, confusion, lethargy, and coma. The mortality is high. Laboratory metabolic abnormalities relate to acute liver dysfunction. The level of CK MM isoenzyme derived from skeletal muscle may be increased 300-fold. The level of CK correlates with prognosis. Salicylates may precipitate the syndrome. Treatment is supportive. The incidence of this syndrome has decreased precipitously over the years, because aspirin is no longer being used to treat children with flulike symptoms.

4. **HIV** may cause subacute or chronic myopathy early or late in relation to the infection. This has been reported to occur among adults but not among children with HIV infection. Proximal, symmetric involvement of lower or upper limbs manifests as weakness with or without atrophy. Concomitant myelopathy or peripheral neuropathy can occur. Serum CK levels may be elevated 10 to 15 times. The syndrome is almost identical to polymyositis. Thus in the evaluation of patients with polymyositis, measurement of HIV titers is recommended. The electrophysiologic and biopsy findings also may be indistinguishable from those of polymyositis. With the advent of protease inhibitors, it appears that the incidence of HIV myopathy with rhabdomyolysis has decreased.

   a. In advanced acquired immunodeficiency syndrome (AIDS), **HIV wasting syndrome** is characterized by marked disproportion between severe muscle mass loss and weakness, which may be mild or even absent. CK level is normal. Biopsy shows atrophy of type II fibers—a common, nonspecific finding in cachexia, immobilization, and malnutrition.

   b. **Prognosis and treatment.** Because of the AIDS epidemic and better management of AIDS, the number of persons with AIDS myopathy has increased. Treatment remains empiric. If the myopathy is mild, a nonsteroidal antiinflammatory agent can be used. Anti–retroviral (zidovudine) therapy can be started if the myopathy progresses.

   c. **Zidovudine myopathy** occurs with long-term use of this medication and results from mitochondrial toxicity in skeletal muscle. Patients report lower-extremity myalgia and proximal weakness. Elevation of CK level increases further after exercise. Symptoms are related to the dosage and duration of zidovudine treatment, often occurring after 1 year of therapy. The myopathy improves once treatment is discontinued. Differentiation from AIDS myopathy can be difficult solely on a clinical basis. Muscle biopsy shows numerous "ragged red fibers," a sign of mitochondrial disease, and its presence supports the diagnosis of zidovudine myopathy. Electron microscopic examination of the biopsy specimen is useful in finding mitochondrial damage. Treatment consists of stopping the medication. Nonsteroidal antiinflammatory agents can be used. Whereas myalgia usually is relieved improve within weeks of discontinuing zidovudine, muscle weakness can persist for months.

III. Parasitic inflammatory myopathy. In North America, **trichinosis, cysticercosis,** and **toxoplasmosis** can cause myopathy. The incidence of these diseases has increased in the AIDS epidemic and with use of various immunosuppressive treatments and conditions. *Trypanosoma cruzi,* the agent of Chagas' disease, predominates in South America, but a few cases have been detected in the United States, mainly attributable to contaminated blood transfusions.

   A. **Natural history, prognosis, and treatment**

   1. **Toxoplasmosis** is a protozoan infection caused by *Toxoplasma gondii.* It is contracted by consuming parasite-infested meat or through contact with cat feces. It also can be acquired transplacentally or through blood transfusion. The infection more severe among patients with AIDS. Myopathy is only one of the manifestations of systemic infection. The course is progressive, subacute, and clinically indistinguishable from that of idiopathic inflammatory myopathy. Fever, myalgia, lymphadenopathy, and neck pain sometimes occur. Serum CK level is elevated. EMG shows the changes observed in polymyositis. The diagnosis of toxoplasmosis is determined with serologic

methods. Muscle biopsy is the definitive test for diagnosing *Toxoplasma* myopathy when tachyzoites or cysts can be identified.

Diagnosing *Toxoplasma* myositis as opposed to other myopathy has significant treatment implications. The treatment of choice is a combination of pyrimethamine and sulfadiazine or trisulfapyrimidines. Pyrimethamine is a folate antagonist, and thus folate should be given to decrease the risk of bone marrow suppression.

2. **Cysticercosis** is contracted by eating uncooked pork or as a result of fecal contamination of food, especially vegetables irrigated with contaminated water. This disease is produced by the larva of the intestinal tapeworm *Taenia solium*. It is found in Mexico, Central America, and the southwestern United States. The disease can occur many years after primary infection. The embryos of the *Taenia* worm invade many tissues, especially skeletal muscle, the central nervous system, and the eye. Involved muscle may contain enlarged and painful nodules. Eosinophilia and eosinorrachia are common. Examination of stool for ova and parasites and detection of antigen in the serum and cerebrospinal fluid (CSF) assist in the diagnosis. Only muscle biopsy can provide the final diagnosis when encysted larvae are detected by means of gross and microscopic inspection and by antigen detection techniques. The muscle pseudohypertrophy is related to the number of larvae present. Calcification of the degenerated cyst is common.

Niclosamide and paromomycin have been effective in removing the adult worm. Praziquantel, commonly used in central nervous system cysticercosis, appears ineffective. Prednisone is used concomitantly to suppress inflammation. The larvae also can be removed surgically.

3. **Trichinosis** is caused by the nematode *Trichinella spiralis*. The larvae infiltrate many tissues, often muscle. The incubation period is 2 to 12 days after ingestion of uncooked pork containing encysted larvae. Often, a prodrome characterized by abdominal pain and diarrhea occurs, followed by fever, myalgia, and proximal muscle tenderness. Examination is remarkable for weakness that can involve extraocular muscles, intercostal muscles, and the diaphragm. Periorbital swelling and ptosis may be found. Myalgia reaches its peak at the third week of illness. Myocarditis also may occur. EMG shows changes supporting acute myopathy. Prominent eosinophilia may reach up to 60%. Antibodies against *T. spiralis* found with flocculation assay can be detected 3 weeks after infection. A definite diagnosis is made by means of identifying the larva at muscle biopsy. An inflammatory, calcified pseudocyst forms in affected muscle.

Albendazole (400 mg three times a day for 2 weeks) is the drug of choice against the larva and the adult worm. This medication should not be used to treat children or pregnant women. For patients with weakness, prednisone (1.0 to 1.5 mg/kg a day) should be used. The prognosis is grave for patients with severe cardiac myositis or encephalitis and those who are immunocompromised.

IV. **Bacterial myositis** is rare but can be life threatening.
  A. **Natural history, prognosis, and treatment**
    1. **Pyomyositis** is a muscle abscess caused by *Staphylococcus aureus*. It should be suspected when a patient with AIDS has localized pain and swelling in a muscle with or without fever or elevation of CK level. When the muscle is examined with ultrasonography, magnetic resonance imaging, or contrast-enhanced computed tomography, an enhancing lesion, often with fluid density, may be appreciated. Systemic antibiotics and local drainage are used. Predisposing factors include muscle trauma and hematogenous spread of bacterial infection, even with negative blood cultures. Pyomyositis should be suspected when any patient has unexplained localized muscle swelling. There may be a paucity of systemic toxicity before sepsis occurs. Aside from HIV infection, risk factors include diabetes, muscle trauma, skin infection, and intravenous drug abuse.
    2. **Lyme disease** can produce myopathy, usually localized to a region adjacent to joint, nerve, or skin lesion. Gallium scans can be diagnostically helpful.

Lyme disease can trigger the appearance of diffuse inflammatory myopathy similar to dermatomyositis, and the spirochete can be found at the muscle biopsy. Antibiotic therapy usually is curative.

3. **Clostridial infection.** Infection with *Clostridium perfringens* can occur after subcutaneous injections in healthy persons. It also can occur through trauma or surgery. Subcutaneous cellulitis with characteristic **crepitus** may ensue. Incubation ranges from hours to 6 weeks. In addition to crepitus, severe local pain, swelling, redness, high fever, rhabdomyolysis, and renal failure can occur. Persons who use intravneous heroin may have clostridial fasciitis and myositis with no systemic toxicity and purplish induration. Contamination with *Clostridium botulinum* among parenteral drug users can produce wound botulism, which affects the neuromuscular transmission apparatus.

4. *Mycobacterium tuberculosis* and *Mycobacterium leprae* can cause myositis. In tuberculosis, the mycobacterium invades the muscle from a neighboring focus or through the blood, resulting in a tuberculous granuloma with painless swelling.

V. **Channelopathy** is a rare disorder characterized by episodes of flaccid muscle weakness that can evolve into paralysis. Attacks usually last hours. Periodic paralysis is either a primary autosomal dominant disorder or a secondary disorder.

A. **Natural history and prognosis**

1. **Primary hypokalemic periodic paralysis** predominates in men. The genetic abnormality is located in chromosome 1q32. It produces missense mutations in voltage-sensing segments of the muscle calcium channel that codes for the $\alpha 1_s$ calcium channel subunit (the dihydropyridine receptor). The dysfunctional $\alpha 1$ subunit of the calcium channel interferes at some point in the membrane signal transfer that activates the ryanodine receptor and subsequent excitation contraction coupling. The muscle is inexcitable, and muscle weakness occurs. The relation between the defects in calcium currents and the hypokalemia-induced attacks of muscle weakness remains puzzling. A lowered extracellular potassium concentration in muscle from patients with hypokalemic periodic paralysis causes membrane depolarization and may reduce calcium release by inactivating sodium channels. Insulin-facilitated potassium influx accounts for the hypersensitivity of patients to insulin infusion and to carbohydrate meals associated with insulin secretion.

This disease affects young and middle-aged persons. Attacks usually occur at night. On awakening, patients may be paralyzed and unable to get out of bed. The flaccid paralysis usually spares the respiratory and cranial muscles, but in very severe cases, respiration is compromised. Often, precipitating factors include high carbohydrate consumption and strenuous physical activity. During attacks, serum potassium level decreases. If serum potassium level is persistently low, the paralysis may be secondary. An ECG may reveal hypokalemic changes, including progressive flattening of T waves, depression of the ST segment, and appearance of U waves. In some families, there is a tendency for the attacks to become more numerous with time. A few patients later have chronic myopathy independent of the severity and frequency of the attacks. EMG does not record normal insertional activity during attacks. The presence of myotonia almost excludes the diagnosis of hypokalemic periodic paralysis.

2. **Secondary hypokalemic periodic paralysis**

a. **Thyrotoxic periodic paralysis** occurs 70 times more often in men than in women 20 to 40 years of age, despite the increased prevalence of hyperthyroidism among women. In nearly all cases, the condition is sporadic and the attacks cease when thyroid function is normalized. Every patient with hypokalemic periodic paralysis needs screening for thyrotoxicosis. This condition is more common in patients of Asian, Hispanic American, and Amerind origin. Symmetric weakness mostly affects the legs. Maximal weakness is more common on awakening. Muscle stiffness and cramps may precede the weakness. Limb paralysis may be severe with sparing of respiratory and bulbar muscles. Previous episodes of mild weakness of short duration are common. Features of hyperthyroidism sometimes are not conspicuous, and the diagnosis is established on suspicion and confirmation with laboratory thyroid panels.

    b. Periodic paralysis secondary to urinary or gastrointestinal potassium loss can result from primary hyperaldosteronism, excessive thiazide therapy, excessive mineralocorticoid therapy for Addison's disease, renal tubular acidosis, the recovery phase of diabetic coma, sprue, laxative abuse, villous adenoma of the rectum, or prolonged gastrointestinal intubation or vomiting.

3. Primary hyperkalemic periodic paralysis produces episodic attacks of weakness accompanied by elevations in serum potassium level (up to 5 to 6 mmol/L). It is often associated with myotonia (inability to relax the muscle) or paramyotonia (muscle stiffness worsened by exercise or cold that gives way to flaccid paralysis) and is inherited in an autosomal dominant manner. It is also called **Gamstorp's disease** or **adynamia episodica hereditaria.** Attacks occur in the first decade of life, usually in the morning before breakfast, and last 20 to 60 minutes. Patients usually have brief periods of generalized weakness. Static weakness is rare. Rest, potassium salts, cold, and stress provoke attacks. Sustained mild exercise may prevent attacks. Ventricular and supraventricular cardiac arrhythmias are dangerous accompanying conditions and necessitate careful monitoring and therapy.

    a. The **pathologic mechanism** is that the abnormal sodium channel of the sarcolemma fails to inactivate. Incomplete inactivation caused by abnormalities of the inactivation gate leads to a sustained influx of sodium, which results in sustained membrane depolarization. Simultaneously, the potassium leaves the sarcoplasm and increases in the serum.

    b. Needle EMG is needed to separate the myotonic (paramyotonia congenita) from the nonmyotonic phenotypes.

    c. Potassium-sensitive periodic paralysis, paramyotonia congenita, and potassium-aggravated myotonia all are caused by **missense mutations** in the voltage-gated sodium channel in adult skeletal muscle. The mutations affect the function of the α1 subunit of the sodium channel encoded by chromosome 17q. The mechanisms by which the mutations produce the various phenotypes (weakness with myotonia, cold-sensitive myotonia, and potassium-sensitive myotonia) are not fully understood. Mutations affecting slow sodium channel inactivation often are associated with episodic weakness, whereas mutations affecting fast channel inactivation are associated with myotonia. Mutant channels may play a role in altered membrane excitability.

4. Andersen syndrome. In some patients with periodic paralysis, cardiac dysrhythmias are important manifestations and sometimes the presenting symptom. Andersen syndrome is a familial disease with young age at onset (first two decades of life), phenotypic variability, and autosomal dominant inheritance. Dysmorphic features vary and include hypertelorism, low-set ears, and a broad nose. A common clinical feature is a prolonged QT interval, but few patients appear with cardiac symptoms. The attacks of weakness occur after a period of rest after exercise. The genetic basis for the syndrome is unknown.

5. Chloride channel mutations produce **myotonia congenita** with dominant and recessive forms (Thomsen and Becker, respectively), and with more myotonia than weakness. More men than women are affected. The dominant form manifests as painless muscle stiffness in adolescence, sometimes occurring after a surprise. Muscle stiffness is relieved after repeated exercise (warm-up), but it returns after rest. Cooling does not produce a significant change. Unlike myotonic dystrophy, the myotonia of myotonia congenita interferes with function. These disorders result from mutations in the chloride channel, usually missense, in the chloride channel gene *CLCN1*. The stiffness and myotonic discharges are caused by repeated muscle membrane depolarization after activation and prevent muscle relaxation. Reducing chloride conductance produces muscle membrane overexcitability. Low chloride conductance interferes with fast repolarization of the T tubule. Chloride channels normally increase the speed of repolarization after the peak of action potential has occurred. When chloride conductance is impaired, the accumulated potassium causes after-depolarization and repeating firing.

B. Prevention and therapeutic approach

1. **Primary hypokalemic periodic paralysis.** Low carbohydrate ingestion and avoidance of strenuous exercise prevent attacks. Mild attacks may not require treatment. For attacks of general paralysis, 0.25 mEq/kg of potassium chloride by mouth in an unsweetened 10% to 25% solution is the preferable therapy. The dose should be repeated every 30 minutes until the weakness is relieved. Muscle strength usually recovers within approximately 1 hour. Patients are encouraged to exercise mildly. Carbohydrate-containing foods and intravenous fluids should be avoided. Intravenous potassium is *not* recommended because of the danger of producing uncontrollable hyperkalemia and should be avoided as much as possible. However, if repeated vomiting precludes administration of oral salts, intravenous potassium can be used carefully with serial ECG monitoring and serum potassium determinations. Potassium dosage should be adjusted for patients with renal disease. Intravenous potassium chloride can be administered in a 5% mannitol solution (20 to 40 mEq/L) or by bolus (0.05 to 0.10 mEq/kg). Glucose and saline diluents should be avoided. Gastrointestinal irritation may occur with oral administration, and phlebitis may accompany intravenous administration.

   For **prevention** of attacks, acetazolamide is the drug of choice at a low starting dosage of 125 mg every other day, which can be increased to 250 mg three times a day. Side effects include increased incidence of nephrolithiasis, paresthesia, anorexia, and metallic taste. Dichlorphenamide, another carbonic anhydrase inhibitor, may be used if acetazolamide fails. The dosage is 25 mg three times a day. In severe cases, patients should eat a low-salt diet and be given the aldosterone antagonist spironolactone (100 mg twice a day) or triamterene (150 mg/d). Both drugs promote renal potassium retention, sodium depletion, and mild acidosis. Patients need periodic renal ultrasound studies, because of the aforementioned risk of renal calculi. Supplemental potassium treatment is contraindicated with the latter two medications. Diazoxide and verapamil also have been used in refractory cases.

2. **Thyrotoxic periodic paralysis.** Control of euthyroid status is imperative. Potassium chloride by mouth can be used to manage acute attacks, and a low-carbohydrate, low-sodium diet may prevent attacks until the patient becomes euthyroid. Acetazolamide is ineffective, sometimes making the disease worse. Propranolol (40 mg four times a day) and other β-adrenergic blocking agents may prevent attacks, possibly by suppressing the adrenergic overactivity induced by hyperthyroidism.

3. **Primary hyperkalemic periodic paralysis**

   a. **Preventive measures** consist of frequent meals rich in carbohydrates, low-potassium diet and avoidance of fasting, strenuous work, and exposure to cold. Slight exercise or ingestion of carbohydrates at the onset of weakness may prevent or abort attacks. Staying in bed longer may precipitate attacks. Patients are advised to rise early and eat a full breakfast.

   b. A thiazide diuretic, acetazolamide, or inhalation of a β-adrenergic agent (metaproterenol or salbutamol) may **abort an attack.** Dilantin (300 mg/d) also can be useful.

   c. For **long-term preventive therapy,** a thiazide diuretic or acetazolamide is recommended at the lowest possible dosage (hydrochlorothiazide, 25 mg every other day).

   d. In **myotonia congenita** the drug of choice is mexiletine, which is structurally similar to lidocaine, and primarily used as an antiarrhythmic agent. It inhibits the sodium current and reduces the rate of increase in the sodium portion of the action potential. The starting dose is 150 mg by mouth twice a day, up to 1,200 mg/d. Adverse effects include elevation of liver enzyme levels, impaired short-term memory, sedation, and hair loss. Mexiletine is contraindicated in the care of patients with second- and third-degree heart block.

VI. Muscular dystrophy is a chronic, hereditary myopathy characterized by a progressive course and characteristic histologic abnormalities. Recent developments in the field of molecular genetics have widened understanding of the pathophysiologic mechanisms of many forms of dystrophy. The most important forms are **X-linked dystrophinopathy**, which includes **Duchenne** and **Becker muscular dystrophy,** and **autosomal-dominant facioscapulohumeral, myotonic, limb-girdle, oculopharyngeal,** and **progressive ophthalmoplegic muscular dystrophy.**

    A. Natural history and prognosis

        1. Dystrophinopathy is a recessive disorder caused by a mutation in the short arm, locus 21, of the X chromosome in the enormous gene that codes for the protein dystrophin. Dystrophin is a filamentous protein present in striated and cardiac muscle and other tissues. Although the role of dystrophin has not been firmly established, anchoring and structural functions have been proposed for this protein. Dystrophin deficiency disrupts membrane localization. The result is tears in the sarcolemma and calcium leak into the muscle fiber, which initiates the process of muscle cell necrosis.

            In the most severe form of dystrophinopathy—Duchenne muscular dystrophy—almost no dystrophin is detected in skeletal muscle at immunohistochemical analysis. In milder allelic forms—phenotypically denominated Becker muscular dystrophy—some muscle fibers express dystrophin, which may be structurally abnormal. Almost all patients with dystrophinopathy are men. Often the disease is caused by spontaneous mutations, which are more common than in other genetic disorders, probably because of the large size of the gene. Approximately 70% of patients with Duchenne and Becker muscular dystrophy have detectable mutations on routine DNA testing of peripheral blood. Deletions of varying sizes can be found in approximately 65% of cases; 5% of patients have gene duplications. *A negative result of a DNA test does not exclude the diagnosis,* because approximately 30% of patients do not have a detectable mutation. The diagnosis in these patients depends on dystrophin analysis at muscle biopsy. In this case, carrier detection in a patient's mother or sisters is impossible. In addition, *negative results of mutation analysis in the mother do not rule out the risk of Duchenne muscular dystrophy affecting future pregnancies.* Even with normal results of a peripheral blood gene, a mutation can be present in a percentage of oocytes (germline mosaicism). All sisters of patients with Duchenne muscular dystrophy must be evaluated independently of the DNA testing of the mother's peripheral blood leukocytes.

           a. Duchenne muscular dystrophy affects children who have noticeable difficulties in walking early in life. Motor developmental delay may be noticeable after the first year, but disease is already present, because muscle necrosis and serum enzyme elevation can be found in neonates. Onset of walking may be delayed past 15 months of age. Signs can usually be recognized before the age of 5 years. They include difficulties in running and climbing stairs. Lower-extremity, lower trunk, and pelvic muscles are affected first.

              Children have hyperlordosis with prominent abdomen and calf pseudohypertrophy. Tiptoe walking is common. Progression is fast. To stand up from the floor, patients use their hands (**Gower's sign**). Joint contractures of the iliotibial bands, hip flexors, and heel cords develop in most patients by 6 to 9 years of age. By the age of 10 years, many of these patients lose the ability to walk or stand and must use a wheelchair. By the midteens they lose upper-extremity function. Mental retardation occurs in 10% of cases. The disease usually is fatal by the end of the second decade. Death usually is related to pulmonary infection, respiratory failure, gastrointestinal complications, or cardiomyopathy. Approximately 8% of female carriers have myopathy of the limb-girdle type. A small number of carriers may also have isolated cardiomyopathy.

The **diagnosis** of Duchenne's muscular dystrophy can be confirmed by an **absence of dystrophin immunostaining** at muscle biopsy. Results of DNA analysis of blood leukocytes with the polymerase chain reaction (PCR) technique are abnormal in more than two thirds of patients with Duchenne muscular dystrophy. Prenatal diagnosis from chorionic villi also is feasible. Fast screening is done by means of measuring serum CK, the level of which is markedly elevated (up to the thousands or tens of thousands of units). The level also is elevated in female carriers. With the advent of molecular diagnosis and in cases with documented family histories, muscle biopsy might not be needed as much as in the past. In less-documented cases, muscle biopsy can be very useful in differentiating this severe disease from others manifesting similarly but carrying a favorable prognosis (congenital myopathy of the nemaline and central core types, for example).

Muscle biopsy specimens from patients with Duchenne muscular dystrophy have abnormal variations in fiber size, fiber splitting, central nuclei, and replacement by fat and fibrous tissues. Dystrophin immunostaining in muscle biopsy is now commonly used to differentiate benign from malignant myopathy. Because of worsening caused by immobilization, it might be preferable to obtain the biopsy specimen from mildly involved rectus abdominis rather than from the gastrocnemius or deltoid muscle. An EMG obtained early in the course of the disease shows findings compatible with those of myopathy. Later, the number of motor units activated decreases, and tissue can even become inexcitable.

    b. Becker's muscular dystrophy is a milder variety of dystrophinopathy in terms of severity and molecular abnormality. Patients may live many decades with mild to moderate symptoms, which can be indistinguishable from those of limb-girdle dystrophy. Onset usually is after 12 years of age. Calf pain during exercise, myoglobinuria, and CK elevation are common findings. Isolated cardiomyopathy may be the sole feature in Duchenne carriers.

2. Emery–Dreifuss muscular dystrophy is an X-linked disease mapping at band Xq28 and characterized by early onset of elbow and ankle contractures followed by weakness and atrophy of humeral and peroneal muscles. This disease has a longer course than does dystrophinopathy. Cardiac involvement is common. Patients experience conduction defects, bradycardia, and heart block, which can lead to syncope or sudden death. Early recognition of this disease can be lifesaving because timed insertion of a pacemaker can prevent a fatal conduction defect. The defective gene, when normal, codes for a protein named *emerin,* which is expressed in skeletal muscle and myocardium. Emerin is a transmembrane protein located on the nuclear membrane in skeletal, cardiac, and smooth muscle and skin cells. The function is unknown.

3. Facioscapulohumeral muscular dystrophy is an autosomal dominant disease that has high penetrance and usually a better prognosis than does Duchenne muscular dystrophy. It affects both men and women and starts before 30 years of age. Ninety-five percent of patients have a demonstrable DNA 4q35 short fragment, which arises from a variable sized deletion in a sequence of a 3.3-kilobase repetitive DNA sequence. Neither the gene nor its product has yet been defined.

Clinically, facial muscles, including the orbicularis oculi, orbicularis oris, and zygomaticus, are affected early, but the disease onset is often difficult to establish, and abnormal features may be taken to be nothing more than family traits. Masseter, temporalis, and extraocular muscles are not involved. Bell's phenomenon and drooping of the lower lip are noticeable. Patients may be unable to whistle. Facioscapulohumeral muscular dystrophy also involves the trapezius, rhomboid, and serratus anterior scapular muscles. Scapular winging is maximized with forward movement because of serratus anterior weakness. Deltoid function and rotator cuff muscles are better preserved, whereas the pectoralis is very atrophic. Patients seek medical attention because of the involvement of the shoulder rather than of the facial muscles. If patients are not disrobed, the diagnosis can be easily missed. Lower-extremity weakness, especially of the anterolateral leg compartment, is found later in the disease.

This disorder has wide phenotypic variability, even within the same family. Some patients remain ambulatory all their lives, whereas others must use a wheelchair, have marked kyphoscoliosis, and die of respiratory insufficiency or infection. The heart usually is spared. Not uncommonly, atrophy and weakness are asymmetric. Trunk weakness may also occur.

4. **Oculopharyngeal muscular dystrophy** is an autosomal dominant disease of late onset that occurs in certain ethnic groups including Jewish Americans, French Canadians, and Hispanic Americans from New Mexico and Colorado. This syndrome manifests as ptosis, progressive dysphagia, rimmed vacuoles in muscle biopsy specimens, and tubulofilamentous inclusions within the striated muscle cell nucleus. The differential diagnosis includes myasthenia gravis and oculocraniosomatic diseases with ragged red fibers (Kearns–Sayre syndrome), which are mitochondrial forms of myopathy characterized by slowly progressive involvement of extraocular musculature, proximal myopathy, peripheral neuropathy, and cardiomyopathy.

5. **Limb-girdle muscular dystrophy** is a heterogeneous collection of both autosomal recessive and autosomal dominant disorders that affect pelvic and upper girdle muscles and spare the face. The onset is between the first and fourth decades of life. Molecular genetic and diagnostic techniques have confirmed the heterogeneity of these disorders. Mutations having been found in at least two different loci (chromosomes 5q and 15q). These diseases progress more slowly than does Duchenne muscular dystrophy, and precise diagnosis often requires referral to a muscle clinic.

6. **Myotonic dystrophy** is the most common muscular dystrophy among adults. Rather than being restricted to the skeletal muscle, it usually represents a multisystemic, autosomal dominant disorder with varied expression. It can also involve the pancreas, gonads, thyroid, myocardium, and brain. Autosomal dominant myotonic dystrophy is produced by a defective gene in chromosome 19 (19q13.2-13.3) that codes for myotonin protein kinase, a ubiquitous enzyme related to protein phosphorylation. The generalized disorder can be explained by the wide distribution of the enzyme. The molecular gene defect is characterized by excessive triple repeats (triplet repeat amplification) of guanine-cytosine-thymine. The length of the repeat is directly correlated with the severity of the disease and inversely correlated with the date of onset.

   a. **Muscle features.** Weakness of facial muscles is typical. The face is hatched and thin with early frontal balding. Ptosis is present but is not as severe as in myasthenia gravis or Kearns–Sayre syndrome. Temporalis and masseter atrophy is characteristic. Sternocleidomastoid weakness is out of proportion to that of shoulder and posterior neck muscles. Limb involvement is predominantly distal and late in appearing. Proximal limb muscles usually are preserved until the late stages. Thus, unlike patients with other forms of dystrophy, patients with myotonic dystrophy usually remain ambulatory. Myotonia is the delay of muscle relaxation after contraction. Often, myotonia is simply a sign that does not elicit symptoms. Seldom do patients report stiffness. Myotonia can be elicited by percussion of the thenar eminence or tongue. Patients often are unable to release the grip after a handshake. Repetitive muscle contractions diminish the myotonia (true myotonia). Clinical diagnosis is supported by the presence of myotonic discharges on an EMG. Molecular diagnosis with the PCR technique can help detect the triple repeat expansion.

   b. **Generalized features.** Many patients have predominant systemic symptoms rather than neuromuscular symptoms. These patients may never be given the diagnosis of myotonic dystrophy. Failure to diagnose the disease can jeopardize patients' medical and preventive care. Common abnormalities include cataracts, tubular testicular atrophy, heart block, and arrhythmias, which can cause sudden death. Whereas severe cardiac arrhythmias may occur in phenotypically mild cases, cardiomyopathy is rare. Constipation and cholelithiasis are related to smooth muscle involvement. Diaphragmatic involvement produces hypoventilation. Hypersomnia is common. Because of the cardiorespiratory compromise, patients are susceptible to complications during surgery and anesthesia. Myotonia can increase with use of depolarizing relaxants. Opiates and barbiturates can induce respiratory failure. Unfortunately, the diagnosis of myotonic dystrophy is sometimes established only after cardiopulmonary complications secondary to general anesthesia have occurred. Mild mental retardation, apathy, and lethargy are not uncommon.

7. **Proximal myotonic myopathy (PROMM)** is an autosomal dominant disorder characterized by progressive weakness, myotonia, and cataracts. Some families link to a locus on the long arm of chromosome 3 but not on chromosome 19. In other families, the locus for PROMM is unknown.

8. **Congenital myotonic dystrophy** is the more severe form that is present since birth. Neonates have bilateral facial weakness, hypotonia, mental retardation, respiratory distress, hydramnios, and reduced fetal movements. The abnormal gene is transmitted exclusively through maternal inheritance.

B. Prevention. For the **dystrophinopathy** (Duchenne and Becker muscular dystrophy), preventive measures comprise prenatal diagnosis, carrier detection, and genetic counseling. Pedigree analysis, serum CK determination, and clinical, routine histologic, and EMG studies are complemented by dystrophin analysis in muscle biopsy, PCR analysis of heterozygotes, and restriction fragment length polymorphism analysis. Fetal abnormalities can be detected with molecular techniques in samples of chorionic villi during early pregnancy (after 8 weeks) or by means of amniocentesis. Analysis of fetal muscle biopsy specimens for dystrophin immunostaining can be performed after 19 weeks of gestation with ultrasound guidance. A known carrier has one chance in two of giving birth to a boy with Duchenne muscular dystrophy or to a carrier girl. Approximately one third of patients, however, do not have family histories. For **myotonic dystrophy,** slit-lamp examination, measurement of insulin, ECG, prenatal care, and thorough cardiopulmonary assessment before surgical procedures can diminish the rate of complications.

C. Therapeutic approach

1. **Duchenne muscular dystrophy**

   a. **Family and patient education** is of utmost importance. The disease causes distress in all aspects of family life. Not only the emotional stress but also the physical and financial limitations imposed by needing to transport and take care of the patient may become insurmountable. The goal is to keep the child ambulatory and functioning at home and at school. If no mental retardation is present, the child can start attending conventional school. Physical adjustments will be needed to compensate for inability to walk and for upper-extremity weakness.

   b. **Physical therapy** is used to preserve mobility and to prevent early contractures, which are common in the flexor muscles of the hips, knees, and ankles. Passive range of motion exercises and adequate orthotics may prolong ambulation but do not stop disease progression. Exercises may be useful in diminishing the risk of obesity, which further impairs ambulation and respiratory function. If patients can no longer walk, they are asked to stand at least 3 hours a day in divided periods. Bed rest is avoided, because weakness can become permanent. Excessive exercise, however, may be detrimental.

   Once patients can no longer walk without assistance, braces, crutches, or surgical procedures are used. Splints can keep the joints in neutral position and are used at night. When the patient must use a wheelchair all the time, contractures and scoliosis worsen. The benefits of scoliosis surgery should be thoroughly counterbalanced against the risks of the procedure and anesthesia. The technique of segmental spinal stabilization of Luque is the method of choice. In general, surgery is used when scoliosis evolves rapidly in combination with restrictive ventilatory failure and when scoliosis has not yet reached 40 degrees. Patients with Duchenne muscular dystrophy are at high risk of side effects of general anesthesia. Succinylcholine or halothane should not be used, because of the risk of episodes that resemble malignant hyperthermia. Adverse effects can be reduced with the use of nondepolarizing muscle relaxants.

  c. **Respiratory therapy.** Breathing exercises or playing wind instruments may improve the quality of life. In later stages, noninvasive intermittent positive-pressure ventilation is useful, especially when patients with very advanced disease retain carbon dioxide and begin to have nightmares. Pulmonary exercises may reduce the propensity for pulmonary infection.

  d. **Medications.** Prednisone (0.75 mg/kg a day) is recommended only for special situations, such as very abrupt deterioration. Prednisone can improve neuromuscular strength after 1 month of treatment. The maximum effect is reached by 3 months. Benefits should outweigh possible side effects, which include insomnia, difficult behavior, and gastrointestinal symptoms. In controlled studies, benefits lasted for 3 years. A low-sodium, low-fat diet should be eaten to prevent weight gain. Zoster immunoglobulin should be given if the child becomes exposed to chickenpox.

  e. **Gene therapy** is still experimental. Myoblast transplantation therapy has succeeded in the *mdx* mouse model but so far has failed in patients. Gene therapy administered through viral vectors or liposomes is being tested in animal models.

  f. Therapy for **Becker muscular dystrophy** follows principles similar to those of therapy for Duchenne disease. In mild cases, thorough follow-up care with prevention of complications may suffice.

2. Management of **Emery–Dreifuss muscular dystrophy** requires careful evaluation of the heart and timely implantation of a pacemaker in many cases to prevent fatal arrhythmias.

3. **Facioscapulohumeral muscular dystrophy.** Physical therapy is empirically recommended. Posterior plastic ankle orthotics can correct foot drop. A motorized wheelchair with adjustable height control is invaluable for patients who cannot walk. For such patients, a brace may provide help for excessive lumbar lordosis and prominent abdomen.

4. In **oculopharyngeal muscular dystrophy,** mild ptosis can be easily managed with the use of special glasses with props. In more severe cases, blepharoplasty with resection of the levator palpebrae muscles may be needed. Dysphagia may be relieved with cricopharyngeal myotomy.

5. In **limb-girdle dystrophy,** the main therapeutic objectives are the general premises described in **V.C.1.**

6. In **myotonic dystrophy,** only when myotonia is disabling or bothersome, phenytoin (100 mg by mouth three times a day) can alleviate myotonia with reasonable efficacy and relatively low risk. Quinine sulfate and procainamide can impair cardiac conduction, because they prolong the PR interval. In general, patients with myotonic dystrophy are not greatly concerned about the myotonia. The main goals are prevention and management of the systemic disease.

VII. Metabolic myopathy comprises a large, heterogeneous group of acquired and inherited disorders the common denominator of which is a metabolic alteration. **Endocrine myopathy, malignant hyperthermia, acid maltase deficiency, McArdle's disease, and carnitine-O-palmitoyltransferase deficiency** are reviewed.

  A. **Natural history, prognosis, and treatment**

  1. **Endocrine myopathy**

    a. **Thyrotoxic myopathy** manifests as weakness and little muscle wasting. Fatigue and heat intolerance also are present. Bulbar and respiratory involvement can occur. Hypokalemic periodic paralysis (see **IV.A.2.a.**) and myasthenia gravis are associated with hyperthyroidism and should be included in the differential diagnosis. Treatment relies on correcting the hyperthyroid state. β-Adrenergic blocking agents may be of help. Glucocorticoids should be used in thyroid storm to block the peripheral conversion of thyroxine in triiodothyronine.

  b. **Hypothyroid myopathy** manifests as enlargement of muscles, weakness, painful cramps, myoedema, and slow-recovery reflexes. This disease is more common among women. Rhabdomyolysis or respiratory muscle involvement may be present. Serum level of CK may be elevated. The diagnosis is supported by abnormal results of thyroid function tests. Treatment is to restore the euthyroid state.

  c. **Steroid myopathy** is characterized by proximal weakness and wasting that are worse in the lower extremities, difficulty in climbing stairs, and a normal CK level. If iatrogenic, the weakness reverses on discontinuation of steroid treatment. Fluorinated corticosteroids, such as dexamethasone and triamcinolone, have greater myopathic potential. EMG reveals normal insertional activity and no spontaneous activity. Treatment includes dose reduction to the lowest possible therapeutic level, conversion to a nonfluorinated steroid, and alternate-dose therapy. However, improvement can take weeks to months. Adequate diet and exercise should help the recovery.

2. **Malignant hyperthermia** is a severe syndrome that occurs during general anesthesia. It is characterized by rapid elevation in body temperature resulting from a fast, uncontrolled increase in skeletal muscle metabolism associated with rhabdomyolysis and by a high mortality. This syndrome is a result of an autosomal dominant susceptibility to general anesthesia, especially to halothane or succinylcholine. Body temperature may climb to 43°C with marked metabolic acidosis, tachycardia, muscle rigidity, disseminated intravascular coagulation, coma, areflexia, and death. CK level increases precipitously, sometimes to 10,000 times the normal value. Myoglobinuria, elevation of various muscle enzymes, and release of muscle potassium also occur.

  a. Prognosis is guarded. Recognition of the syndrome is important in instrumenting rapid treatment, which can diminish the mortality. The pathogenesis is related to malfunction of the calcium channel of the sarcoplasmic reticulum (the **ryanodine** receptor). The abnormal ryanodine receptor may accentuate calcium release. The gene for the ryanodine receptor maps to chromosome 19 (13-1). Malignant hyperthermia can occur in association with dystrophinopathy and central core congenital myopathy.

  b. **Neuroleptic malignant syndrome** manifests as high fever, rigidity, tachycardia, and rhabdomyolysis. However, it has a slower onset than does malignant hyperthermia, over days to weeks, it is not familial, and it usually is triggered by drugs that block central dopaminergic pathways, such as phenothiazines, lithium, and haloperidol (Haldol; Ortho-McNeil, Spring House, PA, U.S.A.) or can occur after discontinuation of levodopa for Parkinson's disease.

  c. **Prevention** includes early diagnosis of impending malignant hyperthermia when symptoms are still few, such as isolated trismus. Greater recognition of the syndrome by anesthesiologists and the availability of dantrolene have reduced morbidity and mortality. The use of barbiturate, nitrous oxide, and opiate-nondepolarizing relaxant anesthetics should not induce malignant hyperthermia.

  d. **Management** of malignant hyperthermia depends on the severity, which is often related to the dosage and duration of the anesthesia. For mild cases, discontinuation of anesthesia may suffice. In more severe cases, correction of acid–base disturbance should be rapidly implemented to save the patient's life. Ventilation should be increased and intravenous sodium bicarbonate (2 to 4 mg/kg) given. Cooling blankets and cold intravenous fluids should be used until the temperature reaches 38°C. Volume loading and diuretics are necessary in the presence of myoglobinuria. Steroids are given for the acute stress reaction. Dantrolene is the specific therapy because it inhibits the calcium release from the sarcoplasmic reticulum. It should be used at 2 mg/kg i.v. every 5 minutes, up to 10 mg/kg, and should correct the associated hyperkalemia. Administration of calcium to correct the hyperkalemia should *not* be undertaken.

3. **Acid maltase deficiency** is an autosomal recessive glycogen storage disease caused by a deficiency in lysosomal α-glucosidase, which normally participates in the metabolism of glycogen into glucose. The infantile form is called Pompe's disease, a generalized glycogenesis with severe cardiomyopathy. Milder cases with little or no heart disease can occur in adults. The genetic abnormality maps to chromosome 17. Infants with Pompe's disease have hypotonia, macroglossia, cardiomegaly, and hepatomegaly. Usually the disease is rapidly fatal. Adults suffer from slowly progressive myopathy with respiratory failure. Diaphragm, biceps, shoulder, and thigh adductor muscles are preferentially affected. Myotonic discharges can be found electrically, but patients usually do not have myotonia. Vacuolar myopathy with high glycogen content is conspicuous. The diagnosis is confirmed by means of leukocyte or urine acid maltase determination. Prenatal diagnosis can be established by means of chorionic villi biopsy. No specific therapy is available. Inspiratory exercises can be of use.

4. **McArdle's disease**, or myophosphorylase deficiency, affects children and adults who have exercise intolerance with myalgia, fatigue and muscle stiffness, myoglobinuria, renal failure, wasting, and seizures. Some patients can tolerate the deficits and learn to avoid the brief, strong exercises that precipitate attacks. Cramps and myoglobinuria usually develop during adulthood. CK level is increased. EMG shows changes supportive of myopathy. The forearm ischemic exercise causes no increase in venous lactate. The disease is autosomal recessive. The gene for muscle phosphorylase maps to chromosome 11. Prognosis is rather benign. Muscle biopsy discloses subsarcolemmal deposits of glycogen at the periphery. The histochemical reaction of the phosphorylase can confirm the diagnosis by being undetectable in patients with McArdle's disease. Experimental therapies with diets and branched-chain amino acids have been tried, but no definite treatment is available.

5. **Carnitine-*O*-palmitoyltransferase deficiency** manifests intermittently with cramps, myalgia, and myoglobinuria. Renal failure resulting from myoglobinuria and respiratory failure may ensue. During attacks, muscle strength is normal. The symptoms are precipitated by exertion. The capacity to perform short, demanding exercise is not impaired. Patients have no warning of the attacks, which usually follow prolonged exercise. Fasting, exposure to cold, high fat intake, viral infections, and general anesthesia can precipitate rhabdomyolysis. The disease is autosomal recessive. The abnormal gene maps to chromosome 1. CK level is normal. No specific therapy is available.

VIII. Toxic myopathy has become more common than the other forms since the introduction of cholesterol-lowering drugs and other medications. Some medications produce direct muscle fiber necrosis, while others produce electrolyte imbalances with rhabdomyolysis. The most important types of toxic myopathy are **necrotizing, autophagic, antimicrotubular, mitochondrial,** and **steroid.**

   A. **Natural history, prognosis, and treatment**

      1. **Toxic necrotizing myopathy.** Cholesterol-lowering drugs include 3-hydroxy-methyl-glutaryl-coenzyme A reductase (3-HMG-CoA reductase) inhibitors such as **lovastatin, simvastatin, pravastatin, atorvastatin, fluvastatin, and cerivastatin**. Onset can be acute or insidious, often with myalgia, occasionally with myoglobinuria, and usually involving the proximal lower-extremity muscles. Patients with renal failure are especially predisposed. Elevated serum CK levels are common, and the EMG findings are abnormal. Muscle fiber necrosis with phagocytosis and small regenerating

fibers are found in serious cases. When the medication is stopped, symptoms tend to resolve in a few weeks to months. The concomitant use of niacin or erythromycin increases the risk of toxic myopathy with these drugs, as does renal and hepatic failure. Asymptomatic elevations of CK level occur in about 1% of patients taking statins. In these patients, the EMG findings usually are normal. **Cyclosporine** and **tacrolimus** have also been associated with toxic myopathy.

2. **Autophagic myopathy** occurs with **chloroquine** and its derivatives for the management of malaria, systemic lupus erythematosus, scleroderma, and rheumatoid arthritis, and with **amiodarone**, for the treatment of cardiac arrhythmias. The myopathy of chloroquine affects the proximal lower-extremity muscles and usually is not very painful. The course is subacute or chronic. The heart can be affected, as can the peripheral nerves (neuromyopathy). Elevation in CK level and myotonic potentials on the EMG can be found. Muscle biopsy shows vacuoles (lysosomes), which stain for acid phosphatase and contain debris and curvilinear structures (autophagic vacuoles). With amiodarone, severe proximal and distal weakness may occur in combination with distal sensory loss, tremor, and ataxia. The treatment is to discontinue the medication.

3. **Antimicrotubular myopathy** is produced by **colchicine** and **vincristine.** This myopathy often is not recognized because the onset can be insidious in patients who may have been taking colchicine for years. The myopathy usually develops with a progressive increase in serum levels of colchicine (rarely measured) in relation to progressive renal failure. Concomitant axonal sensorimotor neuropathy occurs. These drugs bind to nerve and muscle tubulin. Weakness may resolve approximately 6 months after discontinuation of the medication. Because of the neuromyopathy, a mixed pattern of denervation and myopathy can be found in electrophysiologic studies. Muscle biopsy shows acid-phosphatase-positive autophagic vacuoles.

4. The effects of **zidovudine** can be indistinguishable from the myopathy of HIV infection. CK levels are normal or mildly elevated. Muscle biopsy may show ragged red fibers suggestive of mitochondrial dysfunction. Unlike HIV-associated myopathy, zidovudine myopathy is not accompanied by a great deal of inflammation. Treatment is to stop zidovudine. The presence of abundant abnormal insertional EMG activity and marked CK elevation suggest inflammatory HIV myopathy. In this case, zidovudine should probably be continued.

5. **Steroid myopathy** appears to affect more women than men (2:1). Doses of prednisone greater than 30 mg/d carry the risk of myopathy. Fluorinated compounds (triamcinolone, betamethasone, and dexamethasone) have a greater risk. Patients have predominantly proximal muscle weakness and atrophy of all limbs, usually with long-term administration, and have concomitant cushingoid features. However, acute toxic myopathy can occur with administration of high-dose intravenous methylprednisolone with or without neuromuscular blocking agents. Serum level of CK usually is normal, and potassium level may be low. EMG findings are normal. Muscle biopsy shows type 2 fiber atrophy, especially type 2B (fast twitch glycolytic). Tapering to an alternate-day regimen, use of "steroid-sparing" drugs (e.g., azathioprine), use of nonfluorinated steroids, and exercise may reduce the incidence of this myopathy. **Finasteride,** used to manage prostatic hypertrophy, can produce generalized myopathy.

Recommended Readings

Askari AD, Huettner TL. Cardiac abnormalities in polymyositis/dermatomyositis. *Semin Arthritis Rheum* 1982;12:208–219.

Banker BQ, Victor M. Dermatomyositis (systemic angiopathy) of childhood. *Medicine* 1966;45: 261–289.

Brooke MH. *A clinician's view of neuromuscular diseases.* Baltimore: Williams & Wilkins, 1986.

Brooke MH, Fenichel GM, Griggs RC, et al. Duchenne muscular dystrophy: patterns of clinical progression and effects of supportive therapy. *Neurology* 1989;39:475–481.

Dalakas MC, ed. *Polymyositis and dermatomyositis.* Boston: Butterworth, 1988.

Dalakas MC. Polymyositis, dermatomyositis, and inclusion-body myositis. *N Engl J Med* 1991; 325:1487–1498.

Dalakas MC, Illa I, Pezeshkpour GH, et al. Mitochondrial myopathy caused by long-term zidovudine therapy. *N Engl J Med* 1990;322:1098–1105.

Dubowitz V, Brooke MH. *Muscle biopsy: a modern approach.* Philadelphia: WB Saunders, 1973.

Ebers GC, George AL, Barchi RL, et al. Paramyotonia congenita and hyperkalemic periodic paralysis are linked to the adult muscle sodium channel gene. *Ann Neurol* 1991;30:810–816.

Emery AEH. *Duchenne muscular dystrophy.* 2nd ed. New York: Oxford University Press, 1993.

Emery AEH, Dreifuss FE. Unusual type of benign X-linked muscular dystrophy. *J Neurol Neurosurg Psychiatry* 1966;29:338–342.

Engel AG. Acid maltase deficiency in adults: studies in four cases of a syndrome which may mimic muscular dystrophy or other myopathies. *Brain* 1970;93:599–616.

Engel AG, Emslie-Smith AM. Inflammatory myopathies. *Curr Opin Neurol Neurosurg* 1989;2:695–710.

Engel AG, Franzini-Annstrong C, eds. *Myology,* 2nd ed. New York: McGraw–Hill, 1994.

Fischbeck KH. The mechanism of myotonic dystrophy. *Ann Neurol* 1994;35:255–256.

Greenlee JE, Johnson WD Jr, Campa JF, et al. Adult toxoplasmosis presenting as polymyositis and cerebellar ataxia. *Ann Intern Med* 1975;82:367–371.

Griggs RC. Periodic paralysis. In: Wilson JD, et al., eds. *Harrison's principles of internal medicine.* 12th ed. New York: McGraw–Hill, 1991:2121.

Griggs RC, Davis RJ, Anderson DC, et al. Cardiac conduction in myotonic dystrophy. *Am J Med* 1975;59:37–42.

Griggs RC, Mendell JR, Miller RG. *Evaluation and treatment of myopathies.* Philadelphia: FA Davis Co, 1995.

Griggs RC, Moxley RT 3rd, Mendell JR, et al. Prednisone in Duchenne dystrophy: a randomized, controlled trial defining the time course and dose response. *Arch Neurol* 1991; 48:383–388.

Griggs RC, Tawil R, Storvick D, et al. Genetics of facioscapulohumeral muscular dystrophy: new mutations in sporadic cases. *Neurology* 1993;43:2369–2372.

Hoffman EP, Brown RH, Kunkel LM. Dystrophin: the protein product of the Duchenne muscular dystrophy locus. *Cell* 1987;51:919–928.

Hoffman EP, Fischbeck KH, Brown RH. Characterization of dystrophin in muscle-biopsy specimens from patients with Duchenne's muscular dystrophy. *N Engl J Med* 1988;318: 1363–1368.

Jablecki CK. Myopathies. In: Brown WF, Bolton CF, eds. *Clinical electromyography,* 2nd ed. Boston: Butterworth–Heinemann, 1993:653–689.

Karpati G, Carpenter S. Idiopathic inflammatory myopathies. *Curr Opin Neurol Neurosurg* 1988;1:806–818.

Kearns TP, Sayre GP. Retinitis pigmentosa, external ophthalmoplegia, and complete heart block. *Arch Ophthalmol* 1958;60:280–287.

Kissel JT, Amato AA, Barohn RJ, et al. Muscle diseases. *AAN Continuum* 2000;6:120–130.

Lange DJ. Neuromuscular diseases associated with HIV-1 infection. *Muscle Nerve* 1994; 17:16–30.

Lotz BP, Engel AG, Nishino H, et al. Inclusion body myositis: observations in 40 patients. *Brain* 1989;112:727–747.

Rowland LP, Layzer RB, DiMauro S. Pathophysiology of metabolic muscle disorders. In: Asbury AK, McKhann GM, McDonald WI, eds. *Disease of the nervous system.* Philadelphia: WB Saunders, 1986:197–207.

Srinivasan AV, Murugappan M, Krishnamurthy SG, et al. Neuroleptic malignant syndrome. *J Neurol Neurosurg Psychiatry* 1990;53:514–516.

Victor M, Hayes R, Adams RD. Oculopharyngeal muscular dystrophy: a familial disease of late life characterized by dysphagia and progressive ptosis of the eyelids. *N Engl J Med* 1962;267:1267–1272.

Walton IN, ed. *Disorders of voluntary muscle.* New York: Churchill–Livingstone, 1981.

48. NEUROMUSCULAR JUNCTION ABNORMALITIES

Robert M. Pascuzzi

I. Myasthenia gravis (MG) is an autoimmune disorder of neuromuscular transmission involving the production of autoantibodies directed against the nicotinic acetylcholine receptors (AChRs). AChR antibodies are detectable in the serum of 80% to 90% of patients with MG. The prevalence of MG is approximately 1 case in 10,000 to 20,000 persons. Women are affected approximately twice as often as men are. Symptoms may begin at almost any age. The peak for women is in the second and third decades and for men is in the fifth and sixth decades. Associated autoimmune diseases such as rheumatoid arthritis, lupus, and pernicious anemia are present in approximately 5% of patients. Thyroid disease occurs in approximately 10% of cases, often in association with the presence of antithyroid antibodies. Approximately 10% to 15% of patients with MG have thymoma. Thymic lymphoid hyperplasia with proliferation of germinal centers occurs in 50% to 70% of cases.

   A. Clinical manifestations
   1. **The hallmark of MG is** fluctuating or fatigable weakness.
   2. **Initial symptoms.** Ocular symptoms are common, 25% of patients initially having diplopia and 25% having ptosis. By 1 month into the course of the illness, 80% of patients have some degree of ocular involvement. Other initial symptoms are bulbar disorders (dysarthria or dysphagia) in 10% of patients, leg weakness (impaired walking) in 10%, and generalized weakness in 10%. Respiratory failure is the initial symptom in 1% of cases.
   3. Patients usually report symptoms resulting from focal muscle dysfunction, such as diplopia, ptosis, dysarthria, dysphagia, inability to work with the arms raised over the head, and disturbance of gait. In contrast, patients with MG tend not to report "generalized weakness," "generalized fatigue," "sleepiness," or muscle pain.
   4. In the classic case, fluctuating weakness worsens with exercise and improves with rest. Symptoms tend to progress later in the day. Many different factors can precipitate or aggravate weakness, such as physical stress, emotional stress, infection, or exposure to medications that impair neuromuscular transmission (see **E.6.**).

   B. **Diagnosis**
   1. A history of **fluctuating weakness** with corroborating findings on examination remains the basis for clinical diagnosis.
   2. **Edrophonium (Tensilon; ICN, Costa Mesa, CA, U.S.A.) test.** The most immediate and readily accessible confirmatory study is the edrophonium test.
      a. To perform the test, choose one or two weak muscles to judge. Ptosis, dysconjugate gaze, and other cranial deficits provide the most reliable end points.
      b. Use a setting in which hypotension, syncope, or respiratory failure can be managed, because patients occasionally decompensate during the test. If the patient has severe dyspnea, do not perform the test until the airway is secure. Insert an intravenous line.
      c. Have intravenous atropine (0.4 mg) readily available in the event of bradycardia or extreme gastrointestinal side effects.
      d. Draw edrophonium (10 mg, or 1 mL) into a syringe, and give 1 mg (0.1 mL) is given as a test dose while checking the patient's heart rate to ensure the patient is not supersensitive to the drug. If no untoward side effects occur after 1 minute, give another 3 mg. Many patients with MG have improved power within 30 to 60 seconds of administration of the initial 4 mg, at which point the test can be stopped. If after 1 minute there has been no improvement, give an additional 3 mg. If there is still no response, give the final 3 mg 1 minute later.
      e. If muscarinic symptoms or signs (sweating, salivation, or gastrointestinal symptoms) develop at any time during the test, assume that enough edrophonium has been given to effect an improvement in strength, and stop the test.

   f. When a placebo effect or examiner bias is of concern, the test is performed in a double-blind, placebo-controlled manner. The 1-mL control syringe contains either saline solution, 0.4 mg of atropine, or 10 mg of nicotinic acid.

   g. Improvement lasts for just a few minutes. When improvement is clear-cut, the test result is positive. If the improvement is questionable, it is best to consider the test result negative. The test can be repeated several times.

   h. Sensitivity of the edrophonium test is approximately 90%.

   i. Specificity is difficult to determine, because improvement following intravenous administration of edrophonium has been reported in other neuromuscular diseases, including Lambert–Eaton syndrome, botulism, Guillain–Barré syndrome, motor neuron disease, and lesions of the brainstem and cavernous sinus.

3. AChR antibodies

   a. The standard assay for receptor-binding antibodies is an immunoprecipitation assay in which human limb muscle is used for AChR antigen. In addition, assays for receptor modulating and blocking antibodies are available.

   b. Sensitivity. Binding antibodies are present in approximately 80% of all patients with MG (50% of patients with pure ocular MG, 80% of those with mild generalized MG, 90% of patients with moderate to severe generalized MG, and 70% of those in clinical remission). By also testing for modulating and blocking antibodies, one can improve the sensitivity to 90% overall.

   c. Specificity is outstanding. False-positive results are exceedingly rare in reliable laboratories. If blood is sent to a reference laboratory, the test results usually are available within 1 week.

4. Electromyography (EMG), electrophysiologic testing

   a. Repetitive stimulation testing to find progressive reduction. The amplitude of the compound muscle action potential (CMAP) is widely available and has variable sensitivity depending on the number and selection of muscles studied and various provocative maneuvers. In most laboratories, however, this technique has a sensitivity of approximately 50% in all patients with MG (lower in patients with mild or pure ocular disease).

   b. Single-fiber electromyography (SFEMG) is a highly specialized technique, usually available in large academic centers, with a sensitivity of approximately 90%. Abnormal single-fiber results are common in other neuromuscular diseases, and therefore the test must be used in the correct clinical context. The specificity of SFEMG is an important issue in that mild abnormalities can clearly accompany a variety of other diseases of the motor unit, including motor neuron disease, peripheral neuropathy, and myopathy. Certainly, disorders of neuromuscular transmission other than MG can have substantial abnormalities on SFEMG. In contrast, receptor antibodies are not present in patients without MG. In summary, the two highly sensitive laboratory studies are SFEMG and receptor antibody analysis; nonetheless, neither test is 100% sensitive.

C. Natural course. Appropriate treatment of a patient with autoimmune MG requires understanding of the natural course of the disease. The long-term natural course of MG is not clearly established other than being highly variable. Several generalizations can be made.

   1. Approximately one half of patients with MG come to medical attention with ocular symptoms, and 80% have such symptoms within 1 month. The initial symptom is bulbar weakness in 10% of patients, limb weakness in 10%, generalized weakness in 10%, and respiratory weakness in 1%. By 1 month, symptoms remain purely ocular in 40%, generalized in 40%, limited to the limbs in 10%, and limited to bulbar muscles in 10%. Weakness remains restricted to the ocular muscles on a long-term basis in approximately 15% to 20% of cases (pure ocular MG).

2. Most patients with initial ocular involvement tend to have generalized weakness within the first year of the disease (90% of those who have generalization have it within the initial 12 months). Maximal weakness occurs within the initial 3 years in 70% of patients. Nowadays death of MG is rare.

3. Spontaneous long-lasting remission occurs in approximately 10% to 15% of cases, usually in the first year or two of the disease.

4. Most patients with MG experience progression of clinical symptoms during the initial 2 to 3 years. However, progression is not uniform, as illustrated by the 15% to 20% of patients whose symptoms remain purely ocular and those who have spontaneous remission.

D. Treatment options

1. **Cholinesterase inhibitors (CEIs)** are safe and effective. They are the first-line treatment of all patients.

    a. Inhibition of acetylcholinesterase (AChE) reduces the hydrolysis ACh, increasing accumulation of ACh at the nicotinic postsynaptic membrane. The CEIs used in MG bind reversibly (as opposed to organophosphate CEIs, which bind irreversibly) to AChE. These drugs cross the blood–brain barrier poorly and tend not to cause central nervous system (CNS) side effects. Absorption from the gastrointestinal tract tends to be inefficient and variable, with oral bioavailability of approximately 10%.

    b. **Muscarinic autonomic side effects** of gastrointestinal cramping, diarrhea, salivation, lacrimation diaphoresis, and, when severe, bradycardia can occur with any of the CEI preparations.

    c. **Cholinergic weakness.** A feared possible complication of excessive use of CEIs is skeletal muscle weakness (cholinergic weakness). Patients receiving parenteral CEI are at the greatest risk of having cholinergic weakness. It is uncommon (although not unheard of) for patients receiving oral CEI to have marked cholinergic weakness even while experiencing muscarinic cholinergic side effects.

    d. **Commonly available CEIs** are summarized in Table 48.1.

    (1) **Pyridostigmine** (Mestinon; ICN) is the most widely used CEI for long-term oral therapy. Onset of effect is within 15 to 30 minutes of an oral dose, peak effect within 1 to 2 hours, and gradual wearing off 3 to 4 hours after administration. The starting dosage is 30 to 60 mg three or four times a day depending on symptoms. Optimal benefit usually occurs with a dosage of 60 mg every 4 hours. Muscarinic cholinergic side effects are common with larger doses.

Table 48.1 Cholinesterase inhibitors

Inhibitor	Unit dose	Average dose
Pyridostigmine bromide tablet (Mestinon)	60 mg tablet	30–60 mg q4–6h
Pyridostigmine bromide syrup	12 mg/mL	30–60 mg q4–6h
Pyridostigmine bromide timespan (Mestinon Timespan)	180 mg tablet	1 tablet twice a day
Pyridostigmine bromide (parenteral)	5 mg/mL ampules	1–2 mg q3–4h (1/30 of oral dose)
Neostigmine bromide (Prostigmin)	15 mg tablet	7.5–15 mg q3–4h
Neostigmine methylsulfate (parenteral)	0.25–1.0 mg/mL ampules	0.05 mg q3–4h
Ambenonium chloride (Mytelase)	10 mg, 25 mg tablets	2.5–5.0 mg q4–6h

Occasional patients need and tolerate more than 1,000 mg/d, dosing as frequently as every 2 to 3 hours. Patients with considerable bulbar weakness often time their doses approximately 1 hour before meals to maximize chewing and swallowing. Of all the CEI preparations, pyridostigmine has the least muscarinic side effects.

(2) Pyridostigmine may be used in several forms alternative to the 60-mg tablet. The syrup may be necessary for children or for patients who have difficulty swallowing pills. Sustained-release 180-mg pyridostigmine (Mestinon Timespan) sometimes is preferred for nighttime use. Unpredictable release and absorption limit its use.

(3) Patients with severe dysphagia or undergoing surgical procedures may need parenteral CEIs. Intravenous pyridostigmine should be given at approximately 1/30 the oral dose.

(4) **Neostigmine** (Prostigmin; ICN) has a slightly shorter duration of action than does pyridostigmine and slightly greater muscarinic side effects.

(5) **Ambenonium** (Mytelase; Sanofi, New York, NY, U.S.A.) has shown no significant advantages over the other CEIs but has been suggested to be of greatest use in managing appendicular weakness. Headache is an additional occasional side effect.

(6) For patients with intolerable muscarinic side effects at the doses of CEIs needed for optimal power, a concomitant anticholinergic drug such as atropine sulfate (0.4 to 0.5 mg by mouth) or glycopyrrolate (Robinul; A.H. Robins, Richmond, VA, U.S.A.) (1 mg by mouth) on an as-needed basis or with each dose of CEI may be helpful.

(7) Patients with mild disease can often be treated adequately with CEIs. However, patients with moderate, severe, or progressive disease usually need more effective therapy.

2. **Thymectomy.** Association of the thymus gland with MG was first noticed at the beginning of the twentieth century, and thymectomy has become standard therapy over the past 50 years. Prospective, controlled trials have not been performed for thymectomy. Nonetheless, thymectomy is generally recommended for patients with moderate to severe MG, especially those who have inadequate control with CEIs and those younger than 55 years. All patients with suspected thymoma undergo surgery.

  a. **Clinical response.** Approximately 75% of patients with MG appear to benefit from thymectomy. The patient's condition may improve or simply stabilize. For unclear reasons, the onset of improvement tends to be delayed by a year or two in most patients (some patients seem to improve 5 to 10 years after surgery). There are no prospective controlled clinical trials of thymectomy in the management of MG.

  b. **Method.** Most centers use the transsternal approach to thymectomy with the goal of complete removal of the gland. The limited transcervical approach has been largely abandoned because of the likelihood of incomplete gland removal. Some centers perform "maximal thymectomy" to ensure complete removal. The procedure involves a combined transsternal and transcervical exposure with en bloc removal of the thymus. Thorascopic removal of the thymus gland has the potential advantage of less postoperative pain, shorter hospital stay, and smaller incisional scar. The best method involves employment of an experienced surgeon and anesthesiologist who have a record of performing the procedure safely and who can ensure that the entire gland is removed.

  c. **Patients who do not undergo thymectomy.** Patients with very mild or trivial symptoms do not undergo surgery. Most patients with pure ocular MG do not undergo thymectomy, although there has been some reported benefit in selected patients. Thymectomy is often avoided in the treatment of children because of the theoretic possibility of impairing the developing immune system. However, reports of thymectomy on children as young as 2 to 3 years have shown favorable results without adverse effects on the immune system. Thymectomy has been largely discouraged in the treatment of patients older than 55 years because of an expected increased morbidity, latency of clinical benefit, and frequent finding of an atrophic, involuted gland. Nonetheless, older patients have been described to have benefited from thymectomy.

  d. Major complications of thymectomy are uncommon as long as the operation is performed at an experienced center with anesthesiologists and neurologists familiar with the disease and with perioperative care of patients with MG. Common, less serious side effects of thymectomy include postoperative chest pain, which can last several weeks, a convalescence of 4 to 6 weeks, and incisional scarring.

3. **Corticosteroids.** No controlled trials have documented the benefits of corticosteroids in the management of MG. However, nearly all authorities have personal experience attesting to the virtues (and complications) of corticosteroid use for patients with MG.

  a. In general, corticosteroids are used to treat patients with moderately to severely disabling symptoms refractory to CEIs. Patients are commonly hospitalized for initiation of therapy to avoid the risk of early exacerbation. Opinions differ regarding the best method of administration.

  b. For patients with severe MG, it is best to begin with high-dose daily therapy of 60 to 80 mg/d by mouth. Early exacerbation occurs in approximately one half of patients, usually within the first few days of therapy and typically lasting 3 or 4 days. In 10% of cases, the exacerbation is severe, necessitating mechanical ventilation or a feeding tube (thus the need to initiate therapy in the hospital). Overall, approximately 80% of patients have a favorable response to steroids (30% attaining remission and 50% enjoying marked improvement). Mild to moderate improvement occurs in 15% of patients, and 5% have no response. Improvement begins as early as 12 hours and as late as 60 days after initiation of prednisone, but most patients begin to improve within the first week or two. Improvement is gradual, marked improvement occurring a mean of 3 months after initiation of treatment and maximal improvement a mean of 9 months afterward. Among patients with a favorable response, most maintain their improvement with gradual dosage reduction at a rate of 10 mg every 1 to 2 months. Reduction that is more rapid usually is associated with a flare-up of the disease. Although many patients can eventually be weaned from steroids and maintain their responses, most cannot. They need a minimum dosage (5 to 30 mg every other day) to maintain the improvement. Complications of long-term high-dose prednisone therapy are substantial, including cushingoid appearance, hypertension, osteoporosis, cataracts, aseptic necrosis, and the other well-known complications of long-term steroid therapy. Older patients tend to respond more favorably to prednisone.

  c. An alternative prednisone treatment involves a low-dose, alternate-day regimen on a gradually increasing schedule in an attempt to avoid early exacerbation. Patients receive 25 mg prednisone on alternate days (AD) with an increase of 12.5 mg every third dose (approximately every fifth day) to a maximum dose of 100 mg AD or until sufficient improvement occurs. Clinical improvement usually begins within 1 month. The frequency and severity of early exacerbation are less than those associated with high-dose daily regimens.

  d. High-dose intravenous methylprednisolone (1 g/d for 3 to 5 days) can provide improvement within 1 to 2 weeks, but the clinical improvement is temporary.

4. **Nonsteroidal immunosuppressive drug therapy**

  a. Azathioprine (Imuran; Glaxo Wellcome, Research Triangle Park, NC, U.S.A.) is a cytotoxic purine analogue frequently used for immunosuppressive management of MG. Experience with azathioprine therapy for MG is extensive but largely uncontrolled and retrospective.

(1) **Dosage.** The starting dosage is 50 mg/d by mouth. Complete blood cell count and liver function tests are performed weekly in the beginning. If the drug is tolerated and the blood results are stable, the dose is increased 50 mg every 1 to 2 weeks with the aim of a maximum dosage of approximately 2 to 3 mg/kg a day (approximately 150 mg/d for an adult of average size).

(2) **Side effects.** When azathioprine is first started, approximately 15% of patients have intolerable gastrointestinal side effects (nausea, anorexia, and abdominal discomfort), sometimes associated with fever, that lead to discontinuation. Bone marrow suppression with relative leukopenia (white blood cell count, 2,500/μL to 4,000/μL) occurs in 25% of patients but is usually not significant. If the white blood cell count decreases to less than 2,500/μL or the absolute granulocyte count decreases to less than 1,000/μL, administration of the drug is stopped, and the abnormalities usually resolve. Macrocytosis is common and of unclear clinical significance. Liver enzyme levels are elevated in 5% to 10% of patients, but this effect usually is reversible, and severe hepatic toxicity occurs in only approximately 1% of cases. Infection occurs in approximately 5%. There is a theoretic risk of malignant disease (based on observations of organ transplant recipients), but this increased risk has not been clearly established for patients with MG.

(3) **Clinical response.** The condition of approximately one half of patients with MG improves with azathioprine. Improvement usually begins approximately 4 to 8 months into treatment. Maximal improvement takes approximately 12 months. Relapse after discontinuation of azathioprine occurs in more than one half of patients, usually within 1 year.

b. **Cyclosporine** is used for patients with severe MG who cannot be adequately treated with corticosteroids or azathioprine.

(1) **Dosage.** The starting dosage is 3 to 5 mg/kg a day given in two divided doses. Blood levels of cyclosporine should be measured monthly (aiming for a level of 200 to 300 ng/mL) along with electrolytes, magnesium, and renal function (in general, serum creatinine level should not exceed 1.5 times the pretreatment level). Blood should be sampled before the morning dose is taken.

(2) **Clinical response.** More than one half of patients improve with cyclosporine. The onset of clinical improvement occurs approximately 1 to 2 months after therapy is initiated, and maximal improvement occurs approximately 3 to 4 months after treatment begins.

(3) **Side effects** include renal toxicity and hypertension. Nonsteroidal antiinflammatory drugs and potassium-sparing diuretics are among the drugs that should be avoided during treatment with cyclosporine. For patients taking corticosteroids, the addition of cyclosporine can lead to a reduction in steroid dosage (although it is usually not possible to discontinue prednisone).

c. **Mycophenolate mofetil** (CellCept; Roche, Nutley, NJ, U.S.A.) inhibits proliferation of T and B lymphocytes by blocking the de novo pathway of purine synthesis. The drug has been widely used in the care of organ transplant recipients. Numerous reports have suggested that the drug may be an effective option for immunosuppression in MG. The usual adult dose is 1 g twice a day. Anecdotal reports of uncontrolled series suggest that when the drug works, the clinical benefits may be seen within 1 to 2 months of the start of therapy. The safety profile is favorable; some patients have diarrhea and leukopenia.

5. **Plasma exchange (plasmapheresis)** removes AChR antibodies and brings about rapid clinical improvement.

a. **Protocol.** The standard course involves removal of 2 to 3 L of plasma every other day or three times a week until the patient's condition improves (usually a total of five or six exchanges).

   b. **Clinical response.** Improvement begins after the first few exchanges and reaches a maximum within 2 to 3 weeks. The improvement is moderate to marked for nearly all patients but usually wears off after 4 to 8 weeks as a result of reaccumulation of pathogenic antibodies.
   c. **Vascular access** requires placement of a central line.
   d. **Complications** include hypotension, bradycardia, electrolyte imbalance, hemolysis, infection, and access problems, such as pneumothorax from placement of a central line.
   e. **Indications** for plasma exchange include any instance in which rapid temporary clinical improvement is needed, including myasthenic crisis (see **I.E.4.**), impending crisis, preoperative stabilization, and suboptimal long-term control of symptoms with other forms of therapy.
6. **High-dose administration of intravenous immune globulin (IVIG)** is associated with rapid relief of MG symptoms (similar to the results with plasma exchange).
   a. **Protocol.** The usual protocol is 2 g/kg spread out over 5 consecutive days (0.4 g/kg per day). Different IVIG preparations are administered at different rates (contact the pharmacy for guidelines).
   b. **Clinical response.** Most patients with MG improve, usually within 1 week of starting IVIG. The degree of improvement is variable. The duration of response, like that of plasma exchange, is limited to approximately 2 to 8 weeks. Some patients need long-term maintenance therapy with 0.4 g/kg every 2 to 4 weeks to maintain the improvement.
   c. **Complications** include fever, chills, and headache, which respond to slowing of the infusion rate and to antihistamines (diphenhydramine). Occasional cases of aseptic meningitis, renal failure, nephrotic syndrome, and stroke have been reported. Patients with selective immunoglobulin A (IgA) deficiency can experience anaphylaxis, which is best avoided by screening for IgA deficiency ahead of time. The cost of the treatment is high, comparable with that of plasma exchange.
E. **General guidelines for management**
   1. Be certain of the diagnosis.
   2. **Patient education.** Provide the patient with information about the natural course of the disease (including its variable and somewhat unpredictable nature). Briefly review the treatment options outlined in **I.D.** pointing out the effectiveness, time course of improvement, duration of response, and complications. Provide the patient with educational pamphlets prepared by the Myasthenia Gravis Foundation of America or the Muscular Dystrophy Association.
   3. **When to hospitalize the patient.** Patients with severe MG can deteriorate rapidly over a period of hours. Therefore, those with dyspnea should be hospitalized immediately in a constant observation or intensive care setting. Patients with moderate to severe dysphagia, weight loss, or rapidly progressive or severe weakness should be admitted urgently. This allows close monitoring and early intervention in the case of respiratory failure, and expedites the diagnostic evaluation and initiation of therapy.
   4. **Myasthenic crisis** (Table 48.2) is a **medical emergency** characterized by respiratory failure from diaphragmatic weakness or severe oropharyngeal weakness leading to aspiration. Crisis can occur in the setting of surgery (postoperative period), in association with acute infection, or after rapid withdrawal of corticosteroids. Some patients, however, have no precipitating factors). Patients should be admitted to an intensive care unit for measurement of forced vital capacity (FVC) and forced expiratory volume in 1 second (FEV_1) every 2 hours. Changes in arterial blood gas values occur relatively late in neuromuscular respiratory failure. There should be a low threshold for intubation and mechanical ventilation. Criteria for intubation include a decrease in FVC to less than 15 mL/kg (or less than 1 L in an average-sized adult), severe aspiration from oropharyngeal weakness, or labored breathing regardless of the measurements. FVC can be estimated at

Table 48.2 The acutely deteriorating myasthenic patient

Myasthenic Crisis	Cholinergic Crisis
Respiratory distress	Abdominal cramps
Respiratory arrest	Diarrhea
Cyanosis	Nausea and vomiting
Increased pulse and blood pressure	Excessive secretions
Diaphoresis	Miosis
Poor cough	Fasciculations
Inability to handle oral secretions	Diaphoresis
Dysphagia	Weakness
Weakness	Worsening with edrophonium
Improvement with edrophonium	

the bedside by means of asking the patient to count aloud on a single deep breath. If the patient can count to 10, FVC is approximately 1 L. If the patient can count to 25, FVC is approximately 2 L. If the diagnosis is not clear-cut, it is advisable to secure the airway with intubation, stabilize ventilation, and only then address the question of the underlying diagnosis. If the patient has been taking a CEI, the drug should be temporarily discontinued to rule out the possibility of cholinergic crisis (Table 48.2).

5. **Correct any underlying medical problems,** such as systemic infection or thyroid disease (hypo- or hyperthyroidism can exacerbate MG).

6. **Drugs to avoid in MG.** Avoid using D-penicillamine, interferon-α, chloroquine, quinine, quinidine, procainamide, and botulinum toxin. Aminoglycoside antibiotics should be avoided unless needed for life-threatening infections. Ciprofloxacin and other fluoroquinolone antibiotics have been reported to aggravate weakness in some patients with MG. Neuromuscular blocking drugs such as vecuronium, pancuronium, and atracurium can produce marked and prolonged paralysis in patients with MG. Depolarizing drugs such as succinylcholine and mivacurium also can have prolonged effects and should be used only by a skilled anesthesiologist who is well aware that the patient has MG. Iodinated radiographic contrast medium [as is used in computed tomography (CT) and intravenous pyelography] may cause acute exacerbation of MG in occasional patients and is best avoided. Although many other drugs have been reported to aggravate MG, the cause and effect relation often is difficult to establish. The Myasthenia Gravis Foundation of America website (*www.myasthenia.org.*) contains a thorough summary of reported adverse drug effects. The clinician and patient should be alert to the possibility that any newly started medication can affect the patient's MG.

F. **Indications for specific therapies** (Table 48.3). Treatment must be individualized. Mild diplopia and ptosis may not be disabling for some patients, but for an airline pilot or a neurosurgeon, mild intermittent diplopia can be critical. In a similar manner, some patients may tolerate side effects better than others do.

1. **Mild or trivial weakness,** either localized or generalized, should be managed with a CEI (pyridostigmine).

2. **Moderate to marked weakness,** either localized or generalized, should initially be managed with a CEI. Even if symptoms are adequately controlled, patients younger than 55 years undergo thymectomy early in the course of the disease (within the first year). Thymectomy usually is not performed for older patients unless the patient is thought to have thymoma. Thymectomy is performed at an experienced center with the clear intent of complete removal of the gland with either a transsternal or a maximal technique. All patients with suspected thymoma (found at CT of the chest) should undergo thymectomy, even if the myasthenic symptoms are mild. Unless thymoma is suspected, patients with pure ocular disease usually are not treated with thymectomy.

Table 48.3 Management of myasthenia gravis

Mild, trivial weakness: cholinesterase inhibitors

Moderate to marked localized or generalized weakness
   Cholinesterase inhibitors, and
   Thymectomy for patients younger than 55 years

If symptoms are uncontrolled with cholinesterase inhibitors, use immunosuppression
   Prednisone if severe or urgent
   Azathioprine if
      Prednisone is contraindicated
      Prednisone has failed
      Excessive prednisone side effects are present

Plasma exchange or intravenous immunoglobulin
   Impending crisis, crisis
   Preoperative boost (if needed)
   Chronic disease refractory to drug therapy

If the above treatment fails
   Search for residual thymus tissue
   Administer cyclosporine or mycophenylate mofetil
   Refer to neuromuscular specialty group

---

   3. If symptoms are inadequately controlled with a CEI, immunosuppression is used. High-dose corticosteroid therapy is the most predictable and effective long-term option. If patients have severe, rapidly progressive, or life-threatening symptoms, the decision to start corticosteroids is clear-cut. Patients with disabling but stable symptoms may instead be treated with azathioprine, especially if the patient is a poor candidate for corticosteroids (such as a patient who is already overweight, has diabetes, or has cosmetic concerns). Patients who do not improve with corticosteroids or have unacceptable complications are given azathioprine.

   4. Plasma exchange is indicated in the following circumstances:
      a. Rapidly progressive, life-threatening, impending myasthenic crisis or actual crisis, particularly if prolonged intubation with mechanical ventilation are judged hazardous.
      b. Preoperative stabilization of MG (such as before thymectomy or other elective surgery) in patients with poorly controlled disease.
      c. Disabling MG refractory to other therapies.

   5. IVIG should be considered an alternative to plasma exchange with the same indications, especially if plasma exchange is not available or vascular access cannot be obtained.

   6. If these options fail, cyclosporine or mycophenolate mofetil should be used.

   7. If control is poor despite appropriate treatment, CT of the chest should be repeated to look for residual thymus. Some patients improve after a second procedure to complete the thymectomy. Check for other medical problems (diabetes, thyroid disease, infection, and coexisting autoimmune diseases).

   8. Referral to a neurologist or center specializing in neuromuscular disease is advised for all patients with suspected MG and can be particularly important in complicated or refractory cases.

 G. Miscellaneous forms of MG
   1. Transient neonatal myasthenia occurs in 10% to 15% of babies born to mothers with autoimmune MG. Within the first few days after delivery, the baby has a weak cry or suck, appears floppy, and occasionally needs mechanical ventilation. Maternal antibodies that cross the placenta late in pregnancy cause this condition. As these maternal antibodies are replaced by the baby's own antibodies, the symptoms gradually disappear, usually within a few weeks, and the baby is normal thereafter. Infants with severe weakness are treated with oral pyridostigmine at 1 to 2 mg/kg every 4 hours.

2. **Congenital MG** is a group of uncommon hereditary disorders of the neuro-muscular junction. The patients tend to have lifelong, relatively stable symptoms of generalized fatigable weakness. These disorders are nonimmunologic, without AChR antibodies, and therefore patients do not respond to immune therapy (steroids, thymectomy, or plasma exchange). Most patients have symptoms from infancy or early childhood and improve with CEI therapy. There are several different types of this disorder, some of which respond to the following treatments.

   a. **Familial infantile myasthenia** is a presynaptic autosomal recessive condition in which infants or young children experience a severe crisis in the setting of systemic infection. These patients appear to have a defect in reuptake of choline by the motor nerve terminal or a defect in synthesis, packaging, or mobilization of ACh at the motor nerve terminal. Such patients generally improve when treated with a CEI.

   b. **Congenital absence of AChE** is a recessively inherited disorder manifesting in infancy or childhood as generalized weakness and hypotonia. Scoliosis and lumbar lordosis are common as these children grow. Nerve conduction studies show a typical double CMAP (also referred to as a *repetitive discharge*) after a single supramaximal stimulus on nerve conduction studies (the absence of AChE leads to slow clearance of ACh from the synapse and the repetitive depolarization of the postsynaptic muscle fiber membrane).

   c. **The slow channel syndrome follows** an autosomal dominant pattern of inheritance with a variable age at onset and severity of symptoms. Because of the prolonged open time of the AChR ion channel, these patients also have a repetitive CMAP following a single stimulus. Cholinesterase inhibitors are ineffective, but some patients improve when treated with quinidine sulfate (a drug that is contraindicated in all other neuromuscular junction disorders).

   d. Another **heterogeneous group** of congenital myasthenic disorders is characterized by **defective AChRs.** Such conditions tend to be sporadic or follow an autosomal recessive pattern of inheritance. Treatment of most patients with congenital MG usually involves a CEI (pyridostigmine) and in some cases 3,4-diaminopyridine.

II. **Lambert–Eaton syndrome (myasthenic syndrome)**

   A. **Clinical features** (Table 48.4). Lambert–Eaton myasthenic syndrome is a presynaptic disease characterized by chronic fluctuating weakness of proximal limb muscles. Symptoms include difficulty walking, climbing stairs, and rising from a

Table 48.4 Lambert–Eaton syndrome: symptoms and signs

Symptoms
Proximal limb weakness
Fatigue or fluctuation of symptoms
Difficulty rising from a sitting position
Difficulty walking, climbing stairs
Dry mouth, metallic taste
Anticholinergic symptoms (e.g., gastrointestinal, bladder)

Clinical Signs
Proximal limb weakness (legs more than arms)
Weakness at bedside examination is mild compared with patient's symptoms and
   level of function
Absent or markedly hypoactive muscle stretch reflexes
Transient improvement in muscle power after exercise
Lambert's sign—the patient forcefully grips the examiner's hand, and over several
   seconds the grip gradually becomes more powerful

chair. In Lambert–Eaton syndrome, there may be some improvement in power with sustained or repeated exercise. Asking the patient to grip the examiner's hand with maximal force typically results in a modest squeeze that gradually becomes more forceful over 5 seconds (Lambert's sign). In contrast, the ptosis, diplopia, dysphagia, and respiratory failure of MG are far less common. Patients with Lambert–Eaton syndrome often report myalgia, muscle stiffness of the back and legs, distal paresthesia, metallic taste, dry mouth, erectile dysfunction, and other autonomic symptoms from muscarinic cholinergic insufficiency. Lambert–Eaton syndrome is rare compared with MG, which is approximately 100 times more common. Approximately one half of patients with Lambert–Eaton syndrome have underlying malignant disease, usually small-cell carcinoma of the lung. In patients without malignant tumors, Lambert–Eaton syndrome is an autoimmune disease and can be associated with other autoimmune disorders. In general, patients older than 40 years are more likely to be men and to have associated malignant disease, especially if they have a history of cigarette smoking. Younger patients are more likely to be women and to have no malignant neoplasm. Symptoms of Lambert–Eaton syndrome can precede detection of the malignant lesion by 1 to 2 years.

B. Diagnosis. The clinical diagnosis is confirmed with EMG, which typically shows low amplitude of the CMAPs and a decrement to slow rates (2 Hz) of repetitive stimulation. After brief exercise, there is marked facilitation of CMAP amplitude. At high rates of repetitive stimulation (>20 Hz), there is an incremental response. Results of SFEMG are markedly abnormal in almost all patients with symptoms. The pathogenesis involves autoantibodies directed against P/Q type voltage-gated calcium channels at cholinergic nerve terminals. These IgG antibodies also inhibit cholinergic synapses of the autonomic nervous system. Approximately 85% of patients with symptoms have these antibodies to voltage-gated calcium channels in serum, providing another useful diagnostic test. The serologic test has a relatively high specificity.

C. Therapy (Table 48.5)

  1. In patients with associated malignant disease, successful management of the cancer can lead to marked alleviation of the symptoms of Lambert–Eaton syndrome.

  2. Symptomatic improvement in neuromuscular transmission may occur with the use of cholinesterase inhibitors such as pyridostigmine.

  3. 3,4-Diaminopyridine. The quaternary ammonium compound 4-aminopyridine increases ACh release by blocking voltage-dependent potassium conductance and thereby prolonging depolarization at the nerve terminal and enhancing the voltage-dependent calcium influx. CNS toxicity may result in seizures, agitation, and confusion. However, a less toxic derivative, 3,4-diaminopyrimidine (DAP), appears to have more limited access to the CNS and therefore to be less toxic. DAP has been clearly shown to improve the condition of most patients with Lambert–Eaton syndrome with relatively mild toxicity. This compound provides the most effective symptomatic treat-

Table 48.5 Management of Lambert–Eaton syndrome

Manage the associated neoplasm
Symptomatic improvement in neuromuscular transmission
Cholinesterase inhibitors (pyridostigmine)
3,4-Diaminopyridine (limited availability)
Immunosuppressive therapy
Corticosteroids
Azathioprine
Plasma exchange
Intravenous immunoglobulin

ment of patients with Lambert–Eaton syndrome, but availability is limited. The drug has not been approved by the U.S. Food and Drug Administration. Referral to a major neuromuscular center that has an Investigational New Drug Application for use of this drug may be necessary. The typical starting dose of DAP is 5 to 10 mg two or three times a day with a gradual increase as needed up to a maximal dose of 100 mg per day (in four divided doses). Combining DAP with low-dose pyridostigmine tends to provide the best symptomatic benefit. Complications of use of DAP include dose-dependent paresthesia, occasional gastrointestinal symptoms, and in rare cases (at high doses), convulsive seizures.

4. **Immunosuppressive therapy** is used for patients with disabling symptoms. Long-term high-dose corticosteroids, azathioprine, plasma exchange, and IVIG all have been used with moderate success. In general, the use of these therapies should be tailored to the severity of the patient's symptoms.

5. **Additional management issues.** For patients older than 40 years, especially those with a history of smoking, even if the evaluation for malignant disease has negative results, it is best to obtain serial chest CT scans every 3 to 6 months to look for small-cell carcinoma of the lung. The symptoms of Lambert–Eaton syndrome can predate the detection of cancer by 1 to 2 years in some patients. For patients younger than 40 years without associated malignant disease, watch carefully for the development of other autoimmune disorders, such as hyperthyroidism.

III. **Botulism**

A. **Classic botulism** occurs after ingestion of food contaminated with botulinum toxin. Consumption of spoiled sausage resulted in an outbreak of this paralytic illness in the 1700s in Germany, leading to the name botulism, derived from the Latin term for sausage, *botulus*. Botulinum toxin blocks ACh release at the presynaptic motor nerve terminal and causes dysautonomia by blocking muscarinic autonomic cholinergic function as well. The intracellular target of botulinum toxin appears to be a protein of the ACh vesicle membrane. The toxin is a zinc-dependent protease that cleaves protein components of the neuroexocytosis apparatus. Eight different toxins have been identified, but disease in humans is caused mainly by types A, B, and E. Type E is associated with contaminated seafood. All types produce similar clinical signs and symptoms, although type A may cause more severe and enduring symptoms. In all three types, the condition can be fatal. Most cases result from ingestion of bottled or canned foods that have not been properly sterilized during preparation, especially home-canned foods. Foods cooked on an outdoor grill and wrapped in foil for a day or two produce an anaerobic environment, which can lead to toxin production. Home-bottled oils also should be considered. Remember "boiled, foiled, or oiled" when thinking through the possible sources.

1. **Clinical features** begin 12 to 48 hours after ingestion of contaminated food. Bulbar symptoms, including diplopia, ptosis, blurred vision, and speech and swallowing difficulties, occur initially and are followed by weakness in the upper limbs and then in the lower limbs. Severe cases produce respiratory failure necessitating mechanical ventilation. The tendency for paralysis to start in the cranial muscles and then descend the body differentiates the presentation from that of Guillain-Barré syndrome, which more often causes ascending paralysis. Botulism produces autonomic dysfunction, including constipation, ileus, dry mouth, and poorly reactive pupils. Some of these autonomic manifestations are seen in most but not all patients. The presence of normal pupils does not exclude the diagnosis of botulism.

2. **Diagnostic tests.** CMAP amplitudes are typically low on motor nerve conduction studies. Repetitive stimulation studies before and after exercise may show a decrement to low rates of repetitive stimulation and postexercise facilitation of the CMAP amplitude. It is wise to send both stool and serum specimens to the laboratory for detection of the toxin. The specimen is injected into the peritoneum of a mouse, and neutralized or inactivated specimen is injected as the control. If the mouse becomes paralyzed and dies, the test

result is considered positive. Toxin is found in blood samples 30% to 40% of the time, whereas stool samples have a somewhat higher yield (thus the need to send both). Newer polymerase chain reaction tests for the organism have been used to screen for the bacteria in food and may soon be available for use by clinicians.

3. **Management**
   a. The patient should be placed in an intensive care setting, and pulmonary function should be monitored with measurement of FVC every 2 to 4 hours. If FVC decreases to less than 1 L or 15 mL/kg or if the patient appears to be having respiratory difficulty, intubation and mechanical ventilation are necessary. The mainstay of management is general supportive care in the intensive care unit with assiduous attention to complications of immobility (e.g., pulmonary, aspiration, skin breakdown, prophylaxis for deep venous thrombosis). Aggressive physical and occupational therapy are required.
   b. **Use of trivalent equine antitoxin** is controversial, because adverse side effects occur in approximately 20% of patients (anaphylaxis and serum sickness). There is some evidence that antitoxin shortens the duration of clinical illness, especially for type E. If the diagnosis can be made within 48 hours of onset, and the toxin is readily available, then treatment with antitoxin is appropriate. If the diagnosis or antitoxin availability is delayed then treatment should center on meticulous supportive care.

4. **Course.** Even with aggressive support, the overall mortality remains approximately 5% to 10%, usually from respiratory or septic complications. The other patients tend to improve over a period of several weeks to several months. For patients who survive, recovery is nearly complete. Several years after the illness, some patients still have subjective fatigue and autonomic abnormalities, including constipation, erectile dysfunction, and dry mouth. Clinical recovery results from brisk sprouting of new motor axons from the nerve terminal with reinnervation of denervated muscle fibers.

B. **Infant botulism** is the most frequently reported form of botulism in recent years. The infant ingests spores of *Clostridium botulinum,* which lodge, germinate, and produce botulinum toxin in the intestinal tract. The typical manifestations are generalized weakness and constipation in an infant between the ages of 6 weeks and 6 months. The weakness may start in the cranial muscles and then descend, causing a weak suck, a poor cry, and reduced spontaneous movement. The cranial muscles are weak, with poor extraocular movements, reduced gag reflex, and drooling. The diagnosis is validated by finding *C. botulinum* in feces. The toxin usually is not detectable in the serum. EMG studies can point to this diagnosis in 80% to 90% of cases. Infantile botulism can range from mild to severe. Management centers on observation and general support, including respiratory stability. There is no evidence that treatment with antibiotics or antitoxin is helpful. The recovery tends to be excellent over the course of weeks to months.

C. **Wound botulism** occurs when toxin produced from *C. botulinum* infects a wound. The symptoms are similar to those of classic botulism except that the onset may be delayed as long as 2 weeks after contamination of the wound. The diagnosis is supported by results of EMG studies, demonstration of toxin in the blood, or finding the organism in the wound. Wounds that lead to botulism include direct trauma, surgical wounds, and wounds associated with drug use (e.g., intravenous and intranasal cocaine). Management of wound botulism includes débridement of the wound, antibiotics (penicillin), and equine antitoxin.

D. **Botulinum toxin injections.** Because botulinum toxin A is being used increasingly to manage focal dystonia and spasticity, it has become apparent that there is risk of symptomatic complications from excess toxin. Not only is the effect local at the site of injection into muscle, but also there is some degree of distant effect as well. Dysphagia is a frequent side effect of botulinum injection for spasmodic dysphonia. It typically lasts for approximately 2 weeks. On occasion, the dysphagia is severe, especially when patients report some degree of pretreatment dysphagia. The clinician should be alert to the development of excessive weakness in the region of local injection or even remote sites, particularly with higher doses of botulinum toxin.

IV. Hypermagnesemia is an uncommon clinical situation associated with the use of magnesium-containing drugs. Magnesium (Mg^{2+}) is contained in some antacids and laxatives. Magnesium sulfate ($MgSO_4$) is used in the management of preeclampsia and eclampsia, for hemodynamic control during anesthesia and the early postoperative period, and in patients depleted of magnesium, as in chronic alcoholism. Normal serum magnesium level is 1.5 to 2.5 mEq/L (2 to 3 mg/dL) and is maintained through exchange with tissue stores in bone, liver, muscle, and brain. Serum magnesium concentration is maintained through renal excretion. Patients with renal failure are predisposed to hypermagnesemia and should avoid magnesium-containing antacids and laxatives. Elevation of serum magnesium levels due to oral use of magnesium-containing compounds is uncommon as long as the patient has normal renal function. In the management of preeclampsia, hypermagnesemia occurs commonly owing to administration of high doses of parenteral magnesium sulfate and at times results in serious side effects in the mother or the newborn.

    A. The **clinical features of hypermagnesemia** correlate fairly well with serum magnesium levels. In the management of preeclampsia, the neuromuscular transmission effects are monitored and used as a limiting factor in dosage. With serum levels greater than 5 mEq/L, the muscle stretch reflexes become reduced. Levels of 9 to 10 mEq/L are associated with absent reflexes and clinically significant weakness. In the management of preeclampsia, muscle stretch reflexes are tested serially, and magnesium administration is stopped if the reflexes disappear. Serum levels between 3.5 and 7 mEq/L usually are associated with no significant adverse effects in preeclamptic women, but clinical weakness is common with levels greater than 10 mEq/L, and death of respiratory failure can occur. Serum levels greater than 14 mEq/L can induce acute cardiac arrhythmia, including heart block and arrest. Additional symptoms from autonomic nervous system involvement include dry mouth, dilated pupils, urinary retention, hypotension, and flushing skin thought to be from presynaptic blockade at autonomic ganglia. Although severe weakness can develop, mental status usually is not directly affected. Extraocular muscles tend to be spared. Reduced level of consciousness can occur indirectly as a result of hypoxia, hypercarbia, or hypotension.

    B. Magnesium interferes with neuromuscular transmission by inhibiting release of ACh. Magnesium competitively blocks calcium entry at the motor nerve terminal. There may also be a milder postsynaptic affect. Clinically, hypermagnesemia resembles Lambert–Eaton syndrome more than it does autoimmune MG. In addition, magnesium can potentiate the action of neuromuscular blocking agents, which has been emphasized in the care of women who undergo cesarean section after treatment with magnesium for preeclampsia. Patients with underlying junctional disorders are more sensitive to magnesium-induced weakness. Patients with MG and Lambert–Eaton syndrome have been found to decompensate in the setting of magnesium use despite normal or only mildly elevated serum levels. Typically, increased MG symptoms occur with parenteral administration of magnesium, but on occasion exacerbation of weakness occurs with oral use. Therefore, parenteral administration of magnesium should be avoided and oral magnesium preparations used with caution in the care of patients with known junctional disease (e.g., myasthenia gravis, Lambert–Eaton syndrome, botulism).

    C. Management of hypermagnesemia depends on the severity of clinical symptoms. Discontinuation of magnesium is the first step. If the patient is extremely weak, administration of intravenous calcium gluconate 1 g over 3 minutes can produce rapid, although temporary, improvement as long as the patient has normal renal function. If hypermagnesemia is more severe or if there are life-threatening side effects such as cardiac arrhythmia or renal failure, hemodialysis is indicated. Patients who have MG or Lambert–Eaton syndrome respond poorly to calcium. Such patients may respond better to a CEI.

V. Tick paralysis
  A. Clinical features. Tick paralysis is one of the eight most common tick-mediated diseases. Although it can affect a variety of species and any age group, it is most often reported among children. Usually the tick bite occurs 5 to 7 days before the onset of symptoms. The female tick then feeds, becomes engorged (such engorgement is facilitated by mating with a male tick), eggs become fertilized, and the female tick produces a neurotoxin, often called *ixobotoxin*. The natural course of the tick encounter is that engorgement of the female tick reaches an end point at which point the female tick releases and eventually deposits its eggs. Children tend to have a day or two of progressive paresthesia and leg weakness with a tendency to fall. Usually, there is no fever. Over the next day or two the weakness tends to ascend and involve axial as well as limb muscles. There is truncal instability. The patient has difficulty with sitting, cannot walk, and becomes areflexic. As the disease progresses over the next day or two the patient may have bulbar weakness and involvement of respiratory muscles. Some patients appear to have encephalopathy. The initial erroneous diagnosis often is Guillain–Barré syndrome.
  B. Diagnostic studies. One of the best diagnostic studies is electroencephalography (EEG) in that an astute EEG technician may first spot the tick in the scalp while placing the electrodes. The nerve conduction studies may suggest peripheral neuropathy with prolonged distal latencies on the motor nerve conduction studies, reduced nerve conduction velocity, and some reduction in amplitude of the sensory and motor responses. Repetitive stimulation studies often are unhelpful.
  C. Treatment. If a tick is detected and removed (usually it is in the hair or scalp), patients typically have dramatic resolution of the weakness over hours to several days. Otherwise, treatment involves general intensive care monitoring and support.
  D. Subtypes of tick paralysis
    1. In Australia, the *Ixodes holocyclus* tick produces a toxin that seems to act similarly to botulinum toxin in impairing the release of ACh at motor nerve terminals. Patients in Australia with exposure to this tick classically have more severe and fulminant paralytic illness than those exposed to North American ticks. In addition, over the first 1 to 2 days after removal of the tick, clinical symptoms often become more pronounced, and the clinical recovery tends to be slower. In Australia, it is generally recommended that *I. holocyclus* antitoxin be given to the patient before removal of the tick and that patients be observed for an extended period of time after tick removal.
    2. In North America, *Dermacentor* ticks—*Dermacentor andersoni* (the North American wood tick) and *Dermacentor variabilis* (the common dog tick)—are of concern for causing paralysis among adults, even though many other tick species can cause tick paralysis in animals. The *Dermacentor* ticks are fairly easy to spot when they are engorged. Tick paralysis is somewhat more common in the spring and summer in the southeast and northwestern United States than it is in autumn and winter.

Recommended Readings

Chaudhry V, Cornblath DR, Griffin JW, et al. Mycophenolate mofetil: a safe and promising immunosuppressant in neuromuscular diseases. *Neurology* 2001;56:94–96.

Cherington M. Botulism. *Muscle Nerve* 1998;10:27–31.

Ciafaloni E, Massey JM, Tucker-Lipscomb B, et al. Mycophenolate mofetil for myasthenia gravis: an open label pilot study. *Neurology* 2001;56:97–99.

Engel AG, Ohno K, Sine SM. Congenital myasthenic syndromes: recent advances. *Arch Neurol* 1999;56:163–167.

Felz MW, Smith CD, Swift TR. A six-year-old girl with tick paralysis. *N Engl J Med* 2000;342: 90–94.

Grattan-Smith PJ, Morris JG, Johnston HM, et al. Clinical and neurophysiological features of tick paralysis. *Brain* 1997;120:1975–1987.

Grob D, Arsura EL, Brunner NG, et al. The course of myasthenia gravis and therapies affecting outcome. *Ann N Y Acad Sci* 1987;505:472–499.

Gronseth GS, Barhon RJ. Practice parameter: thymectomy for autoimmune myasthenia gravis (an evidenced-based review): report of the Quality Standards Subcommittee of the American Academy of Neurology. *Neurology* 2000;55:7–15.

Jaretsky A, Barohn RJ, Ernstoff RM, et al. Myasthenia gravis: recommendations for clinical research standards. *Neurology* 2000;55:16–23.

Pascuzzi RM. Myasthenia gravis: a clinical trials perspective. In: Biller J, Bogousslavsky J, eds. *Clinical trials in neurological practice*. Boston, Butterworth–Heinemann, 2001;293–310.

Sanders DB, Massey JM. A randomized trial of 3-4 diaminopyridine in Lambert-Eaton myasthenic syndrome. *Neurology* 2000;54:603–607.

www.myasthenia.org. Website of the Myasthenia Gravis Foundation of America. Contains an up-to-date review of adverse drug effects in myasthenia gravis.

49. MIGRAINE, CLUSTER, AND TENSION HEADACHES

James R. Couch, Jr.

I. **Migraine therapy**
   A. **Algorithm for approach to the treatment of a patient with migraine**
      (Fig. 49.1). Migraine is essentially a clinical diagnosis and not one that is associated with specific laboratory or radiologic tests. It is a diagnosis of exclusion in which the physician must rule out other possible causes of the headache process.
      Table 49.1 outlines the process of developing a headache profile. This profile, by enabling the physician to compare the patient's headaches with established headache profiles, can be useful in establishing the diagnosis and developing an approach to treatment.
   B. **Migraine therapy**
      1. Therapies for migraine can be divided into symptomatic and prophylactic or preventive therapies. Symptomatic therapy can be further subdivided into nonspecific therapies and specific abortive therapy. An algorithm for migraine therapy is presented in Fig. 49.2.
         Symptomatic therapies for migraine are oriented primarily toward relief of pain. Pain is the symptom that brings most patients to seek medical help. Nausea and vomiting are the next most common symptoms that lead patients to seek medical help, and antinauseants may often be part of a successful migraine treatment regimen. Successful management of the pain and nausea of migraine usually produces remission of the entire migraine syndrome. Typically, the various symptoms of migraine syndrome tend to occur together. In some cases, migrainous neurologic or gastrointestinal symptoms occur in the absence of pain, a syndrome known as *migraine sans migraine.* There are, however, occasional examples of prolonged migrainous aura that do not respond to antimigraine therapy.
      2. **Nonspecific symptomatic therapy**
         a. **Analgesics.** The simplest therapy for migraine is a nonsteroidal antiinflammatory drug (NSAID), such as aspirin, ibuprofen, or naproxen, all of which are available in over-the-counter preparations and may be effective for a large number of patients, many of whom are never seen by physicians. At times, larger dosages of NSAIDs, such as 800 mg of ibuprofen, 600 mg of fenoprofen, or 500 mg of naproxen, can be effective in relieving migraine. Addition of an antinauseant such as promethazine or hydroxyzine (25 to 50 mg) may be helpful in relieving the gastrointestinal symptoms of migraine as well as extending the effect of the analgesic medication.
            Acetaminophen is an analgesic but has no antiinflammatory action. Some patients find 500 to 1,000 mg of acetaminophen effective for migraine.
         b. **Minor narcotics.** The next step is to use minor narcotics such as codeine (30 to 60 mg), hydrocodone (5 to 7.5 mg), oxycodone (5 mg), or propoxyphene (65 mg) to relieve pain. As with the NSAIDs, use of 25 mg of promethazine or hydroxyzine with the minor narcotic extends the effect of the narcotic and helps relieve the gastrointestinal symptoms of migraine.
         c. **Narcotic agonist–antagonist.** A narcotic agonist–antagonist medication such as butorphanol (Stadol; Bristol-Myers Squibb, Princeton, NJ, U.S.A.) at 2 to 4 mg intramuscularly or nalbuphine (Nubain; Dupont, Wilmington, DE, U.S.A.) at 10 mg intramuscularly is the next step in nonspecific pain relief. These narcotic agonist–antagonist medications stimulate opiate receptors at low doses but become narcotic antagonists and can elicit withdrawal syndromes at higher doses.
         d. **Major narcotics.** If these medications are ineffective, use of a stronger narcotic, such as meperidine (25 to 100 mg) or morphine (5 to 15 mg), may be indicated. These agents usually are given intramuscularly but can be given intravenously at lower dosages. Use of an antinauseant

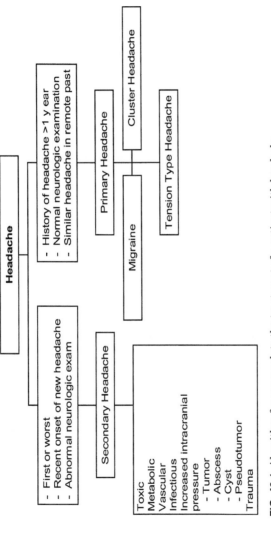

FIG. 49.1 Algorithm for approach to the treatment of a patient with headache.

Table 49.1 Key features of a headache profile (complete a profile for each type of headache)

Frequency of headache in terms of number per week, month, year, or even day

Duration of headache in terms of hours or days

Intensity of headache
  Mild: does not interfere with activity
  Moderate: interferes with activity to some extent but more than 50% of usual activity is possible
  Severe: some activity is possible but less than 50% of activity is carried out
  Disabling: patient must go to bed with the headache

Symptoms associated with headache
  General symptoms: photophobia, phonophobia, osmophobia
  Gastrointestinal and other autonomic symptoms
  Neurologic symptoms
  Mood changes
  Other symptoms

Precipitating factors for headache
  Exogenous: exposure to fumes, solvents, foods, weather changes, for example
  Endogenous: relation to menstrual cycle
  Psychological

Age at onset of headache and course over time

Family history of headache

often extends the effect of the narcotic and allows it to be effective at a lower dose. Promethazine or hydroxyzine at 25 to 75 mg usually is quite effective as an adjuvant agent when given with a narcotic. By and large, the use of narcotics should be limited to patients who have only occasional severe headaches that are refractory to other nonspecific analgesic approaches or to the specific abortive therapies discussed in **I.B.3.**

  e. **Dopamine antagonists.** Occasionally an antinauseant such as meto-clopramide (10 mg), prochlorperazine (10 mg), or droperidol (2.5 to 5 mg over 2 to 5 minutes every 3 to 4 hours) given intravenously is helpful by itself. This approach should be considered before narcotics are used.

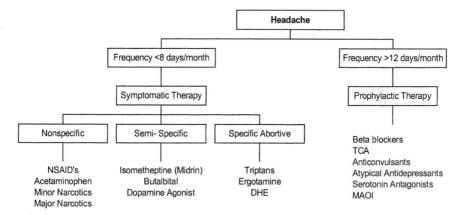

FIG. 49.2 Use of symptomatic and prophylactic therapy for headache. *DHE,* dihydroergotamine; *MAOI,* monoamine oxidase inhibitor; *NSAID's,* nonsteroidal antiinflammatory drugs; *TCA,* tricyclic antidepressant.

3. **Specific symptomatic (abortive) therapies for migraine** generally are not analgesics or narcotics. That is, they do not stimulate the opiate receptors and are not reversible with naloxone. These medications appear to provide specific antimigraine effects but to have no effect on other types of pain. However, the serotonin 5HT-1-B and 1-D receptor agonists, such as triptans and dihydroergotamine (DHE), may produce temporary relief in patients with headaches of inflammatory or vascular–inflammatory origin related to subarachnoid hemorrhage or meningitis.

Current theory suggests that abortive medications work by means of stimulation of the serotonin 5HT-1-B and 5HT-1-D receptors. These are presynaptic receptors on blood vessels (1-B) or central neurons (1-D). Stimulation of presynaptic receptors depolarizes the synapse and reduces transmitter release. Thus stimulation of presynaptic 5HT-1-B receptors on trigeminal nerve endings decreases release of substance P, calcitonin gene-related peptide, and neuropeptide Y on cranial vessels and decreases neurovascular inflammation. Similar presynaptic effect at 5HT-1-D central receptors may alter pain transmission in the trigeminocaudal nucleus or other pain transmission or modulating sites and alter pain transmission and perception.

a. **Ergotamine,** which was isolated from the rye fungus in 1925, was the first abortive medication. The pharmacologic properties of ergotamine are complex. Ergotamine stimulates most of the aminergic receptors and as a result has many pharmacologic actions. Table 49.2 outlines the use of ergotamine. Ergotamine stimulates the 5HT-1-B and 5HT-1-D receptors as intensely as does sumatriptan.

Ergotamine can cause coronary vasoconstriction. There have been several reports of myocardial infarction associated with ergotamine use. Ergotamine can cause vasoconstriction in the digits. This usually is a relatively insignificant finding. With long-term use of ergotamine, however, peripheral cyanosis, acroparesthesia, and peripheral neuropathy all may result. It is unclear whether these findings are related to microvascular constriction, including constriction of vasa nervorum, or whether there is a separate direct neurotoxic effect of ergotamine.

Between 50% and 80% of patients who take ergotamine respond to this medication. For some patients with intermittent migraine, ergotamine may be all that is necessary to control the headache. In other patients,

Table 49.2 Use of ergotamine

PRINCIPLES

Use ergotamine early in the headache to achieve maximal effect; later use may be ineffective
Do not exceed recommended dosage
May be given as a pill, sublingual preparation, or suppository

ORAL THERAPY

1 mg at onset of headache
1 mg at 30 minutes if needed
1 mg/h up to 6 mg/d
Maximum of 6 mg/d or 10 mg/wk

THERAPY BY SUPPOSITORY (USUAL SUPPOSITORY IS 2 MG)

2 mg at onset
May repeat in 1 hour if needed; may repeat again in 6–12 h
Maximum of three suppositories (6 mg) per day, or five suppositories (10 mg) per week
Suppositories can be cut into halves or fourths. Some patients may respond to as little as 0.5 mg of ergotamine given by suppository.
Precaution: Ergotamine is potentially habituating and can precipitate rebound–withdrawal headache in a habituated patient. Because of a long life at tissue receptors, as little as 1 mg every other day may produce a habituation–withdrawal cycle.

the response is relatively inadequate or the extent of side effects is great enough that different or additional medications are required.

Ergotamine provides a degree of psychic stimulation along with its other effects and thus can be abused. **Ergotamine abuse** can cause a habituation–withdrawal headache. This type of headache cannot be brought under control without discontinuing the ergotamine.

The **pharmacodynamics** of ergotamine are deceiving. The serum half-life of the medication is only 2 hours. If, however, the digital vasoconstrictive effect is used to assay ergotamine activity, a single dose of ergotamine in a naive subject may produce digital vasoconstriction for up to 7 days. Even if a patient is taking ergotamine as seldom as every other day, there still is a potential that the drug will lead to habituation–withdrawal or rebound–withdrawal headaches.

b. **Triptans.** The triptans are a new class of medications developed from research on serotonin. Recent investigations into **serotonin** have identified four classes of receptors. **The 5HT-1** receptors are presynaptic receptors. The **5HT-2** are postsynaptic receptors. The **5HT-3** receptors are related to the g-protein system, and **5HT-4** receptors are related to transporter function. The triptans are agents that are 5HT-1-B, 1-D receptor agonists with lesser effects on the 5HT-1-F and 1-A receptors. These medications have been found to have a remarkable affect on the symptomatic relief of migraine. They can abort the migraine attack and produce significant relief for 60% to 70% of patients and complete relief for 25% to 40% of patients. These medications have revolutionized symptomatic therapy for migraine.

(1) **Mechanism of action.** The triptans, through the 5HT-1-B receptor, have a very strong effect on constriction of the intracranial arteries. The arterial activity is highly cerebroselective, but there is also a minimal coronary vasoconstrictive effect (see **I.B.3.b(3)**).

The 5HT-1-D receptor is a neuronal receptor with representation on neurons in the trigeminocaudal nucleus as well as locus ceruleus, dorsal raphe nucleus, and other brain stem structures. Some triptans (rizatriptan, zolmitriptan, and naratriptan) are central nervous system (CNS) penetrant, whereas sumatriptan and ergot derivatives are not supposed to cross the blood–brain barrier. Because all triptans have similar CNS side effects, it is postulated that during the migraine attack, the blood–brain barrier is opened, and drugs such as sumatriptan with lower lipophilicity and CNS penetration can enter the CNS during the attack. This may be the reason the CNS side effects of drowsiness, dizziness, and fatigue occur with all triptans.

Whether the major effect of the triptans in stopping migraine is peripheral through 5HT-1-B receptors on trigeminovascular nerve endings or central through the 5HT-1-D endings on CNS neurons is unclear. Perhaps the antimigraine effect requires both.

(2) **Clinical trials.** The first trials on use of sumatriptan occurred in the mid 1980s. Most clinical trials were completed after the research criteria of the International Headache Society (IHS) were developed. These trials were conducted with the IHS criteria for patient identification and standardization. These criteria allowed studies to be conducted across national and cultural lines and to achieve consistency of research method.

To understand the results, it is necessary to understand the method (Fig. 49.3). In the trials, patients with migraine either with or without aura were identified. Patients were asked to treat one headache or several headaches, depending on the study. The patients were asked to rate their headaches in terms of pain intensity as none, mild, moderate, or severe. Patients were asked to wait until the pain was at least moderate before taking the medication.

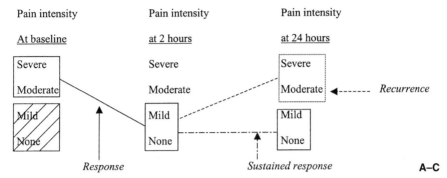

Pain intensity

At baseline

Pain intensity

at 2 hours

Pain intensity

at 24 hours

Response   *Sustained response*   **A–C**

FIG. 49.3 Method for trials of headache therapy since 1988. **A:** At baseline, pain is measured as severe, moderate, mild, or none and measured with the same scale at times up to 24 hours. **B:** Initial medication is taken only when pain is severe or moderate. **C:** The terms *response, recurrence,* or *sustained response* are defined diagrammatically.

Pain level was then reported by the patient on the same scale at 30, 60, 90, and 120 minutes after taking the medication, response at 2 hours being the primary end point. In many studies, response 4 and 24 hours after taking the medication was also reported; however, rescue medication was permitted after 2 hours, so the value of a 4-hour measurement is less clear. The criterion for success was generally achieving mild or no headache at 2 hours from an initial level of moderate or severe headache. Typically, a more stringent criterion of pain free at 2 hours was also reported.

Some patients had recurrence of headache. Recurrence was defined as having reoccurrence of severe or moderate headache after being in response with mild or no headache (Fig. 49.3). This created some confusion in that a patient had to be in response to have recurrence. The recurrence rate with the placebo was often relatively low, but then the placebo response was likewise relatively low. It has been suggested that the term *complete response* would be better. Complete response is defined as headache diminishing to mild or no headache and then never worsening to severe or moderate over a 24-hour period.

Table 49.3 lists the currently available medications as well as eletriptan which is expected to be available in 2001. Two other triptans, almotriptan and frovatriptan, also may be approved in the near future. Table 49.4 gives basic pharmacodynamic data on the triptans and their metabolism.

Table 49.5 summarizes the data for the five triptan medications showing the percentage of patients who achieved response and the percentage who achieved pain-free status. In general, the triptans produced a response (mild or no headache) in 60% to 70% of patients when given as an oral tablet, and pain-free status was achieved by 27% to 41% of patients, depending on the medication. To date, head to head studies have been conducted with zolmitriptan and sumatriptan, rizatriptan and sumatriptan. There have been small differences in the overall response that have not been statistically significant. From a clinical standpoint, however, it appears there is significant idiosyncrasy in the response of individuals to triptans. In the clinic, it is more important that individual patients may respond well to one triptan and less well to another. The reasons for the idiosyncratic differences are still unclear; nevertheless,

Table 49.3 Currently available triptans: usual dose and suggested maximum daily dose

Drug and route of administration	Marketed single dose (mg)	Usual dose (mg)	Usual maximum daily dose (mg)
ORAL (BY DATE OF INTRODUCTION)			
Sumatriptan tablets	25, 50, 100	50	200
Zolmitriptan	2.5, 5	2.5	10
Rizatriptan	5, 10	10	20
Naratriptan	2.5	2.5	10
Eletriptan[a]	(40, 80)	(40)	(160)
Almotriptan	12.5	12.5	25
NASAL SPRAY			
Sumatriptan	20	20	40
Frovatriptan	2.5	2.5	7.5
SUBCUTANEOUS			
Sumatriptan	6	6	12
Dihydroergotamine[b]	1	1	3

[a] Dose information is based on anticipated dosing guidelines pending approval by the U.S. Food and Drug Administration.
[b] Not a triptan, but affects the serotonin 1-B and 1-D receptors equally well.

failure of one triptan does not necessarily mean failure of all other triptans. If a patient has an inadequate response to a triptan, it is always worthwhile to try the other representatives of this group of medications.

(3) **Adverse effects** of the triptans are summarized in Table 49.6. This represents a compilation of a large number of studies. In general, the CNS symptoms of somnolence, fatigue, asthenia, and dizziness are the most common and the most troublesome. Chest pain occurs in a significant number of patients. It is thought to be related to stimulation of esophageal receptors, which causes esophageal spasm, but cardiac origin must be ruled out.

The major adverse event for the triptans relates to the cardiac system. There are rare 5HT-1-B receptors on coronary arteries. It has been shown that triptans can cause approximately 20% constriction of coronary arteries. If the patient has an underlying coronary atherosclerotic lesion, this 20% constriction can be enough to occlude the vessel. There have been myocardial infarctions reported with the triptans and with ergotamine and DHE. Patients who may be given triptans, ergotamines, or DHE should be screened for car-

Table 49.4 Pharmacokinetics of the triptans

Drug	t_{max} (h)	Bioavailability (%)	Serum half-life (h)	Metabolism and excretion
Sumatriptan	2	14	2	MAO-A
Rizatriptan	1	45	2–3	MAO-A
Zolmitriptan	2.5	40	3	MAO-A
Naratriptan	3.5	70	6	Renal (cytochrome P-450)
Eletriptan[a]	2.8	50	4–5	Cytochrome P-450–3A4
Frovatriptan[a]	1.7	70	25	Renal/hepatic
Almotriptan	2	70	4	Renal, MAO-A

[a] U.S. Food and Drug Administration approval anticipated 2001. t_{max}, time to reach maximum concentration; MAO, monoamine oxidase.

Table 49.5 Metaanalytic summary and comparison of response at 2 hours to orally administered triptans at usual recommended doses

Drug and dose	Percentage response at 2 hours (Sev/Mod → Mild/None)	Percentage achieving pain free (Sev/Mod → None)
Sumatriptan 50 mg	62	33
Zolmitriptan 2.5 mg	67	33
Rizatriptan 10 mg	71	41
Naratriptan 2.5 mg	58	27
Eletriptan 40 mg[a]	65	27
Eletriptan 80 mg[a]	75	33
Almotriptan	60	35
Frovatriptan	40	N/A

Pain was initially rated as severe, moderate, mild, or none by the patient before administration and then 30, 60, 90, and 120 minutes after ingestion of the tablet. For these studies, pain had to be moderate or severe before therapy. Response was considered reduction of pain to mild or none. Reduction to pain free also is given.

These data are from a metaanalysis of study results available in 1999 and earlier and do not represent studies with head-to-head comparisons of drugs.

[a] Approval anticipated in 2001.

diac disease. If there is any doubt, the patient needs a more extensive cardiac evaluation. Patients with cardiac disease should not take triptans.

Other adverse events like the therapeutic effect are relatively idiosyncratic. If a patient has a significant event with one triptan, this does not necessarily guarantee that the patient will have the same effect with another triptan. The trial of other triptans is indicated if one causes significant side effects.

Overuse of triptans can produce rebound withdrawal headaches. Triptan should be limited to no more than 3 days per week and in general no more than two or three doses a day.

(4) **Administration.** Table 49.3 provides the usual dose and the usual maximum daily dose of the four available triptans and of one expected to be released soon. Sumatriptan has the widest range of dosage forms with oral, nasal spray, and subcutaneous formulations. All are available as tablets for oral administration. Response onset within 30 to 60 minutes is usual. More than 80% response has been obtained 2 hours and peak response 4 hours after administra-

Table 49.6 Adverse events with triptans

	ST 50 mg	ZT 2.5 mg	RT 10 mg	NT 2.5 mg	ET 40 mg	ET 80 mg	AT	FT
Somnolence	5%	5%	8%	2%	4%	6%	1%	2%
Fatigue, asthenia	3%	3%	7%	2%	3%	6%	N/A	5%
Dizziness	5%	3%	9%	2%	6%	6%	1%	8%
Paresthesia	1%	6%		2%	3%	5%	1%	4%
Throat pain	N/A	N/A	N/A	2%	N/A	N/A	N/A	N/A
Chest pain	<1%	5%	3%	2%	2%	5%	<1%	2%
Nausea	N/A	11%	6%	5%	N/A	N/A	2%	2%

N = 800 1,167

ST, sumatriptan; ZT, zolmitriptan; RT, rizatriptan; NT, naratriptan; ET, eletriptan; AT, almotriptan; FT, frovatriptan.

tion. Dosing can be repeated in more than 1 hour; the usual limit is two doses a day, although more can be used at times (see Table 49.3, Maximum daily dose).

The rapidly melting tablet of rizatriptan and zolmatriptan has achieved good acceptance owing to convenience. Sumatriptan nasal spray can be used when the patient is too nauseated to take a tablet. The response to nasal spray is similar in time course to that of sumatriptan tablets. Subcutaneous sumatriptan (6 mg per dose) has the fastest onset of effect with initial relief in 10 to 20 minutes, 70% to 75% of patients respond within 1 hour, and 80% within 2 hours. For patients who awaken with severe headache or who have very rapid onset of headache, this is a very useful preparation.

c. **DHE.** Dihydroergotamine mesylate (DHE, or DHE 45) is an agonist for most aminergic receptors, including the 5HT-1, 5HT-2, catecholamine, and dopamine receptors. It is equipotent to sumatriptan as a 5HT-1-D agonist.

Given intravenously, 1 mg of DHE is as potent as subcutaneous sumatriptan in migraine relief. Table 49.7 outlines the protocol used by Raskin. Given intravenously, DHE can produce relief in 15 to 30 minutes. DHE has so far not been found to produce habituation–withdrawal or rebound–withdrawal headache.

DHE has a half-life of 10 hours. There is accumulation of metabolites over time with repeated dosing. The results of an uncontrolled study by Belgrade et al. suggested that 70% to 80% of patients had good relief with intravenous DHE and that 50% of those were headache free. Raskin's group and later Silberstein used DHE in the management of intractable migraine or status migrainous with good results. The protocol in Table 49.7 is repeated every 8 hours for 2 to 4 days or until the patient is headache free. If, however, the patient does not respond to the first two or three doses, other approaches should be taken.

DHE is primarily a venoconstrictor, whereas ergotamine has a greater effect on arterioles. The side effects of DHE are similar to those of ergotamine but are less intense. The incidence of peripheral and coronary vasospasm is much lower with DHE than with ergotamine.

DHE also can be used as a 1-mg intramuscular or subcutaneous injection. Studies have shown a slower onset of action but 60% to 70% good

Table 49.7 Dihydroergotamine (DHE) and isometheptene (Midrin)

DIHYDROERGOTAMINE (DHE)
i.v. use (Raskin protocol):
   Metoclopramide or prochlorperazine 10 mg i.v. over the course of 60 seconds
   Wait 5 minutes to allow distribution
   DHE 0.5 mg i.v. over the course of 60 seconds
   Wait 3–5 minutes
   May repeat 0.5 mg i.v. if no relief
Repeat: may repeat every 8 hours for up to 4–6 days
Side effects: chest pressure, anxiety, speeding or dissociation of thoughts, and nausea
s.c. or i.m. use: 1 mg, may be used without antinauseant
Repeat: may repeat every 8 hours, but for longer-term use, suggest once a day
Evaluate for coronary disease before use of DHE. Obtain electrocardiogram for all patients older than 50 years. Do not use for patients at risk of myocardial infarction.

ISOMETHEPTENE (MIDRIN)
   Use: capsules at onset; repeat hourly if needed up to 6 capsules a day
   Repeat: maximum of 6 capsules a day or 10 capsules a week
   Side effects: drowsiness, bad taste, and (rarely) elevated blood pressure

headache relief. Patients may be trained to give their own injections and thus use the medication at home. DHE by nasal spray is effective 50% to 60% of the time.

    d. Isometheptene (Midrin; Carnrick, Cedar Knolls, NJ, U.S.A.) is a combination of 65 mg of isometheptene mucate, a weak catecholamine agonist; 100 mg of dichloralphenazone, an antihistamine; and 325 mg of acetaminophen. The receptor pharmacologic properties have not been studied, but this medication appears to have an abortive antimigraine action. The dosage schedule is presented in Table 49.7. Side effects are very few, and tolerance has not been reported. Some patients respond well to isometheptene. As with other abortive medications, isometheptene should not be used for daily therapy. Use should be limited to no more than 2 or 3 days a week.

    e. Cost. Table 49.8 presents the costs of drugs used in symptomatic therapy for headache. Average wholesale and retail prices are given. There is a wide variation in cost. The patient's resources must be taken into account when the drugs are prescribed.

  4. Preventive antimigraine therapy. The concept of prevention of migraine rather than symptomatic therapy for individual headaches dates from the late 1950s. Although earlier attempts at preventive therapy had been made with various medications, the first successful preventive medication was **methysergide.** The concept of preventive medication is to provide the patient who is having frequent headaches with a medication that will prevent the headaches from occurring. For this type of medication to work, the assump-

Table 49.8 Costs of medications for acute migraine treatment (all treatments per headache)

Medication	Dosage	AWP/dose
Isometheptene (Midrin)	1 capsule, then 1/h (max 5 q12h)	$1.94
Acetaminophen/isometheptene/ dichloralphenazone		.94
Fiorinal tabs, Fiorinal caps	1–2 q4h (max 6/h)	2.98
Aspirin/caffeine/butalbital tabs		.27
Stadol NS spray	1 spray/nostril; repeat once in 3–5 h	10.00[a]
Dihydroergotamine (DHE 45)	1 mg i.m.; repeat up to twice at 1-h intervals (3 mg)	10.68
Cafergot	1 rectal suppository; can repeat once at 1 h	8.20
Ergotamine 2 mg/caffeine	100 mg	5.48
Ergotamine 1 mg/caffeine	100 mg 2 tabs, then 1 q30min 4 times prn (max 6)	3.39
Sumatriptan (Imitrex)	6 mg i.m.; repeat once at 4 h if needed	39.00[b]
Sumatriptan 50-mg tablets	See Table 49.3	16.00
Rizatriptan 10 mg	See Table 49.3	15.40
Zolmitriptan 2.5 mg	See Table 49.3	14.73
Naratriptan 2.5 mg	See Table 49.3	15.53
Almotriptan 12.5 mg	12.5 mg	10.98
Frovatriptan 2.5 mg	2.5 mg	t.b.d.

AWP, average wholesale price; t.b.d., to be determined.
[a] Based on 2-mg dose (1 mg per spray, 12 sprays/bottle)
[b] Sold as a kit with two doses. AWP $77.77.

tion of "critical factors" must be made. This could be theoretically envisioned as follows. Migraine is a state that depends on a trigger precipitating an event. This event leads to a cascade of physiologic changes, which develop into the migraine headache. If this cascade can be interrupted, the migraine headache can be prevented.

The mechanism of migraine prophylaxis remains speculative. It has been suggested that stimulation of the 5HT-2 receptor is related to the migraine-preventive effect. Because the exact mechanism of migraine is unknown, the mechanism by which 5HT-2 receptor stimulation may prevent migraine also is unknown.

a. **General principles of preventive therapy.** The decision to use or not to use preventive medication is based on the following factors (Table 49.1): (1) frequency of migraine, (2) intensity of migraine, (3) duration of headache, (4) the patient's willingness or desire to try the prophylactic approach, and (5) extent and tolerability of side effects of the medication. Occurrence of three or four headaches per month or more than 8 days per month with headache typically are reasonable thresholds for consideration of prophylactic therapy. Two severe headaches lasting 4 days each per month would prompt many patients to consider prophylactic therapy. On the other hand, four headaches of 4 hours each per month would likely result in a request for symptomatic therapy.

It is not uncommon for patients to have significant side effects. Weight gain, sedation, and impaired thinking can occur as side effects with most of these agents. For each patient, the therapeutic benefit must be balanced against the extent of side effects to maximize the overall therapeutic result.

The drugs that have been most successful in migraine prevention are the anti-serotonin drug methysergide, β-adrenergic blocking agents, tricyclic antidepressant agents, and valproic acid. Other drugs for this purpose include other anticonvulsants (gabapentin, topiramate), newer antidepressants [trazodone, nefazodone, selective serotonin reuptake inhibitors (SSRI)], cyproheptadine (an antihistamine with a tricyclic structure), and calcium channel blocking agents.

The preventive medications have numerous side effects and are not well tolerated by all patients. The usual procedure is to start with a small dose and build up the dose gradually until either a therapeutic effect or limiting side effects are observed. Monotherapy should be attempted and explored before combinations of prophylactic medications are tried.

The effective prophylactic antimigraine agents are outlined in Table 49.9. These agents are considered by classes. The cost of these agents is presented in Table 49.10.

b. **β-Blocking agents.** The β-adrenergic blocking agent propranolol was approved for migraine prophylaxis in 1974. The β-adrenergic blocking agents without intrinsic sympathomimetic activity (ISA) appear to have a preventive antimigraine effect. Those with ISA appear to have a minimal effect on migraine prophylaxis. Propranolol is discussed as the representative of this group.

The pharmacology of propranolol is complex. As a nonspecific β-adrenergic blocking agent, it has many pharmacologic effects, including decrease in blood pressure, heart rate, and cardiac contraction; inhibition of bronchodilation, and decrease in the gluconeogenic response among diabetic patients taking insulin. Propranolol also has an antianxiety effect in small doses and has been used to diminish panic attacks and to control stage fright.

Propranolol has been found most effective in the treatment of patients with intermittent migraine. In propranolol studies that were controlled and blinded, approximately 50% to 55% of patients improved more than 50%.

The **side effects** of propranolol include fatigue or a lack of energy, sedation, and weight gain. Orthostatic hypotension and syncope can occur if

Table 49.9 Prophylactic antimigraine agents

β-Adrenergic blocking agents	Range of effective dose (mg/d)		Usual effective dose (mg/d)
Nonspecific β-blockers	Propranolol	20–360	80–240
	Nadolol	40–160	40–80
	Timolol	10–40	20–30
Specific β₁ blocking agents	Atenolol	25–150	50–100
	Metoprolol	25–150	50–100
Tricyclic antidepressants	Amitriptyline	25–300	75–150
	Doxepin	25–300	75–150
	Nortriptyline	10–150	50–100
	Imipramine	25–250	75–150
	Protriptyline	10–60	20–40
Tricyclic antihistamine	Cyproheptadine	4–40	12–24
Calcium channel blocking agents	Verapamil	80–480	120–240
Nonsteroidal antiinflammatory agents	Naproxen	500–1,000	500–1,000
Monoamine oxidase inhibitor	Phenelzine	15–90	30–60
Antiserotonin agent	Methysergide	2–8	4–6
γ-Aminobutyric acid agonist	Divalproex	500–2,000	500–1,000

the hypotensive effect is too great. The slowing of heart rate is occasionally great enough that heart rate decreases to less than 50 beats/min. At this rate, the patient may have great difficulty performing usual activities.

Because of the negative chronotropic and inotropic effects of propranolol, patients may find their capability for exercise diminished. This usually is a problem only when maximum exercise tolerance is tested. Some patients, however, find fatigue or dyspnea with carrying out simple activities of daily living. In patients with limited cardiac reserve, propranolol can induce cardiac failure or worsen existing failure. If these side effects are intolerable or dangerous, propranolol should be discontinued.

The dose of propranolol can vary from as little as 20 to 30 mg/d to as much as 480 mg/d. In most patients who respond to propranolol, doses of 80 to 240 mg/d provide good headache prophylaxis. There is not a dose–response relation but rather an apparently idiosyncratic relation between dosage and headache relief. The usual **method of initiating propranolol therapy,** as with all other prophylactic medication, is to start with a relatively low dose and then increase the dose gradually to a point at which the patient has either relief from headaches or significant side effects, whichever comes first. Typically, a dose of 20 mg twice a day is tolerated initially. The dosage can be advanced 20 mg every third day to a maximum of 40 mg three times a day. The dose usually can then be increased 40 mg every week or every month until the maximum dose is reached.

Three contraindications should be considered: (1) propranolol should not be given to patients with diabetes, because it masks the response to hypoglycemia, (2) propranolol can precipitate asthmatic reactions in patients with actual or latent asthma, and (3) propranolol can enhance or precipitate depression, and this may be severe.

Other β-blocking agents without ISA appear to be equivalent to propranolol in potency and range of effectiveness (Table 49.9). Although some of these agents may have desirable properties such as longer half-life, there has been very little evidence that use of one β-blocking agent without ISA is better than any other. Typically, if one β-blocking agent fails, better results are seldom obtained with trials of other β-blockers.

Table 49.10 Cost of medication: migraine prophylaxis, 1-month supply

Medication	Daily dose (mg)	Tablet size (mg)	No. of tablets per month	AWP
Methysergide (Sansert; Novartis, East Hanover, NJ)	4	2	60	$102.60
Propranolol (Inderal, Wyeth-Ayerst Laboratories, Philadelphia, PA)	240	80	90	90.32
Propranolol (generic)	240	80	90	20.69
Amitriptyline (Elavil; Zeneca Pharmaceuticals, Wilmington, DE)	50	50	30	20.67
	100	50	60	41.55
Amitriptyline (generic)	50	50	30	2.32
	100	50	60	4.70
Doxepin (Sinequan; Pfizer Inc., New York, NY)	50	30		19.09
	100	50	60	36.18
Doxepin (generic)	50	50	30	5.99
	100	50	60	12.10
Divalproex (Depakote; Abbott, Abbott Park, IL)	750	250	90	67.29
Verapamil (Calan; G. D. Searle & Co., Chicago, IL)	80	90	—	44.64
	240 (sustained release)	30	—	40.78
Verapamil (generic)	80	90	—	5.07
	240 (sustained release)	30	—	34.86

AWP, average wholesale price.

c. **Tricyclic antidepressants (TCAs)** have been generally favored for chronic tension-type headache and chronic daily headache with migraine and tension features, whereas the β-adrenergic blocking agents have typically been more effective for pure intermittent migraine. TCAs may be effective for intermittent migraine as well. I have found amitriptyline and doxepin the two most effective TCAs in migraine prevention. The other agents listed in Table 49.9 are relatively less effective. Some patients, however, are found to respond to other tricyclic agents when amitriptyline and doxepin have failed. Although no studies have been performed on this subject, anecdotal experience suggests that some patients may respond better to doxepin than to amitriptyline, or vice versa. If only a modest response is obtained to one of the agents, it usually is worthwhile to try the other to see whether it has better therapeutic efficacy.

The **pharmacologic properties** of TCAs are complex. These agents inhibit reuptake of serotonin and norepinephrine at nerve endings and have anticholinergic, β-adrenergic blocking, and sedative effects.

For amitriptyline, a starting dosage of 10 to 50 mg at bedtime usually is tolerated. The dosage may be increased 10 to 25 mg every 1 to 2 weeks to a maximum of 300 mg/d. The dosage is determined by either (1) good headache relief or (2) occurrence of unacceptable side effects. The response to TCAs, like that to propranolol, is more idiosyncratic and not closely related to blood levels. If the patient has no side effects and no relief, continue to increase the dose. At doses more than 200 mg/d, amitriptyline level should be measured. If the tricyclic level of amitriptyline plus nortriptyline or doxepin plus nordoxepin exceeds 300 mg/mL, the dose should be decreased. Typically, the dose should be divided, one half at bedtime and the other half in divided doses during the day. Giving the entire dose at bedtime may work well for some patients, but others may have recurrence of headache in afternoon or evening with this regimen.

The typical side effects of the TCAs are drowsiness and the anticholinergic effects of dry mouth, constipation, difficult or slowed urination, blurred vision, and weight gain. Most patients accommodate to the drug with dosage adjustment and slow progression of dose. Anxiety and paradoxic stimulation with difficulty sleeping occur among 2% to 5% of patients. Tardive dyskinesia has been reported in rare instances. TCAs may lower seizure threshold. Amitriptyline and imipramine have been associated with sudden death in rare cases. These drugs have rarely been associated with fatal arrhythmias. To date, doxepin has not been reported to have cardiac side effects. For patients older than 50 years or who have risk factors for cardiac disease, an electrocardiogram is recommended before these agents are administered. This precaution is also recommended for most of the preventive antimigraine agents listed in Table 49.9.

Combinations of amitriptyline in doses of 75 to 150 mg/d and propranolol at 80 to 160 mg/d have been used by headache experts to manage migraine. Some patients experience a significant additive effect.

d. **Cyproheptadine.** Pharmacologically, cyproheptadine has a tricyclic structure, but its major effect is that of an antihistamine. Cyproheptadine produced more than 50% improvement in 45% to 50% of subjects in two trials. The potential side effects and potential toxic problems of cyproheptadine are the same as those of amitriptyline, although cyproheptadine usually has fewer side effects than does amitriptyline. Doses of 12 to 24 mg/d are the usual effective dose in those who respond. Doses up to 40 mg/d can be tried if not limited by side effects.

e. **Valproic acid (VPA)** was first reported to be effective in the management of migraine in 1987. This led to several controlled trials in which approximately 50% of subjects treated with VPA had more than 50% improvement. VPA has become a major preventive antimigraine agent.

The formulation of divalproex sodium (Depakote; Abbott, Abbott Park, IL, U.S.A.) has a higher tolerability than does VPA per se. The latter formulation is associated with a high incidence of nausea and gastric irritation. The major side effects of VPA as divalproex sodium are weight gain, tremor, and hair loss. These symptoms remit when VPA is discontinued. Sedation and difficulty thinking may be seen in occasional patients.

Alterations of liver function by changes in carnitine metabolism occur and can result in an elevated level of ammonia in the blood. Hepatotoxicity can occur and is a greater risk in the setting of polytherapy. Children are at greater risk than are adults, and the extent of potential hepatotoxicity in adults is unknown. VPA also may be associated with bone marrow suppression, but this occurs rarely if at all.

The dosage of divalproex sodium is 250 mg once or twice a day initially with an increase to 500 mg three times a day if needed. Higher dosages usually are not effective when a dose of 1,500 mg/d does not give relief.

f. Methysergide is a serotonin receptor blocking agent, although it also has significant potency for blocking norepinephrine receptors. Methysergide is effective for migraine prophylaxis, 50% to 55% of subjects reporting more than 50% relief. Methysergide, however, has a very high side-effect profile. The most common side effects are nausea and abdominal cramping, which occur among 10% of 20% of patients. Other acute side effects include coolness of the digits as a result of vasoconstriction, acroparesthesia, neuropathy, limb edema, rashes, and psychiatric side effects consisting of dissociation of thoughts, anxiety, nervousness, and, rarely, hallucinations.

Among patients who have taken methysergide for prolonged periods (more than 2 years), inflammatory fibrosis can develop in the retroperitoneal area, in the lungs, or in the myocardium., Patients so affected typically are those who have taken methysergide uninterruptedly for more than 2 years and often for as long as 5 years. In rare instances, this reaction has occurred with less than 2 years of therapy. It is recommended that methysergide be given for no more than 6 months at a time without at least a 1-month drug holiday. Usually the patient receives the medication for 5 months, takes a 1-month holiday, and then resumes treatment for another 5 months.

Methysergide should be started at 2 mg/d and increased 2 mg/d to a level of 2 mg three times a day.

Patients should be monitored periodically for elevation of serum creatinine. Some authorities recommend that periodic intravenous pyelograms or CT scans of the kidney with contrast be taken as part of the monitoring process.

Comment: For migraine prophylaxis, propranolol, amitriptyline, cyproheptadine, valproic acid, and methysergide have typically been the most effective. In a compilation of studies performed to determine the extent to which patients had at least 50% improvement, the results showed that 58% of a group of 1,500 patients taking methysergide, 55% of a group of 100 patients taking amitriptyline, 51% of a group of 210 patients taking propranolol, 48% of a group taking divalproex, and 48% of a group of 50 patients taking cyproheptadine reached this criterion in various double-blind studies in a comparison of medication versus placebo. No definite dose–response relation has been found for any prophylactic antimigraine medication. The prophylactic antimigraine response appears idiosyncratic as far as is currently known.

g. Other preventive antimigraine agents

    (1) Anticonvulsants. Gabapentin and topiramate along with VPA herald a new approach to migraine prophylaxis. In addition to being anticonvulsants, all three have significant potency in migraine prophylaxis as well as mood stabilization properties. They all can be used to manage manic depressive illness, depression, phobias, and panic disorders. All of these psychiatric conditions entities occur two to three times as often among migraineurs as among those who do not have migraines.

        (a) Gabapentin is approved for use as an add-on anticonvulsant but has found greater use in the management of neuropathic pain and headache and also may be used in mood disorders. For migraine, the effective dose may range from 300 to 4,000 mg/d. Typically a starting dose is 100 to 300 mg/d and may be advanced every 3 to 7 days to 900 to 1,800 mg/d. The major side effects are sedation, difficulty thinking, and weight gain. If there are no side effects and an inadequate therapeutic effect at 1,800 mg/d, the dose may be increased in 300-mg increments to 3,200 mg/d. The patient should be reevaluated before taking a higher dose.

        (b) Topiramate. In the use of topiramate as an antimigraine drug, doses of 50 to 200 mg/d are typical, although 300 mg/d occasionally is needed. Start with 25 mg at bedtime and advance by 25 mg/d each week. After 100 mg at bedtime, use small doses during the day so that 25% to 33% of the dose is given in the morning and the balance at bedtime. **Side effects** of topiramate are mainly sedation, difficulty thinking, difficulty with word finding, and tingling paresthesia in the limbs. Weight loss is a frequent side effect; it averaged 5 to 7 pounds (2 to 3 kg) in studies of use to treat patients with epilepsy. This side effect may improve patient acceptance. The weight loss is more prominent among overweight patients and can range from 5 to 30 pounds (2 to 14 kg) but plateaus after 2 to 3 months.

Comment: For the anticonvulsants that have migraine prophylactic activity, there appears to be a "window" effect. The antimigraine dose typically is at the low end of the anticonvulsant dose. Moving above the usual upper dose gives no further benefit and worsens side effects and headache. The same "window effect" also occurs with TCAs, methysergide, and propranolol.

- **(2) Newer antidepressant agents.** Trazodone and nefazodone in doses of 100 to 400 mg/d have antimigraine activity in some cases. The high-affinity SSRIs fluoxetine, paroxetine, and sertraline have had anecdotal reports of antimigraine effect but most results of controlled studies are negative. If depression is a major factor and has not responded to a TCA or mood-stabilizing anticonvulsant, use of an SSRI to manage depression can be beneficial. The SSRI can be used with a TCA.
- **(3) Calcium channel blocking agents** generally have been disappointing in their effects in migraine prophylaxis. Initial expectations for these agents were high, but the calcium channel blocking agents have shown low effectiveness in double-blind studies against placebos. There appears, however, to be a smaller group of patients who respond well to calcium channel blocking agents. These patients often have tachyphylaxis after 2 or 3 months taking the medication and need a period of at least 1 month off the medication to restore responsiveness.

  The representative of this group is verapamil. When verapamil is effective, it usually is at a dose of 80 to 240 mg/d. Verapamil typically is more effective when used as the regular formulation and less effective as a slow-release agent or long-acting agent. Usually 80 mg three times a day is a reasonably effective dosage. The dosage may be increased to 120 mg four times a day if tolerated.
- **(4) Clonidine,** an α-agonist, once was thought to be an agent with a bright future in migraine prophylaxis. Several trials of clonidine have been performed, but none has found significant potential. I have had rare patients who have been refractory to other medications and have also responded to clonidine.
- **(5) Monoamine oxidase inhibitors (MAOIs)** have been studied primarily in an anecdotal manner. Phenelzine has been used most commonly. Because of the risk of paradoxic hypertension and the need for a special diet low in tyramine, MAOIs are used only when other drugs have failed. Occasionally, patients may respond to phenelzine at 15 to 30 mg three times a day. The reader is referred to drug compendia for pharmacologic properties and side effects.

- **h. Cost of therapy.** The preventive or prophylactic antimigraine medications vary widely in cost. Table 49.10 reviews the costs of 1-month supplies of these medications at their usual daily doses. The average wholesale price is presented.

II. Cluster headache therapy and management
- **A. Symptomatic therapy.** The therapies for cluster headache can be divided into symptomatic and prophylactic approaches (Fig. 49.4). Symptomatic treatment

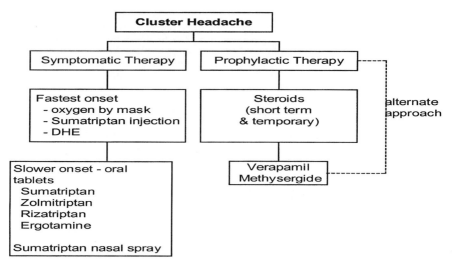

FIG. 49.4 Therapy for cluster headache.

can be further subdivided into nonspecific analgesic medications and specific abortive medications.

1. **Analgesic or narcotic nonspecific medications** generally are a very ineffective way of managing cluster headache. Because of the usual brief duration of the cluster headache and gastroparesis during the headache, analgesic medications usually do not have time to be fully absorbed and become effective by the time the headache terminates. Even for more prolonged headaches, when the medications have time to be effective, the results usually are poor with oral or injected medications. Analgesic and narcotic medications typically provide relatively little relief to patients with cluster headaches.

2. **Abortive medications** include subcutaneous sumatriptan, DHE, and other triptans as well as oxygen.

    a. **Sumatriptan** at a dose of 6 mg subcutaneously usually produces rapid and predictable relief from cluster headache. It is the standard symptomatic therapy for cluster headache. Patients can take sumatriptan for periods of several weeks without having a rebound headache. Studies of oral sumatriptan also have shown fair to good effectiveness, but onset of effect usually is at least 30 minutes.

    b. **Ergotamine** as a therapy for cluster headache can be given by means of pill or suppository. Cluster headache is associated with relative gastroparesis that slows absorption of ergotamine. Nevertheless, studies by Kudrow showed that ergotamine by mouth can be effective in producing pain relief in approximately 10 minutes. The dosage guidelines for ergotamine in cluster headache are similar to those for migraine.

    c. **DHE** given as a subcutaneous or intramuscular injection can produce good relief of cluster headache. Onset of action is within 5 to 10 minutes of administration with a dosage of 1 mg intramuscularly.

    d. **Oxygen** delivered with a mask at a rate of 2 to 3 L/min can produce good relief from cluster headache with onset of effect in a few minutes. Typically, the patient must continue oxygen administration for 15 to 30 minutes. In a large number of patients, the headache recurs soon after oxygen administration is discontinued.

B. **Prophylactic therapy** for cluster headache often is preferable. Because of the stereotyped nature of the headache, its tendency to occur in cycles, and the frequency of headaches during the cycles, patients usually prefer a preventive approach if possible.

1. **Steroids.** Corticosteroids are highly effective in temporary prophylaxis of cluster headache. The most commonly used steroid preparation is prednisone, although equipotent dosages of other corticosteroid preparations have the same degree of activity. For this reason, the recommendations are given in terms of dosage of prednisone.

   The doses of prednisone reported to be effective in cluster headache vary from 10 to 100 mg/d. Typically, a higher dose of 60 to 100 mg is needed to initiate steroid therapy. This dose is maintained for 2 to 3 days or until the cluster headache remits (maximum 7 days). The steroids are then tapered over 1 to 2 weeks. As steroid dosage is tapered, it is common for the cluster headaches to recur below doses of or equivalent to 15 to 20 mg of prednisone per day. As a result, steroids usually are best used for temporary prophylaxis and for gaining control of the cluster headache. Verapamil, methysergide, or another preventative medication is used for longer-term prophylaxis, usually the approximate duration of the usual cluster headache cycle.

   Steroids may not be used for prolonged periods without risk of significant side effects. The side effects, well known to physicians, include increased fragility of blood vessels and skin, osteoporosis, aseptic necrosis of the head of the femur, obesity, myopathy, and psychosis.

2. **Methysergide** was the first medication to demonstrate a prophylactic effect among patients with cluster headache. Kunkel, when reporting on this treatment in 1952, wrote that 70% of patients responded well in the first cycle or cluster treated, 48% of the group responded the second time, and 25% responded the third time. Although there have been few formal studies, my experience has been similar to that of Kunkel. Doses of methysergide vary from 4 to 8 mg/d. Side effects of methysergide are outlined in **I.B.4.f.**

3. **Calcium channel blocking agents.** Verapamil, a calcium channel blocking agent, has been shown to have a prophylactic effect in cluster headache. Because of the lower incidence of side effects, it has become the preferred agent for prophylaxis. Doses of verapamil vary from 120 to 960 mg/d depending on the patient and whether the patient has side effects of bradycardia, hypotension, or constipation. The results with verapamil are generally similar to those of methysergide, with a tendency for subsequent cycles of therapy to diminish in effectiveness. Verapamil should not be used if the patient had sick sinus syndrome, atrioventricular block, or Wolff–Parkinson–White syndrome if there is left ventricular failure.

4. **Combined therapy.** A therapeutic approach combining steroids and either verapamil or methysergide has provided good results in my experience. The patient typically is treated with prednisone at 60 to 100 mg/d for 3 days with a rapid taper of 20 mg every 2 days until the prednisone is discontinued. At the same time that prednisone is started, the patient starts taking verapamil at a dosage of 80 mg three times a day or methysergide 2 mg two or three times a day. The verapamil or methysergide is then continued for 60 to 90 days. This combined therapy has achieved good results in 70% to 80% of first-time trials. In therapy for subsequent cycles, however, the effectiveness of verapamil and methysergide may diminish, as indicated in **II.B.2. and 3.**

   There are several reports of use of divalproex or topiramate to treat patients with cluster headache. More work has to be done but my anecdotal experience has not been very favorable.

   The routine medications for prevention of migraine headache are relatively ineffective for cluster headache. Relatively poor results are obtained with β-adrenergic blocking agents, TCAs, cyproheptadine, or clonidine.

III. **Chronic cluster headache**

   A. **Medications.** Chronic cluster headache is a very difficult problem. This refers to typical cluster headaches whose cycle lasts longer than 6 months without remission. The headaches may occur from several per week to several per day. Lithium has been reported to be effective in several studies. The typical dose is

600 to 1,200 mg/d to control the blood level at 0.6 to 1.2 mEq/L. The usual signs of lithium toxicity include confusion, disorientation, drowsiness, seizures, thirst, and rashes. Patients should be warned about, and observed for development of, these side effects. Blood levels should be monitored if lithium is to be used. When lithium is successful, tachyphylaxis often develops over time. When this occurs, it is necessary to discontinue the lithium and restart it after 4 to 6 weeks to restore responsiveness.

Combinations of steroids with either verapamil or methysergide, and occasionally TCAs or MAOIs, may be beneficial in managing chronic cluster headache.

   B. **Surgical therapy.** For patients who have chronic cluster headaches that do not respond to any medical therapy, surgery on the trigeminal nerve has been somewhat effective. Two procedures have been prescribed—trigeminal gangliotomy by radiofrequency lesioning and preganglionic nerve-root section. Both of these procedures produce numbness and diminished sensation in the distribution of the trigeminal nerve. Patients who have undergone these procedures often find that they still have sensations as if they were having cluster headaches but no longer have the pain. To date, no serious complications have occurred in the small series recorded. Longer-term follow-up data are still inadequate to determine whether these procedures will produce long-term relief.

IV. **Tension-type headache and chronic daily headache**
   A. **Acute intermittent tension-type headache.** For acute, intermittent tension-type headache, use of an analgesic or NSAID such as ibuprofen, naproxen, or acetaminophen usually suffices. For more intense tension headaches, a combination of butalbital (50 mg) and an analgesic such as aspirin (Fiorinal; Novartis, East Hanover, NJ, U.S.A.) or acetaminophen (Fioricet; Novartis) may be very helpful. At times, addition of a muscle relaxant in a low dosage, such as 2 mg of diazepam or 50 mg of orphenadrine may be helpful. Very often, however, a patient with pure tension headache does not see a physician for medication unless the tension headache becomes severe or develops into a migraine. Use of butalbital compounds or benzodiazepines must be undertaken with great care. These are potentially habituating compounds and can easily be overused. Overuse leads to a drug-induced rebound–withdrawal headache.
   B. **Chronic tension-type headache**
      1. **Chronic daily headache with migraine and tension features.** For chronic tension headache, a different situation exists. Chronic tension headaches typically have combined symptoms of tension and migraine headaches and fit into the category of combination tension–migraine or mixed chronic daily headache, or transformed migraine. This is the most common and most treatable type of chronic daily headache. The first-approach therapy typically is to use tricyclic antidepressant agents. Any of the other preventive antimigraine agents also can be used. The antimigraine, anticonvulsant agents, divalproex, gabapentin, and topiramate have been used frequently. Not infrequently, therapies combining a TCA with one of the other medications may be attempted, although there are relatively few standard data on response to these combination regimens. For this type of patient, it is necessary to limit access to habituating medication. Because of the chronicity of the pain problem, patients are likely to overuse medications that are potentially habituating. This overuse can lead to a rebound–withdrawal (habituation–withdrawal) type of headache. In these situations, the medication becomes part of the problem instead of part of the solution.
      2. **Pure chronic tension-type headache** with no associated migrainous features of photophobia, phonophobia, nausea, vomiting, diarrhea, or neurologic symptoms. These patients typically have a continuous mild-to-moderate headache that is worrisome, nagging, and uncomfortable but does not limit activity. Some patients with pure chronic tension-type headache may respond to the preventative antimigraine agents but usually do not. Tizanidine in a dose of 8–24 mg/d may be helpful to some patients. A four times a day schedule usually is used. Physical measures such as biofeedback or physical therapy may work occasionally. Studies are in progress to evaluate botulinum toxin injections, but it is too early to predict success here.

V. Guidelines for referring patients with headaches. Many headache patients are treated capably by primary care physicians, but additional opinions and specialized care sometimes are needed. One of the questions often asked is when a patient should be referred to a headache specialist. Situations that may require referral include the following:

1. New, unexplained headache
2. New, unexplained neurologic findings
3. Poor response to the treatments with which the physician is comfortable
4. A situation in which the referring physician is uncomfortable with the patient for medical or psychological reasons
5. Presence of comorbid medical or psychiatric conditions for which therapy is beyond the physician's expertise

The first area of consideration is a new, unexplained headache. If the patient has a headache that is severe enough to cause continual problems and the treating physician is unable to find an adequate cause, the patient probably should be referred to a specialist with greater knowledge of headaches.

If the patient has new and progressive neurologic findings that cannot be explained with results of available tests and with insight, the patient should be seen by a headache specialist.

The third situation deals with treatment of the headache. If the primary physician is unable to provide the patient with adequate relief, referral should be considered. If the pain can be relieved only by increasing the dose of an analgesic or narcotic medication and the possibility looms that the patient may have habituation–withdrawal headache in response to that medication, the patient should be referred.

If the physician simply feels uncomfortable with the situation and believes that his or her skills may be inadequate to help the patient, referral is advised. The difficult headache patient usually has a very chronic pain problem, which can be exacerbated by psychological factors. If the patient is manifesting a marked degree of chronicity and if communication and trust between the patient and the physician begin to break down, referral is indicated.

Patients with chronic diseases often "doctor shop" to see whether another physician can provide a better level of treatment. If a patient asks for a referral, it is best to proceed with the referral. The patient will respect the physician for assisting him or her in continuing the search for pain relief. The physician's ready agreement to refer the patient demonstrates to the patient that the physician's first concern is the patient's well-being.

There are several specialized headache centers throughout the country. The American Headache Society and the American Council of Headache Education can provide patients with information about these centers. The address for both organizations is 19 Mantua Rd, Mt. Royal, NJ 08061.

Recommended Readings

Belgrade MJ, Ling LJ, Schleevogt MB, et al. Comparison of single-dose meperidine, butorphanol, and dihydro-ergotamine in the treatment of vascular headache. *Neurology* 1989;39: 590–592.

Burstein R, Yarnitsky D, Goor-Aryeh I, et al. An association between migraine and cutaneous allodynia. *Ann Neurol* 2000;47:614–624.

Cady RK, Lipton RB, Hall C, et al. Treatment of mild headache in disabled migraine sufferers: results of the SPECTRUM study. *Headache* 2000;40:792–797.

Callahan M, Raskin N. A controlled study of dihydroergotamine in the treatment of acute migraine headache. *Headache* 1986;26:168–171.

Couch J. Cluster headache: characteristics and treatment. *Semin Neurol* 1982;2:30–40.

Couch J. Medical management of recurrent tension-type headache. In: Tollison CD, Kunkel RS, eds. *Headache diagnosis and treatment.* Baltimore: Williams & Wilkins, 1993:151–162.

Couch J. Complexities of presentation and pathogenesis of migraine headache. In: Cady RK, Fox AW, eds. *Treating the headache patient.* New York: Marcel Dekker, 1995:15–40.

Couch J, Hassanein RS. Amitriptyline in migraine prophylaxis. *Arch Neurol* 1979;36: 695–699.

Couch J, Micieli G. Prophylactic pharmacotherapy. In: Olesen J, Tfelt-Hansen P, Welch KMA, eds. *The headaches.* New York: Raven Press, 1993:537–542.

Edmeads J, Johnson FN. The adverse event and tolerability profile of zolmitriptan. *Rev Contemp Pharmacother* 2000;11:119–132.

Ferrari MD, Saxena PR. Clinical and experimental effects of sumatriptan in humans. *Trends Pharmacol Sci* 1993;14:129–133.

Goadsby PJ. Serotonin receptor agonists in migraine. *CNS Drugs* 1998;10:271–286.

Goadsby PJ, Lipton RB. Newer triptans: emphasis on rizatriptan. Neurology. 2000;55 [Suppl 2]:S8–S14.

Goadsby PJ, Peatfield R. Zolmitriptan in the acute treatment of migraine: an overview. Rev. Contemp Pharmacother. 2000;11:91–97.

Hargreaves RJ, Shepheard SL. Pathophysiology of migraine: new insights. *Can J Neurol Sci* 1999;26[Suppl3]:S12–S19.

Hoffert MJ, Couch JR, Diamond S, et al. Transnasal butorphanol in the treatment of acute migraine. *Headache* 1994;35:65–69.

Humphrey PPA, Feniuk W. Mode of action of the anti-migraine-drug sumatriptan. *Trends Pharmacol Sci* 1991;12:444–445.

Kudrow L. Plasma testosterone levels in cluster headache: preliminary results. *Headache* 1976;16:28–31.

Kunkle EC, Pfeiffer JB Jr, Wilhoit WH, et al. Recurrent brief headache in "cluster" pattern. *Trans Am Neurol Assoc* 1952;77:240–243.

Lipton RB, Stewart WF, Cady R, et al. Sumatriptan for the range of headaches in migraine sufferers: results of the SPECTRUM. *Headache* 2000;40:783–791.

Lipton RB, Stewart WF, Stone AM, et al. Stratified care vs step care strategies for migraine. *JAMA* 2000;284:2599–2065.

Lovshin L. Treatment of histaminic cephalgia with methysergide (UML-491). *Dis Nerv Syst* 1963;24:3–7.

Mathew N. Clinical subtypes of cluster headache and response to lithium therapy. *Headache* 1978;18:26–30.

Mathew NI, Saper JR, Silberstein SD, et al. Migraine prophylaxis with divalproex. *Arch Neurol* 1995;52:281–286.

Moskowitz MA. Neurogenic versus vascular mechanisms of sumatriptan and ergot alkaloids in migraine. *Trends Pharmacol Sci* 1992;13:307–311.

Nappi G, Johnson FN. The clinical efficacy of zolmitriptan. *Rev Contemp Pharmacother* 2000; 11:99–118.

Silberstein SD. The pharmacology of ergotamine and dihydroergotamine. *Headache* 1997; 37[Suppl]:S15–S25.

Silberstein SD. Practice parameter: evidence-based guidelines for migraine headache (an evidence-based review). *Neurology* 2000;55:754–762.

Silberstein SD, Young WB. Safety and efficacy of ergotamine tartrate and dihydroergotamine in the treatment of migraine and status migrainosus. *Neurology* 1995;45:577–584.

Storer RJ, Goadsby PG. Microiontophoretic application of serotonin agonists inhibits trigeminal cell firing in the cat. *Brain* 1997;37:2253–2257.

Subcutaneous Sumatriptan International Study Group. Treatment of migraine attacks with sumatriptan. *N Engl J Med* 1991;325:316–321.

Tfelt-Hansen P, Johnson ES. Nonsteroidal anti-inflammatory drugs in the treatment of the acute migraine attack. In: Olesen J, Tfelt-Hansen P, Welch KMA, eds. *The headaches*. New York: Raven Press, 1993:305–311.

Tfelt-Hansen P, Teall J, Rodriquez F, et al. Oral rizatriptan versus oral sumatriptan: a direct comparative study in the acute treatment of migraine. *Headache* 1998;38:748–755.

Weiller C, May A, Limmroth V, et al. Brain stem activation in spontaneous human migraine attacks. *Nature Med* 1995;1:658–660.

Williamson DJ, Hargreaves RJ, Hill RG, et al. Intravital microscope studies on the effects of neurokinin agonists and calcitonin gene-related peptide on dural vessel diameter in the anesthetized rat. *Cephalalgia* 1997;17:518–524.

Young WB, Mannix L, Adelman JU, et al. Cardiac risk factors and the use of triptans: a survey study. *Headache* 2000;40:587–591.

50. CHRONIC PAIN

Bette G. Maybury

Chronic pain has been described by various pain authorities as pain lasting longer than 1, 3, or 6 months or pain that persists past the "usual" time for a given disorder to heal. Certain chronic or degenerative diseases by their very nature include chronic pain as part of the illness. The International Association for the Study of Pain defines chronic pain as pain that is present for 3 months. Chronic pain is a serious health problem. It contributes to physical, psychological, and psychosocial impairment at great cost to patients, their families, and society. This chapter discusses management of types of pain in general terms.

I. **Types of chronic pain**
   A. **Neuropathic pain**
      1. **Symptoms.** Neuropathic pain may have more than one aspect in a given person. Characteristics frequently described include burning, ripping, throbbing, aching, squeezing, prickling, lancinating, shocklike, or jabbing. The painful symptoms may be associated with numbness, weakness and atrophy, fasciculations, and muscle cramps. Restless leg occurs with some types of neuropathic pain.
      2. **Etiology**
         a. **Polyneuropathy** (see Chapter 46, II.)
            (1) Metabolic, such as diabetes mellitus or uremia
            (2) Nutritional, such as vitamin deficiency, alcoholism
            (3) Toxic, such as heavy metals, organic compounds, medications
            (4) Vasculitic or inflammatory, such as rheumatoid arthritis, systemic lupus erythematosus, Guillain–Barré syndrome, chronic inflammatory demyelinating polyneuropathy
            (5) Infectious, such as human immunodeficiency virus infection
            (6) Malignant, such as paraneoplastic disorders
            (7) Inherited, such as hereditary sensory motor neuropathy, such as Fabry's disease
            (8) Ischemic e.g., Peripheral vascular disease.
            (9) Idiopathic
         b. **Mononeuropathies/mononeuropathy multiplex**
            (1) Metabolic, such as diabetic amyotrophy.
            (2) Vasculitic or inflammatory, such as collagen vascular disease, polyarteritis nodosa, sarcoidosis
            (3) Infectious, such as herpes zoster, infectious mononucleosis, leprosy
            (4) Malignant, such as direct or metastatic invasion
            (5) Traumatic, surgical
            (6) Idiopathic
   B. **Musculoskeletal pain**
      1. **Symptoms.** Musculoskeletal pain can include deep or superficial aching, throbbing, burning, or tenderness, which can be diffuse or local. The pain frequently is associated with muscle spasms, stiffness, and decreased range of motion.
      2. **Etiology**
         a. Arthritis
         b. Fibromyalgia and myofascial pain
         c. Myopathy
         d. Trauma, aftermath of surgical procedure
         e. Metabolic bone or muscle disease
   C. **Psychological and psychosocial pain.** Depression, anxiety, and insomnia frequently accompany chronic pain. Patients may markedly decrease physical activity or withdraw socially. Treatment to reverse or diminish these symptoms and behaviors is imperative to prevent a vicious circle of increasing pain, dysfunction, and impairment. For some patients, psychological or psychosocial dysfunction may be the primary cause of the chronic pain rather than a secondary

condition. In either situation, a formal psychological or psychiatric evaluation and ongoing treatment can be helpful. Most patients are amenable to this recommendation if approached in a positive manner. Acknowledgment by the primary physician that psychological and emotional stress is to be expected with chronic pain allows the patient to accept intervention to improve coping with the illness.

II. Management of chronic pain
A. Removal of causative agent or management of underlying disease
B. Medications
1. **Opioids** (Table 50.1). If possible, opioids should be avoided in the management of benign chronic pain. In reality, they sometimes are necessary. Guidelines include use of the following:
   a. Preparations with least abuse potential and least side effects; oral dosage if possible. Long-acting agents are best.
   b. Lowest dose needed for analgesia (concomitant use of a nonsteroidal antiinflammatory drug [NSAID] often greatly potentiates efficacy)
   c. Scheduled doses with monitoring for abuse, such as multiple pharmacies or physicians
   d. Therapy for side effects such as constipation or nausea The opioid medications exert their effect by interaction with several types of opioid receptors in both the peripheral and the central nervous system. They not only produce analgesia but also may have side effects of sedation, respiratory depression, nausea, cognitive impairment, pruritus, dizziness, hypotension, constipation, and urinary retention. Avoid concomitant use of pure opioid agonist and agonist–antagonist medications or use of agonist–antagonist after long-term use of a pure agonist.
2. **NSAIDs** (Table 50.2) are thought to produce their analgesic and antiinflammatory effects through inhibition of prostaglandin production. Other nonprostaglandin effects are likely, and central effects have been postulated as well. Use of a given NSAID should be dictated by patient response in regard to efficacy and side effects. Sequential trials of different medications are warranted because effectiveness varies from one person to another. Medication trials should last approximately 4 weeks unless side effects intervene. NSAIDs should be taken with food. Side effects include heartburn,

Table 50.1 Equivalent opioid dosages

Medication	Dose (mg)	
	Intramuscular	Oral
PURE AGONISTS		
Morphine	10	30
Codeine	130	200
Hydrocodone	—	5–10
Hydromorphone	1.5	7.5
Meperidine	100	300
Methadone	1	3
Oxycodone	—	30
Propoxyphene hydrochloride	—	300
Propoxyphene napsylate	—	400
Fentanyl transdermal	25 µg/h = 45 mg morphine sustained release	
AGONISTS–ANTAGONISTS		
Butorphanol	2	2 (nasal spray)
Pentazocine	60	180[a]

[a] Oral analgesia is weak and unpredictable.

Table 50.2 Nonsteroidal antiinflammatory drug daily dosages

Medication	Maximum daily dose (mg)	Dosing schedule
Acetylsalicylic acid	6,000	q.i.d.
Celecoxib	400	b.i.d.
Choline magnesium trisalicylate	6,000	q.d.–b.i.d.
Diclofenac	200	t.i.d.
Diflunisal	1,500	b.i.d.
Etodolac	1,200[a]	t.i.d.
Fenoprofen	3,200	q.i.d.
Flurbiprofen	300	t.i.d.
Ibuprofen	3,200	q.i.d.
Indomethacin	200	t.i.d.
Ketoprofen	300	t.i.d.
Meclofenamate	400	b.i.d.
Meloxicam	15	q.d.
Nabumetone	2,000	q.d.–b.i.d.
Naprozen, naprozen sodium	1,500/1,375	b.i.d.
Oxaprozin	1,200	q.d.
Piroxicam	20	q.d.
Rofecoxib	50	q.d.–b.i.d.
Sulindac	400	b.i.d.
Tolmetin	2,000	q.i.d.
Ketorolac[b]	40	q.i.d.

[a] For patients weighing 60 kg or less, maximum dosage is 20 mg/kg.
[b] Not recommended for continuous long-term use.
q.i.d., four times a day; b.i.d., twice a day; q.d.–b.i.d., once or twice a day; t.i.d., three times a day; q.d., every day.

bloating, flatulence, diarrhea, gastric ulceration and bleeding, hepatic and renal dysfunction, and inhibition of platelet aggregation.

3. **Antidepressants** (Table 50.3). Use of antidepressants as pain medication should be explained to the patient to avert suspicion that "the doctor just thinks I'm depressed." The mechanism of action of pain medication is unknown but is likely multifactorial, such as decreased synaptic transmission, potentiation of endogenous opioids, improved sleep, and antidepressant effect. In general, lower doses are needed for management of pain than for management of depression. Begin with a low dose (e.g., a tricyclic at 10 to 25 mg) and titrate upward as needed and tolerated. Side effects include sedation, dry mouth, constipation, orthostatic hypotension, urinary retention, dizziness, confusion, and weight gain. Use of antidepressants can unmask latent mania in persons with bipolar disorder. Amitriptyline sometimes paradoxically causes agitation rather than sedation. Substituting doxepin may circumvent this problem. Concomitant use of monoamine oxidase inhibitors with antidepressants should be avoided.

4. **Anticonvulsants** (Table 50.4). The mechanism of action of anticonvulsants probably is decreased synaptic transmission. Various mechanisms may include ion channel blocking, increase in inhibitory neurotransmitters, and decrease in excitatory neurotransmitters. These are the most useful medications for lancinating, jabbing pain. Side effects include sedation, nausea, dizziness, ataxia, and diplopia. Bone marrow suppression and hepatic dysfunction occur rarely. Development of generalized rash necessitates immediate discontinuation. Complete blood cell count with differential, platelet count, and liver enzyme levels should be monitored at intervals. A modest, but stable, elevation of γ-glutamyl transferase level may occur and is no cause for concern.

Table 50.3 Antidepressant daily dosages

	Dosage (mg)	
Medication	As a pain reliever	As an antidepressant
More Sedating		
Amitriptyline	10–150 q.h.s.	150–250 q.h.s.
Doxepin	10–150 q.h.s.	150–250 q.h.s.
Imipramine	10–150 q.h.s.	150–250 q.h.s.
Trazodone[a]	25–300 q.h.s.	200–400 q.h.s.
Less Sedating		
Buproprion[a]	75–150 b.i.d.	75–150 b.i.d.
Desipramine[a]	10–100 q.a.m.	100–250 q.a.m.
Nortriptyline	10–75 q.h.s.	75–100 q.h.s.
Protriptyline[a]	5–10 t.i.d.–q.i.d.	5–10 t.i.d.–q.i.d.
Newer Agents		
Citalopram (SSRI)	Insufficient data	20–40 q.d.
Fluoxetine (SSRI)	Insufficient data	20–60 q.d.
Fluvoxamine (SSRI)	Insufficient data	150 b.i.d.
Mirtazapine[b]	Insufficient data	15–45 q.d.
Nefazodone	Insufficient data	100–300 q.d.
Paroxetine (SSRI)	Insufficient data	20–40 q.d.
Sertraline (SSRI)	Insufficient data	50–200 q.d.
Venlafaxine	Insufficient data	25–75 t.i.d.

[a] Less anticholinergic.
[b] Rare agranulocytosis.
q.h.s., at bedtime; b.i.d., twice a day; q.a.m., every morning; t.i.d., three times a day; q.i.d., four times a day; q.d., every day; SSRI, selective serotonin reuptake inhibitor.

a. **Phenytoin.** Start with 300 mg daily with further increases as needed and tolerated. Steady-state blood levels may take as long as 2 weeks to be reached. Loading may be accomplished by giving 1,000 mg orally in divided doses over 12 to 24 hours. Unique side effects include gingival hyperplasia, hirsutism, and acne. Lymphadenopathy, fever, and arthralgia occur rarely. Late complications are uncommon but can include peripheral neuropathy, osteoporosis, and cerebellar atrophy. Supplementation with calcium and vitamin B are recommended for long-term use.

b. **Carbamazepine.** Start with 100 mg twice a day and increase the daily dose 100 mg every 3 days up to 200 mg three times a day or until relief of symptoms or occurrence of side effects. Leukopenia is common but

Table 50.4 Anticonvulsant daily dosages

Medication	Dose (mg)	Dosing schedule
Carbamazepine	200–600	t.i.d.
Gabapentin	300–3,600	t.i.d.
Lamotrigine	100–600	b.i.d.
Oxcarbazepine	300–1,200	b.i.d.
Phenytoin	300–400	b.i.d.
Sodium valproate	250–1,000	b.i.d.–t.i.d.
Topiramate	30–400	b.i.d.

t.i.d., three times a day; b.i.d., twice a day.

white blood cell counts as low as 2,500/μL with absolute granulocyte count greater than 1,000 per μL are acceptable. Hyponatremia can develop and limit use. Concomitant use of propoxyphene, erythromycin, or cimetidine markedly increases carbamazepine level.

c. **Sodium valproate.** Start with 125 to 250 mg twice a day and increase the daily dose 125 mg every 3 to 4 days to symptom relief or side effects. If gastrointestinal side effects are troublesome at the lowest dose, use of 125-mg sprinkles may circumvent the problem. Addition of baclofen may augment effectiveness. Weight gain and peripheral edema are relatively common side effects. At higher doses, tremor or hair loss may develop. Thrombocytopenia is not uncommon and is dose related, usually resolving with decreases in dose.

d. **Gabapentin.** Start with 300 mg daily and increase to 300 mg two or three times a day as needed and tolerated. Further increases to as much as 1,600 mg three times a day may be helpful. Side effects are uncommon and include sedation, dizziness, weight gain, and ataxia. The first three can be minimized by slower increases in dose. If necessary, 100-mg capsules are available to start at lower dose. Because gabapentin has low protein binding and renal clearance, it has fewer drug interactions than do other anticonvulsants. It is particularly effective for sympathetic nervous system–mediated pain (reflex sympathetic dystrophy or complex regional pain syndrome type I).

e. **Lamotrigine.** Start with 25 to 50 mg daily for 2 weeks and increase to 25 to 50 mg twice a day for another 2 weeks. Thereafter increase the daily dose 50 to 100 mg weekly. If lamotrigine is used concomitantly with valproic acid, decrease the dose with slower titration (25 mg every other day for 2 weeks, 25 mg a day for 2 weeks, then weekly 25-mg to 50-mg increases in daily dose to a maximum of 150 mg daily). A serious rash necessitating hospitalization can develop. There have been rare deaths due to Stevens–Johnson syndrome or toxic epidermal necrolysis. If a rash develops, prompt discontinuation is recommended. Other side effects include cognitive and behavioral changes, dizziness, and imbalance.

f. **Topiramate.** Start with 15 to 25 mg daily and increase the daily dose 15 to 25 weekly. Side effects include psychomotor slowing, word-finding difficulty, mood disturbance, sedation, fatigue, dizziness, and imbalance. Low dosing and slow titration decrease the likelihood of side effects. Weight loss is common. The risk of kidney stones increases twofold to fourfold. Increased fluid intake is recommended, and concomitant use of carbonic anhydrase inhibitors should be avoided.

g. **Oxcarbazepine.** Start with 150 mg twice a day and increase the dose to 300 mg twice a day after 1 week. Thereafter the daily dose can be increased 600 mg on a weekly basis. Side effects include psychomotor slowing, sedation, fatigue, dizziness, and ataxia. Hyponatremia may develop.

5. **Neuroleptic agents** (Table 50.5). In addition to central effects, neuroleptics are believed to decrease peripheral sensory transmission. Many practitioners prefer to avoid neuroleptics because of the danger of tardive dyskinesia with long-term use. The lower doses used for pain treatment make this less likely but do not guarantee tardive dyskinesia will not develop. Elderly patients are at higher risk. Other side effects include parkinsonian symptoms, dystonia, cognitive impairment, sedation, and orthostatic hypotension. Neuroleptics can cause myocardial depression and potentiate cardiac arrhythmias in susceptible patients. Less common are bone marrow suppression, hepatic toxicity, and neuroleptic malignant syndrome. In general, the atypical neuroleptics are associated with fewer side effects and appear less likely to cause tardive dyskinesia. Medication for extrapyramidal side effects should be used only if the symptoms occur. Diphenhydramine 10 to 25 mg three times a day has fewer anticholinergic side effects than does benztropine 1 to 6 mg daily or trihexyphenidyl 2 to 10 mg daily.

Table 50.5 Neuroleptic daily dosages

Medication	Dose (mg)	Dosing schedule
Dopamine Antagonists		
Chlorpromazine	10–50	q.h.s.
Fluphenazine	1–3	q.h.s.
Haloperidol	1–3	q.h.s.
Perphenazine	1–5	q.h.s.
Thioridazine	10–75	q.h.s.
Trifluoperazine	1–5	q.h.s.
Serotonin–Dopamine Antagonists (Atypical Neuroleptics)		
Clozapine[a]	12.5	q.h.s.
Olanzapine	2.5	q.h.s.
Quetiapine	2.5	q.h.s.
Risperidone	0.25	q.h.s.

[a] Risk of agranulocytosis and seizures.
q.h.s., at bedtime.

6. **Anxiolytic agents** (Table 50.6). Anxiety frequently accompanies chronic pain and must be managed to achieve optimum pain relief. Anxiolytic treatment decreases the need for escalating doses of other medications. Long-term use of benzodiazepines should be avoided if possible. Benzodiazepines may be needed in the acute phase until serotonergic medication takes effect. If benzodiazepines are needed long term, long-acting agents such as clonazepam are preferred. Side effects of benzodiazepines include sedation and cognitive impairment, and there is risk of abuse. Physical dependence occurs, and medication must be discontinued gradually to avoid excessive dysphoria and possible seizures.

7. **Muscle relaxants** (Table 50.7) are most suited for short-term use. They may be more effective for chronic pain if used intermittently. Both baclofen

Table 50.6 Anxiolytic daily dosages

Medication	Dose (mg)	Dosing schedule
Benzodiazepines		
Alprazolam	0.5–3	b.i.d.–t.i.d.
Chlordiazepoxide	15–30	t.i.d.
Clonazepam	0.25–0.5	b.i.d.
Clorazepate	7.5–30	b.i.d.
Diazepam	4–40	b.i.d.–q.i.d.
Lorazepam	1–6	b.i.d.–t.i.d.
Oxazepam	10–15	q.d.
Nonbenzodiazepines		
Buspirone[a]	15–60	b.i.d.
Fluoxetine[a]	10–40	q.a.m.
Hydroxyzine	100–400	q.i.d.
Paroxetine[a]	20–40	q.p.m.
Venlafaxine[a]	75–225	t.i.d.

[a] Avoid concomitant use of monoamine oxidase inhibitors.
b.i.d., twice a day; t.i.d., three times a day; q.i.d., four times a day; q.d., every day; q.a.m., every morning; q.p.m., every evening.

Table 50.7 Muscle relaxant daily dosages

Medication	Dose (mg)	Dosing schedule
Baclofen	60–80[a]	t.i.d.–q.i.d.
Carisoprodol	1,050–1,400	t.i.d.–q.i.d.
Cyclobenzaprine	20–40	b.i.d.–t.i.d.
Diazepam	6–40	t.i.d.–q.i.d.
Metaxalone	2,400–3,200	t.i.d.–q.i.d.
Methocarbamol	4,000–4,500	t.i.d.–q.i.d.
Orphenadrine	200	b.i.d.

[a] Start with 5 mg b.i.d. and titrate upward.
t.i.d., three times a day; q.i.d., four times a day; b.i.d., twice a day.

and diazepam must be discontinued slowly from high doses. Sedation is a common side effect and can limit use. A bedtime dose only sometimes is helpful, particularly in the care of patients with primarily nocturnal muscle spasm or morning muscle stiffness and difficulty sleeping.

   8. Other agents
   a. Quinine sulfate 300 mg at bedtime for cramps and restless legs
   b. Lidocaine 5% patch
   c. Carbidopa/levodopa 12.5/50 to 25/100 mg for cramps and restless legs
   d. Clonidine 0.1 mg/d has intrinsic analgesic effect and potentiates opioids both endogenous and exogenous.
   e. Capsaicin 0.025% to 0.075% topical cream applied to affected area three or four times a day. Mechanism is thought to be depletion of substance P. Expect initial increase in pain for 2 to 4 weeks as substance P is released. If the agent is discontinued, substance P reaccumulates. and pain recurs.
   f. Calcium channel blockers may be effective for metabolic myopathy and sympathetic mediated pain.
      (1) Verapamil 40 to 160 mg three times a day
      (2) Nifedipine 10 to 30 mg three times a day
   h. Mexiletine 100 to 300 mg three times a day
   9. Nerve or trigger point anesthetic blockade
C. Nonpharmacologic modalities
   1. Physical and occupational therapy. Massage, heat and cold, ultrasound, exercise, and bracing
   2. Electrical stimulation. Transcutaneous electrical nerve stimulation (TENS), dorsal column or thalamic stimulators. The classic proposed mechanism of action of TENS is that large-fiber stimulation closes a sensory "gate" opened by excessive firing of small, pain-carrying fibers. TENS is a noninvasive but relatively expensive modality. Application of electrodes by an experienced practitioner for optimum effect increases the likelihood of success. Contraindications include use of a cardiac pacemaker, pregnancy, and patient inability to properly use the device.
   3. Psychological intervention
      a. Personal or family counseling or both
      b. Behavior modification
      c. Biofeedback or relaxation training or both
         An important aspect of the management of chronic pain is prevention, if possible. This includes thorough evaluation, avoidance of unnecessary surgery, and aggressive management of acute pain. Once chronic pain is established, multiple strategies should be used, if needed, to promote the best patient outcome.
III. Referrals. Consider referral to an anesthesiologist experienced in pain management for trigger-point injection or peripheral nerve, epidural, or sympathetic blockade. Referral to a psychiatrist or psychologist experienced in pain management is indicated for patients

with prominent symptoms in this area that require more counseling or support than can be provided in a general practice setting. It is also warranted for patients who do not respond well to psychotropic medications. A physiatrist can be helpful in the management of musculoskeletal pain, which can accompany neurologic disease or injury that results in weakness with resultant strain on compensating muscles. If a patient remains disabled and dysfunctional, referral to a multidisciplinary pain center should be considered.

Recommended Readings

Loeser JD, Butler SH, Chapman CR, et al., eds. *Bonica's management of pain.* Philadelphia: Lippincott Williams & Wilkins, 2001.

Cailliet R. Pain: mechanisms and management. Philadelphia: FA Davis Co, 1993.

Kaplan HI, Sadock BJ. Synopsis of psychiatry. Baltimore: William & Wilkins, 1997.

Tollison CD, Satterthwaite JR, Tollison JW, eds. Handbook of pain management. Philadelphia: Lippincott Williams & Wilkins, 2001.

Warfield CA, Fausett HJ, eds. Manual of pain management. Philadelphia: Lippincott Williams & Wilkins, 2001.

Warfield CA., ed. Principles and practice of pain management. New York: McGraw-Hill, 1993.

51. COMPLEX REGIONAL PAIN SYNDROME

R. Venkata Reddy

The nomenclature for the pain syndromes commonly called **reflex sympathetic dystrophy** or **causalgia** has changed because not all patients seem to have sympathetically maintained pain and not all have dystrophy. A recent taxonomy developed by the International Association for the Study of Pain (IASP) suggested the terms **complex regional pain syndrome** type I (CRPS type I) for reflex sympathetic dystrophy and CRPS type II for causalgia. The sole differentiating criterion between CRPS type I and type II is the presence of a known nerve injury in CRPS type II. According to the IASP, CPRS type I is a syndrome that usually develops after an initiating noxious event, is not limited to the distribution of a single nerve, and is apparently disproportionate to the inciting event. It is associated at some point with evidence of edema, changes in skin blood flow, abnormal sudomotor activity in the region of the pain, or allodynia (pain caused by a stimulus that normally does not provoke pain), or hyperalgesia (an exaggerated response to a stimulus that is normally painful). CRPS type I is associated with a variety of precipitating factors (Table 51.1). Trauma is the most common precipitating event in the development of CRPS type I, an estimated 5% of traumatic cases resulting in CRPS type I.

I. **Pathophysiology.** The pathophysiologic mechanism is unknown. Various hypotheses put forth over the years include peripheral mechanisms, central mechanisms, or psychogenic factors.
   A. **Peripheral mechanisms** do not address the issues of spread of pain beyond a dermatomal territory and pain occurring in patients without nerve injury. They are of four types.
      1. After an inciting event, a subset of **C-polymodal nociceptors** develop sensitivity to sympathetic stimulation and thus may be stimulated by noradrenalin. An alternative explanation is that noradrenalin may act indirectly through release of prostaglandins, which stimulate the nociceptors.
      2. Sympathetic efferents cause abnormal activation of peripheral nociceptors.
      3. Aberrant nerve sprouts are generated at the site of injury and develop into neuromas.
      4. Artificial synapses form at the site of nerve injury and allow "ephaptic" transmission between sympathetic efferent and sensory afferent fibers.
   B. **Central mechanisms** are of two types.
      1. Self-sustaining loops of abnormal interneuronal firing in the dorsal horn, after being propagated by a peripheral irritative focus, giving rise to ascending projections of pain and descending sympathetic hyperactivity
      2. Long-term sensitization or "wind-up" of wide-dynamic-range neurons in the spinal cord resulting from ongoing nociceptive stimulation from the periphery. The sensitized wide-dynamic-range neurons then respond to activity in large diameter A-mechanoreceptors, which are activated by light touch. The pain threshold is reduced and previously subthreshold stimuli are then perceived as painful.
   C. **Psychogenic factors.** A major problem in the diagnosis and management of CRPS is the lack of properly controlled comparison of placebo with sympathetic blockade. Furthermore, a fair number of patients with neuropathic pain seem to improve with injections of placebo. In some patients, the symptoms may be conversion–somatization of an underlying psychiatric condition, because these patients seem to respond to cognitive psychotherapy.
II. **Diagnosis and course**
   A. **Diagnosis**
      1. **IASP diagnostic criteria.** The IASP criteria include:
         1. The presence of an initiating noxious event or a cause of immobilization
         2. Continuing pain, allodynia, or hyperalgesia with which the pain is disproportionate to any inciting event.
         3. Evidence at some time of edema, changes in skin blood flow, or abnormal sudomotor activity in the region of the pain.
         4. Diagnosis excluded by the existence of conditions that would otherwise account for the degree of pain and dysfunction

Table 51.1 Precipitating factors in the development
of complex regional pain syndrome type I

Soft-tissue injury	Malignancy
Fracture	Arthritis
Sprain	Bursitis
Joint dislocation	Peripheral nerve injury
Operative procedures	Carpal tunnel release
Immobilization with a cast or splint	Venipuncture
Arthroscopic surgery	Myocardial infarction
Brachial plexopathy	Polymyalgia rheumatica
Radiculopathy	Myelopathy
Stroke	Dental extraction
Spinal cord injury	Prolonged bed rest
Drugs (isoniazid, phenobarbital, ergotamine, cyclosporine)	

Criteria 2 through 4 must be satisfied.

A study validated the IASP diagnostic criteria for CRPS but showed the CRPS criteria have inadequate specificity and are likely to lead to overdiagnosis. The investigators proposed the following **modified research diagnostic criteria** for CRPS:

1. Continuing pain disproportionate to any inciting event
2. At least one symptom in each of the four following categories:
   Sensory: hyperesthesia
   Vasomotor: temperature asymmetry, skin color changes, skin color asymmetry, or a combination of these signs
   Sudomotor, edema: edema, sweating changes, sweating asymmetry, or a combination of these symptoms
   Motor/trophic: decreased range of motion, motor dysfunction (weakness, tremor, dystonia), trophic changes (hair, nail, skin), or a combination of these symptoms
3. At least one sign in two or more of the following categories
   Sensory: evidence of hyperalgesia to pin prick or allodynia to light touch
   Vasomotor: evidence of temperature asymmetry, skin color changes, asymmetry, or a combination of these signs
   Sudomotor/edema: evidence of edema, sweating changes, sweating asymmetry, or a combination of these symptoms
   Motor/trophic: evidence of decreased range of motion, motor dysfunction (weakness, tremor, dystonia), trophic changes (hair, nail, skin), or a combination of these symptoms

These research criteria may help prevent overdiagnosis of CRPS and may improve the ability to differentiate CRPS from other types of neuropathic pain.

2. The diagnosis of CRPS type I is generally made on the basis of **history and clinical findings.** The varying degrees of clinical features are summarized in Table 51.2. CRPS type I is being recognized with increasing frequency among children. The lower extremities are more commonly affected than are the upper extremities. The female preponderance of this condition is much greater among children than among adults. Patients typically are pubertal adolescent girls.

The therapeutic response to **sympathetic neural blockade** should be carefully evaluated to identify the responders to this diagnostic procedure. The pain-relieving effect should outlast the expected 6- to 12-hour effect of the local anesthetic.

3. **Differential diagnosis.** CRPS type II (causalgia), unrecognized local lesion (e.g., fracture, strain, sprain), traumatic vasospasm, cellulitis, Raynaud's disease, thromboangiitis obliterans, thrombosis, diabetic painful neuropathy, painful root syndrome, and gout

Table 51.2 Clinical features of complex regional pain syndrome type I

Feature	Example
Autonomic deregulation	Temperature, vasomotor, and sudomotor instability
Blood flow alterations	Hyperhydrosis, hypohydrosis, edema, and discoloration
Sensory abnormalities	Hyperalgesia (increased response to a stimulus that is normally painful), burning pain, hyperpathia (prolonged painful sensation to touch), allodynia (pain resulting from a stimulus that is normally painless, e.g., touch), and dysesthesia (unpleasant abnormal sensation)
Motor dysfunction	Weakness, tremor, and dystonia
Trophic changes	Skin thinning, hair loss, brittle nails, and changes in structure of both superficial and deep tissues
Psychological disturbances	Anxiety, depression, and suicidal ideation
Radiologic changes	Patchy osteoporosis, soft-tissue edema, and articular erosion

4. **Methods** used to aid in difficult-to-diagnose cases of and various severities of CRPS type I include radiography and scintigraphy.
   a. **Radiography.** Plain radiographs may show patchy osteopenia in one half of all patients. Plain radiography remains useful in detecting or excluding other bony abnormalities.
   b. **Scintigraphy.** A three-phase technetium bone scan (TPBS) is helpful in confirming the diagnosis and staging of CRPS type I. It helps detect physiologic changes rather than anatomic details with a sensitivity of 60% and a specificity of 86%. TPBS findings also can be abnormal in patients with osteomyelitis, stress fracture, degenerative arthritis, bone infarction, malignant tumors, osteoma, Reiter's disease, and thoracic outlet syndrome. A TPBS is used in three ways.
      (1) **Blood flow phase.** Rapid-sequence images of the involved extremity are obtained after intravenous injection of a radionuclide tracer to evaluate the vascularity of a region.
      (2) **Blood pool phase.** Images are obtained immediately after the blood flow phase to evaluate regional perfusion, including that of soft tissue.
      (3) **Bone scan phase.** Static images are obtained 2 to 3 hours after initial injection to detect abnormal osteoblastic activity, reflected locally as increased periarticular uptake in the affected extremity.
B. **Course.** CRPS type I is a dynamic process that can progress through three stages.
   1. **Stage 1 (acute).** The pain is described as aching or burning, aggravated by physical contact or emotional upset, and typically restricted to a vascular or peripheral nerve or root territory. Some patients report abnormal spontaneous sensations (paresthesia) or burning distal pain. Hyperalgesia may be present, as may allodynia to light touch, thermal stimulation, deep pressure, or joint movement. Tissue swelling and local vascular, bony, and trophic changes occur in the affected part. Radiography may show diffuse bony changes. TPBS may reveal increased radionuclide uptake in all phases. Stage 1 usually occurs 1 to 3 months after injury.
   2. **Stage 2 (dystrophic)** is characterized by spontaneous burning pain radiating proximally or distally from the site of injury and associated with pronounced hyperpathia (prolonged painful sensation to touch), decreased hair growth, brittle nails, and indurated edematous tissue. Radiography may show patchy osteoporosis. TPBS shows normalization in the blood flow and blood pool phases. The bone scan phase remains intense. Stage 2 usually occurs 3 to 6 months after injury.

3. **Stage 3 (atrophic).** Pain tends to subside or diminish in intensity. The skin is cool, thin, and shiny. Irreversible trophic changes occur with subcutaneous atrophy and wasted fingertips. Radiographs may show severe patchy osteopenia. TPBS shows reduced blood flow and blood pool phases and bone scan phase normalization. Stage 3 usually occurs 6 months to years after injury.

III. **Prevention** is best accomplished through early recognition and treatment. The unnecessary use of braces, casts, splints, and immobilization should be avoided. If CRPS type I is suspected, **heat** rather than cold should be applied. Alcohol is better avoided because it affects temperature regulation and may aggravate soft-tissue damage by increasing hyperoxide activity in the area of damage.

IV. **Management.** CRPS type I remains one of the most perplexing chronic pain syndromes to manage. The treatment goals early in the course of the disease are cessation of aberrant sympathetic hyperactivity or hypoactivity, desensitization of normal sensory pathways transmitting pain, and maintenance of normal musculoskeletal function. Reasonable approaches for the management of upper- and lower-extremity CRPS type I are presented in algorithms in Figs. 51.1 and 51.2.

A. **Pharmacologic therapy**
1. **Antiinflammatory agents.** Proposed mechanisms of the actions of nonsteroidal antiinflammatory drugs (NSAIDs) in the prevention of CRPS type I include reduced swelling with increased mobility of muscles and joints, inhibition of prostaglandin synthesis causing reduced sensitivity of pain receptors, and thromboxane inhibition causing interference with vasoconstriction.

Administration of NSAIDs usually is begun in the care of patients with early, mild symptoms, particularly when an inflammatory process (e.g., arthritis) is a component of the painful condition. Regardless of the agent chosen, the dosage should be maximized for optimal control of pain. NSAIDs are of minimal beneficial value, however, in the management of long-standing CRPS type I.

An intravenous regional blockade technique with **ketorolac** at a dose of 60 mg in saline solution or 0.5% lidocaine to volumes of 40 mL in the upper extremity and 50 mL in the lower extremity has produced prolonged pain relief with no serious side effects in some patients.

2. **Antidepressants** are effective adjuvants and are commonly used in CRPS type I. They have direct analgesic effects. Proposed mechanisms include: (1) potentiation of descending inhibitory pain-modulating pathways by blockade of presynaptic reuptake of the neurotransmitters serotonin and norepinephrine, (2) a neuronal membrane-stabilizing effect, (3) alterations in adrenergic, anticholinergic, and adenosinergic effects, and (4) a synergistic effect with opioid analgesics through bioavailability enhancement. The direct antidepressant and sedative effects are beneficial in managing the depressive and anxious states that patients with chronic pain are likely to experience. No clear-cut results of studies show a significantly higher quality of analgesia for any one antidepressant, hence the choice of drug depends on the patient's medical profile and previous response to antidepressants.

a. **Amitriptyline** is the prototype tricyclic antidepressant and is the most widely used. Its propensity for norepinephrine reuptake blockade is greater than that for serotonin. Two weeks of treatment may be needed before the analgesic effect is observed. Treatment should begin with small doses of 10 to 25 mg at bedtime. The dose should be increased 10 to 25 mg every 1 to 2 weeks while the patient is examined for side effects until a beneficial effect is achieved or a maximum of 150 mg is reached.

b. Antidepressants can interfere with the reuptake mechanism of bretylium, an agent commonly used in an intravenous regional sympathetic blockade technique. Antidepressant therapy should be discontinued for at least 2 weeks before initiation of an intravenous bretylium block.

c. **Complications** of antidepressant use include sedation, orthostatic hypotension, dry mouth, blurred vision, and urinary retention.

3. **Systemic corticosteroids.** In addition to having antiinflammatory effects, corticosteroids may have inhibitory effects on spontaneous neural discharge.

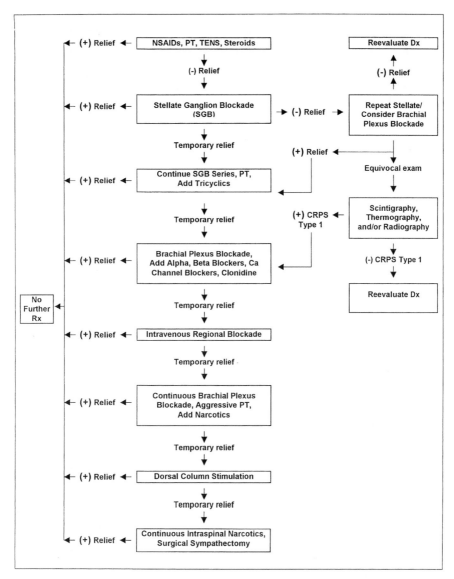

FIG. 51.1 Upper-extremity complex regional pain syndrome algorithm. *NSAID*, nonsteroidal antiinflammatory drug; *PT*, physical therapy; *TENS*, transcutaneous electrical nerve stimulation; (+), present; (–), absent; *Dx*, diagnosis; *Rx*, treatment; *Ca*, calcium; *CRPS*, complex regional pain syndrome.

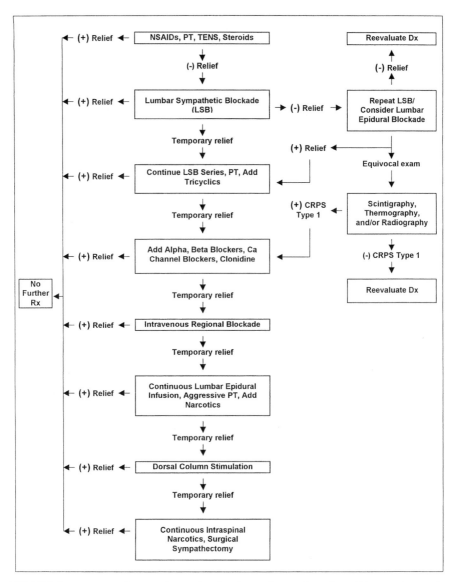

FIG. 51.2 Lower-extremity complex regional pain syndrome algorithm. Abbreviations as in Fig. 51.1.

The effects are only temporary, and these agent do not inhibit the sympathetic reflex mechanism in CRPS type I.

    a. A standardized regimen of high initial dosage and subsequent tapering of dosage consists of **prednisone** (or an equivalent) at 15 mg four times a day, 10 mg four times a day, 10 mg three times a day, 10 mg twice a day, 15 mg every morning, 10 mg every morning, and 5 mg every morning for 4 days each.

    b. Injections of depot steroids directly into inflamed muscles and joints may greatly reduce pain in an affected extremity and serve adjunctively as a therapy for CRPS type I.

    c. Potential **harmful effects** of steroids include osteoporosis, hyperglycemia, adrenal suppression, glucose intolerance, and sodium and water retention.

4. Narcotic analgesics rarely are needed in the management of CRPS type I. Intermittent use of narcotic analgesics as a prophylactic measure may be beneficial before exercise therapy. In severe, dystrophic stages associated with long-standing pain not controlled with other medical therapy or nerve block procedures, narcotic analgesics may become a necessary adjunct to long-term care. In such cases, administration by means of an intrathecal morphine pump (see **IV.F.2.**) may be appropriate. The risks of tolerance and dependence that attend long-term narcotic use must be carefully weighed against the benefits.

5. Calcium channel blockers are used to manage in CRPS type I for their peripheral vasodilatory effects as well as their antagonistic effects with norepinephrine on arterial and venous smooth muscles.

    a. Nifedipine has the most vasodilatory effect of all the calcium channel blockers. A hypothermic extremity, as typically observed in CRPS type I, is an appropriate indication.

    b. Side effects of calcium channel blockers include an increase in pain, hypotension, myocardial depression, and cold intolerance as a result of peripheral vasodilatation.

6. α_2-Agonists have been studied in recent years to determine their analgesic effects on chronic pain states.

    a. Clonidine, a centrally acting α_2 agonist, decreases sympathetic outflow and vasodilatation. Clonidine administered transdermally by means of application of a patch inhibits norepinephrine release from peripheral presynaptic adrenergic terminals. Clinically, it produces substantial reduction in hyperalgesia in response to mechanical stimuli confined primarily to the skin beneath the patch. Reports of systemic analgesic effects of clonidine are conflicting. Therefore, this agent may be most useful for patients with CRPS type I limited to only small areas. The recommended method of application is to place a patch over an area of allodynia, starting with 0.1 mg placed every 3 days and increasing the dosage in 0.1-mg increments every 12 days, to a dose of 0.3 mg. The skin should be checked for desensitization underneath the patch on replacement, and tolerance of side effects should be documented before the dosage is increased. The localized analgesia effect typically occurs within 36 to 48 hours and subsides within 1 week of discontinuance.

    b. Clonidine administered in a 300-mg dose within the epidural space produces effective analgesia for patients with refractory CRPS type I, but long-term relief has not been fully addressed.

    c. Significant **side effects** of clonidine include hypotension, bradycardia, and sedation.

7. α_1-Antagonists have been shown to be of some help to patients with CRPS type I.

    a. Terazosin, an oral α_1-antagonist, appears to be effective for some patients and can be used in a once daily dosing regimen.

    b. Terazosin can be started at 1 mg at bedtime and titrated slowly upward to 3 mg at bedtime.

       c. Use of α-blockers is limited by their prominent side effects of hypotension, reflex tachycardia, fatigue, and dizziness.

   8. Anticonvulsants stabilize abnormal hyperexcitability in both peripheral and central neurons and are thus hypothesized to inhibit excessive discharge of regional sympathetic nerves. Phenytoin at a dosage of 100 mg four times a day or carbamazepine at 200 mg three times a day may be used for management of dysesthesia.

   9. Calcitonin, given parenterally or intranasally, is widely used for CRPS type I pain in the United Kingdom. It has analgesic activity and inhibits bone resorption activity.

B. Physical therapy is a useful adjunct in the management of CRPS type I. It is used to control and minimize dystrophic changes in muscles and joints. Compliance increases if adequate pain relief can be achieved before initiation of physical therapy.

   1. Range-of-motion and stretching exercises are used for progressive stretching of restrictive tissue for maintenance of flexibility.

   2. Strengthening exercises entail progressive resistance to the musculoskeletal system to maintain strength and coordination of the muscles. These exercises include isotonic, isometric, isokinetic, and aerobic exercises. If a lower extremity is involved, the therapy should focus on a gradual increase in the weight-bearing capability of the limb.

   3. Deep friction massage is useful as a desensitization technique in the care of patients who can tolerate such manipulation.

   4. Physical therapy has been reported by many to be the mainstay of treatment of children.

C. Psychotherapy. Patients with CRPS type I experience a range of behavioral changes, including depression, anxiety, suicidal ideation, and drug addiction. Patients in whom these traits develop at or before the time of injury are considered at higher risk of development and maintenance of symptoms of CRPS type I. Therefore all such patients should be considered for psychological consultation. **Psychotherapeutic** management of CRPS type I includes counseling and cognitive-behavioral techniques.

   1. Counseling is a means whereby the patient is helped to cope with the pain, irrespective of how well it may be controlled with pharmacologic or physical treatments. The services of a psychiatrist, psychologist, or social worker are used when appropriate.

   2. Cognitive-behavioral techniques include biofeedback, relaxation, and hypnosis.

D. Transcutaneous electrical nerve stimulation (TENS). According to the gate theory put forth by Melzack and Wall in 1965, painful transmission from the periphery carried by afferent C fibers causes a loss of interneuronal large-diameter A-fiber inhibition in the dorsal horns of the spinal cord. Both sets of fibers synapse on interneurons in the substantia gelatinosa of laminae II and III before secondary fibers transmit across the midline to ascending tracts and eventually synapse in the thalamus and higher cortical centers. TENS is thought to provide pain relief by closing this gating mechanism through preferential stimulation of large-diameter A fibers and inhibition of the smaller fibers within the substantia gelatinosa or by causing the release of endorphins, enkephalins, or both. Overall, TENS relieves symptoms of CRPS type I for most children but only for approximately 25% of adults.

E. Sympathetic blockade. The mechanism of continued pain relief from sympathetic blockade is not completely understood. The relief of symptoms of early CRPS type I through inhibition of sympathetic activity seems to be a paradoxic effect if one considers that this stage is typically characterized by sympathetic hypoactivity consisting of vasodilation, redness, warmth, and sweating. Possible explanations for this effect include blockade of afferent nerve fibers transmitting pain, blockade of efferent fibers eliminating sensitization of nociceptors, and inhibition of localized vasospasm.

   Sympathetic blockade can be performed on the cervical sympathetic chain, primarily the stellate ganglion, for head, neck, and upper-extremity dystrophy and on the lumbar sympathetic chain for lower-extremity dystrophy. For sympathetic blockade to be used as a therapeutic intervention, several criteria should be met. First, the blockade should demonstrate a desired effect. Efficacy is assessed subjectively by the degree of pain relief and objectively by the degree of functional improvement of the extremity. Second, the effect should last longer than the known duration of the local anesthetic. Third, the patient must be willing to continue a series of sympathetic blockades for the therapy to be effective.

Once a sympathetic blockade has been shown effective, a series of frequent blocks is performed. Initially, the interval between procedures should roughly equal the time it takes for the pain to return and limit rehabilitation. This typically equates to intervals ranging from daily to no more than weekly. After the first three to five blockades, the time interval is extended to approximately 1.5 times the period of pain relief and improved function. Medical therapy, physical therapy, and desensitization techniques are used in conjunction. As long as the patient's condition continues to improve, this therapy is continued. Resolution of symptoms typically occurs with four to eight blocks. If pain remains after sympathetic blockade, the diagnosis of CRPS type I should be reconsidered.

The patient's condition is considered refractory if pain relief is incomplete or if the painful condition returns after a series of sympathetic blockades has been performed.

1. **Stellate ganglion block.** The stellate ganglion is the irregularly shaped ganglionic mass derived from fusion of the inferior cervical and first thoracic sympathetic ganglia. Preganglionic fibers destined for the upper extremity originate from upper thoracic segments to approximately T8. Stellate ganglion block involves instillation of local anesthetic at the anterior tubercle of C6. These blockades are repeated one to three times a week, up to 10 in a series, until a long-term effect is achieved. If pain relief remains inadequate, a brachial plexus block or intravenous regional bretylium block is attempted.

   a. **Indications.** CRPS type I and CRPS type II of the upper extremity are the two most common indications for stellate ganglion block.

   b. **Complications.** Most injections result in Horner's syndrome and temporary hoarseness. Bilateral stellate ganglion blocks is not recommended because of the possibility of bilateral recurrent laryngeal nerve paralysis and loss of cardioaccelerator activity. Block of the phrenic nerve results in temporary paralysis of a hemidiaphragm. Injections into the vertebral artery may result in seizures or cerebral air embolism. Intradural injections can result in unconsciousness, respiratory paralysis, seizures, and sometimes cardiovascular collapse. Other complications include brachial plexus block, pneumothorax, and osteitis of the transverse process.

2. **Lumbar sympathetic block.** The abdominal portion of the sympathetic trunk that supplies the lower extremities is anterolateral to the vertebral bodies of L1-3 along the medial margin of the psoas major muscle. Blockade of the lumbar sympathetic nerves can be performed with a spinal, epidural, or peripheral nerve block, but relief after lumbar sympathetic blockade most clearly delineates the cause of the pain as sympathetically mediated.

   a. **Indications** include sympathetically mediated pain, postherpetic neuralgia, phantom limb pain, and stump pain.

   b. **Complications** of lumbar sympathetic blockade include back pain, somatic nerve block, intraspinal anesthesia, intravascular injection, kidney trauma, and bowel perforation.

3. **Intravenous regional sympathetic blockade.** Bretylium, like guanethidine, selectively inhibits peripheral sympathetic nerve transmission by entering the preganglionic nerve endings by means of active transport and displacing norepinephrine from its storage sites. Its concentration builds up at these sites and prevents reuptake of norepinephrine and release of any remaining norepinephrine in response to neuronal stimulation. The norepinephrine depletion results in impairment and eventual loss of sympathetic adrenergic nerve function. This blockade lasts for many hours, for days, and sometimes for weeks because of the strong binding and slow elimination of the drug. In

sufficient concentration, guanethidine can cause permanent damage to the norepinephrine reuptake pump.

   a. Indications. Intravenous regional sympathetic blockade with bretylium or guanethidine remains an alternative for patients who do not respond to block procedures. This procedure is less invasive than blocks and can be performed by physicians unfamiliar with the use of regional anesthesia. It is also useful for patients for whom regional anesthesia is contraindicated.

   b. Complications. Placement of an Esmarch bandage and tourniquet on an extremity may be intolerable to a patient with painful CRPS type I. Agent not taken up by the tissue on release of the tourniquet may enter the systemic circulation and cause hypertension and tachycardia. Orthostatic hypotension can result from the chemical sympathetic blockade. Bretylium in high concentrations has local anesthetic and neuromuscular blocking properties. These drugs should not be administered to patients taking monoamine oxidase inhibitors or to patients with known pheochromocytoma. Other side effects include dysrhythmia, dizziness, diarrhea, edema, and nausea.

F. Other therapies for CRPS type I

   1. Dorsal column stimulation (DCS) has become a widely accepted mode of therapy for refractory CRPS type I. The mechanisms of DCS are explained by the gate-control theory of pain and an increase in production of endogenous endorphins.

   a. Indications. DCS is indicated for patients with chronic intractable pain. Patient-selection criteria include failure of conservative therapies, absence of drug abuse or history of psychological disorders, absence of contraindication to spinal implantation, and a successful trial of DCS with temporary electrodes.

   b. Complications include infection, arachnoiditis, a high long-term failure rate, and mechanical failure.

   2. Intraspinal opioid programmable pump. Preganglionic sympathetic intermediolateral columns of the spinal cord are modulated by projection from multiple supraspinal nuclei, including the nucleus raphae magnus. Intrathecal administration of morphine may be effective in relieving refractory CRPS type I by increasing nucleus raphae magnus inhibition of sympathetic outflow, in addition to its inhibitory effects on nociceptive neurons. Moreover, continuous intrathecal administration of morphine with a programmable pump allows stable cerebrospinal fluid concentrations. The result is fewer episodes of pain breakthrough or drug overdose. Intrathecal therapy also may reduce the overall dosage requirements and delay the development of tolerance.

   a. Indications. The intraspinal opioid programmable pump is reserved for treatment of patients with CRPS type I who are unresponsive to all other forms of less invasive measures. A successful trial of intrathecal morphine placed percutaneously is required.

   b. Complications. An important disadvantage of an intraspinal opioid infusion pump is the high cost of implanting and maintaining the device. In addition, physical tolerance and dependence complicate therapy for many patients. Other problems of intraspinal opioid programmable pump therapy include infection, arachnoiditis, mechanical failure, unremitting breakthrough pain, and opioid tolerance and dependence.

G. Surgical sympathectomy. For upper-extremity CRPS type I, surgical sympathectomy involves extensive ablation of the thoracic sympathetic ganglia from T1 to T6 or T7 through a transthoracic approach. Surgical sympathectomy for lower-extremity CRPS type I involves ablation of the lumbar sympathetic chain from L1 to L4. The pain relief derived from surgery may be inadequate or transient owing either to incomplete sympathetic denervation or to subsequent nerve regeneration.

   1. Indications. Surgical sympathectomy usually is reserved for patients with CRPS type I who have been able to obtain definite but only temporary relief from repeated sympathetic nerve blocks and remain incapacitated by the disease.

2. Complications. Potential morbidity, including wound complications, permanent Horner's syndrome, and painful neuralgia, warrants exhaustive physical, pharmacologic, and psychological therapy before consideration of surgical sympathectomy.

V. Referrals. Patients with CRPS type I should be referred to a specialist in chronic pain treatment or a neurologist if: (1) signs and symptoms remain persistent despite a 6-week trial of conservative measures, (2) pain is severe and intractable any time after the inciting event, (3) a new-onset neurologic deficit is noted, or (4) signs and symptoms have spread to other parts of the body.

Recommended Readings

Besson JM, Chaouch A. Peripheral and spinal mechanisms of nociception. *Physiol Rev* 1987; 67:67–186.

Bonica JJ. Causalgia and other reflex sympathetic dystrophies. In: JJ Bonica, ed. *The management of pain.* Philadelphia: Lea & Febiger, 1990:220–243.

Bruehl S, Harden RN, Galer BS, et al. External validation of IASP diagnostic criteria for complex regional pain syndrome and proposed research diagnostic criteria. *Pain* 1999;81: 147–154.

Chaturvedi SK. Phenytoin in reflex sympathetic dystrophy. *Pain* 1989;36:379–380.

Cline MA, Ochoa J, Torebjork HE. Chronic hyperalgesia and skin warming caused by sensitized C-nociceptors. *Brain* 1989;112:621–647.

Davis KD, Treede RD, Raja SN, et al. Topical application of clonidine relieves hyperalgesia in patients with sympathetically maintained pain. *Pain* 1991;47:309–317.

Demangeat JL, Constantinesco A, Brunot B, et al. Three-phase bone scanning in reflex sympathetic dystrophy of the hand. *J Nucl Med* 1988;29:26–32.

Doupe J, Cullen CH, Chance CQ. Post-traumatic pain and the causalgic syndromes. *J Neurol Neurosurg Psychiatry* 1944;7:33–48.

Geertzen JH, de Bruijn H, de Bruijn-Kofman AT, et al. Reflex sympathetic dystrophy: early treatment and psychological aspects. *Arch Phys Med Rehabil* 1994;75:442–446.

Gobelet C, Waldburger M, Meier JL. The effect of adding calcitonin to physical treatment on reflex sympathetic dystrophy. *Pain* 1992;48:171–175.

Hord AH, Rooks MD, Stephens BO, et al. Intravenous regional bretylium and lidocaine for treatment of reflex sympathetic dystrophy: a randomized, double-blind study. *Anesth Analg* 1992;74:818–821.

Kanoff RB. Intraspinal delivery of opiates by an implantable, programmable pump in patients with chronic, intractable pain of nonmalignant origin. *J Am Osteopath Assoc* 1994;94: 487–493.

Lynch ME. Psychological aspect of reflex sympathetic dystrophy: a review of the adult and pediatric literature. *Pain* 1992;49:337–347.

Melzack R, Wall PD. Pain mechanisms: a new theory. *Science* 1965;150:971–975.

Merskey H, Bogduk N. Complex regional pain syndromes (CRPS). In: *Classification of chronic pain: descriptions of chronic pain syndromes and definitions of pain terms,* 2nd ed. Seattle: IASP Publications, 1994:40–43.

Payne R. Neuropathic pain syndromes, with special reference to causalgia and reflex sympathetic dystrophy. *Clin J Pain* 1986;2:59–73.

Prough DS, McLeskey CH, Poehling GG, et al. Efficacy of oral nifedipine in the treatment of reflex sympathetic dystrophy. *Anesthesiology* 1985;62:796–799.

Raja SN. Reflex sympathetic dystrophy: pathophysiological basis for therapy. *Pain Digest* 1992;2:274–280.

Rauck RL, Eisenach JC, Jackson K, et al. Epidural clonidine treatment for reflex sympathetic dystrophy. *Anesthesiology* 1993;79:1163–1169.

Roberts WJ. A hypothesis on the physiological basis for causalgia and related pains. *Pain* 1986;24:297–311.

Stanton-Hicks M, Janig W, Hassenbusch S, et al. Reflex sympathetic dystrophy: changing concepts and taxonomy. *Pain* 1995;63:127–133.

Verdugo RJ, Ochoa JL. Placebo response in chronic, causalgiform, "neuropathic" pain patients: study and review. *Pain Rev* 1994;1:33–46.

Wilder RT, Berde CB, Wolohan M, et al. Reflex sympathetic dystrophy in children. *J Bone Joint Surg Am* 1992;74:910–919.

52. PRIMARY CENTRAL NERVOUS SYSTEM TUMORS

Bertrand C. Liang
Diane M. Liang

Approximately 20,000 **primary central nervous system (CNS) tumors** are diagnosed each year in the United States. These tumors tend to affect younger patients and are the second most frequent cause of cancer-related death among children, the third most frequent cause of cancer-related death among patients 15 to 35 years of age, and the fourth most frequent cause of cancer-related death among patients 36 to 45 years of age. However, the incidence of the histologically more malignant tumors seems to be rising, especially among the elderly.

Primary CNS tumors are thought to arise from precursor cells to nervous system elements. In tumor cells, an accumulation of aberrant genetic events allows dysregulation of differentiation and growth; the result is neoplastic proliferation. This proliferation results in the development of a mass, which becomes clinically apparent with neurologic symptoms. This chapter discusses some of the more frequent tumors, including **glioma** (astrocytoma, anaplastic astrocytoma, glioblastoma, and oligodendroglioma), **primitive neuroectodermal tumor** (medulloblastoma), **ependymoma**, and **meningioma**. Also discussed is **primary CNS lymphoma,** which is being seen with increasing frequency in the immunocompromised and immunocompetent population.

   I. Glioma is the most common intracranial tumor, comprising about 60% of all primary CNS neoplasms. Although there are several grading systems currently in use, the three-tiered classification system has become the most popular. Astrocytoma is the most well-differentiated and lowest-grade tumor. Anaplastic astrocytoma is an intermediate-grade tumor, and glioblastoma is the most malignant and poorly differentiated glioma. The most malignant form, glioblastoma, is the most common, representing 50% to 60% of cases of glioma diagnosed. Most studies of all grades of glioma show either no sex preponderance or a slight male bias. These tumors do not tend to be inherited, except in a few rare syndromes (e.g., neurofibromatosis, Li–Fraumeni syndrome, tuberous sclerosis, and ataxia–telangiectasia). No definite environmental association of these tumors has been found in comparisons of urban and rural populations.

   A. Astrocytoma
      1. Course of disease. Approximately 30% of cases of glioma diagnosed are astrocytoma. This low-grade neoplasm tends to occur among younger patients, typically in the fourth decade of life or earlier. There is a paucity of prospective information regarding the course of astrocytoma. Retrospective analysis has shown age to be an important predictive factor; younger patients, especially those younger than 20 years, have the highest 5-year survival rate. The incidence of malignant transformation and response to therapy are not well known. Total surgical resection and good postoperative performance status have been associated retrospectively with prolonged survival. One exception to the lack of information on low-grade tumors is **pilocytic astrocytoma,** which occurs most often in children and occasionally in adults. With only surgical intervention, these tumors have an excellent prognosis and only rarely transform to malignant neoplasms. Other tumors that fit into the rubric of low-grade astrocytoma include **ganglioglioma** and **neurocytoma.** These tumors tend to behave in a benign manner and to require only surgical intervention.
      2. Therapy. Except as noted, no prospective studies have evaluated the efficacy of therapeutic intervention in low-grade astrocytoma. It is accepted that surgical excision is a reasonable initial approach to these tumors, although any further therapy is based only on anecdotal or retrospective analyses. Currently there are no generally accepted guidelines for radiation therapy for low-grade astrocytoma, although many clinicians believe that for some older patients, treatment with high-dose radiation (6,000 cGy) is appropriate. At least initially, chemotherapy is not believed to play a part in treatment of these patients because of the slow growth of these tumors.

However, many astrocytomas progress to higher-grade neoplasms, in which case therapy is referable to the more malignant tumor (see **I.B.** and **I.C.**). Follow-up computed tomography (CT) or magnetic resonance imaging (MRI) typically is performed every 6 months and when the patient has clinical changes.

3. **Prognosis.** Patients with astrocytoma who have the best prognosis are young, have undergone gross total tumor resection, and have minimal or no postoperative neurologic or other deficits. Among these patients, the 5-year survival rate is greater than 80%. Further specific prognostic assessment in other patient subgroups is difficult, but at least a fraction of astrocytomas in such patients progress to higher-grade neoplasms that necessitate other types of therapy. For any patient with a diagnosis of astrocytoma (with the exception of pilocytic astrocytoma, ganglioglioma, and neurocytoma), continual follow-up evaluation is necessary, because malignant transformation can occur at any time.

B. **Anaplastic astrocytoma**

1. **Course of disease.** Anaplastic astrocytoma is diagnosed much less frequently than are its lower- and higher-grade counterparts. Part of the reason for this revolves around the pathologic criteria for anaplastic astrocytoma compared with those for glioblastoma (anaplasia without necrosis in the specimen). Even with these criteria, there may still be an overestimation of the incidence of anaplastic astrocytoma because of sampling errors that occur when specimens from subtotal resection or stereotactic biopsy are sent to pathologists for review. It has been estimated that as many as 30% of tumors diagnosed as anaplastic astrocytoma at stereotactic biopsy are of higher grade (glioblastoma). Apart from difficulties with histologic grading, few prospective analyses of these tumors have been performed. Retrospective studies have shown anaplastic astrocytoma to occur typically in the fifth decade of life, usually with a long (more than 1 year) history of neurologic symptoms. The most important favorable prognostic factors include young age and good performance status. Surgery has not been found to influence survival, perhaps because anaplastic tumors tend to be diffusely infiltrating. A high percentage of these tumors recur at higher pathologic grade.

2. **Therapy.** Patients with anaplastic astrocytoma need a multidisciplinary approach similar to that used for glioblastoma.

   a. **Surgery and corticosteroids.** Surgery should be considered if the diagnosis is in question, if there would be benefit from cytoreduction (reduction of mass effect), or if surgery is indicated because of emergency clinical conditions. Surgery does not seem to affect survival per se. Corticosteroids may be necessary to decrease symptoms of increased intracranial pressure. Dexamethasone often is given at a starting dosage of 4 mg four times a day, titrated for relief of symptoms. Doses greater than 32 mg/d are rarely useful. Minimizing doses of corticosteroids because of known side effects should be an important goal after radiation treatment.

   b. **Radiation therapy** is an important aspect of management of anaplastic astrocytoma, with a current recommended dose of approximately 6,000 cGy. The fractionation schedule of radiation therapy usually ranges from 180 to 200 cGy/d. Focal radiation of 4,500 cGy within a 3-cm margin with a boost of 1,500 cGy for the 1.5-cm margin surrounding the area of enhancement of the tumor has been found as effective as whole-brain irradiation. Highly focused radiation, such as stereotactic radiosurgery may be of palliative benefit at recurrence.

   c. **Chemotherapy.** Anaplastic astrocytoma is managed with both adjuvant and recurrent chemotherapy. Adjuvant chemotherapy (given within 2 weeks after the completion of radiation) usually consists of a combined regimen of procarbazine (60 mg/m^2 by mouth on days 8 to 21), lomustine (CCNU; 110 mg/m^2 by mouth on day 1), and vincristine (PCV; 1.4 mg/m^2 intravenously [i.v.] on days 8 and 29) every 6 to 8 weeks for 1 year or until tumor recurrence. At recurrence, high-dose intravenous carmustine

(BCNU; 250 mg/m^2) is administered every 6 to 8 weeks until further tumor progression. Administration of these drugs requires that specific laboratory values and clinical cautions be assessed periodically (see **VI.B.** and Tables 52.1 and 52.2). Further therapy after this point usually revolves around phase I or phase II drugs or other experimental therapies. Consultation with a neurooncologist often is necessary. Follow-up CT or MRI evaluation should be performed 6 weeks after completion of radiation therapy and before each cycle of chemotherapy.

3. **Prognosis.** With implementation of surgery, radiation therapy, and chemotherapy, patients with anaplastic astrocytoma have a median survival period of more than 3 years. Typical time to first tumor recurrence is approximately 2.5 years, and time to death after progression is 8 months. Patients younger than 40 years have the highest likelihood for response to treatment and prolonged survival. Few patients older than 60 years respond to this multimodal approach to therapy, and patients in this age group have the highest incidence of serious side effects. Clinical judgment and careful consideration of the patient's wishes are necessary before any decision regarding therapeutic intervention, especially chemotherapy.

C. **Glioblastoma**

1. **Course of disease.** Glioblastoma is the most frequently diagnosed primary CNS neoplasm. Its course, unlike those of astrocytoma and anaplastic astrocytoma, is well defined. This tumor is the most malignant of the gliomas and has a poor prognosis with inexorable progression to death. Patients with glioblastoma usually come to medical attention in the sixth decade of life with a short history (less than 6 months) of neurologic symptoms. The best predictors of survival and response to chemotherapy are the same as those for anaplastic astrocytoma—patient age and performance status. A shorter duration of symptoms before diagnosis has been associated with longer survival periods. Currently it is unclear whether extent of surgery is an important prognostic factor.

2. **Therapy** for glioblastoma is similar to that for anaplastic astrocytoma. Maximal surgical debulking usually is suggested for patients who can undergo the procedure safely. Subsequent high-dose radiation therapy (6,000 cGy or

Table 52.1 Chemotherapy dosages and monitoring laboratory tests

Drug	Dosage	Laboratory tests
BCNU	200–250 mg/m^2	CBC, electrolytes, BUN, creatinine, liver function tests,[a] pulmonary function tests[b]
Procarbazine	PCV: 50–100 mg/m^2 Alone: 150 mg/m^2	CBC, electrolytes, liver function tests
CCNU	100–150 mg/m^2	CBC, electrolytes, BUN, creatinine, liver function tests, pulmonary function tests
Vincristine	1.0–1.4 mg/m^2	CBC, electrolytes, BUN, creatinine, urinalysis
Cyclophosphamide	15 mg/kg	CBC, electrolytes, BUN, creatinine, urinalysis
Methotrexate (with leucovorin)	i.a.: 2.5 g i.v.: 1 g/m^2 i.t.: 12 mg	CBC, electrolytes, BUN, creatinine, liver function tests, urinalysis
Ara-C	3 g/m^2	CBC, electrolytes, BUN, creatinine, liver function tests

[a] Liver function tests include aspartate (AST) and alanine (ALT) aminotransferase and bilirubin.
[b] Pulmonary function tests should include diffusion coefficient.
BCNU, carmustine; CBC, complete blood cell count; BUN, blood urea nitrogen; PCV, vincristine; CCNU, lomustine; i.a., intraarterial; i.v., intravenous; i.t., intrathecal; Ara-C, cytarabine.

Table 52.2 Treatment toxicity

Treatment	Toxicity
Radiation Therapy	
Acute	Worsening of neurologic symptoms, symptoms of increased intracranial pressure
Early delayed	Somnolence, fatigue, worsening of neurologic symptoms
Late delayed	Worsening of neurologic symptoms, radiation necrosis
Chemotherapy[a]	
BCNU, CCNU	Pulmonary fibrosis, hepatic necrosis, encephalomyelopathy
Procarbazine	Malignant hypertension (sensitivity to amines)
Vincristine	Sensorimotor neuropathy, SIADH, diminished levels of phenytoin
Cyclophosphamide	Hemorrhagic cystitis, water retention, alopecia
Methotrexate	Hepatic dysfunction, renal failure, stomatitis, motor neuropathy
Ara-C	Cholestasis, mucositis

[a] Hematologic/infection (all).
BCNU, carmustine; CCNU, lomustine; SIADH, syndrome of inappropriate secretion of antidiuretic hormone; Ara-C, cytarabine.

more) is as described for anaplastic tumors (see **I.B.2.b.**). Adjuvant chemotherapy with carmustine usually is initiated within 2 weeks after completion of radiation treatment and is given every 6 to 8 weeks. Recurrence is managed with procarbazine, CCNU, and vincristine, high-dose oral procarbazine alone (each cycle consisting of 150 mg/m^2/day for 28 days, followed by a 28-day rest), or experimental therapy. Consultation with a neurooncologist is necessary at this point. CT or MRI should be performed before each cycle of chemotherapy.

3. The **prognosis** for patients with glioblastoma is poor. Patients treated with surgery alone have a median survival time of 14 to 26 weeks. The addition of radiation therapy increases the survival period to 40 weeks. Administration of chemotherapy with nitrosoureas such as procarbazine and carmustine further increases the median survival time to 50 weeks and increases the proportion of patients surviving 18 months. Nevertheless, with multimodality therapy, the median survival time is less than 1 year and fewer than 15% of patients survive 2 years.

D. **Oligodendroglioma**
1. **Course of disease.** Oligodendroglioma arises from presumed oligodendroglial precursors and usually manifests in the fourth or fifth decade of life. These tumors occur in proportion to the volume of white matter, and hence the frontal lobes are the areas most frequently affected. There is an inconsistent relation between histologic grade and malignant behavior. Few data are available regarding the frequency of malignant degeneration, although it is well known that some oligodendrogliomas transform into glioblastomas. Better prognostic factors include relatively benign histologic features, postoperative radiation therapy, complete surgical resection, and good preoperative and postoperative performance status. Close follow-up care is necessary in the treatment of these patients, especially given the long-term survival of particular subsets.
2. **Therapy.** Management of the different types of oligodendroglioma is evolving. Maximal surgical excision is considered the initial step in management of these tumors. Radiation therapy can follow surgery in a manner similar to that of anaplastic astrocytoma or glioblastoma. Although there is no strict relation between histologic anaplasia and malignant potential, most neurooncologists suggest that patients with anaplastic oligodendroglioma be treated with multiagent chemotherapy, that is, procarbazine, CCNU, and vin-

cristine. Patients with nonanaplastic oligodendroglioma typically are observed without further therapy after radiation therapy and are given multiagent chemotherapy only at recurrence. For the first year, MRI or CT should be performed before administration of chemotherapy and every 6 to 8 weeks for anaplastic tumors or every 3 months for nonanaplastic oligodendroglioma. If there is no evidence of recurrence, imaging can be performed every 6 months thereafter.

   3. The **prognosis** for oligodendroglioma is more favorable than that for either anaplastic astrocytoma or glioblastoma. Overall, the median survival period is more than 5 years, and the 10-year survival rate is 24%. Selected patients with the particularly good prognostic factors noted in **I.D.1.** have the likelihood of longer survival.

II. Primitive neuroectodermal tumor (PNET)

   A. Course of disease. PNETs are primarily neoplasms of children. These tumors constitute the most frequently diagnosed soft-tissue malignant tumors in the pediatric ages but account for fewer than 1% of all adult tumors. In adults, the median age at diagnosis is 24 years. The most often diagnosed PNET is medulloblastoma, which typically occurs in the posterior fossa. There is a male-to-female ratio of 2 : 1. These tumors are graded according to the Chang criteria (TM system), although there is no influence per se on prognosis. Medulloblastoma can metastasize throughout the craniospinal axis, as well as outside the nervous system, for as long as 10 years after the initial diagnosis. Bone, lymph nodes, lung, pleura, liver, and breast are the most frequent sites of seeding outside the nervous system. Prolonged survival is associated with high-dose posterior fossa radiation accompanied by additional radiation therapy to the entire brain, spinal cord, and coverings as well as with early treatment. There may be improved survival among female patients. The extent of surgery is important in relapse-free, but not overall, survival.

   B. Therapy. Maximal surgical resection and radiation are the mainstays of therapy for medulloblastoma. Radiation doses of 5,200 to 5,500 cGy to the posterior fossa and 3,600 cGy to the remaining neuraxis are considered appropriate and have been associated with prolonged progression-free survival, particularly in low-stage disease. Management of recurrent disease typically revolves around chemotherapy, although the most beneficial regimen has yet to be defined. However, most neurooncologists recommend a multidrug protocol with drugs such as the nitrosoureas, a platinum-based compound, and steroids. Consultation is required to determine the most current regimen. Imaging studies should be performed after radiation therapy and before each cycle of chemotherapy. Because recurrences are not uncommon, follow-up evaluation of these patients, including periodic radiographic examinations, should be performed for at least 10 years after completion of therapy.

   C. Prognosis. With maximal treatment (radiation being paramount in importance), the 5-year survival rate is 50% to 76%, and the 10-year survival rate is 33% to 60%. Recurrence, when it is found, is typically in the posterior fossa. Some patients with more extensive tumors may benefit from chemotherapy in either an adjuvant or a recurrence setting. Those patients with metastatic lesions, especially outside the nervous system, have a worse prognosis than do those who have solitary recurrences in the posterior fossa.

III. Ependymoma

   A. Course of disease. Ependymoma, like PNET, is a tumor of the young and is uncommon in adults. The tumor arises most frequently in the central canal of the spinal cord or the filum terminale as well as in white matter adjacent to a ventricular surface. Like medulloblastoma, ependymoma tends to seed throughout the nervous system, although the likelihood of such seeding is defined by the grade of the tumor. Ependymoma is graded in a variety of ways but can be most conveniently divided into differentiated (low-grade, myxopapillary) and anaplastic (high-grade) ependymoma. Anaplastic tumors are most often associated with neuraxial spread. A particular subtype of ependymoma, ependymoblastoma, has an especially high frequency of seeding. However, the usual area of recurrence for all ependymomas is the primary site, although seeding can accompany local treatment failure in the higher grades. Better prognostic factors include low grade, treatment with surgery with little residual tumor remaining postoperatively, and high-dose radiation therapy.

B. Therapy. Evaluation of the entire nervous system and cerebrospinal fluid for malignant cells often is recommended in the management of ependymoma. Maximal surgical resection and radiation therapy are the necessary initial treatments, because local control of disease is a major predictor of outcome. For low-grade tumors, a dose of 5,400 cGy to the primary tumor is considered standard, with no additional treatment of the rest of the nervous system. For anaplastic tumors, 5,400 cGy is applied to the primary tumor site and 3,500 to 4,000 cGy to the neuraxis. Chemotherapy is given at recurrence, although only anecdotal data on the most beneficial regimen are available. Hence, the chemotherapeutic protocol to be followed for recurrence therapy should be determined in consultation with a neurooncologist to determine the most current regimen. Imaging should be performed after radiation therapy and before each chemotherapeutic intervention. Continual follow-up evaluation is necessary because of the possibility of late recurrence.

C. Prognosis. Patients with ependymoma of low grade treated maximally with surgery, radiation, and chemotherapy have a 5-year survival rate of 60% to 80%. Higher-grade disease has a significantly worse prognosis: 10% to 47% of patients survive for 5 years. As with medulloblastoma, seeding carries a worse prognosis.

IV. Meningioma

A. Course of disease. Meningioma is a common nervous system tumor, constituting approximately 15% of all CNS neoplasms. There is a slight female preponderance. Although the peak age at diagnosis is 45 years, asymptomatic tumors are common in older adults as well. These neoplasms grow slowly and typically are benign in behavior. However, the recurrence rate for totally resected tumors is still 10%. Fifteen percent of meningiomas recur if a dural attachment remains after surgery, and 39% recur if only subtotal resection can be accomplished. These tumors occur most frequently in the parasagittal and falx regions, and can be associated with inherited syndromes (e.g., neurofibromatosis). Malignant meningioma, which is rare, has anaplastic pathologic features and behavior and necessitates continual monitoring and treatment.

B. Therapy. Surgical removal is the therapy of choice for meningioma. Cauterization or embolization has been performed on particularly vascular tumors to ease removal. Radiation and chemotherapy play no role in the management of typical meningioma, although malignant tumors may necessitate these additional interventions. Imaging studies should be performed yearly for at least 3 years and if symptoms develop.

C. The **prognosis** for meningioma is good. Tumors can recur, however, and recurrence necessitates additional surgery or, for malignant meningioma, radiation therapy and chemotherapy.

V. Primary CNS lymphoma

A. Course of disease. Primary CNS lymphoma (PCNSL) is a rare tumor in the immunocompetent population, comprising less than 2% of all brain tumors and extranodal lymphomas. Pathologically, these tumors are typically non-Hodgkin's B-cell tumors, although T-cell tumors are occasionally found. The incidence of PCNSL has been rising, both in the immunocompetent population and, primarily, because of the increasing population of patients with acquired immunodeficiency syndrome (AIDS). Moreover, other immunocompromised patients such as recipients of renal transplants are acquiring PCNSL with increasing frequency. Other immunodeficiency diseases reported in association with PCNSL include Wiskott–Aldrich syndrome, agammaglobulinemia, and ataxia–telangiectasia. Although concurrent non-Hodgkin's lymphoma at other extranodal sites is uncommon in these patients, staging evaluation of a patient found to have PCNSL should include radiographic imaging (CT or MRI) of the chest, abdomen, and pelvis as well as examination of a bone marrow aspirate. Because PCNSL can occur in ocular and meningeal tissues, slit-lamp and cerebrospinal fluid examinations should be performed. Finally, human immunodeficiency virus testing should be performed on all patients with a diagnosis of PCNSL. Combination chemotherapy and radiation therapy has been found to prolong survival significantly in comparison with surgery and radiation alone.

B. **Therapy.** Use of biopsy alone to establish the diagnosis of PCNSL is the sole surgical intervention required. No additional benefit is derived from subtotal or total resection of any visualized mass. Radiation therapy can be given either initially after biopsy or at recurrence after adjuvant chemotherapy. The optimal regimen has yet to be defined, but combination therapy with both radiation and chemotherapy has been successful in prolonging median survival to more than 40 months, although in some regimens leukoencephalopathy and cognitive changes have been found. Although treatment of patients AIDS and PCNSL has shown tumor regression, ultimately there has been no increase in overall survival rate among these patients.

In the management of PCNSL, the two most successful regimens have entailed large doses of chemotherapy. In the first, disruption of the blood–brain barrier with mannitol has been used with efficacy. Intravenous cyclophosphamide (15 mg/kg) and intraarterial methotrexate (2.5 g) are administered with the disruption, oral leucovorin (20 mg every 6 hours) is given 36 hours after completion of the infusion of methotrexate and continued for 5 days, and procarbazine (100 mg/d by mouth) and dexamethasone (24 mg/d by mouth) are given for 14 days after the disruption. This cycle is repeated every 28 days for 1 year. Radiation therapy is given at relapse. In the second regimen, chemotherapy is combined with radiation therapy as adjuvant treatment. Dexamethasone (16 mg/kg by mouth) is given until an Ommaya reservoir has been placed, and then intravenous administration of methotrexate (1 g/m²) is begun, given on days 1 and 8. Intrathecal methotrexate (12 mg through the Ommaya reservoir) is administered on days 1, 4, 8, 11, 15, and 18 with a dexamethasone taper. Whole-brain radiation (4,000 cGy) with a cone-down boost (1,440 cGy) is then given. Three weeks later, cytarabine (Ara-C; 3 g/m²) is given intravenously for 2 days and repeated 3 weeks later. Both regimens have high response rates; the median survival period is more than 40 months. Imaging (preferably MRI) should be performed before each intervention and every 6 to 8 weeks thereafter.

C. The **prognosis** for PCNSL is better than that for the malignant glial tumors. With radiation and chemotherapy, the median survival of patients with PCNSL can be expected to be greater than 3.5 years. Although each of the regimens described in **V.B.** has been associated with limited side effects, some studies of high-dose chemotherapy with radiation for PCNSL have shown both leukoencephalopathy and cognitive changes with treatment. Thus, careful assessment and follow-up evaluation of neurologic status is extremely important. Patients with AIDS respond to such regimens; however, prognosis in that patient population is related to the underlying disease.

VI. **Treatment toxicity**

A. **Radiation toxicity** can be conveniently classified according to the time of presentation into **acute reactions, early delayed reactions,** and **late delayed reactions.**

1. **Acute reactions** occur during the course of treatment. They consist of symptoms of increased intracranial pressure or worsening of existing neurologic symptoms. These symptoms usually are mild and transient and are thought to result from radiation-induced edema. Occasionally it is temporarily necessary to administer a corticosteroid or to increase the dose.

2. **Early delayed reactions** occur several weeks to months after completion of radiation treatment. These reactions may manifest as worsening symptoms or as increasing somnolence and fatigue. It is believed that these symptoms are caused by temporary inhibition of myelin synthesis. Although this syndrome is typically temporary and mild, there have been reports of severe reactions necessitating intensive medical support. Careful consideration is necessary to avoid interpreting an early delayed reaction as a treatment failure without enlargement of tumor mass on images.

3. **Late delayed reactions** may occur months to years after completion of radiation therapy. The main type of late delayed reaction is radiation necrosis, which can mimic tumor recurrence in that it can be progressive, irreversible, and fatal. Higher doses of external beam radiation, used in treating patients with glioblastoma and with stereotactic radiosurgery, are most frequently associated with radiation necrosis. This effect may be a result of damage to small and medium-sized arterioles or a direct effect on glial cells. Radiation necrosis is difficult to diagnose without biopsy. Use of a variety of anatomic (MRI and CT) and functional (positron emission tomography and single photon emission CT) imaging modalities has not facilitated reliable differentiation of necrosis from tumor recurrence. Management of suspected or confirmed radiation necrosis usually entails surgery; however, only total resection (compared with biopsy) is clinically beneficial. There is anecdotal evidence that anticoagulants (heparin and warfarin) may be useful therapy for radiation necrosis at dosages used in stroke management.

B. **Chemotherapy toxicity.** All drugs used in the management of glioma can cause myelosuppression, which in the case of the alkylating agents, is typically delayed and cumulative. Because of this, weekly blood counts, measurement of electrolytes, including calcium and magnesium, and liver function tests should be performed weekly during each cycle. Procarbazine inhibits monoamine oxidase and thus predisposes patients to autonomic sensitivity. Avoidance of foods containing high amounts of tyramine (e.g., red wine, cheese, and tomatoes) and of any sympathomimetic drugs (tricyclic antidepressants, hypnotics, antihistamines, narcotics, and phenothiazines) is necessary during therapy. The nitrosoureas (carmustine and lomustine) can cause hepatic necrosis and pulmonary fibrosis, which are related to cumulative dosing (more than 1,500 mg/m^2). Current recommendations include avoiding nitrosourea therapy in the care of patients with marked pulmonary disease and monitoring of pulmonary function tests every few cycles. Nitrosoureas should be discontinued when a cumulative dose of 1,500 mg/m^2 is attained. Vincristine causes sensorimotor neuropathy and can produce changes in mental status, result in the syndrome of inappropriate secretion of antidiuretic hormone (SIADH), and diminish levels of phenytoin. Methotrexate–leucovorin may be associated with stomatitis. Cytarabine has been shown to cause cholestasis and mucositis in some patients. Cyclophosphamide can cause a hemorrhagic cystitis, water retention, and alopecia. Table 52.1 lists the chemotherapeutic interventions, dosages, and laboratory values that have to be monitored, usually weekly, while these drugs are being given. Table 52.2 gives the possible side effects of therapy among patients with glial tumors.

VII. **Ancillary support**

A. **Diagnosis and recurrence.** With the exception of the more benign tumors (e.g., meningioma, pilocytic astrocytoma, ganglioglioma, and neurocytoma), most primary CNS tumors recur and necessitate terminal care. Because cancer, especially cancer of the brain, is such a devastating diagnosis, it is important to realize and understand the anxiety of the patient and family. Most neurooncologists are members of a multidisciplinary team of physicians, nurses, and social workers who specialize in the care of patients with brain tumors and their families. Each member of the health care team should speak with the patient and concerned family members and provide both practical and emotional support. A mutual understanding of the disease and management of long-term expectations provides a better overall working relationship and maximizes the quality of life for the patient and family. At recurrence, the patient and family may need additional support.

These issues can be addressed by either the nursing or social work staff in addition to the physician. Patient care concerns have to be especially identified in this aspect of treatment. Education is a particularly important aspect of patient care. It includes teaching the patient and family about chemotherapeutic intervention, daily medications, and specific nutritional or equipment requirements. Support staff can act as facilitators in identification and accessing of community resources and services such as home care nursing and cancer support groups.

B. Terminal care. In the United States, once terminal care is needed, it is appropriate to contact local hospice services. Hospice provides the patient and family with emotional support, respite care, equipment, and supply services when death is imminent. The importance of hospice care, in conjunction with frequent contact with the health care team, cannot be overemphasized because of the emotional consequences of such an impending loss. This combination of care can be helpful in making the patient as comfortable as possible and can aid in the transition of the family after death.

Recommended Readings

Balmaceda C. Advances in brain tumor chemosensitivity. *Curr Opin Oncol* 1998;10:192–200.

Bloom HJG, Bessell EM. Medulloblastoma in adults: a review of 47 patients treated between 1952 and 1981. *Int J Radiat Oncol Biol Phys* 1990;18:761–772.

DeAngelis LM, Yahalom J, Heinemann MH, et al. Primary CNS lymphoma: combined treatment with chemotherapy and radiotherapy. *Neurology* 1990;40:80–86.

DeAngelis LM, Yahalom J, Thaler HT, et al. Combined modality therapy for primary CNS lymphoma. *J Clin Oncol* 1992;10:635–643.

Garton GR, Schomberg PJ, Scheithauer BW, et al. Medulloblastoma: prognostic factors and outcome of treatment—review of Mayo Clinic experience. *Mayo Clin Proc* 1990;65: 1077–1086.

Glantz MJ, Burger PC, Herndon JE 2nd, et al. Influence of the type of surgery on the histologic diagnosis in patients with anaplastic gliomas. *Neurology* 1991;41:1741–1744.

Grant R, Liang BC, Page MA, et al. Age influences chemotherapy response in astrocytomas. *Neurology* 1995;45:929–933.

Hubbard JL, Scheithauer BW, Kispert DB, et al. Adult cerebellar medulloblastomas: the pathological, radiographic, and clinical disease spectrum. *J Neurosurg* 1989;70:536–544.

Kaplan RS. Complexities, pitfalls, and strategies for evaluating brain tumor therapies. *Curr Opin Oncol* 1998;10:175–178.

Kortmann RD. Postoperative neoadjuvant chemotherapy before radiotherapy as compared to immediate radiotherapy followed by maintenance chemotherapy in the treatment of medulloblastoma in childhood: results of the German prospective randomized trial HIT '91. *Int J Radiat Oncol Biol Phys* 2000;46(2):269–279.

Levin VA, Silver P, Hannigan J, et al. Superiority of post-radiotherapy adjuvant chemotherapy with CCNU, procarbazine, and vincristine (PCV) over BCNU for anaplastic gliomas: NCOG 6G61 final report. *Int J Radiat Oncol Biol Phys* 1990;18:321–324.

Liang BC, Thornton AF Jr, Sandler HM, et al. Malignant astrocytomas: focal tumor recurrence after focal external beam radiation therapy. *J Neurosurg* 1991;75:559–563.

Liang BC, Weil M. Locoregional approaches to therapy with gliomas as the paradigm. *Curr Opin Oncol* 1998;10:201–206.

Liang BC, Grant R, Junck L, et al. Primary central nervous system lymphoma: treatment with multiagent systemic and intrathecal chemotherapy with radiation therapy. *Int J Oncol* 1993;3:1001–1004.

Louis DN. A molecular genetic model of astrocytoma histopathology. *Brain Pathol* 1997;7;(2): 755–764.

Neuwelt EA, Goldman DL, Dahlborg SA, et al. Primary CNS lymphoma treated with osmotic blood-brain barrier dysruption: prolonged survival and preservation of cognitive function. *J Clin Oncol* 1991;9:1580–1590.

Newton HB, Junck L, Bromberg J, et al. Procarbazine chemotherapy in the treatment of recurrent malignant astrocytomas after radiation and nitrosourea failure. *Neurology* 1990;40:1743–1746.

Packer RJ. Chemotherapy for medulloblastoma/primitive neuroectodermal tumors of the posterior fossa. *Ann Neurol* 1990;28:823–828.

Reddy AT, Packer RJ. Pediatric central nervous system tumors. *Curr Opin Oncol* 1998;10: 186–193.

Rempel SA, Molecular biology of central nervous system tumors. *Curr Opin Oncol* 1998;10: 179–185.

Robertson PL, Zeltzer PM, Boyett JM, et al. Survival and prognostic factors following radiation therapy and chemotherapy for ependymomas in children: a report of the Children's Cancer Group. *J Neurosurg* 1998;88; 695–703.

Thomas DGT, ed. *Neuro-oncology: primary malignant brain tumors*. Baltimore: Johns Hopkins University Press, 1990.

Thomas PR, Deutsch M, Kepner JL, et al. Low-stage medulloblastoma: final analysis of trial comparing standard-dose with reduced-dose neuraxis irradiation. *J Clin Oncol* 2000;18: 3004–3011.

Whitaker SJ, Bessell EM, Ashley SE, et al. Postoperative radiotherapy in the management of spinal cord ependymoma. *J Neurosurg* 1991;74:720–728.

Yung, WKA, Albright RE, Olson J, et al. A phase II study of temozolemide vs. procarbazine in patients with glioblastoma multiforme at first relapse. *Br J Cancer* 2000;83;(5):588–593.

53. NERVOUS SYSTEM COMPLICATIONS OF CANCER

Alok Pasricha and Jack M. Rozental

Neurologic complications of cancer can be metastatic, treatment related, or remote (paraneoplastic). They can cause substantial cognitive and motor disability or death, even while systemic disease may seem under control. Timely recognition and aggressive management of some complications can have a beneficial effect on the patient's quality and length of life. In most instances, management of nervous system complications is palliative, so quality-of-life judgments may be more important than longevity in making therapeutic decisions.

I. **Metastasis to the brain parenchyma**
  A. Approximately 20% of patients cancer eventually have metastatic disease to the central nervous system (CNS), but only one half of those have symptoms. Metastasis accounts for most tumors identified in the CNS.
    1. The tumors that cause 75% of brain metastasis are lung (50%), breast (15%), and melanoma (10%); gastrointestinal and other malignant pelvic tumors such as those of the prostate and ovary cause another 10%.
    2. Approximately 50% of metastatic lesions are single.
    3. Approximately 20% of patients have two metastatic lesions.
    4. Patients with breast, gastrointestinal, and pelvic tumors tend to have single brain lesions.
    5. Patients with lung cancer, melanoma, and tumors of unidentified origin usually have multiple metastatic lesions.
    6. CNS structures are colonized in rough proportion to their relative mass.
      a. Most metastatic lesions localize to the frontal and parietal lobes, and few (1%) to the brainstem.
      b. Metastatic lesions prefer the arterial border zones of the major vessels (anterior middle and middle posterior cerebral arteries) presumably because of decreased vascular caliber and flow.
  B. Among metastatic lesions from pelvic (prostate, ovary, uterus) and gastrointestinal tumors, approximately 50% are to the posterior fossa. Only 10% of other primary tumors metastasize to the posterior fossa.
  C. **Management**
    1. The brain has no lymphatic vessels nor can it expand within the skull; therefore edema contributes to the mass effect and increased intracranial pressure (ICP) produced by tumors.
    2. Increased ICP from an intracranial tumoral mass is managed with dexamethasone 10 mg intravenously (i.v.) followed by 4 mg i.v. or orally four times a day for maintenance.
    3. For a patient with minimal deficit, treatment can begin with dexamethasone 4 mg orally four times a day.
    4. If the initial steroid dose is inadequate, the dosage of dexamethasone can be increased to 6, 8, or more milligrams intravenously or orally four times a day.
    5. Clinical improvement should become apparent within 24 to 48 hours of treatment, continue for several days, then plateau.
    6. Administration of dexamethasone should be tapered as tolerated after the patient's condition is stable and the patient has begun more definitive therapy.
  D. **Steroids** should be used carefully.
    1. An antacid regimen should be started with the steroid as prophylaxis against gastric bleeding, ulceration, or perforation.
    2. Stevens–Johnson syndrome can occur in a patient taking a steroid and anticonvulsants who is receiving brain irradiation.
  E. Patients in extremis from increased ICP may need an osmotic diuretic such as mannitol 20% solution 1 g/kg i.v., which acts within minutes. A bladder catheter should be used.
    1. Smaller doses of mannitol (0.25 to 0.5 g/kg) can be repeated, but ICP must be monitored.

2. Only short-term hyperosmolar therapy is useful for the following reasons.
  a. When serum sodium concentration increases to more than 160 mEq/L, the treatment stops being useful.
  b. Dehydration can lead to cardiovascular collapse.
  c. A rebound increase in ICP occurs despite continued treatment, especially upon rehydration.
3. Patients given osmotic diuretics need a bladder catheter.

F. **Hyperventilation** causes ICP to decrease rapidly. Hyperventilation and osmotic diuretics should be used only if precisely indicated and if a definitive end point is first established.

G. **Seizures**
1. Between 15% and 30% of patients with brain metastasis have seizures.
2. Status epilepticus is managed in the standard manner with intubation (if indicated) and intravenous anticonvulsants.
  a. The drug of choice for patients having a seizure when they arrive for treatment is phenytoin (Dilantin; Pfizer, New York, NY, U.S.A.), intravenously or orally. Most patients can start at the usual maintenance dosage of 300 mg/d orally.
  b. If a patient has had several seizures in the preceding hours, load with 15 to 20 mg/kg (1,000 to 1,200 mg) i.v. or divided into three or four oral doses over 12 to 24 hours.
  c. **Therapeutic levels**
    (1) If the loading dose is administered i.v., therapeutic levels (10 to 20 mg/dL) are reached at the end of the infusion.
    (2) If the load is administered orally all at once, a therapeutic level is reached in 4 to 6 hours.
    (3) If the oral dose is divided, it takes 24 hours to reach therapeutic level.
    (4) If only a maintenance schedule is initiated, it takes 4 to 7 days to reach a therapeutic level.
  d. If seizures continue, the phenytoin dose and blood level can be increased beyond the customary therapeutic range until dose-related toxicity occurs.
  e. Patients who have subsequent seizures almost invariably have subtherapeutic drug levels.
3. If seizures can not be controlled, use carbamazepine (Tegretol; Novartis, East Hanover, NJ, U.S.A.) titrated up to 200 mg orally three or four times a day or valproic acid. One of several newly approved anticonvulsants, such as gabapentin (Neurontin; Pfizer) or lamotrigine (Lamictal; Glaxo Wellcome, Research Triangle Park, NC, U.S.A.), also can be considered.
4. Except for patients with melanoma (50% of whom have seizures), there is no consensus regarding the use of prophylactic anticonvulsants in the care of patients with brain metastasis.
5. Posterior fossa metastasis is not epileptogenic.
6. Dexamethasone and phenytoin have complex interactions.
  a. Each can increase the required dose of the other.
  b. When phenytoin, dexamethasone, and whole-brain irradiation are used concurrently, the risk of erythema multiforme and erythema multiforme bullosa (Stevens–Johnson syndrome) increases.

H. **Surgical management**
1. A patient with minimal disability, a single, circumscribed, accessible lesion, inactive systemic disease, and a long interval between diagnosis of the primary tumor and brain metastasis is the ideal candidate for surgery.
2. A shunt is indicated for obstructive hydrocephalus.
3. In as many as 10% of cases, an intracranial mass in a patient with cancer is not a metastatic lesion. The differential diagnosis includes the following:
  a. Primary CNS tumor
  b. Abscess, demyelinating plaque
  c. Arteriovenous malformation
    Therefore biopsy is advisable if it can be performed safely.

4. Current areas of controversy are as follows.
   a. **Reoperation.** A second surgical procedure may be indicated for metastatic lesions that recur in the original tumor bed with minimal further parenchymal invasion.
   b. **Excision of multiple metastatic masses.** If one or two of several metastatic lesions are symptomatic or life-threatening, palliative resection should be considered.

I. Radiation therapy

1. Radiation is the primary therapy for brain metastasis.
   a. Dosages range from 30 to 40 Gy in 180- to 200-cGy fractions to whole brain over 2 to 4 weeks.
   b. Patients with radiosensitive tumors may benefit from a boost to the tumor bed.
   c. Acute complications of radiation are few (mild headache, hair loss and asthenia) if dexamethasone is administered concurrently.
   d. Toxic effects of radiation therapy include the following.
      (1) **Leukoencephalopathy.** Radiation encephalopathy can be divided according to the time of onset after exposure into acute, early delayed, and delayed.
      (2) **Acute encephalopathy** occurs within a few days of exposure. Patients experience headache, nausea, and changes in mental status. These may be related to increased ICP. Steroids in high doses help. This complication is especially common if steroids do not accompany the radiation dose.
      (3) **Early delayed encephalopathy** is probably caused by demyelination and starts 14 to 120 days after exposure. Features are headache and drowsiness. Brainstem signs including ataxia, diplopia, dysarthria may be present. Spontaneous recovery in a few weeks in usual.
      (4) **Delayed radiation encephalopathy** occurs several months to years after the exposure. It can manifest as diffuse cerebral atrophy or as focal deficits with increased ICP. At pathologic examination, necrosis is seen. It is caused by either direct radiation damage or vascular changes that may be due to microangiopathy or accelerated atherosclerosis.
      (5) **Myelopathy.** Transient radiation myelopathy may occur in patients within the first year of exposure. It is usually self-limiting. Signs include Lhermitte's sign (a shock-like sensation down the back to the legs when the neck is flexed) and paresthesia. Demyelination may be found at pathologic examination.
      (6) **Delayed severe myelopathy** resembling cord compression that progresses to paraplegia or quadriplegia can occur after 1 year. MRI findings usually are normal. Necrosis and atrophy may be found at pathologic examination. No specific treatment exists; corticosteroids may help temporarily.
      (7) **Plexopathy.** Radiation-induced plexopathy can occur soon after treatment and must be differentiated from direct neoplastic involvement of the plexus. Clues to radiation damage include doses greater than 6,000 cGy, lack of pain, lack of lymphedema or induration of the supraclavicular fossa, and presence of myokymic discharges on an electromyogram (EMG).
   e. CNS tolerance to radiation is inversely proportional to the volume irradiated.
2. **Prophylactic cranial irradiation** is controversial because although it decreases the incidence of subsequent brain metastasis from small-cell lung cancer (SCLC), it does not have a significant effect on patient survival.
3. **Stereotactic radiosurgery** (either linear accelerator based or "gamma knife") is a noninvasive technique that delivers a single large fraction or several smaller fractions of ionizing radiation to a well-defined, limited

intracranial target with a sharp peripheral dose fall-off. The result is minimal exposure to normal surrounding brain.

    a. A 10 to 25 Gy fraction can be administered as a boost either before or after conventionally fractionated radiation to tumor volumes of up to 30 cm^3 (maximum tumor diameter of approximately 4 cm).

    b. To remain within brain tolerance parameters, the dose varies inversely with collimator size and number of isocenters.

    c. Initial clinical data suggest that tumor control rates greater than 80% can be achieved with complete response rates of approximately 40%.

    d. Tumors with volumes smaller than 2 cm^3 may respond better than those with volumes larger than 10 cm^3.

  4. Brachytherapy

    a. A series of catheters are stereotactically implanted directly into the tumor bed and afterloaded with high-activity iodine-125 or iridium-192.

    b. The target includes the contrast-enhancing tumor and a 1-cm margin.

      (1) The target receives 45 to 60 Gy of radiation at a dosage rate of 40 to 50 cGy per hour.

      (2) The dose delivered to surrounding normal tissue decreases by the square of the distance from the source.

      (3) The therapeutic ratio improves at continuous low dosage rates because tumors are less able to repair sublethal damage and the radiosensitivity of hypoxic cells depends less on oxygen.

  5. A patient with radiation necrosis has acute or subacute neurologic deterioration and signs and symptoms of a mass lesion.

    a. Neither computed tomography nor magnetic resonance imaging (MRI) can help differentiate a necrotic mass from recurrent tumor.

    b. Necrosis can be managed conservatively with steroids.

    c. Resection is indicated if neurologic deterioration continues, escalating steroid doses become necessary, or intolerable steroid toxicity develops.

J. Chemotherapy

  1. Chemotherapy is not routinely indicated for management of CNS metastasis.

    a. Most tumors are relatively drug resistant.

    b. CNS metastasis most frequently occurs in patients with advanced cancer who have undergone unsuccessful chemotherapy.

  2. Chemotherapy may be considered in some cases.

    a. A patient with a chemosensitive tumor, a good performance status, and inactive systemic disease with CNS metastasis that recurs after radiation with or without surgery.

    b. CNS metastasis from SCLC, breast cancer, lymphoma, and germ cell tumors may respond to chemotherapy with response rates comparable with those of the systemic tumor.

K. Cerebellar metastasis

  1. The signs are gait or limb ataxia, nystagmus, and papilledema.

  2. The symptoms are instability of gait, headache, dizziness, vomiting, and double vision.

  3. Initial treatment considerations are the same as for supratentorial metastasis, that is, dexamethasone and irradiation.

  4. Acute complications of irradiation are more common with cerebellar than with supratentorial metastasis; therefore, dexamethasone should be started at least 48 hours before radiation therapy is initiated.

  5. The risk of brain herniation after lumbar puncture is greater among patients with posterior fossa masses.

  6. The indications for resection are the same as for supratentorial metastasis, but any sign of clinical instability or deterioration, an expanding mass, hydrocephalus, or lack of response to dexamethasone should prompt consideration of immediate neurosurgical intervention.

II. Pituitary apoplexy

  A. This condition is acute panhypopituitarism from a metastatic lesion in the sella turcica or the pituitary gland that causes necrosis or hemorrhage of the gland. It also can be caused, however, by a pituitary adenoma of sufficient severity to produce signs of compression of parasellar structures or signs of meningeal irritation.

B. The syndrome is characterized by headache, ophthalmoplegia, bitemporal hemianopsia or amaurosis, encephalopathy, or coma.

C. Pituitary apoplexy is life threatening when the patient becomes unable to maintain blood pressure despite treatment with fluids and pressors.

D. *This condition is an emergency.* Treatment consists of high doses of a corticosteroid: dexamethasone 6 to 12 mg i.v. every 6 hours. Surgical decompression may be needed.

III. Metastasis to the skull base. The hallmark of metastasis to the skull base is involvement of the cranial nerves as they exit through the basal foramina. Most primary tumors are from the breast, lung, or prostate. Five major syndromes are recognized.

A. Orbital syndrome manifests as dull, continuous, progressive pain over the affected eye with proptosis, external ophthalmoplegia, and blurred vision. There is decreased sensation over the distribution of the first division of the trigeminal nerve (cranial nerve V).

B. Parasellar syndrome (cavernous sinus metastasis) manifests as unilateral frontal headache and ophthalmoplegia. The patient may have decreased sensation over the distribution of the first division of cranial nerve V. If sinus thrombosis occurs, there is chemosis, edema of the eyelid and forehead, proptosis, and papilledema with retinal hemorrhage. This is a cause of Tolosa–Hunt syndrome. In both parasellar and orbital syndrome, steroids are warranted before radiation therapy to prevent acute vision loss from radiation-induced edema.

C. Middle fossa syndrome (gasserian ganglion) is signaled by pain, numbness, or paresthesia over the distribution of the second or third divisions of cranial nerve V. The initial presentation may be a numb chin or lip syndrome. Pterygoid and masseter weakness and abducens palsy are late complications. Sixty-five percent of these lesions are from breast cancer and 15% from lymphoproliferative tumors. Fifty percent of patients have mandibular metastasis, 15% have skull base lesions, and 20% carcinomatous meningitis.

D. Jugular foramen syndrome manifests as hoarseness and dysphagia (cranial nerve X) with or without pain (cranial nerve IX or X). Examination may reveal asymmetric palatal elevation (cranial nerve IX), weakness of the ipsilateral sternocleidomastoid and trapezius muscles (cranial nerve XI), and Horner's syndrome (sympathetic). Weakness and atrophy of the tongue may be found if cranial nerve XII is compromised by extension of the tumor to the adjacent hypoglossal canal.

E. Occipital condyle syndrome manifests as stiff neck and severe occipital pain that increases with neck flexion. There are dysarthria and dysphagia from unilateral involvement of cranial nerve XII in approximately one half of cases.

IV. Dural metastasis can cause headache or underlying venous sinus thrombosis and may invade the parenchyma. Subdural effusion with tumor cells is usually associated. Breast and prostate tumors are most commonly implicated.

V. Spinal epidural metastasis

A. Metastatic epidural spinal cord compression occurs in 5% to 10% of patients with cancer. *It is a neurooncologic emergency.* Metastatic compression occurs more frequently than compression by primary spinal cord tumors.

B. Prognosis. The most important determinant is neurologic performance status at presentation.

1. Of ambulatory patients, 90% remain so after treatment, and they have a 75% probability of surviving 1 year.

2. Only 50% of paraparetic and 13% of paraplegic patients with "radiosensitive" tumors become ambulatory after treatment.

3. Fewer than 10% of nonambulatory patients survive 1 year.

4. Once sphincter control is lost, it is unlikely to be regained.

5. Once neurologic dysfunction begins, paraplegia and loss of sphincter control follow within hours. Once established, the neurologic deficit usually is irreversible.

C. Epidural tumor must be suspected on clinical grounds and must prompt timely confirmation and treatment.

    1. Approximately 60% of epidural metastatic lesions arise from prostate, lung, breast, and kidney cancer.

    2. Approximately 50% of adults with acute transverse myelopathy have spinal cord compression from epidural metastasis. In one half of those patients, it is the initial manifestation of cancer, and in one half of those, the primary tumor is in the lung.

D. Presentation

    1. Approximately 95% of patients with epidural tumor have progressive axial pain with or without a radicular or referred component.

    2. Some weakness and sensory disturbance are present in 80% of patients.

    3. Almost 60% of patients have sphincter dysfunction, a poor prognostic sign that implies bilateral cord or root damage.

E. Site of involvement

    1. In approximately 85% of epidural tumors from solid cancers, the bony vertebral column is the site of metastasis. Metastatic lesions never involve the intervertebral disks or transgress the dura.

        a. The vertebral body is involved in 45% of cases.

        b. The posterior arch and pedicle are involved in 40%.

        c. The entire vertebra is involved in 15%.

    2. Between 50% and 70% of lesions involve the thoracic spine.

    3. Twenty percent to 30% involve the lumbosacral spine.

    4. Ten percent to 20% involve the cervical spine.

    5. At least one third of patients with breast and prostate cancer have metastatic lesions at multiple levels.

    6. Most patients with lung cancer have metastatic lesions at only one level.

F. There are **three mechanisms of metastatic epidural spinal cord compression.**

    1. Most common is hematogenous spread to the vertebra, which has vascularized bone marrow and growth factors.

    2. Second is through Batson's plexus, which is the vertebral venous plexus. The Batson's veins are valveless and allow tumor seeding when intraabdominal pressure increases, as in coughing, sneezing, or a Valsalva maneuver.

    3. Tumor also may reach the epidural space by means of direct invasion of a paravertebral mass through the intervertebral foramen. This is the mechanism of 75% of cases of cord compressions from lymphoma.

G. Diagnosis. A neuroimaging study should be performed in all cases of suspected epidural tumor to establish the diagnosis, the upper and lower limits of tumor invasion, and whether tumor exists at discontinuous levels.

    1. MRI is the imaging modality of choice for confirmation, visualization of extent of disease, and treatment planning. Because disease often is multifocal within the vertebral column, the entire spine should be visualized.

    2. Non–contrast-enhanced T1-weighted images are obtained first and followed by contrast-enhanced and T2-weighted images. This is because contrast enhancement can obscure subtle vertebral metastasis.

    3. Gadolinium enhancement is, however, helpful for detection of epidural, intradural, and intramedullary processes.

    4. The typical findings are multiple foci of low signal intensity on T1-weighted images. Collapse and destruction of vertebral bodies and sparing of the adjacent disk are common. Fat suppression techniques increase sensitivity.

    5. On plain radiographs of the spine, pedicle changes are seen before vertebral bodies because the pedicle is compact bone. The most common findings are pedicle erosion, paravertebral soft-tissue shadow, and vertebral collapse or dislocation.

    6. The findings on plain radiographs correlate with vertebral metastasis in examinations of 85% to 95% of patients with epidural compression from solid tumors but in only one third of patients with lymphoma.

H. Initial management
1. If cord compression is suspected, or upon confirmation, a 100-mg i.v. bolus of dexamethasone is administered and followed by 24 mg i.v. every 6 hours.
2. Maintenance dosage of dexamethasone (4 mg i.v. or orally every 6 hours) is instituted and then tapered as tolerated.
3. Steroids rapidly decrease vasogenic edema and promote clinical improvement. Steroids rarely produce a dramatic reversal of established neurologic disability, but the prognosis is better when they do.
4. The bladder should be catheterized for measurement of postvoid residual volume, and an indwelling catheter should be inserted if necessary.
5. Prophylaxis against deep venous thrombosis and a stool-softening regimen should be started.

I. Although the intent of therapy remains **palliative,** several treatment options are available.
1. **Decompressive laminectomy** works only temporarily and fails for the following reasons:
    a. Metastatic tumor generally is located in the vertebral body (that is, anterior to the spinal cord) and not in the neural arch.
    b. **Laminectomy** can contribute to spinal instability.
2. **Anterior vertebral body resection**
    a. Must be coupled with surgical stabilization of the spine.
    b. Operative morbidity (10%) is caused by nonhealing, breakdown, or infection of the wound and failure to stabilize the spine.
3. **Radiation** alone is the procedure of choice for radiosensitive tumors.
    a. A total 20 to 40 Gy dose divided over 10 fractions is the usual treatment
    b. The port should encompass two vertebral bodies above and two below the epidural defect and any discontinuous lesions.
    c. Radiation is indicated promptly after the diagnosis is made and should follow administration of dexamethasone.
    d. If surgery is performed first, radiation should follow after the wound heals.
    e. The tumors that most commonly produce epidural metastasis—those of the lung, breast, and prostate and lymphoma—are likely to respond to radiation.
    f. If neurologic deterioration continues, surgical intervention should be considered.
    g. The complications of radiation therapy are
        (1) Bone marrow depression
        (2) Radiation myelopathy or syrinx (6 to 18 months after therapy)
        (3) Risk of a subacute syndrome characterized by Lhermitte's sign several weeks after radiation
4. **Laminectomy plus radiation.** There is no evidence that combining laminectomy with radiation results in a better outcome than does radiation alone.
5. **Epidural tumors** do not respond rapidly enough to chemotherapy to warrant use of this modality in acute situations.
6. **Recurrent spinal epidural metastasis**
    a. **Local metastatic lesions** develop within two vertebral bodies of a previous lesion and within 3 months of the original diagnosis. They represent a failure of tumor control at the margin of the radiation port.
    b. **Distant metastatic lesions** develop three or more vertebral bodies from a previous lesion and 15 months or longer after the original diagnosis.
    c. Patients who previously responded to radiation therapy may be considered for repetition of irradiation. They may benefit but not survive to experience the consequences of exceeding spinal cord radiation tolerance.

VI. Leptomeningeal metastasis
A. Leptomeningeal metastasis occurs when tumor cells invade the arachnoid and pia mater either focally or multifocally.
1. It develops in as many as 70% of patients with leukemia and 5% to 8% with non-Hodgkin's lymphoma. Among the solid tumors, adenocarcinoma of the

breast, lung, and gastrointestinal tract and melanoma are common. Breast cancer is the most common.

  2. Primary CNS tumors, including ependymoma and medulloblastoma, when untreated have a high incidence of leptomeningeal metastasis.
  3. Most primary CNS lymphomas are parenchymal and can lead to leptomeningeal spread.

B. **Pathology.** Typical pathologic features are
  1. Sheetlike layers of tumor cells
  2. Infiltration of cranial or spinal nerve roots
  3. Parenchymal invasion through the Virchow and Robin spaces that is more prominent along the ventral brain surface

C. **Presentation**
  1. The clinical features are attributable to involvement of the cerebrum or the spinal or cranial nerves.
  2. The initial feature may be hydrocephalus with no intracranial mass lesion.
  3. Chronic, worsening, unremitting headache or somatic pain may be present without apparent cause.
  4. Extraocular nerve palsy, seventh cranial nerve, fifth cranial nerve, and eighth cranial nerve involvement can occur.
  5. Involvement of lumbosacral nerve roots giving rise to **cauda equina syndrome** with weakness and sensory loss can occur.
  6. The major differential diagnosis is bacterial or fungal meningitis.

D. **Diagnosis**
  1. **Lumbar puncture** should be performed in all cases. The results are abnormal in more than 95% of cases.
  2. Lumbar puncture may reveal lymphocytic pleocytosis, low glucose level (one third of cases), elevated protein level, or malignant cells. Cerebrospinal fluid (CSF) pressure may be high.
  3. Positive cytologic findings are present in only one half cases on the first tap, and several taps may be needed. Cytologic tests should be performed on a cytospin sample, not on stained smears. CSF samples should be processed immediately after withdrawal to prevent cell lysis.
  4. Markers such as carcinoembryonic antigen, β_2 microglobulin and lactate dehydrogenase can be used for follow-up evaluation of the CSF once the initial diagnosis has been made with a cytologic examination.
  5. **MRI** is the radiologic modality of choice. Gadolinium-enhanced MR images show linear enhancement on the surface of nerve roots and spinal cord.
  6. MRI findings may be abnormal even in the absence of initial positive cytologic findings or spinal symptoms. Treatment can be initiated on the basis of MRI findings.

E. **Initial treatment**
  1. In the decision to treat, the systemic disease status and likelihood of successful palliation should be considered.
  2. Dexamethasone rarely provides symptomatic improvement and should be tapered after more definitive treatment is initiated.

F. **Craniospinal radiation**
  1. Either 30 Gy to the entire neuraxis or 24 Gy in 10 to 15 fractions to the most symptomatic areas usually is administered.
  2. Irradiating the entire neuraxis rarely controls leptomeningeal disease, and it can aggravate or produce severe bone marrow depression. Most patients are unable to tolerate a complete course. Total cranial spinal axis radiation therapy is thus used mainly for meningeal leukemia.

G. **Intrathecal chemotherapy**
  1. This modality is useful because tumor diffusely infiltrates the leptomeninges.
  2. After systemic administration, most drugs reach CSF concentrations between 1% and 25% of the plasma concentration. Hence, the dose intensity of treatment in the CSF is decreased, and the patient becomes predisposed to CNS failure.

3. The volume of distribution in the CSF is small, so high concentrations can be achieved with small drug doses.
4. Drug clearance half-lives tend to be longer in the CSF than in plasma, maximizing exposure.
5. Intrathecal chemotherapy can be used alone or with neuraxis irradiation.
6. The first few doses can be administered by means of lumbar puncture, but if continued, this mode of administration can lead to an epidural hematoma, CSF leaks, and virtual subdural or epidural compartments through which drug can be lost.
7. Other constraints to delivery through lumbar puncture relate to the dynamics of CSF flow, which is craniocaudal, tends to bypass the ventricles, is affected by patient position, and may be severely disturbed in the presence of meningeal tumor with or without increased ICP.
8. A ventricular catheter with subcutaneous (Ommaya) reservoir should be implanted for drug delivery.
   a. The most serious, but uncommon, complication of use of Ommaya reservoirs is infection. Therefore, proper sterile technique should be followed with each use.
   b. Fever, headache, lethargy, and CSF extravasation around the reservoir are signs of infection of an Ommaya reservoir.
9. Only approximately one half patients with leptomeningeal cancer secondary to solid tumors respond to treatment, as opposed to approximately three fourths of patients with lymphoma or leukemia.
10. Methotrexate is the most commonly used drug for intrathecal management of solid tumors. Cytosine arabinoside may be added to methotrexate for lymphoma or leukemia.

VII. Metastasis to the spinal cord parenchyma
A. Treatment
1. Treatment is palliative.
2. Dexamethasone is the initial emergency treatment and should be followed by irradiation of the entire cord.
3. Because approximately 75% of cases are secondary to lung and breast cancer and lymphoma, some clinical improvement can be expected, especially if the patient is treated before a myelopathy develops.
4. Surgical decompression accomplishes little because the disease is intrinsic to the spinal cord, and resection of the lesion itself generally is not feasible.

VIII. Metastasis to the peripheral nervous system
A. Presentation
1. Pain, numbness, paresthesia, or weakness
2. Must be differentiated from radiation plexopathy
3. Pain, paresthesia, and weakness are more frequent with neoplastic involvement than with radiation plexopathy.
4. Horner's syndrome is frequent with metastasis to the brachial plexus.

B. Treatment
1. Aggressive pain relief is imperative.
2. Nonnarcotic drugs fail early, and adequate doses of narcotics should be prescribed.
3. If narcotics fail, several anesthetic or neurosurgical procedures are available.
4. Radiation or chemotherapy is instituted as appropriate.

IX. Neurologic complications of chemotherapy
A. Most cytotoxic drugs are capable of nervous system toxicity.
B. Important reasons for recognizing iatrogenic toxicity are as follows:
1. Drug-induced complications can obscure or mimic the presentation of metastasis, paraneoplastic syndromes, or primary neurologic disease.
2. Neurotoxicity can contribute to morbidity, disability, and death.
3. Neurotoxicity can result from metabolic derangement of therapy or cancer-induced end-organ failure.
4. The offending agent can be recognized during treatment with a multiple-drug regimen.

C. **Common complications attributable to chemotherapy**
   1. **Peripheral neuropathy**
      a. Chemotherapeutic agents commonly implicated in development of neu-ropathy are vinca alkaloids (vincristine, vinblastine), cisplatin, and paclitaxel (Taxol; Bristol-Myers Squibb, Princeton, NJ, U.S.A.).
      b. **Cisplatin.** Peripheral neuropathy is the dose-limiting side effect. Large-fiber sensory polyneuropathy is common, as is ototoxicity, especially if the cumulative dose exceeds 400 mg/m^2. Symptoms include paresthesia, proprioceptive loss, and ataxia. Autonomic symptoms such as gastro-paresis and vomiting are frequent. Neuropathy may develop even months after the drug is stopped (coasting). Most patients improve spontaneously if the total dose is less than 500 mg/m^2.
      c. **Paclitaxel.** Dose-related sensory neuropathy occurs with doses greater than 200 mg/m^2. Painful paresthesia, multimodality sensory loss, ataxia, and mild distal weakness are common. Loss of the distal muscle stretch reflexes is almost universal. Neurotrophins have prevented this neu-ropathy in animal models.
      d. **Docetaxel** causes dose-dependent polyneuropathy similar to that caused by paclitaxel.
      e. **Vinca alkaloids.** Length-dependent sensorimotor neuropathy is the dose-limiting side effect. Neurotoxicity is related to tubulin binding, which interferes with axonal microtubule assembly. Vincristine pro-duces mild neuropathy in almost all patients at conventional doses. Autonomic dysfunction that manifests as gastroparesis, urinary reten-tion, constipation, and ileus is an early manifestation. In rare instances, cranial nerve involvement such as facial sensory loss, facial weakness, or recurrent laryngeal palsy occurs. Reduction in dose or early with-drawal leads to complete recovery. Glutamic acid or ORG 2766, a corti-cotropin-derived synthetic peptide has been reported to reduce the severity of the neuropathy.
      f. **Etoposide** is a semisynthetic derivative of podophyllotoxin used to manage SCLC and lymphoma. It has been reported to cause axonal neu-ropathy in as many as 10% of cases.
      g. **Suramin** is used as an investigational antineoplastic drug for refractory malignant tumors. It leads to two distinct patterns of neurotoxicity that may be dose limiting. It can cause either length-dependent axonal poly-neuropathy (30% to 50% of cases) or subacute demyelinating polyradicu-loneuropathy resembling Guillain–Barré syndrome (15% of cases). Inhibition of nerve growth factor may be an important mechanism in the development of neuropathy, which occurs after peak plasma concentra-tion increases to more than 350 μg/mL. Improvement after plasma-pheresis has been reported.
   2. **Transient, dose-dependent myalgia** may occur several days after admin-istration of paclitaxel or vincristine.
   3. **CNS complications**
      a. The prototype drug for CNS complications is methotrexate.
      b. Route of administration, dosage, and simultaneous use of methotrexate with other neurotoxic therapy (particularly cranial irradiation) can cause additive or synergistic toxicity.
      c. Intrathecal methotrexate produces aseptic meningitis within a few hours after administration (lasts several days and subsides without sequelae) and transient or permanent myelopathy.
      d. Leukoencephalopathy is a delayed effect of either intrathecal or high-dose systemic administration. It can occur in as many as 45% if methotrexate is combined with cranial irradiation or other neurotoxic drugs.
      e. High-dose methotrexate can produce an acute, self-limited neurologic syndrome characterized by encephalopathy (seizures, delirium, confu-sion) or, sometimes, a stroke-like syndrome of unknown causation.
   4. **Cerebellar toxicity**
      a. Purkinje cells are very sensitive to chemotherapy.

        b. Cerebellar toxicity occurs in 8% to 50% of patients given high-dose cytarabine (doses >48 g/m^2).

            (1) Symptoms occur within 24 to 48 hours as nystagmus and mild ataxia followed by a florid encephalopathic and ataxic syndrome.

            (2) Patients may improve within 1 week and recover completely within 2 weeks.

            (3) The pathogenesis of this syndrome relates to the minimal amounts of cytidine deaminase (which inactivates cytarabine) in the CNS.

        c. **5-Fluorouracil** causes abrupt cerebellar dysfunction in as many as 7% of patients a few days to months after the start of treatment. The dysfunction resolves after the drug is discontinued. Cerebellar dysfunction is likely with schedules that entail one or more weekly boluses of more than 15 mg/kg of 5-fluorouracil.

    5. The following simple treatment strategies are of value.

        a. Physical and occupational therapy can be the determinant between a functional and a disabled patient.

        b. An ankle–foot orthosis for foot drop may preserve the patient's ability to walk or help avoid tripping.

        c. Neuropsychologic therapy may assist in the management of cognitive disability from leukoencephalopathy.

X. Other complications

  A. Neuropathic pain. The characteristic symptoms of injury to the nervous system—spontaneous pain and allodynia—imply a neuropathic pain syndrome. This is different from nociceptive pain felt in the viscera or somatic areas because of excessive stimulation of nociceptors under normal conditions. There is evidence to suggest that up-regulation of sodium channels and N-methyl-D-aspartate (NMDA) receptors play an important role. The common neuropathic pain syndromes are as follows.

    1. Brachial plexus pain. Tumor invasion of the brachial plexus from breast carcinoma leads to pain most referable to the C8-T1 distribution. Pain precedes neurologic findings by months. Management of the underlying tumor relieves pain in approximately 50% of cases; however, if pain returns, an exhaustive search for tumor recurrence must be undertaken.

    2. Lumbar plexus pain. The lumbar plexus is commonly involved in extension of pelvic and colon tumors or metastasis from distant tumors. Pain felt in the distribution of one or more nerve roots is the first symptom and is followed by weakness and sensory loss. Bowel and bladder involvement usually occurs late.

    3. Base of skull metastasis. Involvement of the trigeminal nerve or the area of the jugular foramen causes pain in the distribution of the nerves involved. Pain in the face may be shock like and may be referable to the orbit or brow area. **Swallow syncope** refers to the occurrence of lightning-like pain on swallowing followed by syncope. It is caused by tumor involving the glossopharyngeal nerve.

    4. Carcinomatous meningitis. Tumor seeding along nerve root sleeves produces radicular pain symptoms.

    5. Postsurgical pain. Five percent to 20% of patients undergoing mastectomy have characteristic postmastectomy pain. The syndrome includes a burning, tight feeling in the upper inner arm and across the chest. This may lead to frozen shoulder because of guarding in the area. Thoracotomy is widely recognized as being very painful in the immediately postoperative period because the intercostal nerves are subjected to direct trauma during the procedure. Radical neck dissection can lead to poorly defined burning stabbing pain because of injury to the cervical nerves.

    6. Radiation injury to peripheral nerves and plexus can have painful sequelae with onset usually delayed for years after exposure. Pain may be the initial presentation of cervical plexus injury, whereas lumbar plexus injury often manifests as weakness. These must be differentiated from tumor recurrence.

7. **Chemotherapy-related pain.** Several chemotherapeutic agents can cause neuropathy that can be painful.
8. **Treatment.** Opioids are considered the mainstay of treatment. Other agents commonly used include tricyclic antidepressants, including tertiary and secondary amines. The mechanism of action is inhibition of reuptake of monoamine neurotransmitters. Anticonvulsants such as carbamazepine and gabapentin also are used. Ketamine and dextromethorphan have been efficacious in experimental models. NMDA receptors have a theoretical role because of the presumed role of excitatory amino acids in perpetuating pain. Systemic administration of local anesthetics has shown promise in experimental models. Corticosteroids have been used in a variety of settings mainly as an adjunct to opioids. No clinical studies have assessed the efficacy of corticosteroids as primary analgesics. Local anesthetics such as capsaicin also can be used. Local depletion of substance P is the presumed mechanism of capsaicin.

B. Encephalopathy
1. **Seizures**
   a. Encephalopathic conditions can cause seizures, and seizures can cause encephalopathy.
   b. A postictal state can mimic encephalopathy; in debilitated, elderly patients it can last 1 week or more.
2. If controllable causes are excluded, management is supportive.

C. CNS infection
1. The most frequently encountered organisms are *Listeria monocytogenes, Cryptococcus neoformans,* and *Aspergillus fumigatus.*
2. Next in frequency are gram-negative rods, *Candida albicans,* and herpes zoster virus.
3. Latent mycobacterial infections can become reactivated.
4. **Presentation**
   a. CNS infections manifest as fever, changes in mental status, and seizures.
   b. Headache and stiff neck can be subtle if the patient is unable to mount an adequate inflammatory response.
   c. In patients with severe leukopenia, the CSF may not be purulent, and the infecting organism may not be readily detectable.
   d. Gram or Ziehl–Neelsen staining of cytospin sediment may reveal the pathogen before culture results turn positive.
5. *Lumbar puncture should be approached with caution* because a patient with increased ICP may have herniation or a patient with thrombocytopenia may have an epidural hematoma.
6. **Treatment** consists of antibiotics and support.
7. **Progressive multifocal leukoencephalopathy (PML)**
   a. PML is CNS infection by an opportunistic papovavirus, the JC virus.
   b. Rare cases go into long-term remission.
   c. PML manifests as changes mental status, speech and vision deficits, and weakness.
   d. Diagnosis is by means of biopsy of a focal (nonenhancing) white-matter brain lesion.
   e. Treatment with adenosine arabinoside (Ara-A) or cytosine arabinoside (Ara-C; cytarabine) is of unproven benefit.

D. Cerebrovascular complications
1. At autopsy, approximately 15% of cancer patients are found to have cerebrovascular disease; one half had had symptoms.
2. Atherosclerosis remains the leading cause of infarction, but only approximately 15% of infarcts are symptomatic.
3. Patients with cancer also may have cerebrovascular disease as a complication of the neoplastic process or its management.
4. Ischemic infarcts, rather than hemorrhages, predominate among patients with carcinoma. Nonbacterial thrombotic endocarditis and intravascular coagulation are frequent causes of symptomatic cerebral infarction in this population.

5. The most frequent causes of intraparenchymal hemorrhage are coagulopathy and hemorrhage into metastatic lesions from melanoma and germ cell tumors.
6. Mucinous cancers may produce infarction from widespread occlusion (by mucin) of any cerebral artery.
7. A large proportion of patients with symptomatic cerebrovascular disease and leukemia experience hemorrhagic infarction.
8. There is no specific therapy for these complications.
9. Chemotherapy, especially with cisplatin, can cause both acute and late vasculoocclusive complications.
   a. Acute vascular occlusion may be related to endothelial injury.
   b. Late occlusion may be related to vasospasm from hypomagnesemia.
10. **Late effects of radiation therapy** include noninflammatory arteriopathy, which causes large- and small-vessel occlusion, mineralizing microangiopathy, and accelerated atherosclerosis.
11. **Dural sinus thrombosis,** particularly of the superior sagittal sinus, is underdiagnosed.
    a. It is frequently asymptomatic and eventually recanalizes.
    b. It is most frequent in patients with leukemia receiving chemotherapy and in patients with coagulopathy or with widespread cancer.
    c. It manifests as headache, seizures, papilledema, focal motor signs, and encephalopathy.
    d. The diagnosis is made by means of angiography, contrast-enhanced computed tomography, MRI, or MR angiography.
    e. Treatment is supportive with or without limited-term anticoagulation if there is no hemorrhage, but this indication is controversial.
12. **Neoplastic angioendotheliosis** or intravascular lymphomatosis is intravascular occlusion of small blood vessels by malignant mononuclear cells.
    a. It is a rare complication of lymphoma.
    b. When the occluded vessels are in the CNS, patients have multifocal deficits and encephalopathy with short-term or subacute progression to death.
    c. This disorder is difficult to differentiate from PML, vasculitis, and multiple emboli.
E. Syncope in patients with head and neck cancer
   1. Manifests in advanced or recurrent disease as syncope accompanied by paroxysmal head and face pain.
   2. An abnormally strong carotid sinus reflex mediates the syncopal attacks.
   3. A relation between the syncope and sudden death exists and should prompt a search for recurrent carcinoma.
   4. Pain is managed with carbamazepine.
   5. Syncope is managed with anticholinergic drugs such as propantheline 15 to 30 mg orally four times a day. Ephedrine 25 mg orally four times a day may be added if there is a vasodepressor component.
XI. **Paraneoplastic syndromes** or remote effects of cancer are thought to originate from production of an antibody to onconeural antigens shared between the tumor and the CNS. The neurologic syndromes can involve any part or parts of both the peripheral and central nervous systems. They must be differentiated from treatment-related toxicity and from metastasis. The anti-neuronal antibodies found in the paraneoplastic disorders are not thought to be directly pathogenic; they should rather be considered as markers for the disorder. There is also evidence that T-cell cytotoxic mechanisms play an important role in nervous system injury. The following paraneoplastic syndromes have been described:
   A. **Paraneoplastic limbic encephalopathy** may develop alone or in association with disorders of other parts of the nervous system—brainstem, cerebellum, or peripheral nerves. The most common associated tumor is SCLC (75% of cases), followed by germ cell tumor, thymoma, and Hodgkin's lymphoma. Neurologic dysfunction often precedes the tumor diagnosis by several months or longer.
      1. **Clinical features**
         a. Most characteristic is a subacute amnestic syndrome with relative preservation of other cognitive functions. Both short-term anterograde and

variable retrograde amnesia are present. Memory deficit may be preceded by weeks of depression, personality changes, and emotional lability. Partial complex seizures are common.

   b. Most patients eventually have manifestations of a more generalized multifocal paraneoplastic encephalomyelitis with signs and symptoms of involvement of brainstem, cerebellum, dorsal root ganglia, spinal cord, and autonomic nervous system.

   c. The course is variable and unpredictable. Most patients' conditions appear to stabilize at a level of severe disability. A few patients become obtunded and comatose.

   2. Diagnosis

   a. Anti-Hu antibodies are present in 50% of patients with SCLC and symptoms suggestive of limbic encephalopathy. The prognosis is better among patients who do not have anti-Hu antibodies.

   b. A new paraneoplastic antibody anti-Ta has been identified in the CSF and serum of patients with this syndrome who have testicular cancer (seminomatous or nonseminomatous).

   c. "Atypical antibodies" including anti-CV2 associated with thymoma and antibodies that stain hippocampal neurons in patients with colon cancer also have been reported.

   d. MRI is of limited help, but T2-weighted images may show abnormalities in the mesial temporal lobes. CSF may have inflammatory changes, including increased protein, moderate pleocytosis, oligoclonal bands, and an increased level of immunoglobulin G (IgG).

B. Paraneoplastic cerebellar degeneration (PCD). Although an unusual syndrome, PCD may be profoundly disabling. The onset of cerebellar degeneration may occur 2 years before the diagnosis of cancer, during the course of the disease, or infrequently after apparent clinical remission. It is more common among women and is associated with adenocarcinoma of the ovary, uterus or adnexa, carcinoma of the breast, SCLC, and less commonly with Hodgkin's lymphoma. In the setting of gynecologic malignant tumors, it usually occurs as an isolated syndrome. In the setting of SCLC, it occurs as a part of more diffuse CNS involvement with paraneoplastic encephalomyelitis.

   1. Clinical features

   a. The most common initial symptom is loss of coordination, which may begin unilaterally. Disease progression usually is subacute over days or weeks. By the time the disorder manifests itself, most patients have severe truncal and gait ataxia. Speech is dysarthric, and head titubation may occur. Vertigo, nausea, and vomiting are common.

   b. Examination usually reveals disorders of ocular motility, including nystagmus, dysmetria, dysconjugate gaze, and occasionally, opsoclonus. Patients often are left with a severe neurologic deficit without much improvement.

   2. Diagnosis

   a. Three major and several minor patterns of antineuronal antibody patterns have been associated with PCD. Only one of these, the anti-Yo antibody (type 1 anti–parietal cell antibody) is strictly associated with PCD and is present exclusively in women with gynecologic or breast carcinoma. The other two, the anti-Hu (type 2, antineuronal nuclear antibody type 1) and the anti-Ri (type 2b, anti-neuronal nuclear antibody type 2) are associated with more complex disorders that may initially be diagnosed as PCD.

   b. The anti-Hu pattern is associated with SCLC and anti-Ri exclusively with breast carcinoma. Newer antibodies include anti-Tr autoantibodies in patients with Hodgkin's disease and anti-CV2 in patients with cancer of the lung. Most patients who have PCD in association with Hodgkin's disease, non–small cell lung cancer, or gastrointestinal carcinoma do not have any demonstrable antineuronal antibodies.

   3. Management. Treatment is unsatisfactory, but the best results are found among patients with no underlying gynecologic malignant tumors. Plasmapheresis or intravenous immunoglobulin is beneficial to fewer than 10% of patients.

C. **Opsoclonus–myoclonus** is a condition characterized by random, chaotic ocular movements. It is reported to occur with a vast variety of tumors, more diverse than in PCD or paraneoplastic encephalomyelitis. It occurs in 2% to 3% of children with neuroblastoma. In most of these cases, the neurologic syndrome leads to discovery of the tumor. Paraneoplastic opsoclonus usually appears as a part of a constellation of symptoms that usually includes ataxia, myoclonus, alteration in mental status, or a combination of these disorders.

   1. **Clinical features.** Eye movements are conjugate, high amplitude, and in all directions of gaze. They are almost continuous and persist during eye opening. Unlike other paraneoplastic disorders, opsoclonus–myoclonus may go into spontaneous remission and be relieved with immunosuppressive therapy or tumor treatment. No clinical features differentiate paraneoplastic from nonparaneoplastic opsoclonus–myoclonus.

   2. **Diagnosis.** The diagnosis is clinical, but patients with opsoclonus and ataxia associated with breast cancer may have anti-Ri antibodies. Patients with SCLC and opsoclonus usually have no detectable antineuronal antibodies. Findings at MRI of the brain usually are normal. Children with opsoclonus need a complete evaluation for neuroblastoma, including nuclear imaging with metaiodobenzylguanidine, which may show tumor in the absence of a radiologic lesion.

   3. **Management.** Corticotropin or corticosteroids produce rapid and dramatic neurologic improvement in at least two thirds of children independently of tumor status. In a number of adult patients with or without antineuronal antibodies, improvement has followed treatment with corticosteroids.

D. **Myelopathy** can occur with multiple-system neurologic involvement, as in paraneoplastic encephalomyelitis, in which case cord involvement is patchy. Necrotizing myelopathy, a distinct clinical entity, also occurs independently. Necrotizing myelopathy can occur in association with a variety of carcinomas and lymphoid tumors without showing predilection for any particular type.

   1. **Clinical features of necrotizing myelopathy**
      a. The usual presentation is subacute onset of bilateral symptoms involving motor, sensory, and sphincter dysfunction with little or no pain. Examination reveals transverse spinal cord dysfunction. Most patients have rapid deterioration with progressively ascending paralysis and death due to respiratory failure.
      b. The **differential diagnosis** of subacute myelopathy in a cancer patient includes intramedullary spinal metastasis and spinal cord injury caused by radiation or by intrathecal chemotherapy, all of which are more common than a paraneoplastic process.

   2. **Diagnosis.** Findings at spinal MRI may be normal or show intramedullary involvement. No antineuronal antibodies have been associated specifically with paraneoplastic necrotizing myelopathy.

   3. **Management.** There is anecdotal evidence of improvement with steroids.

E. **Motor neuron disease.** Lower motor neuron signs are the predominant manifestation of as many as 25% of cases of multifocal paraneoplastic encephalomyelitis. It is unclear, however, how often pure motor neuron disease is a paraneoplastic syndrome. There is no convincing evidence that nonhematogenous neoplasms occur in patients with amyotrophic lateral sclerosis any more frequently than would be expected in an age-matched control population. Most of the patients have SCLC. The prevalence of plasma cell dyscrasia among patients with motor neuron disease is higher than among controls; however, most of these patients have monoclonal gammopathy of undetermined significance.

   1. **Clinical features.** Patchy weakness, fasciculations, and atrophy are the usual manifestations. Patients also may have alteration in mental status, cerebellar ataxia, and brainstem findings.

   2. **Diagnosis.** Anti-Hu antibodies may or may not be present.

3. **Management.** Scattered cases of improvement are reported after plasma exchange and administration of corticosteroids and alkylating agents such as melphalan.

F. **Stiff person syndrome.** Muscle stiffness or rigidity can occur in the setting of several paraneoplastic disorders and reflect either central or peripheral nervous system dysfunction. A syndrome resembling stiff person syndrome can be associated with a variety of neoplasms, including SCLC, Hodgkin's disease, and carcinoma of the breast or colon.

1. **Clinical features.** Patients have increasing aching and rigidity of the axial and proximal limb muscles that usually are asymmetric at onset and occasionally are severe painful spasms. They may occur spontaneously or be precipitated by movement or sensory stimuli. Some patients have a fixed posture or opisthotonus in the later stages.

2. **Diagnosis.** A needle EMG shows continuous firing of motor units during the spasm. Most patients have serum and CSF antibodies against the synaptic vesicle–associated protein amphiphysin. Carcinoma of the breast and SCLC are the most commonly associated tumors. Anti-amphiphysin antibodies are not specific for this syndrome; they have been found in patients with limbic encephalopathy, cerebellar degeneration, or sensory neuronopathy.

3. **Management.** Some patients report improvement after tumor treatment and therapy with prednisone.

G. **Retinal degeneration (carcinoma-associated retinopathy)** is a heterogenous disorder with varying tumor associations and different pathophysiologic mechanisms. More than 90% of patients have SCLC. Melanoma is the other associated tumor. Visual symptoms precede discovery of the tumor in most instances by as long as 2 years.

1. **Clinical features.** Blurring or dimming of vision, which is frequently bilateral, is a common symptom. Night blindness also is common, especially with melanoma. Positive symptoms such as sparkles and shimmering lights may be present. Examination reveals an afferent pupillary defect in most patients and mild to moderate arteriolar narrowing, but otherwise the examination findings are unremarkable.

2. **Diagnosis.** An EMG can be useful in the evaluation of patients with visual loss. The most common antibody is polyclonal IgG anti-CAR antibody. These antibodies react with the calcium-binding protein recoverin. Some patients may have antibodies against unidentified retinal proteins. Many patients with cancer-associated retinopathy have no detectable antineuronal antibody.

3. **Management.** Most patients have mild to moderate improvement with 60 to 80 mg of prednisone within days. Management of the tumor appears to have no significant effect on the condition.

H. **Neuropathy**

1. **Subacute sensory neuronopathy.** More than 90% of patients have SCLC. Other neoplasms include carcinoma of the breast, prostate, and colon and lymphoma. In most cases, neurologic symptoms precede the discovery of the tumor by months to up to 2 years.

a. **Clinical features.** Development is subacute, and symptoms may begin in the face, trunk, or abdomen or be unilateral. The earliest symptoms are patchy numbness and paresthesia that may spread. Examination usually reveals involvement of all modalities of sensation with loss of reflexes and flexor plantar responses and preserved strength if subacute sensory neuronopathy is the isolated or predominant paraneoplastic syndrome. Pseudoathetoid posturing of extremities may be seen. The condition of most patients stabilizes at a severe level of disability.

b. **Diagnosis**

(1) Most patients have anti-Hu antibodies in the serum and CSF, usually in association with SCLC.

(2) Nerve conduction studies reveal reduced or absent sensory action potentials and normal or borderline motor conduction velocities. Some patients may have features of both axonal and demyelinating neuropathy.

       (3) CSF examination usually reveals pleocytosis with mononuclear predominance, an increased protein level and intrathecal IgG synthesis, and oligoclonal bands.

       (4) In patients with known cancer, neuropathy usually is related to the toxic effects of chemotherapy, metastasis, and nutritional deficits. Common chemotherapeutic agents drugs implicated are cisplatin, paclitaxel, docetaxel, and vinca alkaloids.

    c. Management. Corticosteroids, plasma exchange, and immune globulin are occasionally effective.

  2. Demyelinating neuropathy associated with neoplasms. There are reports of acute, predominantly motor polyradiculoneuropathy occurring in the setting of a number of neoplasms, especially lymphoma. The CSF and electrodiagnostic findings resemble those of Guillain–Barré syndrome. Several cases of sensorimotor neuropathy fulfilling the criteria for chronic inflammatory demyelinating polyneuropathy have been documented among patients with lymphoma. The neuropathy may precede the diagnosis of the tumor by several years.

  3. Lambert–Eaton myasthenic syndrome (LEMS). In approximately 50% of cases, this syndrome is associated with carcinoma, most commonly SCLC. It is now thought to be an autoimmune disorder triggered by the cancer. Malignant growth may not be present at onset and may not be discovered for up to 2 years.

    An antibody for the P/Q type voltage-gated calcium channel (VGCC) is found in most patients with LEMS. SCLC commonly expresses an array of VGCCs thought to be important in the development of LEMS in patients with lung cancer. An EMG reveals an incremental response at high frequencies (10 to 50 Hz), increased jitter on a single-fiber EMG, unstable motor units, and blocked conduction.

    In patients with cancer, Lambert–Eaton myasthenic syndrome responds to management of the cancer. In the absence of cancer-specific treatment, all therapies have little or no benefit. Cholinesterase inhibitors, guanidine hydrochloride, aminopyridines, and immunosuppressants are helpful in the treatment of patients without cancer.

Recommended Readings

Byrne TN. Spinal cord compression from epidural metastases. *N Engl J Med* 1992;327: 614–619.

Cybulski GR. Methods of surgical stabilization for metastatic disease of the spine. *Neurosurgery* 1989;25:240–252.

Delatrre JY, Krol G, Thaler HT, et al. Distribution of brain metastases. *Arch Neurol* 1988; 45:741–744.

Dropcho EJ, Dalmau J, Greenlee JE, et al. Paraneoplastic disorders. *Continuum* 1999;5(6).

Graus F, Rogers LR, Posner JB. Cerebrovascular complications in patients with cancer. *Medicine* 1985;64:16–35.

Greenberg HS, Deck MDF, Vikram B, et al. Metastasis to the base of the skull: clinical findings in 43 patients. *Neurology* 1981;1:530–537.

Mehta MP, Rozental JM, Levin AB, et al. Defining the role of radiosurgery in the management of brain metastases. *Int J Radiat Oncol Biol Phys* 1992;24:619–625.

Posner JB. *Neurologic complications of cancer.* Philadelphia: FA Davis Co, 1995.

Rottenberg DA, ed. *Neurological complications of cancer treatment.* Boston: Butterworth–Heinemann, 1991.

Rozental JM. Neurologic complications of cancer. In: Brain MC, Carbone PP, eds. *Current therapy in hematology–oncology,* 5 ed. St Louis: Mosby–Year Book, 1995:587–600.

Willson JKV, Masaryk TJ. Neurologic emergencies in the cancer patient. *Semin Oncol* 1989; 16:490–503.

54. NEUROTOXICOLOGY

Daniel E. Rusyniak

Neurotoxicology is defined as the study of adverse reactions on the central nervous system (CNS) or peripheral nervous system (PNS) from acute or chronic poisoning. A variety of compounds exist that are known to be toxic, as do some that are potentially toxic. Neurotoxic syndromes can mimic a variety of neurologic diseases. Neurotoxins can be classified into one of three categories:

1. **Drugs.** Prescription and illicit drugs
2. **Chemicals.** Industrial, household and abused agents
3. **Environmental.** Biologic agents and naturally occurring chemicals

Establishing causation is paramount to the correct diagnosis and the treatment of any patient with a suspected neurotoxic syndrome. Causation may be established by applying the principles established by Sir Austin Bradford Hill in differentiating association from causation in epidemiologic studies and applying them to the patient with a neurotoxic disorder. Not all of the following are required in every case:

1. **Exposure.** Confirming an exposure occurred is best done with quantitative methods on either biologic fluids (blood, urine, hair) or in the environment (air, water). At times, historical features alone may be adequate.
2. **Temporality.** Determining whether exposure occurred before or concurrent with symptoms. Some toxins have long latent periods before symptoms develop.
3. **Dose–response.** In general the higher the dose and longer the exposure, the greater is the severity of symptoms.
4. **Similarity to reported cases.** Symptoms should be similar to those reported in the literature
5. **Improvement as exposure is eliminated.** With a few exceptions, most neurotoxic syndromes are alleviated after the toxin is eliminated, although it can take months to years.
6. **Existence of animal model.** Animal models of toxicity are helpful in establishing causation; however, they may not be available or applicable.
7. **Other causes eliminated.**

This overview is not intended to be an exhaustive review of the topic of neurotoxicology. It is intended as a quick reference of toxins clinicians are most likely to encounter or those of historical significance. For more detailed work on the topic, see the recommended readings.

I. **Peripheral nervous system, neuromuscular junction, and muscle toxins**
   A. **Peripheral neuropathy.** Toxic peripheral neuropathy most commonly is axonopathy, is symmetric, has an acute or subacute onset, and involves the distal axons of the lower extremities first.
      1. **Heavy metals**
         a. **Arsenic**
            (1) **Sources.** Ground and well water, seafood (organic arsenic), industrial, and homicidal agents
            (2) **Route of exposure.** Ingestion is most common.
            (3) **Systemic signs.** Gastrointestinal (nausea, vomiting, diarrhea), dermatitis, larger exposures may result in multisystem organ failure, including cardiovascular collapse, renal failure, hepatitis, and pancytopenia.
            (4) **Physical examination findings.** Hypopigmented followed by hyperpigmented lesions on trunk and limbs, and palmoplantar keratosis, hepatomegaly, garlic odor on breath. Mees lines (transverse semilunar white bands across the nails) may be present in only 5% of cases and may take as long as 40 days to develop.
            (5) **Neurologic manifestations**
               (a) **CNS.** In severe poisoning, encephalopathy, coma, and seizures occur.
               (b) **PNS.** Severe poisoning may cause ascending paralysis and pain and paresthesia similar to those of Guillain-Barré syndrome.

Chronic or less severe poisoning manifests as painful distal sensorimotor axonopathy.

(6) Diagnosis

    (a) Laboratory

        (i) 24-hour urine. The standard of reference. Useful for recent exposures (<30 days). The normal result is <50 µg/L or <100 µg/24 hours. False-positive results are common owing to seafood ingestion (nontoxic organic arsenic) and often necessitate repetition of testing after abstaining from seafood.

        (ii) Blood. Less reliable owing to short half-life of arsenic. Normal result is <7 µg/dL.

        (iii) Hair. Useful for chronic or remote exposures. Normal result is <1 mg/kg.

        (iv) Cerebrospinal fluid (CSF). Can show an increase in protein and red blood cells.

    (b) Radiographs. May show radiopacities in the gastrointestinal tract if ingestion is recent.

    (c) Nerve conduction velocity (NCV) studies after severe acute exposure may show findings of proximal demyelination characteristic of acute inflammatory demyelinating polyneuropathy along with distal, motor and sensory axonopathy. In less severe exposure or chronic exposure, sensory distal axonopathy is greater than motor distal axonopathy.

    (d) Electrocardiography in rare instances shows a prolonged QT interval with risk for torsades de pointes.

(7) Treatment

    (a) Removal of exposure

    (b) If material is retained in the gastrointestinal tract, consider either whole-bowel irrigation or use of cathartics.

    (c) Begin chelation therapy before confirmation if clinical presentation is highly suggestive.

        (i) Dimercaptosuccinic acid (DMSA) is an oral agent useful in the treatment of subacutely or chronically poisoned patients with working gastrointestinal tracts. The dosage is 10 mg/kg by mouth three times a day for 5 days then twice a day until the urinary arsenic level is less than 50 µg/L per 24 hours. Complications include a transient increase in results of liver function tests.

        (ii) British anti-Lewisite (BAL) is useful in severe exposures when oral therapy cannot be given or the patient has ileus. The dosage is 3 to 5 mg/kg intramuscularly (i.m.) every 4 to 6 hours until urinary arsenic level is less tan 50 µg/kg per 24 hours. Complications include pain over the injection site, hypertension, febrile reactions, and agitation.

        (iii) Dimercaptoproprane-1-sulfonate (DMPS) is not currently approved by the U.S. Food and Drug Administration. The dosage is 100 mg by orally or intravenously (i.v.) three times a day.

b. Lead

    (1) Sources. Lead-based paint (houses painted before 1978), soil, ceramic glaze, gun ranges, battery manufacturing, industry, retained foreign bodies, ethnic folk remedies.

    (2) Route of exposure. Ingestion or inhalation

    (3) Systemic signs. Abdominal pain, anorexia, constipation, anemia, nephropathy (Fanconi's syndrome), hypertension, and rarely gout

    (4) Physical examination findings. Bluish black lines around gums (lead lines).

(5) Neurologic manifestations

(a) CNS. Encephalopathy, coma, visual perceptual defects, and seizures more common among children. Children may have signs of increased intracranial pressure (bulging fontanel or papilledema)

(b) PNS. Peripheral neuropathy more common among adults. It manifests as motor axonopathy of the arms greater than the legs and extensors greater than flexors (foot or wrist drop). It can be symmetric or asymmetric. Results of NCV studies often are normal but may show decreased conduction velocity.

(6) Diagnosis

(a) Laboratory

(i) Blood lead. The standard for testing. Normal result is <10 μg/dL

  Children. Levels >10 μg/dL necessitate investigation. Levels >45 μg/dL necessitate chelation.

  Adults. Levels >40 μg/dL necessitate removal from worksite. Levels >70 μg/dL necessitate chelation.

(ii) Complete blood cell count. Microcytic anemia with basophilic stippling.

(iii) CSF. May have increased opening pressure, pleocytosis, and elevated protein level.

(b) Radiographs. May see lead lines in children at growth plates and retained radiopaque material in gastrointestinal tract

(7) Treatment

(a) Remove from exposure

(b) If material is retained in gastrointestinal tract, consider either whole bowel irrigation or use of cathartics

(c) Chelation therapy

(i) DMSA. May use as sole agent in treatment of patients able to take drugs orally. The dosage is 10 mg/kg by mouth three times a day for 5 days then three times a day for 14 days. Wait 1 week and repeat measurement of lead level. Start for children at levels >45 μg/dL or for adults with symptoms and levels >70 μg/dL. Continue until level is <25 μg/dL in children or 30 μg/dL in adults.

(ii) BAL 3 to 5 mg/kg i.m. four times a day for patients unable to take oral medications

(iii) Ethylenediaminetetracetic acid (EDTA) 35 to 50 mg/kg every day i.v. continuous infusion as combination therapy with BAL. Start 4 hours after initiation of BAL therapy.

c. Other metals

(1) Thallium. Used as homicidal agent. Manifestations of toxicity are similar to those of arsenic poisoning. Other findings include constipation, alopecia totalis, and rapid onset of peripheral neuropathy (48 hours to 1 week). Physical examination may reveal Mees' lines and blackened hair roots under low-power light microscopic examination.

(2) Cisplatin. Used in chemotherapy. Toxicity manifests as distal symmetric paresthesia that may not occur for months after exposure. NCV studies show sensory neuronopathy.

(3) Gold salts. Used in rheumatoid arthritis, associated rarely with seizures and encephalopathy. Toxicity manifests as distal symmetric sensorimotor polyneuropathy.

2. Solvents

a. n-hexane, methyl-*n*-butyl ketone (MBK), 2,5-hexanedione.

(1) Sources. May be a component of glue, varnish, cement, and ink

(2) Route of exposure. Inhalational, abused (huffing or bagging)

(3) **Systemic signs.** Anorexia, weight loss, renal tubular acidosis if mixtures contain toluene

(4) **Physical examination.** Solvent odor on breath

(5) **Neurologic manifestations.** Distal weakness, paresthesia, sensory loss, and areflexia. NCV studies may show motor more than sensory polyneuropathy with reduced sensory and motor amplitudes and prolonged motor conduction velocity.

(6) **Diagnosis**

    (a) Clinical history and physical examination findings

    (b) **Sural nerve biopsy.** Axonal degeneration, demyelination, and paranodal axonal swelling with neurofilament accumulation.

(7) **Treatment.** Removal from the source results in improvement, although symptoms may progress for a time after exposure (coasting).

  b. Other solvents. Methyl-ethyl-ketone alone does not cause peripheral neuropathy but synergistically worsens the effects of n-hexane, MBK, or hexanedione. Other solvents that cause peripheral neuropathy include carbon disulfide, which causes distal axonal neuropathy and psychosis, and acrylamide monomer, which causes distal sensorimotor polyneuropathy.

3. Pesticides

  a. Sources. Pesticides containing organophosphates or carbamates, chemical warfare agents.

  b. Route of exposure. Ingestion, inhalation, dermal contact

  c. Systemic signs. Cholinergic excess: vomiting, diarrhea, lacrimation, salivation, diaphoresis, bronchospasm, bronchorrhea, miosis, bradycardia, or tachycardia

  d. Neurologic manifestations

    (1) **CNS.** Decreased mental status, seizures

    (2) **PNS**

      (a) **Nicotinic.** Excess acetylcholine at first depolarizes then depresses nicotinic receptors at the neuromuscular junction resulting in fasciculations and cramping followed by flaccid paralysis.

      (b) **Intermediate syndrome.** Proximal muscle weakness, including respiratory symptoms, beginning 1 to 4 days after cholinergic phase

      (c) **Organophosphate-induced delayed neurotoxicity.** Occurs 1 to 4 weeks after organophosphate poisoning and manifests as symmetric, distal, predominantly motor polyneuropathy. NCV studies reveal denervation of affected muscles along with reduced amplitude and prolonged conduction velocity.

  e. Diagnosis

    (1) History and physical examination findings

    (2) **Plasma cholinesterase.** Less specific but readily available with rapid turnaround time. A decrease in level by 50% of baseline or serial increasing levels after poisoning indicate exposure.

    (3) **Red blood cell cholinesterase.** More specific but long turnaround time. A decrease of 25% of baseline level indicates exposure.

  f. Treatment

    (1) Remove from exposure and decontaminate the skin with soap and water.

    (2) Respiratory and cardiovascular support

    (3) **Atropine** initial dose of 2 mg i.v. and then double dose every 5 to 10 minutes until drying of respiratory secretions.

    (4) **Pralidoxime** initial dose of 1.5 g i.v. over 30 minutes and then infusion of 500 mg/h until resolution of muscle weakness.

    (5) **Diazepam** 10 mg or lorazepam 2 mg i.v. for seizures with repetition of dosage as needed for control.

4. Gases

    a. Nitrous oxide. Chronic inhalational abuse or repetitive anesthesia exposures can deplete bioavailable cobalamine (vitamin B_{12}) with the development of a myeloneuropathy. Symptoms include both sensorimotor polyneuropathy and upper motor neuron findings. Magnetic resonance imaging (MRI) of the spinal cord may show increased signal intensity in the posterior and lateral columns on T2-weighted images.

    b. Ethylene oxide. Chronic workplace exposure in industry or through the sterilization of hospital supplies can result in symmetric distal sensorimotor polyneuropathy.

5. Pharmaceuticals

    a. Dapsone. Chronic use in dermatologic and rheumatologic disorders may result in a motor neuropathy characterized by weakness and atrophy in the upper more than the lower extremities. NCV studies show motor axonopathy.

    b. Pyridoxine. Sensory neuropathy can occur from either large acute doses or excessive long-term use. Permanent sensory neuronopathy has been reported after massive doses (>50 g) over a short time.

    c. Other pharmaceuticals associated with peripheral neuropathy include amiodarone, colchicine, dideoxycytidine, hydralazine, isoniazid, metronidazole, nitrofurantoin, and thalidomide.

B. Toxins affecting ion channels

  1. Ciguatera poisoning

    a. Sources. Ingestion of reef fish (barracuda, sea bass, parrot fish, red snapper, grouper, amber jack, kingfish, and sturgeon)

    b. Mechanism of action. Prolongation of sodium channel opening

    c. Systemic signs. Abdominal pain, vomiting and diarrhea, bradycardia, hypotension.

    d. Neurologic manifestations. Headache, dysesthesia and paresthesia of mouth, hands and feet, hot–cold reversal (cold objects cause burning sensation).

    e. Diagnosis. Based on the clinical symptoms and history. Samples of fish can be sent out for further testing.

    f. Treatment. Supportive care, mannitol 1 g/kg i.v. over 30 minutes has been suggested as an effective treatment if given early.

  2. Tetrodotoxin poisoning

    a. Sources. Ingestion of puffer or globefish

    b. Mechanism of action. Blocks sodium channels

    c. Systemic signs. Vomiting, hypotension, respiratory arrest

    d. Neurologic manifestations. Paresthesia of the mouth and extremities followed by paralysis of voluntary and respiratory muscles

    e. Diagnosis. History of puffer fish ingestion and clinical features

    f. Treatment. Supportive care

  3. Other toxins affecting ion channels. Grayanotoxin (rhododendron, sodium channel opener), scorpion toxin (sodium channel opener), saxitoxin (shellfish, sodium channel blocker).

C. Toxins affecting neuromuscular junction

  1. Black widow spider venom

    a. Sources. Black widow spider (*Latrodectus mactans*)

    b. Mechanism of action. Increased release of acetylcholine and norepinephrine

    c. Systemic signs. Hypertension, nausea, diaphoresis, restlessness

    d. Neurologic manifestations. Diffuse muscle spasms and rigidity (may be misdiagnosed as acute surgical abdomen)

    e. Diagnosis. History and clinical examination

    f. Treatment. Intravenous opiates for pain control and benzodiazepines for muscle relaxation. In severe cases antivenin (equine-based antiserum) can be given, but it carries risk of anaphylaxis and must be used with caution.

2. Botulism
  a. Sources
    (1) Food. Ingestion of food contaminated with preformed toxin
    (2) Infant. Ingestion of foods (honey) contaminated with *Clostridium botulinum* spores
    (3) Wound. Wounds infected with the bacterium *C. botulinum*
  b. Mechanism of action. Inhibits fusion of presynaptic vesicles and prevents release of acetylcholine
  c. Systemic signs. Sore throat, dry mouth, vomiting, and diarrhea followed by abdominal distention and constipation
  d. Neurologic manifestations. Descending motor paralysis including ophthalmoplegia, dysphagia, mydriasis (only 50%), skeletal and respiratory muscles
  e. Diagnosis
    (1) Difficult to differentiate from Miller Fisher syndrome. Ataxia, paresthesia, areflexia, and elevated CSF protein are more common in Miller Fisher syndrome.
    (2) Laboratory. Confirmation of *C. botulinum* in serum, stool, gastric contents, wound culture, food specimens, or positive mouse bioassay
    (3) Electromyography. Facilitation (progressively increasing amplitude) may be present on repetitive nerve stimulation (50/sec) in 60% of cases
  f. Treatment
    (1) Supportive care and antibiotics (wound botulism)
    (2) Trivalent antiserum. Obtain from the Centers for Disease Control and Prevention (404) 639-2888.
3. Other toxins affecting the neuromuscular junction include the venom of the funnel web spider (increases acetylcholine release), saliva from the tick *Ixodes holocyclus* (prevents acetylcholine release), hypermagnesemia (prevents acetylcholine release), venom from cobra, coral snake, mamba, and Mojave rattlesnake (blocks acetylcholine nicotinic receptors)

C. Myopathy
  1. Immobility. Toxins that cause depressed mental status or coma can cause extended periods of immobility. Prolonged compression of muscular compartments can impair delivery of oxygen and nutrients and cause subsequent muscle breakdown and rhabdomyolysis. Examples include alcohol, barbiturates, benzodiazepines, and narcotics.
  2. Excess activity. Toxicity that cause excessive energy use can result in a supply and demand imbalance. This can be the direct effect of the drug or secondary to fighting against restraints. Excessive consumption of adenosine triphosphate results in muscle breakdown and rhabdomyolysis. Examples include amphetamines, cocaine, phencyclidine (PCP), and anticholinergic drugs.
  3. Myotoxins
    a. Hypokalemia. Drugs that cause total body potassium depletion can cause muscle breakdown and rhabdomyolysis. Examples include toluene and amphotericin B (renal tubular acidosis), glycyrrhizinic acid in licorice (increases mineralocorticoid activity), and long-term use of diuretics.
    b. Metabolic poisons. Compounds that interfere with the production of adenosine triphosphate can result in muscle breakdown and rhabdomyolysis. Examples include cyanide, hydrogen sulfide, salicylates, dinitrophenol, chlorophenoxy herbicides (2,4-D), and carbon monoxide.
    c. Direct-acting myotoxins. Numerous agents exist that have direct toxic effects on the muscle that result in myopathy and rhabdomyolysis. Examples include ethanol, heroin, corticosteroids, antimalarials, ε-aminocaproic acid, 3-hydroxy-3-methylglutaryl coenzyme A (HMG-CoA) reductase inhibitors (e.g., lovastatin), and snake bites.

II. Central nervous system toxins
A. Acute delirium
1. **Anticholinergic syndrome.** Occurs from blocking central and peripheral muscarinic receptors
   a. **Sources.** Pharmaceuticals: tricyclic antidepressants, antihistamines, skeletal muscle relaxants (cyclobenzaprine), phenothiazines, antipsychotics (olanzapine), benztropine, carbamazepine, amantadine, class-1a antiarrhythmics, scopolamine. Plants: jimson weed, nightshades, mandrake.
   b. **Systemic signs.** Dry mouth, mydriasis, dry axilla, hypoactive bowel sounds, urinary retention, tachycardia, flushed skin, low-grade fever
   c. **Neurologic manifestations.** Acute delirium with visual hallucinations, increased motor activity (picking at bed sheets), mumbling tangential speech pattern
   d. **Treatment**
      (1) **Charcoal** 1 g/kg by mouth if the patient is awake and is not at risk of aspiration and if ingestion is within 1 to 2 hours
      (2) **Benzodiazepines.** Repeat intravenous doses for agitation and tachycardia
      (3) **Butyrophenones** (haloperidol or droperidol) in addition to benzodiazepines for patients with severe agitation and acute psychosis
      (4) **Physostigmine** may be useful as a diagnostic tool in differentiating anticholinergic syndrome from other neurologic causes (e.g., encephalitis). Because of its short half-life and potential complications, physostigmine is generally not recommended for treatment. The dosage is 1 to 2 mg slow i.v. push over 10 minutes. Complications are seizures, arrhythmia, and cholinergic crisis. Contraindicated in the care of patients with unknown ingestions, bradycardia, or ingestions increasing risk of seizures (tricyclic antidepressants).
      (5) Intravenous hydration and serial measurement of creatine kinase for rhabdomyolysis
2. **Sympathomimetic syndrome.** Occurs from an increase in central and peripheral catecholamines
   a. **Sources.** Pharmaceuticals: ephedrine, phenylpropanolamine, methylphenidate, phentermine. Illicit drugs: cocaine, amphetamines, methamphetamine, methylenedioxymethamphetamine (ecstasy). Plants: ma huang.
   b. **Systemic signs.** Tachycardia, hypertension, diaphoresis, mydriasis, fever, chest pain, myocardial infarction, and ventricular arrhythmia
   c. **Neurologic manifestations.** Psychomotor agitation, seizures, mania, tactile hallucinations (formication), increased muscle tone, increased reflexes with clonus, impaired cognition and chronic psychiatric symptoms (chronic abuse), hyponatremia-induced cerebral edema, ischemic or hemorrhagic stroke
   d. **Treatment**
      (1) **Charcoal** 1 g/kg by mouth if the patient is awake and is not at risk of aspiration and if ingestion is within 1 to 2 hours
      (2) **Benzodiazepines.** Repeat intravenous doses for seizures, agitation, tachycardia, hypertension, and chest pain. Avoid use of β-blockers secondary to unopposed α-stimulation and vasospasm.
      (3) **Butyrophenones** (haloperidol or droperidol) in addition to benzodiazepines for patients with severe agitation and acute psychosis
      (4) Intravenous hydration and serial measurement of creatine kinase for rhabdomyolysis
      (5) Active cooling of hyperthermic patients
3. **Serotonin syndrome.** Occurs from increase in central serotonin level with subsequent increase release in central and peripheral catecholamine levels. Typically occurs in patients taking more than one serotoninergic agent.

    a. Sources. Pharmaceuticals: Selective serotonin reuptake inhibitors (fluoxetine), tricyclic antidepressants, monoamine oxidase inhibitors, meperidine, dextromethorphan, tramadol, triptans, amphetamines, L-tryptophan, and lithium. Plants: (St. John's wort)

    b. Systemic signs. Tachycardia, hypertension, diaphoresis, mydriasis, hyperthermia

    c. Neurologic manifestations. Agitation, confusion, hallucinations, increased motor tone and activity (lower more than upper extremity), hyperreflexia with lower extremity clonus.

    d. Treatment

        (1) Charcoal 1 g/kg by mouth if the patient is awake and is not at risk of aspiration and if ingestion is within 1 to 2 hours

        (2) Benzodiazepines. Repeat intravenous doses for agitation, tachycardia, and hypertension

        (3) Cyproheptadine (4 to 8 mg by mouth) can be used for its antiserotonergic effects

        (4) Intravenous hydration and serial measurement of creatine kinase for rhabdomyolysis

4. Hallucinogens

    a. Sources. Anticholinergic agents: See **III.A.1.** Illicit drugs: lysergic acid diethylamide (LSD), mescaline, PCP, ketamine. Plants: morning glory, nutmeg. Mushrooms: *Amanita muscaria* mushrooms, psilocybin mushrooms. Animals: bufotoxin from *Bufo* toads.

    b. Systemic signs. Tachycardia, hypertension, diaphoresis, mydriasis

    c. Neurologic manifestations. Visual hallucinations, increased motor activity, hyperreflexia

    d. Treatment

        (1) Charcoal 1 g/kg by mouth if the patient is awake and is not at risk of aspiration and if ingestion is within 1 to 2 hours

        (2) Benzodiazepines. Repeat intravenous doses as needed for agitation

        (3) Butyrophenones (haloperidol or droperidol) in addition to benzodiazepines for patients with severe agitation and acute psychosis

        (4) Intravenous hydration and serial measurement of creatine kinase for rhabdomyolysis

5. Withdrawal syndromes result in a hyperadrenergic state with symptoms similar to those of sympathomimetic syndrome

    a. Benzodiazepines, barbiturates, and **ethanol** can cause a life-threatening withdrawal syndrome characterized by a hyperadrenergic state (tachycardia, hypertension, diaphoresis, piloerection, fever), nausea, vomiting, diarrhea, altered mental status, hallucinations, and seizures. Management of acute symptoms involves repeated intravenous doses of benzodiazepines (high doses at times) followed by scheduled oral benzodiazepines for prevention.

    b. Baclofen can cause a life-threatening withdrawal syndrome characterized by disorientation, hallucinations, fever, hypotension, rebound spasticity, seizures, and coma. Treatment involves oral or intrathecal baclofen and benzodiazepines.

    c. γ-Hydroxybutyrate (GHB). Abrupt discontinuance of chronically abused GHB compounds results in a withdrawal syndrome similar to benzodiazepine and ethanol withdrawal. Treatment is with intravenous or oral benzodiazepines and supportive care.

6. Wernicke's encephalopathy. Characterized by altered mental status (global confusional state), ataxia, and ophthalmoplegia (nystagmus, sixth-cranial-nerve palsy, conjugate palsy, vestibular paresis, pupillary abnormalities) in persons with chronic alcoholism or patients with other thiamine deficiency states (e.g., hyperemesis gravidarum, anorexia nervosa, malignant tumor of the gastrointestinal tract, pyloric stenosis, inappropriate parenteral nutrition). Although classically diagnosed with the triad of mental confusion (66% of patients), staggering gait (51% of patients), and ocular abnormalities (40% of patients), Wernicke's encephalopathy can occur in the absence of some or all of the symptoms. Diagnosis is by clinical features and improvement with treatment. MRI findings of bilateral, symmetric changes involving the periventricular regions in the brainstem (cerebral aqueduct, fourth ventricle), third ventricle and thalamus, mamillary body shrinkage, and decreased serum thiamine levels support the diagnosis. Treatment is with intravenous thiamine (100 mg) and magnesium followed by daily thiamine and multivitamin supplementation.

B. **Subacute encephalopathy**
   1. **Bismuth.** Long-term use of bismuth salts for ostomy odor or in the management of peptic ulcer disease can manifest as subacute progressive encephalopathy. Patients have symptoms of progressive dementia and delirium, ataxia, severe myoclonus, and in rare instances, seizures. Symptoms may not occur until after weeks or years of continued use. Other symptoms include dark stools and dark staining of the gums. This syndrome can be mistaken for Creutzfeldt–Jakob disease or other progressive forms of encephalopathy and can be fatal if not diagnosed. Treatment involves stopping the drug and providing supportive care.
   2. **Lithium.** Chronic use or acute overdose of lithium salts can manifest as progressive encephalopathy. Patients come to medical attention with tremor, altered mental status, ataxia, myoclonus, and in rare instances, seizures. Other symptoms include nausea, vomiting, diabetes insipidus, hypothyroidism, and renal failure. An elevated serum lithium level supports the diagnosis. Treatment involves correcting hyponatremia and in selected cases hemodialysis.
   3. **Aluminum.** Long-term use of aluminum phosphate binders or aluminum-contaminated dialysates in the care of patients with renal failure can result in progressive encephalopathy. Patients come to medical attention with agitation, confusion, myoclonus, coma, or seizures. Some die before treatment can be instituted. Other symptoms include osteomalacia and microcytic hypochromic anemia. Treatment involves removal of sources of aluminum and for some patients, chelation with deferoxamine.
   4. **Carbon monoxide.** Patients with carbon monoxide poisoning may have a syndrome known as **delayed neurologic sequelae.** This occurs 4 to 30 days after exposure and manifests as altered mental status, personality changes, memory loss, difficulty concentrating, and encephalopathy. Physical examination findings may include hyperreflexia, frontal release signs (glabella, palmar grasp), masked facies, and parkinsonian features. Treatment consists of supportive care. MRI findings include bilateral globus pallidus infarcts and demyelination of subcortical white matter. Neuroimaging may show abnormalities involving the centrum semiovale, putamen, thalamus, caudate nucleus, hippocampus, and hypothalamus.

C. **Coma and CNS depression.** Many toxins causing CNS depression and coma can mimic brain death, including loss of brainstem reflexes. Many of these toxins have long half-lives, so clinical criteria of brain death do not apply.
   1. **Sedative hypnotics**
      a. **Sources.** Ethanol, benzodiazepines, barbiturates, central-acting muscle relaxants, chloral hydrate, buspirone, zolpidem, baclofen, clonidine, antihistamines, and numerous antidepressants and antipsychotics.
      b. **Systemic signs.** Pressure sores, hypotension, bradycardia, hypothermia
      c. **Neurologic manifestations.** Somnolence, coma, areflexia, nystagmus, amnesia
      d. **Treatment**
         (1) **Charcoal** 1 g/kg by mouth if the patient is awake and is not at risk of aspiration and if ingestion is within 1 to 2 hours
         (2) Supportive care
         (3) The use of **flumazenil,** a benzodiazepine antagonist, is generally not recommended because of increased risk of seizures.

2. Opioids, opiates

    a. Sources. Pharmaceuticals: hydrocodone, oxycodone, morphine, hydromorphone, propoxyphene, meperidine, fentanyl, methadone. Illicit drugs: heroin, designer opioids

    b. Systemic signs. Hypotension, bradycardia, bradypnea, pulmonary edema, track marks on skin, skin abscesses, decreased bowel sounds, cyanosis

    c. Neurologic manifestations. Coma, miosis, areflexia, and seizures (meperidine and propoxyphene). Seizures from meperidine are the result of elevated levels of normeperidine (a major metabolite of meperidine). Risk factors for normeperidine seizures are renal failure and chronic dosing. Naloxone (Narcan; Endo Pharmaceuticals, Chadds Ford, PA, U.S.A.) does not reverse meperidine- or propoxyphene-related seizures.

    d. Treatment

        (1) Supportive care

        (2) Naloxone 0.1 to 1 mg i.v. push followed by 1 mg every minute until reversal of respiratory depression or maximum of 10 mg. Complications include acute opioid withdrawal.

3. GHB

    a. Sources. GHB, γ-butyrolactone, butanediol (used for mood enhancement, sleep induction, and by body builders for purported increased growth hormone release)

    b. Systemic signs. Bradycardia, hypotension, hypothermia, nystagmus, vomiting

    c. Neurologic manifestations. Areflexic coma (typically short duration—less than 6 hours with rapid reversal), normal or miotic pupils, seizures

    d. Treatment

        (1) Supportive care

4. Carbon monoxide

    a. Sources. Automotive exhaust, smoke inhalation, faulty heaters, external heating sources, propane- and gas-powered tools and vehicles

    b. Systemic signs. Tachycardia, hypotension, chest pain, dyspnea, myocardial infarction, cardiac arrhythmia, flushed skin, pressure sores, nausea, vomiting

    c. Neurologic manifestations. Headache, confusion, cognitive deficits, coma, seizures, stroke, parkinsonism (delayed complication), delayed sequelae (see **III.B.4.**)

    d. Diagnosis

        (1) Laboratory. Carbon monoxide levels are indicative of exposure but are not reliable predictors of toxicity or symptoms. The normal result is <5% for nonsmokers and <10% for smokers.

    e. Treatment

        (1) Removal from source of carbon monoxide

        (2) 100% oxygen through a non-rebreather for 6 to 12 hours if symptoms are mild or moderate

        (3) Indications for hyperbaric oxygen therapy

            (a) Loss of consciousness

            (b) Coma or persistent neurologic deficit

            (c) Myocardial ischemia or ventricular dysrhythmia

            (d) Hypotension or cardiovascular compromise

            (e) Pregnancy with any of the above, levels >20%, or signs of fetal distress

5. Cocaine washout syndrome occurs among abusers of cocaine or other stimulants, the increased use of which decreases the level of CNS catecholamines. This results in symptoms of depressed mental status, confusion, or coma (unresponsive to stimuli, including intubation). Patients may have disconjugate gaze. Other physical examination findings, vital signs, and laboratory findings generally are normal. Symptoms may last for 8 to 24 hours, and treatment is supportive. This should always be a diagnosis of exclusion.

D. Cerebellar disorders
  1. Toluene–solvent abuse syndrome
    a. Sources. Toluene-containing paint thinner, paint stripper, and glue
    b. Route of exposure. Inhalational: huffing (inhaling soaked rags) or bagging (inhaling from bags containing solvent)
    c. Systemic signs. Abdominal pain, anorexia, weight loss, gastritis, possible renal tubular acidosis (hypokalemia and acidosis), rhabdomyolysis, hepatitis, solvent odor on breath
    d. Neurologic manifestations. Tremor of the head and extremities, ataxia, staggering gait, cognitive deficits, personality changes, optic nerve atrophy, hearing loss, loss of smell, extremity spasticity, and hyperreflexia
    e. Diagnosis
      (1) Laboratory. Elevated serum toluene levels and urine hippuric acid levels confirm exposure.
      (2) Imaging. MRI of the brain often shows cerebellar and cerebral atrophy. Evidence of white-matter disease can be seen with increased signal intensity on T2-weighted images in the periventricular, internal capsular, and brainstem pyramidal regions.
      (3) Electrophysiologic studies. Brainstem auditory evoked response testing may show sparing of early components and loss or decrement of the late components (waves III and IV). Abnormal pattern visual evoked cortical potentials and prolonged P100 peak latency may occur in patients with toxic optic neuropathy caused by toluene abuse.
    f. Treatment
      (1) Supportive care
      (2) Drug rehabilitation
  2. Mercury poisoning
    a. Sources
      (1) Elemental. Thermometers, chemistry kits, barometers, dental amalgam makers, photography
      (2) Inorganic. Vinyl chloride manufacturing, disinfectants, calomel
      (3) Organic. Seafood, treated grains, germicidal agents
    b. Route of exposure. Inhalation, ingestion, dermal contact
    c. Systemic signs
      (1) Elemental. Metal fume fever (dyspnea, fever, chills), stomatitis, pneumonitis, hypertension, anorexia
      (2) Inorganic. Hemorrhagic gastroenteritis, renal failure, acrodynia (erythema and edema of hands and feet, rash, diaphoresis, tachycardia, hypertension)
      (3) Organic. Dermatitis
    d. Neurologic manifestations
      (1) Elemental. Tremor, insomnia, memory loss, emotional lability, depression, psychosis, constricted vision, peripheral neuropathy, ataxia
      (2) Organic. Ataxia, tremor, visual field constriction, paresthesia, neurasthenia, hearing loss, dysarthria, cognitive deficits. In utero exposure results in fetal malformations, microcephaly, cerebral palsy, blindness, and deafness.
    e. Diagnosis
      (1) Laboratory
        (a) 24-hour urine. Levels do not correlate well with symptoms and are not useful in organic mercury exposure. Normal result is <20 µg/L, toxicity >150 µg/L, false-positive results common with recent seafood ingestion.
        (b) Blood mercury. Useful in organic exposures because 90% is eliminated in bile. Normal result is <5 µg/L. False-positive results are common with recent seafood ingestion.
        (c) Hair. Less reliable, may have some role in establishing remote exposure to methyl mercury.

(2) Neuroimaging

(a) MRI. Characteristic neuropathologic changes have been described in patients with Minamata disease. Typical abnormalities involve the visual cortex, cerebellar vermis and hemispheres, and postcentral cortex.

f. Treatment

(1) Inorganic

(a) DMSA. 10 mg/kg by mouth three times a day followed by 10 mg/kg by mouth twice a day for 14 days. Then repeat measurement of mercury level.

(b) BAL 3 to 5 mg/kg per dose every 4 hours i.m. for 2 days followed by 2.5 to 3 mg/kg per dose i.m. every 6 hours for 2 days then 2.5 to 3 mg/kg per dose every 12 hours for 7 days if patient is unable to take oral medication.

(c) DMPS. Not approved in United States. Oral dose: 100 to 300 mg three times a day.

(2) Organic

(a) BAL. Not recommended because of increased CNS concentrations of mercury

(b) DMSA. See **III.D.2.f.(1)(a).**

3. Antiepileptics. Numerous antiepileptic agents, including phenobarbital, diphenylhydantoin, and carbamazepine, in elevated concentration or acute overdose manifest as the predominantly cerebellar findings of ataxia, nystagmus, and CNS depression.

4. Ethanol. Both acute intoxication and chronic abuse of ethanol can result in cerebellar findings of ataxia, tremor, and altered mental status. One must consider Wernicke's encephalopathy when any patient with chronic alcoholism has changes mental status and ataxia not related to acute intoxication.

E. Parkinsonism

1. 1-Methyl-4-phenyl-1,2,3,6-tetrahydroyridine (MPTP), a byproduct of the production of a synthetic analogue of meperidine, was responsible for the acute development of parkinsonism in 7 users. This syndrome was characterized by the rapid (24 to 72 hours) development of end-stage parkinsonism with tremor, rigidity, bradykinesia, and postural instability, masked facies, and decreased blink rate. Investigation of the mechanism of toxicity has led to the development of an animal model for Parkinson's disease.

2. Manganese. A parkinsonian-like illness has been described among miners or workers exposed to manganese oxide and among those who have ingested potassium permanganate. This syndrome is the result of degradation of the globus pallidus. It begins with a prodrome of nonspecific symptoms (insomnia, irritability, muscle weakness) and progresses to psychiatric manifestations (hallucinations, emotional lability, delusions) and finally to classic parkinsonian features of tremor, gait disturbance, masked facies, bradykinesia, and rigidity.

3. Neuroleptic drugs. The use of neuroleptic agents, including phenothiazines and butyrophenones, has been associated with the acute development of parkinsonian symptoms. Cessation of the neuroleptic typically results in resolution of symptoms within a few weeks. Prolonged use of neuroleptics can result in tardive dyskinesia with choreiform movements of the face, tongue, and limbs. If recognized early, most symptoms of tardive dyskinesia resolve within 5 years.

4. Carbon monoxide, cyanide, hydrogen sulfide. Agents that inhibit the mitochondrial respiratory chain can cause development of bilateral globus pallidus infarction and subsequently a parkinsonian syndrome. This typically results from a combination of hypotension and hypoxia in severe poisoning and can have neuropsychiatric manifestations (see **III.B.**) or more classic parkinsonism.

F. Seizures. Toxins cause seizures by one of the four following mechanisms: decrease in the seizure threshold of a patient with an underlying seizure disorder, direct effects on the CNS, withdrawal seizures, or metabolic derangement. Most toxin-related seizures are generalized tonic–clonic. Most patients with toxin-induced seizures can be treated with standard seizure algorithms. The exception is that treatment is successful more often with benzodiazepines and barbiturates then with diphenylhydantoin.

1. **Stimulants** (see also **III.A.2.**)
   a. **Sources.** Cocaine, amphetamines, methamphetamines
   b. **Mechanism of toxicity.** Thought to be secondary to increased levels of CNS catecholamines with subsequent neuronal excitation. Also can cause vasculitis, vasospasm, and accelerated atherosclerosis and increase risk of both ischemic and hemorrhagic stroke with the associated seizure risk.
   c. **Treatment**
      (1) **Diazepam** 10 mg or lorazepam 2 mg i.v. for seizures with repeat doses as needed for control
      (2) **Phenobarbital** 20 mg/kg i.v. at rate of 25 to 50 mg/min
2. **Cholinergics** (see also **II.A.3.**)
   a. **Sources.** Organophosphate and carbamate insecticides, chemical warfare agents
   b. **Mechanism of toxicity.** Thought to be increased CNS concentration of acetylcholine with secondary release of glutamate
   c. **Treatment**
      (1) **Diazepam** 10 mg or lorazepam 2 mg i.v. for seizures with repeat doses as needed for control
      (2) **Phenobarbital** 20 mg/kg i.v. at rate of 25 to 50 mg/min
      (3) **Atropine** 2 to 4 mg i.v. for signs of cholinergic excess
      (4) **Pralidoxime** 1.5 g i.v. over 30 minutes for nicotinic symptoms
3. **γ-Aminobutyric acid (GABA) antagonists**
   a. **Sources.** Tricyclic antidepressants, phenothiazines, flumazenil, chlorinated hydrocarbons, hydrazines, cephalosporins, ciprofloxacin, imipenem, penicillins, isoniazid, steroids, clozapine, olanzapine, cicutoxin (water hemlock), picrotoxin (fish berries), wormwood (absinthe)
   b. **Mechanism of action.** Direct or indirect inhibition of $GABA_A$ receptors or decreased synthesis of GABA through inhibition of either glutamic acid decarboxylase or pyridoxal kinase (isoniazid, hydrazines)
   c. **Treatment**
      (1) **Diazepam** 10 mg or lorazepam 2 mg i.v. for seizures with repeated doses as needed for control
      (2) **Phenobarbital** 20 mg/kg i.v. at rate of 25 to 50 mg/min
      (3) **Pyridoxine** for isoniazid or hydrazine overdose. The amount of pyridoxine administered should be equivalent to the estimated amount of isoniazid ingested. It can be given intravenous push to patients with severe symptoms or as an intravenous infusion. If an unknown amount of isoniazid has been ingested, 5 g can be given empirically.
4. **Glutamate agonists**
   a. **Sources.** Domoic acid (shellfish), ibotenic acid (*A. muscaria* mushrooms), β-*N*-oxalylamino-L-alanine (BOAA found in legumes of the genus *Lathyrus*)
   b. **Mechanism of action.** Direct agonists at glutamate receptors [*N*-methyl-D-aspartate (NMDA), α-amino-3-hydroxy-5-methyl-4-isoxazolepropionic acid (AMPA)]
   c. **Other clinical features.** Patients with lathyrism from BOAA have spastic paraplegia.
   d. **Treatment**
      (1) **Diazepam** 10 mg or lorazepam 2 mg i.v. for seizures with repeat doses as needed for control
      (2) **Phenobarbital** 20 mg/kg i.v. at rate of 25 to 50 mg/min
5. **Antihistamines**
   a. **Sources.** First-generation (sedating) antihistamines (diphenhydramine, chlorpheniramine, brompheniramine)

  b. Mechanism of action. Central histamine-1 receptor antagonism
  c. Other clinical features. See anticholinergic syndrome (**III.A.1.**).
  d. Treatment
    (1) **Diazepam** 10 mg or lorazepam 2 mg i.v. for seizures with repeated doses as needed for control
    (2) **Phenobarbital** 20 mg/kg i.v. at rate of 25 to 50 mg/min.
6. **Adenosine antagonists**
  a. Sources. Theophylline, caffeine, theobromine, pentoxifylline, carbamazepine
  b. Mechanism of action. Antagonism of presynaptic A1 receptors, which prevents inhibition of glutaminergic neurons, and A2 receptors, which cause cerebral vasoconstriction.
  c. Other clinical features
    (1) The manifestations of theophylline toxicity are similar to those of sympathomimetic syndrome (see **III.A.2.**).
    (2) The manifestations of carbamazepine toxicity are similar to those of anticholinergic syndrome (see **III.A.1.**).
  d. Treatment
    (1) **Phenobarbital** 20 mg/kg i.v. at rate of 25 to 50 mg/min for altered mental status, CNS agitation, theophylline levels greater than 100 µg/mL, or seizures
    (2) **Diazepam** 10 mg or lorazepam 2 mg i.v. for seizures with repeated doses as needed for control
    (3) **Hemodialysis** for theophylline or caffeine overdose with seizures.
7. **Withdrawal seizures**
  a. Sources. Ethanol, benzodiazepines, barbiturates, baclofen
  b. Mechanism of action. Prolonged use thought to result in down-regulation of GABA receptors and up-regulation of glutamate receptors
  c. Other clinical features. Delirium, hallucinations, tachycardia, hypertension, fever, autonomic instability, hypertonicity (baclofen)
  d. Treatment
    (1) **Diazepam** 10 mg or lorazepam 2 mg i.v. for seizures with repeated doses as needed for control
    (2) **Phenobarbital** 20 mg/kg i.v. at rate of 25 to 50 mg/min
    (3) **Baclofen** should be given to patients thought to have baclofen withdrawal. In general, oral dosage of baclofen should be restarted at the previous rate, or the baclofen pump should be refilled.

Recommended Readings

Goldfrank LR, Flomenbaum NE, Lewin NA, et al. *Goldfrank's toxicologic emergencies,* 6th ed. Stamford, CT: Appleton & Lange, 1998.

Haddad LM, Shannon MW, Winchester JF. *Clinical management of poisoning and drug overdose,* 3rd ed. Philadelphia: WB Saunders, 1998.

Klassen CD. *Casarett and Doull's toxicology,* 5th ed. New York: McGraw–Hill, 1996.

Spencer PS, Schaumburg HH. *Experimental and clinical neurotoxicology,* 2nd ed. New York: Oxford University Press, 2000.

55. SLEEP DISORDERS

Phyllis C. Zee

Sleep problems and disorders are prevalent in the general population, and it is estimated that approximately 30% of the U.S. population regularly suffers from insomnia. Sleep problems influence health-related quality of life and chronic medical and neurologic conditions. Patients who report disturbed sleep generally describe one or more of three types of problems—insomnia, excessive daytime sleepiness (EDS), and abnormal motor activities, complex behaviors, or disturbed sensations during sleep.

The *International Classification of Sleep Disorders (ICSD)* lists 84 sleep disorders. The *ICSD* has the following four major categories: dyssomnia—that is, disorders of initiating and maintaining sleep and disorders of excessive sleepiness; parasomnia; disorders associated with medical or psychiatric disorders; and proposed sleep disorders. To assist the clinician in diagnosing sleep disorders, a differential diagnosis–based classification adapted from the *ICSD* is used in this chapter.

I. Insomnia is the inability to fall asleep, the inability to maintain sleep, the perception of inadequate sleep or nonrestorative sleep. The three main categories of insomnia are psychophysiologic insomnia, idiopathic insomnia, and sleep state misperception.
   A. Psychophysiologic insomnia
       1. Course. For the diagnosis of psychophysiologic insomnia to be made, a patient has to have sleep difficulties that substantially affect daytime functioning and have a learning or conditioning component that typically involves one or more of the following: daily worries about not being able to fall asleep or stay asleep accompanied by intense efforts to fall asleep each night; paradoxic improvement away from the usual sleep environment (e.g., in another room of the house or away from home); and somatized tension and anxiety associated with bedtime and the subject of sleep. The most difficult differential diagnosis is with generalized anxiety disorder, in which anxiety is pervasive and involves most aspects of daily life rather than exclusively the inability to sleep. Differentiation from affective disorders also is important.
       2. Treatment and outcome. A varied individualized approach is indicated for most patients. A combined treatment approach involving good sleep hygiene, behavioral therapy, and medications is most effective. Although pharmacologic intervention has an important role in the management of insomnia, it is not the basic, long-term approach. A 4- to 8-week trial of sleep hygiene counseling, behavior modification, and judicious use of hypnotics is recommended. If insomnia does not improve after this period of treatment, referral to a sleep specialist should be considered and nocturnal polysomnography performed to determine an underlying medical or psychiatric or psychological disease.
           a. Behavioral therapy. There are four important factors in sleep hygiene. The first factor includes circadian rhythm and the structuring of sleep–wake cycles. The second factor involves physiologic changes in sleep that accompany aging. The third factor is the important effects on sleep exerted by social and recreational drugs such as nicotine, caffeine, and alcohol. The fourth factor concerns conditions and activities that promote arousal during sleep time. Sleep hygiene instructions that address these four areas are listed in Table 55.1.

           The most widely used behavioral therapy program in the management of insomnia includes a combined program of relaxation techniques, stimulus–control therapy, and sleep restriction therapy. Relaxation techniques may include progressive muscle relaxation, biofeedback, deep breathing, meditation, guided imagery, and other techniques to control cognitive arousal. These techniques are first taught during training sessions and then practiced daily for 20 to 30 minutes by the patient at home, usually around bedtime. **Stimulus–control therapy** is useful in the management of conditioned insomnia. This technique is an attempt

Table 55.1 Sleep hygiene instructions.

Homeostatic Drive for Sleep

Avoid naps, except for a brief 10- to 15-minute nap 8 hours after arising; check with your physician first, because in some sleep disorders naps can be beneficial.

Restrict sleep period to average number of hours you have actually slept per night in the preceding week. Quality of sleep is important. Too much time in bed can decrease quality on the subsequent night.

Get regular exercise every day, preferably 40 minutes in the afternoon. It is best to finish exercise at least 3 hours before bedtime.

Have a warm, non-caffeine-containing drink, which can help you relax as well as warm you.

Take a warm bath 90–120 minutes before bedtime and wear warm socks to help lower body temperature.

Circadian Factors

Keep a regular out-of-bed time (do not deviate more than 1 hour) 7 days a week.

Do not expose yourself to bright light if you have to get up at night.

Expose yourself to bright light, either outdoor or artificial, during the day.

Drug Effects

Do not smoke to get yourself back to sleep.

Do not smoke after 7:00 P.M.; give up smoking entirely.

Avoid caffeine entirely for a 4-week trial period; limit caffeine use to no more than three cups no later than 10:00 A.M.

Avoid alcoholic beverages after 7:00 P.M. Alcohol can fragment sleep over the second half of the sleep period.

Arousal in Sleep Setting

Keep clock face turned away, and do not find out what time it is when you wake up at night.

Avoid strenuous exercise after 6:00 P.M.

Do not eat or drink heavily for 3 hours before bedtime. A light bedtime snack may help.

If you have trouble with regurgitation, be especially careful to avoid heavy meals and spices in the evening. Do not retire too hungry or too full. You may have to raise the head of your bed.

Keep your room dark, quiet, well ventilated, and at a comfortable temperature throughout the night.

Use a bedtime ritual. Reading before lights-out may be helpful if it is not occupationally related.

Learn to use simple self-hypnosis when you wake at night. Do not try too hard to sleep; instead, concentrate on the pleasant feeling of relaxation.

Use stress management and relaxation techniques in the daytime.

Be sure your mattress is not too soft or too firm and that your pillow is of the right height and firmness.

Use a sleeping pill only occasionally.

Use the bedroom only for sleep; do not work or do other activities that lead to prolonged wakefulness.

to break the conditioning by teaching the patient to associate the bedroom with sleep behavior. The instructions for stimulus—control behavioral therapy are listed in Table 55.2. Sleep restriction therapy involves curtailment of time in bed to a few hours per night until the patient learns to use the time in bed for sleeping.

  b. Hypnotic drugs. The most widely used prescription hypnotics are the benzodiazepines. Two new classes of hypnotics, imidazopyridines (e.g., zolpidem) and pyrazolopyrimidines (zaleplon) have been introduced for the management of insomnia. These medications are indicated for occasional sleepless nights to break the vicious circle of patients' needing

Table 55.2 Stimulus–control behavioral therapy

Go to bed only when sleepy. Stay up until you are really sleepy, then return to bed. If sleep still does not come easily, get out of bed again. The goal is to associate bed with falling asleep quickly.

Use the bed only for sleeping. Do not read, watch television, or eat in bed.

If unable to sleep, get up and move to another room.

Repeat the preceding step as often as necessary throughout the night.

Set the alarm and get up at the same time every morning, regardless of how much you slept during the night. This helps the body acquire a constant sleep–wake rhythm.

Do not nap during the day.

---

sleep so desperately they become tense, which perpetuates the insomnia. The choice of hypnotic may depend on the nature of the sleep problems. For example, if the predominant problem is falling asleep, a fast-acting, short-half-life hypnotic may be preferable. If the problem is frequent awakenings and sleep maintenance insomnia, a longer-acting hypnotic may be more effective.

Hypnotics that are long acting as well as those that contain active metabolites can cause "hangover" side effects in the morning. Continued use of hypnotics on a daily basis should be avoided, because they usually lose their effects (necessitating escalation of dosage), and may produce rebound insomnia when withdrawn. Rebound insomnia and development of tolerance may occur less frequently with zolpidem and zaleplon than with benzodiazepines. However, both zaleplon and zolpidem lack significant anxiolytic properties at the usually prescribed dosages and therefore are not useful in the treatment of persons with insomnia who may benefit from the anxiolytic effects of hypnotics. The most widely used prescription hypnotics and their properties are listed in Table 55.3. Although patients with chronic insomnia rarely become "great" sleepers after treatment, most can manage the predisposition to insomnia by using the combination of sleep hygiene, behavioral treatment, and occasional hypnotics.

B. Idiopathic insomnia

1. **Course.** Idiopathic or primary insomnia is a lifelong inability to sleep, presumably associated with a predisposition for insomnia resulting from abnormality of the sleep–wake cycle or autonomic activity. Patients with this condition are a heterogeneous group. Most have been poor sleepers since childhood, and the insomnia, although it persists over the entire life span, can be aggravated by stress and tension. Patients with idiopathic insomnia may have atypical reactions to stimulants and sedatives.

   Idiopathic insomnia often is accompanied by other factors, such as poor sleep hygiene or psychiatric disorders. Therefore, there tends to be a continuum from

Table 55.3 Benzodiazepine hypnotics pharmacologic

Drug	Onset of action (min)	Duration of action (h)	Active metabolites	Recommendation dose (mg)
Estazolam	15–30	6–8	Yes	1–2
Flurazepam	15–30	8–10	Yes	15–30
Quazepam	15–30	8–10	Yes	7.5–15
Temazepam	40–60	6–8	No	15–30
Triazolam	15–30	3–4	No	0.125–0.25
Zaleplon	15–30	~1	No	5–10
Zolpidem	15–30	3–6	No	5–10

idiopathic insomnia to psychophysiologic insomnia to insomnia associated with psychiatric problems.

2. **Diagnosis.** A diagnosis of idiopathic insomnia is made when there is no clear emotional or other trauma believed to have initiated the insomnia. Psychiatric and medical causes must be ruled out. The severity of the insomnia is such that waking function is impaired.

3. **Treatment and outcome.** There is no consistent approach to management of idiopathic insomnia, because each case is different and a highly empirical approach may be necessary. Some patients respond to treatment with heterocyclic antidepressants, such as amitriptyline or trazodone at bedtime. Effective dosages vary greatly, ranging from low (25 mg) to high (200 mg). In addition to medication, referral for supportive psychological treatment often is necessary, as is good sleep hygiene.

C. **Sleep state misperception**

1. **Course.** It is not uncommon for patients to overestimate sleep latency and underestimate total sleep time. In sleep state misperception, this tendency is extreme. Patients who claim not to sleep at all typically sleep several hours when studied in the laboratory.

2. **Diagnosis.** Sleep state misperception is suggested when a patient reports persistent insomnia, although sleep duration and quality are normal. This condition can be diagnosed only in the laboratory, because one needs to document that sleep is normal.

3. **Treatment and outcome.** Confronting and reassuring patients with the fact that their sleep is normal and that they sleep longer than they think they do and behavioral treatments (see **I.A.1.a.**) are effective.

D. **Insomnia associated with psychiatric disorders**

1. **Course.** Psychiatric conditions are major causes of insomnia. Results of epidemiologic studies suggest that as many as 57% of persons with insomnia have a psychiatric condition or will have one within 1 year. The underlying condition usually is a mood disorder, anxiety disorder, somatoform disorder, personality disorder, or schizophrenia. It is rare to encounter a patient with a mood disorder who does not also have sleep–wake problems. Sleep in major depression is characterized by early morning awakening (2 to 4 hours after sleep onset) and frequent nocturnal awakening with inability to reinitiate sleep. The incidence of insomnia among patients with anxiety disorders is high. The typical symptoms are difficulty with sleep initiation and, to a lesser degree, nocturnal awakenings. Tiredness is common, but napping is unusual. Patients with anxiety disorders are susceptible to conditioning factors that produce psychophysiologic insomnia.

2. **Treatment and outcome.** Treatment should first address the underlying psychiatric disorder. For major depressive disorders, this involves use of antidepressants or selective serotonin reuptake inhibitors (SSRIs). An antidepressant with sedative properties is favored over a less sedating one for patients with insomnia. Administration 30 minutes before bedtime also aids in promoting sleep. Amitriptyline, trimipramine, doxepin, trazodone, nefazodone, and mirtazapine are the most sedating, whereas protriptyline and SSRIs such as fluoxetine have stimulating effects that may worsen insomnia. Antidepressants with anxiolytic properties are useful in the treatment of anxious, depressed patients and facilitate psychotherapeutic or pharmacologic treatment. Anticholinergic side effects of tricyclic antidepressants (cardiotoxicity, urinary retention, erectile dysfunction, and dry mouth) limit the usefulness of these agents, particularly by the elderly.

The management of intense anxiety may require supportive psychotherapy with pharmacotherapy. The benzodiazepines and some antidepressants, such as paroxetine, are the medications of choice for an anxiolytic effect. The choice of the type of benzodiazepine is individualized according to the predominant symptoms. For example, if the main problem is difficulty initiating sleep, a single bedtime dose of a drug with an intermediate duration, such as alprazolam, lorazepam, or oxazepam, may be preferred over use of longer-acting agents such as flurazepam and chlordiazepoxide. The latter two may be more useful in providing anxiolytic and hypnotic relief to patients with sleep maintenance insomnia. If this condition is suspected, referral to a sleep specialist or psychiatrist is recommended for evaluation of the underlying psychiatric disorder.

II. Insomnia associated with circadian rhythm disorders

A. **Course.** Circadian rhythms are generated by a neural clock located in the suprachiasmatic nucleus of the hypothalamus. Disruption of biologic timing results in circadian rhythm disorders that are most often associated with patients' reports of insomnia. Circadian rhythm disorders are characterized by essentially normal sleep that is not synchronized with conventional environmental light–dark cycles and periods of sleep. Diagnosis requires specialized assessment, including use of a sleep diary, and a careful history interview to elicit the appropriate major diagnostic criteria.

The most common sleep disturbances associated with disruption of circadian rhythmicity are the **sleep phase syndromes. Delayed sleep phase syndrome (DSPS)** is persistent inability to fall asleep until the early morning hours (1 to 3 A.M., and sometimes later). If allowed, the patient would sleep until the late morning or early afternoon (10 A.M. to 2 P.M.). When the patient is forced to rise at 7 or 8 A.M., sleep is curtailed, and daytime sleepiness develops. Despite the daytime sleepiness, patients find that in the evening they become more alert and remain unable to fall asleep until the early morning hours. **Advanced sleep phase syndrome (ASPS)** is characterized by early evening sleep onset (8 to 9 P.M.) and early morning awakening (3 to 5 A.M.). Although DSPS predominates at younger ages and ASPS at older ages, both syndromes can be chronic and result in sleep problems throughout life. Because many features of the sleep of patients with depression (early morning awakening) resemble those of ASPS, depression must be considered in the differential diagnosis.

Another type of circadian rhythm disorder encountered in practice is **irregular sleep–wake pattern.** This condition differs from the phase disorders in that there is loss of circadian rhythmicity, which results in the lack of a long, consolidated sleep period. Sleep usually is broken into short sleep periods or naps during the course of 24 hours. Irregular sleep–wake patterns occur among patients with Alzheimer's disease and among other elderly persons in nursing homes.

B. **Treatment and outcome**

1. The traditional treatment is **chronotherapy,** a behavioral technique in which bedtime is systematically delayed (for DSPS) or advanced (for ASPS) in 3-hour increments each day until the desired sleep phase is achieved. The patient is then instructed to maintain the newly established bedtime rigidly. Although this approach works, it is an arduous procedure, and maintenance of the effect has been difficult.

2. A new approach in the treatment of sleep phase disorders is **bright light therapy.** Light intensity greater than 2,500 lux is considered bright. Appropriately timed bright light exposure can alleviate DSPS and ASPS. Exposure to bright light in the early morning results in an advancement of circadian phase, whereas exposure to light in the evening delays circadian rhythms. For management of DSPS, exposure to light usually is scheduled for 1 to 2 hours in the morning (6 to 8 A.M.). For ASPS, light exposure is recommended in the evening, approximately 2 to 4 hours before scheduled bedtime. Despite high rates of success in achieving the desired sleep phase under immediate treatment, many patients do not continue the light regimen and have a relapse. Some patients are able to maintain a normalized phase without maintenance of light exposure for as long as several months, whereas others drift back toward the pretreatment phase within a few days.

3. **Melatonin** has been shown to shift the phase of circadian rhythms in humans. Several studies are underway to determine the effectiveness of melatonin in the management of DSPS.

4. Management of irregular sleep–wake patterns and associated behavioral problems in this group of patients is a challenge. Treatment with sedative–

hypnotics is prevalent in nursing homes. These medications have side effects that may not be well tolerated by older patients. Some promising studies have indicated that structured activity programs, morning exposure to bright light and evening melatonin may alleviate these sleep–wake and behavioral disorders. An initial evaluation by a sleep specialist and ophthalmologic consultation are recommended before bright light therapy is initiated. The cost of light units ranges from $150 to $300.

III. Disorders of excessive sleepiness. Sleepiness severe enough to affect activities of daily living is estimated to be present among 30% of the population and is most commonly caused by self-imposed restriction of sleep. However, approximately 4% to 5% of the population has EDS as a result of a sleep disorder. Sleepiness is excessive and an indication of a sleep disorder when it occurs at undesirable times, such as while driving and during social activities. EDS can be divided into two types—extrinsic and intrinsic. Some extrinsic causes include environmental factors, drug dependency, sleep-disordered breathing, and movement disorders during sleep. The more common types of intrinsic hypersomnia usually are associated with primary central nervous system (CNS) disorders such as narcolepsy and idiopathic hypersomnia.

    A. Narcolepsy

        1. Course. Narcolepsy is a manifestation of a dissociation between wakefulness and sleep, particularly rapid eye movement (REM) sleep. The onset usually occurs in adolescence or young adulthood, and men are affected more often than are women. Studies have shown a strong genetic association between narcolepsy and the DR2 DQw1 (DR15 Dqw6 under the new nomenclature) human leukocyte antigen (HLA). Evidence has shown **lower levels of the neuropeptide orexin (hypocretin) in the cerebrospinal fluid** of patients with narcolepsy and cataplexy, indicating orexin deficiency in the pathophysiologic mechanism of narcolepsy.

        2. Clinical features. Narcolepsy is a syndrome characterized by EDS, irresistible sleep attacks, cataplexy, sleep paralysis, and hypnagogic hallucinations. All patients must have pathologic levels of daytime sleepiness, and the presence of cataplexy is pathognomonic for narcolepsy. Moreover, nocturnal sleep often is disrupted for patients with narcolepsy. Decreased quality and quantity of nocturnal sleep exacerbate the EDS even further.

        3. Diagnosis. In addition to the clinical history, nocturnal polysomnography and multiple sleep latency testing are performed to establish a diagnosis of narcolepsy. Shortened mean sleep latency and the presence of sleep-onset REM sleep in the naps can help confirm the clinical diagnosis. If the results of sleep studies are inconclusive, results of HLA typing may provide additional aid in establishing the diagnosis.

        4. Treatment and outcome. Treatment approaches to narcolepsy emphasize control of narcoleptic symptoms to allow optimal social and professional productivity by maintaining the patient's alertness throughout the day. Choice of treatment must take into account that narcolepsy is a lifelong disorder and that patients will have to take medications for many years. Clinicians are not unanimous in their approach to management of narcolepsy. The drug treatments recommended in this chapter form a reasonable guideline for the treatment of most patients with narcolepsy.

            a. The drugs commonly used to manage EDS and sleep attacks are the **CNS stimulants** methylphenidate, dextroamphetamine, pemoline, and modafinil. Because of frequent side effects, such as irritability, tachycardia, elevated blood pressure, and nocturnal sleep disturbance, amphetamines are no longer the first-line treatment. The use of methylphenidate is preferable because of its lower incidence and severity of these side effects. Pemoline, another stimulant with a long half-life and slower onset of action, is less effective than methylphenidate but is well tolerated. Modafinil is a stimulant medication recently approved in the United States for the management of narcolepsy. Modafinil has several advantages over other stimulants in that it has fewer cardiovascular side effects and the prescription can be refilled. Medications used in the management of EDS and the dosages are listed in Table 55.4. Drugs with

Table 55.4 Commonly used narcolepsy drugs currently available

Drug	Usual dosage[a]
Stimulants	
Dextroamphetamine	5–60 mg/d
Methamphetamine	20–25 mg/d
Methylphenidate	10–60 mg/d
Modafinil	200–400 mg/d
Pemoline	37.5 mg/d
Adjunct-Effect Drug[b]	
Protriptyline	2.5–10 mg/d
Drugs for Management of Auxiliary Effects	
Tricyclic antidepressants with atropinic side effects	
Clomipramine	25–200 mg/d
Desipramine	25–200 mg/d
Imipramine	25–200 mg/d
Protriptyline	2.5–20 mg/d
Antidepressant without atropinic side effects	
Fluoxetine	20–60 mg/d
Experimental Drugs or Drugs Available in Few Countries	
γ-Hydroxybutyrate	—

[a] Occasionally, depending on clinical response, the dosage may be outside the usual dosage range. All drugs administered orally.
[b] Adjunct–effect drugs improve excessive daytime sleepiness if associated with a stimulant.

norepinephrine-releasing properties have the greatest impact on sleepiness. However, even at the highest recommended doses, no drug brings persons with narcolepsy to a normal level of alertness.

b. The management of cataplexy, sleep paralysis, and hypnagogic hallucinations involves **tricyclic antidepressant medications.** Protriptyline and clomipramine have been used widely, often with good results. Other tricyclic medications, such as imipramine, desipramine, and amitriptyline, also are effective; however, anticholinergic side effects (particularly erectile dysfunction) limit the ability of many patients to tolerate these medications, particularly if high doses are needed to control cataplexy. Fluoxetine is somewhat less effective for cataplexy, but it has the advantage of being a mild stimulant. An example of an initial regimen for narcolepsy among adults is provided in Table 55.5.

c. A third approach to the management of narcolepsy is to **improve the nocturnal sleep** of persons with narcolepsy. Improvement of nocturnal sleep not only decreases EDS but also may help cataplexy. Nocturnal sleep disturbances may be related to periodic limb movements of sleep (PLMS), which frequently occur among patients with narcolepsy. They may, however, also be a complication of treatment with stimulants and tricyclic medications. Management of PLMS with a dopamine agonist drug such as 10 to 100 mg carbidopa/levodopa (Sinemet; DuPont, Wilmington, DE, U.S.A.) or a benzodiazepine such as 0.5 mg clonazepam may be helpful.

d. **Nonpharmacologic treatment**—scheduled short naps and support therapy—must be emphasized. Short naps of 15 to 20 minutes three times during the day help maintain alertness. Patients with narcolepsy often experience social and professional difficulties owing to sleepiness and cataplexy. Narcolepsy can result in unemployment, rejection by friends, and depression. For these reasons, it is important to encourage

Table 55.5 Example of an initial treatment plan for narcolepsy in adults

---

Avoidance of shifts in sleep schedule.

Avoidance of heavy meals and alcohol intake.

Regular timing of nocturnal sleep: 10:30 P.M. to 7:00 A.M.

Naps. Strategically timed naps, if possible (e.g., 15 minutes at lunchtime and 15 minutes at 5:30 P.M.)

Medication. The effects of stimulant medications vary widely among patients. The dosing and timing of medications should be individualized to optimize performance. Additional doses, as needed, may be suggested for periods of anticipated sleepiness.

    Modafinil: 200 mg/d (200 mg on awakening or 100 mg twice a day)

      If difficulties persist: may increase modafinil to 400 mg/d

    Methylphenidate: 5 mg (three or four tablets) or 20 mg SR in morning (on empty stomach)

      If difficulties persist:

        methylphenidate (SR): 20 mg in morning

5 mg after noon nap

5 mg at 4:00 P.M.

    If no response:

      Dexedrine spansule (SR): 15 mg at awakening

5 mg after noon nap

5 mg at 3:30 or 4:00 P.M. (or 15 mg at awakening and 15 mg after noon nap)

    For cataplexy:

      Clomipramine at 75–125 mg *or*

      Protriptyline at 10–20 mg *or*

      Imipramine at 75–125 mg

SR, sustained-release tablet.

patients with narcolepsy to join support groups and to provide referral for psychotherapy when needed.

    5. Side effects of stimulant medications. Hypertension, abnormal liver function, alterations in mood, and psychosis are the most commonly reported complications of stimulant therapy for narcolepsy. Moreover, tolerance and, less frequently, addiction may be observed with drugs such as amphetamines. Interestingly, with high dosages of amphetamines (100 mg/d), a paradoxic effect of increased sleepiness may result. This paradoxic effect disappears with reduction of the daily dosage. Other common side effects include increased jitteriness, verbal aggressiveness, "racing thoughts," increased heart rate, tremor, and involuntary movements.

  B. Idiopathic CNS hypersomnia

    1. Course. Idiopathic CNS hypersomnia is a disabling illness. It is characterized by excessive daytime sleepiness, but there are no clearly defined sleep attacks or other features associated with narcolepsy. The age at onset varies from adolescence to middle age. The symptoms are lifelong, with some worsening in old age.

    2. Clinical features. Patients report sleepiness throughout the day associated with prolonged naps that are not refreshing. Automatic behaviors may occur during periods of drowsiness. These behaviors often are inappropriate, and patients usually do not have any recollection of these events. Patients have severe difficulty awakening in the morning.

    3. Diagnosis. It is important to differentiate CNS hypersomnia from narcolepsy and nocturnal sleep disorders such as sleep-disordered breathing or periodic movements of sleep, which are associated with daytime sleepiness. Therefore, the diagnosis is made by means of elimination of other causes of daytime sleepiness. Polysomnography should be performed to rule out these possibilities, and multiple sleep latency testing should be performed to document the level of objective daytime sleepiness.

4. **Treatment and outcome.** Because multiple etiologic factors may be responsible for CNS hypersomnia and because of the relative lack of understanding of the pathophysiologic mechanism, treatment is symptomatic and the response is variable. Behavioral therapies and sleep hygiene instructions should be recommended but have only modest positive effect. The only medications that provide partial relief of excessive sleepiness are stimulant drugs. The most commonly recommended medications are pemoline, methylphenidate, dextroamphetamine, and modafinil. Tricyclic antidepressants, selective serotonin reuptake inhibitors, clonidine, bromocriptine, amantadine, and methysergide have been used with varying success. Sometimes combinations of these drugs yield better control of sleepiness. Even with the highest recommended dose, complete control of daytime sleepiness is seldom achieved in this group of patients. Therefore, prescribing more than 60 mg of methylphenidate or 40 mg of dextroamphetamine does not provide significant additional symptomatic relief. The patient should be advised not to drive or engage in potentially dangerous activities that require high levels of alertness.

IV. **Parasomnia** is a group of conditions that occur during sleep or are associated with arousal from sleep. These conditions include enuresis, sleepwalking, night terrors, dream anxiety attacks, nocturnal complex seizures, and REM behavior disorder. The ones that are most often encountered in adult clinical practice are discussed.

A. **Non-REM parasomnia.** Sleepwalking and sleep terrors are episodic behaviors that occur as arousals from non-REM stages of sleep, usually when the patient is coming out of slow-wave sleep. Because sleepwalking (somnambulism) and sleep terrors (pavor nocturnus) among adults are most often associated with each other, the key features are discussed together.

1. **Course.** The prevalence of sleepwalking and sleep terrors is estimated at approximately 6% of the population. These types of parasomnia are most frequent among children and often disappear by adolescence. These behaviors may be considered normal among children, but for a large number of persons, they persist into adulthood. Patients may report a family history of parasomnia.

2. **Clinical features.** During these episodes, patients exhibit stereotyped behaviors, such as talking, sitting up, and getting up to walk. These episodes are potentially dangerous, because patients may bump into walls and windows or fall down stairs. With sleep terrors, extreme autonomic discharge and screaming are present. Patients usually have only vague recollections of these events and are confused if awakened.

3. **Diagnosis.** For adults, thorough evaluation of abnormal nocturnal behavior should be performed to differentiate non-REM parasomnia from other pathologic entities and from side effects of medications.

4. **Treatment and outcome.** Therapy for non-REM parasomnia includes several approaches consisting of preventive measures, psychological interventions, and medications.

a. **Preventive measures and psychological intervention.** Preventive measures are taken to avoid serious injury during episodes of sleepwalking. The patient should be advised to locate the bedroom on the first floor, lock windows and doors, cover windows and glass doors with heavy draperies, and remove hazardous objects from the house.

Hypnosis and psychotherapy have also been used in the management of parasomnia. Hypnosis has been shown helpful, at least for a short time, to young adults. The need for psychotherapy depends on the association of psychological factors with the parasomnia. Psychotherapy has been used most widely to treat young adults for sleep terrors. Most cases of parasomnia increase in severity and frequency with psychological stress. Therefore, in addition to psychotherapy, relaxation programs, such as progressive muscle relaxation and biofeedback, may be beneficial.

      b. Medications. The benzodiazepines—most commonly clonazepam, alprazolam, and diazepam—have been used. In the management of sleep terrors, tricyclic antidepressants (particularly imipramine) have been used either alone or in combination with benzodiazepines to provide control of symptoms. In addition, several studies have shown that treatment with carbamazepine (Tegretol; Novartis, East Hanover, NJ, U.S.A.) may be beneficial. An example of an initial therapeutic approach is to start with clonazepam (0.5 to 1.0 mg) approximately 30 minutes before bedtime. If the response is inadequate, the dose should be increased by balancing the side effects, which include confusion and daytime drowsiness, particularly in the care of the elderly. A secondary line of treatment includes initiation of low doses of tricyclic antidepressant drugs or carbamazepine at bedtime.

          Results of management of non-REM parasomnia are poorly documented. However, the little information in the literature indicates that response to combinations of pharmacologic and nonpharmacologic therapies is excellent. As many as 70% of adult patients report disappearance of the symptoms after various lengths of time.

B. REM sleep behavior disorder (RBD)

    1. Course. REM sleep is normally accompanied by muscle atonia. There are, however, pathologic conditions, such as RBD, in which there is a loss of REM atonia or excessive motor activation during sleep. Patients with this disorder most commonly report vigorous sleep behaviors that are accompanied by vivid dreams. These behaviors may be quite violent and result in serious injury. RBD occurs in both acute and chronic forms. The **acute form** usually is associated with toxic–metabolic etiologic factors, most commonly, drug withdrawal states, particularly delirium tremens. Loss of REM atonia also may occur among patients taking medications that suppress REM sleep, such as tricyclic antidepressants and fluoxetine. The **chronic form** usually occurs among older adults. It has been seen in association with various brainstem abnormalities, extrapyramidal neurologic disorders, and medical conditions (Parkinson's disease, progressive supranuclear palsy, Shy–Drager syndrome, multiple systems atrophy, brainstem stroke, brainstem tumor, demyelinating disease, and medication toxicity or withdrawal) or is idiopathic. The differential diagnosis of RBD includes non-REM parasomnia, sleep apnea, periodic movements of sleep, nocturnal seizures, and nocturnal rhythmic movements. It is important to recognize this condition and differentiate it from other nocturnal behaviors, because RBD can be managed effectively.

    2. Treatment and outcome. Management of RBD involves pharmacologic therapy and interventions that address issues concerning environmental safety.

      a. The most effective **drug therapy** is clonazepam at a dosage of 0.5 to 1.0 mg at bedtime. Clonazepam may be taken earlier (1 to 2 hours before bedtime) by patients who report sleep-onset insomnia or morning drowsiness as a result of the medication. Clonazepam is effective in 90% of cases, and there is little evidence of abuse and infrequent tolerance in this group of patients. Beneficial effects are observed within the first week of treatment. Typically, treatment with clonazepam results in control of vigorous, violent sleep behaviors, but mild to moderate limb movement, sleeptalking, and other complex behaviors may persist. Discontinuation of treatment usually results in recurrence of symptoms. There have been few reported cases of successful treatment with desipramine, carbidopa/levodopa, or clonidine.

      b. Environmental safety is an important issue in the management of RBD. Patients should be advised to remove potentially dangerous objects from the house, to pad hard and sharp surfaces around the bed, to cover windows with heavy draperies, and even to place the mattress on the floor to avoid falling out of bed. The combination of drug therapy and

implementation of safety precautions offers safe and effective management of RBD.
  c. Nocturnal seizures should be considered in the differential diagnosis of many forms of parasomnia. If the history suggests a seizure disorder or if symptoms are not controlled, **referral** to a neurologist or sleep specialist for further evaluation is recommended.
C. **Restless legs syndrome (RLS) and PLMS**
  1. **Course.** RLS is characterized by creeping, crawling, and disagreeable sensations in the lower and occasionally in the upper extremities associated with irresistible movements of the extremities. The symptoms are present at rest and are relieved by movements such as stretching, rubbing, and walking. Lying down in bed and falling asleep is a major problem for patients with RLS. Dysesthesia and the need to move the lower extremities are the most severe at bedtime and often are associated with sleep-onset insomnia. Many patients also report severe dysesthesia and leg jerks in the middle of the night with difficulty returning to sleep.

  Most patients with RLS also have periodic limb movement disorder (PLMD). However, PLMD can occur without RLS and has its own diagnostic category. It is characterized by stereotyped repetitive rhythmic movements (lasting 0.5 to 5.0 seconds with an intermovement interval of 20 to 40 seconds) of the legs (commonly, dorsiflexion of the foot) and occasionally may also involve the upper extremities. PLMD usually is more frequent during the first half of the night but can be present throughout sleep. Movements may be associated with sleep disruption. If numerous, the movements can result in nocturnal awakenings and excessive daytime sleepiness. The prevalence of PLMD increases with age, from 5% among those younger than 50 years to 44% among those 65 years and older.

  For most patients with RLS or PLMD, the cause is unknown and therefore termed **idiopathic.** In many cases, RLS is familial. However, both RLS and PLMD may be associated with anemia resulting from iron, folic acid, or vitamin B_{12} deficiency; neuropathy; myelopathy; rheumatoid arthritis; thyroid dysfunction; and uremia. Results of studies suggest that RLS is associated with alteration in cerebrospinal fluid ferritin levels. Furthermore, PLMD may be induced or exacerbated by tricyclic antidepressants as well as by withdrawal from a variety of hypnotic agents. The existence of these conditions should be entertained in the differential diagnosis of PLMD so that patients receive the appropriate therapy. If these conditions are suspected, referral to the appropriate specialist is recommended.
  2. **Treatment.** The four major classes of drugs that have been shown to be effective in the management of RLS and PLMD are dopaminergic drugs, benzodiazepines, anticonvulsants, and opioids.
    a. Several studies have shown that dopaminergic medications are effective and considered a first line for the management of RLS and PLMS. Although carbidopa/levodopa was initially widely used, the risk of rebound symptoms decreased its overall effectiveness in many patients. Carbidopa/levodopa (25 mg/100 mg) is given at bedtime, and the dosage is increased progressively until a therapeutic effect is obtained. Usually a dose of carbidopa/levodopa (50 mg/200 mg) is sufficient to control RLS and PLMD. A second administration during the day may be necessary if patients report an increase in leg movements in the morning. Treatment with controlled-release carbidopa/levodopa (Sinemet CR) may also alleviate the rebound effect. The side effects of levodopa treatment are generally minimal. The major side effects are rebound symptoms of dysesthesia or leg movements during the day. Dyskinesia associated with long-term levodopa treatment, as observed among patients with Parkinson's disease, are uncommon in this group of patients. The newer dopamine agonist medications, such as pramipexole, pergolide, and ropinirole have been shown effective in the management of RLS and PLMD. Many sleep specialists recommend starting therapy with a dopamine

agonist medication such as pramipexole (0.125 to 0.25 mg) in the evening.

b. The **anticonvulsant** gabapentin (starting with 100 to 300 mg), either alone or in combination with the dopamine agonist medications, also relieves the symptoms of RLS and PLMD

c. Several **benzodiazepines,** including clonazepam, nitrazepam, lorazepam, and temazepam, have been found to improve the nocturnal sleep of patients with RLS and PLMS. Of these, clonazepam is the most widely used. The therapeutic action of clonazepam most likely results from its ability to decrease the number of arousals caused by leg movements. The usual starting dosage of clonazepam is 0.5 to 1.0 mg at bedtime for management of PLMS. Management of RLS may require additional doses to control symptoms during the day. Because benzodiazepines are CNS depressants, they may aggravate sleep apnea, particularly among older persons.

d. **Opioids** are highly effective in the management of RLS and PLMS. However, the risks of abuse, addiction, and tolerance limit their clinical use. In severe cases refractory to other treatments, intermittent therapy with opioids provides some relief. Other proposed treatments include carbamazepine, clonidine, and baclofen.

V. Sleep-disordered breathing. The most commonly encountered types of abnormal nocturnal breathing are the sleep apnea and hypopnea. Sleep apnea is cessation of breathing for at least 10 seconds caused by obstruction of the upper airway (obstructive sleep apnea), loss of respiratory effort or rhythmicity (central apnea), or a combination of the two (mixed apnea). Hypopnea is a decrease in airflow, which can be obstructive or central in origin. Most patients with sleep apnea have combinations of the central and obstructive types, which suggests that the mechanisms of the different types of sleep apnea overlap.

A. Central sleep apnea

1. **Course.** Patients with central sleep apnea constitute less than 10% of all patients with sleep apnea who undergo studies in sleep laboratories. Therefore, only a few studies have been reported, which limits knowledge of this disorder. Little information is available regarding the cardiovascular sequelae of central sleep apnea. The most common finding is sinus arrhythmia with bradycardia. Oxygen desaturation in patients with central sleep apnea tends to be generally mild to moderate compared with that in patients with obstructive sleep apnea. Although the cause of central sleep apnea in most cases is unknown, it has been associated with certain diseases that should be considered in the differential diagnosis and management of this disorder. These diseases include central alveolar hypoventilation (Ondine's curse), obesity hypoventilation (pickwickian) syndrome, congestive heart failure (Cheyne–Stokes breathing pattern), autonomic dysfunction (Shy–Drager syndrome, familial dysautonomia, and diabetes mellitus), neuromuscular disorders (muscular dystrophy, myasthenia gravis, and motor neuron disease), and brainstem lesions.

2. **Treatment** of patients with central sleep apnea is limited and not satisfactory. Studies regarding treatment usually have involved small numbers of patients, and very few have addressed the long-term efficacy of the proposed treatments.

   a. One approach is noninvasive nocturnal ventilation delivered by means of a nasal mask with a volume- or pressure-cycled ventilator. This approach is used to manage only the most severe cases of central alveolar hypoventilation or in the care of patients with neuromuscular disorders.

   b. For patients with medical or neurologic conditions known to be associated with central sleep apnea, the condition should be managed specifically and the central apnea reassessed. However, if the problem persists or if a cause is not found, several pharmacologic agents can be used. Acetazolamide, a carbonic anhydrase inhibitor, has been shown to control central sleep apnea. In a small number of patients, acetazolamide has been shown to reduce substantially the number of episodes of central apnea. The recommended dosage is 250 mg four times a day. Even fewer studies address the long-term efficacy of this treatment. The side effects associated with mild metabolic acidosis usually are well tolerated by this group of patients.

    c. Other medications, such as theophylline, naloxone, and medroxyprogesterone acetate, have been used with varying degrees of success. Tricyclic antidepressants, particularly clomipramine, have been used successfully to treat a small number of patients. Because none of these medications has been studied systematically, more precise recommendations regarding their use are currently not available.

    d. Some patients with central sleep apnea have been shown to benefit from therapy with nasal continuous positive airway pressure (CPAP). This type of therapy is most beneficial to obese patients who also have signs of upper airway obstruction with predominantly central apnea. Nasal CPAP also has been shown effective in the treatment of patients with congestive heart failure in whom central apnea and periodic breathing are observed during sleep. Finally, oxygen therapy has been useful in managing central apnea.

B. Obstructive sleep apnea (OSA)

    1. Course. The initial symptoms of OSA syndrome are loud snoring, excessive sleepiness, fatigue, morning headaches, memory problems, alterations in mood, and episodes of apnea witnessed by the bed partner. OSA is associated with considerable morbidity, including sleep fragmentation, daytime sleepiness that may lead to vehicular and industrial accidents, nocturnal hypoxemia, and cardiovascular as well as cerebrovascular sequelae (e.g., stroke, right heart failure, and hypertension). OSA is generally caused by upper airway obstruction resulting from obesity and skeletal and soft-tissue abnormalities. Examination of the nose and throat may indicate a possible cause. However, some patients with OSA may have normal findings at physical examination.

    If OSA is suspected, **polysomnography** should be performed to ascertain the severity of the breathing disorder, which will determine the appropriate therapy. Some patients who have symptoms indistinguishable from those of OSA may have predominantly sleep hypopnea. sleep hypopnea syndrome should be managed in the same manner as sleep apnea syndromes.

    The **apnea–hypopnea (AH) index** (number of respiratory events per hour of sleep) is used to measure sleep-disordered breathing. An index of 5 is generally accepted as the upper limit of the normal range. An AH index greater than 20 has been shown to result in increased mortality. Therefore, all patients with indexes greater than 20 should be treated. Patients who have milder indexes but whose respiratory events are accompanied by moderate to severe oxygen desaturation and who have additional risk factors such as hypertension, history of heart disease, high cholesterol level, and cigarette smoking also should be treated.

    2. Therapy. The approach to management of obstructive sleep apnea and hypopnea syndromes involves both general measures and interventions that address specific abnormalities. For most patients, nasal CPAP is the most effective medical therapy for control of sleep apnea.

        a. General measures for identifying and addressing coexistent lifestyle issues that exacerbate OSA should be part of treatment of all patients. Although difficult to achieve, weight loss is an important factor in the treatment of obese persons with apnea. Sleep apnea generally improves with weight loss and may even be abolished with weight loss of 40 to 50 pounds (18 to 23 kg). In addition to dietary control, this approach requires an exercise program and psychological counseling for long-lasting results. Unfortunately, results indicate that most patients regain the weight within 2 years. If sleep-disordered breathing is more prominent in the supine position, positional therapy to avoid sleep in the supine position is very useful.

Alcohol, hypnotic drugs, and other CNS depressant drugs interfere with the arousal response that terminates apneic episodes. Therefore, patients should avoid alcohol use and should not take hypnotics or sedatives.

If a specific cause for upper-airway obstruction is found, an otorhinolaryngologic or maxillofacial evaluation is recommended for possible surgical intervention and trials of orthodontic devices, including tonsillectomy or adenoidectomy for enlarged tonsils or adenoids and correction of retrognathia or micrognathia. Results indicate that dental devices may be useful to patients with mild to moderate sleep apnea who have some degree of retrognathia or micrognathia. If chronic rhinitis is found, nasal steroid sprays may be beneficial.

   b. **Nasal CPAP.** If no specific cause of upper airway obstruction is found, nasal CPAP is the treatment of choice. This treatment is effective for most patients with obstructive apnea and hypopnea. The level of CPAP should be determined by means of titration of the therapeutic pressure in a sleep laboratory, respiratory data being obtained in all sleep stages. Nasal CPAP requires patency of the nasal airway. Therefore this procedure may not be effective for patients with severe nasal obstruction. The most common causes of intolerance of nasal CPAP are nasal symptoms, dryness, discomfort from the mask, and social and psychological factors of having to use this appliance during sleep. Added humidification often alleviates dryness and associated nasal congestion. With higher pressures, bilevel positive airway pressure (BiPAP) may be a more comfortable alternative to CPAP. Most home care companies provide both nasal CPAP and BiPAP services.

   Although improvement of symptoms, including daytime sleepiness, may be observed within 1 or 2 days of treatment with nasal CPAP, maximal improvement may not occur for several weeks. Follow-up studies indicate that long-term compliance with nasal CPAP is a substantial problem, many patients not using CPAP throughout the night and on a daily basis. Compliance increases with close follow-up care. Follow-up visit should be scheduled 1 month after the start of CPAP and every 6 months thereafter.

   If a patient with sleep apnea also has low baseline oxygen saturation during the day or during sleep, referral to an internist or pulmonologist is recommended.

   c. **Uvulopalatopharyngoplasty** is a surgical procedure in which excess soft tissue of the soft palate, uvula, and sometimes the tonsils and adenoids, is removed. A recent advance in this type of approach is laser-assisted uvuloplasty. The advantages are that the laser procedure is office based and that the amount of tissue removed can be titrated to effect. However, the efficacy of these procedures in the management of sleep apnea is variable. It is estimated that these surgical approaches are effective approximately 50% of the time for amelioration of sleep apnea but are more effective for snoring. Thus patients may continue to have silent obstructive apnea after surgery.

   d. **Drug therapy.** When nasal CPAP is not an option, patients with mild to moderate OSA may benefit from drug therapy. Protriptyline at a dosage of 10 mg at bedtime with upward adjustment depending on response and side effects may be an alternative treatment. Drug therapy is generally unsatisfactory for management of OSA.

Recommended Readings

ASDC Case Series Committee. Diagnosis, treatment and follow-up of about 8,000 sleep-wake disorder patients. In: Guilleminault C, Lugaresi E, eds. *Sleep / wake disorders: natural history, epidemiology and long-term evolution.* New York: Raven Press, 1983:87–97.

Bootzin RR, Epstein D, Wood JM. Stimulus control instructions. In: Hauri P. *Case studies in insomnia.* New York: Plenum Publishing, 1991.

Coccagna G. Restless legs syndrome/periodic movements in sleep. In Thorpy MJ, ed. *Handbook of sleep disorders.* New York: Marcel Dekker, 1990:457–478.

Coleman RM, et al. Epidemiology of periodic movements during sleep. In: Guilleminault C, Lugaresi E, eds. *Sleep/wake disorders: natural history, epidemiology and long-term evolution.* New York: Raven Press, 1983:217–229.

Czeisler CA, Richardson GS, Coleman RM, et al. Chronotherapy: resetting the circadian clocks of patients with delayed sleep phase insomnia. *Sleep* 1981;4:1–21.

Diagnostic Classification Steering Committee. *International classification of sleep disorders: diagnostic and coding manual.* Rochester, MN: American Sleep Disorders Association, 1990.

Ekbom KA. Restless legs syndrome. *Neurology* 1960;10:868–873.

Guilleminault C. Sleep disorders. In: Frederiks JAM, ed. *Handbook of clinical neurology: clinical neuropsychology.* New York: Elsevier, 1985:129–145.

Guilleminault C. Amphetamines and narcolepsy: use of Stanford database. *Sleep* 1993;16: 199–201.

Guilleminault C, Faull KF. Sleepiness in non-narcoleptic, nonsleep apneic EDS patients: the idiopathic CNS hypersomnolence. *Sleep* 1982;5:S175–S181.

Hauri P, Fisher J. Persistent psychophysiologic (learned) insomnia. *Sleep* 1986;9:38–53.

Issa F, Sullivan C. Reversal of central sleep apnea using nasal CPAP. *Chest* 1986;90:163–171.

Kavey NB, Whyte J, Resor SR Jr, et al. Somnambulism in adults. *Neurology* 1990;40:749–752.

Kryger MH, Roth T, Dement WC. Principles and practice of sleep medicine. Philadelphia: WB Saunders, 2000.

Langdon N, Shindler J, Parkes JD, et al. Fluoxetine in the treatment of cataplexy. *Sleep* 1986;9:371–372.

Mahowald MW, Ettinger MG. Things that go bump in the night: the parasomnias revisited. *J Clin Neurophysiol* 1990;7:119–143.

Mitler M, Erman M, Hajdukovic R. The treatment of excessive somnolence with stimulant drugs. *Sleep* 1993;16:203–206.

Moldofsky H, Musisi S, Phillipson EA. Treatment of case of advanced sleep phase syndrome by phase advance chronotherapy. *Sleep* 1986;9:61–65.

National Institute of Mental Health, Consensus Development Conference. Drugs and insomnia: the use of medications to promote sleep. *JAMA* 1984;251:2410–2414.

Reynolds CF III, Shipley JE. Sleep in depressive disorders. In: Hales RE, Frances AJ, eds. *Psychiatry update: the American Psychiatric Association annual review.* Vol 4. Washington, DC: American Psychiatric Press, 1985:341–351.

Sanders MH, Kern N. Obstructive sleep apnea treated by independently adjusted inspiratory and expiratory positive airway pressures by nasal mask. *Chest* 1990;98:317–324.

Schenck CH, Mahowald MW. Motor dyscontrol in narcolepsy: rapid eye movement (REM) sleep without atonia and REM sleep behavior disorder. *Ann Neurol* 1992;32:3–10.

Schenck CH, Bundlie SR, Ettinger MG, et al. Chronic behavioral disorders of human REM sleep: a new category of parasomnia. *Sleep* 1986;9:293–308.

White D, Zwillich CW, Pickett CK, et al. Central sleep apnea: improvement with acetazolamide therapy. *Arch Intern Med* 1982;142:1816–1819.

Zee PC and Grujic, Z. Neurological diseases associated with disturbed sleep and circadian rhythms. In: Turek FW, Zeem PC, eds. *Neurobiology of sleep and circadian rhythms.* New York: Marcel Dekker, 1999.

Zorick F, Roehrs T, Conway W, et al. Effects of uvulopalatopharyngoplasty on the daytime sleepiness associated with sleep apnea syndrome. *Bull Eur Physiopathol Respir* 1983;19: 600–603.

Zorick FJ, Roth T, Hartze KM, et al. Evaluation and diagnosis of persistent insomnia. *Am J Psychiatry* 1981;138:769–773.

56. DIZZINESS AND VERTIGO

B. Todd Troost

Dizziness and **vertigo,** particularly dizziness, represent one of the most common problems presenting to the primary care physician. Although dizziness usually is benign and readily controllable, some forms are life threatening and necessitate immediate attention and action. Isolated rotary vertigo usually is a manifestation of peripheral vestibular or inner ear dysfunction. For example, in the setting of upper respiratory infection, acute rotary vertigo without associated double vision, perioral numbness, limb weakness, or ataxia usually is a benign, self-limited condition that should be managed conservatively.

On the other hand, for patients with diplopia or other brainstem signs, attention should be given to the possibility of brainstem or cerebellar infarction. Immediate computed tomography or, preferably, magnetic resonance imaging (MRI) should be performed to rule out a developing cerebellar stroke, which may require immediate surgical intervention. Cardinal features suggesting central nervous system (CNS) abnormalities are history, associated symptoms, and posterior fossa signs of (1) direction-changing nystagmus, (2) ataxia, (3) weakness, and (4) falling in the direction of the most prominent nystagmus.

Dizziness may be very vaguely described, including reports of unsteadiness, light-headedness, and instability (Table 56.1). It may be produced by a variety of conditions, including peripheral vestibulopathy (inner ear), systemic disorders such as postural hypotension or the nonspecific effects of drugs or cardiac arrhythmia, and CNS disorders.

The major causes of dizziness and vertigo are otologic or peripheral vestibular, central neurologic, and systemic or medical (Table 56.2). Vertigo is the illusion or hallucination of movement. If the sensation is of rotary vertigo, the cause almost always is the peripheral vestibular apparatus, that is, the inner ear or labyrinth. Because the inner ear is anatomically juxtaposed to the cochlea or hearing apparatus, auditory symptoms often are present, as in Ménière's disease.

The sensation of balance and the ability to maintain posture depend on input from three major sensory systems—the inner ear, the eyes, and proprioceptive input from the peripheral nerves. Hearing also is important, because auditory cues aid postural stability. All the sensory information must be integrated by the brain and coordinated by the cerebellum and motor pathways of the CNS to maintain posture and ambulation.

I. **Otologic or peripheral vestibular causes of vertigo**
   A. **Benign paroxysmal positional vertigo (BPPV)**
   1. **Course and prognosis.** BPPV is characterized by brief attacks of vertigo produced by changes in head position. BPPV may follow previous attacks of labyrinthitis or head trauma. This disorder is caused by loose particles in the posterior semicircular canal of the inner ear. BPPV constitutes at least 50% of all cases of vertigo. The frequency increases with age, and this disorder is estimated to be present, at one time or another, in 40% of patients 70 years or older. It usually is benign and self-limiting, disappearing spontaneously. Many patients, however, have recurrent attacks of BPPV over months or even many years, which can be disabling. Specific intervention in the form of exercise therapy is needed to reposition the particles so that attacks no longer occur.
   2. **Prevention.** There is no specific method for preventing BPPV. Individual attacks are prevented by avoiding specific provocative head positions.
   3. **Therapeutic approach.** The primary therapeutic option is one form or another of exercise therapy. The severity of individual attacks and the accompanying nausea may be lessened by medical therapy, but such therapy does not prevent future attacks. Exercise therapy is indicated for all patients with BPPV. There are two general approaches to therapy—a single treatment session in an outpatient office setting and a series of exercises performed by the patient at home.
      a. **Office single-treatment approach** (Epley maneuver). Among the single-treatment approaches are the canalith repositioning maneuver and its modifications. One standard protocol is presented. This technique works best for patients for whom a specific head position, such as with

Table 56.1 Symptoms represented by the term *dizziness*

Vertigo	Swaying	Staggering
Unsteadiness	Twisting	Weaving
Imbalance	Blurring vision	Moving
Spinning	Disorientation	Tilting
Floating	Poor equilibrium	Listing
Fainting	Bouncing	Rocking
Feeling faint	Falling	Oscillating
Giddiness	Swimming	Rolling
Lightheadedness		

From Troost BT. Dizziness and vertigo. In: Bradley WG, Daroff RB, Fenichel GM, et al., eds. *Neurology in clinical practice,* 3rd ed. Boston: Butterworth–Heinemann, 2000:239–251.

the left ear down, produces attacks of vertigo. Often the examiner notices characteristic rotary vertical nystagmus accompanying the vertigo when the head is placed in the offending position (Figs. 56.1 and 56.2).

Treatment protocol for the left ear

(1) The patient is moved quickly from a seated position back over the end of the examination table with the head extended and turned approximately 45 degrees with the left ear down. (In each position in this protocol, nystagmus can be induced as a result of the change from the previous head position.) The patient is kept in this position until the nystagmus or symptoms subside—typically for 10 to 15 seconds.

(2) The head is slowly rotated so that the right ear is turned 45 degrees down; the head is kept extended.

(3) The head and body are rotated to the right until the patient is facing downward. This position is maintained for approximately 15 seconds.

(4) The patient is brought up gradually to a seated position with the head turned to the right.

Table 56.2 Major causes of vertigo

Otologic or Peripheral Vestibular Causes of Vertigo
Benign paroxysmal positional vertigo
Labyrinthitis or vestibular neuronitis
Ménière's disease
Ototoxicity
Perilymphatic fistula
Tumors involving the eighth cranial nerve

Central Neurologic Causes of Vertigo
Brainstem ischemia and infarction
Basilar artery migraine
Seizures
Multiple sclerosis
Chiari malformation

Medical or Systemic Causes of Vertigo
Postural hypotension
Cardiac arrhythmia
Metabolic causes: hypoglycemia and hypothyroidism
Drug effects
Multiple afferent sensory loss

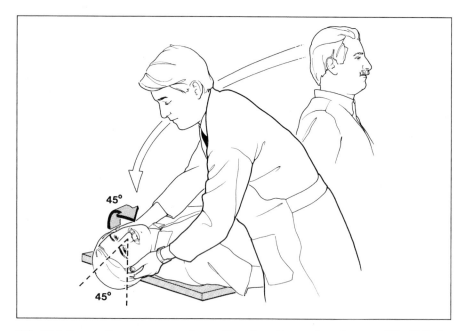

FIG. 56.1 Provocative maneuvers for positional vertigo and nystagmus (Dix–Hallpike maneuver). The patient is abruptly moved from a seated position to one with the head hanging 45 degrees below the horizontal and rotated 45 degrees to one side and is then observed for benign paroxysmal positional nystagmus (BPPN). The maneuvers are repeated with the head straight back and turned to the other side. (From Troost BT, Patton JM. Exercise therapy for positional vertigo. *Neurology* 1992;42:1441–1444, with permission.)

      (5) The head is turned forward with the chin slightly depressed.

          Some authorities recommend that the patient remain upright as much as possible over the next 24 to 48 hours. Another variation is to apply a handheld mechanical oscillator to the head in each position. The overall success rate of this single treatment is reported to be 50% to 75%.

    b. Home exercise therapy (Brandt–Daroff technique). The patient is first instructed carefully about the type of exercise to be performed (Fig. 56.3).

      Treatment protocol for either ear

      (1) In a seated position, on the edge of a couch or bed, the patient is asked to lie quickly on one side, placing the worst ear (if this can be determined) down first (Fig. 56.4). The patient is asked to move rapidly from the sitting position and to rest the head on a pillow or other support. The patient should not move so forcefully as to produce a neck injury.

      (2) The patient then returns rapidly to an upright seated position and remains there for 30 seconds or until the symptoms subside.

      (3) The patient rapidly lies down on the other side and remains there for approximately 30 seconds or until the symptoms subside.

      (4) The patient then returns to the upright seated position. This constitutes a single repetition.

          Ten to 20 repetitions should be performed three times each day. Each session lasts approximately 30 minutes. Some patients have intense symptoms at the onset of the BPPV, including vomiting.

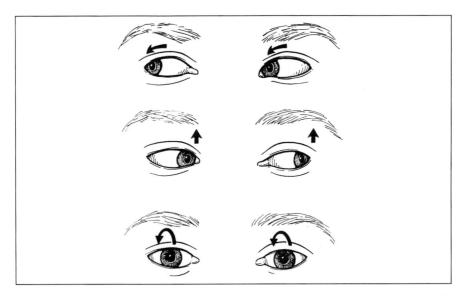

FIG. 56.2 In benign paroxysmal positional nystagmus, the nystagmus fast phase is horizontal–rotary directed toward the bottom ear when gaze is directed toward the ear that is down **(top).** The nystagmus fast phase is upward toward the forehead when gaze is directed to the ear that is up **(center).** With the eyes in the central orbital position, the nystagmus fast phase is vertical upward and rotary toward the ear that is down **(bottom).** (From Troost BT, Patton JM. Exercise therapy for positional vertigo. *Neurology* 1992;42:1441–1444, with permission.)

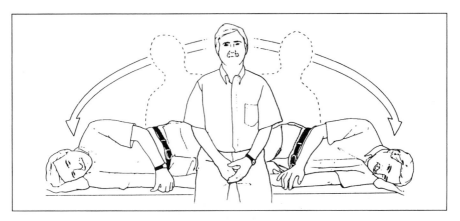

FIG. 56.3 Exercise therapy. The patient begins in the seated position and then leans rapidly to the side, placing the head on the bed or table. The patient remains there until the vertigo subsides and then returns to the seated upright position, remaining there until all symptoms subside. The maneuver is repeated to the opposite side, completing one full repetition. Ten to 20 repetitions should be performed three times a day. (From Troost BT, Patton JM. Exercise therapy for positional vertigo. *Neurology* 1992;42:1441–1444, with permission.)

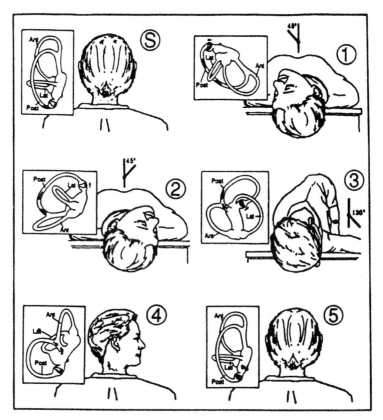

FIG. 56.4 Positioning sequence for left posterior semicircular canal shows orientation of left labyrinth and gravitating canaliths. *S (start)*, Patient is seated with operator behind patient. Oscillation is started. *1*, Head is placed over end of table, 45 degrees to left, with head extended. (Canaliths gravitate to center of posterior semicircular canal.) *2*, Head is rotated 45 degrees to right; head is kept well extended in process of coming from position 1. (Canaliths reach common crus.) *3*, Head and body are rotated until facing downward 135 degrees from supine. (Canaliths traverse common crus.) *4*, Patient is brought to sitting position; head is kept turned to right in process of coming from position 3. (Canaliths enter utricle.) *5*, Head is turned forward with chin down approximately 20 degrees. (From Epley JM. Fine points of canalith repositioning procedure for treatment of BPPV. *Insights Otolaryngol* 1994;9:7, with permission.)

These patients may need hospital admission or hydration in an outpatient setting with concurrent administration of vestibular suppressant medications. It is clear that patients who experience extreme discomfort during these maneuvers will not be likely to pursue them on their own outside the office or hospital setting. Most patients are willing to perform exercises at home. This protocol is particularly useful for patients with BPPV who have (1) bilateral BPPV, (2) uncertainty as to which ear is involved, or (3) failure of single office treatment protocols.

Recovery can be quite rapid, occurring during the first few days of exercise therapy. Some patients have progressive improvement over weeks or months, which suggests that the vestibular system may adapt to the abnormal perturbation causing the symptoms.

4. **Expected outcome.** Approximately 50% of patients who have well-defined vertigo and nystagmus in certain head positions have improvement after the single treatment maneuver. Variations include the use of a handheld oscillator or longer duration at each single position. The home set of maneuvers, known as Brandt–Daroff maneuvers, may produce a very rapid improvement in a few days but can take weeks or even months to produce a cure. Progressive improvement should be noticed by the patient within the first few weeks. It is estimated that approximately 20% of patients have recurrences within the first year, and either of the maneuvers described earlier may be repeated with a high expectation of further improvement. The overall success rate of exercise therapy approaches 90%, even among patients who have had symptoms for years.

5. **Referral.** Persistence of BPPV after repeated exercise therapy of either general type has failed indicates the need for referral to an otolaryngologist or neurootologist. Rare instances of persistent disabling positional vertigo unresponsive to exercise therapy may necessitate a surgical approach—either sectioning of the nerve to the posterior semicircular canal or a surgical canal plugging operation. Most cases of BPPV are readily diagnosed. Most of the patients do not need expensive evaluation that includes MRI. If the diagnosis is unclear, it is less expensive to refer the patient to specialists in the area, who can make the diagnosis on the basis of history and careful physical examination without the need for neuroimaging procedures.

B. **Labyrinthitis.** Peripheral vestibulopathy encompasses disorders such as vestibular neuronitis, labyrinthitis, and viral neurolabyrinthitis. **Vestibular neuronitis,** by strict definition, is characterized by a single episode or recurrent episodes of true vertigo lasting from hours to days and often associated initially with vomiting. When the condition is associated with hearing loss, the entire labyrinth is assumed to be involved, and the term **labyrinthitis** is used. Despite this technical distinction, many neurootologists, otologists, and neurologists use the terms *vestibular neuronitis* and *labyrinthitis* interchangeably whether or not auditory symptoms are present. In such patients, the vertiginous sensation may be worsened by head movement but not necessarily by a particular head position. Whether isolated viral involvement of the vestibular nerves is the cause of acute or episodic vertigo is controversial. Many authorities prefer the terms *acute peripheral vestibulopathy* and *recurrent peripheral vestibulopathy.* In the acute phase, most patients have sudden and severe vertigo, nausea, and vomiting without any hearing disturbance or facial weakness.

1. **Course and prognosis.** In general, the prognosis is good. At least 90% of patients have only a single attack with no apparent residual deficit.

2. **Prevention.** There is no specific preventive therapy for acute inner ear inflammation. However, patients with middle ear infections or otitis media should be treated with appropriate antibiotic therapy to prevent spread to the inner ear.

3. **Therapeutic approach.** Therapy is outlined for symptomatic management of acute dizziness presumed caused by labyrinthitis. Classes of drugs are listed in Table 56.3.

Although most of the drugs used for dizziness are loosely referred to as *vestibular suppressants,* it is often unclear which agent will be effective in a given patient and what its true mechanism of action is likely to be. The primary vestibular afferent system can be suppressed directly or indirectly through the inhibitory portion of the major vestibular efferent system. An important function of some agents may be to act on other sensory systems such as proprioceptive or visual input to the vestibular nuclei of the brainstem.

Many of the agents commonly used are empiric. Few controlled studies have investigated the response of patients with presumed peripheral vestibular dysfunction. Therapy with many of the drugs used by physicians for treating such patients is based on studies of the prevention of motion

Table 56.3 Medical therapy for vertigo

Antihistamines
Meclizine (Antivert, Pfizer Inc., New York, NY; Bonine, Pfizer Inc. Consumer Health
  Care Group, New York, NY)
Cyclizine (Marezine, OTC)
Dimenhydrinate (Dramamine)
Promethazine (Phenergan, Wyeth–Ayerst Laboratories, Philadelphia, PA)

Anticholinergics
Scopolamine (hyoscine)
Atropine

Sympathomimetic
Ephedrine

Antiemetics
Trimethobenzamide (Tigan, Roberts Pharmaceutical Corporation, Eatontown, NJ)
Prochlorperazine (Compazine, SmithKline Beecham Pharmaceuticals, Philadelphia, PA)

"Tranquilizers"
Diazepam (Valium, Roche Products)
Prazepam (Verstran, Centrax)
Haloperidol (Haldol, Ortho-McNeil Pharmaceutical, Raritan, NJ)
Chlorpromazine (Thorazine, SmithKline Beecham)

Combination Preparations and Others
Scopolamine with ephedrine
Scopolamine with promethazine
Ephedrine with promethazine
Buclizine hydrochloride (Bucladin)
Cyclandelate (Cyclospasmol)
Diuretics
Diet

sickness among healthy persons or of the various regimens used by otologists to treat patients with Ménière's disease. Each class of drugs is discussed separately.

   a. Antihistamines (Table 56.4) are among the agents most commonly
   used in the management of dizziness. The drug usually used initially is
   meclizine hydrochloride in dosages up to 50 mg three times a day.
   Because the main side effect of antihistamines is drowsiness, the smallest dosage should be used initially, even as low as 12.5 mg two or three
   times a day.
      For dizziness, the antihistamines in the histamine-1 (H_1) antagonist
   group are used. The H_1 blockers, effective in motion sickness, may act by
   means of central antagonism of acetylcholine, as does scopolamine. An
   excellent drug as a second choice is promethazine, a phenothiazine with
   the strongest acetylcholine-blocking action. The usual starting dosage is
   25 mg three times a day, but if this produces drowsiness and still has a
   positive effect, the dosage can be reduced to 12.5 mg three times a day.
   b. Anticholinergics (Table 56.5) that block the muscarinic effect of acetylcholine have been widely used and studied for the prevention of motion
   sickness. Atropine acts centrally to stimulate the medulla and cerebrum,
   but the closely related alkaloid scopolamine is more widely used.
      Transdermal delivery of scopolamine may prevent or mitigate the nau-
   sea and vomiting associated with motion sickness but not the dizziness.
   In general, transdermal scopolamine is not useful for patients with
   acquired vestibulopathy. Frequent side effects are blurred vision and dry

Table 56.4 Antihistamines for dizziness

Generic name	Trade name	Dosage[a]
Ethanolamines		
Diphenhydramine hydrochloride	Benadryl (Parke–Davis, Morris Plains, NJ)	50 mg q.d.–b.i.d.
Dimenhydrinate	Dramamine	50 mg q.d.–b.i.d.
Piperazines		
Cyclizine hydrochloride	Marezine	50 mg q.d.–b.i.d.
Meclizine hydrochloride	Antivert, Bonine	25–50 mg t.i.d.
Phenothiazine		
Promethazine hydrochloride	Phenergan	25–50 mg/d

[a] Usual adult starting dosage can be increased by a factor of 2 or 3 with drowsiness as the most common side effect.
q.d.–b.i.d., once or twice a day; t.i.d., three times a day.

mouth, in addition to occasional confusion. Some patients have great difficulty when they try to discontinue the use of scopolamine patches. A side effect of low-dose scopolamine or atropine is transient bradycardia (4 to 8 fewer beats/min) associated with the peak action of oral scopolamine at 90 minutes and diminishing thereafter.

    c. **Sympathomimetics** have been used in the management of motion sickness, particularly in combination with anticholinergics. The sole agent in this class that may have an application in combination with other drugs is ephedrine. Tolerance may develop after a few weeks of treatment.

    d. **Antiemetics** (Table 56.6) may be used when the patient has prominent nausea. Many of the antihistaminic and anticholinergic drugs listed in Tables 56.3 and 56.4 are also used for their antiemetic actions. Prochlorperazine (Compazine; GlaxoSmithKline, Research Triangle Park, NC, U.S.A.) should be used with caution, particularly by the intramuscular route, because of the high incidence of dystonic reactions. Because promethazine (Phenergan; Wyeth-Ayerst, Philadelphia, PA, U.S.A.) has a marked antiemetic effect, it is particularly useful when there is prominent nausea.

Table 56.5 Anticholinergics for dizziness

Generic name	Trade name	Dosage[a]
Scopolamine	Donphen[a]	1 tablet t.i.d.
Scopolamine	Donnatal (A.H. Robins Company, Inc., Richmond, VA)[a]	1 tablet t.i.d.
Scopolamine hydrobromide tablets	—	0.45–0.50 mg q.d.–b.i.d.
Scopolamine	Transderm-V1 (Novartis Consumer Health, Inc., Summit, NJ)	0.5-mg patch, change every 3 days

[a] The combination preparations Donphen and Donnatal each contain a mixture of atropine alkaloids with approximately $\frac{1}{4}$ g (15.0–16.2 mg) of phenobarbital.
t.i.d., three times a day; q.d.–b.i.d., once or twice a day.

Table 56.6 Antiemetics

Generic name	Trade name	Dosage[a]
Trimethobenzamide	Tigan	250 mg q.d.–b.i.d. orally 200 mg q.d.–b.i.d. rectally
Phenothiazines		
Promethazine	Phenergan	12.5–25.0 mg t.i.d.–q.i.d. orally 12.5–25.0 mg suppository
Prochlorperazine	Compazine	5–10 mg t.i.d.–q.i.d. orally 25-mg suppository

[a] Interactions with other drugs and extrapyramidal side effects, especially with Compazine, should promote caution.
q.d.–b.i.d., once or twice a day; t.i.d.–q.i.d., three or four times a day.

    e. Tranquilizers (Table 56.7) is the general name given to drugs from different classes that have central and probably peripheral effects. Such drugs include benzodiazepines, butyrophenones, and phenothiazines. Diazepam is one of the most widely prescribed drugs for the management of dizziness. Many physicians believe it should *not* be the first choice, primarily because of the risk of habituation and depression, and because it can be the actual cause of dizziness. Nonetheless, diazepam remains the first choice of many otoneurologists and otologists. Other longer-acting benzodiazepines can be helpful for certain patients, but no study has substantiated the effectiveness.

    Haloperidol in low oral doses (0.5 mg three times a day) is effective for many patients with peripheral vestibular dysfunction who are not helped by other antidizziness medications.

    f. Combination preparations, including agents listed in Table 56.3, are frequently useful, particularly the combination of ephedrine and promethazine. Some other agents and regimens used primarily in the medical management of Ménière's disease are listed in the same table. Low-sodium diets and diuretics have been helpful to some patients. In the belief that in some cases, an effect on blood supply to the peripheral end organ may be a

Table 56.7 "Tranquilizers" for dizziness

Generic name	Trade name	Dosage
Benzodiazepines		
Diazepam	Valium	5–10 mg q.d.–t.i.d.
Prazepam	Verstran	10 mg/d
Butyrophenone		
Haloperidol	Haldol	0.5–1.0 mg q.d.–b.i.d.[a]
Phenothiazines		
Promethazine hydrochloride	Phenergan	25–50 mg/d
Chlorpromazine	Thorazine	10–50 mg/d[b]

[a] Very low dose compared with antipsychotic levels. Patients should be observed for dystonia.
[b] Usual precautions for phenothiazines. My colleagues and I have not used chlorpromazine for dizziness, but it is used as an adjunct by some.
q.d.–t.i.d., once to three times a day; q.d.–b.i.d., once or twice a day.

factor, agents such as cyclandelate have been used. The general approach to acute or chronic vestibulopathy is first to use an antihistamine such as meclizine hydrochloride. If this is not helpful, the next step is to use promethazine. If this is ineffective, low doses of diazepam can be tried if it is kept that use of benzodiazepines carries risk of habituation. Most of these medications are relatively inexpensive. Single drugs such as antihistamines are less expensive than are the combination preparations.

4. **Expected outcome.** It should be expected that some patients with peripheral vestibular dysfunction will respond to medical therapy with significant lessening of symptoms. Medication may have to be taken daily by patients with chronic peripheral vestibulopathy.

5. **Referrals.** Patients who do not respond to medical therapy need referral to a neurootologist or a neurologist.

C. **Ménière's disease**
1. **Course and prognosis.** Ménière's disease is characterized by attacks of severe vertigo and vomiting, tinnitus (often described as roaring), fluctuating hearing loss, ill-described aural sensations of fullness and pressure, and spontaneous recovery in hours to days. Most often, the patient has a sensation of fullness and pressure along with decreased hearing and tinnitus in a single ear. These symptoms are followed by severe vertigo attacks that reach peak intensity within minutes and slowly subside over hours with a persistent sense of disequilibration for days after an acute episode. On some occasions, patients with Ménière's disease experience such severe attacks that they suddenly fall to the ground. Consciousness is not lost in such episodes, although awareness of surroundings may be altered by the intensity of the accompanying sensation.

Ménière's disease usually develops between the ages of 30 and 50 years and is slightly more common among women than among men. The prognosis is for progressive reduction in hearing along with increasing frequency of attacks. Although some patients' stabilizers "burn out," they are left with residual hearing loss but no subsequent attacks of severe vertigo. Approximately 50% of cases of Ménière's disease become bilateral. The hearing loss often progresses to a moderated deficit and then stabilizes.

2. **Prevention.** There is no specific intervention or therapy that prevents the development of Ménière's disease.

3. **Therapeutic approach**
   a. The usual first-line treatment of patients with Ménière's disease is **vestibular medications** such as those described in **I.B.** All these forms of therapy have, for certain patients, lessened the severity of attacks and have provided successful treatment of many patients. However, a subset of patients are unresponsive to standard medical therapy, and surgical intervention must be considered for them.
   b. **Labyrinthectomy** or **vestibular nerve section** is a main mode of therapy. Medical labyrinthectomy may be performed with aminoglycoside drugs—those particularly destructive to the peripheral vestibular hair cells in the inner ear. In this procedure, a drug such as gentamicin is injected through the tympanic membrane with the idea that there will be selective destruction of vestibular hair cells but relative sparing of hearing. A new approach involves direct injection of gentamicin directly into the posterior semicircular canal. Although surgical labyrinthectomy usually is a last resort for patients who have clearly defined severe attacks of Ménière's disease that are unresponsive to medical therapy, gentamicin therapy, a relatively benign procedure, is now being used earlier in the course of the illness with excellent results.
   c. Various **shunting procedures** have been used in the management of Ménière's disease, such as an endolymphatic shunt from the inner ear to the mastoid.
   d. The indication for **surgical therapy** is complete failure of medical treatment. There are no specific contraindications to labyrinthectomy

depending on the general state of the patient's health, but the procedure has certain limitations and pitfalls. Labyrinthectomy should generally be limited to patients who have severe reduction or complete loss of hearing, because patients lose hearing after labyrinthectomy. Selective posterior fossa sectioning of the vestibular nerve may spare hearing. Complications of the procedure are the usual ones for any surgical procedure, such as postoperative infection and leakage of cerebrospinal fluid with subsequent meningitis.

4. **Expected outcome.** It is expected that many patients will respond favorably to medical treatment with less severe attacks of vertigo. Therapy does not prevent progressive hearing loss. Surgical therapy for unilateral Ménière's disease is expected to be curative. The patient is subsequently free of attacks after an initial period of days to a few weeks then experiences increased disequilibration resulting from loss of vestibular input on one side. Patients who undergo bilateral surgical procedures, although they may be free of future attacks of severe vertigo, have a persistent state of some dysequilibrium and have difficulty making rapid turns. There is also a sensation of movement of the visual environment with rapid head movement, known as *oscillopsia*.

5. **Referrals.** Patients with suspected Ménière's disease should be referred to an otologist.

D. **Ototoxicity**

1. **Course and prognosis.** The usual cause of bilaterally reduced vestibular function is treatment with ototoxic antibiotics, particularly gentamicin. The patient experiences severe ataxia and oscillopsia. The prognosis for complete recovery is only fair. Bilateral complete loss of vestibular hair cells is highly unusual. Some recovery is to be expected; however, it usually takes months or even years.

2. **Intervention.** Diligent monitoring of aminoglycoside levels during therapy is extremely useful in avoiding ototoxicity. Some patients are unusually sensitive, and treatment should be stopped, except for a life-threatening illness, at any sign of imbalance or vertigo during therapy. Extreme caution should be used in treating patients with renal dysfunction, because aminoglycosides are excreted through the kidneys. A major reduction in aminoglycoside dosage should be made for patients with concomitant renal insufficiency. It is therefore important that any patient considered for aminoglycoside therapy undergo careful assessment of renal function before the treatment is begun.

3. **Therapeutic approach.** The primary therapeutic option is to avoid the occurrence of ototoxicity. No specific therapy is available once ototoxicity has occurred. Further reduction of vestibular function with medications such as those used to manage labyrinthitis generally are not helpful, although an occasional patient with bilateral, but asymmetric, aminoglycoside ototoxicity may experience modest improvement.

4. **Expected outcome.** As mentioned in **B.3.,** some patients experience modest relief from the use of vestibular suppressant medication, but significant improvement is unusual.

5. **Referrals.** Patients with bilaterally reduced vestibular function should be referred to an otologist or a neurologist specializing in balance disorders.

E. **Perilymphatic fistula** usually follows barotrauma, as in scuba diving, or a blow to the ear resulting in a rupture between the fluid in the semicircular canals and the middle ear.

1. **Course and prognosis.** Patients experience extreme pressure sensitivity with attacks of vertigo or imbalance and ataxia associated with increased pressure in the ear. On occasion, symptoms are exacerbated by certain head positions. Small perilymphatic fistulas may close spontaneously.

2. **Prevention.** During deep-sea diving, careful monitoring of pressure is mandatory to protect the inner ear from barotrauma. Ear protection should be worn in any situation in which there may be aural trauma.

3. **Therapeutic approach.** When perilymphatic fistula is diagnosed, the initial treatment should be prolonged bed rest with avoidance of sudden increases in

pressure, such as from a Valsalva maneuver. Rest promotes spontaneous sealing of the fistula. Persistence of symptoms after 2 weeks of bed rest, however, should lead to surgical exploration of the inner ear with an attempt to localize and seal the fistula. The surgical technique includes occlusion of the fistula, usually with biologic material such as muscle. Most surgical patients are kept at bed rest for 2 weeks with strict avoidance of activities that might reopen the fistula, such as coughing or straining at stool. A limitation is an inability to find the exact location of the fistula during surgical exploration lest an inadvertent new rupture be caused by the procedure itself.

   4. **Expected outcome.** Most patients experience relief either with bed rest or with surgical therapy. Reexploration may be necessary.
   5. **Referrals.** Patients with suspected perilymphatic fistula should be immediately referred to an otolaryngologist.

F. **Tumors involving the eighth cranial nerve**
   1. **Course and prognosis.** Tumors of the cerebellopontine angle rarely manifest solely as episodic vertigo. The most common tumor in this location results from a proliferation of Schwann cells, hence the name **schwannoma.** Most of these tumors arise under the vestibular portion of the eighth cranial nerve within the internal auditory canal. They enlarge progressively, deform the internal auditory canal, and compress adjacent neural structures, such as the acoustic portion of the eighth cranial nerve, the facial nerve, the trigeminal nerve, and eventually the brainstem and cerebellum. The most common symptoms associated with eighth-nerve tumors are progressive unilateral sensorineural hearing loss and tinnitus. Intermittent vertigo occurs in approximately 20% of patients, but a symptom of imbalance or disequilibration is more common, approaching 50%. The prognosis for untreated tumors of the cerebellopontine angle is determined by the type of tumor and the rate of growth. Ultimately, untreated tumors affect hearing and vestibular function. As they enlarge, the tumors involve nerves such as the seventh cranial nerve and compress the brainstem. Surgical intervention is needed.
   2. **Prevention.** There is no specific means of preventing tumors of the cerebellopontine angle, but prevention of subsequent neurologic damage can be accomplished with early diagnosis. Any patient with progressive unexplained unilateral hearing loss, with or without vertigo, needs neuroimaging studies to detect or rule out the presence of a tumor.
   3. **Therapeutic approach.** The primary therapeutic option is surgery. Small tumors can be approached through the ear by an otolaryngologist or through the posterior fossa by a neurosurgeon. Monitoring of seventh and eighth nerve function during surgery may allow preservation of function. Once a tumor is suspected, the patient needs high-resolution MRI with contrast enhancement of the posterior fossa. It is less expensive to proceed immediately to a focused neuroimaging study and referral to an appropriate specialist than to delay until the tumor has grown considerably.
   4. **Expected outcome.** Tumors involving the eighth nerve inevitably progress and causing losses of hearing, balance, and other cranial nerve functions, as discussed earlier. Prognosis for benign tumors detected early and operated on is excellent.
   5. **Referrals.** Patients believed to have eighth-nerve tumors should be referred to neurosurgeons or otolaryngologists specializing in neurootology.

II. **Central neurologic causes of vertigo**
   A. **Brainstem ischemia and infarction**
      1. **Course and prognosis.** Vertigo, including brief episodes of isolated vertigo, may be caused by posterior circulation disturbance. The posterior circulation supplies blood to the brainstem, the cerebellum, and the peripheral vestibular apparatus. It is not surprising that vertebrobasilar ischemia may be accompanied by vertigo. In general, brainstem transient ischemic attacks (TIAs) should be accompanied by neurologic symptoms or signs in addition to vertigo before a clear-cut diagnosis is entertained. Symptoms include transient clumsiness, weakness, loss of vision, diplopia, perioral numbness, ataxia, drop attacks, and

dysarthria. The prognosis after a definite posterior circulation TIA is uncertain. It is estimated that at least one third of patients have strokes within 3 years. Therefore, prevention and therapy are paramount.

2. Prevention. All risk factors for ischemic stroke should be evaluated, including hypertension, hyperlipidemia, diabetes, and smoking. The patient also needs evaluation for possible cardiac sources of emboli. It is clear that the best therapy for stroke is prevention.

3. Therapeutic approach. Once an actual infarction has occurred, therapy is primarily supportive. Therapeutic approaches are directed at preventing future TIAs and preventing actual infarction. The first-line therapy is antiplatelet drugs, including aspirin and ticlopidine. In situations in which there is increasing frequency of TIAs or a suspected source of emboli, the patient should be hospitalized, and intravenous heparin may be given. Patients with suspected cardiac sources of emboli are candidates for long-term warfarin therapy. A history of gastric ulcers or bleeding is a contraindication to anticoagulation. Therapy for ischemic cerebrovascular disease is discussed in Chapter 36, **II.**

4. Expected outcome. The appropriate therapy for diminishing risk factors may significantly reduce the likelihood of permanent defects resulting from infarction. Some patients may have strokes despite therapy.

5. Referrals. Any patient believed to have brainstem ischemia and infarction should be referred for a complete neurologic and neurovascular evaluation.

B. Basilar artery migraine

1. Course and prognosis. This condition usually is diagnosed among young women who have episodic events such as diplopia, dysarthria, vertigo, ataxia, and bilateral visual loss followed by diffuse throbbing headache. There may be a family history of "sick headache." When vertigo is followed by diffuse headache, this condition should be considered. Prognosis is variable, some episodes disappearing spontaneously. Rare patients, however, may have brainstem infarction, so intervention is paramount.

2. Prevention. Prophylactic therapy for migraine may eliminate attacks, but overall is less successful than for migraine without aura (common migraine).

3. Therapeutic approach. There are two general approaches to therapy for migraine. One is immediate abortive treatment with agents such as ergotamines or sumatriptan. However, when there are significant neurologic symptoms, prophylactic therapy with calcium channel blockers, β-blockers, amitriptyline, or methysergide should be considered. Migraine therapy is presented in Chapter 49, **II.**

4. Expected outcome. Ideally, basilar artery migraine should be controlled with prophylactic therapy so that the patient has no attacks with accompanying neurologic symptoms such as vertigo.

5. Referrals. Patients with neurologic symptoms precipitating or accompanying migraine attacks should be referred to a neurologist for treatment.

C. Seizures

1. Course and prognosis. Seizures are a rare cause of isolated vertigo. There is alteration of consciousness or accompanying features with complex partial seizures (such as lip smacking, drooling, or even associated motor activity). Even if there are some episodes of isolated vertigo, sooner or later most patients have episodes of clear alteration of consciousness. The prognosis at that point depends on the cause of the seizure. The prognosis is worse if there is a tumor and is generally much better if there is a small cortical scar that can be removed surgically.

2. Prevention. There is no specific prevention for the onset of seizures, but individual patients may find certain precipitants that can be avoided such as alcohol or sleeplessness.

3. Therapeutic approach. Primary therapy for recurrent seizures is properly selected antiepileptic drugs. Therapy for seizure disorders is covered in Chapters 38, **II.** and 39, **II.**

4. **Expected outcome.** Ideally, patients are treated completely with anticonvulsant therapy. Complex partial seizures can be refractory and even require surgical intervention.

5. **Referrals.** Once a diagnosis of seizure disorder has been made, the patient is often referred to a neurologist.

D. **Multiple sclerosis**

1. **Course and prognosis.** Multiple sclerosis is diagnosed primarily on the basis of a history of different neurologic signs or symptoms in the CNS that are separated in time. For example, a patient may have an episode of vertigo at one time and an attack of optic neuritis at another time. Clinical diagnosis usually is confirmed with MRI. Multiple sclerosis tends to progress, new neurologic signs and symptoms occurring over many years. Prognosis depends on the extent of the neurologic involvement.

2. **Prevention.** There is no known specific preventive therapy for multiple sclerosis, but severity of individual attacks can be lessened with therapy.

3. **Therapeutic approach.** Therapy for multiple sclerosis includes immediate treatment with intravenous methylprednisolone sodium succinate (Solu-Medrol; Pharmacia & Upjohn, Kalamazoo, MI, U.S.A.) and a variety of interventions designed to prevent future attacks and progression. Therapy for multiple sclerosis is discussed in Chapter 40, **II.**

4. **Expected outcome.** It is believed that with appropriate therapy, individual attacks can be lessened in severity and future attacks lessened by regimens discussed in Chapter 40, **II.**

5. **Referrals.** Patients with suspected or known multiple sclerosis are often referred to neurologists.

E. **Arnold–Chiari malformation**

1. **Course and prognosis.** The adult type of Arnold–Chiari malformation is brainstem or cerebellar herniation through the foramen magnum. The condition usually manifests as unsteadiness or vertigo and down-beating nystagmus, particularly on sideward gaze. Ocular oscillation may produce a sense of tumbling when the patient looks to the side. The course is progression of all symptoms. The patient may begin to experience sudden headache with coughing as the brainstem compression progresses over years.

2. **Prevention.** No remedial action can slow the progression of the illness.

3. **Therapeutic approach.** Once a symptomatic condition has been identified, surgical intervention should be decompression of the posterior fossa.

4. **Expected outcome.** Surgical intervention usually halts progression of the brainstem signs and symptoms and may alleviate them.

5. **Referrals.** Once symptomatic Arnold–Chiari malformation has been identified through the use of MRI, the patient often is referred to a neurologist, who may then refer the patient for neurosurgical intervention.

III. **Medical or systemic causes of vertigo and dizziness**

A. **Postural hypotension**

1. **Course and prognosis.** Patients usually describe the symptom complex of postural hypotension as light-headedness rather than a sensation of spinning. Episodes usually are associated with changes in posture such as from lying to standing but may take several minutes to develop. There may be an accompanying graying-out of vision or even actual fainting. The course and prognosis depend on the specific cause if postural hypotension is the result of an autonomic neuropathy, because in diabetes it tends to worsen progressively with time. If it is the result of a medication such as an antihypertensive medication, major improvements can be achieved by changing the drug regimen.

2. **Prevention.** There is no known specific preventive therapy for autonomic neuropathy. Careful monitoring of blood pressure usually can prevent postural hypotension caused by an antihypertensive medication.

3. **Therapeutic approach.** Therapy for postural hypotension resulting from autonomic neuropathy is difficult. Some episodes may be prevented by use of elastic stockings or pantyhose. Sodium-retaining steroids such

as fludrocortisone (Florinef; Bristol-Myers Squibb, Princeton, NJ, U.S.A.) may be helpful, but care must be taken not to produce congestive heart failure.

4. Expected outcome. The outcome depends on the specific cause, but when the disorder is a medication side effect, the expectation is that it can be ameliorated.

5. Referrals. Patients with postural hypotension resulting from autonomic system failure often are referred to neurologists specializing in autonomic neuropathy. Difficult-to-treat patients with hypertension should be referred to internists or primary care physicians.

B. Cardiac arrhythmia

1. Course and prognosis. Once presyncope or syncope with light-headedness due to cardiac arrhythmia has been diagnosed through monitoring, the usual history is worsening attacks. The prognosis is for further attacks and even life-threatening periods of asystole.

2. Prevention. Medications that can interfere with cardiac arrhythmia, such as β-blockers, should be avoided.

3. Therapeutic approach. Patients with cardiac arrhythmia as the cause of dizziness may be treated with antiarrhythmics or pacemakers under the direction of a cardiologist.

4. Expected outcome. With proper identification and management, most cardiac arrhythmias can be controlled.

5. Referrals. Patients with cardiac arrhythmias are referred to cardiologists.

C. Metabolic causes of dizziness and vertigo, including hypoglycemia and hypothyroidism

1. Course and prognosis. Metabolic causes of dizziness are unusual and often difficult to diagnose. The symptom complex usually is not spinning vertigo but is vague episodes of disequilibration. This specific prognosis depends on the exact cause and correction of the metabolic condition.

2. Prevention. Episodic hypoglycemia can be prevented with frequent small meals or regulation of oral hypoglycemic or insulin therapy when it occurs in patients with diabetes.

3. Therapeutic approach. Therapy for endocrine disorders producing disequilibration depends on the specific metabolic abnormality identified. Therapy is directed at correcting the metabolic anomaly.

4. Expected outcome. Correction of the metabolic abnormality usually is beneficial with lessening of dizziness or disequilibration.

5. Referrals. Patients with identified metabolic abnormalities suspected of causing disorders of equilibrium should be referred to internists or endocrinologists.

D. Drug effects

1. Course and prognosis. Disorders of balance are produced by a variety of medications, particularly anticonvulsants, hypnotics, and some tranquilizers. Unless medication specifically affects blood pressure to produce light-headedness, the symptom complex is described as unsteadiness or incoordination. Patients have persistent symptoms as long as they continue to take the drugs.

2. Prevention depends on the awareness that certain medications, including those used to manage dizziness (such as benzodiazepines), may have medication side effects.

3. Therapeutic approach. The general approach is gradual withdrawal, whenever possible, of the medication believed to be producing the side effects. In the case of antiepileptic drugs, which are needed to control seizure disorders, alternative antiepileptic drugs can be used. Very gradual reductions in benzodiazepines may be needed if there is a problem of habituation.

4. Expected outcome. There usually is marked relief of symptoms of dizziness and disequilibration once offending medications have been replaced or withdrawn.

5. Referral. Patients taking antiepileptic drugs who have ataxia or disequilibration should be referred to a neurologist. When other medications, such as hypnotics, sedatives, or tranquilizers, are believed to be possible causes of disequilibration, they can be selectively decreased or eliminated by the primary care provider.

E. Multiple afferent sensory loss

1. **Course and prognosis.** In the elderly, a constellation of sensory deficits, such as combined hearing loss, visual loss, age-related vestibular change, and peripheral neuropathy, as well as a significant sense of disequilibration, unsteadiness, and falls, can occur. All of these sensory systems work together to produce a sense of stability and balance. The ultimate prognosis depends on factors that are correctable. For example, cataract removal may greatly enhance balance.

2. **Prevention.** Awareness that multiple sensory deficits may produce unsteadiness among the elderly should promote specific endeavors to correct the remedial problems and improve function.

3. **Therapeutic approach.** Specific interventions such as cataract removal or proper refractive correction can improve vision, and hearing aids may improve auditory sensitivity. A specific therapeutic maneuver that can improve balance is the use of a "dragging cane." Proprioceptive input from the cane being moved across the ground may greatly improve postural stability. Depending on the degree of disequilibration, some patients may be forced to use other assistive devices such as walkers.

4. **Expected outcome.** When specific sensory deficits are improved, there may be a significant improvement in balance.

5. **Referrals.** Patients with marked visual problems should be referred to ophthalmologists and those with auditory disorders to otolaryngologists.

Recommended Readings

Amarenco P. The spectrum of cerebellar infarctions. *Neurology* 1991;41:973–979.

Caplan LR. *Stroke: a clinical approach,* 2nd ed. Boston: Butterworth–Heinemann, 1993.

Colledge NR, Barr-Hamilton RM, Lewis SJ, et al. Evaluation of investigations to diagnose the cause of dizziness in elderly people: a community based controlled study. *BMJ* 1996; 313:7880–7892.

Derebery MJ: The diagnosis and treatment of dizziness. *Med Clin North Am* 1999;83:163–177.

Epley JM. The canalith repositioning procedure: for treatment of benign paroxysmal positional vertigo. *Otolaryngol Head Neck Surg* 1992;107:399–404.

Froehling DA, Silverstein MD, Mohr DN, et al. Does this dizzy patient have a serious form of vertigo? *JAMA* 1994;271:385–388.

Furman JM, Cass SP. Benign paroxysmal positional vertigo. *N Engl J Med* 1999;341: 1590–1596.

Halmagyi, GM, Cremer PD: Assessment and treatment of dizziness. *J Neurol Neurosurg Psychiatry* 2000;68:129–134.

Hoffman RM, Einstadter D, Kroenke K. Evaluating dizziness. *Am J Med* 1999;107:468–478.

Oas JG, Baloh RW. Vertigo and the anterior inferior cerebellar artery syndrome. *Neurology* 1992;42:2274–2279.

Ooi WL, Barrett S, Hossain M, et al. Patterns of orthostatic blood pressure change and their clinical correlates in the frail, elderly population. *JAMA* 1997;277:1299–1304.

Troost BT. Dizziness and vertigo. In: Bradley WG, Daroff RB, Fenichel GM, et al., eds. *Neurology in clinical practice,* 3rd ed. Vol. 1. Boston: Butterworth–Heinemann, 2000:239–251.

Troost BT, Arguello L. Hearing loss and tinnitus without dizziness and vertigo. In: Bradley WG, Daroff RB, Fenichel GM, et al., eds. *Neurology in clinical practice,* 3rd ed. Vol. 1. Boston: Butterworth–Heinemann, 2000:733–742.

Troost BT, Patton JM. Exercise therapy for positional vertigo. *Neurology* 1992;42:1441–1444.

57. NEUROLOGIC DISEASES IN PREGNANCY

Kathleen B. Digre
Michael W. Varner

Pregnancy is common. In the United States, there are 4,000,000 live births per year. At any given time, 10% of all women of reproductive age are pregnant. It is thus common to see neurologic conditions occur in association with pregnancy. Furthermore, physiologic changes in pregnancy can mimic neurologic diseases and can affect the severity of neurologic signs and symptoms. Not only can neurologic conditions be affected by pregnancy, but also treatment frequently must be altered to accommodate a developing fetus. Finally, pregnancy-specific conditions can present with neurologic symptoms and signs.

I. **Normal physiologic changes in pregnancy**
   A. **Cardiovascular**
      1. Increase (30% to 50%) in cardiac output
      2. Increase (30% to 50%) in blood volume
      3. Midpregnancy decrease in blood pressure
   B. **Pulmonary**
      1. Increase (20% to 30%) in minute volume
      2. Increase in respiratory rate
   C. **Renal**
      1. Increase (30% to 50%) in renal blood flow
      2. Decreased serum level of blood urea nitrogen and creatinine (due to increased renal clearance)
   D. **Gastrointestinal**
      1. Decreased motility
      2. Elevated alkaline phosphatase level (placental). Other results of liver function tests are normal.
      3. Increased cytochrome P-450 activity
   E. **Hematologic**
      1. Decreased hematocrit (20% to 30% increase in red blood cell volume but 30% to 50% increase in blood volume)
      2. Increased white blood cell count
      3. Decreased platelet count
   F. **Coagulation factors**
      1. Increased levels of plasminogen, fibrinogen, and factors VII, VIII, IX, and X
      2. No change in factor V, antithrombin III, or platelet adhesion
      3. Thrombophilia (e.g., factor V Leiden mutation) is more likely to produce thromboembolic complications.
   G. **Connective tissue.** Thickening and fragmentation of reticular fibers with mild hyperplasia of smooth muscle cells
   H. **Hormonal changes.** Progressive increase in estrogens and progesterone until delivery.
   I. **Evaluating neurologic conditions in pregnancy** (Table 57.1)
   J. U.S. Food and Drug Administration risk factor classification of drugs in pregnancy
      1. **Class A.** Controlled studies show no risk to fetus in first trimester; fetal harm is remote.
      2. **Class B.** No controlled studies have been completed, but there are no known risks.
      3. **Class C.** Studies on animals may show effects on fetuses, but no results of controlled studies are available. The drug can be used if the risk is justified.
      4. **Class D.** There are risks, but the drug may be used if serious disease or life-threatening conditions exist.
      5. **Class X.** Human and animal studies show risk. The risk of use outweighs any benefit.
II. **Seizure disorders in pregnancy**
   A. **Frequency.** 1.0% of the population

Table 57.1 Evaluating neurologic conditions in pregnancy

Test	Risk to mother	Risk to fetus	Contraindications
MRI	None	None known	Metal, cardiac pacemaker, otologic implant
MRI with gadolinium (risk category C)	None	None known	Same as above
CT	None	Minimal[a]	None
CT with contrast enhancement	None	Minimal[a]	Allergy to contrast medium
Angiography	Minimal in most centers	Minimal[a]	Allergy to contrast medium
Lumbar puncture	None	None	Incipient herniation or mass lesion
Ultrasonography	None	None	None
EEG	None	None	None
NCV/EMG	None	None	None
Tensilon test	Minimal	Minimal	Heart failure
Visual fields	None	None	None
Dilated eye examination	None	None with punctal occlusion	Incipient glaucoma
Fluorescein angiography	None	Minimal	Allergies

[a] Abdominal shielding.
MRI, magnetic resonance imaging; CT, computed tomography; EEG, electroencephalography; NCV, nerve conduction velocity; EMG, electromyography.

> **1.** 2.8 million persons in the United States, including 1.1 million women of reproductive age
> **2.** In an unselected population, frequency is 7 to 8 per 1,000 deliveries.

B. Heredity
> **1.** 2% to 5% if parent has idiopathic epilepsy
>> **a.** Relatively higher if the parent is the mother
>> **b.** Relatively lower if the parent is the father
> **2.** No significant transmission if disease is acquired

C. Course of disease in pregnancy
> **1.** The best figures for disease activity during pregnancy are as follows:
>> **a.** Improved, 22%
>> **b.** Exacerbated, 24% (most likely to occur in the first trimester)
>> **c.** No change, 54%
> **2.** Postulated mechanisms for changes in frequency during pregnancy include:
>> **a.** Physiologic
>>> **(1)** Hormonal (estrogens decrease and progestins increase seizure threshold)
>>> **(2)** Metabolic (increased cytochrome P-450 activity)
>> **b.** Sleep deprivation
>> **c.** Noncompliance (e.g., maternal fear of birth defects from taking medications)
>> **d.** Pharmacokinetic decreases in drug levels
>>> **(1)** Impaired absorption
>>> **(2)** Increased volume of distribution
>>> **(3)** Decreased albumin concentration
>>> **(4)** Reduced plasma protein binding
>>> **(5)** Increased drug clearance

        e. Folate supplementation
        f. Stress, anxiety
        g. Alcohol or other drug use
    3. Seizure frequency during pregnancy does not correlate with
        a. Maternal age
        b. Seizure type
        c. Drug regimen
        d. Seizure frequency in previous pregnancies
    4. Fetal risks with generalized convulsive seizure
        a. Physical injury from maternal abdominal trauma
        b. Hypoxic–ischemic injury due to maternal hypoxia

D. Therapeutic options
    1. Pharmacologic
        a. Be certain of the diagnosis.
        b. Be familiar with and use the few drugs that are the most effective for the various types of seizures.
    2. Surgery in general should be addressed before or after pregnancy.
    3. General
        a. Maintain daily habits (meals, sleep, minimize stress).
        b. Avoid alcohol and sedatives.
        c. Avoid hazardous situations.
        d. Avoid ketogenic diet.

E. Drug dosages, plasma levels, and clinical management
    1. Anticonvulsant drug levels decline during pregnancy in almost all women. This does not equate with a need to increase dosage.
        a. Free (non-protein-bound) drug level equates best with clinical status (seizure control and side effects). Should be obtained in pregnancies complicated by persistent or recurrent seizures or side effects.
        b. Total drug level. Usual laboratory result. Sufficient if the patient has good clinical control.
        c. With the exception of valproic acid, the average decline in free levels is less than that for total levels.
    2. Frequency of measurement of levels
        a. Ideally, preconceptional total and free levels should be obtained and optimized.
        b. Obtain non-protein-bound (free) levels every trimester (3 months), and again 4 weeks before term when
            (1) Seizure types do not interfere with activities of daily living.
            (2) The epilepsy is well-controlled.
        c. Obtain monthly free levels when
            (1) Uncontrolled seizures interfere with activities of daily living during the year before conception.
            (2) Previously controlled seizures recur during pregnancy.
            (3) Seizures are controlled but total drug levels decrease more than 50% on routine screens.
            (4) Troublesome or disabling side effects develop.
            (5) Lack of compliance is suspected or confirmed.
        d. Always check levels post partum and adjust dosage because levels often increase as the physiologic effects of pregnancy resolve within 10 to 15 days after delivery.
    3. Changing drug dosage
        a. Reasons not to change dosage
            (1) Total drug levels are declining in a woman with well-controlled seizures, unless there are greater than 30% decline in free levels and a history of poor control.
            (2) A woman taking two or more drugs discovers that she is pregnant (the time to change to monotherapy is before conception).
        b. Reasons to change dosage
            (1) Increased numbers of tonic–clonic seizures

      (2) Complex partial or other seizure types that interfere with activities of daily life, and the patient wants better control

      (3) A decline of more than 60% in total level (75% for valproic acid) or a decline of more than 30% in free levels in a seizure-free patient who has had seizures within the year before becoming pregnant

      (4) Troublesome or disabling side effects

      (5) It is reasonable to consider a change from polytherapy to monotherapy.

   c. Discontinuation of monotherapy should ideally be accomplished before conception but can be considered cautiously during pregnancy if a patient has been seizure free for more than 2 years, has normal findings at neurologic examination, normal electroencephalographic findings, no structural brain disorder, and no history of prolonged convulsive seizures.

4. Antiepileptic drugs used in pregnancy (Table 57.2)

5. Other drugs to add or consider for patients with epilepsy

  a. Folic acid

      (1) Requirements may be further increased because of malabsorption, competitive metabolism, and increased hepatic metabolism.

      (2) Increased supplementation may precipitate seizures by lowering anticonvulsant levels.

      (3) Best advice is to maintain usual supplementation.

      (4) Compelling evidence links the folic acid antagonism properties of anticonvulsants to relatively increased risk of fetal neural tube defects in women taking anticonvulsants during the first trimester (neural tube defects form, or do not form, 26 to 28 days after conception). *Women of reproductive potential should take continuous folic acid supplementation (400 μg/d) whether or not they are considering pregnancy.*

  b. Vitamin K should be administered (10 mg by mouth every day) to all pregnant women receiving antiepileptic drugs beginning 4 weeks before expected delivery until birth to minimize the risk of neonatal hemorrhage.

  c. Vitamin D

      (1) Anticonvulsants can induce clinical osteomalacia and rickets or, more commonly, asymptomatic hypocalcemia.

      (2) Unlikely to be of clinical significance for well-nourished women

      (3) Not routinely supplemented

6. Epilepsy teratogenesis

  a. Should be discussed with all epileptic women of reproductive age

  b. Other factors that may explain the increased incidence of anomalies in infants of epileptic mothers are as follows:

      (1) Increased incidence of anomalies in infants of epileptic mothers not taking medication. The only anomalies that are more common in phenytoin-exposed fetuses are hypertelorism and digital hypoplasia.

      (2) Increased incidence of characteristic malformations in infants of epileptic fathers, described as being intermediate between treated and untreated epileptic mothers

      (3) A specific metabolic defect (epoxide hydrolase deficiency) more common in persons with epilepsy may predispose to damage in some cases.

         (a) Teratogenic in animals

         (b) Inherited as autosomal codominant

         (c) Correlates highly with the incidence of fetal anomalies

      (4) Epilepsy may represent an underlying genetic disease.

      (5) The defects may result from an anticonvulsant-mediated relative folate deficiency. (Folate antagonists are known abortifacients and teratogens.) Women of reproductive potential should take continuous folic acid supplementation (400 μg/d) whether or not they are considering pregnancy.

(text continues on page 776)

Table 57.2 Drugs used in epilepsy

Drug	Indication	Dosage	FDA category	Side effects
Phenobarbital	Generalized seizures	1–2 mg/kg a day; 90–120 mg/d	D	Sedation
Phenytoin	Generalized seizures	4–5 mg/kg a day; 300–600 mg/d	D	Gingival hyperplasia and hirsuitism
Fosphenytoin	Status epilepticus	Maximum 100–150 mg PE/min i.v. (i.m. option available)	D	—
Primidone	Generalized and partial complex seizures	500–2,000 mg/d in 2 or 3 divided doses	D	Fatigue, depression, nausea; folate deficiency
Carbamazepine	Generalized and partial complex seizures	10–30 mg/kg a day divided t.i.d. or q.i.d.; maximum 1,600 mg/d	C	Diplopia, dizziness, headache, nausea
Oxcarbazepine	Partial complex seizures	Initial: 600 mg/d divided b.i.d. Maintenance: 1,200 mg/d divided b.i.d.	C	Hyponatremia, rash
Valproic acid	Generalized and myoclonic seizures	15–60 mg/kg a day	D	1% neural tube defect
Valproate i.v.	Status epilepticus, difficult-to-control seizures	Loading dose of 20 mg/kg in 100 mL NS over 1 h Maintenance 15 mg/kg a day divided t.i.d.	D	Thrombocytopenia, injection site erythema
Lamotrigine	Generalized Seizures Adjunctive therapy for partial seizures	Starting dose: 25 mg b.i.d.	C	Insomnia or drowsiness, rash and nausea

Drug	Indication	Dosage	FDA category	Side effects
Ethosuximide	Absence seizures	500–1,500 mg/d given as 1 or 2 doses	C	Nausea, vomiting, anorexia, agitation, headache
Felbamate	Partial onset with secondary generalization Mostly used in Lennox–Gastaut syndrome	300–400 mg t.i.d.	C	Aplastic anemia, liver failure
Gabapentin	Adjunctive for partial seizures	300–600 mg t.i.d.	C	Fatigue
Tiagabine	Partial and tonic–clonic seizures	30–50 mg/d in divided doses	C	Dizziness and sedation
Vigabatrin[a]	Partial seizures, secondary tonic–clonic seizures	2 g/d	No FDA category	Sedation
Topiramate	Adjunctive, partial, and tonic–clonic seizures	12.5–25 mg/d with gradual increase to 6 mg/kg or 400 mg/d	C	Mental dullness, renal calculi
Zonisamide	Partial, generalized, or myoclonic seizures	Initial: 100–200 mg/d divided b.i.d. Maintenance: 400–800 mg/d	C	Hypersensitivity reaction, nephrolithiasis
Levetiracetam	Partial or generalized seizures	Initial: 1,000 mg/d divided b.i.d. Maintenance: 1,000–3,000 mg/d divided b.i.d.	C	Fatigue, weakness
Trimethadione	Generalized seizures	—	X, absolutely contra-indicate	—

[a] Not approved in the United States at present.
FDA, U.S. Food and Drug Administration; i.v., intravenous; i.m., intramuscular; t.i.d., three times a day; q.i.d., four times a day; b.i.d., twice a day; NS, normal saline solution.

7. **Anticonvulsant teratogenesis** should be discussed with all epileptic women of reproductive age.
   a. Fetal anticonvulsant syndrome occurs in 3% to 5% of epileptic women and can occur in association with use of any anticonvulsant medication. The relative risk is dose dependent. This syndrome is being seen with decreasing frequency as fewer women receive polytherapy and more receive monotherapy.
      (1) Craniofacial and digital dysmorphic changes
      (2) Growth deficiency
      (3) Microcephaly
      (4) Cardiac defects
      (5) Mental retardation
   b. Anticonvulsants and neural tube defects
      (1) Risk is 1% to 2% for valproic acid. It is less than 1% for other anticonvulsants. However, these risks are higher than the 0.1% population-wide risk in the United States.
      (2) The relative risk is dose related.
      (3) If the medications are necessary for seizure control, the patient should be offered maternal serum α-fetoprotein and ultrasound screening.
      (4) Women of reproductive age who are taking anticonvulsants should take folate supplements.
   c. Trimethadione is clearly teratogenic and is contraindicated in pregnancy.
8. **Breast-feeding**
   a. Most anticonvulsants cross into breast milk, although at low levels. Ratios between concentrations in breast milk and serum are as follows:
      (1) Phenytoin, 0.10
      (2) Carbamazepine, 0.41
      (3) Phenobarbital, 0.39
   b. **Contraindications** to breast-feeding are as follows:
      (1) Poorly controlled maternal seizures
      (2) Rapid somnolence on the part of an initially hungry infant, which suggests a drug effect

F. **Onset of seizures during pregnancy: differential diagnosis**
   1. Tumor
      a. Tumors are especially likely to manifest in the first trimester, because this is when the pregnancy-associated increase in extracellular fluid begins.
      b. Meningioma tends to expand during pregnancy (response to the progressive increases in estrogen and progesterone).
   2. **Intracranial hemorrhage**
   3. **Cortical venous thrombosis,** especially late in pregnancy and in the immediate puerperium
   4. **Gestational epilepsy**
      a. A diagnosis of exclusion
      b. Represents only a small fraction of all women who have initial seizures while pregnant
   5. **Rule out eclampsia.** The most common multisystem disease in late pregnancy is preeclampsia or eclampsia.

G. **Status epilepticus** during pregnancy (follow guidelines for nonpregnant patients)
   1. Less than 1% of all pregnant epileptic women
   2. Not an indication for termination of pregnancy
   3. Management should include the following:
      a. Hospitalization
      b. Securing the airway
      c. Intravenous access for normal saline solution and B vitamins
      d. Baseline laboratory studies including electrolytes, complete blood cell count, glucose, calcium, and arterial blood gases

    e. Maternal and fetal vital signs, including electrocardiography (ECG) and fetal heart rate monitoring

    f. Glucose bolus (50 mL of D50)

    g. Thiamine (100 mg intramuscularly or intravenously [IV])

    h. Begin diazepam (5 to 15 mg i.v. in 5-mg boluses) or lorazepam (0.1 mg/kg i.v., not to exceed 2 mg/min) and fosphenytoin (150 mg/min) or phenytoin 18 to 20 mg/kg i.v., not to exceed 50 mg/min, with ECG and blood pressure monitoring, administered in non-glucose-containing fluids).

    i. If seizures persist, intubate and begin either phenobarbital (20 to 25 mg/kg i.v., not to exceed 100 mg/min). Alternatives include lorazepam, midazolam, propofol, or intravenous valproic acid.

    j. If seizures still persist, institute general anesthesia with halothane and neuromuscular junction blockade.

III. Headache

  A. The most common headache diagnoses are as follows:

    1. Migraine (with or without aura) occurs in 10% to 20% of women of child-bearing age.

      a. Unilateral or bilateral throbbing headaches associated with photophobia, phonophobia, nausea, or vomiting; exacerbated by activity

      b. Particularly prominent in women of reproductive age

    2. Tension-type headache is very common.

      a. Increases through the day, local soreness, frequently begins in the neck or back of the head; usually bilateral; may be relieved with activity

      b. Not associated with nausea or vomiting

      c. May be episodic (fewer than 15 days/month) or chronic (more than 15 days/month)

  B. Genetics of migraine. Thought to be inherited. Hemiplegic migraine is autosomal dominant associated with calcium channel abnormalities on chromosomes 1 and 19.

  C. Course of migraine in pregnancy

    1. The condition of most women with migraine improves when the woman is pregnant. This is especially true of the following:

      a. Menstrual migraine

      b. Migraine onset at menarche

    2. Approximately 10% to 20% of headaches worsen or have the initial onset during pregnancy, usually in the first trimester.

    3. Migraineurs have no increased risk of complications during pregnancy, but headaches usually recur near term and in the puerperium.

    4. Multiparous migraineurs may have an increase in headaches in the third trimester, whereas primiparous women report less headache activity in pregnancy and the puerperium.

  D. The **differential diagnosis** of headache or migraine occurring for the first time in pregnancy includes:

    1. Intracranial hemorrhage

    2. Cerebral venous thrombosis

    3. Intracranial hypertension (increased intracranial pressure)

    4. Stroke (carotid or vertebral artery dissection)

    5. Brain tumor

    6. Severe preeclampsia

  E. Therapeutic options

    1. Nonmedication treatment

      a. Avoidance of dietary and environmental trigger factors

      b. Biofeedback, relaxation therapy, massage

      c. Physical therapy

      d. Heat or ice packs

    2. Acute medication treatment principles

      a. Prevention of nausea (Table 57.3)

      b. Management of pain (Table 57.4)

      c. Sedation (Table 57.5)

Table 57.3 Acute migraine treatment in pregnancy: nausea prevention

Drug	Dosage (mg)	FDA schedule	Side effects
Promethazine	25–75 p.o., p.r., i.m.	C: trimester 1	—
		B: trimester 2, 3	—
Hydroxyzine	25–75 p.o., i.m.	C	Fatigue
Prochlorperazine	10–25 p.o., p.r., i.m., i.v.	C	Dystonic reaction
Trimethobenzamide	200–250 p.o., p.r.	C	—
Chlorpromazine	25 p.o., p.r., i.m., i.v.	C	Dystonic reaction
Metoclopramide	5–10 i.m., i.v.	B	Dystonic reaction

FDA, U.S. Food and Drug Administration; p.o., orally; p.r., rectally; i.m., intramuscularly; i.v., intravenously.

> **3. Prophylactic treatment.** In general, avoid daily medications, but if headaches are too severe or interfere excessively with life, daily treatment may be needed. In general, monotherapy should be attempted. The lowest dosage should be encouraged (Table 57.6).

IV. Tumors
- **A. Incidence**
  1. Probably less than 100 per year nationwide
  2. Pregnancy does not increase the risk of brain tumors but does increase the likelihood of symptoms.
  3. The types of tumors are identical to those observed in nonpregnant women of the same age, primarily glioma (32%), meningioma (29%), acoustic neuroma (15%), and others (24%).
- **B. Clinical features**
  1. Headache
  2. Nausea and vomiting
  3. Focal deficits or seizures
- **C. Diagnosis**
  1. Magnetic resonance imaging (MRI) with contrast enhancement (gadolinium)
  2. Computed tomography (CT) with contrast enhancement
- **D. Treatment**
  1. Dexamethasone (risk factor C)
     - **a.** Dosage: 6 mg every 6 hours or 4 mg every 4 hours
     - **b.** Problems: gastrointestinal; cushingoid changes with prolonged use
  2. Mannitol (risk factor C) for acute swelling
- **E. Pituitary tumors**
  1. **Course of disease**
     - **a. Microadenoma** rarely is symptomatic (5%).
     - **b. Macroadenoma** is symptomatic in 15% to 35% of cases.
  2. **Visual field** evaluation must be performed for macroadenoma.
  3. **Treatment**
     - **a.** Bromocriptine (risk factor C) may be taken throughout pregnancy if the tumor enlarges.
     - **b.** If vision is threatened, surgical treatment is appropriate.
  4. **Sheehan's syndrome** involves pituitary infarction, frequently associated with tumor.
     - **a.** Manifests as inability to lactate, hypopituitarism, hypothyroidism
     - **b.** Treatment involves steroid and thyroid replacement.
  5. **Lymphocytic hypophysitis** mimics pituitary adenoma and suprasellar masses because it manifests as endocrinologic abnormalities, headaches, and a suprasellar mass at imaging. Lymphocytic hypophysitis occurs in pregnant and postpartum women. Biopsy often is needed to make the diagnosis. Steroid treatment with dexamethasone (category C) often is helpful.

V. Pseudotumor cerebri (idiopathic intracranial hypertension) is characterized by increased intracranial pressure not caused by an intracranial space-occupying lesion demon-

Table 57.4 Acute migraine treatment in pregnancy: pain treatment

Drug	Dosage (mg)	FDA schedule	Side effects
Acetaminophen	350–500	B	—
Aspirin	325–650	C	Bleeding, diathesis, in utero closure of ductus arteriosus, oligohydramnios
Caffeinated compounds	—	B	—
Butalbital-acetaminophen	—	C	Possible neonatal withdrawal with heavy use
Isometheptene	Two at onset, then one per hour to maximum of five per 24 hours	C	—
NSAIDs[a]			
Ibuprofen	200–800	B	Bleeding diathesis, oligohydramnios, in utero closure of ductus arteriosus
Naproxen	200–500	B	Bleeding diathesis, oligohydramnios, in utero closure of ductus arteriosus
Triptans			
Sumatriptan	25–100 p.o. 20 n.s. 6 s.c.	C	Contraindicated in coronary artery disease
Zolmitriptan	2.5–5 p.o.	C	Contraindicated in coronary artery disease
Naratriptan	1.25–2.5 p.o.	C	Contraindicated in coronary artery disease
Rizatriptan	10 p.o.	C	Contraindicated in coronary artery disease
Narcotic (use with antiemetic)			
Butorphanol	—	B	Respiratory depression, nausea
Meperidine	50–100	B	Respiratory depression, nausea
Ergotamine (DHE or ergotamine)	Avoid	X	Possible abortifacient

[a] NSAIDs, nonsteroidal anti-inflammatory drugs. Use in pregnancy should be restricted to less than 48 hours (more than 48 hours of consecutive therapy is associated with progressive risk of in utero closure of the ductus arteriosis, renal damage, and platelet dysfunction).
FDA, U.S. Food and Drug Administration; p.o., orally; n.s., nasal spray; s.c., subcutaneously.

Table 57.5 Acute migraine treatment in pregnancy: sedation

Drug	Dose (mg)	FDA schedule	Side effects
Chloral hydrate	500–1,500	C	—
Pentobarbital	—	D	Withdrawal
Hydroxyzine, promethazine	25–75	C	—
Meperidine (plus antiemetic)	—	B	—
Diazepam	5–10	D	Lethargy
Lorazepam	—	D	
Clonazepam	0.5–1.0	C	—
Chlorpromazine	25–50	C	Dystonic reaction; decreased blood pressure

FDA, U.S. Food and Drug Administration.

strated at MRI or CT. Pregnancy does not cause pseudotumor cerebri. However, this disorder can occur during pregnancy. Pregnancy does not by itself cause visual loss. Pseudotumor cerebri does not cause miscarriage.

A. **Symptoms and signs**
 1. Headache is the most common symptom (more than 90% of cases). Patients are otherwise alert and healthy.
 2. Transient visual obscuration
 3. Papilledema in almost all cases
 4. Cranial nerve VI palsy and possibly cranial nerve VII palsy in some cases
 5. Obesity

Table 57.6 Migraine prophylaxis in pregnancy

Drug	Dosage (mg)	FDA schedule	Side effects, comments
β-Blockers			
Propranolol hypotension	20–80	C	IUGR,[a] prematurity,
Nadolol	10–40	C	IUGR
Timolol	10–30	C	IUGR
Tricyclic Antidepressants			
Amitriptyline in pregnancy	10–75	C, D	Limb deformities; considered by some to be the best
Nortriptyline	10–75	D	—
Imipramine	10–75	D	—
Desipramine	10–75	C	—
Cyproheptadine	4 t.i.d.	B	Weight gain; occasionally effective
Calcium Channel Blockers			
Verapamil	80–240	C	Constipation
Nifedipine	10–30	C	Decreased blood pressure
Amlodipine	2.5–5	C	—
Anticonvulsant			
Gabapentin	100–300	C	Fatigue

[a] Contraindicated drugs: methysergide, valproic acid.
FDA, U.S. Food and Drug Administration; IUGR, intrauterine growth retardation; tid, three times a day.

B. Differential diagnosis of papilledema and no mass lesion in pregnancy
1. Venous thrombosis (most important)
2. Venous hypertension
3. Meningitis
4. Syphilis

C. Evaluation must include an imaging procedure (MRI and MR venography), cerebrospinal fluid with opening pressure, and cerebrospinal fluid constituents. Because the greatest threat to the patient is visual loss, visual acuity and visual field examinations must be performed frequently.

D. Treatment options
1. **Medical treatment**
   a. Weight loss (restriction of weight gain is better than substantial weight loss)
   b. Frequent lumbar puncture
      (1) Safe
      (2) Painful, often difficult
   c. Acetazolamide (500 to 2,000 mg) after the first trimester (risk C)
   d. Furosemide (Lasix; Aventis, Bridgewater, NJ, U.S.A.) (risk C)
   e. Chlorthalidone (risk B)
   f. Steroids (prednisone, methylprednisolone)
2. **Surgical treatment**
   a. Optic nerve sheath decompression is the preferred procedure to save vision.
   b. Lumbar peritoneal shunt can be difficult for pregnant patients.

VI. Cerebrovascular disease

A. Stroke or vascular occlusion. Attributable risk of ischemic stroke or intracerebral hemorrhage in pregnancy or the puerperium is 8.1/100,000 pregnancies. The causes of stroke during pregnancy are listed in Table 57.7.
   1. Arterial
      a. Characteristically manifests as paresis but without altered consciousness or seizures
      b. Represents 90% of strokes during pregnancy
   2. **Venous**
      a. Characteristically manifests as headache, seizures, increased intracranial pressure, and alteration of consciousness
      b. Represents 80% of strokes during puerperium
   3. **Intracranial hemorrhage** characteristically manifests as sudden onset of headache, loss of consciousness, and accompanying signs of neck stiffness and altered blood pressure.
   4. **Diagnosis**
      a. CT and MRI (newer techniques of diffusion and perfusion may show early injury)
      b. Angiography
      c. Cardiac evaluation (transesophageal echocardiography—look also for right to left shunt)
      d. Appropriate laboratory studies. The factor V Leiden mutation is now thought to be associated with at least one half of all cases of venous thromboses among white women. Consider protein C or protein S deficiency (may be falsely depressed simply because of pregnancy), antithrombin III, antiphospholipid antibodies, platelets, fibrinogen, homocysteine levels.
   5. Treatment is directed at the underlying cause; treatment should be individualized.
      a. **Heparin,** unfractionated or low molecular weight (risk category C), does not cross the placenta and can therefore be used safely during pregnancy.
      b. **Warfarin** (risk category D) crosses the placenta and is contraindicated during pregnancy. However, it can be used during breast-feeding.
      c. **Low-dose aspirin** (<80 mg/d) (risk category C) can be used safely in pregnancy when clinically indicated.

Table 57.7 Causes of stroke in pregnancy

Arterial occlusive disease
  Thrombotic cause
    Atherosclerotic
    Fibromuscular dysplasia
  Embolic source
    Cardiac
      Peripartum cardiomyopathy
      Mitral valve prolapse
      Rheumatic heart disease
      Endocarditis (infective and nonbacterial)
      Paradoxic embolus
      Atrial fibrillation
      Carotid or vertebral artery dissection
    Amniotic or air embolism (acute fulminant cardiovascular collapse)
Venous occlusive disease
  Hypercoagulable state (antithrombin III, protein S or protein C deficiencies, factor V
    Leiden deficiency, hyperhomocysteinemia)
  Infection
Drug abuse
Hypotensive disorders
  Watershed infarction
  Sheehan's pituitary necrosis
Hematologic disorders
  Lupus anticoagulant, Sneddon's syndrome
  Thrombocytopenic purpura
  Sickle cell disease
  Protein C, antithrombin III, protein S deficiencies
  Hyperhomocysteinemia
  Factor V Leiden deficiency
Arteritis and angiopathy
  Systemic lupus erythematosus
  Infectious arteritis (syphilis, tuberculosis, meningococcal)
  Cerebral angiitis
  Takayasu's arteritis
  Postpartum cerebral angiopathy
  Fibromuscular dysplasia and dissection
Intracerebral hemorrhage
  Eclampsia and hypertensive disorders
  Venous thrombosis
  Choriocarcinoma
  Arteriovenous malformation
  Vasculitis
  Infective endocarditis
  Drug abuse
  Hematologic disorders
  Moyamoya disease
  Tumors
Subarachnoid hemorrhage
  Aneurysm (saccular, mycotic)
  Arteriovenous malformation (cerebral, spinal cord)
  Eclampsia
  Vasculitis
  Choriocarcinoma
  Venous thrombosis

Table 57.7 *Continued*

Other
  Carotid cavernous fistula
  Dural vascular malformation
  Carotid and vertebral arterial dissection (fibromuscular dysplasia)

From Digre KB, Varner MW. Diagnosis and treatment of cerebrovascular disorders in pregnancy. In: Adams HP, ed. *Handbook of cerebrovascular diseases*. New York: Marcel Dekker, 1993:255–286, with permission of Marcel Dekker with subsequent modifications.

        d. Management of acute stroke with tissue plasminogen activator is not currently recommended.
        e. Manage elevation of homocysteine levels with folate.
  B. Cerebral venous thrombosis
    1. Occurs primarily post partum. The signs and symptoms are as follows:
      a. Headache
      b. Seizures
      c. Hemiplegia
      d. Papilledema
      e. Obtundation and coma, especially in internal cerebral vein thrombosis
    2. Diagnosis is now optimum by means of MRI and MR venography; angiography or venography occasionally is needed.
    3. Treatment
      a. Correction of predisposing factors (infection, dehydration)
      b. Control of seizures
      c. Use of antiedema agents when appropriate
      d. Anticoagulation (see **VI.A.5.a.** through **c.**)
    4. Risk factors are as follows:
      a. Cesarean delivery
      b. Hypertension
      c. Infection other than pneumonia or influenza
      d. Drug abuse, especially cocaine, methamphetamines, intravenous drug abuse
  C. Postpartum cerebral angiopathy is a rare cause of a stroke-like syndrome characterized by seizure and focal neurologic deficits. Reversible cerebral vasoconstriction is found at angiography. Medications such as ergot alkaloids (e.g., ergonovine, bromocriptine, ergotamine) and certain vasoconstrictive agents (isometheptene, sympathomimetic drugs) have been reported to cause the disorder. Treatment has been mainly supportive.
  D. Hematologic disorders
    1. Antiphospholipid antibody syndrome is associated most frequently with recurrent miscarriage, fetal growth restriction, and severe preeclampsia and eclampsia.
    2. Sickle cell disease
    3. Deficiencies of antithrombin III, or protein C or S
    4. Thrombophilia, especially factor V Leiden mutation
  E. Subarachnoid hemorrhage. Table 57.8 presents the differentiating causes.
    1. Intracranial aneurysm
      a. Thought to be present in 1% of all women of reproductive age
      b. A significant contributor to maternal mortality
      c. Rupture probably equally likely throughout pregnancy
      d. More likely to occur in older, parous women
      e. Diagnosis requires CT, lumbar puncture to look for red blood cells, and angiography.
      f. Optimum outcomes with surgical correction

Table 57.8 Differentiating causes of subarachnoid hemorrhage

Clinical feature	Aneurysm	Arteriovenous malformation	Eclampsia
Age (y)	25–37 (increases with age)	15–20 (younger)	Any age
Headache	Severe	May be severe	60% frontal
Parity	Multiparous	Primiparous	Both
Epigastric pain	–	–	+
Nausea, vomiting	+/–	+/–	+
Trimester	3rd	3rd	2nd, 3rd
Loss of consciousness	⅓–⅔	⅓–⅔	All
Nuchal rigidity	Prominent	May be present	Rare
Seizure	15%–30%	Present	100%
Hypertension	30%–50%	After bleed	90% >140/90 mm Hg
Proteinuria	30%	14%	All
Focal weakness	20%	Frequent	Rare
Cerebrospinal fluid	Blood	Blood	Clear, some blood
Recurrent hemorrhage	Less than 2 weeks	+	No
Subsequent pregnancy	Risk is low if mother treated	Highly likely if untreated	May recur especially with predisposing causes
Prognosis	Mother treated: 11% maternal mortality and 5% fetal mortality Untreated: 63% maternal mortality and 27% fetal mortality	Recurrence untreated: 32% maternal mortality	Good if mother delivers. Fetus: variable, depends on gestational age

From Digre KB, Varner MW. Diagnosis and treatment of cerebrovascular disorders in pregnancy. In: Adams HP, ed. *Handbook of cerebrovascular diseases.* New York: Marcel Dekker, 1993:274, with permission.
–, not present; +, present; +/–, present or absent.

    g. Avoid nitroprusside because of its cyanide effect on the fetus. Hypertension can be controlled with verapamil or nimodipine.
    h. Vaginal delivery should be anticipated after successful clipping unless obstetric contraindications exist. If delivery occurs before clipping, cesarean section or forceps delivery with epidural anesthesia is indicated.
    i. Vasospasm can be managed with nimodipine. Volume expansion must be monitored, because pregnant women are relatively more prone to pulmonary edema (decreased osmotic pressure).
    j. Outcome
        (1) Grades 1 through 3: with expedited surgery, 95% successful outcome expected
        (2) Grade 4: 45% to 75% mortality
        (3) Fetal outcome: 27% mortality rate without surgery
    k. Subsequent pregnancies after successful clipping have a good prognosis.
    l. Asymptomatic aneurysm should be managed if larger than 7 mm in diameter.
  2. Arteriovenous malformation
    a. Characteristically occurs in younger women who have had fewer pregnancies

    b. Diagnosis requires CT, lumbar puncture, and angiography.

    c. The aneurysm should be corrected, if possible, surgically or with embolic therapy.

    d. Stereotactic radiation therapy is not indicated during pregnancy.

    e. Delivery is vaginal with epidural anesthesia and low-outlet forceps.

F. Eclampsia, severe preeclampsia

  1. Definition

    a. Complicates 5% to 7% of pregnancies

    b. Severe preeclampsia. One or more of the following is present: persistent blood pressure >160/110 mm Hg, >5 g proteinuria in 24 hours, oliguria (<500 mL/24 hours), elevated results of liver function tests, thrombocytopenia, persistent visual disturbances or headache, epigastric pain, pulmonary edema, fetal growth restriction not explainable by other causes.

    c. Eclampsia. Seizures or coma in a woman with preeclampsia in whom no other explanation can be found.

    d. HELLP syndrome. A form of severe preeclampsia characterized by *h*emolysis, *e*levated results of *l*iver function tests, and *l*ow *p*latelet count.

  2. Symptoms and physical findings

    a. Headache, dizziness, scotomata, nausea, vomiting, abdominal pain

    b. Generalized edema

    c. Funduscopic findings: segmental vasospasm, serous retinal detachment

    d. Neurologic finding: hyperreflexia

    e. Bedside testing: Visual acuity, Amsler grid for detection of scotomata

  3. CT and MRI findings

    a. CT. Edema and hypodense lesions 75%, hemorrhage 9%

    b. MRI

      (1) Severe preeclampsia. Deep white-matter signals on T2-weighted images

      (2) Eclampsia. Signals on T2-weighted images at gray matter–white matter junctions, particularly in the parietal–occipital areas; cortical edema, hemorrhage; looks very much like hypertensive encephalopathy or reversible white-matter deficit.

  4. Electroencephalogram is abnormal for 80% of patients with eclampsia (slowing most common)

  5. Treatment

    a. Delivery

    b. Magnesium sulfate

      (1) Administered in a 4 to 6 g loading dose followed by 2 g/h i.v.

      (2) Found to be superior to intravenous diazepam and phenytoin in randomized controlled trials

      (3) Side effects include weakness, diplopia, ptosis, blurred vision, nausea, vomiting, and respiratory depression. *Use with caution in the care of patients with reduced renal clearance or neuromuscular diseases such as myasthenia gravis.*

      (4) Neurologic findings of magnesium toxicity include diminished deep tendon reflexes, ptosis, diminished accommodation.

    c. Decrease blood pressure when necessary with an antihypertensive medication such as hydralazine or labetalol.

    d. Control seizures if not controlled with an anticonvulsant such as diphenylhydantoin (fosphenytoin) only if magnesium sulfate is unsuccessful.

    e. Manage cerebral edema or herniation with hyperventilation, steroids, or mannitol after delivery.

  6. Postpartum eclampsia (one third of eclamptic convulsions do not begin until after delivery, usually within 24 to 48 hours after delivery). Usually defined as within 7 days of delivery. Late postpartum eclampsia can occur up to 10 to 14 days after delivery. Consider the possibility of stroke, venous thrombosis, or reversible angiopathy if late postpartum eclampsia is diagnosed.

  7. Outcome

    a. The maternal mortality rate is 1% to 5%.

    b. The perinatal mortality rate is 13% to 30%

8. Complications
  a. Intracranial hemorrhage, frequently from uncontrolled hypertension
  b. Congestive heart failure, frequently from iatrogenic fluid overload
  c. Intrahepatic hemorrhage
VII. Multiple sclerosis (MS)
  A. MS does not affect pregnancy per se, or vice versa. Although recent studies do show that there maybe increased relapses post partum, especially in the first 6 months post partum, pregnancy does not affect the rate of disability.
    1. Patients who have sphincter disturbances or paraplegia may experience increased difficulty during pregnancy.
    2. There is no evidence of direct genetic transmission of MS.
    3. MS does not occur more frequently in pregnancy.
    4. Patients with MS have fewer pregnancies.
  B. There is an increased incidence of exacerbations (in the relapsing–remitting form) in the first 6 months post partum.
  C. Management of acute MS in pregnancy (Table 57.9)
    1. Steroids (see Chapter 40, **V.B.1.**)
    2. The interferons and copolymer are not yet recommended in pregnancy, although patients who were pregnant have used the medications without fetal harm.
VIII. Paraplegia
  A. Pregnancy is associated with increased risk of
    1. Urinary tract infection
    2. Pressure sores
  B. Labor progresses normally. Maternal perception depends on the level of the block.
    1. Above T10, painless
    2. Below T10, painful
  C. Autonomic hyperreflexia
    1. Occurs only if the block is at or above T5-6
    2. Develops in association with excessive activity of any viscus (e.g., labor)
    3. Characteristic signs and symptoms

Table 57.9 Drugs used in the management of multiple sclerosis (MS)

Drug	Use in MS	FDA category	Side effects
Immediate Treatment			
IV Solumedrol	Acute exacerbations	C	Anxiety, gastro-intestinal distress
Interferon β-1a (Avonex)	Prevention of exacerbations (relapsing–remitting)	C	Fatigue, malaise, low fever
Interferon β-1b (Betaseron)	Prevention of exacerbations (relapsing–remitting)	C	Fatigue, malaise
Glatinamer acetate (Capaxone)	Prevention of exacerbations (relapsing–remitting)	B	Fatigue
Methotrexate	Chronic progressive	X, do not use	—
Azathioprine	Chronic progressive	D	—
Symptomatic Management of MS Comorbidities			
Baclofen	Spasticity	B	—
Amantadine	Fatigue	B	—

       a. Throbbing headache
       b. Hypertension
       c. Reflex bradycardia
       d. Sweating
       e. Nasal congestion
       f. Cutaneous vasodilatation and piloerection above the level of the lesion
    4. Symptoms are caused by the sudden release of catecholamines, so treatment may include reserpine, atropine, clonidine, glyceryl trinitrate, or hexamethonium.
    5. May be misdiagnosed as preeclampsia

IX. Root lesions and peripheral neuropathy
  A. Lumbar disk
    1. Signs and symptoms are the same as in nonpregnant patients.
    2. Generally treated nonoperatively. Consider surgery if there are:
       a. Bilateral symptoms
       b. Disturbance of sphincter function
  B. Carpal tunnel syndrome
    1. Pain and paresthesia commonly are worse at night and tend to be worse in the dominant hand.
    2. Tinel's sign
    3. Symptoms usually respond to nocturnal wrist splinting and resolve within 3 months post partum.
  C. Bell's palsy
    1. Facial paresis of lower motor neuron type when no other specific etiologic agent can be found. Signs and symptoms include
       a. Abrupt onset, often with pain around the ear
       b. Feeling of facial stiffness and pulling to one side
       c. Difficulty closing the eye on the affected side
       d. Taste disturbances
       e. Hyperacusis
    2. Approximately three times more likely to occur during pregnancy, primarily in the third trimester or immediately post partum.
    3. Steroids are probably effective if given within the first 5 to 7 days. Surgery is ineffective.
  D. Other forms of cranial nerve palsy
    1. Cranial nerve IV: reported rarely to occur; mechanism similar to cranial nerve VII or VI palsy
    2. Cranial nerve VI
  E. Meralgia paresthetica
    1. Causes numbness in the lateral aspect of the thigh
    2. Usually resolves within 3 months post partum
  F. Sciatica and back pain. Lumbosacral disk surgery should be reserved only for progressive atrophy or bowel or bladder dysfunction.
  G. Guillain–Barré syndrome
    1. Causes are not generally affected by pregnancy.
    2. Labor and delivery are otherwise normal.

X. Myasthenia gravis
  A. Variable weakness and fatigability of skeletal muscles resulting from defective neuromuscular transmission (reduced acetylcholine receptors in the neuromuscular junction)
  B. Does not affect labor progress, except for voluntary efforts in the second stage
  C. Certain drugs should be avoided, including
    1. Ester anesthetics: tetracaine (Pontocaine; Sanofi Winthrop, New York, NY, U.S.A.), chloroprocaine (Nesacaine; AstraZeneca, Wilmington, DE, U.S.A.)
    2. Curare (and other nondepolarizing muscle relaxants)
    3. Halothane (Fluothane; Wyeth-Ayerst, Philadelphia, PA, U.S.A.)
    4. Aminoglycoside antibiotics
    5. Quinine and quinidine
    6. Magnesium sulfate. The antidote is edrophonium (Tensilon; ICN, Costa Mesa, CA, U.S.A.), not calcium.

D. Treatment
  1. Antepartum
      a. Pregnancy per se does not affect the severity of preexisting disease.
      b. Perinatal mortality is increased because of increased risk of premature delivery as well as neonatal myasthenia.
      c. Pharmacologic management of myasthenia gravis is not altered by pregnancy.
  2. Intrapartum
      a. Oral medications should be discontinued at the onset of labor and the intramuscular equivalents continued until oral medications can again be ingested. Equipotent dosages are as follows:
          (1) Neostigmine 0.5 mg i.v.
          (2) Neostigmine 0.7 to 1.5 mg intramuscularly
          (3) Neostigmine 15 mg by mouth
          (4) Pyridostigmine 60 mg by mouth
      b. Analgesia and anesthesia for labor require the utmost caution because of the risks of respiratory depression and aspiration.
      c. Myasthenia gravis does not affect the progress of labor and is not an indication for cesarean section.
  3. Post partum
      a. Exacerbations are more likely to occur post partum and tend to be sudden and severe in onset.
      b. Women with severe disease or whose babies have symptoms after nursing should not breast-feed.
      c. Most women return to preconceptional oral dosage with modest increases in dose to allow for the additional stresses of early parenthood.
E. Neonatal myasthenia
  1. Occurs in 10% to 15% of cases
  2. Results from transplacental transfer of maternal antibody against acetylcholine receptors
XI. Myotonic dystrophy
  A. Clinical characteristics
      1. Autosomal dominant
      2. Weakness and wasting in muscles of face, neck, and distal limbs
      3. Myotonia of hands and tongue
      4. Variable age at onset. The condition sometimes is diagnosed in mothers only after an affected child is born.
      5. Predisposition to cardiac arrhythmia
      6. Treatment
          a. Dystrophy: none
          b. Myotonia: phenytoin (Dilantin; Pfizer, New York, NY, U.S.A.), quinine, procainamide
  B. Effects on pregnancy
      1. Increased risk of spontaneous abortion
      2. Increased risk of premature labor and polyhydramnios
      3. Normal first stage of labor
      4. Normal response to oxytocin
      5. Prolonged second stage of labor
  C. Labor management
      1. Outlet forceps
      2. Regional anesthesia
      3. Avoid succinylcholine.
          a. Can cause hyperthermia
          b. Nonpolarizing agents are safe.
XII. Parkinson's disease in pregnancy is rare because the age at which most patients have the disease is past childbearing years. However, pregnancy has been successfully accomplished in patients with Parkinson's disease
  A. Pregnancy may adversely affect Parkinson's in that there may be exacerbations soon after pregnancy

   B. Drugs used in Parkinson's disease
   1. Levodopa (schedule C)
   2. Amantadine can increase risk of complications and malformations
   3. Other drugs

Recommended Readings

Batocchi AP, Majolini L, Evoli A, et al. Course and treatment of myasthenia gravis during pregnancy. *Neurology* 1999;52:447–452.

Berg G, Hammar M, Moller-Nielsen J, et al. Low back pain during pregnancy. *Obstet Gynecol* 1988;71:71–75.

Bernardi S, Grasso MG, Bertollini R, et al. The influence of pregnancy on relapses in multiple sclerosis: a cohort study. *Acta Neurol Scand* 1991;84:403–406.

Birk K, Ford C, Smeltzer S, et al. The clinical course of multiple sclerosis during pregnancy and the puerperium. *Arch Neurol* 1990;47:738–742.

Branch DW. Antiphospholipid antibodies and pregnancy: maternal implications. *Semin Perinatol* 1990;14:139–146.

Briggs GG, Freeman RK, Yaffe SJ. *Drugs in pregnancy and lactation,* 5th ed. Baltimore: Williams & Wilkins, 1998.

Carr SC, Gilchrist JM, Abuelo DN, et al. Antenatal treatment of myasthenia gravis. *Obstet Gynecol* 1991;78:485–489.

Chanceller MD, Wroe SJ. Migraine occurring for the first time during pregnancy. *Headache* 1990;30:224–227.

Cornelissen M, Steegers-Theunissen R, Kollee L, et al. Supplementation of vitamin K in pregnant women receiving anticonvulsant therapy prevents neonatal vitamin K deficiency. *Am J Obstet Gynecol* 1993;168:884–888.

Crawford P, Appleton R, Betts T, et al. Best practice guidelines for the management of women with epilepsy. The Women with Epilepsy Guidelines Development Group. *Seizure* 1999;8:201–217.

Damek DEM, Shuster EA. Pregnancy and multiple sclerosis. *Mayo Clin Proc* 1997;72: 977–989.

Davis RK, Maslow AS. Multiple sclerosis in pregnancy: a review. *Obstet Gynecol Surv* 1992; 47:290–296.

Dias MS, Sekhar LN. Intracranial hemorrhage from aneurysms and arteriovenous malformations during pregnancy and the puerperium. *Neurosurgery* 1990;27:855–866.

Digre KB, Varner MW. Diagnosis and treatment of cerebrovascular disorders in pregnancy. In: Adams HP, ed. *Handbook of cerebrovascular diseases.* New York: Marcel Dekker, 1993: 255–286.

Digre KB, Varner MW, Osborn AG, et al. Cranial MR imaging in severe preeclampsia versus eclampsia. *Arch Neurol* 1993;50:399–406.

Gilmore J, Pennell PB, Stern BJ. Medication use during pregnancy for neurologic conditions. *Neurol Clin* 1998;16:189–205.

Hagell P, Odin P, Vinge E. Pregnancy in Parkinson's disease: a review of the literature and a case report. *Mov Disord* 1998;13:34–37.

Holcomb W, Petrie R. Cerebrovascular emergencies in pregnancy. *Clin Obstet Gynecol* 1990; 33:467–472.

Kerrison JB, Lee AG. Acute loss of vision during pregnancy due to a suprasellar mass. *Surv Ophthalmol* 1997;41:402–408.

Kittner SJ, Stern BJ, Feeser BR, et al. Pregnancy and the risk of stroke. *N Engl J Med* 1996; 335:768–774

Lanska DJ, Kryscio RJ. Risk factors for peripartum and postpartum stroke and intracranial venous thrombosis. *Stroke* 2000;31:1274–1282.

Malone FD, D'Alton ME. Drugs in pregnancy: anticonvulsants. *Semin Perinatol* 1997; 21:114–123.

Mas JL, Lamy C. Stroke in pregnancy and the puerperium. *J Neurol* 1998;245:305–313.

Maymon R, Fejgin M. Intracranial hemorrhage during pregnancy and puerperium. *Obstet Gynecol Surv* 1990;45:157–179.

Morrell MJ. Guidelines for the care of women with epilepsy. *Neurology* 1998;51[Suppl 4]:S21–S27.

Nygaard I, Bartscht K, Cole S. Sexuality and reproduction in spinal cord injured women. *Obstet Gynecol Surv* 1990;45:727–732.

Omtzigt JCG, Los FJ, Grobbee DE, et al. The risk of spina bifida aperta after first-trimester exposure to valproate in a prenatal cohort. *Neurology* 1992;42:119–125.

Perry K. The diagnosis and management of hemoglobinopathies during pregnancy. *Semin Perinatol* 1990;14:90–102.

Plauche WC. Myasthenia gravis in mothers and their newborns. *Clin Obstet Gynecol* 1991; 34:82–99.

Practice parameter: management issues for women with epilepsy (summary statement). Report of the Quality Standards Subcommittee of the American Academy of Neurology. *Epilepsia* 1998;39:1226–1231.

Rosa F. Spina bifida in infants of women treated with carbamazepine during pregnancy. *N Engl J Med* 1991;324:674–677.

Scharff L, Marcus DA, Turk DC. Headache during pregnancy and in the postpartum: a prospective study. *Headache* 1997;37:203–210.

Silberstein SD. Headaches and women: treatment of the pregnant and lactating migraineur. *Headache* 1993;33:533–540.

Simolke G, Cox S, Cunningham FG. Cerebrovascular accidents complicating pregnancy and the puerperium. *Obstet Gynecol* 1991;78:37–42.

Turrentine MA, Braems G Ramirez MM. Use of thrombolytics for the treatment of thromboembolic disease during pregnancy. *Obstet Gynecol Surv* 1995;50:534–541.

Thomas S. Neurological aspects of eclampsia. *J Neurol Sci* 1998;155:37–43.

Uknis A, Silberstein SD. Review article: migraine and pregnancy. *Headache* 1991;31:372–374.

Varner MW, Digre KB. Myasthenia gravis. In: Coulam CB, Faulk WP, McIntyre JA, eds. *Immunological obstetrics*. London: Norton, 1992:666–676.

Wand JS. Carpal tunnel syndrome in pregnancy and lactation. *J Hand Surg* 1990;15:93–95.

Yerby MS, Freil PN, McCormich K. Antiepileptic drug disposition during pregnancy. *Neurology* 1992;42:12–16.

Zahn CA, Morrell MJ, Collins SD, et al. Management issues for women with epilepsy: a review of the literature. *Neurology* 1998;51:949–956.

58. THE ABCs OF NEUROLOGIC EMERGENCIES

James D. Fleck
José Biller

This chapter is designed to be a very brief reference for common neurologic emergencies. In general, we presume an accurate diagnosis has been made and concentrate on acute therapy. Although not comprehensive, this guide should allow you to care for a patient with the following problems for the first few hours to days.

I. **Elevated Intracranial Pressure (ICP)**
   A. 30-degree head-up neutral position
   B. Avoid hypotonic solutions
   C. If ICP monitor has been placed, maintain cerebral perfusion pressure at 70 to 80 mm Hg
   D. Mannitol (20% solution) 1.0 g/kg intravenous (i.v.) bolus followed by 0.25 to 0.5 g/kg every 4 to 6 hours
   E. Corticosteroids (if vasogenic edema)
   F. Hyperventilation to PCO_2 of 30 to 35 mm Hg (initial target)
      1. Typically loses effectiveness in 24 to 48 hours
      2. Reported to be a 4% change in cerebral blood flow for every 1 mm Hg change in PCO_2
      3. Hyperventilation to a PCO_2 <30 mm Hg only as a last resort for uncontrolled elevated ICP or impending herniation
   G. Sedation and paralysis if necessary
   H. Cerebrospinal fluid (CSF) drainage if necessary
   I. Barbiturates

II. **Coma**
   A. Thorough general and neurologic examination
   B. ABCs: maintain airway, breathing, circulation
   C. Intravenous fluids: normal saline solution
   D. Manage hypoglycemia with 50 mL of 50% glucose i.v. Consider Thiamine 100 mg i.v. before glucose.
   E. Consider naloxone 0.4 to 2.0 mg i.v. for opiate overdose.
   F. Consider flumazenil 0.2 mg i.v. for benzodiazepine overdose.
   G. Blood tests: arterial blood gases, glucose, electrolytes, calcium, magnesium, phosphorus, blood urea nitrogen (BUN), creatinine, liver enzymes, ammonia, complete blood cell count, urinalysis, blood and urine toxicology screens, thyroid function.
   H. If focal neurologic signs, deep coma, or history of head trauma, consider therapy for elevated ICP with hyperventilation and mannitol.
   I. Emergency head imaging: typically unenhanced computed tomography (CT) of the head
   J. Consider lumbar puncture if suspected central nervous system (CNS) infection or suspected subarachnoid hemorrhage with normal findings on head CT.
   K. Electroencephalography (EEG)

III. **Status Epilepticus (Generalized convulsive status epilepticus)**
   A. ABCs: maintain airway, breathing, circulation
   B. Intravenous line with normal saline solution
   C. Reduce temperatures >39°C with cooling blankets
   D. Consider 100 mg thiamine i.v.
   E. Consider 50 mL of 50% glucose i.v.
   F. Lorazepam 0.1 mg/kg i.v. at 2 mg/min, maximum of 8 mg in adults *or* diazepam 0.2 mg/kg i.v. at ≤5 mg/min up to a total dose of 20 mg
   G. Phenytoin 20 mg/kg i.v. (at <50 mg/min in adults) *or* fosphenytoin 20 mg phenytoin equivalents (PE) per kilogram i.v. (at ≤150 PE/min)
   H. If seizures continue, one can give additional bolus of phenytoin 10 mg/kg or fosphenytoin 10 mg PE/kg
   I. Intubation, airway protection, and possibly ventilatory support
   J. Phenobarbital 20 mg/kg i.v. (<100 mg/min)

    K. If seizures still continue, use pentobarbital, midazolam, propofol, thiopental, or inhalational general anesthesia
      1. Goal is burst-suppression pattern on EEG
      2. Pentobarbital loading with 5 to 10 mg/kg i.v., maintenance 1 to 3 mg/kg per hour
      3. Midazolam: loading with 0.2 mg/kg i.v. (slow i.v. bolus); infusion at 0.75 to 10 μg/kg per minute
      4. Propofol: loading with 1 to 2 mg/kg i.v.; infusion 2 to 10 mg/kg per hour
      5. Thiopental: loading with 3 to 4 mg/kg i.v.; 50 to 150 mg/h

IV. Bacterial Meningitis
    A. Treat within 30 minutes of arrival for medical care
    B. Manage elevated ICP
    C. Control seizures
    D. Manage complications (subdural empyema, brain abscess, acute hydrocephalus, vasculitis, vascular spasm, venous thrombosis, hyponatremia)
    E. No universally accepted standard for duration of treatment
    F. Empiric antibiotic treatment of immunocompetent patients with community-acquired meningitis: Ceftriaxone or cefotaxime *plus* vancomycin *plus* dexamethasone 0.15 mg/kg i.v. every 6 hours for 4 days (American Academy of Pediatrics recommendation for infants and children—first dose to be given before or within 4 hours of antibiotic). See Table 58.1 for antibiotic doses.
    G. Consider ceftazidime if *Pseudomonas* infection is suspected
    H. Consider ampicillin if *Listeria* infection is suspected, as in an immunocompromised host
    I. Chemoprophylaxis of meningococcal and *Haemophilus influenzae* infection with rifampin

V. Herpes Simplex Encephalitis
    A. Fluid and ICP management
    B. Seizure control
    C. Acyclovir i.v. 10 mg/kg every 8 hours for 14 to 21 days; adjust dose to patient's renal function

VI. Brain Abscess
    A. If there is no clear etiologic factor, administer ceftriaxone (Table 58.1) *plus* vancomycin (Table 58.1) *plus* metronidazole 500 mg every 6 hours in adults and 7.5 mg/kg every 8 hours in children
    B. Sulfa drugs for Nocardial infection
    C. Ceftazidime if gram-negative aerobes are suspected
    D. Surgical treatment

VII. Cerebral Toxoplasmosis
    A. Pyrimethamine: loading dose of 100 to 200 n g then 75 to 100 mg/d *plus* folinic acid 10 to 15 mg/d *plus* Sulfadiazine 6 to 8 mg/d
    B. If patient is allergic to sulfa drugs, substitute clindamycin 2,400 to 4,800 mg/d.

VIII. Ischemic Stroke: Within 3 Hours of Onset
    A. Unenhanced head CT does not show hemorrhage

Table 58.1 Antibiotic therapy for bacterial meningitis

Antibiotic	Total daily dose (dosing interval)	
	Adults	Children (older than 2 mo)
Ceftriaxone	4 g (q12h)	100 mg/kg (q12h)
Cefotaxime	8 g (q4h)	225 mg/kg (q6h)
Vancomycin	2 g (q6h)	40–60 mg/kg (q6h)
Ceftazadime	6 g (q8h)	125–150 mg/kg (q8h)
Ampicillin	12 g (q4h)	200–300 mg/kg (q6h)

B. Intravenous recombinant tissue plasminogen activator (rt-PA) 0.9 mg/kg, maximum dose of 90 mg
    1. Ten percent of dose as initial bolus and rest of dose infused over 60 minutes
C. Exclusion criteria
    1. Stroke or serious head trauma in last 3 months
    2. Major surgery within 14 days
    3. History of intracranial hemorrhage
    4. Systolic blood pressure >185 mm Hg or diastolic blood pressure >110 mm Hg
    5. Aggressive treatment to decrease blood pressure
    6. Rapidly improving or minor symptoms
    7. Symptoms suggestive of subarachnoid hemorrhage
    8. Gastrointestinal or genitourinary bleeding in last 21 days
    9. Arterial puncture at noncompressible site in preceding 7 days
    10. Seizure at onset of stroke
    11. Anticoagulants or heparin used within preceding 48 hours and elevated partial thromboplastin time (PTT) or prothrombin time (PT) greater than 15 seconds
    12. Platelet count <100,000/μL
    13. Glucose <50 mg/dL or >400 mg/dL
D. No antiplatelet agents or anticoagulants within first 24 hours of treatment
E. Avoid hypertension (>180/105 mm Hg) during and after treatment

IX. Management of Intracranial Bleeding after Thrombolytic Therapy
    A. Stop thrombolytic
    B. Draw blood to measure hematocrit, hemoglobin, PT and international normalized ratio (INR), aPTT, platelet count, and fibrinogen and for type and cross match
    C. Emergency unenhanced head CT
    D. Prepare for administration of 6 to 8 units of cryoprecipitate containing factor VIII
    E. Prepare for administration of 6 to 8 units of platelets
    F. Arrange hematology and neurosurgery consultations

X. Management of Intracranial Bleeding Associated with Oral Anticoagulant Therapy with Warfarin
    A. Discontinue warfarin
    B. Vitamin K 10 mg subcutaneously or 10 to 20 mg slow i.v. injection
    C. Fresh frozen plasma 10 to 20 mL/kg *or* prothrombin complex concentrate (50 units of factor IX/kg body weight) containing high concentrations of the vitamin K–dependent coagulation factors II, VII, IX, and X. Prothrombin complex concentrate may cause pathologic thrombosis.
    D. Neurosurgery consultation

XI. Subarachnoid Hemorrhage
    A. Unenhanced head CT
    B. Lumbar puncture if CT findings are normal
    C. Four-vessel cerebral angiography
    D. Avoid blood pressure elevations
    E. Nimodipine 60 mg enterally every 4 hours for 21 days
    F. Sedation, bedrest
    G. Anticonvulsants
    H. Management of elevated intracranial pressure
    I. Stool softeners
    J. Neurosurgery consultation

XII. Cerebellar Hemorrhage
    A. ABCs: maintain airway, breathing, and circulation
    B. Neurosurgery consultation
    C. Ventriculostomy for acute hydrocephalus
    D. Consider craniotomy with removal of hemorrhage

XIII. Acute Spinal Cord Injury
    A. Methylprednisolone 30 mg/kg i.v. bolus followed by 5.4 mg/kg per hour infusion for 23 hours
        1. Start within 8 hours of injury

XIV. Metastatic Epidural Spinal Cord Compression
    A. Dexamethasone: optimal dose of corticosteroid is uncertain (100 mg bolus *or* 10 mg bolus followed by 16 to 96 mg/d in divided doses)

    B. Consider radiation therapy
    C. Consider surgical intervention:
        1. If worsening deficits during or following radiotherapy
        2. If radioresistant tumor
        3. If spinal instability
    D. Pain control with narcotic analgesics
    E. Venous thromboembolism prophylaxis for nonambulatory patients

XV. Guillain–Barré Syndrome
    A. Nerve conduction studies including F waves
    B. Lumbar puncture looking for albuminocytologic dissociation
    C. Intubation if respiratory compromise: forced vital capacity (FVC) <15 mL/kg
    D. Monitoring for autonomic disturbances
    E. Plasma exchange: total 200 to 250 mL/kg over 1 to 2 weeks *or* immunoglobulin 0.4 g/kg i.v. per day for 5 days

XVI. Myasthenic Crisis
    A. Careful monitoring of airway, swallowing, and respiration
    B. Intubation when FVC <15 mL/kg
    C. Consider edrophonium (Tensilon) test
    D. Optimize anticholinesterase dose
        1. If there is concern about anticholinesterase toxicity, stop anticholinesterase
    E. Manage concurrent infections
    F. Plasma exchange *or* immunoglobulin 0.4 g/kg i.v. a day for 5 days

XVII. Acute Dystonic Reaction
    A. Stop causative agent
    B. Diphenhydramine 50 mg i.v.
    C. Benztropine 1 to 2 mg i.v.
    D. Typically follow with oral anticholinergic agent for 2 weeks, especially if long-acting dopamine receptor blocking agent was causative agent

XVIII. Neuroleptic Malignant Syndrome
    A. Immediate withdrawal of all neuroleptics or dopamine-depleting agents or re-institution of previously withdrawn dopaminergic therapy
    B. Hydration and maintenance of adequate urine flow
    C. Alkalinization of urine if myoglobinuria
    D. Lowering of elevated body temperature
    E. Bromocriptine 2.5 to 5.0 mg four times a day, increase four times a day dose until response occurs (maximum 50 mg/d)
    F. Dantrolene 1 to 10 mg/kg a day in divided doses
    G. Other possible agents for treatment include amantadine and carbamazepine
    H. For severe psychosis during treatment, consider electroconvulsive therapy

XIX. Acute Serotonin Syndrome
    A. Discontinue all serotonergic drugs
    B. Cyproheptadine 4 to 8 mg three times a day
    C. Other possible treatments include methysergide, propranolol, and chlorpromazine

XX. Giant Cell Arteritis, Temporal Arteritis
    A. Immediate sedimentation rate
    B. Oral prednisone 1 to 2 mg/kg every day *or* 1 g/d methylprednisolone i.v. for 3 days followed by oral prednisone 1 to 2 mg/kg a day, especially if there are visual symptoms or visual loss
    C. Superficial temporal artery biopsy

XXI. Central Retinal Artery Occlusion
    A. Ocular massage
    B. Breathing 95% oxygen and 5% carbon dioxide
    C. Lowering of intraocular pressure with acetazolamide intravenously or orally
    D. Anterior chamber paracentesis
    E. Aspirin
    F. Consider intraarterial thrombolysis (<12 hours)

Recommended Readings

Biller J, Chair. Asconapé J, Kase CS, et al. Iatrogenic neurology. *Continuum* 2001;7:1–224.

Chamberlain MC, Kornanik PA. Epidural spinal cord compression: a single institution's retrospective experience. *Neuro-oncology* 2000;192:120–123.

Johnson RT, Griffin JW, eds. *Current therapy in neurologic disease,* 5th ed. St Louis: Mosby, 1997.

Roos K, ed. *Central nervous system infectious diseases and therapy.* New York: Marcel Dekker, 1997.

Ropper AH, ed. *Neurological and neurosurgical intensive care,* 3rd ed. New York: Raven Press, 1993.

Wijdicks E. *Neurologic catastrophes in the emergency department.* Boston: Butterworth–Heinemann, 2000.

APPENDIX: CLINICAL SIGNS AND ANCILLARY DIAGNOSTIC STUDIES FOR DELIRIUM

John C. Andrefsky and Jeffrey I. Frank

Etiologic factor	Clinical comments	Laboratory diagnosis	Neuroimaging and other diagnostic studies
Systemic infection (including sepsis, pneumonia)	Can cause ↓ LOC; fever; hypotension; tachycardia; symptoms and signs of local infection	**Laboratory:** ↑ peripheral WBC; metabolic acidosis (sepsis); respiratory alkalosis and hypoxia (pneumonia); pyuria (urinary tract infection)	
Bacterial meningitis	Can cause ↓ LOC; HA; NR; seizures; rarely FNF; fever; hypotension; tachycardia	**Laboratory:** ↑ peripheral WBC **Lumbar puncture:** ↑ WBC 100–100,000 cells/mL; neutrophils 85%–95%; protein usually >100 mg/dL; glucose <50% serum; (+) Gram stain and cultures; ↑ CSF pressure	**CT:** early—normal; late—enlarged ventricles secondary to communicating hydrocephalus **MRI:** early—T1WI with gadolinium with meningeal enhancement
Tuberculous meningitis	Can cause ↓ LOC; ocular palsy; HA; NR; FNF; evidence of systemic tuberculosis; cough; weight loss	**Laboratory:** ↓ serum sodium (SIADH) **Lumbar puncture:** ↑ WBC 50–500 cells/mL; early—neutrophils and lymphocytes; late—lymphocytes; protein 100–200 mg/dL; glucose <40 mg/dL; (+) culture (may take weeks to become positive); ↑ CSF pressure	**CT:** plaque-like dural thickening or dural calcifications around basilar cisterns
Cryptococcal meningitis	Subacute onset of HA; NR may be lacking; ataxia; spastic paraparesis; usually without FNF; fever; cough if respiratory involvement	**Laboratory:** ↓ serum sodium (SIADH) **Lumbar puncture:** ↑ WBC <500 cells/mL usually lymphocytes; ↑ protein; glucose <50 mg/dL; (+) culture; (+) India ink preparation and cryptococcal antigen; ↑ CSF pressure	**CT:** usually not useful, but can identify hydrocephalus when present **MRI:** T2WI with multifocal basal ganglia and midbrain hyperintensities that represent cryptococcomas
Lyme disease	Subacute onset of meningoencephalitis; HA; NR; N/V; somnolence; behavioral changes; depressed mood; seizures; cranial nerve palsy; rash called *erythema chronicum migrans* after tick bite as first manifestation	**Laboratory:** ELISA shows positive IgM in 90% of patients if serum tested in acute and convalescent periods **Lumbar puncture:** ↑ WBC up to 3,000 cells/mL, usually lymphocytes; ↑ protein up to 400 mg/dL; glucose normal	**CT, MRI:** normal to extensive white-matter lesions; both superficial and deep; discreet and confluent; indistinguishable from multiple sclerosis and acute disseminated encephalomyelitis
Meningeal syphilis	Confusion may occur any time within 2 years of inoculation; cranial nerve palsies; NR; N/V	**Laboratory:** (+) RPR suggests active syphilis, but high false-negative and false-positive rate; (+) MHA-TP or	**CT:** can identify hydrocephalus when present

Condition	Clinical features	Laboratory / Lumbar puncture	Imaging
	if hydrocephalus present; seizures; afebrile	FTA-ABS implies previous syphilitic infection. **Lumbar puncture:** ↑ WBC 200–300 cells/mL, mostly lymphocytes; ↑ protein 40–200 mg/dL, glucose normal; (+) CSF VDRL, but high false-negative rate	
Tertiary syphilis	Insidious onset of confusion 15–20 y after inoculation; dementia; Argyll Robertson pupils; dysarthria; myoclonic jerks; action tremor; seizures	**Laboratory:** see Meningeal syphilis. **Lumbar puncture:** ↑ WBC 10–200 cells/mL, mostly lymphocytes; ↑ protein 40–200 mg/dL, but (+) CSF VDRL, but high false-negative rate	
Herpes simplex encephalitis	Confusion over days; ocular palsy; occasional NR; ataxia; seizures; hemiparesis; fever	**Lumbar puncture:** ↑ WBC 10–500 cells/mL (usually <200), mostly lymphocytes; ↑ RBC up to the thousands; ↑ protein; normal to slightly ↓ glucose; virus is rarely isolated from the CSF, but PCR can be helpful	**CT:** early—normal or with low attenuation in the temporal lobe with mass effect. **MRI:** early—T1WI with gyral edema; T2WI with high signal intensity in the temporal lobe. **EEG:** PLEDs (2–3 per second) over the temporal regions
Progressive multifocal leukoencephlopathy	Confusion over days to weeks; dementia; aphasia; hemiparesis; quadraparesis	**Lumbar puncture:** usually normal but may have mildly ↑ protein	**CT:** nonenhancing areas of low attenuation in white matter. **MRI:** T2WI with multifocal oval or round supratentorial and infratentorial white-matter hyperintesities
Human immunodeficiency virus infection	Subacute onset of confusion; slowly or rapidly progressing dementia; ataxia of gait and limbs; seizures	**Laboratory:** (+) HIV serology. **Lumbar puncture:** normal or have mild lymphocytosis and mildly ↑ protein	**CT:** with atrophy and multiple areas of low attenuation in deep white matter. **MRI:** T2WI—diffuse, patchy, or confluent increased signal lesions
Brain abscess	HA; signs of ↑ CSF pressure; focal or generalized seizures; fever during suppurative phase	**Laboratory:** ↑ peripheral WBC. **Lumbar puncture:** moderately ↑ WBC, mostly neutrophils; moderately ↑ RBC; ↑ protein; normal glucose; (+) cultures (50% of patients)	**CT:** early—normal or with subcortical low attenuation that later is better defined; (+) ring enhancement with contrast. **MRI:** early—T2WI with subcortical hypointensity; late—central area becoming hyperintense; T1WI with gadolinium with intense rim enhancement

continued

Etiologic factor	Clinical comments	Laboratory diagnosis	Neuroimaging and other diagnostic studies
Epidural abscess	NR; fever; malaise	**Laboratory:** ↑ peripheral WBC **Lumbar puncture**[a]**:** mildly ↑ WBC; mildly ↑ protein; cultures usually normal	**CT:** large volume of fluid between cranium and dura; contrast may enhance dura and detectability of more subtle epidural fluid collections
Subdural empyema	Confusion preceded by HA; can cause ↓ LOC; aphasia; NR; N/V; focal seizures; hemiplegia; hemianesthesia; fever; malaise	**Laboratory:** ↑ peripheral WBC **Lumbar puncture:** ↑ WBC 50–1,000 cells/mL, mostly neutrophils; ↑ protein 75–300 mg/dL; normal glucose	**CT:** low attenuation crescentic extraaxial fluid collections **MRI:** T2WI with a mildly hyperintense collection; gadolinium-enhanced T1WI with a surrounding membrane
Toxoplasmosis	Acute onset of confusion; usually asymptomatic; retinochoroiditis; NR; myoclonus; asterixis; seizures; neurologic manifestations common in patients with AIDS; can have fever; splenomegaly; if immunocompromised: myositis; fever; rash; myocarditis; pneumonitis; malaise; hepatomegaly	**Laboratory:** (+) serum antibody to toxoplasmosis **Lumbar puncture**[a]**:** ↑ WBC, mostly lymphocytes; ↑ protein	**CT:** solitary or multiple ring-enhancing masses with contrast **MRI:** T1WI—multifocal hypointense lesions that are hyperintense on T2WI; T1WI with gadolinium—usually prominent rim enhancement of the lesions
Subacute spongiform encephalopathy (Creutzfeldt–Jakob disease)	Subacute delirium with rapid progression; behavioral changes; depression; myoclonic jerks lateralized at first then generalized; sleep disturbances; fatigue; weight loss	**Lumbar puncture:** normal; prion protein 14-3-3	**EEG:** early—diffuse and nonspecific slowing; late—stereotyped high-voltage slow and sharp waves on a flat background **Brain biopsy:** diffuse loss of neurons and vacuoles within glial cells and neurons
Whipple's disease	Subacute confusion; supranuclear ophthalmoplegia; oculomasticatory myorhythmia; myoclonus; ataxia; seizures; hypersomnia; fever; weight loss; abdominal pain; hyperpigmentation; lymphadenopathy	**Laboratory:** anemia; biopsy of jejunal mucosa has macrophages filled with PAS-positive material **Lumbar puncture:** usually normal or ↑ WBC to 400 cells/mL, mostly monocytes; moderately ↑ protein; CSF histiocytes or macrophages laden with PAS-positive material often present	

Systemic lupus erythematosus	Confusion and ↓ LOC most often occur late in course; seizures; cranial neuropathy; FNF	**Laboratory:** (+) ANA test **Lumbar puncture:** ↑ WBC 5–50 cells/mL, mostly lymphocytes; mildly ↑ protein 50–100 mg/dL; usually normal glucose; ↑ CSF pressure rarely increased	**MRI:** multifocal areas of hyperintensity on T2WI, mainly periventricular and subcortical white matter; some lesions may enhance **Angiography:** normal; small-vessel disease; large-vessel arteriopathy; or fusiform aneurysm
Acute disseminated encephalomyelitis	Acute onset of confusion; can cause ↓ LOC; HA; NR; myoclonic movements; choreoathetosis; ataxia; if spinal cord involvement then paraplegia; quadriplegia; ↑ or ↓ deep tendon reflexes; variable degrees of bowel and bladder dysfunction; fever; often postinfectious	**Lumbar puncture:** ↑ WBC 20–200 cells/mL, mostly lymphocytes; mildly ↑ protein <100 mg/dL; normal glucose; ↑ CSF pressure (50% of patients)	**MRI:** T2WI with multifocal subcortical hyperintense foci; not all lesions enhanced with gadolinium
Hypernatremia and hyperosmolality	Temporal profile of onset is variable; can cause ↓ LOC; hypotension and tachycardia, particularly when associated with volume-depleted state	**Laboratory:** confusion usually with serum osmolality ≥320 mOsm/kg water	
Hyponatremia and hypoosmolality	Variable onset of confusion; can cause ↓ LOC; myoclonus; seizures; generalized weakness	**Laboratory:** confusion usually with serum sodium <120 mEq/L	
Central pontine myelinolysis	Confusion due to severe electrolyte disturbance (hyponatremia); extreme hyperosmolality or rapid correction of hyponatremia causes syndrome characterized by subacute quadriplegia, variable pseudobulbar palsy, and locked-in syndrome	**Laboratory:** recent extreme hyperosmolality or rapid correction of hyponatremia of <130 mEq/L **Lumbar puncture:** normal (50% of patients) or mildly ↑ monocyte count; ↑ CSF pressure; ↑ protein	**CT:** normal or low-attenuation white matter changes and central pontine cavitation **MRI:** T1WI with hypointense lesions and T2WI with hyperintense lesions; mostly nonenhancing; the presence of pontine and basal ganglia lesions is specific for this disorder

continued

Etiologic factor	Clinical comments	Laboratory diagnosis	Neuroimaging and other diagnostic studies
Hypokalemia	Areflexic paralysis; generalized weakness; cardiac arrhythmias; paralytic ileus; renal tubular damage; rhabdomyolysis; myoglobinuria	**Laboratory:** serum potassium <2.0 mEq/L	
Hypercalcemia	Confusion; can cause ↓ LOC; depression; proximal weakness; restless leg syndrome; cardiac arrhythmias, asystole	**Laboratory:** confusion usually with calcium level >12 mg/dL; but variable symptomatic threshold	
Hypophosphatemia	Can cause ↓ LOC; paresthesia; seizures; generalized weakness; myocardial, hepatic, erythrocyte, leukocyte, and platelet dysfunction	**Laboratory:** confusion usually with serum phosphate <0.1 mg/dL	
Hypermagnesemia	Hypotension; bradyarrhythmias; asystole	**Laboratory:** curare-like effects if serum magnesium >10 mEq/L	
Hypomagnesemia	Can cause ↓ LOC; N/V; paresthesia; seizures; generalized weakness; paralytic ileus; fatigue	**Laboratory:** confusion usually with serum magnesium <0.1 mEq/L	
Respiratory acidosis	See Hypercapnia		
Metabolic acidosis	Confusion due to cause of metabolic acidosis; can cause ↓ LOC; mild diffuse muscle hypertonus; cardiac depression	**Laboratory:** if uncomplicated metabolic acidosis, ABG will have pH <7.35 and HCO$_3$ <24 mEq/L; symptomatic usually when pH <7.24	
Respiratory alkalosis	Lightheadedness; paresthesia; circumoral numbness	**Laboratory:** if uncomplicated respiratory alkalosis, ABG will have pH >7.45 and PCO_2 <40 mm Hg	
Metabolic alkalosis	Tetany; neuromuscular irritability; cardiac depression with severe alkalosis	**Laboratory:** if uncomplicated metabolic alkalosis, ABG will have pH >7.45 and HCO$_3$ >24 mEq/L	

Diabetic ketoacidosis	Can cause ↓ LOC; hyperosmolar state contributes to symptom complex; HA; N/V; generalized weakness; abdominal pain	**Laboratory:** variable symptomatic threshold	
Hyperosmolar nonketotic hyperglycemia	Can cause ↓ LOC; severe dehydration; similar to hypernatremia	**Laboratory:** confusion usually with serum osmolality >320 mOsm/kg water, but variable symptomatic threshold	
Hypoglycemia	Can cause ↓ LOC; HA; myoclonic twitching; seizures; nervousness; trembling; sweating; hunger	**Laboratory:** confusion usually with levels <30–40 mg/dL	
Hypercapnia	Can cause ↓ LOC; papilledema; HA asterixis; action tremor; course twitching of muscles; seizures	**Laboratory:** if uncomplicated respiratory acidosis, ABG will have pH <7.35 and PCO_2 >40 mm Hg	
Hypoxia	Can cause ↓ LOC; poor judgment; shortness of breath; cyanosis	**Laboratory:** confusion may be present with PO_2 <55 mm Hg	
Hypotension	Can cause rapid ↓ LOC; cyanosis	**Vital signs:** onset of confusion usually with systolic BP <60 mm Hg; may be higher in hypertensive patients	
Uremia	Confusion may be episodic; can cause ↓ LOC; irritability; apathy; muscular twitching; asterixis; tetany; fatigue	**Laboratory:** confusion usually related to the rapidity of renal failure and not to clear thresholds **Lumbar puncture:** mildly ↑ WBC; mildly ↑ protein	**EEG:** triphasic waves or diffuse slowing
Hepatic encephalopathy	Early: confusion with agitation Late: ↓ LOC; signs of ↑ CSF pressure; myoclonus; asterixis; FNF are rare; icteric sclera; spider telangiectasia; caput medusae; ascites; splenomegaly; jaundice	**Laboratory:** hypoglycemia; hyperammonemia; ↑ PT; elevated liver enzymes **Lumbar puncture:** if protein is ↑, search for another cause; ↑ CSF glutamine	**EEG:** triphasic waves or diffuse slowing

continued

Etiologic factor	Clinical comments	Laboratory diagnosis	Neuroimaging and other diagnostic studies
Reye's syndrome	Onset of confusion is rapid, as is progression to ↓ LOC; confusion preceded by 1 wk of vomiting, fevers, and upper respiratory infections	**Lumbar puncture:** usually acellular; normal protein; ↓ glucose; ↑ CSF pressure	
Pancreatic encephalopathy	Acute onset of confusion; can cause ↓ LOC; agitation; hallucinations; dysarthria; N/V; quadriplegia; midabdominal pain; upper abdominal tenderness	**Laboratory:** serum amylase usually increases later and may remain elevated for several days	
Acute intermittent porphyria	Confusion resolves over days to weeks and precedes the severe cases of polyneuropathy; psychosis; ocular palsy; facial paralysis; hypertension; tachycardia; colicky pain	**Laboratory:** ↑ urinary δ-aminolevulinic acid and porphobilinogen **Lumbar puncture:** normal or mildly ↑ protein	
Hyperthyroidism	Subacute onset of confusion; agitation; emotional lability; tremor; seizures; proximal weakness; heat intolerance; palpitations; tachycardia; atrial fibrillation; fatigue; weight loss	**Laboratory:** abnormal thyroid function tests **Lumbar puncture:** normal, occasionally ↓ protein	
Hypothyroidism	Confusion may be mild; can cause ↓ LOC; paranoia; confabulation; ataxia; peripheral neuropathy; delayed relaxation of deep tendon reflexes; cold intolerance; bradycardia; periorbital swelling; hair loss	**Laboratory:** abnormal thyroid function tests **Lumbar puncture:** normal, occasionally ↑ protein	
Cushing's syndrome	Psychosis; depression; hallucinations; proximal muscular weakness; hypertension; obesity; hirsutism; incessant activity or immobility	**Laboratory:** abnormal dexamethasone suppression test	**CT:** cerebral atrophy

Condition	Clinical features	Laboratory / Imaging
Adrenal cortical insufficiency	Irritability; seizures generalized weakness; hypotension; fatigue; weight loss; skin hyperpigmentation	**Laboratory:** abnormal cortisol stimulation test
Pituitary apoplexy	Acute onset of confusion; can cause ↓ LOC; acute HA; bilateral amaurosis; ophthalmoplegia	**CT:** enlarged sella with infarction of pituitary tumor; hemorrhage in and above the sella; often misread as normal **MRI:** T2WI—hyperintensities surrounding the third ventricle and aqueduct; T1WI with gadolinium—enhancement of the above areas and the mammillary bodies
Wernicke's encephalopathy	Signs of alcohol withdrawal; loss of long-term memory; anterograde amnesia; confabulation; ocular palsy; gaze palsy; nystagmus; gait ataxia; peripheral neuropathy; dyspnea; postural hypotension; precipitated or aggravated by glucose load in malnourished; prevented with thiamine supplement	**Laboratory:** low transketolase activity and elevated blood pyruvate **Lumbar puncture:** normal or mildly ↑ protein
Pellagra	Acute onset of confusion; depression; myelopathy involving posterior and lateral columns; fatigue; scaly dermatitis; diarrhea	**Laboratory:** decreased excretion of urinary N-methyl-nicotinamide
Vitamin B_{12} deficiency	Confusion usually begins after spinal cord involvement; depression; paranoia; general weakness and paresthesia can progress to ataxic paraparesis; bowel and bladder dysfunction	**Laboratory:** megaloblastic anemia; low vitamin B_{12} level (usually <200 pg/mL); ↑ serum methylmalonic acid **Lumbar puncture:** usually normal or mildly ↑ WBC or mildly ↑ protein
Acute alcohol intoxication	Can cause ↓ LOC; unrestrained behavior; incoordination; atrial flutter; acute gastritis; diuresis	**Laboratory:** confusion usually with level >200 mg/dL but variable symptomatic threshold

continued

Etiologic factor	Clinical comments	Laboratory diagnosis	Neuroimaging and other diagnostic studies
Acute alcohol withdrawal (delirium tremens)	Onset of delirium usually 2–4 d after cessation of alcohol and is fairly acute; agitation; dilated pupils; seizures (7–48 h after cessation of alcohol); fever; tachycardia; perspiration	**Laboratory:** alcohol level does not have to be 0 mg/dL for withdrawal to occur	
Opioid intoxication	Constricted pupils; N/V; hypothermia; bradycardia; respiratory depression; constipation	**Laboratory:** (+) drug screen	
Cocaine intoxication	Agitation; psychotic behavior; pupillary dilatation; N/V; seizure; tachycardia; bradycardia; cardiac arrhythmias; respiratory depression; nares may have erosions	**Laboratory:** (+) drug screen	
Amphetamine intoxication	Same as cocaine; except no psychomotor agitation, but maladaptive behavior or psychological change may be present	**Laboratory:** (+) drug screen	
Phencyclidine intoxication	Can cause ↓ LOC; nystagmus; dysarthria; muscle rigidity; tremor; hyperacusis; ataxia; seizure; decreased responsiveness to pain; ↑ BP; tachycardia	**Laboratory:** (+) drug screen	
Sedative–hypnotic, barbiturate intoxication	Can cause ↓ LOC; slurred speech; nystagmus; incoordination; unsteady gait; hypothermia; hypotension; respiratory depression	**Laboratory:** (+) drug screen; if barbiturate is suspected, check level	

Barbiturate withdrawal	Delirium follows convulsive phase; withdrawal begins ~12 h after last dose; if chronically intoxicated, withdrawal can take 48–72 h; tremor; insomnia; generalized seizures occur 7 days from last dose; fever; tachycardia	**Laboratory:** check barbiturate level
Benzodiazepine intoxication	Onset of delirium is during or soon after ingestion of drugs; can cause ↓ LOC; hostile behavior; slurred speech; hypotension; syncope	**Laboratory:** (+) drug screen
Benzodiazepine withdrawal	Onset of confusion is 2–3 d after last dose with short acting drugs or 5–6 d with long acting ones; anxiety; dysphoria; N/V; tremor muscle twitches; occasional seizures; intolerance for bright lights and loud noises; sweating	**Laboratory:** (+) drug screen
Lithium intoxication	**Level 1.5–2.0:** onset of confusion; N/V; nystagmus; slurred speech; ataxia; dizziness; abdominal pain **Level >2.0:** can cause ↓ LOC; clonic limb movement; seizure; syncope; circulatory failure	**Laboratory:** ↑ peripheral WBC, ↑ sodium, magnesium, calcium, and glucose levels; ↓ potassium and phosphorous levels
Carbon monoxide poisoning	**10–30% carboxyhemoglobin:** HA; N/V **30–40% carboxyhemoglobin:** confusion; severe HA; dizziness **>50% carboxyhemoglobin:** can cause ↓ LOC; seizure; shock; tachypnea	**Laboratory:** elevated carboxyhemoglobin level **CT:** low attenuation in the watershed regions, especially in the basal ganglia and parasagittal regions **MRI:** T2WI—hyperintensities in the watershed regions; T1WI with gadolinium with striking enhancement

continued

Etiologic factor	Clinical comments	Laboratory diagnosis	Neuroimaging and other diagnostic studies
Subarachnoid hemorrhage	Confusion may occur with the original hemorrhage, associated vasospasm, or hydrocephalus; acute onset HA; NR; N/V; ↑ BP; tachycardia	**Laboratory:** check PT, PTT, DIC profile and platelet count **Lumbar puncture:** ↑ RBC; ↑ protein; ↓ glucose; ↑ CSF pressure (50% of patients)	**CT:** high attenuation following the course of the gyri; may be localized but usually diffuse, especially within the cisterns; frequently misread as normal **Angiography:** usually diagnostic of aneurysm or AVM
Acute subdural hematoma (<3 d)	Confusion may appear at the time of trauma or be delayed as hematoma enlarges; can cause ↓ LOC; aphasia; seizure; hemiparesis	**Laboratory:** check PT, PTT, and platelet count **Lumbar puncture:** unnecessary with modern imaging	**CT:** high attenuation crescent-shaped fluid collection over the underlying hemisphere **MRI:** hyperacute—T1WI isointense and T2WI isointense to hyperintense hemorrhage; acute—T1WI isointense to moderately hypointense hemorrhage; T2WI very hypointense hemorrhage
Subacute (3 d to 3 wk) and chronic (>3 wk) subdural hematoma	Variable onset of confusion; may be intermittent; can cause ↓ LOC; dementia; HA; TIA-like episodes; seizures	**Laboratory:** check PT, PTT, and platelet count **Lumbar puncture:** unnecessary with modern imaging	**CT:** subacute—nearly same attenuation as underlying cortex; chronic—low attenuation compared with enhancing membrane; may be loculated **MRI:** subacute—hyperintensity on both T1WI and T2WI; chronic—variable; T1WI usually isointense to hypointense; T2WI hyperintense
Epidural hematoma	Confusion may appear acutely after trauma or may appear after a lucid interval; can cause rapid ↓ LOC; HA; FNF	**Lumbar puncture:** unnecessary with modern imaging	**CT:** high-attenuation biconvex mass with mass effect **MRI:** acute—T1WI with isointense epidural mass, T2WI with hyperintense epidural mass
Concussion	Confusion occurs after head injury with subsequent resolution; HA; N/V	**Lumbar puncture:** normal	**CT:** normal

Contusion	Onset of confusion after injury; can have progressive brain swelling with ↓ LOC; FNF; fever; tachycardia	**Lumbar puncture:** unnecessary with modern imaging	**CT:** early—normal or with patchy ill-defined low-attenuation frontal or temporal lesions mixed with smaller high-attenuation foci of petechial hemorrhage; edema; contusions may enhance; common locations are inferior frontal and anterior temporal lobes **MRI:** acute—T1WI with some hyperintense signal abnormalities (hemorrhage), T2WI with multiple superficial hyperintense signal abnormalities on T2WI
Transient ischemic attack	Confusion begins with the onset of ischemia; FNF may be present depending on the areas of the brain affected with full resolution of deficits; see Cerebral infarction for specific areas	**Lumbar puncture:** normal	Imaging studies are normal
Cerebral infarction	Confusion begins with the onset of the stroke; HA; large-vessel occlusions; visual field deficit if posterior cerebral arteries are involved Localizations that can be associated with confusion: 1. Parahippocampal–fusiform–lingual gyri on either side of the brain 2. Right posterior parietal region 3. Right prefrontal region 4. Bilateral PCA territories 5. Transient confusion if left PCA involved	**Lumbar puncture:** unnecessary with modern imaging	**CT:** early—normal or with sulcal effacement and loss of gray–white junction; late—with low attenuation in a specific vascular territory **MRI:** early—T1WI with brain swelling; T2WI with hyperintensity after 8 h

continued

Etiologic factor	Clinical comments	Laboratory diagnosis	Neuroimaging and other diagnostic studies
Intracerebral hemorrhage	Confusion begins with the onset of the hemorrhage; HA; see Cerebral infarction for localizations which can be associated with confusion	**Laboratory:** check PT, PTT, and platelet count **Lumbar puncture:** unnecessary with modern imaging	**CT:** area of high attenuation representing the hematoma; degree of mass effect related to size and location of hematoma **MRI:** see Acute subdural hematoma for intensities of the hematoma on T1WI and T2WI
Vasculitis	Usually subacute confusion; HA; aphasia; FNF	**Lumbar puncture:** normal or ↑ WBC; ↑ protein; glucose usually normal; CSF pressure can be normal, ↓, ↑	**CT:** multiple areas of low attenuation
Cerebral venous sinus occlusion	Subacute onset of confusion; can cause ↓ LOC; aphasia; papilledema; signs of ↑ CSF pressure; HA; seizures; FNF	**Lumbar puncture:** if idiopathic, normal or ↑ protein; if septic thrombophlebitis, CSF similar to meningitis; if hemorrhagic infarction, ↑ RBC; ↑ CSF pressure if thrombosis is acute	**CT:** without contrast: with high attenuation in sinus representing thrombus; with or without cortical or subcortical hemorrhage; with contrast: sinus with low attenuation with enhancement around thrombus (empty delta sign); possible focal area of low attenuation representing area of venous infarction **MRI:** acute—T1WI with isointense clot; subacute—T1WI or T2WI with hyperintense clot **MR venography:** no flow in occluded sinus
CNS tumors	Onset of confusion subacute and progressive; irritability; abulia; aphasia; signs of ↑ CSF pressure; seizures	**Lumbar puncture:** all values variable and depend on histologic type of tumor, location, and presence of ↑ CSF pressure and hemorrhage	**CT, MRI:** results variable and depend on histologic tumor type, location, and presence of ↑ CSF pressure and hemorrhage
Metastasis	Onset of confusion can be acute or subacute; FNF common	**Laboratory:** Serum tumor markers may be used to diagnose primary tumor if not known	**CT, MRI:** results are variable; metastatic lesions can occur anywhere in the CNS; most are isodense with adjacent brain; may have mass effect and significant edema; most strongly enhance; may have associated hemorrhage; MR signal intensity of metastatic lesions varies

Carcinomatosis	Onset of confusion can be acute or subacute; HA; backache; cranial nerve palsy and radiculopathy common; hydrocephalus in 50% of patients	**Lumbar puncture:** ↑ WBC, usually lymphocytes; ↑ protein; ↓ glucose; (+) CSF cytology; may have ↑ CSF pressure	**CT:** may be normal; may have meningeal enhancement after administration of contrast material **MRI:** abnormalities seen in 33%–66% of patients; tumor appears as enhancing lines or small nodular deposits along the cortical surface; diffuse meningeal enhancement may be seen
Limbic encephalitis	Onset of confusion is subacute; dementia; retentive memory defect; depression; agitation; anxiety; hallucinations; seizures	**Laboratory:** systemic evidence of carcinoma; usually oat cell carcinoma of the lung **Lumbar puncture:** ↑ WBC 10–50 cells/mL, mostly lymphocytes; mildly ↑ protein	**CT:** usually normal **MRI:** high signal intensities in the medial temporal lobe; almost identical to herpes simplex encephalitis
Generalized seizure (absence)	Onset of confusion is with the seizure or postconvulsive; can cause ↓ LOC; automatism; myoclonic jerks	**Laboratory:** if seizure remains focal, no lab abnormalities; if generalized tonic–clonic, then ↑ peripheral WBC; metabolic acidosis **Lumbar puncture:** may have mildly ↑ WBC if done within 72 h of a generalized tonic–clonic seizure, assuming no recent CNS injury, infection, or stroke	**CT, MRI:** results are variable and depend on the cause of the seizure **EEG:** interictal—may be normal; ictal—with generalized 3 per second spike and wave
Partial seizure	Onset of confusion with onset of seizure; auras; illusions; hallucinations; anxiety; fear; automatism; persistence of complex acts; amnesia; may see secondary generalization; ↑ BP; tachycardia; ↓ respirations	**Laboratory:** if seizure remains focal, no lab abnormalities; if generalized tonic–clonic, then ↑ peripheral WBC; metabolic acidosis **Lumbar puncture:** may have mildly ↑ WBC if done within 72 h of a generalized tonic–clonic seizure; assuming no recent CNS injury, infection, or stroke	**CT, MRI:** results are variable and depend on the cause of the seizure **EEG:** interictal—may be normal or with intermittent spikes or sharp waves; ictal—may be normal or with repetitive focal spike discharges
Postconvulsive (after generalized or complex partial seizures)	Confusion occurs after a seizure; duration of confusion is variable; aphasia; postconvulsive paralysis	**Lumbar puncture:** see Generalized seizure and Partial seizure for results	**CT, MRI:** results are variable and depend on the cause of the seizure **EEG:** diffuse or focal slowing

continued

Etiologic factor	Clinical comments	Laboratory diagnosis	Neuroimaging and other diagnostic studies
Hypertensive encephalopathy	Rapid onset of confusion and ↑ BP; can cause ↓ LOC; papilledema; HA; N/V; seizures; visual disturbances	**Lumbar puncture:** ↑ protein usually <100 mg/dL; ↑ CSF pressure in many cases	**CT:** generalized cerebral edema as manifested by loss of gray–white junction, diffuse loss of sulci and cisternal spaces, small ventricles
Beclouded dementia	Patients have dementia and ↑ confusion secondary to another etiologic factor; signs of dementia	**Laboratory:** abnormal results depend on etiologic factor	**CT, MRI:** results are variable and depend on the cause of the dementia; diffuse atrophy and ex vacuo hydrocephalus usually are seen
Postoperative delirium	Onset of confusion after surgery; fever; hypothermia; BP changes; tachycardia	**Laboratory:** electrolyte abnormalities; anemia; hypoxemia; or multiple etiologic factors may be present	**CT, MRI:** results are variable and depend on the cause
Cardiac bypass	Onset of confusion is after surgery; ↓ LOC, FNF may be present	**Laboratory:** multiple etiologic factors may be present	**CT, MRI:** may show mild generalized edema or be consistent with cerebral infarction
Temperature dysregulation	Onset of confusion may occur from inciting pathologic condition; consider all causes of temperature dysregulation	**Laboratory:** multiple etiologic factors may be present, especially medications, drug overdoses, or CNS lesion	**CT, MRI:** results are variable and depend on the cause

Sensory deprivation	Onset of confusion may occur after period of deprivation	**Laboratory:** consider additional pathologic conditions
Sleep deprivation	Onset of confusion may occur after period of deprivation	**Laboratory:** consider study to rule out sleep apnea as a contributing cause; blood and urine drug screen
Hydrocephalus	Onset of confusion may occur within minutes or over days to months depending on the cause; ↓ LOC common; sixth-nerve and upgaze palsy common; deep tendon reflexes may be increased	**Laboratory:** serum studies may be useful depending on the cause **Lumbar puncture:** see Chapter 1, **III.D.1.** for contraindications; may be useful when chronic CNS infection is a possibility	CT: dilated ventricular system with loss of sulci and cisternal spaces as CSF pressure increases; pattern of ventricular dilatation may help with diagnostic considerations

CT, MRI: results are variable and depend on the contributing cause

Subject Index

Page numbers followed by *f* refer to figures. Page numbers followed by *t* refer to tables.